NUTRITION AND METABOLISM IN PATIENT CARE

JOHN M. KINNEY, M.D.
Professor Emeritis in Surgery, Columbia University
Visiting Professor, Rockefeller University
Attending in Medicine and Surgery
St. Luke's-Roosevelt Hospital Center, New York

K.N. JEEJEEBHOY, M.B., B.S.
Professor of Medicine, University of Toronto
Chief of Gastroenterology
Toronto General Hospital, Toronto

GRAHAM L. HILL, M.D.
Professor and Chairman
University Department of Surgery
Auckland Hospital, Auckland

OLIVER E. OWEN, M.D.
Professor of Medicine
Temple University School of Medicine
Program Director, General Clinical Research Center
Temple University Hospital, Philadelphia

1988
W.B. SAUNDERS COMPANY
Harcourt Brace Jovanovich, Inc.
Philadelphia • London • Toronto
Montreal • Sydney • Tokyo

W. B. SAUNDERS COMPANY
Harcourt Brace Jovanovich, Inc.

West Washington Square
Philadelphia, PA 19105

Library of Congress Cataloging-in-Publication Data

Nutrition and metabolism in patient care.

1. Diet therapy. 2. Nutrition. 3. Metabolism.
I. Kinney, John M., 1921–   . [DNLM: 1. Diet
Therapy. 2. Metabolism. 3. Nursing Care.
4. Nutrition. WB 400 N97455]
RM216.N835   1988   615.8′54   87-16358
ISBN 0-7216-1156-7

Editor: Albert Meier
Designer: W. B. Saunders Staff
Production Manager: Carolyn Naylor
Manuscript Editor: Mark Coyle
Illustration Coordinator: Lisa Lambert
Indexer: Angela Holt

Nutrition and Metabolism
in Patient Care   ISBN   0–7216–1156–7

Last digit is the print number:
9   8   7   6   5   4   3   2   1

To Our Wives

CONTRIBUTORS

E. Victor Adlin, M.D.
Associate Professor of Medicine, Temple University School of Medicine; Attending Staff, Temple University Hospital, Philadelphia, PA
Edema and Hypertension

J. Wesley Alexander, M.D., Sc.D.
Professor of Surgery, University of Cincinnati; Director of Research and Attending Surgeon, Shriners Burn Institute; Attending Surgeon, University Hospital; Consulting Surgeon, The Christ Hospital, and Children's Hospital Medical Center, Cincinnati, OH
Nutritional Management of the Infected Patient

Anders Alvestrand, M.D.
Associate Professor, Karolinska Institute, Stockholm; Assistant Head Physician, Department of Renal Medicine, Huddinge University Hospital, Huddinge, Sweden
Renal Diseases

Jeffrey Askanazi, M.D.
Associate Professor, Albert Einstein College of Medicine of Yeshiva University; Associate Attending in Anesthesiology, Montefiore Medical Center, New York, NY
Respiratory Diseases

Alun H. Beddoe, M.Sc., Ph.D.
Chief Physicist, Department of Medical Physics, Otago Hospital Board, Dunedin, New Zealand
Dimensions of the Human Body and Its Compartments

William R. Beisel, M.D.; F.A.C.P.
Adjunct Professor, Department of Immunology and Infectious Disease, School of Hygiene and Public Health, The Johns Hopkins University, Baltimore, MD
Metabolic Response to Infection

Jonas Bergström, M.D.
Professor of Renal Medicine, Karolinska Institute, Stockholm; Director, Chairman, Department of Renal Medicine, Huddinge University Hospital, Huddinge, Sweden
Renal Diseases

Palmer Q. Bessey, M.D.
Associate Professor of Surgery, and Chief, Section of Trauma, Burns, and Critical Care, Department of Surgery, University of Alabama at Birmingham; Attending Surgeon, University of Alabama Hospital; Staff Surgeon, Surgical Service, Veterans Administration Hospital, Birmingham, AL
The Burned Patient

Michael R. Bye, M.D.
Assistant Professor of Pediatrics, Albert Einstein College of Medicine of Yeshiva University; Director, Division of Pediatric Pulmonary Medicine, Montefiore Medical Center, New York, NY
Cystic Fibrosis

George F. Cahill, Jr., M.D.
Professor of Medicine, Harvard Medical School, Boston, MA; Vice President, Howard Hughes Medical Institute, Bethesda, MD
Starvation: Some Biological Aspects

Yvon A. Carpentier, M.D.
Associate Professor of Surgery, University of Brussels; Head, Division of Clinical Nutrition, Hopital Universitaire Saint-Pierre, Brussels, Belgium
The Intensive Care Patient

Katie Casper, B.S.
Research Assistant, Columbia University School of Medicine, St. Luke's–Roosevelt Hospital Center, New York, NY
Heart Diseases

Britton Chance, D.Sc.
Emeritus University Professor, University of Pennsylvania, Philadelphia, PA
Phosphorus Magnetic Resonance Spectroscopy as a Probe of Nutritional State

Ranjit K. Chandra, M.D., F.R.C.P.(C)
Professor of Pediatric Research, Medicine, and Biochemistry, Memorial University of Newfoundland; Consultant Pediatrician and Director of Immunology, Janeway Child Health Centre, St. John's, Newfoundland, Canada
Food Allergy; Immunity and Infection

Lydia A. Conlay, M.D., Ph.D.
Assistant Professor of Anesthesia, Harvard Medical School; Assistant Anesthetist, Massachusetts General Hospital, Boston, MA
Nutrients and Brain Function

John M. Daly, M.D.
Jonathan E. Rhoads Professor of Surgical Science, University of Pennsylvania School of Medicine; Chief, Division of Surgical Oncology, Hospital of the University of Pennsylvania, Philadelphia, PA
Neoplastic Diseases

Mukesh B. Desai
Resident in Surgery, University of Toronto, Toronto, Ontario, Canada
Peptic Ulcer

John T. Devlin, M.D.
Assistant Professor, University of Vermont College of Medicine; Attending in Medicine and Coordinator, Nutrition Support Committee, Medical Center Hospital of Vermont, Burlington, VT
Exercise

R. Philip Eaton, M.D.
Chief, Division of Endocrinology and Metabolism, University of New Mexico Hospital, Albuquerque, NM
Hyperlipoproteinemia

David H. Elwyn, Ph.D.
Senior Research Scientist, Albert Einstein College of Medicine of Yeshiva University and Montefiore Medical Center, New York, NY
The Intensive Care Patient

Allan J. Erslev, M.D.
Distinguished Professor, Thomas Jefferson University, Philadelphia, PA
Anemias

C. Richard Fleming, M.D.
Professor of Medicine, Mayo Medical School, Rochester, MN; Consultant in Gastroenterology, Mayo Clinic, Jacksonville, FL
Nutritional Options

Peter Fürst, M.D., Ph.D.
Professor and Chairman, University of Hohenheim, Institute for Biological Chemistry and Nutrition, Stuttgart, Federal Republic of Germany
The Intensive Care Patient

John Galloway, M.D.
Assistant Professor of Surgery, Emory University School of Medicine, Atlanta, GA
Heart Diseases

Paul E. Garfinkel, M.D., F.R.C.P.(C)
Professor and Vice Chairman, Department of Psychiatry, University of Toronto; Psychiatrist-in-Chief, Toronto General Hospital, Toronto, Ontario, Canada
Eating Disorders

David M. Garner, Ph.D.
Professor of Psychiatry, University of Toronto; Director, Research Division, Department of Psychiatry, Toronto General Hospital, Toronto, Ontario, Canada
Eating Disorders

Susan A. Goldstein, Ph.D.
Research Fellow, Division of Critical Care Medicine, Department of Anesthesiology, Montefiore Medical Center, New York, NY
Respiratory Diseases

William H. Goodson, III, M.D.
Associate Professor of Surgery, University of California, San Francisco; Attending Staff, Moffitt and Long Hospitals, University of California, San Francisco, Hospitals, San Francisco, CA
Wound Healing

T. Flint Gray, B.S.
Senior Medical Student, Emory University School of Medicine, Atlanta, GA
Heart Diseases

Gordon R. Greenberg, M.D., F.R.C.P.(C)
Associate Professor of Medicine, University of Toronto; Staff Gastroenterologist, Toronto General Hospital, Toronto, Ontario, Canada
Inflammatory Bowel Disease

Joan E. Harrison, M.D., F.R.C.P.(C)
Professor of Medicine, University of Toronto; Staff Physician, Toronto General Hospital, Toronto, Ontario, Canada
The Skeletal System

Steven B. Heymsfield, M.D.
Associate Professor, Columbia University School of Medicine; Director, Human Body Composition Laboratory and Weight Control Unit, Obesity Research Center, St. Luke's–Roosevelt Hospital, New York, NY
Heart Diseases

Graham L. Hill, M.D.
Professor and Chairman, University Department of Surgery, Auckland Hospital, Auckland, New Zealand
Dimensions of the Human Body and Its Compartments; The Perioperative Patient

Robert D. Hoff, M.D.
Staff, George Baptist Hospital, Atlanta, GA
Heart Diseases

Edward S. Horton, M.D.
Professor of Medicine, University of Vermont College of Medicine; Attending in Medicine, Medical Center Hospital of Vermont, Burlington, VT
Exercise

Nancy N. Huang, M.D.
Professor Emeritus, Department of Pediatrics, Temple University School of Medicine; Attending Staff, St. Christopher's Hospital for Children, Philadelphia, PA
Cystic Fibrosis

Thomas K. Hunt, M.D.
Professor of Surgery, University of California, San Francisco; Attending Staff, Moffitt and Long Hospitals, University of California, San Francisco, Hospitals, San Francisco, CA
Wound Healing

Frank L. Iber, M.D., M.A., B.S.
Professor of Medicine and Chief of Gastroenterology, Stritch College of Medicine, Loyola University of Chicago; Chief of Gastroenterology, Hines Veterans Administration Hospital and Foster McGaw Hospital, Chicago, IL
Alcohol-Associated Diseases

K. N. Jeejeebhoy, M.B., B.S.
Professor of Medicine, University of Toronto; Chief of Gastroenterology, Toronto General Hospital, Toronto, Ontario, Canada
Nutrient Metabolism; Peptic Ulcer; Short Bowel Syndrome; The Functional Basis of Assessment

David J. A. Jenkins, M.D., Ph.D.
Professor, Department of Medicine and Department of Nutritional Sciences, University of Toronto; Staff Physician, Division of Endocrinology, St. Michael's Hospital; Associate Physician, Division of Gastroenterology, Toronto General Hospital, Toronto, Ontario, Canada
Diseases of the Colon

Barry D. Kahan, Ph.D., M.D.
Professor of Surgery and Director of Immunology and Organ Transplantation, University of Texas Medical School, Houston, TX
The Renal Transplant Patient

Harvey L. Katzeff, M.D.
Assistant Professor of Medicine, Cornell University Medical College; Adjunct Attending, Rockefeller University Hospital, New York, NY; Assistant Attending, North Shore University Hospital, Manhasset, NY
Endocrine Diseases

John M. Kinney, M.D.
Professor Emeritus in Surgery, Columbia University; Visiting Professor, Rockefeller University; Attending in Medicine and Surgery, St. Luke's–Roosevelt Hospital Center, New York, NY
Energy Metabolism: Heat, Fuel and Life; Respiratory Diseases; The Intensive Care Patient

Vladimir Kvetan, M.D.
Assistant Professor of Anesthesiology and Medicine, Albert Einstein College of Medicine of Yeshiva University; Director, Critical Care Medicine, Department of Anesthesiology, Montefiore Medical Center, New York, NY
Respiratory Diseases

Sally A. Lederman, Ph.D.
Assistant Professor of Public Health Nutrition, Columbia University School of Public Health, New York, NY
Pregnancy and Lactation

Sum P. Lee, M.D., Ph.D., F.R.A.C.P.
Associate Professor of Medicine, University of Washington School of Medicine; Gastroenterologist, Veterans Administration Medical Center, Seattle, Washington
Diseases of the Liver and Biliary Tract

Michael J. McMahon, Ch.M., Ph.D., F.R.C.S.
Senior Lecturer in Surgery, University Department of Surgery, General Infirmary; Consultant Surgeon, General Infirmary and Chapel Allerton Hospital, Leeds, England
Diseases of the Exocrine Pancreas

Kenneth G. McNeill, M.A., D.Phil.
Professor of Physics, University of Toronto; Special Staff Member, Toronto General Hospital, Toronto, Ontario, Canada
The Skeletal System

Donna Muller, Ph.D., R.D.
Nutritionist, Pulmonary Section, St. Christopher's Hospital for Children, Philadelphia, PA
Cystic Fibrosis

Hamish N. Munro, M.D., D.Sc.
Senior Scientist, USDA Human Nutrition Research Center on Aging at Tufts Medical School; Professor of Medicine, Tufts Medical School, Boston, MA; Professor of Nutrition, Tufts University, Medford, MA; Adjunct Professor of Physiological Chemistry, Massachusetts Institute of Technology, Cambridge, MA
Aging

Jennifer Nelson, M.S., R.D.
Coordinator, Section of Clinical Dietetics; Home Enteral Nutrition Coordinator, Mayo Clinic, Rochester, MN
Nutritional Options

Oliver E. Owen, M.D.
Professor of Medicine, Temple University School of Medicine; Program Director, General Clinical Research Center, Temple University Hospital, Philadelphia, PA
Regulation of Energy and Metabolism; Obesity

Judy Palmer, M.D.
Attending Staff, Children's Hospital at Stanford, Palo Alto, CA
Cystic Fibrosis

Shakuntla Puri, M.D.
Post-Doctoral Fellow in Immunology, Janeway Child Health Centre, St. John's, Newfoundland, Canada
Food Allergy

Richard S. Rivlin, M.D.
Chief, Nutrition Service, Memorial Sloan-Kettering Cancer Center; Professor of Medicine and Chief, Nutrition Division, New York Hospital–Cornell Medical Center, New York, NY
Endocrine Diseases

Gary Rodin, M.D., F.R.C.P.(C)
Associate Professor of Psychiatry, University of Toronto; Staff Psychiatrist, Toronto General Hospital, Toronto, Ontario, Canada
Eating Disorders

Pedro Rosso, M.D.
Professor of Pediatrics, Pontificia Universidad Catolica de Chile, Santiago, Chile
Pregnancy and Lactation

Daniel V. Schidlow, M.D.
Associate Professor of Pediatrics, Temple University School of Medicine; Chief of Pulmonary Section, St. Christopher's Hospital for Children, Philadelphia, PA
Cystic Fibrosis

Charles R. Shuman, M.D.
Professor of Medicine, Temple University School of Medicine; Staff Physician, Metabolic Division, Temple University Hospital, Philadelphia, PA
Diabetes Mellitus

David B. A. Silk, M.D., F.R.C.P.
Co-Director, Department of Gastroenterology and Nutrition, Central Middlesex Hospital, London, England
Malabsorption

Robin C. Spiller
Senior Registrar, Central Middlesex Hospital, London, England
Malabsorption

Ezra Steiger, M.D., F.A.C.S.
Assistant Clinical Professor of Surgery, Case Western Reserve University; Staff Surgeon and Head, Section of Surgical Nutrition, Cleveland Clinic Foundation, Cleveland, OH
Enterocutaneous Fistulas

Riyad Tarazi, M.D.
Cardiac Transplantation Fellow, University of Minnesota, Minnesota Heart and Lung Institute, Minneapolis, MN
Enterocutaneous Fistulas

Arleen K. Thom, M.D.
Research Fellow, Division of Surgical Oncology, University of Pennsylvania, Philadelphia, PA; Resident in Surgery, Robert Wood Johnson School of Medicine, Camden, NJ
Neoplastic Diseases

Charles T. Van Buren, M.D.
Professor of Surgery and Associate Director, Organ Transplant Division, University of Texas Medical School, Houston, TX
The Renal Transplant Patient

Richard L. Veech, M.D.
Chief, Laboratory of Metabolism and Molecular Biology, National Institute of Alcohol Abuse and Alcoholism, Rockville, MD
Phosphorus Magnetic Resonance Spectroscopy as a Probe of Nutritional State

Douglas W. Wilmore, M.D.
Professor of Surgery, Harvard Medical School; Director, Nutrition Support Services, Brigham and Women's Hospital, Boston, MA
The Burned Patient

Myron Winick, M.D.
R. R. Williams Professor of Nutrition and Professor of Pediatrics, Columbia University College of Physicians and Surgeons; Attending Pediatrician, Presbyterian Hospital, New York, NY
Pregnancy and Lactation

FOREWORD

The maintenance of a proper food intake has been a cornerstone in the care of patients throughout the centuries. However, many diseases, as well as severe injury, alter the function of the gastrointestinal tract and reduce appetite, which results in progressive malnutrition. The nutritional therapy for such patients has changed dramatically over the past 25 years as the result of many factors. Among these has been the increasing awareness of the extent of malnutrition in patients entering the hospital and of the fact that malnutrition has been found to become worse during hospitalization. In order to improve the nutritional therapy of hospitalized patients, the components of a normal diet have been carefully defined and then combined into solutions that could be safely given by vein, or as specialized nutritional support into the intestinal tract. Once such products were introduced, it became apparent that the nutritional condition of any given patient depends not only on the level of nutritional support, but on the metabolic changes that accompany disease and injury. Nutrition and metabolism are thus intimately connected and interacting. Some of the metabolic changes in various conditions appear to be useful for survival, while other reactions become deleterious if excessive or overly prolonged. The amounts and proportions of nutrients that are supplied should aim to support, or modify, the metabolic events in a beneficial way.

Clinical interest in the interaction of nutrition and metabolism was at a low ebb for many years. However, the recent upsurge of interest and knowledge in these fields has suggested the need for a new clinical reference text. The four editors of this book are well known scientists with vast knowledge of nutrition and metabolism in various clinical conditions. They have been successful in compiling a single volume sharply focused on patient care with due reference to the relevant nutritional and metabolic background. These editors represent individual expertise in energy metabolism, gastrointestinal disease, body composition, and endocrinology, as well as extensive experience in the nutritional support of hospitalized patients. All chapters are written by medical scientists who have made valuable contributions to our knowledge of a particular area of nutrition or metabolism.

An attractive component of this book is that it covers nutritional and metabolic issues related to conditions in both the fields of internal medicine and surgery. The approach to nutritional support differs to some extent between the representatives of nutritional science, internal medicine, and surgery. The editors have endeavored to emphasize the fundamental knowledge that is common to each of these approaches.

I am certain that this book will not only be useful in the care of today's patient, but that it will also act as a stimulus to promote necessary research in the field which will become tomorrow's patient care.

ARVID WRETLIND

PREFACE

The field of nutrition is in an interesting phase in relation to medical practice and to the growth of medical science. More than ever before, medical practice must incorporate nutritional considerations. However, it is difficult to remain familiar with the growing science of nutrition when the physician is also faced with the challenge of keeping up to date in many other rapidly expanding areas. At the same time, public awareness of nutrition is steadily increasing in the affluent developed countries, where the popular life-style now emphasizes physical conditioning together with increasing attention to diet. This attitude is strengthened by the growing recognition in the lay press of the role of diet in heart disease and of various medical problems associated with obesity.

Current books on nutrition have not focused on the correlation with metabolism. It is increasingly clear that what is optimum nutrition for a given patient depends upon his underlying metabolic status, as well as on his primary diagnosis. This book, therefore, is an effort to combine nutrition and metabolism, including the influence of the conventional hormones and selected evidence on the growing array of tissue and cell mediators.

Nutrition has traditionally been considered the province of physicians working with certain medical diseases, all of them chronic in nature. The surgeon, prior to the advent of TPN, usually dealt with acute, short-term kinds of treatment; the relatively long-term effects of nutrition were not considered. The surgeon tended to worry about malnutrition only insofar as it was seen to threaten wound healing. The introduction of TPN and of specialized enteral nutrition has greatly improved the care of gastrointestinal disease. It has also provided a tremendous stimulus to investigation of the proper role of nutrition in acute forms of therapy for other surgical diseases and injuries. However, there have been few books that have attempted to present the nutrition and metabolism of acute, as well as chronic, clinical problems.

This book has been divided into four sections. The first section provides basic information on the normal human body and the elements of nutrition. The first chapter deals with energy metabolism with more than the usual historical emphasis, since the interrelationships of the concepts of heat, fuel, and life have been closely interwoven with the growth of our understanding of nutrition. A chapter on the control of metabolism assumes special importance since metabolic control does much to determine optimum nutrition for a particular patient. The chapter on body composition presents state-of-the-art information to promote understanding of the underlying significance of changes in body weight, both during the onset of malnutrition and during subsequent nutritional therapy.

The second section of the book reports on nutritional considerations that arise when variations occur in the otherwise normal individual: aging, physical activity, pregnancy, and so forth.

The third section is concerned with a variety of clinical conditions both medical and surgical, acute as well as chronic. Classically, certain diseases have enlisted the attention of those interested in nutrition, particularly hyperthyroidism, diabetes, renal disease, and obesity. The problem of atherosclerosis has focused much recent attention on diet in relation to heart disease. However, less attention has been paid to the effect of nutrition on the function of the heart and the lungs, as highlighted in chapters in this book. The delicate balance that exists between the compromised function of the heart, or the lungs, and the increased demand for gas exchange, associated with aggressive nutrition, is a unique example of how organ physiology can be improved with better nutrition and how it can also be threatened by improper nutrition. The chapters on nutrition and immunity and the ones on the nutritional therapy of injury and infection highlight the growing interest in the mechanisms of inflammation and immunity and on the ways that these are influenced by nutrition. The chapters on the lung and on cancer also lend special insight into the interrelationships of inflammation, immunity, and nutrition. These are but some examples of how the effectiveness of nutrition needs to be monitored in terms of the function of cells and tissues, as well as monitored for the restoration of normal body weight and body composition.

The field of clinical nutrition has been held back by the lack of generally accepted and readily available measurements for nutritional assessment. Failure to agree on such measurements is the result of lack of adequate data on the sensitivity, precision, and cost of each measurement, when used for assessing nutritional status. Therefore, the fourth section includes a chapter dealing with this problem. Computerized data banks are now allowing hospitals to arbitrarily identify patients at risk from malnutrition and then to compare evidence of their improvement with the cost of whatever nutritional support is provided. Escalating concern about improving hospital nutrition has even reached the regulatory organizations, both governmental agencies and the Joint Commission for Hospital Accreditation. Good hospital nutritional practice can be expected to undergo outside review in the future, much as having a safe bacteriological environment and a properly run pharmacy are scrutinized today. At the same time, there is increasing evidence of hospitals seeking physicians with training and certification in nutrition to provide leadership roles in improving the nutritional care of hospitalized patients. The final chapter deals with considerations involved in the choice of techniques of enteral and parenteral nutritional support.

We believe that this book will be of importance in advancing the role of nutrition in the care of patients with disease and injury at a time when the science of nutrition is expanding rapidly, while at the same time the increased expenditures for improved medical care have come under critical scrutiny.

We offer most sincere thanks to the contributing chapter authors. By catching the spirit of what we set out to accomplish, each of them has helped to make our task as editors both pleasant and informative.

JOHN M. KINNEY
K. N. JEEJEEBHOY
GRAHAM L. HILL
OLIVER E. OWEN

CONTENTS

I

HUMAN METABOLISM AND ITS REGULATION AND MEASUREMENT

1

ENERGY METABOLISM: HEAT, FUEL AND LIFE

JOHN M. KINNEY

The concept of energy exchange in the human body may be difficult to think of as important in understanding and treating disease and injury. This is because energy that enters the body in the chemical bonds of food undergoes an interlocking series of steps, each one of which represents a problem of supply and demand. Various medical disciplines are concerned with selected parts of energy exchange, such as nutrition, intermediary metabolism, ventilation, circulation, cellular energetics, tissue and organ work, or processes of heat loss. Taken together these constitute a dynamic system whose quantitative relationships are subject to measurement or at least reasonable estimation.

The common measurements of nutritional status performed on hospitalized patients relate to concentrations, particularly in the blood or urine. Only a limited number of clinical measurements are available that indicate the rate of an important process. This is particularly true in energy metabolism, for which there are no routine measurements in clinical care that document the rate of energy expenditure, heat production, or the associated levels of ventilation and circulation that must provide for the amount of gas exchange needed to support this energy transfer. A further limitation in considering energy exchange as part of medical practice is the lack of an easily measured part of the body (the metabolic body size) that is responsible for energy utilization and heat production in the body. It is reasonable to hope that new technology will streamline and simplify measurements of both energy expenditure and body composition, so that they may be considered together as important parts of the mainstream of medical practice.

The simple definition of an engine is a device that consumes fuel to perform work. The energy that does not appear as work is dissipated as heat. The human body may be considered as a machine that does its own maintenance and powers a convective system that distributes fuel and oxygen to the local sites of utilization and removes the waste products as well as the heat. In addition to the internal maintenance of tissues and the regulation of energy balance, the body may move and do work. The healthy body maintains relatively large stores of organic materials, which can be utilized for reserve energy, while body heat reserves are relatively limited in relation to the normal rate of heat production. The human machine has an optimum range for body composition and also an optimum operating temperature, or body heat content. However, the range for the former can vary considerably, while the range for the latter is protected within narrow limits. The ability of normal humans to think, move, and work without delay or prior preparation illustrates a unique degree of independent energy utilization. This constant and ready availability of energy underlies animal life in general and human life in particular ways.

The concept of energy as the ability to perform work is relatively difficult to grasp in comparison with the associated tissue fuels, which can be seen, weighed, and otherwise recognized by the senses. Despite the problems of defining energy, current discussions of food intake are most commonly referred to in terms of calories, and malnutrition is most often described as a lack of caloric intake. This is in contrast to ancient history, when the understanding of life was related to body temperature and, therefore, to heat production. The methods by which early man produced heat were considered to be involved with vital processes that could not be understood and thus provided an easy excuse for the failure to search for explanations of energy and heat metabolism.

Major concepts of energy were established during the century between 1750 and 1850. Much less attention has been paid to the preceding century, when many of these major concepts in energy were partially recognized but incompletely understood. The limitations on the understanding of energy during the century before 1750 were partly the result of poor, or nonexistent, equipment for making crucial measurements. However, an equally important limitation was caused by widely accepted, but erroneous, concepts, the most outstanding of which had to do with "phlogiston." This widely accepted concept prevented otherwise outstanding experimentation from making a proper contribution to the advancement of scientific understanding.

Many of the major concepts of energy were important milestones in the growth of human biology. The following three were especially noteworthy: (1) the recognition that heat content was separate from temperature provided an important insight into the behavior of heat in all materials, including human tissues; (2) the idea that respiration was the same basic process as combustion illuminated our understanding of all animal life; and (3) the understanding that the processes of heat production and heat loss in the human body obeyed the laws of thermodynamics did much to free biology from vitalistic concepts and to establish living processes as appropriate subjects for scientific study.

There is now growing attention to measuring energy expenditure and heat production in various pathological situations where the measurements may deviate to an unknown degree from standard tables, which are commonly referred to in energy measurements. Many of the laws and concepts that have been established in regard to energy metabolism have been demonstrated only in certain well-defined circumstances. Our classical knowledge of energy metabolism may not be complete, and factors that are not currently defined may be important in explaining the human variability in maintaining body weight on a given food intake, or in performing a given amount of work at a fixed energy cost. There is greater awareness of factors related to body weight and food metabolism, when compared with the relatively limited information about heat production and its relationship to heat loss. This chapter is an effort to present considerations that apply to thermal, as well as to the substrate, aspects of human life.

The past 15 years have seen a resurgence of interest in human energy metabolism. Some types of obesity may be the result of metabolic abnormalities that affect energy storage. The introduction of parenteral and enteral nutritional support for the hospitalized patient has emphasized that calorie intake should be provided in the light of measured or estimated energy expenditure. New clinical interest in energy metabolism has stimulated manufacturers to design and market equipment for the simplified bedside measurement of gas exchange. This attention to measuring energy expenditure for practical clinical purposes has brought about greater awareness of the magnitude and importance of interrelationships between food, work, and heat in the normal human body. It has become apparent that the human body deals with energy as two matched balances: a substrate balance between food intake and the oxidation of fuel versus a thermal balance between heat production and heat loss. The substrate balance involves the input and output of relatively large body energy stores, while the thermal balance involves the input and output of very limited stores of body heat. Therefore, excesses of food intake produce obesity only if sustained over months or years, while increasing heat production plus decreasing heat loss can produce a major fever in minutes to hours. The delicate matching that the normal body maintains between the substrate balance and thermal balance is obviously of extremely high priority. This is handled with such efficiency that most physicians take it for granted as part of the "wisdom of the body." It seems reasonable to expect that medical practice of the future will discover that disease and injury disturb the integration of the substrate balance with the thermal balance, and that future intensive care of the critically ill patient will require monitoring of each of these balances to minimize the metabolic stress that may arise when they cease to operate at optimum levels.

It is an interesting commentary on current attitudes toward energy metabolism to compare modern medicine with animal husbandry or the automotive industry. Government funds, both in the United States and in Europe, have been allocated in much larger amounts for the study of animal energetics and the efficient use of food for animal growth than for comparable studies in man. The design and development of more sophisticated auto engines has involved advanced studies of fuel combustion and heat dissipation. The local automobile service station is apt to adjust the carburetor settings in terms of the optimum analysis of the exhaust gases. Some state laws demand measurement of the exhaust gases to detect undesirable levels of products of incomplete fuel combustion. These examples suggest that energy measurements are utilized despite the cost when economic gains are obvious, whereas energy measurements in medicine lack the corresponding economic stimulants.

Normal life may be defined as the conversion of energy to perform meaningful work at an acceptable metabolic cost. Illness and injury may be defined as energy conversion, work requirements, or metabolic costs that have now become excessive. Therefore, death may be defined as the irreversible loss of the ability to use energy to perform sufficient work in one or more vital organs.

HISTORY

Vitalism and Body Heat

The concept of life being associated with a "vital force," or a vital heat, dates back to the earliest cultures. It was once thought that a spirit inhabited the living body and was responsible for the production of vital heat and that disease occurred when the healthy spirit was dispossessed by an evil spirit. Those who believed in vitalism felt that life represented a new and foreign principle, or substance, imposed on materials that constituted the body. Through most of its history vitalism has been a philosophical concept that was independent of natural science. The early Greeks endowed water, fire, and earth with the life-creating principle.[1] Hippocrates, who gave to Greek medicine its scientific spirit, felt that the essence of life was an "ether," a subtle fire, existing from the beginning of time, that was present in air and all matter. This ether was similar to the "pneuma" described in the works of Plato. To some the pneuma had the attributes of a material substance comparable to oxygen, while to others it was an intangible material essential to all of life. The Hippocratic school believed that the ether, or pneuma, entered the body through the lungs and was carried throughout the body in the blood, sustaining vital action of life forces. By 300 B.C., this vital force had been separated into two parts: the vital spirits that resided in the heart and the animal spirits that resided in the brain.

Aristotle believed that the innate heat of the heart was the source of life and that all of its powers were related to nutrition, sensation, movement, and thought. He believed that an animal might live when other parts of the body were cool, but that it would die as soon as the heat was lost from the heart. He therefore equated the heart with the soul, which was set aglow with fire. In locating this vital force in the heart, Aristotle gave this organ a preeminence in body functions that required that other aspects of body function be subservient to this source of life. He also believed that nature had created the brain as a counterbalance to the heart and to the heat that it contained. He believed that in man the large size of the brain was due to the large amount of heat and blood contained in the human heart. His views on vital heat, together with later contributions by Galen, formed the strongest and longest-lived biological doctrine that medicine has ever known. As late as the 18th century, vital heat was utilized in explanations by the foremost physicians and physiologists of the time.

Galen believed in the importance of anatomical research to explain physiological function and therefore the source of life. He believed that venous blood originating in the liver traveled to the right side of the heart, where a separation took place, the living portion proceeding to the left side of the heart and the dead portion moving to the lungs, where it underwent refreshment under the influence of the life-giving pneuma. These beliefs, based on Greek speculation and grafted onto Roman thought, influenced successive generations of scientists and physicians for 1500 years (Fig. 1–1).

Avicenna, author of the Canon of Medicine, an immense encyclopedia that codified medical knowledge in the 11th century, also emphasized the importance of vital heat. This internal heat was equated with physical vitality and was differentiated from external heat, which was thought to be harmful to bodily health.

Until the early years of the 17th century, efforts were made to clarify the distinction between fire and vital heat. Jean Fernel wrote, "Innate heat is not the same nature as fire. It comes from a different source from fire." He argued that life was possible because of innate heat, but that innate heat was different from external heat, which was derived from fire. He believed that vital heat entered man at the very moment that the embryo became an independent individual, which he set at around 40 days before birth. He thus concluded that death was synonymous with the loss of innate heat from the body.

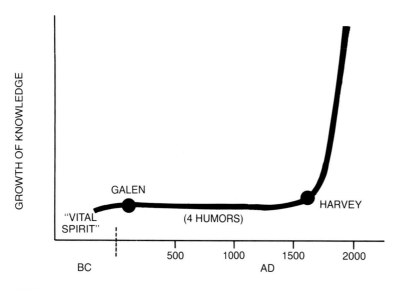

FIGURE 1-1. *The growth of knowledge regarding body heat, fuel and life is shown as a diagram to emphasize the lack of change for approximately 1500 years.*

William Harvey and Vitalism

The 1600's represented a period of dramatic transition in the history of science. This was particularly true for astronomy and physics, as well as for chemistry and biology. The concept of vital heat, as developed by the early Greek physicians, had remained substantially unchanged since 100 A.D. William Harvey stood at the threshold not only of modern medicine, but of a modern approach to science in general.[1] It is of particular interest that Harvey's early notebooks stressed the great importance of heat to sustain life and the necessity of cooling and ventilation for the continued production of vital heat. He felt that heat was necessary for the digestion of food and for the nourishment of life processes. He noted that the movement of animals was affected by internal warmth, since "warmer things are more agile, and colder things more lazy," which he believed was true for all species.

Harvey's doctrine of the circulation of blood depended upon the concept of innate heat for much of his theory. He was aware that if an artery was occluded, the distal tissues would be cold and lifeless. Thus, as blood moved through the extremities it would cool and thicken and have to return to the heart to be warmed. Harvey considered the heart to be "the innate fire and the beginning of life." He also believed that the blood passing from the right heart was saved from "bubbling to excess" by its contact with the expired air in the lungs before being returned to the left heart. Therefore, these cyclic processes provided the means by which the two extremes of hot and cold could be balanced, maintaining a normal body temperature.

However, in later writings Harvey indicated a change in attitude toward the nature of the body's innate heat.[2] In earlier publications, he had compared body heat to an ordinary flame, or fire, but later he cited Aristotle, who maintained that innate heat is not fire and does not derive from fire. Harvey then began to link internal heat closely to blood, maintaining that it had no existence apart from blood. Although the belief in the heat of the blood still had a touch of vitalism, Harvey had in essence reduced the heat of the blood to a property of the blood. He was certain that heat was closely related to the maintenance of life, but became progressively more careful about his analogies to fire and to limiting the origins of vital heat to the heart.

Rene Descartes attempted to establish an alternate physiology, consistent with his general view of the mechanics of nature.[1] According to his view, the heart was little more than a container where the blood was heated by some natural process akin to fermentation. Descartes believed that his interpretation of innate heat was successful in illustrating the living body as a machine. The warmth of the heart he believed was somehow responsible for generating animal spirits, which continually rose from the heart to the brain and from there through the nerves to the muscles, accounting for the motion of the body.

Descartes saw the whole body as a machine, but the chemists of the 17th century sought to apply chemical theory to various physiological functions. Instead of assuming that heat was inherent in the living body, or that heat was the basis of a whole array of physiological activities, they examined each function and sought a chemical basis to explain it. A pioneer in these attempts was van Helmont. He rejected the idea that innate heat was a vital factor, or even essential to life. He noted that frogs and fish remained cool, while being as alive as warm-blooded mammals. He believed that the death of warm-blooded animals did not occur because heat was lost, but rather that heat disappeared because the animal was dead. In support of this belief, he noted the heart of a cold-blooded frog beats in a manner similar to those of other animals, demonstrating that there was no innate heat in the heart responsible for its expansion and contraction. The concepts of van Helmont were singularly important because he was seeking a specific cause for the production of animal heat and refused to consider the warmth of the animal as a vital, or inherent, quality. His concepts removed animal heat as the major vital factor, thus setting investigators free to study vital heat independently and develop new theories to account for it (Fig. 1–2).

Air, Heat, and Life

William Harvey was not only a pioneering investigator, but while at Oxford he developed around him a remarkable group of early physiologists. Three of these men, Robert Boyle, Robert Hooke, and John Mayow, introduced a conceptual framework involving animal heat, respiration, and combustion.[2] During the last four decades of the 17th century, these men and their colleagues carried out experiments demonstrating that atmospheric air, or some part of it, was involved in a similar manner in both combustion and respiration. In both processes, they noted that heat was produced. Thus, it appeared that while respiration was not in fact important for cooling the lungs, it was somehow responsible for the production of vital heat. Boyle and Hooke experimented with a vacuum pump and showed that neither a flame nor a chick could survive in a vacuum. Hooke then opened the thorax of a dog, removed its diaphragm, and showed that the dog remained alive when the lungs were supplied fresh air by means of a bellows.[2] Thus, the important feature of breathing was a supply of fresh air and not the mechanical action of the organs involved. Additional studies suggested that atmospheric air contained a quality that allowed it to support respiration and combustion, and that when this quality

was exhausted the air became useless for this support. Mayow proposed that a portion of the air, important for the maintenance of life, was made up of nitrous particles, or "ariel nitre." Thus, in 1668, the Oxford group had published the hypothesis that something contained in the air was necessary for respiration and that it behaved in a process similar to that which had been described for combustion.

An important direct measurement of the heat of the heart was made by Giovanni Borelli in Italy. He utilized a thermometer to measure the temperature of different organs in a living stag and found the liver, lungs, and intestines to have the same degree of warmth as the heart. Borelli thus concluded that the heart could not contain either fire or flame.

The nature of physiological explanation changed during the 17th century, and the concept of animal heat reflected these changes. At the beginning of the century, innate heat was thought to arise in the heart, but at the end of the century not only was a causal explanation sought for heat production, but that explanation was very similar to the general theory of combustion.

Body Temperature and Body Heat

Hermann Boerhaave was one of the most influential physicians of the early 18th century, and his teachings in Leiden influenced the direction of medicine in many countries. He believed in a mechanical explanation for the production of animal heat, believing that blood flow through the lungs caused friction to be a chief source of that heat. In an effort to investigate the cooling function of the air, Boerhaave asked Gabriel Fahrenheit to utilize improved thermometers to measure how great a degree of heat in

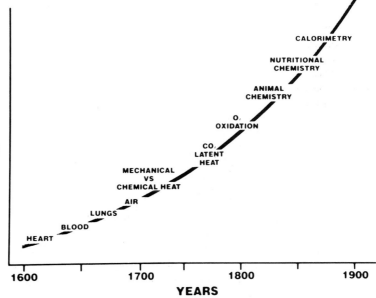

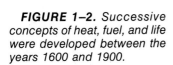

FIGURE 1–2. *Successive concepts of heat, fuel, and life were developed between the years 1600 and 1900.*

ambient air could be endured by animals.[3] While he did not develop any original concepts concerning the source of innate heat, his teachings emphasized the need for quantitative measurement in medical care and his influences stimulated the development of thermometry in medical practice.

Respiration and Combustion

Ancient man had probably recognized that where a fire could not burn, an animal could not live. Boyle and other investigators realized that a similar alteration in terms of the volume of air was caused by combustion and respiration. The last half of the 18th century saw dramatic advances, owing to the recognition of the relation between specific components of air entering and leaving the body and the production of animal heat.

Joseph Black recognized a similarity in the products of combustion and breathing, both of which produced a gas that he named "fixed air." He never published his reflections on animal heat and its association with respiration. However, his concepts were published from the lecture notes of his students.[4] Black as a Professor of Medicine befriended a young instrument maker, James Watt, who had been asked to repair a museum model of the Newcomen steam engine.[5] Conversations between Black and Watt may have contributed to Black's doctrine of latent heat being associated with a change of state (from ice to water and from water to vapor) and to the realization that different substances have characteristically different capacities for heat.[6] He believed heat to be "inseparably necessary to the very existence of vegetables and animals," and also believed that the process of spontaneous evaporation greatly contributed to the ability of animals to withstand the heat of tropical climates.

An English minister, Joseph Priestley,[7] and a Swedish apothecary, Joseph Scheele, independently produced a gaseous material from a simple chemical reaction that was later shown to be oxygen. Unfortunately, both men were unable to recognize the significance of their experiments because of their belief in the presence of a fictitious material, "phlogiston," which they thought was released upon heating.

In 1777, Antoine Lavoisier in France presented two papers on the source of animal heat.[8] He speculated that respiration and combustion were similar and that perhaps respiration might be capable of generating animal heat. Lavoisier reported experiments that indicated that five sixths of the air breathed in by an animal was incapable of supporting either respiration or combustion, and that only one sixth consisted of "pure air." This latter air had been called "dephlogisticated" by Priestley, who noted that it was necessary for both respiration and combustion. Lavoisier suggested that highly respirable air was converted to "fixed air" by the burning of powdered charcoal, so that perhaps the same process occurred in the lungs during respiration. He wrote, "La respiration est donc une combustion."

The Early 1800's

The early part of the 19th century was characterized by many confrontations between physiologists and chemists. The rapid development of methods for identifying and analyzing organic compounds made it essential to investigate such vital phenomena as respiration, digestion, and nutrition in the light of this new chemical knowledge. Those who were trained as chemists sought to treat biological problems by an extension of the methods they had found to be successful in their own discipline. This was in contrast to investigators accustomed to dealing with organisms by anatomical studies or vivisection. The chemical approach was defined most clearly in the efforts of Lavoisier and by his followers, who sought to extend the theory of respiration that he had put forward at the end of the 18th century. Some Parisian chemists in the early 19th century were engaged in experiments to determine whether the heat actually produced by an animal matched the heat theoretically due to the chemical reactions of respiration. However, two well-known physiologists of the time, François Magendie of France and Johannes Müller of Germany, both doubted the adequacy of Lavoisier's theories. Many biologists of this period questioned the adequacy of a given chemical process to account for animal heat and even questioned any chemical explanation of related biological phenomena. When Claude Bernard began his physiological training, he was quickly exposed to both the prominence and the doubts concerning the chemical theory of respiration and animal heat production. He developed a growing conviction that chemical theories were useful only when they were coupled with direct animal experimentation.

During the 1840's, biochemical thought was being led by the brilliant German chemist, Justus Liebig, and his French counterpart, Jean-Baptist Dumas.[9] Various differences developed into acrimony between these two leaders in European chemistry. An extended confrontation developed between them over the source of animal fat. Liebig maintained that the formation of fat from sugar was possible in the animal body, while Dumas maintained that there was "preformed fat" even in corn, which could provide the fat found in the animal body. Boussingault, a French colleague of Dumas, undertook a massive effort in 1844 to use detailed analysis of food intake and carcass analysis of farm animals to support Dumas' view of the source of animal fat.[9] However, by the end of the following year, his experiments had proved, in both the goose and the pig, that animals could form fat from other classes of food.

Liebig has often been considered to be the father

of the modern methods of organic analysis. He copied the principle of Boussingault's balance method in order to account for the rate of exchange of carbon compounds in the animal economy, and applied to the problems of biology the advantages of the new organic chemistry which he himself was creating.[10]

The word "energy" was being used at the beginning of the 19th century to refer to mechanical energy. Its relationship to heat depended upon which theory of heat one believed in. One popular theory was that heat was synonymous with motion. This concept influenced the studies of Benjamin Thompson, who was later made Count Rumford because of his experiments with heat.[11] His observation of the heat generated when cannons were being bored represented a cornerstone in the belief that heat was the result of motion. Chemists were seeking a theory that would apply to the expansion of materials on heating and during changes of state. Lavoisier had proposed a caloric theory that attempted to explain all phenomena of heat in terms of an elastic fluid or "igneous fluid." Joseph Black examined the contemporary theories and decided to reject the concept that heat was based on motion and to accept the idea that heat, or "caloric," was in fact a fluid with particles that were self-repulsive. This idea provided an obvious explanation for expansion of this material on heating and contraction on cooling. However, many biologists felt that the explanation of heat remained unsatisfactory.

The work of Hermann von Helmholtz, a towering scientific personality, influenced all branches of 19th century science from theoretical mechanics to applied physiology.[11] He was trained as a physician and had spent several years in the laboratory of Müller. When he addressed the problem of "vital forces," and especially that of vital heat, he argued that vital forces were, like other forces, being conserved in nature and that, as all phenomena were reducible to mechanics, vital forces could be considered as mechanical forces. The mathematical treatment of this argument led to his famous publication in 1847, "On the Conservation of Force." The conservation of energy appeared to be a multiple discovery that burst forth among various European scientific investigators related to two independent groups that were working in England and Germany between 1840 and 1855. The English group, originating with James Prescott Joule, was preoccupied by problems of the efficiency of conversion between the various "mechanical powers." The German investigators, Helmholtz and Julius Mayer, were troubled by the physiological problem of "animal heat" and their work resulted in the formulation of the law of the conservation of energy. At the begining of the 19th century, the central concepts in physics were related to space, time, mass, and force, but by the end of the 19th century the central concepts were expressed in terms of space, time, mass, and energy.

The Late 1800's

Pioneering contributions in metabolism and nutrition came from Germany during the second half of the 1800's, particularly from the school established by Carl von Voit.[10] Max von Pettenkofer was a professor of medical chemistry at Munich and one of his first students was Voit, whose name is associated with his teacher in the Pettenkofer-Voit respiration apparatus. Voit expanded studies of physiology and metabolism as related to nutrition, whereas Pettenkofer moved away from these studies into experimental hygiene. This early respiration calorimeter was able to measure carbon dioxide output, although oxygen consumption could not be measured. Nevertheless, it was possible to establish the daily carbon balance as well as nitrogen balance of the human subject. One of the early contributions of Voit was to establish that nitrogen in the air did not play a significant role in protein metabolism in the body. Urinary urea was found to be proportional to protein destruction.

Max Rubner was trained in the laboratories of Voit and extended many of the concepts of his teacher in nutrition and metabolism.[12] The apparatus for quantitative evaluation of carbon dioxide production provided extensive opportunity for examining the metabolism of the principal foodstuffs in animals and man. Rubner built a self-registering calorimeter that combined measurements of expired carbon dioxide with the nitrogen excreted in the urine and feces. This work was the background for the law of constant heat sums, which states that in a chemical reaction the heat produced or absorbed is the same irrespective of the pathway providing the end products. Rubner measured the varying influence of foods on energy production and found that a difference existed between carbohydrates, fats, and protein, which he termed "specific dynamic action." He proposed the standard caloric values for the major foodstuffs that are still in use today. He also became impressed with the fact that energy metabolism resulted in heat and that heat had to be lost through the surface of the body. Therefore, calculations of the body surface area seemed to bear a linear correlation with the energy metabolism of the animal. This was the origin of the "law of surface area," which is discussed later under the components of metabolic rate. Rubner also presented evidence that fat, carbohydrate, and protein are interchangeable in terms of their calorie equivalents, contributing to the heat production of the body. He also performed classic studies in a dog in which the direct measurement of heat production was shown to agree well with the indirect calculations from gas exchange, thus supporting the fact that the animal body followed the law of the conservation of energy.

In the period from 1895 to 1910, many investigators who had received their early training in Germany set up their own laboratories elsewhere in Europe or in the United States, with a continuing interest in the study of calorimetry. W. O. Atwater, an American nutritionist who had studied under Voit, joined forces with the physicist E. B. Rosa and constructed a large calorimeter capable of measuring the amount of heat given off by a man confined in it for prolonged periods.[13] This apparatus confirmed Rubner's experiments and demonstrated that the energy expended by a man in doing work, such as bicycle riding, was exactly equal to the heat released by the metabolism of food being oxidized in the body. The physiologist F. G. Benedict extended Atwater's work by the construction of special facilities in the nutrition laboratory of the Carnegie Institute in Boston. Advanced equipment made possible the simultaneous measurement of total gas exchange and heat production. Such work was also extended in the physiological laboratories at Cornell University Medical College under the direction of Graham Lusk.[14] This facility had a small respiration calorimeter suitable for animals and small human subjects. In addition, the Russell Sage Institute of Pathology constructed a respiration calorimeter in Bellevue Hospital for the determination of energy metabolism in various disease states. The Russell Sage calorimeter was under the direction of Eugene DuBois, a colleague of Lusk and also a close friend of Max Rubner. These measurements of energy expenditure in hospitalized patients demonstrated the increased energy metabolism associated with different kinds of fever, but they are best remembered for confirmation of the usefulness of measuring basal metabolism in the diagnosis and treatment of disease of the thyroid gland.

During the 1920's there was a major shift away from energy metabolism and calorimetry. Biochemists were becoming interested in enzyme function, and nutritionists were busy searching for new vitamins.[10] Interest in calorimetry became relegated to the hospital measurement of the BMR as an indicator of thyroid function. This remained as a standard measurement in hospital laboratories until approximately 1950. At that time, new chemical methods for measuring materials in the urine and the blood related to thyroid metabolism caused hospitals to abandon use of the basal metabolic rate and therefore to terminate the last remaining quantitative approach to energy expenditure in patients.

The measurement of human energy expenditure received only limited attention from 1920 to 1970. Renewed interest in energy expenditure then arose from two particular sources, one related to surgical patients and the other to a medical disorder. The common association of weight loss with acute surgical disease and injury was attributed to a state of hypermetabolism of unknown degree. The introduction of parenteral and enteral nutrition support stimulated the desire to adjust energy intake to energy expenditure. In medicine, the search for the understanding of obesity has stimulated ongoing studies of diet-induced thermogenesis, since an abnormality of this process might account for increased energy storage.

HEAT METABOLISM AND DIRECT CALORIMETRY

Body Temperature

From a thermodynamic standpoint, the body does not expend energy, but merely converts it from one form to another. The final form into which energy is converted is heat, which cannot be used for the performance of work in a biological system and ultimately leaves the body to return to the environment. Thus, the human body takes in energy in a highly organized form as food and returns an equivalent amount of energy to the environment as heat. This overall concept of the human body as a continuous energy exchange device is represented in Figure 1–3 as a "black box" with the entry of energy as food and its exit as heat. The associated gas exchange represents the substrate oxidation and heat production. Therefore, the energy balance of the body represents two matched balances that must proceed simultaneously: a substrate balance that determines body composition and thermal balance that determines body heat content, as indicated in Figure 1–4. The exchange of heat between the human body and its environment is accomplished at such a rate and direction as to preserve an almost constant internal body temperature of 37° C. Skin temperature, for example, may fluctuate from 20 to 40° C. However, prolonged exposure to cold or hot environments causing local temperatures as low as 18° C or as high as 45° C is usually associated with both pain and tissue injury.

The development of heat metabolism was dependent upon the availability of reliable and convenient devices for thermometry. Sanctorius is generally credited with having written about a thermometer in 1611 to determine the presence of fever by an oral measurement.[3] Fahrenheit was stimulated by the great physician Boerhaave to develop a more useful clinical thermometer, and this resulted in having a thermometer with a series of gradations based on three fixed points: zero as the temperture of a mixture of ice, water, and salt; 32° as the temperature of ice and water without the salt; and 96° as a person's oral temperature. Later, Celsius utilized a temperature scale with zero for the freezing point of water and 100° for the boiling point of water. Thus, since the middle 1700's an instrument has been available for the accurate recording of body temperature during periods of both health and disease (Fig. 1–5). However, it was not until 100 years later that Carl Wunderlich was instrumental in establishing the practice of accurately monitoring and

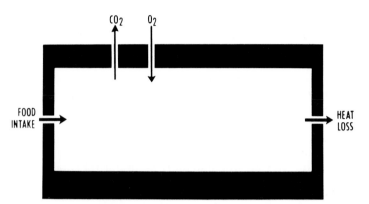

FIGURE 1–3. The human body can be regarded in simple terms as a continuous energy exchange device.

recording the body temperature in illness. He concluded that temperatures below 38° C were probably normal and that those above that represented fever. He noted that children tended to respond to infection with greater fevers than did adults and that old people often had a depressed febrile response. Later, Carl von Liebermeister suggested that fever was not the result of an inability of the organism to regulate body temperature, but that the organism was simply regulating its body temperature at a higher level. The past century has seen many experiments involving the physiological and behavior reponses of intact organisms and also studies involving electrical recording of neuronal activities, all of which support Liebermeister's claim made over 100 years ago that during fever heat regulation is adjusted to a higher level.

The tissues and organs of the human body appear to have optimum function when the temperature is close to 37° C. In 1865, Claude Bernard[15] noted that the protection of the temperature of the "milieu interieur" was critical for life. The temperature of pe-ripheral tissues such as skin and subcutaneous tissue are generally cooler than visceral temperatures and subject to much wider fluctuations. It is important to recognize that there is no single normal temperature but that a range of temperatures exists for healthy persons. A normal oral temperature averages approximately 36.7° C and can vary by as much as 0.5° C, whereas the corresponding range for rectal temperature is usually approximately 0.6 to 0.7° C higher than oral temperatures. In resting man, temperatures above the normal range are potentially more dangerous than those below it, since the normal human temperature is only a few degrees below the temperature at which tissue destruction occurs. During vigorous exercise the internal body temperature may increase in a normal person to levels of 39 or even 40° C.

In view of the vulnerability of the tissues to temperatures that differ appreciably from 37° C, human evolution has been associated with the development of an elaborate mechanism for regulating body temperature. To accomplish the regulation of human temperature two distinct control systems have been

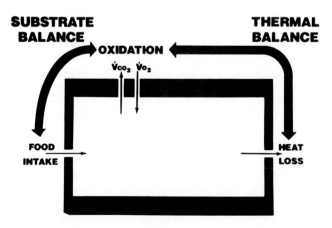

FIGURE 1–4. Human energy exchange represents two coordinated balances: a substrate balance, which has received considerable study, and a thermal balance, which has received much less attention in clinical care.

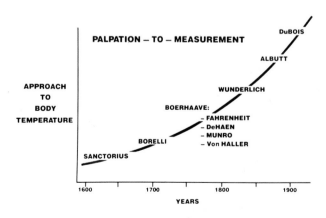

FIGURE 1–5. The growth of understanding in human energy and heat metabolism depended in part upon the gradual development of reliable and convenient thermometry.

employed: behavioral regulation involving the conscious voluntary use of all available means, and physiological regulation, employing the involuntary responses of the body to maintain constant temperatures. Figure 1–6 is taken from Hardy[16] and shows the environmental temperatures on earth and in near space as related to physiological and behavioral regulation of body temperature. Phylogenetically, behavioral regulation is a much older system. Many species control body temperature within rough limits by moving into more favorable thermal environments. Therefore, thermal regulatory response to temperature is the sum of behavioral and physiological activity. Behavioral regulation is important, but the permitted deviations in the value of the control temperature are great. The addition of physiological regulation to behavioral regulation provides both the precise control and the ability to handle greater deviations in environmental temperature.

In the resting or sedentary human, the changes in body heat content normally take place in the peripheral tissues. With cold exposure, selective vasoconstriction reduces the supply of blood to the skin and peripheral tissues, diverting blood to the organs of the viscera. In resting humans, most heat is produced in the body core, that is, the trunk, viscera, and brain, even though these tissues amount to only approximately one third of the entire body mass.

The heat that is supplied from the central organs must escape from the body surface; thus, the vasomotor system provides a unique means of control of heat loss. During activity the principal site of heat production shifts to the muscles.

Routes of Heat Loss

The human body exchanges heat with its surroundings through four main channels: radiation, conduction, convection, and vaporization.[17] Radiative heat loss involves the exchange of thermal energy between objects through a process that depends only upon the temperatures and the nature of the surfaces of the radiating objects. Therefore, the flow of heat by radiation does not depend upon the presence of an intervening medium, and heat will pass by the process of radiation from a hot object to a cooler object through a vacuum. For a normal naked person sitting quietly in an environment of 25° C, radiative heat loss will amount to 50 to 70 per cent of the entire heat loss. Not all of the body surface is effective in radiation exchange with the environment, because some surfaces exchange energy with other skin areas. A standing man with his arms at his sides has an effective radiating area of about 75 per cent of the total, while with the arms and legs extended the value may go as high as 85 per cent. In the tightly curled up position the radiating area can be reduced in 50 per cent of the total body surface area.

Conduction is the term applied to the flow of heat from one object to another without the physical transfer of material. Heat is conducted from internal tissues within the body to the skin surface and from the skin through the thin layer of air with which it is in contact, or into cooler objects such as the floor or clothing that may touch the skin. Of all the routes of heat exchange between the body and its environment, conduction is the one with which we are most familiar; our experience dates back to early childhood when the lessons of hot and cold were first learned. The direction of heat flow is always toward the lower temperature. For the resting human, heat exchange by conduction of heat from solid objects is usually small, and this factor is often neglected in heat balance calculations. It is perhaps desirable to think of insulation rather than conduction, because insulation represents the resistance to air flow. If there is a series of insulators, such as several layers of clothing, the total insulation is the sum of the resistance of each layer. The insulation value of a man's ordinary winter suit is referred to as one "clo" unit. The efficiency in insulation of various forms of clothing can be characterized by their clo units. The greatest insulators are the natural ones of animals, such as feathers and fur. These materials trap a highly insulating layer of air and prevent disturbance of this layer of warm air on the surface of the

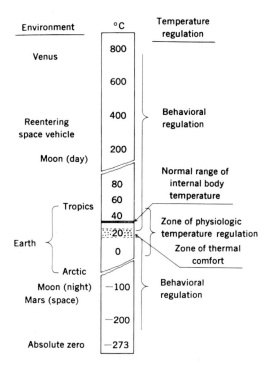

FIGURE 1–6. *The range of environmental temperature is shown in relation to physiological and behavioral regulation of body temperature. (From Hardy JD, Bard P. Body temperature regulations.* In *Mountcastle VB (ed). Medical Physiology. Vol. 2. 13th ed. St. Louis, CV Mosby, 1974.)*

body. Fat is a good insulator, and its role in the resistance to conduction of heat from the internal organs to the skin is important physiologically. The thicker layer of subcutaneous fat that women have in comparison to men provides greater insulation and reduces heat loss on exposure to cold.

Convection is the type of heat transfer that depends upon the existence of a fluid or gaseous medium between hot and cold objects. Thus, heat can be lost owing to extremes of warm air rising from the skin and passing into the cooler environment as a result of natural convection. The rate of heat loss from the skin by convection will of course depend on the skin and air temperatures as well as the air velocity. Convective heat transfer by the blood stream to the skin is of great physiologic importance and is under the control of the sympathetic nervous system. For each liter of blood at 37° C that flows to the skin and returns to the body core at 36° C, the body loses approximately 1 kcal of heat. The increased heat production associated with vigorous exercise is accompanied by an increase in blood flow to the skin of up to tenfold, providing efficient heat loss from the body. The term conductance is applied to the combined effect of the two heat transfer channels: conduction of heat through the muscle and fat layers, and convective heat transfer by the blood. Calculations of conductance are often based on the assumption that all the body heat is produced in the body core, conducted to the skin, and then transferred into the environment.

Benedict and other investigators since Rubner have pointed out that evaporative heat loss represents about 25 per cent of the metabolic heat carried away from the body as a result of water being evaporated from the skin and the lungs. This compares with approximately 60 per cent of heat loss due to radiation under normal conditions, and the combination of conduction and convection accounting for approximately 15 per cent. Although an equation can be written that combines the four major channels of heat loss in the human body, it can seldom be profitably used. Under most conditions, the thermal characteristics of the environment cannot be properly measured. However, for carefully controlled environments, the heat loss equations become simple, since the physiological reactions of man are known and can often be predicted by physical measurements.

Evaporative heat loss occurs when water is converted into vapor at body temperature; 0.6 kcal of heat per gram of water is absorbed in the process. Thus, evaporating water from the skin is an efficient way of losing heat even in an environment hotter than the skin. In this case the evaporative heat loss would have to take care of both the metabolic heat production and the heat absorbed by the radiation and convection from the hot environment. The body is always losing some heat by evaporation from the skin and respiratory tract, even in very cold weather when the physiological problem is how to retain body heat. At ambient temperatures below 30° C, the evaporative heat loss is fairly constant at around 12 to 15 gm of water per square meter per hour, one quarter to one half of this being due to the loss of moisture in breathing and the remainder to the slow transudation of water through the almost dry skin. At 30° C the evaporative heat loss amounts to about 25 per cent of the total heat loss. Above 30° C the evaporative heat loss increases with rising ambient temperature, and active sweating is stimulated to take care of the decreased heat loss due to radiation and convection. When the environmental and skin temperatures are equal, there can be no heat loss by radiation and convection, since the thermal gradient is zero. In such cases, usually in an ambient temperature of 35 to 36° C, all heat loss must be due to whatever evaporation is possible.

The secretory activity of sweat glands is under the control of sympathetic innervation. During exercise, sweating in humans is even more important than for the resting or sedentary individual because the rates of heat production can reach high values during heavy work and heat must be eliminated rapidly. To provide for this high heat flux, it is first necessary to stimulate the vasomotor system to transfer the heat from the muscles and the body core to the skin, and secondly, in all except the most cold environments, the sweat glands must be activated so as to eliminate the heat from the skin surface. During exercise the internal body temperature must rise to some degree in order to activate vasodilatation and transfer heat to the skin. The controlling system for regulation of heat balance involves detection of temperature, transmission of the information to some integrating network, provision of the set point or preferred temperature information, comparison of the set point and temperature signals, production of deviation or error signals, and transmission of the error signals to the appropriate effector mechanisms for shivering, sweating, and/or vasomotor action.

Direct Calorimetry

Rubner conducted extensive studies on the chemical composition of different foods and on gas exchange in animals, which led to the construction of an animal calorimeter that could accurately measure the amount of heat produced by a dog in 24 hours.[14] The amount of heat calculated from gas exchange measurements corresponded closely to the measured amount of heat lost in the calorimeter. These results were regarded as a demonstration of the truth of the law of the conservation of energy. Following Rubner, Atwater[13] and Rosa utilized their large calorimeter to confirm Rubner's experiments and demonstrate that the energy expended by a man, either at rest or doing work, was exactly equal to the energy set free by metabolism in the body.

Benedict extended Atwater's work in the nutrition laboratory of the Carnegie University Medical College in New York City, and in the respiration calorimeter constructed at the Bellevue Hospital where human disease was studied under the direction of DuBois.[14]

The Atwater-Rosa respiration calorimeter could measure both gas exchange and simultaneous heat production in man. Original respiratory measurements were based on the volume of carbon dioxide expired, but later the volume of oxygen inspired was added to the measurements to obtain the respiratory quotient.

The construction and operation of large direct calorimeters used for the study of heat production has been described in detail by a number of writers. The chambers are essentially airtight boxes of various sizes, some of which are large enough to permit the subject to move about and to exercise on a bicycle ergometer. The walls of the chamber are insulated in various ways and heated to a constant temperature to prevent any heat loss from the chamber to the room. Webb[18] has pointed out that there are essentially five types of calorimeters for direct measurement of heat loss. They are air flow, water flow, gradient layer, compensating heater, and storage calorimeters. The physical form may be a small room or chamber, or a box, or a bath, or a suit. The common form of calorimetry prior to World War II involved heat loss from the subject by conduction and radiation, which was absorbed by water flowing through copper tubes in a system that allowed the difference in temperature of the water entering and leaving the chamber to be multiplied by the volume of water flowing per unit time.

Benzinger[19] perfected the gradient layer calorimeter, which has certain advantages for measuring heat loss. This is based on an inner and an outer cylinder separated by an air space of fixed dimensions. Thermocouples attached to the walls of the inner and outer chambers measure the temperatures of the walls very accurately. The outer wall is maintained at a temperature close to that of the room by electric fans, and the inner wall is warmed by the heat loss from the subject. A temperature gradient is thus established between the inner and outer walls that is proportional to the rate of heat loss. The principle is that once a steady state of heat flow is reached between the inner and outer surfaces of the wall of the calorimeter, the integrated difference, or gradient, of temperatures between the inner and outer surfaces of this layer is proportional to the rate of total heat loss, or heat gain, from any source within the cavity. During change from one constant heat flow rate to another, the temperature gradient shows a rapid exponential rise or fall to a new level, which then represents the new steady heat flow rate. If the wall is constructed of thick layers of material, there will be a high gradient and the steady state will be reached very slowly. Thin layers will reach a steady state more rapidly but have a less sensitive response. The integrated response is also independent of the manner in which heat is transferred to the layer, whether by conduction, convection, radiation, or condensation of the water vapor that had previously been generated at the surface of the heat source.

Webb and associates[20] modified a space suit designed for use by astronauts, in order to measure heat output directly. Since the astronauts would be in a vacuum environment, and since their insulated space suits were made with reflective outer surfaces to minimize radiant heat exchange, they were thermally insulated, losing body heat only to a water-cooled undergarment. This suggested that with proper instrumentation and control, the space suit could be made to perform as a direct calorimeter. The Webb suit consists of layers of down and quilted polyester, which gives the assembly a high insulation value. Next to the skin, the subject wears a union suit made up of elastic mesh incorporating a network of small plastic tubing that is distributed over the whole body except for the face, hands, and soles of the feet. By measuring the change in water temperature across the suit plus the flow rate of the water, one can calculate the rate of heat loss from the body when correction factors are applied for other routes of small heat loss. Rectal and skin temperatures were measured throughout an experiment to follow any change in body heat content. The suit could be combined with indirect calorimetry including a full face mask through which air was drawn from the room at a fixed and constantly measured flow rate. The mix of exhaled and ambient air passed to the equipment cart where a small sample was drawn through a mixing chamber and then analyzed for CO_2 and O_2 content. Twenty-four-hour studies of healthy men revealed a correspondence between indirect and direct calorimetry of ± 3 per cent, as long as the men were resting and eating approximately what was required for a steady state. Thermal comfort was maintained by adjusting the water temperature at the suit inlet so that the subject was never chilling, never sweated, and was kept on the warm side of the vasomotor zone of thermoregulation. The unique aspect of this equipment is that the subject can wear the suit with both direct and indirect calorimetry measurements being made throughout not only during the waking day but during sleep as well. During the day, subjects can sit in comfortable chairs, read, play cards, eat meals at a table, and exercise on a bicycle ergometer.

Information on nine direct calorimeters that are currently in use has been assembled by van Es.[21] The design of chambers for direct calorimetry is limited by size so as to detect accurate signals of heat loss and to allow the subject to be as active as in normal life. The ventilation for such chambers varies from 50 to 200 L per minute. As simultaneous gas exchange measurements are made, it is obvious that the higher the rate of ventilation, the more the gas exchange of the individual being studied will be diluted by the air flow through the chamber; thus the instruments for measurement of O_2 and CO_2 must be more sensitive in order to achieve satisfactory accuracy.

From the time of Rubner, it has been accepted that the law of conservation of energy is true for humans and that the indirect calorimetry calculations of heat production and the direct measurement of heat loss will agree. Excellent agreement has been reported by Head and associates[22] using a calorimeter designed for clinical studies (Fig. 1–7). However, this agreement is true only for a steady state, and during many circumstances where there is either exercise or food intake, there will be a period of some hours thereafter in which the heat production will be seen to exceed the heat loss. This has led to the recommendation that measurements of direct and indirect calorimetry be conducted for a minimum of 24 hours if at all possible.

Body Temperature and Energy Expenditure

It has been pointed out by Kluger[23] that most terrestrial animals regulate their temperature somewhere between 35 and 42° C. The upper thermal limit for survival is around 45° C, where proteins begin to be denatured. The regulation of body temperature within this range appears to be due to the effects of temperature on biochemical reactions that provide benefit to the organism. The physics of heat exchange between an organism and the environment are most suitable at this level of body temper-

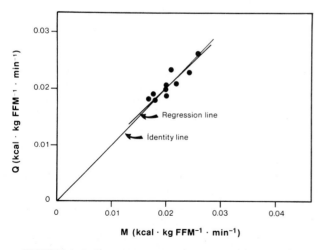

FIGURE 1–7. The close correspondence of heat release (Q), measured by direct calorimetry, to heat production, measured by indirect calorimetry, using equipment employed in a hospital for clinical studies. (From Heymsfield SB, Head CA, McManus CB III, et al. Am J Clin Nutr 1984; 40:116–130. © Am J Clin Nutr. American Society for Clinical Nutrition. Reproduced with permission.)

ature. Kluger has emphasized that living organisms can be separated between ectotherms, whose body temperature is dominated by the ambient temperatures, and endotherms, which regulate their body temperature as humans do at approximately 37° C. This thermoregulatory reflex requires a sensory input and a control center for integration, which is present in both endotherms and ectotherms. However, the difference lies in the effector arm, since endotherms have the metabolic machinery to generate sufficient amounts of internal heat to raise core temperature as needed. Human metabolic heat production at a neutral environmental temperature of about 30° C can be expected to be approximately 70 kcal per hour.

It is generally believed that fever can be beneficial when it is involved as part of stimulating host defense against infection. There have been relatively few recent studies concerning energy expenditure in the presence of fever. However, extensive studies were performed over 60 years go by DuBois and co-workers on basal metabolism in various fevers.[24] The relation between the basal metabolism rate and body temperature was measured in six different fevers, and the average value indicated that there was a 13 per cent increase in the metabolic rate for each degree centigrade of rectal temperature, which would correspond to approximately 7 per cent degree Fahrenheit. DuBois noted that previous information for a number of chemical reactions, where the temperature was plotted against the rate of chemical reaction, showed that the temperature coefficients tended to average between 2 and 3.5. In their clinical studies they had found that practically all of the fever experiments fell within these limits and that the average line had a temperature coefficient of 2.3. An objection to this type of analysis relates to considering the human body as simply a single compartment of enzymes whose reaction rates are increased in linear fashion above normal body temperature. It is obvious that many other biological changes are part of the response to fever and that many influences on heat balance must be considered in attempting to determine the optimum body temperature.

Ambient Temperature and Energy Expenditure

Careful control of heat loss mechanisms is a fundamental characteristic of all homeotherms. At raised environmental temperatures, or lower body temperatures, the usual direction of heat flow from the body core to the exterior becomes reversed and heat storage, rather than heat loss, takes place with a concomitant rise in core temperature. Such a reversal in the usual direction of heat flow must be temporary and reversible, or death will ensue from overheating. If heat production is plotted against environmental temperature, the area of lowest heat production is referred to as the thermoneutral zone and is formally defined as the range of ambient temperature within which metabolic rate is at a minimum and within which temperature regulation is achieved by physical processes alone, the individual being in thermal equilibrium with the environment. This thermoneutral zone is bounded by an upper and a lower critical temperature. The upper critical temperature is the ambient temperature above which thermoregulatory evaporative heat loss is recruited. The lower critical temperature is the ambient temperature below which the rate of metabolic heat production of a resting thermoregulating individual increases to maintain thermal balance. The "comfort" zone, or the zone of thermoneutrality, is a similar but slightly wider area than what has just been described as a neutral thermal environment. The zone of minimal heat production has also been defined as the range of environmental temperature over which heat production is kept at a minimum by a combination of vasodilatation, postural change, and increased evaporative heat loss.

The relationship between metabolic heat production and environmental temperature is summarized in Figure 1–8.[25] It is evident that the lowest sustained heat production is at an environmental temperature, referred to as the thermoneutral or "comfort" zone, which is bounded by critical temperatures below which thermoregulation is achieved by increasing heat production and above which there is inevitable body heating. The lower critical temperature stimulates the extra heat associated with shivering, while the upper critical temperature causes evaporative cooling due to sweating.

GAS EXCHANGE AND INDIRECT CALORIMETRY

The production of heat, or energy, by the human body can be measured by the use of both direct and indirect calorimetry. Each of these techniques has its particular advantages and disadvantages. Since energy is utilized in the human body by means of chemical reactions, it is possible to evaluate energy utilization from the measurement of the substances consumed and the products formed (Fig. 1–9).

The measurement of energy expenditure is referred to as calorimetry in which energy is measured as heat, being one of the most conveniently handled forms of energy. Energy can neither be created nor be destroyed, and therefore the energy content of any system can be increased or decreased only by the amount of energy that is added to or subtracted from the system. The units for energy are the same units used to express work. Energy is defined as the capacity for performing work, and work is the transference of energy by a process involving the movement of a solid body through space. Work is expressed as the force acting upon a body to produce motion, times the distance through which it acts. Various units are used for expressing work. The most common are calories, both small and large. Whenever "calories" are discussed without qualification, reference is made to the "large Calorie" or kilocalorie, which is defined as the amount of heat required to raise the temperature of 1 kg of water by 1° C. Another term used for expressing the energy equivalent is the kilogram-meter, which is the amount of work performed when a body of given weight is moved against gravity through a known distance. An additional unit of energy, the joule, has

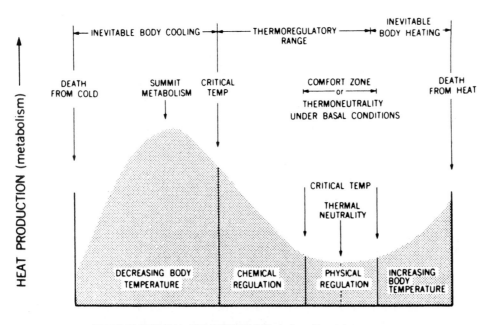

FIGURE 1–8. Heat production is shown to vary with environmental temperature, emphasizing the relatively small capacity in man to compensate for elevated environmental temperature. (From Sinclair, JC (ed). Temperature Regulation and Energy Metabolism in the Newborn. New York, Grune and Stratton, 1977.)

been proposed to serve as the common denominator for adding the quantities of different forms of energy. One joule = 10^7 ergs, and 4.18 joules = 1 small calorie. Kleiber[26] published a spirited article opposing the use of the joule to substitute for the calorie in malnutrition.

Methodology

Measuring energy expenditure indirectly utilizes the known proportionality between O_2 consumption and CO_2 production.[27] This method for measuring energy expenditure is often referred to as "respiratory calorimetry" or as "respiratory metabolism." It can be performed by an open circuit method, where the subject is permitted to breathe air from the outside, while his expired air is collected in either a special gas meter or other container for volumetric measurement. This gas volume is corrected for standard conditions and is analyzed for its O_2 and CO_2 content, with the subsequent calculations of O_2 consumption and CO_2 production. In the use of the closed-circuit method, the subject is completely shut off from the outside air and breathes through a closed system. The respirometer contains pure oxygen. As the gas is expired by the subject, the CO_2 is constantly removed as it passes through a CO_2 trapping material such as soda lime. The decrease in the gas volume in this closed system in related to the rate of O_2 consumption, from which the metabolic rate can then be calculated.

Equipment for indirect calorimetry has commonly been attached to the subject or patient with a tight-fitting mask or with a mouthpiece and noseclip. Because many individuals are uncomfortable with anything tight on the face or in the airway, a transparent plastic head canopy with a plastic neck seal has been designed that allows the subject or patient to lie comfortably for prolonged periods as a uniform flow of air is ventilating the canopy and passes through tubing to equipment that continuously measures flow and the concentration of O_2 and CO_2.[28] Such a head canopy can be utilized with portable gas exchange equipment initially designed for use with a mouthpiece and noseclip.[29] The flow-through system of the head canopy provides greater comfort than the mouthpiece and noseclip; however, it places greater demands on the gas analyzers for sensitivity and reliability. Special equipment can be utilized to balance the air flow into and out of the head canopy, thus making it possible to translate the pressure changes within the canopy due to the patient's ventilation into a continuous electrical signal representing the simultaneous measurement of spirometry together with gas exchange.[30]

The difficulties of obtaining sufficient accuracy in measurements of indirect calorimetry are not properly appreciated, according to Tobin and Hervey.[31] It is important to recognize that gas exchange, which is measured from expired air taken at the airway and not diluted by air ventilating a canopy or a respiration chamber, will have the highest concentration of CO_2 and the largest decrease in O_2 content, while the air required for ventilation of a chamber will reduce the absolute changes in O_2 and CO_2 that need to be measured and therefore places greater emphasis on the sensitivity and precision of the analytical equipment.

To obtain 2 per cent accuracy with a flow-through method of indirect calorimetry, differences in gas concentration of the order of 0.5 per cent have to be measured to 0.01 per cent. Weissman and co-workers[29] reached similar conclusions when validating the use of a flow-through head canopy with equipment that had been designated for measurement with a mask or mouthpiece.

A mathematical analysis of gas exchange measurements for indirect calorimetry has been presented by Cole and co-workers.[32] These workers em-

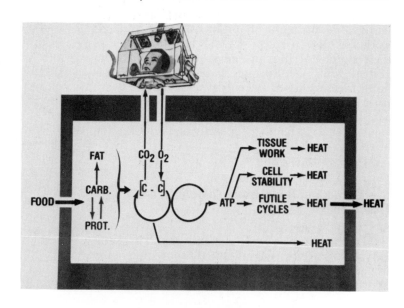

FIGURE 1–9. *The human body is constantly required to integrate energy intake, intermediary metabolism, gas exchange, fuel oxidation, tissue and organ work, heat production, and heat loss. The human body is not a "heat engine" in which heat can be used to perform work, yet heat produced from one stimulus appears to be interchangeable with heat produced from another stimulus in order to satisfy thermoregulatory demands for the protection of an optimum body heat content.*

phasize that throughout the history of indirect calorimetry, the analysis of gas exchange has been subject to simplifications and approximations. Mathematical expressions are presented to show that short-term measurements in large respiration calorimeters can have greatly improved precision if these equations can be solved with a sufficiently fast response time. They note that with the power of modern computers there seems little justification in the continued use of the simplifications and approximations that are part of the common calculations in indirect calorimetry.

The use of conventional indirect calorimetry is seldom applied to studies that extend over more than a few hours. Therefore, extrapolation of such data is open to question when one attempts to estimate daily energy expenditure, which includes normal activity, nutrition, and sleep. The general concepts, based on a measurable balance of energy in and energy out, are well established, but the demonstration of this balance is most convincing when the subject or patient is being studied for a sufficiently long period of time. Several groups have built respiration chambers that offer an opportunity for continuous studies lasting 24 hours or longer.[21] This allows the measurement of energy and nutrient balance by the use of an airtight room that forms part of an open circuit indirect calorimeter.

Van Es[21] pointed out that many investigators, who had established the early standards for basal metabolic rate, ended up with a "normal" variability of ±15 per cent. However, he noted that in his laboratory the prediction of 24-hour energy expenditure with a respiration chamber, and normalized for fat-free body mass, showed a variability of only ±5 per cent. Therefore, van Es proposed that a 24-hour period of measurement be adopted as a minimum standard for the measurement of energy expenditure, whether by calorimetry, gas exchange, or both measured together.

It is of interest that 24-hour gas exchange measurements were carried out by Pettenkofer[33] in 1862 using a respiration chamber. Atwater and co-workers[13] also used prolonged measurements in their studies of human energy expenditure from 1897 to 1905. Van Es states that no new data on 24-hour measurements of energy expenditure were presented between 1905 and 1971. Jequier and Schutz[34] have recently emphasized the particular value of such a chamber for studying the utilization of specific foods.

Gas Exchange, Respiratory Quotients, and Tissue Fuel

Of all the types of chemical bonds found in chemistry, only one type is significant as a source of energy for animals. This is the bond between carbon and hydrogen in compounds of nutritional value (car-

bohydrates, edible fats, and certain amino acids), where there is release of energy in biological reactions as the carbon and the hydrogen are oxidized to CO_2 and water. The sum total of all the processes of growth, repair, and reproduction can be summarized in the word "metabolism," which derives from a Greek term meaning "change." Thus, one may say that the metabolism of carbohydrate and fat permits the body to carry on its work of energy exchange. The value of the energy supplied in food is determined by burning a measured quantity of pure material in a bomb calorimeter.[34] This device is placed in a known amount of water at a certain temperature. After combustion of the material inside the bomb, the resulting rise in the temperature of the water is multiplied by the specific heat of water and by the volume of the water in liters to obtain the caloric value of the material.

The general formula for carbohydrate oxidation may be written as:[34]

$$C_6H_{12}O_6 + 6\ O_2 \rightarrow 6\ CO_2 + 6\ H_2O$$

The respiratory quotient (RQ) in this process is the ratio of six volumes of CO_2 to six volumes of oxygen, which equals 1.00.

In the oxidation of fat, extra molecular O_2 is required not only for the oxidation of carbon, but also for the oxidation of hydrogen. For this reason the RQ is a value less than unity. The oxidation of a sample triglyceride (tripalmitin) may be indicated as follows:

$$2\ C_{51}H_{98}O_6 + 145\ O_2 \rightarrow 102\ CO_2 + 98\ H_2O$$

The RQ then is the ratio of 102 volumes of CO_2 to 145 volumes of O_2, which equals 0.703.

The oxidation of protein is more difficult to calculate because some of the oxygen and carbon of the constituent amino acids remain combined with nitrogen and are excreted as nitrogenous products in the urine and feces. In addition, the composition of proteins may vary somewhat. However, an average protein would be oxidized with 138.18 grams of O_2 associated with the production of 152.17 grams of CO_2. Converting these quantities into volumes, the RQ for protein is 77.52 L of CO_2 over 96.70 L of O_2, which equal 0.802.

The process of lipogenesis, in which fatty acids are derived from glucose, has a very high RQ. If one considers a lipid produced as a triglyceride that has equal molar amounts of palmitic, stearic, and oleic acids, this compound might be $C_{55}H_{104}O_6$. One might then write the following equation:

$$13.5\ C_6H_{12}O_6 + 3\ O_2 \rightarrow C_{55}H_{104}O_6 \\ + 26\ CO_2 + 29\ H_2O$$

The RQ from this reaction is then 26 over 3, or 8.67.

The conversion of gas exchange to calories of heat production per unit of time involves assigning a fraction of the total O_2 consumption to the oxidation of each of the three foodstuffs. The first step in the calculations of indirect calorimetry involves the calculation of protein oxidation from urinary nitrogen excretion. The associated O_2 consumption and CO_2 production from this protein oxidation is then subtracted from the total gas exchange, leaving the nonprotein RQ to be calculated from the remaining gas exchange. The proportions of fat and carbohydrate oxidized during the period of gas exchange measurements are determined from the nonprotein RQ, using any of the widely published tables. The scale of RQ going from 0.7 to 1.0 can then be related to the kilocalories per liter of O_2 utilized, where the RQ of 0.70 is equal to 4.686 kilocalories and an RQ of 1.0 has a value of 5.047 kilocalories per liter of O_2 utilized.

The conversion of total RQ to nonprotein RQ represents a change of only a few per cent of energy expenditure; therefore the conversion is sometimes ignored.[35]

When very high carbohydrate loads are given, as is sometimes done with high-carbohydrate total parenteral nutrition, the nonprotein RQ may go up as high as 1.2, or even 1.3, as the result of a significant amount of glucose being converted into fatty acids with a correspondingly high RQ. The calculation of substrate oxidation from measurements of gas exchange has recently been reviewed by Bursztein and others[36] and by Frayn.[37]

The calculation of the BMR is simply an abbreviated form of indirect calorimetry in which the O_2 consumption is measured under basal conditions, which are usually defined as those existing in a subject who has had no food intake for the prior 5 hours and who has been lying quietly for at least 30 minutes in a thermoneutral environment. The measurement is commonly made for 10 to 15 minutes and is then converted to values that are often expressed as kcal of energy expenditure per hour, utilizing an assumed RQ of 0.82.

Calorimetry and Physical Activity

The influence of mechanical work on energy expenditure was of great interest to early workers in the field of calorimetry. The following paragraph from Lusk[14] summarizes much of the early research in this field:

The source of mechanical work must be from metabolism, for mechanical energy cannot be derived from nothing. The necessary energy might be obtained in one of two ways, either at the expense of a proportionate reduction in the quantity of heat liberated by the resting organism, or by an increase in the amount of the metabolism. In the former case work would diminish the heat production and might cool the tissues, which is not observed to take place. If work were done at the expense of increased metabolism, and if this increase were completely converted into mechanical effect, then the heat production of the organism might remain the same as in the resting state. If, however, the result of mechanical effort be a stimulation of metabolism to the extent of not only enabling the body to do work but also causing it to produce more heat than when at rest, then the tendency of the tissues must be to grow warmer, perhaps with a resulting outbreak of sweat to reduce the body temperature through physical regulation. The last named is the actual process.

The fuel for muscular work has intrigued investigators since the days of Lavoisier and his discovery that oxygen consumption was increased by mechanical exercise. Pettenkofer and Voit[38] presented laboratory data that indicated that protein metabolism was not appreciably affected by muscular work. Experiments by Rubner[39] demonstrated that there was a summation of the extra heat production associated with simultaneous mechanical work. These two stimuli to thermogenesis thus appear to be completely separable entities. Rubner also showed[40] that the energy expenditure during work is independent of the surrounding temperature or environmental conditions. However, the extra heat produced by mechanical work can substitute for the extra heat that results from exposure to a cold environment. Thus, the human body is not a "heat engine" in which heat can be used to perform work, yet heat produced from one stimulus appears to be interchangeable with heat produced from another stimulus in order to fulfill the thermoregulatory demands for the maintenance of an optimum body heat content.

Because of the difficulties in measuring energy expenditure by direct calorimetry and because of the importance of learning about energy expenditure during normal activities, field studies have been conducted during various forms of physical activity using a portable meter (the Kofranyi-Michaelis respirometer).[27] This device, worn on the back with a harness, consists of a dry gas meter for measuring the total volume of expired air and is connected to an aliquoting device containing a 100-ml rubber bag that continuously removes samples from each breath of expired air. Gas analysis is performed on the aliquots of expired air that are trapped in the rubber bladder. Data from such measurements have to include the energy cost of wearing the meter, unless the meter is set at the side of the subject or carried by another individual during physical activity. There are a number of problems connected with the prolonged measurement of expired air for gas exchange. The patient or subject must wear cumbersome collection devices. Large-bore tubing must be attached to these devices to connect them with expired air collection, or measuring equipment. Because of these encumbrances the performance of an activity may be altered. This objection, however, is now being reduced by the development of miniaturized components. Another frequent problem is the imposed limitation on working conditions.

The lack of satisfactory ways to measure energy

expenditure in free-living humans has prompted an indirect approach to measurement of long-term CO_2 production. Approximately 20 years ago, Lifson and McClintock[41] observed that hydrogen and oxygen isotopes in body water were eliminated at different rates and that the difference between those rates was proportional to CO_2 production. Thus, it appeared that it was possible to measure the energy expenditure in free-living subjects by measuring the elimination rates of the separate isotopes when water labeled with both deuterium and ^{18}O was administered to a subject.[42] Schoeller and Webb[43] studied five healthy adults for 5 days, comparing the nearly continuous measurement of respiratory gas exchange with the doubly labeled water method. The values from gas exchange being measured directly were 6 per cent less than those obtained by the water method, with a coefficient of variance of 8 per cent. A subsequent study conducted 10 days after starting total parenteral nutrition in four adult subjects with inflammatory bowel disease indicated an estimated error of 5 per cent in the calculated change in body energy stores, utilizing metabolic balance studies over a 14-day period. Further studies are needed to establish the validity of the method in various clinical conditions.

The Fick principle can be modified to calculate the O_2 consumption of acutely ill patients if one is able to measure cardiac output and has knowledge of the O_2 content of arterial and mixed venous blood.[44] However, efforts to utilize these measurements to obtain O_2 consumption have shown significant variability, and since the necessary blood samples are not readily available in patients, other than in the ICU setting, these techniques have not achieved wide popularity.

These problems have led to the use of proportional physiological responses such as heart rate or pulmonary measurements. Physical activity may be measured indirectly through the use of activity diaries or surveys and by activity-related means, such as pedometers or cumulative heart beats. With any method, the instruments must be properly calibrated and the psychological, sociological, and physiological variables that may alter measurement accuracy must be considered. Also such factors as body size, growth and development, sex, climate, disability, occupation, and the use of leisure time must be considered in the total assessment of energy expenditure.

Five methods to assess the energy expenditures of individuals indirectly over any prolonged period of time have been reviewed by Buskirk and co-workers.[45] These are: (1) the assessment of caloric intake required to maintain body weight over a period of time; (2) an activity questionnaire-interview; (3) a diary of time activities maintained every minute, or 5 minutes, by the subject or an observer (accompanied by a determination of O_2 consumption for each major activity); (4) continuous indirect calorimetry with measurements of O_2 consumption and/or CO_2 production; and (5) the establishment of individual O_2 consumption–heart rate regression lines, with subsequent continuous monitoring of heart rate.

Evaluation of the heart rate method for sensing energy expenditure has several problems related to it, including the fact that there is much variability between individuals in the relationship between O_2 consumption and heart rate. The accuracy of the method is enhanced if individual relationships can be developed in a setting closely approximating the natural one. By using incremental heart rate, the increase over that measured during rest, or by using the relative value in the range from rest to maximal work, one can reduce some of the variation between individuals. Although the accuracy of the heart rate method has been questioned by some investigators, several workers have used it for extensive studies.

A simpler method for the indirect measurement of energy expenditure involves measuring the rate of pulmonary ventilation. By measuring the minute volume of ventilation for representative activities, the average ventilation can be related to O_2 consumption and energy expenditure. Such devices as Douglas bags, spirometers, and flow meters can be used to measure pulmonary ventilation. The technique's major disadvantage is that a mask and flow meter must be transported.[46]

Estimates of the accuracy and practicality of various methods for activity assessment and daily energy expenditure indicate that the most accurate methods are usually the most impractical. Therefore, a compromise must be made with the experimental goals. The prepared diary may be acceptable for activity assessment; for daily energy expenditure assessment, monitoring the pulmonary ventilation may also be acceptable. Durnin[47] has presented a critique of field studies attempting to measure energy expenditure in population groups.

The measurement of gas exchange as part of the clinical management of patients with varying kinds of disease and injury is receiving increasing attention.[48] This development has some similarities to the introduction of the flame photometer for the measurement of serum sodium and potassium during the 1950's and the introduction of blood gas electrodes in the 1960's. In each case, reliable instrumentation had to be developed before knowledge gained from research equipment could be applied to patient care. At the same time, a large body of clinical experience could be obtained only after the new instrumentation became available. This early phase of the learning curve for most physicians produced a separation into two groups, the enthusiasts and the skeptics. Each group went to extremes, so that some physicians carried out measurements that were unnecessary and made no contribution to patient care, while others failed to gain experience with the new measurements and therefore were slow to appreciate the clinical conditions in which such information could be of great importance to patient care.

TRADITIONAL COMPONENTS OF METABOLIC RATE

During the decade from 1920 to 1930, there seemed to be a growing conviction that the factors that determined whole-body energy expenditure, or metabolic rate, had been defined for both animals and humans. The steady growth of knowledge in this field over the previous century had seemed to establish the total metabolic rate as follows:

$$TMR = BMR + SDA + physical\ activity$$

The basal metabolic rate, or BMR, was generally accepted to be the metabolic rate of the postabsorptive individual who was resting quietly in a thermoneutral temperature. The specific dynamic action, or SDA, had been well established by Rubner and was considered to be only a small proportion of the energy expenditure that was normally spent in daily activity. The energy expenditure during many types of activity had already been measured.

Metabolic Body Size

The metabolic rate or heat production per unit time, and in particular the basal metabolic rate of humans, was generally expressed in kilocalories per square meter of body surface. These units were based on the theory that with differing body size, the metabolic rate was proportional to the respective surface areas. Kleiber[49] reviewed this theory, called the surface law, and the following information is taken from this review. Rubner, in 1883, noted a systematic decrease of the metabolic rate umit weight of fasting dogs when the weight was corrected from that of little dogs of 3 kg to large animals of 31 kg. When the metabolic rate was expressed per square meter of body surface, however, the effect of body size disappeared. From this and similar observations, Rubner deduced his simple rule that fasting homeotherms produce daily 1000 kcal of heat per square meter of body surface. Voit published a table of seven species showing the surface law of metabolic rate to be true for large and small animals, including humans. Many workers calculated the surface area of animals and humans assuming that they were spheres with a density of 1 kg per liter. The surface area of such a sphere in square decimeters is 4.84 × wt to the 2/3 power, when weight is expressed as kilograms. Considering that animals are not really spheres, Meeh, in 1879, substituted for the factor 4.84 a term, k, which is constant only within a group of similarly shaped animals but differs according to the shape of the animal. A set of these constants was

provided by Lusk in his later work. The surface of man averages 12.3 square decimeters per unit of the 2/3 power of body weight. For slim people the Meeh constant would be higher and for stout people lower than this average. DuBois and DuBois[50] developed a formula in 1916 that allowed the calculation of the surface area of stout and slim human beings more accurately than the Meeh formula:

Surface area = 71.84
× weight to the 0.425 power
× length to the 0.725 power

Kleiber considered this formula to be dimensionally correct for any size. The DuBois formula as calculated from weight and height is well defined within one species, but in comparing humans and smaller animals, for example, one would have to rely on the ill-defined concept of "true" body surface. In attempting to avoid the assumptions involved in the surface law and ill-defined terms related to the body surface area, Harris and Benedict[51] derived the following prediction equations empirically:

For men: Heat production = 66.473 + 13.7516W + 5.003s − 6.775a
For women: Heat production = 655.0955 + 9.5634W + 1.8496s − 4.6756a

"W" equals weight in kilograms, "s" is height in centimeters, and "a" is age in years, and the equations give the total heat production in kilocalories per day.

Consolazio and colleagues[27] noted that for many years the standards of Aub and DuBois[52] and Boothby and co-workers[53] were frequently used by clinicians even though they were high compared with the actual basal metabolic rate. These values were assumed to be high because some of the data collected by the authors were the result of first tests performed on untrained subjects. Other workers in the field have shown that the training of subjects by repeating tests for several days can decrease the BMR levels by 8 to 10 per cent.

Robertson and Reid[54] went to extremes in computing their standard tables, using only the lowest values on repetitive tests. They collected data on successive days until there was no further fall in the heat production. The lowest value was then taken as the true basal metabolic rate. This approach has been criticized by many workers in the field. Fleisch[55] tabulated the values for kilocalories per hour per square meter from 24 sets of standards. He calculated the arithmetic mean for each age group and then weighted the values for the total number of subjects. These values are 8.5 per cent below the Mayo clinic standards published by Boothby and co-workers.[53]

The multiple regression equations developed by Harris and Benedict in 1919 have been widely used for predicting daily caloric needs of hospitalized patients. These equations require knowledge of the weight, height, age, and sex of the patient or subject. Two assumptions are required: that 24-hour basal energy expenditure can be predicted from a 5- to 15-minute measurement in the early morning, and that O_2 consumption and CO_2 production can be reliably translated into the rate of energy expenditure.

Kleiber has observed that the Harris-Benedict equations deal with well-defined quantities such as weight, height, and age, while the DuBois prediction seems to be more acceptable to clinicians, as well as physiologists, because it has a rational physiological meaning. After further analysis Kleiber[49] concluded:

For all practical purposes one may assume that the mean standard metabolic rate of mammals is 70 × 3/4 power of their body weight in kilograms per day or about 3 times the 3/4 power of their body weight in kilograms per hour.

The basal rate of oxygen consumption within any species is roughly proportional to body weight to the 0.67 power. This seems to make some intuitive sense, since both the surface area and the cross-sectional area of body forms scaled by isometry are proportional to the 0.67 power of the body volume. However, Kleiber in 1932 first made the observation that the basal metabolic rate, whether measured by the rate of food consumption, oxygen consumption, or heat production, varies in an even more regular and repeatable way when the comparison is made not only within a species but between species of mammals. This relationship, which has come to be known as Kleiber's law, states that the metabolic rate between species is proportional to the weight to the 0.75 power over a range of animals from mice to elephants. The Kleiber relationship between size and metabolic rate is also relevant to human development. Wilkie[56] noted that the basal rate of oxygen consumption in the newborn rises in about 6 hours from a rate of 3.5 ml/kg, which is appropriate for an animal the size of the mother, to approximately 7 ml/min/kg, which is appropriate for the mass of the baby. While the fetus is within its mother it behaves from an energy point of view as if it were simply one of her organs, turning over at the relatively low metabolic intensity determined by her weight. Within 36 hours after birth, the rates at which all of its enzymes act and the rate of activity of its mitochondria have changed, speeding up its cellular processes sufficiently to bring it to that point on the human segment of the Kleiber line determined by its own weight as a separate small individual.

Specific Dynamic Action

Lavoisier and Seguin noted that during the digestion of a meal the rate of oxygen consumption rose.[8] This response was noted by workers during the following century and termed the "work of digestion." Rubner fed bones to dogs and found no increase in the metabolic rate, while Benedict and Emmes,[57] in 1912, and later Borsook,[58] in 1936, showed that intravenous injection of amino acids increased metabolic rate to the same extent as oral ingestion did. The work of digestion was thus no longer a valid explanation for increased metabolic rate after food intake. Rubner showed in animal studies that the increase in energy expenditure following food ingestion was not due to the mechanical work of the intestinal tract, but was attributable to metabolic activity in the liver and glandular tissue. In order not to commit himself to a definite explanation, Rubner created the term "specific dynamic action" for the increased metabolic rate following food intake.[49]

Many investigators had believed that the most clearly evident specific dynamic action of food ingestion was related to the ingestion of amino acids, while that associated with carbohydrate or with fat ingestion was considered to be small or insignificant. Some investigators had assumed that the specific dynamic action was somehow related to the mass action of amino acids themselves, while others felt that the catabolism of these amino acids, that is the deamination and metabolism of the carbon residues of amino acids, contributed the effect. Wilhelmj and co-workers[59] stated that the most suitable manner of expressing the relation between specific dynamic action and administered amino acid was as calories per millimole of amino acid deaminated. This no longer assumed that urinary nitrogen indicated complete oxidation of the nitrogen-free residue of protein, but only that nitrogen in the urine was a measure of deamination of amino acids. Borsook and Winegarden[60] noted a correlation between an increase in metabolic rate and a corresponding increase in urinary nitrogen excretion.

Fuel for Physical Activity

The relationship of work, heat, and the oxidation of organic substances in the body was already clear to Lavoisier and Seguin in 1792, long before Helmholtz had formulated the law of conservation of energy in 1847. The source of animal work, like the source of animal heat, was clearly the chemical energy released when organic compounds were catabolized.[49] Lavoisier and Seguin measured human work efficiency and noted that 36.8 L of oxygen was consumed above the resting level for 5867 kilogrammeters of physical work, the latter being the equivalent of 13.8 kcal, yielding a net efficiency of 8 per cent for muscle work. Helmholtz had calculated a gross efficiency of 20 per cent, similar to the gross efficiency measured with horses.[49]

During the early 1800's, it was widely believed that protein was a special fuel for muscle work. Fick and Wislicenus[61] tested this hypothesis in 1868 on a climb in the Swiss Alps. They demonstrated that only a minor part of the energy expended for their muscular work could have been derived from the breakdown of protein. Krogh and Lindhard[62] noted that with carbohydrate as a fuel, the efficiency of muscular work was 10 per cent better than with the breakdown of fat. The first experiments in which the effect of work upon the total metabolism of man was demonstrated were conducted by Pettenkofer and Voit.[14] Their subject was a healthy workman who performed 9 hours of exercise on an ergometer each day during two study periods, one during starvation and one during consumption of a medium mixed diet. These early experiments clearly showed that mechanical work did not increase the protein metabolism, even in starvation, but that the power to perform physical work was apparently supplied by an increased metabolism of nonprotein materials. Experiments by Atwater and Benedict[63] were the first to demonstrate that mechanical work is done at the expense of a dynamic equivalent of metabolism, an important confirmation of the law of the conservation of energy.

Experiments conducted by Rubner and later reported by Lusk[14] have shown that there is a summation of function as regards the extra heat production due to the specific dynamic action of protein and the extra heat production resulting from mechanical work. The two factors appeared to be completely separable entities.

RESURGENCE OF INTEREST IN METABOLIC RATE

The three major factors that determine human daily energy expenditure—basal metabolic rate, specific dynamic actions of foods, and physical activity—were formerly thought to be well established and not deserving of further study. This undoubtedly contributed to the lack of research in this area during the period from 1920 to 1960. Since that time there has been a resurgence of interest in whole-body energy metabolism leading to re-examinaton of all three of the major factors contributing to daily energy expenditure.

Metabolic Body Size: Shifting Attitudes

The past two decades have produced advances in the measurement of body composition that might be expected to delineate the metabolic body size and provide a better reference for energy expenditure measurements. Unfortunately, the new techniques for body composition are not readily available for bedside use, and physicians have been left to decide whether to use body weight, or some related calculation, for expressing measured energy expenditure. The physician must then select which of the time-

honored publications of normal data will be utilized as the standard for the measurement performed on his patient.

Long and associates[64] observed that the results calculated from the Harris-Benedict equation were in close agreement with those obtained by gas exchange analysis in normal males and females. However, Daly and co-workers[65] recently conducted a study of the basal energy expenditure of 201 healthy adult men and women, using both direct and indirect calorimetry, and reported that the Harris-Benedict equations overestimated the measured expenditure by 10 to 15 per cent. These authors also report on 15 other studies in which measured basal energy expenditure in healthy, lean individuals could be compared with a value predicted from the Harris-Benedict equation. A striking range of results was obtained, from +19 to −14 per cent. The reasons for the variability could not be determined, but the variability emphasized the importance of standardized measurement procedures with carefully calibrated equipment.

Data from 223 subjects, which provided the basis for the Harris-Benedict equations, were analyzed by Cunningham.[66] Body weight and age were used with the prediction equation of Moore and colleagues[67] (for calculation of total body water). The estimated lean body mass was found to be the best single predictor of BMR, while the influence of sex and age added little to the estimation. These findings suggested that estimations of BMR based on body surface area owed their usefulness to a hidden correlation to lean body mass in each sex. This would be in agreement with Benedict's suggestion, made in 1915, that the "active body mass" determined the BMR.

Body weight or total body mass encompasses two major compartments, body fat and lean body mass. Grande[68] suggested that much of the variation in reports of normal basal metabolic rate could be eliminated if BMR were expressed in units of fat-free body mass or active tissue mass. For persons of a given sex and age the basal oxygen consumption appears to be correlated to about the same extent with fat-free body weight and with calculated surface area. The utility of fat-free body weight as a standard of reference becomes evident when persons of different sex and age are compared. For both males and females, from 20 to 60 years of age, a single value can be used to indicate the normal metabolic rate. The single value of 4.4 ml of oxygen per minute (or about 1.3 calories per hour) per kilogram of fat-free body weight can be used instead of the customary tables and graphs based on the artificial concept of surface area as a determinant of basal metabolism. The "active protoplasmic mass," referred to without measurement by various investigators over the past century, appears to be similar to the "body cell mass" estimated by Moore and co-workers from the isotope dilution measurements of total exchangeable potassium.[67] The body cell mass may represent from one third to two thirds of the total body weight, but it accounts for essentially all of the energy consumption and heat production.

Roza and Shizgal[69] reanalyzed data from measurements by Harris and Benedict, converting body weight, age, and sex to total body water, then to extracellular water and intracellular water, to K_e, and finally to body cell mass, utilizing the regression equations of Moore and colleagues.[67] The Harris-Benedict equations predicted resting energy expenditure with a precision of 14 per cent in normally nourished individuals, but were unreliable in the malnourished patient. The resting energy expenditure was directly related to body cell mass and was independent of age and sex.

The cellular protein of the body is commonly regarded as the machinery of the body. Thus, there has been interest in the new technique of neutron activation analysis for measurements of body nitrogen. Such a measurement can be calculated from the mean value for healthy people if one is dealing with a normal subject. Standard deviation of individual values can be improved by predicting body nitrogen from the fat-free mass and can be improved even more by predictions from measurements of body potassium. The experience with seven systems, utilizing both delayed and prompt gamma analysis, has been presented by Beddoe and co-workers.[70] These authors emphasize that cellular hydration may or may not be associated with changes in body cell protein in various states of depletion and illness. If one is able to measure both total body nitrogen and total body potassium, it is possible to derive values for the muscle and nonmuscle nitrogen as discussed by Burkinshaw and co-workers[71] and Cohn and associates.[72] Unfortunately, there is no established method for separating the amount of extracellular protein in supporting structures from the intracellular protein, which is presumably related to the actively metabolizing cell mass.

Weir[35] published a modification for computing metabolic rate in which it was pointed out that utilizing the total O_2 consumption and CO_2 production without correction for nitrogen excretion introduced errors that were a matter of only a few per cent. The relative lack of influence of protein oxidation on caloric expenditure has to do with two factors: (1) the average protein oxidation is only 10 to 20 per cent of the metabolic fuel that is being oxidized, and (2) the RQ for protein oxidation is fairly close to the middle of the range for fat and carbohydrate oxidation.

Heusner[73] recently presented a detailed review of body size and energy metabolism, extending Kleiber's concept that energy expenditure was proportional to the body weight taken to the 2/3 or 3/4 power. However, this approach has special value only when comparing species with a broad range of body weights.

There has been an increased use of the lean body mass or the fat-free mass as the metabolic size for expressing energy expenditure. This concept appears reasonable except for the lack of widespread methodology for measuring body fat (anthropometry or densitometry) or lean body mass (calculated from measuring total body water). However, extensive new data presented in Chapter 2 suggest that the biologic heterogeneity in a population of adult men and women results in body weight being as good a reference for energy expenditure as other measures such as fat-free mass.

Diet-Induced Thermogenesis

Because of the growing attention to the matter of diet-induced thermogenesis, there has been a tendency to suggest that patients or subjects do not change their body weight to any major degree despite considerable differences in caloric consumption. Forbes[74] has reviewed two venerable papers (Neumann in 1902 and Gulick in 1922) whose authors served as their own experimental subjects. The body weight of both investigators did indeed vary with their energy intake and did so in a systematic fashion. The daily changes in body weight were not large, yet they were large enough to reflect changes in energy intake, confirming that body weight does respond to modest as well as to profound alterations in energy intake.

Recent discussions of this subject often start with attention to non-shivering thermogenesis or cold-induced thermogenesis. When exposed to cold, mammals usually increase their heat production, not only by an increase in muscle activity (shivering thermogenesis), but also by some non-shivering mechanism (non-shivering thermogenesis). After acclimation to cold, certain species of animals kept at temperatures as low as 4° C can dispense with shivering and succeed in maintaining a normal body temperature solely by cold-induced thermogenesis. Although such animals consume and oxidize a large quantity of food, they do not become obese, since the large food intake is needed to provide the additional heat required to maintain body temperature. The existence of this cold-induced metabolic process and its mediation by the sympathetic nervous system led James and Trayhurn[75] to propose that perhaps some cases of obesity were due to a defective response to non-shivering thermogenesis. Brown adipose tissue has long been recognized as a heat-producing organ and known to be involved in some way in the response to altered ambient temperature in small animals. However, its small size in comparison with the total amount of adipose tissue in adult animals raised questions as to whether it could have a major heat-producing role for the entire body. Previous studies on the capacity of brown adipose tissue to contribute to cold-induced thermogenesis were based on measurements of blood flow, which have since been shown to underestimate the heat-producing capacity.[76] Newer evidence for a link between the thermogenic functioning of brown adipose tissue and the overall energy balance in experimental animals has led to a number of questions concerning the potential importance of this tissue for energy balance in adult humans.

It was formerly thought that, in humans, brown adipose tissue was present only in the newborn infant and steadily decreased in amount with progressive age. Scattered reports have suggested that adult humans may continue to have significant amounts of brown adipose tissue, which had previously been unrecognized because the tissue was not evident in the presence of large amounts of white adipose tissue. In addition, there is no good biochemical marker for brown adipose tissue. Functional brown adipose tissue has been recognized by surface thermography in newborn infants and also in adults. Infrared thermograms of the backs of adult subjects showed increased skin temperature in the paraspinal areas.[77] James and Trayhurn[78] have observed that given the dominance of the thermal regulatory thermogenesis in small animals and the biological importance of substrate supply to brown adipose tissue in both mice and human infants, it would not be surprising if brown adipose tissue retained its biological function into adult life in humans, as in the mouse, responding to the inflow of fuel and reacting particularly to a supply of fat, which requires little in the way of metabolic processing before being suitable for heat generation.

The administration of 100 g of glucose to normal human subjects is associated with a rise in plasma norepinephrine concentrations and with signs of cardiovascular stimulation as compared with a control noncaloric liquid.[79] The increase in plasma norepinephrine is greater and more sustained in healthy elderly individuals than in normal young subjects. The rise appears to begin at 30 minutes and peaks at 60 minutes in young subjects and at 120 minutes in elderly subjects. The differences in the plasma norepinephrine response in young and elderly subjects cannot be attributed to changes in norepinephrine clearance.[80] The increase in plasma norepinephrine concentration is associated with increases in pulse rate in the elderly, pulse pressure in young and old, and the product of heart rate times systolic blood pressure in both the young and the old. An increase in oxygen consumption occurs in association with the rise in plasma norepinephrine level after glucose administration. The rise in plasma norepinephrine concentration, the signs of cardiovascular stimulation, and the increase in oxygen consumption, all provides evidence for sympathetic stimulation following glucose ingestion.[81]

Krebs[82] suggested that the energy losses following administration of protein were somehow linked to urea production. However, studies by Garrow and Hawes[83] did not demonstrate any association between the amount of urea produced and the increase in metabolic rate after a meal. This led these authors to suggest that the increase in metabolism following a protein meal was perhaps more related to protein synthesis than to protein catabolism. Ashworth[84] studied metabolic rates during recovery from protein-calorie malnutrition and found that the metabolic response to a meal was not necessarily dependent on the protein intake.

The thermic response to food and to cold were formerly thought to be independent. However, in animals in which brown adipose tissue is the main organ responsible for non-shivering thermogenesis, it has been found that the thermogenic activity can be stimulated by feeding. Stock and Rothwell[85] have proposed that brown adipose tissue may perform a regulatory function in response to overfeeding. These authors and others have studied rats that have become obese when eating a highly palatable cafeteria diet instead of the normal rat chow. Under these circumstances the brown adipose tissue of the rats showed a marked increase in weight, together with a substantial increase in thermogenesis. This response is remarkably similar to that shown by cold-induced thermogenesis, and both types of response are felt to involve stimulus of the sympathetic nervous system. Landsberg and Young[81] have presented evidence that diet-induced changes in sympathetic nervous system activity may underlie some of the changes in organ function that accompany alterations in nutritional status. Utilizing measurements of norepinephrine turnover rate to estimate sympathetic activity in denervated organs of experimental animals, fasting has been shown to suppress and overfeeding has been shown to stimulate the sympathetic nervous system. Studies from this laboratory have reported a significant fall in urinary norepinephrine excretion during a 3-day fast in normal weight human subjects. This is in direct contrast to the increase in urinary norepinephrine excretion observed in acutely ill surgical patients at a time when they were receiving high levels of glucose and amino acids as parenteral nutrition.[86]

Diet-induced thermogenesis can be divided into obligatory and adaptive components. Obligatory thermogenesis, formerly known as "specific dynamic action," is the energy cost of digestion, absorption, and the inner conversion of food substrates, and is thought to be due largely to the synthesis of protein and fat from carbohydrate. This is in contrast to adaptive diet-induced thermogenesis (originally named Luxuskonsumption), which represents the dissipation of energy over and above that associated with basal metabolic activity and the obligatory diet-induced thermogenesis (Fig. 1–10).[87] Adaptive thermogenesis is stimulated by the ingestion of a meal, a part of which is oxidized to produce this, and may account for as much as 10 or 15 per cent of the energy expenditure. Recently, there has been considerable controversy regarding the existence of

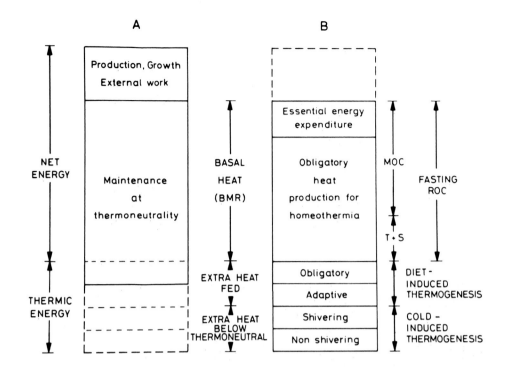

FIGURE 1–10. *The utilization of metabolizable energy is represented in terms of energy balance (Column A) and thermal balance (Column B). MOC, minimal oxygen consumption; ROC, resting oxygen consumption; T + S, = resting muscle tone and sympathetic activity. (From Girardier L, Stock MJ (eds). Mammalian Thermogenesis. London, Chapman and Hall, 1983.)*

adaptive diet-induced thermogenesis in both humans and other mammals. The concept that the body is able to control its weight and energy content and hence to dispose of the excess consumed energy comes partly from studies in which individuals have been shown to maintain a constant body weight despite different levels of energy intake. The evidence for adaptive diet-induced thermogenesis relies upon the demonstration of an apparent discrepancy between estimates of energy intake as food, energy expenditure, and the energy storage or change in body fat. Unfortunately, most of these studies have not involved actual measurements of energy balance. Stock and Rothwell[85] have suggested that the capacity for diet-induced thermogenesis enables an animal to consume adequate quantities of a poor-quality diet in order to obtain sufficient essential nutrients without compromising energy balance by depositing the excess energy intake as fat. The capacity for diet-induced thermogenesis appears to be principally influenced by genetic background and age, with lean strains of animals having a greater capacity than fatter strains and young animals being more thermogenic and resistant to excess weight gain than old animals.

Observations on individuals who habitually consume either very large or very small amounts of food have led to additional speculation concerning diet-induced thermogenesis. It has been known for some time that there is a twofold range in the customary energy intake of adult humans who are similar in all other respects (age, sex, weight, occupation, and so forth). One is forced to conclude that humans, like other animals, have the capacity to raise diet-induced thermogenesis independently of demands made by tissue synthesis and can therefore compensate for intakes in excess of requirements.

A variety of studies over the past decade have shown an increasing number of similarities between cold-induced thermogenesis and diet-induced thermogenesis. This list now includes increases in food intake, metabolic rate, sympathetic activity, thermogenic and lipolytic responses to norepinephrine, inhibition by beta receptor antagonists and by oxygen deficiency, and increases in brown adipose tissue size and cell number. In addition, studies on the in vivo metabolic rates of various tissues have shown that all of the diet-induced changes in thermogenic capacity are due, at least in the rodent, to the increased activity of brown adipose tissue. The mitochondria of brown adipose tissue appear to be unique in that they are physiologically uncoupled when the tissue is active. Oxidation of substrates therefore produces large amounts of heat and only small amounts of ATP. The level of oxidation can also proceed at very high rates because when it is uncoupled from phosphorylation, the tissue is no longer controlled by the availability of ADP for the synthesis of ATP. The uncoupling of brown adipose tissue mitochondria is due to a "proton" conductance pathway in the inner mitochondrial membrane.[88] The activity of the pathway is increased in animals exhibiting both cold-induced and diet-induced thermogenesis, and there is now little doubt that it is an important and powerful source of heat in brown adipose tissue.

Lipogenesis versus Thermogenesis

Hibernation is a process that not only causes a surge of heat production upon awakening but also has been associated with previous excessive energy storage. Migrating birds have been found to store large amounts of fat before prolonged overseas flights, in which survival is dependent upon prolonged exercise without food intake. Thus, an important area for future study of energy metabolism is how animals, and perhaps humans, control the balance between lipogenesis and thermogenesis. Is it possible that the weight loss and hypermetabolism of human illness and injury represents an initial shift in this balance toward thermogenesis and that the later, or anabolic, phase of convalescence represents a shift from thermogenesis to lipogenesis?

Physical Activity

Despite an extensive literature over the past century on energy expenditure related to varying forms of physical activity, there has been renewed interest in the efficiency of physical work and whether this can contribute to the apparent differences in energy expenditure of people with similar life-styles. Waterlow[89] has reviewed the question of metabolic adaptation to low intakes of energy and protein and has discussed the efficiency of physical work in terms of mechanical efficiency and physiological efficiency.

The study of mechanical efficiency is usually performed by having a subject exercise on something like a bicycle ergometer so that the mechanical work done can be related to the gas exchange occurring at that time. The mechanical efficiency of healthy men studied in this way is found to be between 26 and 30 per cent. In spite of the care to control conditions for such studies, there is considerable variability between subjects. Measuring the amount of mechanical work done in many kinds of physical activities becomes relatively complicated. The variability in response to exercise may be related to a different pattern of muscle fiber types adapted to different speeds of work. Komi and associates[90] performed muscle biopsies on well-trained athletes. There was a positive correlation between the proportion of slow-twitch fibers and the $\dot{V}O_2$ at the anaerobic threshold, a measure of maximum working capacity. Slow-twitch fibers are said to be more efficient than fast-twitch fibers, in terms of mechanical force development per unit ATP used. Waterlow[89]

offered the hypothesis that a possible mechanism of adaptation in muscle is a relative preservation of slow-twitch fibers and perhaps more generally the achievement of an optimum pattern of a person's physical activity related to a particular life-style.

The physiological efficiency of physical activity may be considered as the energy expended during work, minus the energy expended at rest, divided by the total energy expended while working. In this way no attempt is made to estimate the actual mechanical work that is done. The energy costs of activities and occupations can be expressed as multiples of the BMR. It has been shown that for walking and running in normal subjects the cost per kilogram appears to be independent of body weight. Gross expenditure per kilogram is therefore probably the most useful parameter for comparisons between individuals, or groups, when one is looking at adaptive changes in working efficiency.

Edmundson[91] reported a study of the working efficiency of farmers in Java, comparing big eaters with small eaters. When the 24-hour intake and the total energy expenditure were measured, an index of "relative efficiency" was calculated as the input divided by the output. This ratio seemed to vary from 0.6 in the large eaters to 1.6 in the small eaters. In a second experiment, Edmundson[92] measured the energy cost of work on a bicycle ergometer and, when the work was set at 100 watts, he found a significantly lower gross energy cost in the small than in the big eaters, although their weights and heights were the same. Norgan[93] has observed that a significant difference in work metabolism appears to arise from a low efficiency in the high intake group rather than a high efficiency in those with a low dietary intake.

Efficiency in the activities of real life may be influenced by unnecessary movements, and abolishing unnecessary movements may be an important form of adaptation to decreased food intake. The speed at which people work may also be important. If there is a given task to be done, is it more economical to perform it slowly or quickly?

The resurgence of interest in metabolic rate has been accompanied by an increasing clinical awareness of the manifold areas where a quantitative idea of energy expenditure can contribute to patient care. Obvious examples are adjusting the reducing diet of the obese patient, or designing the correct caloric intake for the acute patient in the intensive care unit. Less obvious, but of equal importance, is following the delicate balance of the patient who needs adequate nutrition to avoid progressive weight loss, yet suffers from compromised lung function so that additional demands for ventilation with overenthusiastic nutrition are poorly tolerated.

Technological advances offer promise of simplifying measurements of both energy expenditure and body composition so that energy supply and demand per unit of body cell mass can someday be a routine part of patient management.

INFLUENCE OF ENERGY ON NITROGEN METABOLISM

Among life processes, the demand for energy has precedence over all other requirements. The proportion of protein intake that is burned to meet the energy needs of the body is increased when protein is in excess or when food intake is inadequate. An undernourished child in a developing country will burn increased amounts of his protein intake because he is "energy deprived," whereas a child in an affluent society will do the same thing because he is eating a high-protein diet. Various animal studies have shown that if food intake is reduced to match the needs for basal metabolism, then the efficiency of protein utilization approaches zero. However, both animals and humans can maintain a satisfactory nitrogen balance on a low protein intake, if total energy intake is high. The effect of energy intake on nitrogen balance has attracted new interest as the result of two factors: the increasing use of parenteral and enteral nutrition for the treatment of various catabolic states, and the nutritional efforts to achieve weight reduction in the severely obese individual without major loss of lean tissue.

It is not surprising that protein precedes energy in the term "protein-energy malnutrition." The persistent idea has been that body protein represents the machinery of the body and that inadequate food intake becomes serious only because there is a loss of, or failure to gain, body protein. Yet it is of little practical value to think of protein in isolation from the rest of food intake, especially in isolation from the intake of energy. Much has been written about the nutritional importance of the amino acid composition of various proteins. However, the efficiency of the utilization of dietary protein may be influenced less by its amino acid composition than by the energy value of the associated intake, because protein can function either as an energy source or as a nutrient for synthesis.

Allison and co-workers[94] showed clearly that the response to dietary protein in dogs depends not only on the level of protein fed, but also on the severity of the energy restriction imposed. Dogs that were more severely restricted in energy intake initially responded in different ways to varying levels of dietary protein, but eventually all of them drifted into negative nitrogen balance, their fat stores presumably exhausted. Those with moderate energy restriction retained considerable nitrogen. Nettleton and Hegsted[95] observed that when normal animals or human subjects were fed energy-restricted diets for short periods of time, the total energy available did not seem to be reduced, presumably because the dietary energy deficit was compensated for by the oxidation of body fat. But it seemed reasonable to expect that the relationship between energy and protein intake would be different when normal animals were compared with those that were chronically deprived. Thus, they studied young rats that were given varying degrees of energy and protein restrictions over 16 days. They found that the change in tissue nitrogen varied with the tissue studied and the time of observation, as well as with the severity of the food restriction. After 8 days, animals fed high levels of protein during the most severe energy restriction showed increases in the gastrocnemius muscle, but losses in liver nitrogen. After 16 days of the same conditions, both tissues had marked nitrogen loss. Nitrogen losses were increased at the lowest level of food intake, whereas the same level of dietary protein was protective of tissue nitrogen when the energy intake was increased.

A curious parallel appears to exist between the resting energy expenditure and the level of nitrogen excretion in an individual on a given level of nutritional intake. Factors that cause increases or decreases in energy expenditure are usually associated with similar changes in nitrogen excretion. The fundamental mechanisms underlying this relationship are poorly understood. Much current knowledge on the effects of energy intake on protein metabolism has been the result of nitrogen balance studies. The responses of whole-body nitrogen metabolism to altered energy supplies appear to be regulated by the pre-existing status of protein metabolism, as well as by the level of the protein intake. This complicates the problem of separating the influence of energy balance and nitrogen balance in normal humans, which separation is particularly difficult in the presence of acute illness or injury.

The parallel behavior of energy expenditure and nitrogen excretion has led to an accepted assumption that increased nitrogen loss represents protein breakdown for nonspecific fuel needs. Fatty acids from adipose tissue provide a large and ready source of two-carbon energy but cannot be used as a source of net production of glucose, glycogen, or carbohydrate intermediates in mammalian tissue. The glucogenic amino acids from body protein represent the major gluconeogenic reserve of the body along with the glycerol released from triglyceride breakdown. Therefore, in clinical conditions in which hypermetabolism and increased nitrogen excretion are associated with tissue breakdown, the increased urea synthesis and excretion are now thought to represent accelerated gluconeogenesis and not simply the need to supply extra two-carbon fragments for general fuel at the expense of protein.

Both the basal metabolic rate and the protein synthesis rate are much higher in small species than in large species. Garlick[96] reported that the synthesis of whole-body protein declines with increased body size, when expressed per unit of body weight, but that the protein synthesis rate is relatively constant among species of widely differing body weights when expressed per unit of surface area or metabolic body size (per kilogram to the 0.7 power). Thus, whole-body protein synthesis shows an approximate correlation with body weight, similar to the correlation that exists with basal metabolism, which is consistent with the idea that a significant portion of energy requirements are associated with protein synthesis. The corollary to this is that variations in protein synthesis may be shown to be an important factor in variations found in total energy expenditures. Reeds and co-workers[97] compared estimates of protein synthesis with heat production in young pigs. Their findings indicate that the minimum proportion of energy expenditure associated with protein synthesis is approximately 15 to 25 per cent of total body heat production. Young and co-workers[98] observed that in human subjects there appears to be a relatively constant relationship between whole-body protein synthesis rates and resting energy expenditure, whether studied in early infancy or in adult life. These authors also observed that there is a broad similarity between the contribution of different organs to whole-body heat production and the contribution by these same organs to whole-body protein synthesis. Young and Munro[99] estimated that muscle protein synthesis accounts for approximately 30 per cent of whole-body protein turnover in young adult men. Assuming that total body protein accounts for about 20 per cent of basal energy metabolism, these authors estimate that about 6 per cent of whole body energy metabolism is associated directly with the protein metabolism of muscle. Kien and co-workers[100] and Bilmazes and associates[101] have reported that the metabolic response to injury is accompanied by increased turnover of muscle protein. These studies were performed on patients in whom presumably there was an increase in energy expenditure.

The influence of reducing physical activity has been studied by Schønheyder and co-workers[102] who used ^{15}N-glycine to measure the protein synthesis rate in subjects who were immobilized for several days in a plaster cast. A negative nitrogen balance as a result of this treatment was found to be associated with a decrease in the rate of protein synthesis, rather than a change in protein breakdown. Young and Torun[103] conclude that between the extremes of major exercise and total inactivity there is a pattern of physical activity and energy expenditure that is consistent with, and necessary for, the maintenance of a satisfactory state of body protein metabolism. It is generally agreed that when total energy expenditure increases owing to muscular work, it does not cause a change in nitrogen balance as long as there is energy equilibrium. Increasing the work load, of course, produces a negative nitrogen balance when there is an energy deficit. In a normal adult with a negative nitrogen balance, increasing the protein intake can still be expected to diminish the nitrogen deficit.

Investigators have long believed that endogenous urinary nitrogen excretion is somehow associated with the rate of resting energy metabolism and that both of these factors are a function of some part of body composition. When deciding on the appropriate intake of energy and nitrogen to provide a satisfactory dietary intake, clinicians usually depend on information from indirect calorimetry and nitrogen balance studies. A value of 2 mg of urinary nitrogen excretion per basal kilocalorie has been accepted as generally applicable to most mammals, when receiving no nitrogen intake. However, experimental studies in humans have usually related urinary nitrogen excretion to body weight. Daily urinary nitrogen loss, with no nitrogen intake, will reach a low level of approximately 37 mg/kg. Other losses include an average fecal loss of 12 mg/kg, percutaneous losses of 3 mg/kg, and 2 mg/kg for other minor losses. Thus, the total nitrogen loss, with no protein intake, amounts to 54 mg/kg or 0.34 g of body protein per kg, which corresponds to 24 g of body protein for a 70-kg man. Since there may be some loss of efficiency in nitrogen utilization, the recommended dietary allowances established by the National Research Council have suggested that the average nitrogen loss be considered to be approximately 70 mg/kg.[104] These estimates of average nitrogen loss have led to the recommendation of a minimal intake of high quality protein amounting to at least 0.5 g/kg of body weight in normal adult individuals.

A large body of literature exists on the influence of nitrogen intake on nitrogen balance. The average U.S. diet is thought to provide an intake of nitrogen that is as much as twice the theoretical minimal requirement. Thus, when nitrogen intake is decreased, the nitrogen equilibrium is preserved by a reduction in synthesis and output of urea, as long as the amino acid intake remains above the minimum level. When nitrogen intake rises above normal levels there is an associated rise in urea output, which establishes equilibrium at a new higher level, often associated with a small but definite rise in blood urea levels.

It has been stated many times that when protein is supplied with inadequate calories, the protein is merely degraded and burned for fuel. The extent to which this concept is true has been challenged by the work of Blackburn and co-workers,[105] who have reported that it is possible to improve nitrogen retention greatly, and even achieve nitrogen equilibrium, by the administration of amino acids by peripheral vein without any associated nonprotein energy source. The metabolic behavior induced by this "protein-sparing therapy" remains controversial, and many investigators continue to believe that the administration of carbohydrates together with amino acids is beneficial. Studies by Calloway[106] have shown progressive improvement in nitrogen retention in normal subjects as their energy intake is increased. Calloway and Spector[107] stated,

To the general principle set forth, that on a fixed adequate protein intake, energy level is the deciding factor in nitrogen balance, and that with a fixed calorie intake the protein level is the determinant, may be added a corollary. That is, at each fixed inadequate protein intake there is an individual limiting energy level beyond which increasing calories without protein, or protein without calories, is without benefit.

The investigation of patients in acute catabolic states with increased resting energy expenditure has consistently shown associated increases in urinary nitrogen excretion. Comparable studies performed in patients with extensive weight loss and tissue depletion demonstrate a reduction in both resting energy expenditure and in nitrogen excretion, if there is no major catabolic stimulus from injury or infection. A study was conducted by Elwyn and co-workers[108] in 10 depleted patients; 6 with secondary sepsis were maintained on parenteral nutrition with a constant intravenous infusion of amino acids (173 mg/kg of body weight) and with three different levels of energy intake as carbohydrate (15.4, 37.6, and 58.5 kcal/kg) given sequentially for 4 days each. The analysis of the nitrogen balance in relation to the energy intake demonstrated a progressive nitrogen-retention of about 1.7 g/1000 kcal. The correlation of nitrogen balance was then plotted against energy balance. A graphic representation of the quantitative relation between nitrogen balance and energy balance has been presented by Kinney and Elwyn.[109,110] The findings from this study have been compared with data reported by Rudman[111] and co-workers and have served to guide further nutritional studies. Although the concept rests on limited experimental evidence and the numbers should be considered only approximations, our group believes that it can serve as a tentative guide to the quantities of nitrogen and energy best suited for treating the depleted patient. Further discussion of this approach is presented in Chapter 38.

Energy should be given to patients in an amount that will meet their energy expenditure and will provide an appropriate rate of fat restoration, if this is required. This is in contrast to planning the intake of nitrogen, which should be given to provide an adequate weight gain on the basis that 1 g of nitrogen is the equivalent of approximately 32 g of hydrated lean body mass. An additional factor to be considered is whether the nonprotein calorie source for the energy intake is made up of carbohydrate or fat. Carbohydrate exerts a specific protein-sparing action above and beyond that seen with the administration of fat. This is commonly thought to be related to the ability of carbohydrate to stimulate the output of insulin. Studies performed with 3-methylhistidine have indicated that carbohydrate administration causes both an increased synthesis and a reduced breakdown of muscle protein, which is typical of the action of insulin.[112]

Peters and co-workers[113] conducted a study in which three energy-to-nitrogen ratios were used with patients requiring total parenteral nutrition, the ratios being 204:1, 163:1, and 102:1 kcal/g of nitrogen. The study was conducted in stable patients without infection in 40-week study periods. The energy-to-nitrogen ratio of 163 kcal/g of nitrogen appeared to be most effective for nitrogen equilibrium in these patients. An energy-to-nitrogen ratio of 102:1 kcal/g was associated with weight loss and a negative nitrogen balance. Conversely, increasing the energy-to-nitrogen ratio to 204:1 kcal/g did not result in improved nitrogen retention for this group of patients. The authors suggest that different energy-to-nitrogen ratios may be appropriate depending upon the underlying disease state.

Rajantie and co-workers[114] reported a study in 20 elderly patients who were randomized following colon resection to receive a conventional energy-to-nitrogen ratio: 201 kcal/g of nitrogen in the first group, and a second group in which fat was added to provide a ratio of 336 calories per g of nitrogen. A positive postoperative nitrogen balance was obtained in both groups, and the authors concluded that a positive nitrogen balance could be obtained with a restricted amino acid supply, if energy was provided in abundance. Rhodes and colleagues[115] presented a study of 20 patients who, after abdominal operations, were given a fixed intake of 2600 kcal per day with a fixed energy-to-nitrogen ratio of 167:1 kcal/g, while another group of patients received a caloric intake that was adjusted according to the previous day's measured metabolic expenditure. These authors reported that the excess calorie intake over expenditure did not correlate with an increased positive nitrogen balance, but that the patients on the varied caloric intake, who were receiving a higher nitrogen intake per calorie, tended to have an increased positive nitrogen balance. They concluded from this study that a fixed intake of 2600 kcal per day was not suitable for adult patients requiring intravenous feeding after abdominal operation, and that the currently prescribed nitrogen intakes were perhaps suboptimal.

Chen and co-workers[116] studied 32 infants and children receiving intravenous nutrition and examined a wide range of energy-to-nitrogen ratios. The intakes given varied from 150 to 400 g of nitrogen, and these investigators found an inverse linear correlation between the blood urea nitrogen levels and the energy-to-nitrogen ratio of the infusate. They observed a similar correlation between the blood urea nitrogen levels and the energy-to-nitrogen ratio in dogs, where blood urea nitrogen could be shown to have decreased down to a ratio of 450 kcal/g of nitrogen. The authors concluded that amino acid is utilized for protein synthesis directly in proportion to the calorie supply and that for the complete utilization of 1 g of nitrogen, a very high energy intake of over 400 kcal of nonprotein calories should be administered. Shaw and co-workers[117] studied 10 nutritionally depleted patients receiving total parenteral nutrition. The patients received, in random order, either a diet with a low nitrogen content or a diet with a high nitrogen content, and a caloric intake that was calculated to represent 1.08 times the total energy expenditure per day. The resting energy expenditure of these patients increased approximately 10 per cent when they changed their dietary intake from only 5 per cent dextrose to the low-nitrogen TPN, and increased again by 10 per cent when they changed to the high-nitrogen TPN. A nitrogen retention of 21 per cent of the increase in nitrogen intake was three times that observed in normal adult subjects. This is consistent with the idea that malnourished patients respond to intravenous nutrition in a manner similar to the dietary response of growing children. Attainment of a markedly positive nitrogen balance, when the energy balance is close to zero, indicates that the lean body mass in depleted patients can be restored without a high energy intake, which insures a strongly positive energy balance.

Providing nutritional support for the ill or injured patient is beginning to be tailored to the body size of each particular patient. The original concept of "hyperalimentation" was arbitrarily established as giving three 1-L bottles per day, each of which contained approximately 1000 kcal of glucose and amino acids. The energy-to-nitrogen ratio happened to be 150 kcal/g nitrogen, which was a convenient ratio, somewhat lower than in the average American diet. The tissue composition of weight loss in acute surgical patients appears to approximate 100 kcal/g of nitrogen lost,[118] but there is no evidence that this ratio is superior for TPN used to treat such patients. Various published studies suggest that there is a TPN range of perhaps 120 to 180 kcal/g of nitrogen where nitrogen retention is roughly equal and that extreme values above and below this range are less effective. It is not surprising that there is not a single most effective ratio, since there are variable energy requirements independent of protein metabolism and protein utilization that involve many pathways with varying energy requirements. Both the calorie intake and the nitrogen intake are most commonly considered today on the basis of administering an amount per unit of body weight.

The source of nonprotein energy will influence the level of nitrogen retention, depending upon the duration of the study and the condition of the patient involved. There are many reports in the literature that suggest that carbohydrate is more efficient than fat in producing nitrogen retention.[119] It has often been assumed that this difference was associated with the ability of carbohydrate to stimulate insulin secretion, which then enhanced amino acid uptake in muscle. A study by Long and co-workers[120] in patients with major burns showed that the nitrogen retention achieved with increasing amounts of carbohydrate was not evident when equivalent energy was provided as fat. Greenberg and co-workers[121] have shown in other patients treated with parenteral nutrition that the apparent advantage of carbohydrate over fat in effecting nitrogen retention was most evident during the first 5 to 7 days of administration and that by the tenth day the nitrogen balance was very similar for the groups receiving carbohydrate or fat. At present, it appears that whatever difference exists between the nitrogen-sparing effects of carbohydrate and of fat is due not only to the endogenous stimulation of insulin secretion, but also to the severity of the stimulus to the catabolism and to the duration of administration of the nutrient.

REFERENCES

1. Mendelsohn E. Heat and Life. The Development of the Theory of Animal Heat. Cambridge, Harvard University Press, 1964: 8–66.
2. Frank RG, Jr. Harvey and the Oxford Physiologists. Berkeley, University of California Press, 1980.
3. van der Star P. The history of thermometry in medicine. Bibl Radiol 1969; 5:1–7.
4. Read J. Joseph Black, M.D. The teacher and the man. *In* Kent A (ed). An Eighteenth Century Lectureship in Chemistry. Glasgow, Jackson, Son & Company, 1950: 78.
5. Robinson E, McKie D (eds). Partners in Science: James Watt and Joseph Black. Cambridge, Harvard University Press, 1970.
6. McKie D, Heathcote NH de V. The Discovery of Specific and Latent Heats. London, Edward Arnold & Company, 1935.
7. Priestley J. Experiments and Observations on Different Kinds of Air. Vol 1. New York, Kraus Reprint Company, 1970.
8. Holmes FL. Lavoisier and the Chemistry of Life. Madison, University of Wisconsin Press, 1985.
9. Holmes FL. Claude Bernard and Animal Chemistry. Cambridge, Harvard University Press, 1974.
10. Leicester HM. Development of Biochemical Concepts from Ancient to Modern Times. Cambridge, Harvard University Press, 1974.
11. Elkana Y. The Discovery of the Conservation of Energy. Cambridge, Harvard University Press, 1974.
12. Cathcart EP. The early development of the science of nutrition. *In* Bourne GE, Kidder GW (eds). Biochemistry and Physiology of Nutrition. Vol 1. New York, Academic Press, 1953: 1.
13. Atwater WO, Benedict FG. A Respiration Calorimeter with Appliances for the Direct Determination of Oxygen. Washington, Carnegie Institute, 1905; 42:193.
14. Lusk G. The Science of Nutrition. 4th ed. New York, Johnson Reprint Corporation, 1976.
15. Bernard C. Lessons on animal heat. *In* Benzinger TH (ed): Temperature, Part I. Arts and Concepts. Stroudsburg, PA, Dowden, Hutchinson & Ross, 1977: 24.
16. Hardy JD, Bard P. Body temperature regulation. *In* Mountcastle VB (ed). Medical Physiology. Vol 2. 13th ed. St. Louis, CV Mosby, 1974: 1305.
17. Winslow CEA, Herrington LP. Temperature and Human Life. Princeton, Princeton University Press, 1949: 27–57.
18. Webb P. Human Calorimeters. New York, Praeger, 1984.
19. Benzinger TH, Huebscher RG, Minard D, et al. Human calorimetry by means of the gradient principle. J Appl Physiol 1958; 12(Suppl 1):1–24.

20. Webb P, Annis JF, Troutman SJ. Energy balance in man measured by direct and indirect calorimetry. Am J Clin Nutr 1980; *33*:1287–1298.

21. van Es AJH. Results of enquiry on calorimetric equipment and experimental routines for studies in which human energy metabolism is followed for 24 h and longer. *In* van Es AJH (ed). Human Energy Metabolism: Report of an EC Workshop. Wageningen, The Netherlands, Euro-Nut Report 1984; *5*:19.

22. Head CA, McManus CB, Seitz S, et al. A simple and accurate indirect calorimetry system for assessment of resting energy expenditure. JPEN 1984; *8*:45–48.

23. Kluger MJ. Fever: Its Biology, Evolution and Function. Princeton, Princeton University Press, 1979: 8–14.

24. DuBois EF. Basal Metabolism in Health and Disease. Philadelphia, Lea & Febiger, 1924: 311–340.

25. Swyer PR: Heat loss after birth. *In* Sinclair JC (ed): Temperature Regulation and Energy Metabolism in the Newborn. New York, Grune & Stratton, 1978: 119.

26. Kleiber M: Joules vs calories in nutrition. J Nutr 1972; *102*:309–312.

27. Consolazio CF, Johnson RE, Pecora LJ: Physiological Measurements of Metabolic Functions in Man. New York, McGraw-Hill, 1963: 1–59.

28. Kinney JM, Morgan AP, Domingues FJ, et al. A method for continuous measurement of gas exchange and expired radioactivity in acutely ill patients. Metabolism 1964; *13*:205–211.

29. Weissman C, Damask MC, Askanzi J, et al. Evaluation of a non-invasive method for the measurement of metabolic rate in humans. Clin Sci 1985; *69*:135–141.

30. Spencer JL, Zikria BA, Kinney JM, et al. A system for the continuous measurement of gas exchange and respiratory functions. J Appl Physiol 1972; *33*:523–528.

31. Tobin G, Hervey GR. Accuracy in indirect calorimetry. *In* van Es AJH (ed): Human Energy Metabolism: Report of an EC Workshop. Wageningen, The Netherlands, Euro-Nut Report 1984; *5*:32.

32. Cole TJ, Murgatroyd PR, Brown D, et al. A rigorous mathematical analysis of gaseous exchange in indirect open-circuit calorimetry. *In* van Es AJH (ed): Human Energy Metabolism: Report of an EC Workshop. Wageningen, The Netherlands, Euro-Nut Report 1984; *5*:37.

33. Pettenkofer M. Ueber die Respiration. Ann Chemie und Pharm Suppl 1862; *2*:1–52.

34. Jequier E, Schutz Y. Long-term measurements of energy expenditure in humans using a respiration chamber. Am J Clin Nutr 1983; *38*:989–998.

35. Weir JB de V. New methods for calculating metabolic rate with special reference to protein metabolism. J Physiol 1949; *109*:1–9.

36. Bursztein S, Saphar P, Glaser P, et al. Determination of energy metabolism from respiratory functions alone. J Appl Physiol 1977; *42*:117–119.

37. Frayn KN. Calculation of substrate oxidation rates in vivo from gaseous exchange. J Appl Physiol 1983; *55*:628–634.

38. Pettenkofer M, Voit C. Zeitsch f Biol 1866; *2*:537.

39. Rubner M. Sitzungsberichte der König. Preuss. Akad d Wissensch 1910; *16*:316.

40. Rubner M. *In* Leyden von. Handbuch der Ernahrungstherapie. Leipzig, 1903: 74.

41. Lifson N, McClintock R. Theory of the use of turnover rates of body water for measuring energy and material balance. J Theoret Biol 1966; *12*:46–74.

42. Schoeller DA. Energy expenditure from doubly labeled water: some fundamental considerations in humans. Am J Clin Nutr 1983; *38*:999–1005.

43. Schoeller DA, Webb P. Five-day comparison of the doubly labelled water method with respiratory gas exchange. Am J Clin Nutr 1984; *40*:153–158.

44. Keil JW, Shepard AP. Continuous measurement of arteriovenous oxygen difference and VO_2 by microcomputer. Am J Physiol 1983; *245*: H178–H182.

45. Buskirk ER, Hodgson J, Blair D: Assessment of daily energy balance: some observations on the methodology for indirect determination of energy intake and expenditure. *In* Kinney JM (ed): Assessment of Energy Metabolism in Health and Disease. Columbus, Ohio, Ross Laboratories, 1980: 113.

46. Ford AB, Hellerstein HK. Estimation of energy expenditure from pulmonary ventilation. J Appl Physiol 1959; *14*:891—893.

47. Durnin JVGA. Indirect calorimetry in man: a critique of practical problems. Proc Nutr Soc 1978; *37*:5–19.

48. Damask MC, Forse AR, Kinney JM. Clinical application of gas exchange measurements. Clin Anaesthesiol 1983; *1*:599–631.

49. Kleiber M: The Fire of Life. Huntington, NY, Robert E. Kreiger, 1975.

50. DuBois D, DuBois EF. Clinical calorimetry. A formula to estimate the approximate surface area if height and weight be known. Arch Intern Med 1916; *17*:836–871.

51. Harris J, Benedict F. A Biometric Study of Basal Metabolism in Man. Washington, Carnegie Institute, 1919; *279*:40–44.

52. Aub JC, DuBois EF. Clinical calorimetry; the basal metabolism of old men. Arch Intern Med 1917; *19*:823–831.

53. Boothby WM, Berkson J, Dunn HL. Studies of the energy metabolism of normal individuals: a standard of basal metabolism with a nomogram for clinical application. Am J Physiol 1936; *116*:468–484.

54. Robertson JD, Reid DD: Standards for the basal metabolism of normal people in Britain. Lancet 1952; *262*:940–943.

55. Fleisch A: Le metabolisme basal standard et sa determination au moyen du "Metabocalculator." Helvet Med Acta 1951; *18*:23–44.

56. Wilkie DR: Metabolism and body size. *In* Pedley TJ (ed). Scale Effects in Animal Locomotion. New York, Academic Press, 1977: 23.

57. Benedict FG, Emmes LE. The influence upon metabolism of non-oxidizable material in the intestinal tract. Am J Physiol 1912; *30*:197.

58. Borsook H. The specific dynamic action of protein and amino acids in animals. Biol Rev 1936; *11*:147–180.

59. Wilhelmj C, Jessie M, Bollman L, et al. Studies of the physiology of the liver. XVII. The effect of the removal of the liver on the specific dynamic action of amino acids administered intravenously. Am J Physiol 1928; *87*:497.

60. Borsook H, Winegarden HM. On the free energy of glucose and tripalmitin. Proc Natl Acad Sci 1930; *16*:559–573.

61. Fick A, Wislicenus J. Recherches sur l'origine de la force musculaire. Annales des Sciences Naturelles. Cinquieme Serie: Zoologie, Paleonthologie. Paris, Victor Masson & Fils, 1868: 257–279.

62. Krogh A, Lindhard J. The relative value of fat and carbohydrate as sources of muscular energy. Biochem J 1920; *14*:290.

63. Atwater WO, Benedict FG. Experiments on the metabolism of matter and energy in the human body. U.S. Department of Agriculture, Bull 36, 1903.

64. Long CL, Schaffel N, Geiger JW, et al. Metabolic response to injury and illness: estimation of energy and protein needs from indirect calorimetry and nitrogen balance. JPEN 1979; *3*:452–456.

65. Daly JM, Heymsfield SB, Head CA, et al. Human energy requirements: overestimation by widely used prediction equation. Am Soc Clin Nutr 1980; *42*:1170–1174.

66. Cunningham JJ. A reanalysis of the factors influencing basal metabolic rate in normal adults. Am J Clin Nutr 1980; *33*:2372–2374.

67. Moore FD, Oleson KH, McMurrey JD, et al. The Body Cell Mass and Its Supporting Environment. Philadelphia, WB Saunders Company, 1963.

68. Grande F. Body weight, composition and energy balance. *In* Olson RE, et al. (eds). Present Knowledge in Nutrition. Washington, The Nutrition Foundation, 1984: 7.

69. Roza AM, Shizgal HM: The Harris Benedict equation reev-

aluated: resting energy requirements and the body cell mass. Am J Clin Nutr 1984; 40:168–182.

70. Beddoe AH, Streat SJ, Hill GL. Evaluation of an in vivo prompt gamma neutron activation facility for body composition studies in critically ill intensive care patients: Results in 41 normals. Metabolism 1984; 33:270–280.

71. Burkinshaw L, Morgan SB, Silverton NP, et al. Total body nitrogen and its relation to body potassium and fat-free mass in healthy subjects. Clin Sci 1981; 61:457–462.

72. Cohn SH, Vaswani AN, Yasumura S, et al. Assessment of cellular mass and lean body mass by noninvasive nuclear techniques. J Lab Clin Med 1985; 106:305–311.

73. Heusner AA. Body size and energy metabolism. Ann Rev Nutr 1985; 5:267.

74. Forbes GB. Energy intake and body weight: a reexamination of two "classic" studies. Am J Clin Nutr 1984; 39:349–350.

75. James WPT, Trayhurn P. Thermogenesis and obesity. Br Med Bull 1981; 37:43–48.

76. Foster DO, Frydman ML. Nonshivering thermogenesis in the rat. II. Measurements of blood flow with microspheres point to brown adipose tissue as the dominant site of the calorigenesis induced by noradrenaline. Can J Physiol Pharmacol 1978; 56:110–122.

77. Rothwell NJ, Stock MJ: A role for brown adipose tissue in diet-induced thermogenesis. Nature 1979; 281:31–35.

78. James WPT, Trayhurn P: Obesity in mice and men. In Beers RF, Basset EG. Nutritional Factors: Modulating Effects on Metabolic Processes. New York, Raven Press, 1981: 123.

79. Young JB, Landsberg L: Fasting, feeding, and the regulation of sympathetic activity. N Engl J Med 1978; 298:1295–1301.

80. Young JB, Rowe JW, Pallotta JA, et al. Enhanced plasma norepinephrine response to upright posture and glucose administration in elderly subjects. Metabolism 1980; 29:532–539.

81. Landsberg L, Young JB. Autonomic regulation of thermogenesis. In Girardier L, Stock MJ. Mammalian Thermogenesis. London, Chapman and Hall, 1983: 99.

82. Krebs HA. The metabolic fate of amino acids. In Munro HN, Allison JB (eds). Mammalian Protein Metabolism. New York, Academic Press, 1964: 125.

83. Garrow JS, Hawes SF. Role of amino acid oxidation in causing specific dynamic action in man. Br J Nutr 1972; 27:211–219.

84. Ashworth A. Metabolic rates during recovery from protein-calorie malnutrition: the need for a new concept of specific dynamic action. Nature 1969; 223:407–409.

85. Stock M, Rothwell N. Obesity and Leanness. London, John Libbery, 1982: 49.

86. Askanazi J, Carpentier YA, Elwyn DH, et al. Influence of total parenteral nutrition on fuel utilization in injury and sepsis. Ann Surg 1980; 191:40–46.

87. Girardier L, Stock MJ. Mammalian thermogenesis: an introduction. In Girardier L, Stock MJ (eds). Mammalian Thermogenesis. London, Chapman and Hall, 1983: 1.

88. Himms-Hagen J: Brown adipose tissue metabolism and thermogenesis. Ann Rev Nutr 1985; 5:69–94.

89. Waterlow JC. Metabolic adaptation to low intakes of energy and protein. Ann Rev Nutr 1986; 6:495–526.

90. Komi PV, Ito A, Sjodin B, et al. Muscle metabolism, lactate breaking point and biochemical features of endurance running. Int J Sports Med 1981; 2:148–153.

91. Edmundson W. Individual variations in work output per unit energy intake in East Java. Ecol Food Nutr 1977; 6:147–151.

92. Edmundson W. Individual variations in basal metabolic rate and mechanical mark efficiency in East Java. Ecol Food Nutr 1979; 8:189–195.

93. Norgan NG. Adaptation of energy metabolism to level of energy. In Panzkova J. Energy Expenditure Under Field Conditions. Prague, Charles University, 1983: 56.

94. Allison JB, Anderson JA, Seeley RD. The determination of the nitrogen balance index in normal and hypoproteinemic dogs. Ann NY Acad Sci 1946; 47:245–271.

95. Nettleton JA, Hegsted DM. Protein-energy interrelations during dietary restriction: effects on tissue nitrogen and protein turnover. Nutr Metab 1975; 18:31–40.

96. Garlick PJ, Clugston GA, Waterlow JC. Influence of low-energy diets on whole-body protein turnover in obese subjects. Am J Physiol 1980; 238:E235–244.

97. Reeds PJ, Wahle KWJ, Haggarty P. Energy costs of protein and fatty acid synthesis. Proc Nutr Soc 1982; 4:155.

98. Young VR, Munro HN, Matthews DE, et al. Relationship of energy metabolism to protein metabolism. Presented at the 4th Congress of the European Society of Parenteral and Enteral Nutrition, Vienna, 1982.

99. Young VR, Munro HN. N-methylhistidine (3-methylhistidine) and muscle protein turnover: an overview. Fed Proc 1978; 37:2291–2300.

100. Kien CL, Rohrbaugh DK, Burke JF, et al. Whole body protein synthesis in relation to basal energy expenditure in healthy children and in children recovering from burn injury. Ann Surg 1978; 187:383–391.

101. Bilmazes C, Kien CL, Rohrbaugh HN, et al. Quantitative contribution by skeletal muscle to elevated rates of whole-body protein breakdown in burned children, as measured by N-methylhistidine output. Metabolism 1978; 27:671–676.

102. Schønheyder F, Heilskov NSC, Oleson K. Isotopic studies on the mechanism of negative nitrogen balance produced by immobilization. Scand J Clin Lab Invest 1954; 6:178–188.

103. Young VR, Torun B. Physical activity: impact on protein and amino acid metabolism and implications for nutritional requirements. Prog Clin Biol Res 1981; 77:57–85.

104. Food and Nutrition Board, National Academy of Sciences, National Council: Recommended Dietary Allowances. Washington, 1980.

105. Blackburn GL, Flatt JP, Clowes GHA, et al. Protein-sparing therapy during periods of starvation with sepsis or trauma. Ann Surg 1973; 177:588–594.

106. Calloway DH. Nitrogen balance of men with marginal intakes of protein and energy. J Nutr 1975; 105:914.

107. Calloway DH, Spector H. Nitrogen balance as related to caloric and protein intake in active young men. Am J Clin Nutr 1954; 2:405.

108. Elwyn DH, Gump FE, Munro HN, et al. Changes in nitrogen balances of depleted patients with increasing infusions of glucose. Am J Clin Nutr 1979; 32:1597–1611.

109. Kinney JM, Elwyn DH. Protein-energy interrelationships. In Selvey N, White PL (eds). Nutrition in the 1980's: Constraints on Our Knowledge. New York, Alan R. Liss, 1981: 179.

110. Elwyn DH. Nutritional requirements of adult surgical patients. Crit Care Med 1980; 8:9–20.

111. Rudman D, Millikan WJ, Richardson TJ, et al. Elemental balances during intravenous hyperalimentation. J Clin Invest 1975; 55:94.

112. Munro HN, Young VR. Urinary excretion of N-methylhistidine (3-methylhistidine): a tool to study metabolic responses in relation to nutrients and hormone status in health and disease in man. Am J Clin Nutr 1978; 31:1608–1614.

113. Peters C, Fischer JE. Studies on calorie to nitrogen ratio for total parenteral nutrition. Surg Gynecol Obstet 1980; 151:1–8.

114. Rajantie J, Kauste A, Holttinen K, et al. Nitrogen utilization during postoperative low nitrogen, high calorie parenteral nutrition. Clin Nutr 1983; 2:41–46.

115. Rhodes JM, Carroll A, Dawson J, et al. A controlled trial of fixed versus tailored calorie intake in patients receiving intravenous feeding after abdominal surgery. Clin Nutr 1985; 4:169–174.

116. Chen WJ, Ohashi E, Kasai M. Amino acid metabolism in parenteral nutrition; with special reference to the calo-

rie:nitrogen ratio and the blood urea nitrogen level. Metabolism 1974; 23:1117–1123.

117. Shaw SN, Elwynd DH, Askanazi J, et al. Effects of increasing nitrogen intake on nitrogen balance and energy expenditure in nutritionally depleted adult patient receiving parenteral nutrition. Am J Clin Nutr 1983; 37:930–940.

118. Duke JH, Jørgensen SB, Broell JR, et al. Contribution of protein to caloric expenditure following injury. Surgery 1970; 68:168–174.

119. Munro HN. Energy intake and nitrogen metabolism. In Kinney JM, Munro HN, Buskirk E (eds). Assessment of Energy Metabolism in Health and Disease. Columbus, Ohio, Ross Laboratories, 1980.

120. Long JM, Wilmore DW, Mason AD, et al. Effect of carbohydrate and fat intake on nitrogen excretion during total intravenous feeding. Ann Surg 1977; 185:417–422.

121. Greenberg GR, Marliss EB, Anderson GH, et al. Protein-sparing therapy in postoperative patients: effects of added hypocaloric glucose or lipid. N Engl J Med 1976; 294:1411.

2

REGULATION OF ENERGY AND METABOLISM

OLIVER E. OWEN

Foods are eaten and their energy content is used to maintain the viability of the body. This transfer of chemical energy through the body as glucose, amino acids, and free fatty acids to maintain body heat and to perform work is highly regulated and influenced by the energy needs of the body, substrate availability, membrane transport, hormone signals, enzyme activity, and other modulators.

This chapter reviews the generation of energy in the mitochondria, the regulatory roles of the cell membrane and transduction of its receptor-hormonal signals, the energy requirements of modern-day humans, macronutrient storage in the whole body, and the flux rates of nutrient fuels among the major organs of the body. It emphasizes data derived primarily from adult humans.

Several textbook chapters[1-4] are recommended for readers wishing additional information. Darnell et al.[4] cite the most useful recent references.

BIOENERGETICS OF ENERGY CONVERSION

The living human is dependent upon organelles, mitochondria, for the supply of energy needed to do the constant work of biosynthesis, ion and solute pumping, and movement. Energy is derived from the oxidation of foodstuffs.

Energy, heat, and work are measured in the same units. Values are usually expressed as kilocalories, abbreviated kcal, and kilojoules, abbreviated kJ. The physiological or biochemical values of macronutrients are given in Table 2–1.

The body effectively transfers high-energy electrons trapped in carbohydrates, fats, and proteins to other forms of energy: chemical (carbohydrates to fats), mechanical (muscular movements), electrical (nerve transmissions), and osmotic (electrolyte concentration gradients). Orderly biochemical oxidations liberate free energy, which can be utilized to perform the aforementioned energy-requiring op-

TABLE 2–1. Physiological Fuel Values

Carbohydrates	4.10 kcal/g	17.0 kJ/g
Pure glucose	3.75 kcal/g	15.7 kJ/g
Fats*	9.30 kcal/g	39.0 kJ/g
Proteins†	4.10 kcal/g	17.0 kJ/g

*An average value for animal and plant lipids.
†Nitrogen excreted as urea.

erations and to generate heat. Heat is dissipated to the environment.

The transfer of free energy from one chemical compound to another occurs in quanta. For example, the transfer of energy from the oxidation of a mole of glucose (~ -8000 kcal/mole) to synthesize a peptide bond requires $\sim +5000$ kcal/mole. The difference between the amount of calories stored in the peptide bond and the amount of calories released from glucose oxidation, ~ -3000 kcal/mole, is immediately surrendered to the environment. Eventually, the stored peptide bond energy is also released as heat into the environment. Thus, the flow of chemical energy from ingested foodstuffs is eventually and irretrievably dissipated to the environment as heat.

The energy contained in foodstuffs has high chemical potential (electron-rich) that can be used to drive an energy-requiring process (endergonic reaction). Electrons are passed along a chain of proteins known as an electron-transport chain, embedded in an ion-impermeable, inner mitochondrial membrane. The energy released by the electron in its descent down the chain is harnessed to generate the cellular batteries, adenosine triphosphate and other nucleotides, needed to drive in vivo energy-requiring biochemical reactions. Thus, the oxidation of glucose, fatty acids, and amino acids (exergonic reactions) releases free energy, most of which is trapped by various nucleotides, adenosine triphosphate (ATP), cytidine triphosphate (CTP), uridine triphosphate (UTP), and guanosine triphosphate (GTP).

The concentrations of ATP in cells range around several millimoles. The concentrations of GTP, CTP, and UTP are typically a tenth or less of those for ATP. The intercellular pools of these nucleotide batteries are interrelated in that ATP rephosphorylates the other nucleotides when they are consumed in the transfer of energy to endergonic reactions. Although ATP is a charged battery packed with chemical energy, it should be recognized that the quantity of ATP needed to equal the caloric value of 14 kg of stored triglycerides (body fat) is about 9090 kg. Thus, this readily available source of energy is not a good depot for energy storage.

In addition to the small and replenishable stores of energy as nucleotide triphosphates, primarily ATP, muscle and brain contain phosphagens (creatine phosphate), which serve as a backup energy source when work demands are high and prompt. Thus, the cleavage of high-energy-yielding pyro-

phosphate bonds in ATP or other nucleotide triphosphates and, in special tissue like muscle and brain, phosphagens drives the body. ATP and its kindred are readily replenished by oxidative metabolism of endogenously stored fuels or exogenously derived nutrients: the transfer of electrons from carbohydrates, fats, and proteins to oxygen generates high-energy phosphate bonds, and the coupling of oxygen utilization to pyrophosphate bond formation is known as oxidative phosphorylation (Fig. 2–1). Oxidative phosphorylation occurs in the inner membrane of the mitochondria, which functions as an energy-conversion machine. Two electrons or hydrogen atoms are removed at each step in a series of reactions necessary to cleave carbon-hydrogen, carbon-carbon, carbon-oxygen, and carbon-nitrogen linkages. The electrons are sequentially transferred to nicotinamide adenine dinucleotide (NAD → NADH) or to flavin adenine dinucleotide ($FADH_2$), ubiquinone, cytochrome c, and oxygen. A molecule of ATP or comparable nucleotide pyrophosphate is generated at each of the latter three transfers. The mechanism for generating ATP (Fig. 2–2) was recently described:[3]

As the high-energy electrons from the hydrogens on NADH and $FADH_2$ are transported down the electron-transport chain in the inner mitochondrial membrane, the energy released as they pass from one carrier molecule to the next is used to pump protons across the inner membrane from the mitochondrial matrix into the intermembrane space. This creates an electrochemical proton gradient across the inner mitochondrial membrane, and the backflow of protons down this gradient is in turn used to drive a membranebound enzyme, ATP synthetase, that catalyzes the conversion of ADP + P_i to ATP, completing the process of oxidative phosphorylation.

The electrochemical gradient across the mitochondrial inner membrane also drives ADP, P_i, substrates, and calcium into the mitochondrial matrix as it drives ATP into the cytosol. As a result the ADP molecules produced by ATP hydrolysis in the cytosol rapidly enter mitochondria for recharging, while the ATP molecules formed in the mitochondrial matrix by oxidative phosphorylation rapidly escape to the cytosol where they are needed.

The turnover rate of pyrophosphate bonds depends upon the energy requirements of the body. In the resting state about 85 per cent of the pyrophosphate bonds in the entire body are consumed and replenished daily. During strenuous, competitive physical activity for a brief period of time this turnover rate can be increased by 10 to 20 times.

The number of molecules of high-energy phosphate bonds produced per number of molecules of oxygen consumed is the phosphate-oxygen ratio (P:O ratio). This ratio varies with the nature of foodstuffs oxidized. In the laboratory it is 2.82 for fat and 3.00 for glucose. The efficiencies at which the free energies released from the oxidization of fuels are trapped in pyrophosphate bonds and the sub-

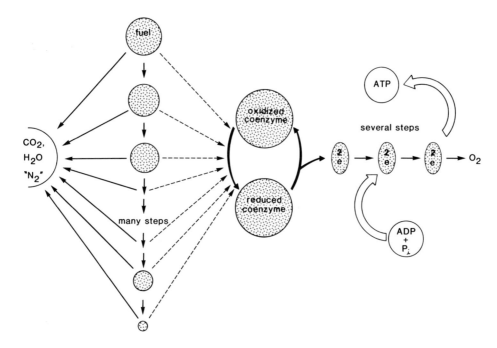

FIGURE 2–1. Oxidative phosphorylation is driven by electron transfer from various substrates to molecular oxygen, and adenosine triphosphate is synthesized. (From Owen OE, Caprio S, Sapir DG, et al. Ketogenesis and metabolic acidosis during diabetic ketoacidosis: new perspectives. In Melchionda N (ed). Recent Advances in Obesity and Diabetes. New York, Raven Press, 1984: 309–318. Reproduced with permission.)

sequent efficiencies at which the free energies released from cleavages of the pyrophosphate bonds are used to perform in vivo functions have not been fully defined (see Chapter 5). However, one possible mechanism for the loss of free energy is at the transfer of ions across the mitochondrial membranes into the cytosolic matrix independent of generating ATP. This uncoupling of oxidative phosphorylation is known to occur in brown adipose tissue for the generation of heat. The significance or magnitude of this uncoupling of electron transport and ATP synthesis, and thus of heat generation, is poorly delineated in humans. One of the reasons for giving the foregoing information in a clinical textbook of nutrition is to lay the foundation of generating useful ATP. Uncoupling electron transport and ATP synthesis augments substrate (glucose, fatty acids, amino acids, etc.) oxidation. Thus, uncouplers, such as lipophilic weak acids (dinitrophenol), could be developed to waste body fuel supplies (stored triglycerides) and induce weight and, specifically, fat loss.

MEMBRANE REGULATION OF TRANSPORT

With a division of labor among the tissues in the human body, elaborate communication systems de-

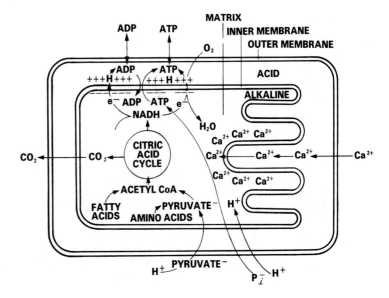

FIGURE 2–2. High-energy electrons contained in fatty acids, amino acids, and carbohydrates are passed to NADH (and $FADH_2$) and then down the electron transfer system localized in the inner mitochondrial membrane. The concentrated protons (H^+) in the intermembrane space create an energy gradient that drives ATP generation.

veloped for the regulation of nutritional supplies for maintaining fuel homeostasis. The simplest exchange of nutrients between tissues occurs at the cell-to-cell level, where the gap junctions are engaged in passing molecules between cells to coordinate their metabolic activities. However, more highly specialized membranous structures have developed for the selective passage of ions, nutrients, and complex molecules among cells and organs.

Cells are enclosed by bilayer phospholipid membranes (plasma membranes) in which are embedded proteins that permit and promote the uptake of glucose, amino acids, fatty acids, ions, and other essential nutrients (Fig. 2–3). Intrinsic plasma membrane proteins catalyze metabolic reactions initiated by simple cellular touch or integrated by hormonal and neuronal stimuli. In addition to a limiting external plasma membrane, cells contain limiting internal membranes that surround individual and specialized structures (organelles). In these membranes the ratio of proteins to lipids varies widely. However, all membranes contain two phospholipid layers, each having hydrophilic and hydrophobic components. The hydrophobic portions face each other and form the inner parts and the hydrophilic portions form the outer parts of the two leaflets or the bilayers of the phospholipid membrane. Cholesterol, with its hydrophobic and hydrophilic regions, is a constituent that tends to reduce the fluidity of the bilayer membranes. Carbohydrates bound to proteins, forming glycoprotein, or to lipids, forming glycolipids, are also abundant in plasma membranes.

Membrane proteins have several important and specific functions. They serve as hormonal receptors, transmitting surface signals to the interior of the cells. They also form various membrane-bound enzymes. Others act as anchors for the cytoskeletal systems of the intracellular components and serve extracellularly to attach cells to each other. Equally important, but aside from nutrition, is that proteins on plasma membranes are specific for tissues, and distinctive membrane proteins give cells their individuality and are largely responsible for conveying the antigenicity of cells. These specific surface proteins are known as HLA antigens in humans. Membrane proteins may be confined to the exterior or interior of the bilayer membrane or may be transmembrane proteins spanning both bilayers and hav-

PHOSPHOLIPID BILAYER MEMBRANE

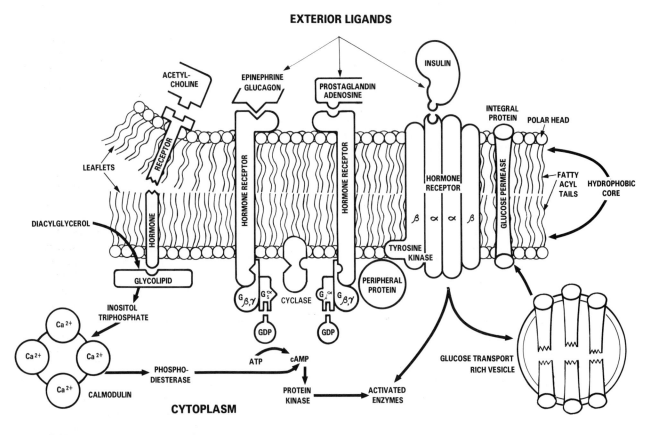

FIGURE 2–3. *The phospholipid bilayer membrane is a complex structure that maintains the intracellular milieu constant and is a fundamental regulator of cellular metabolism. It has outer (polar head) and inner (polar head) surfaces and central cores (hydrophobic cores), and integral peripheral proteinaceous components.*

ing regions on both sides of the membrane. Membrane proteins interacting with the central or hydrophobic portion of the membrane are referred to as integral proteins. Membrane proteins that do not interact with the hydrophobic core of the bilayer phospholipid leaflets are known as peripheral proteins. These peripheral proteins reside on the inner or outer membrane wall. Many, but not all, of the proteins located in the bilayer lipid layer are able to migrate or move in the membranes as though they are floating in the lipids of the membrane.

All closed phospholipid bilayer membranes are asymmetrical in that they have an external and an internal surface. Every molecule of a substance resides on the same side of the membrane. In general, glycolipids and glycoproteins (with their oligosaccharides) are attached on the extracytoplasmic (external) surface and enzymes are bound on the cytoplasmic (internal) surface. The asymmetry is essential for executing the functioning of membranes (Fig. 2–3).

Some small molecules involved in metabolism cross the bilayer phospholipid membranes by simple or passive diffusion. For example, the oxygen needed to permit oxidative metabolism and the waste carbon dioxide and urea passively diffuse in or out, respectively, across membranes. Concentration gradients, travel distances, and solubilities dictate passive diffusion rates.

Some ions and other small molecules (glucose, amino acids, fatty acids) are actively transported across the membranes. These energy-requiring systems are facilitated at special places in the membranes known as transport sites or zones, which are highly regulated by specific membrane transport proteins collectively known as transporters or permeases. Large protein molecules (albumin and globulin) are transported across the membranes as engulfed particles.

The active transporters of glucose and amino acids (and fatty acids) are composed of unique sets of proteins specific for individual classes of macronutrients and other complex molecules. There are maximum rates (V_{max}) for transporting molecules or macronutrients bound specifically to their transporters. In addition, there are concentrations of molecules, for example glucose or amino acid, that allow one-half maximum transport rates across cell membranes, and these concentrations are described by constants (K_m). Thus, facilitated transport is specific for a molecule (or ion) that binds to its unique transport protein(s) and has a maximum transfer rate. These highly selective membrane transport proteins have specificities similar to those of enzymes.

After a macronutrient, such as glucose or amino acid, is transported across the cell membranes, it can undergo phosphorylation, another energy-requiring reaction, which functionally traps the activated nutrient inside the cell for further metabolism.

The active transport of ions across cell membranes is of interest to the nutritionist because maintaining ionic gradients across membranes requires a large portion of the energy released from foods. The Na^+, K^+ ATPase transport system exchanges intracellular Na^+ for extracellular K^+; the calcium transport system pumps Ca^{2+} out of the cell, or in the case of muscle, from the cytosol into the sarcoplasmic reticulum; the proton transport system concentrates hydrogen ions between the mitochondrial membranous layers in the lysosomal vesicles and in the stomach lumen. The Na^+, K^+, Ca^{2+}, and H^+ transport systems are the only ones known to be coupled directly to ATP hydrolysis. However, the transport of some other substances is also energy-requiring.

The transmembrane movement of glucose and amino acids (and probably fatty acids) is driven indirectly by the intracellular hydrolysis of ATP because the transport of these substances is coupled to the gradient generated by pumping Na^+. Coupled movement of substances can be in the same direction, e.g., Na^+ and glucose and/or amino acids move inwardly together (symport), or in opposite directions, e.g., Na^+ moves inwardly and Ca^{2+} moves outwardly (antiport). Water flows with the movement of ions and molecules across cell membranes. Thus, the concentration of solutes between compartments drives water movement. Another mechanism that moves water through membranes and junctions is the hydrostatic pressure.

Ions, gases, nutrients, waste products, and water are not the only substances transported across the various membranes of cells and their organelles. Cells import and export large molecules, especially proteins. Secretion of molecules (insulin, glucagon, etc.) is accomplished by exocytosis in which intracellular vesicles fuse with the cell membranes and contents of the vesicles are extruded into the extracellular spaces. Uptake of macromolecules is accomplished by phagocytosis, in which particles are attached to the surface of plasma membranes and thereafter are engulfed by invagination of the membrane. Specific proteins bind as ligands to receptors on plasma membranes and undergo internalization. This process is referred to as receptor-mediated endocytosis (Fig. 2–4). It allows the selective uptake of proteins and other small particles delivered to plasma membranes by circulating blood and other extracellular fluids. The binding of proteins to receptors either on the plasma membranes or organelle membranes is specific not only for the proteins but also for the cell types (tissues), and internalization of receptor-ligands requires energy. The binding sites of a ligand to its receptor and the affinity (high or low) of the ligand for its receptors can be measured. Receptors become concentrated on plasma membranes to form areas known as coated pits. These depressed surface areas with receptors coated with ligands internalize by endocytosis. Vesicles bud off the plasma membranes housing numerous receptor-ligand complexes. The receptors in

ENDOCYTOSIS

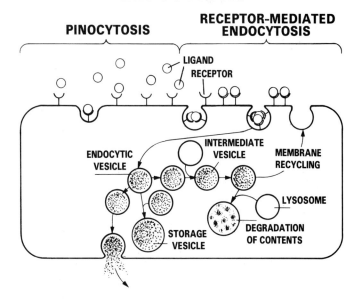

FIGURE 2–4. *The processes of endocytosis and exocytosis transport substances across membranes. Ligands bind to receptors, allowing selective uptake of proteins and other small particles, which become engulfed and metabolized. Remnants are extruded. Some substances simply pass unchanged through cells.*

the vesicles become uncoupled from the ligands and recycle to the surface of the plasma membranes while the ligand fuses with a lysosome and undergoes degradation or enters the cytoplasm for another fate. In the case of the low-density lipoprotein (LDL) enriched with cholesterol esters, catabolism of the receptor uncoupled ligand, LDL, produces cholesterol, fatty acids, and amino acids, which are freed and become available for the various metabolic pathways of these nutrients. Similar systems are involved in iron and vitamin B_{12} metabolism. However, it should be noted that most nutrients do not need to travel via the lysosomal pathways.

The quantities of plasma membrane receptors internalized as receptor-ligand vesicles are enormous and require amounts of energy that would be prohibitive if recycling of surface receptors did not occur. The proteins as well as the phospholipid components of plasma membrane receptors are recycled.

Endocytosis and exocytosis are important for transporting nutrients in plasma to tissue since the junctions between endothelial cells lining capillaries are very tight and normally do not allow the free passage of plasma (or water). Small vesicles on the blood side of thin endothelial cells rapidly bud off the plasma membrane (endocytosis) and carry engulfed plasma with carbohydrates, amino acids, fatty acids, vitamins, minerals, and other substances across the cells, fuse with the plasma membranes of the tissue side, and release (exocytosis) their contents into the interstitial fluids in contact with the various cells of organ systems. The transfer time is about 1 minute, and the volume of plasma with its life-supporting nutrients that can be transported is about 100 or more times what could be moved in the absence of these shuttling vesicles.[5]

Plasma or organelle membrane receptors can be divided into two groups based on whether the major function of the receptor is to transmit information that modifies cell behavior and metabolism (class I receptors) or whether the major function is to remove substrates from the extracellular fluids (class II receptors).[6] In general, hormones are the ligands that bind to class I receptors. These receptors may be randomly distributed on the cell surface, and the ligand-receptor complex is independent of divalent cations (Ca^{2+}). Receptor-ligand complexes internalize, resulting in the loss of surface receptors and thus desensitization to the ligands or down-regulation of the receptors.[6] Internalized receptors have different fates in that they may be catabolized or recycled to the surface of the membranes. Usually nutrients (lipoproteins, minerals, and vitamins) are the ligands that bind to class II receptors. The formation of receptor-ligand complexes is dependent on pH and generally on divalent cation (Ca^{2+}). The receptor can be randomly distributed over the membrane surface but may be localized in coated pit areas. Following internalization, all class II receptors recycle to the cell surface, whereas the ligand can be used for synthetic purposes (cholesterol), degraded, stored (fatty acids and amino acids), or passed through the cell (capillary endothelium) for use by other tissues.

HORMONAL REGULATION OF METABOLISM

Hormones are released from endocrine glands to regulate target cells. Hormones that travel through the blood stream regulate distant target cells by endocrine signals, whereas hormones that travel between adjacent cells regulate by paracrine signals.

Hormones that circulate in the blood and travel through extracellular fluids can be classed as (1) water-soluble molecules (insulin, glucagon, epidermal growth factor, growth hormone, insulin-like growth factors I and II, cholecystokinin, epinephrine, norepinephrine, prostaglandins, etc.), which move freely in biological fluids and bind to plasma membranes to immediately initiate the transduction of their signals, or (2) lipid-soluble molecules (cortisol, aldosterone, estrogens, testosterone, thyroxine, triiodothyronine, etc.), which travel in aqueous fluids on carrier proteins from which they dissociate, diffuse across the plasma membrane, interact with receptor proteins in the cytosol or nucleus, and slowly initiate the transduction of their signals by modifying the rate of synthesis of specific messenger RNA's.

The large peptides (insulin, glucagon, growth hormone, insulin-like factors I and II, etc.) or small amines (epinephrine, norepinephrine) occupy their unique docking sites to form receptor-ligand complexes that within milliseconds trigger short-lived chain reactions leading to subsequent bioregulatory responses. Some hormone-receptor complexes (those involving glucagon, epinephrine, etc.) convey signals following the activation of adenylate cyclase at the inner surface of the plasma membrane. Adenylate cyclase converts ATP to cyclic AMP, a water-soluble second messenger that diffuses through the cell-activating protein kinases that in turn phosphorylate other intracellular proteins, especially enzymes. Phosphorylated enzymes are generally much more energized than unphosphorylated enzymes. A stimulatory ligand bound to a receptor can induce several hundred molecules of cyclic AMP before the hormone dissociates from the receptor. This obviously amplifies hormonal signals.

Additional members of the receptor-ligand-second messenger unit are interlinking stimulatory and inhibitory G proteins. G proteins, so called because they bind guanine nucleotides, act as transducers of information across cell membranes. They differ in that one G protein ($G_s\alpha$) interconnects the stimulating hormones (epinephrine, glucagon, ACTH, and vasopressin) and the other ($G_i\alpha$) interconnects the inhibitory hormones (prostaglandins) to adenylate cyclase.[7]

Cyclic AMP can also be regulated by undergoing degradation via phosphodiesterases. These degrading phosphodiesterases are responsive to the intracellular Ca^{2+} that binds to calmodulin, a ubiquitous Ca^{2+} binding protein and a subunit of phosphorylase. Intracellular Ca^{2+} concentration is regulated by hormonal and/or neuronal controls. In muscle, for example, it has been demonstrated that the neurotransmitter (acetylcholine)-receptor complex causes elevation of cytoplasmic Ca^{2+}, which activates glycogen phosphorylase kinase to stimulate the enzyme, glycogen phosphorylase, that catalyzes the conversion of glycogen to glucose-6-phosphate. This reaction can be magnified through another route in which catecholamine and beta-adrenergic (epinephrine) augmentation of the cyclic AMP cascade also activates glycogen phosphorylase.

Cell behavior is also regulated or influenced by inner surface cell membrane inositol phospholipid metabolites. The binding of hormones and/or neurotransmitters to their receptors activates phospholipase, which triggers the hydrolysis of phosphatidylinositol-4,5-bisphosphate and the release of inositol-1,4,5-triphosphate into the cytoplasm and diacylglycerol, which remains in the plane of the membrane. An interesting aspect of this ligand-receptor–initiated reaction is that both the triphosphate and diacylglycerol function as second messengers to activate separate cellular processes. Inositol triphosphate causes the release of Ca^{2+} from a compartment of the endoplasmic reticulum. The other metabolite, diacylglycerol, activates a protein kinase, protein kinase C, that phosphorylates certain proteins. The activation of protein kinase C by diacylglycerol is a complex process that requires Ca^{2+} and phosphatidylserine as cofactors. The degradation of diacylglycerol yields arachidonic acid, yet another intracellular signal.[7]

Insulin is the cardinal hormone that regulates the concentrations of fuels, specifically glucose, in the blood. Insulin receptors, located on the surface of most cells, are composed of two α and two β subunits.[8] When insulin is linked to its receptor, the tyrosine residue of the receptor becomes phosphorylated; thus the insulin receptor is itself an insulin-dependent tyrosine kinase.[8,9] An unconfirmed report links the tyrosine kinase activity of the insulin-activated receptor to phospholipase C–liberated inositol triphosphate and diacylglycerol from plasma membrane glycolipids.[7,10] The intracellular concentration of cyclic AMP falls in most tissues. Regardless of the exact mechanisms, many signals are transmitted from the insulin-receptor complex to promote activities of several plasma membrane permeases and cytoplasmic enzymes. Insulin rapidly stimulates translocation of glucose from the extracellular fluids to the cytoplasm of many tissues.[8] The binding of insulin to its receptor recruits vesicles with many glucose permeases that are located just beneath the plasma membranes. Insulin stimulates cells, causing the glucose-rich permease vesicles to fuse with the plasma membrane and augment glucose transport many fold. This ligand-receptor activation also stimulates glycogen, protein, and lipid synthesis. It suppresses gluconeogenesis, proteolysis, lipolysis, and ketogenesis.[11] Glucagon counteracts the roles of insulin.[12]

Cyclic AMP, cytoplasmic Ca^{2+}, inositol triphosphates, diacylglycerol, and insulin-dependent tyrosine kinase modify the activities of specific enzymes that control the rates of catabolism or anabolism of carbohydrates, fats, and proteins by stimulating (or suppressing) the actions of cyclic AMP–dependent enzymes called protein kinases. The protein kinases transfer their terminal phosphate groups of ATP to serine, threonine, or tyrosine of substrate enzymes.[7] These enzymes are specialized to catalyze biological reactions. They are extraordinarily specific for substrates and have catalytic powers that supersede anything designed by humans. They introduce the elements of water (hydrolases) or phosphoric acid (phosphorylases) at specific bond sites, transfer a group from one substrate to another (transferases), cause oxidation-reduction reactions (oxidoreductases), add to double bonds (lyases), induce isomerization of substances (isomerases), and form bonds with ATP cleavage (ligases). Some enzymes work independently to induce reactions, whereas others need cofactors. A cofactor may be a metal (Zn^{2+}, Mg^{2+}, Mn^{2+}, Cu^{2+}, K^+, or Na^+) or a vitamin (thiamine, riboflavin, nicotinic acid, pantothenic acid, pyridoxine, vitamin B_{12}, vitamin A, vitamin D). The active enzyme–cofactor complex is called the holoenzyme; when the cofactor is removed, the inactive remainder is called an apoenzyme.[13]

Thus, closed membranes limit cells and their organelles. They are semipermeable and have numerous chores to do in permitting, promoting, or excluding ions and macro- and micronutrients. The selectivity of the limiting membranes enables the cell to maintain a relatively constant internal milieu. The biological membranes are dynamic structures whose components, including the phospholipid bilayers, transporters, and receptors, and their second messengers, protein kinases and enzymes, undergo rapid and reversible rearrangements in response to intracellular and extracellular nutrient, hormonal, or neuronal signals. These dynamic responses are energy-dependent, but oxidative metabolism of nutrients yields the energies for cellular (whole-body) survival, growth, and reproduction. The total energy demands of these biological processes are equal to whole-body energy requirements.

WHOLE-BODY METABOLISM

Whole-body energy requirements are measured directly by determining the amount of body heat generated in a body calorimeter (direct calorimetry) and indirectly by determining the respiratory exchange rates of oxygen and carbon dioxide and the urinary excretion rate of nitrogen (indirect calorimetry). From these techniques it has been learned that the total daily caloric requirements of humans are dictated by their body size and state of activity. Although definitions of metabolic states differ, the lowest or basal metabolic requirement (BMR) is considered in this chapter to occur transiently during the early morning hours of deep sleep.[14] In clinical practice this transient basal rate has little influence on total energy requirements. Furthermore, the BMR is impractical to measure. Another state of metabolism is the resting metabolic rate (RMR), which is considered in this chapter to occur while an individual is lying quietly during the awake hours. It is frequently stated, but inadequately documented,

that the RMR is the best predictor of overall caloric requirements and usually accounts for 65 to 70 per cent of daily energy expenditure.[15] It is not widely appreciated that the RMR of adult humans varies from about 800 to 3000 kcal per day.[16,17] Obviously, the range is greater if infants and children are included. Superimposed on this wide range of resting energy requirements are those associated with exercise. Physical activity usually accounts for about 20 to 30 per cent of the daily caloric expenditure.[18] However, the quantity of energy used for physical activity has a large variance. Competitive athletes can consume 10 to 20 times their RMR for minutes to hours during forceful exercise. Although smaller quantities of fuels are expended by those unable to participate in such strenuous activities, considerable amounts of energy can be used during exercise periods by anyone capable of doing augmented physical activity. The role of exercise on energy requirement, body composition, and changes in body weight is reviewed in Chapter 11.

The usual values given for resting metabolic rates are based on three large and authoritative studies done during the first half of this century. In 1919, Harris and Benedict published their classic monograph on RMR of males and females.[19] They developed regression formulas for predicting the RMR of men and women based on height, weight, age, and sex. DuBois and DuBois measured the body surface area (BSA) of humans and derived a formula for calculating BSA based on height and weight.[20] Boothby et al. (Mayo Foundation) studied males and females[21] and reported in 1922 that the RMR could best be predicted from BSA.[22] Between 1930 and 1950, Robertson and Reid studied males and females and derived regression formulas for predicting RMR based on sex, age, and BSA.[23]

Although there are additional early studies pertaining to RMR, values in tables widely used for predicting RMR are smoothed means derived from these three studies and are expressed as calories per m^2 of BSA per hour or day for men and women of given ages.[24]

More recent studies have shown that the Harris and Benedict equations overestimate the measured RMR in morbidly obese humans[25] and in malnourished patients.[26] When calculations are made for adults to adjust for differences in the active protoplasmic tissue, the sex, age, and nutritional status of an individual[25,27,28] have little direct influence on RMR. These conclusions are based on a reanalysis of the Harris and Benedict subjects, on studies of obese or ill humans, and on other studies.[25–28] However, only recently have systematic reappraisals of the caloric requirements of modern-day humans been done.[16,29] The resting metabolic caloric requirements (RMR) of 44 healthy lean and obese women, some of whom were trained athletes, and 60 healthy lean and obese men were found to be different from those given in the classic tables and prediction equations.[16,26,29] The caloric expenditure, measured by indirect calorimetry, was related to the body composition, determined by skinfold thickness and densitometric techniques. The ages of the women ranged from 18 to 65 years and body weights from 43 to 143 kg;[16] the men ranged in ages from 18 to 82 years and in body weight from 60 to 171 kg.[29] In these new studies stepwise and multiple regression analyses were used to determine whether one or several variables of weight, height, age, or body compositional components best predicted the RMR of males or females (Table 2–2).

First it was noted that body compositional variables reflecting active protoplasmic tissue such as weight, body surface area, fat-free mass (by skinfold thickness or densitometry), lean body mass, and body cell mass are all highly interrelated (Table 2–2). Therefore, it is extremely difficult if not impossible currently to identify which of these variables most accurately reflects active protoplasmic tissue. Nonetheless, the variables most highly, but comparably, correlated with the measured RMR are weight, body surface area, lean body mass, body cell mass, and fat-free mass (by densitometry or skinfold thickness). However, combinations of variables in stepwise regression analysis to predict RMR gave values comparable to weight alone in predicting the RMR of humans. Since weight is the most easily and accurately measured variable and is highly correlated with RMR of both women and men, it is a good variable to use if estimates of RMR are needed for humans.[16,29] This does not deny the existence of minor differences among variables that reflect active protoplasmic tissues, specifically fat-free mass (lean body mass) and RMR. Nonetheless, at this time, the weight of an individual is the most practical measurement available and a good variable to use for predicting the RMR.

The recommendation that weight be used to predict RMR, if direct measurement cannot be made, questions the claim that RMR correlates best with lean body mass.[27,28,30–36] Although this may be true, it should be recognized that the resting energy requirements of various aerobic "lean" tissues are vastly different per unit mass.[37,38] In normal-weight adults brain (which is mostly lipids rather than proteins) and liver together constitute only 4 to 5 per cent of total body weight but are collectively responsible for about 40 per cent of the RMR.[38,39] Muscle composes 35 to 40 per cent of body weight but accounts for only about 20 per cent of the RMR.[38,39] Adipose tissue normally constitutes about 15 to 25 per cent of body weight but accounts for only 2 to 5 per cent of RMR.[38,39] These disproportionate rates of energy requirements per unit mass of different tissues partly explain why weight correlates about as well with RMR as do the bulk masses of active protoplasmic tissue with their heterogeneous metabolic requirements. These same considerations should be extended to obese and athletic humans. Although

the absolute RMR is greater the heavier the woman or man,[16,29,30] there is reduced energy expenditure per kilogram of body weight for men and women as weight increases. Large variations in body weight occur, not because of differences in the amounts of high-energy-requiring brain and liver masses, but because of large differences in the amounts of moderate-energy-requiring skeletal muscle masses, especially in athletes, or because of huge differences in the amount of low-energy-requiring adipose tissue masses, especially in obese humans. In essence, a major portion of the RMR in adults is relatively constant because of brain and liver metabolism; the increases in RMR per kilogram of body weight depend primarily on other body components, particularly skeletal muscle and adipose tissue.

Figure 2–5 displays the relationships among measured RMR and body weight of modern-day humans. The slopes of the regression lines for the RMR and weight for healthy nonathletic lean and obese women as well as those for lean and obese men are statistically indistinguishable. Therefore, single regression lines (equations) with their 95 per cent confidence limits are used for predicting the RMR of nonathletic healthy lean and obese women (RMR = 795 + 7.18 × kg wt) and men (RMR = 879 + 10.20 × kg wt). Note that both sexes have wide 95 per cent confidence limits, reflecting the fundamental fact that the caloric requirements of men and women have broad ranges: people are heterogeneous in regard to their caloric requirements. This observation needs general recognition. Included in Figure 2–5 are the relationships for a few world-class competitive athletic women. The regression line for the athletic women (RMR = 50.4 + 21.1 × kg wt) is different from that for the nonathletic women, and the 95 per cent confidence limits for the regression line for the athletes are narrow.

It should be emphasized that owing to the large variations in measured RMR the predicted RMR may over- or underestimate the actual (measured) RMR of nonathletic women by 21 to 33 per cent and nonathletic men by 18 to 29 per cent. On the other hand, it appears that close estimates can be made for female athletes. The predicted RMR of a well-trained competitive athlete estimates actual RMR within 8 to 10 per cent. Athletic women have greater increases in RMR per gain in body weight than nonathletic women (Fig. 2–5). Body weight is also more highly correlated with RMR among women athletes (r = 0.94) than among the nonathletes (r = 0.74). Comparable data for athletic men are not available.

Gender is a factor considered to have important influences on the RMR. Differences in body composition may be responsible for this influence. Figure 2–6 shows the relationship between RMR and fat-free mass measured and calculated from densitometry (FFMD) for women and men with weights ranging from 43 to 171 kg and ages ranging from 18 to 82 years. The slopes of the RMR regression

TABLE 2–2. Resting Metabolic Rate, Body Composition Variables, and Anthropometric Measurements: Correlation Coefficients

	RMR	AGE	HT	WT	BSA	BMI	LBM	BCM	FFMD	FATMD	FFMSF	FATMSF
All Women (n = 44)												
AGE	0.06											
HT	0.41	0.00										
WT	0.74	0.28	0.33									
BSA	0.77	0.29	0.51	0.98								
BMI	0.67	0.31	0.05	0.96	0.88							
LBM	0.77	0.18	0.30	0.95	0.94	0.93						
BCM	0.77	0.08	0.31	0.93	0.92	0.91	0.99					
FFMD	0.71	0.07	0.53	0.84	0.90	0.72	0.83	0.83				
FATMD	0.66	0.22	0.06	0.96	0.91	0.98	0.91	0.90	0.68			
FFMSF	0.78	−0.05	0.52	0.92	0.94	0.82	0.87	0.88	0.95	0.82		
FATMSF	0.69	0.24	0.17	0.98	0.93	0.98	0.93	0.92	0.77	0.99	0.82	
Athletes (n = 8)												
AGE	−0.20											
HT	0.80	0.06										
WT	0.96	−0.11	0.80									
BSA	0.95	−0.04	0.92	0.97								
BMI	0.68	−0.26	0.20	0.76	0.58							
LBM	0.96	−0.33	0.75	0.97	0.93	0.77						
BCM	0.94	−0.43	0.70	0.94	0.90	0.77	0.99					
FFMD	0.84	−0.14	0.71	0.95	0.90	0.77	0.93	0.91				
FATMD	0.47	−0.02	0.33	0.25	0.30	0.07	0.25	0.24	−0.05			
FFMSF	0.85	0.24	0.72	0.93	0.90	0.59	0.82	0.75	0.95	0.56		
FATMSF	0.62	−0.60	0.37	0.49	0.46	0.34	0.63	0.68	0.40	0.80	0.13	
Nonathletes (n = 36)												
AGE	0.02											
HT	0.41	0.02										
WT	0.74	0.22	0.38									
BSA	0.75	0.23	0.55	0.98								
BMI	0.66	0.24	0.08	0.95	0.88							
LBM	0.75	0.12	0.33	0.95	0.93	0.93						
BCM	0.75	0.01	0.33	0.93	0.91	0.91	0.99					
FFMD	0.69	0.06	0.52	0.89	0.93	0.77	0.85	0.85				
FATMD	0.70	0.09	0.13	0.97	0.92	0.98	0.93	0.92	0.76			
FFMSF	0.77	−0.12	0.52	0.95	0.96	0.85	0.90	0.91	0.95	0.87		
FATMSF	0.71	0.16	0.21	0.98	0.94	0.98	0.94	0.92	0.82	0.99	0.87	
Nonathletic Men (n = 60)												
AGE	−0.31											
HT	0.28	−0.18										
WT	0.75	−0.21	0.25									
BSA	0.75	−0.23	0.49	0.96								
BMI	0.68	−0.18	−0.04	0.95	0.85							
LBM	0.74	−0.46	0.32	0.92	0.93	0.86						
BCM	0.72	−0.63	0.32	0.85	0.86	0.79	0.98					
FFMD	0.76	−0.40	0.52	0.85	0.92	0.72	0.91	0.88				
FATMD	0.61	−0.04	0.02	0.93	0.82	0.95	0.76	0.68	0.59			
FFMSF	0.78	−0.38	0.56	0.91	0.93	0.78	0.90	0.87	0.97	0.66		
FATMSF	0.55	0.01	0.19	0.93	0.85	0.94	0.80	0.69	0.68	0.97	0.69	
A/H	0.22	0.44	−0.08	0.21	0.19	0.24	0.15	0.01	0.09	0.25	0.08	0.46

RMR, resting metabolic rate; HT, height; WT, weight; BSA, body surface area; BMI, body mass index; LBM, lean body mass; BCM, body cell mass; FFMD, fat-free mass by densitometry; FATMD, fat mass by densitometry; FFMSF, fat-free mass by skinfolds; FATMSF, fat mass by skinfolds; A/H, abdominal/hip ratio.

lines for women and men are different when RMR is plotted against body weight (Fig. 2–5). However, there is no difference between the slopes for RMR and fat-free mass of men (RMR = 290 + 22.3 × FFMD kg) and women (RMR = 334 + 19.7 × FFMD kg) (Fig. 2–6). These findings are consistent with the fact that healthy adult men have less stored, inert triglycerides than women per unit of body weight. Thus, the influence of sex is negated when fat-free mass is used to calculate the predicted RMR.[28] However, it should be recognized that actual measurement of body fat-free mass is difficult; sep-arate formulas for men and women are used to calculate fat-free mass by skinfold thickness[40] (see Chapter 4), and the formulas used are based on questionable theory. Lastly, accuracy of measurement may be dependent upon the evaluator.[40]

An important fact to be extracted from the literature and demonstrated in Figures 2–5 and 2–6 is that per unit of body weight or of fat-free mass the RMR may vary twofold. Different caloric requirements among adult males and females are independent of leanness and obesity.

In the classic studies done during the first half of

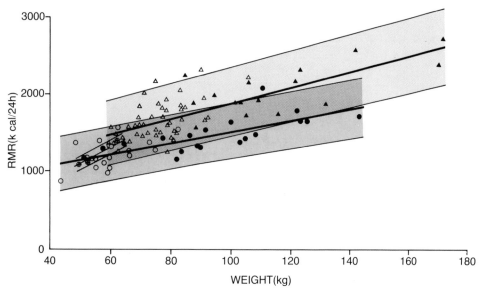

FIGURE 2–5. *The RMR (kcal/24 hr) are contrasted against the weights (kg) of the 44 lean (○) and obese (●) healthy women, 8 of whom were athletes (⊕), and 60 lean (△) and obese (▲) healthy men.*

the century, age was another factor regarded as a regulator of the RMR. However, the inverse influence of age on the RMR of today's healthy women ($-2.9 + 2.3 \times$ age yr) and men ($-3.3 + 1.8 \times$ age yr) is present but small and statistically insignificant.[29] Thus, in healthy adults with normal physical and mental functions, age can generally be regarded as having little or minor influence on RMR. This claim, however, must be guarded because age can be associated with brain dysfunction. As noted above, normally the central nervous system consumes about 20 per cent of the RMR, and the liver consumes an additional 20 per cent.[38] Some of the energy requirements of the liver are used to synthesize glucose (and ketone bodies) for the nervous

system.[38–41] Thus, a large portion of the RMR can be directly or indirectly related to the metabolic requirements of the nervous system. Losses of this high-energy-requiring tissue due to diseases associated with age (especially strokes) have an impact on the RMR. Muscle losses accompanying age can also decrease the RMR (see Chapter 7).

The new prediction regression formulas based on weight (Fig. 2–5) for lean and obese humans show that the old prediction regression formulas of Harris and Benedict,[19] Mayo Foundation,[21] and Cunningham[28] systematically overestimate the RMR of women and men. These discrepancies arise in part from the trivial influence of age on the RMR of today's women and men. Figure 2–7 shows the pre-

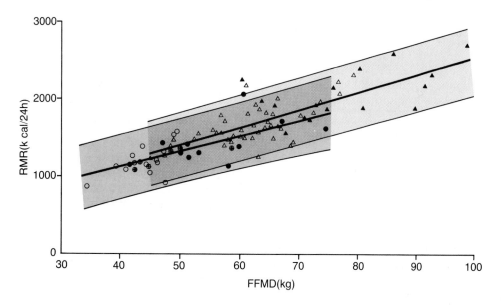

FIGURE 2–6. *The RMR (kcal/24 hr) are contrasted against the fat-free masses (FFMD) by densitometry for 44 lean (○) and obese (●) healthy women, 8 of whom were athletes (⊕), and 60 lean (△) and obese (▲) healthy men.*

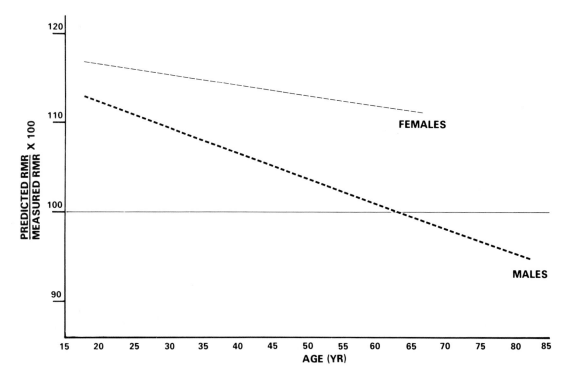

FIGURE 2–7. *The measured RMR of women and men, displayed as 100 per cent, are contrasted against the predicted RMR for women and men based upon the Harris-Benedict equation.*

dicted RMR from the Harris and Benedict equations plotted against age and recently measured and reported RMR.[29] The classic and most commonly used prediction equations of Harris and Benedict greatly overestimate the RMR of young women and men, break even at 64 years for men, and slightly underestimate the RMR of elderly men. Thus the influence of age in the classical equations as well as the tables[23] used for predicting the RMR is exaggerated for today's adults in developed nations.

Using weight as the variable, easily and accurately measured, and eliminating age simplifies prediction of resting metabolic requirements. To be sure, the usefulness in a given subject of any prediction equation derived from a population with large 95 per cent confidence limits is questionable, but actual measurement of metabolic requirements is not always practical.

FASTING METABOLISM

Oxidation of fuels is influenced by body mass and nutritional state. Figure 2–8 shows a two-dimensional surface generated from resistant regression lines showing the nature and quantity of fuels oxidized after an overnight 12- to 13-hour fast by healthy humans who are lean to obese.[29] The progressive increase in the RMR from the lightest to the heaviest man is accompanied by a progressive decrease in the nonprotein respiratory quotient (RQ). The percentage of the RMR provided from glucose oxidation derived from glycogenolysis decreases

only slightly, but the quantity provided from fat oxidation derived from lipolysis triples as the weight of adults triples. Thus, the percentages of carbohydrate, protein, and fat oxidized to meet the resting energy requirements after an overnight fast are influenced by body mass. Larger bodies need more fuels, and usually there is a lot more free fatty acid stored as triglycerides and readily available to meet the energy demands than there is glucose stored as glycogen. Furthermore, the bulk of the body tissues preferentially oxidize fatty acids over glucose during fasting, even though enough of both fuels is available.

The influences of feasting and fasting are diametrically opposed. Feasting is associated with a rapid, transient rise in energy utilization (see below) and fasting is associated with a gradual decline in energy requirements (Fig. 2–9). Part of this diminution in caloric requirements is associated with the loss of body mass, much of which is muscle and other active protoplasmic tissues. However, there is an additional decrease that is out of proportion to mass reduction and causes alterations in the ratio of active to inactive thyroid hormones. The total reduction in caloric requirements following several weeks of fasting or prolonged periods of consuming a hypocaloric diet is much less than is generally acknowledged (see Chapter 9).

NUTRIENT AND HORMONAL REGULATION OF POSTPRANDIAL METABOLISM

The postprandial state is also associated with augmented energy expenditure. This heightened met-

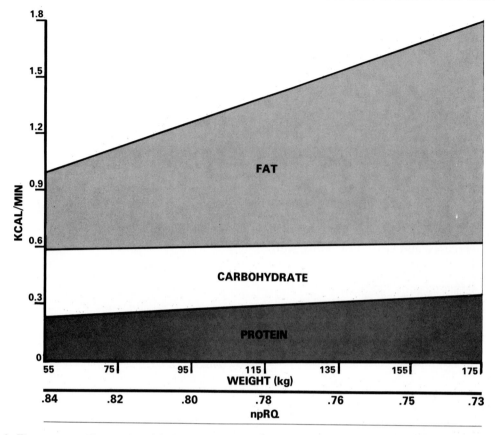

FIGURE 2–8. *The nature and quantity of fuels oxidized in healthy lean and obese males. The nonprotein RQ decreases as body weight increases.*

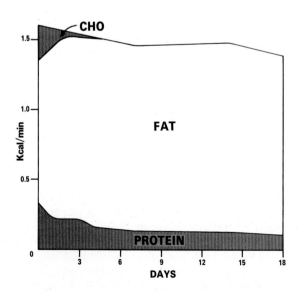

FIGURE 2–9. *Nature and quantity of fuels oxidized during prolonged starvation in four healthy, obese subjects.*

abolic state accompanying food ingestion was initially denoted as the specific dynamic action of food but is currently referred to as the thermic effect of food (TEF) or synonymously as dietary induced thermogenesis. In humans, TEF has been divided into obligatory energy expenditure associated with eating, digesting, absorbing, and storing food[42] and facultative energy exenditure associated with hormone secretion,[43,44] Na+, K+ ATPase pump activity,[45] protein synthesis,[46] and substrate recycling.[47,48] TEF is usually considered to account for about 10 to 15 per cent of the total daily energy requirements. However, the percentage varies tremendously, depending upon the nature and quantity of nutrients ingested.

TEF is another component of energy expenditure that has been recently re-evaluated. Several investigators have reported that the rise in metabolic rate that follows food ingestion is reduced in obese humans, suggesting that obese people have an increased metabolic efficiency that results in augmented storage of nutrients in body fat, but other researchers have failed to show a difference in the TEF between lean and obese humans.[16,18,30,49–58] This question is addressed at length in Chapter 8.

The nature and quantity of fuels oxidized after eating mixed meals quickly fluctuate. In the resting state following an overnight fast, eating a large breakfast meal containing 43 per cent carbohydrate, 42 per cent fat, and 15 per cent protein induces rapid changes in macronutrient oxidative rates. Figure 2–10 shows three-dimensional response surfaces generated from resistant regression lines relating the nature and quantity of fuels oxidized. There are threefold increases in carbohydrate oxidation rates and slight but significant increases in protein oxidation rates during the postprandial period. The increases in postprandial oxidation rates for carbohydrate and protein are progressively delayed as body weight and food intake increase. A reciprocal relationship between carbohydrate and lipid postprandial oxidation rates develops: as postprandial carbohydrate oxidation increases, lipid oxidation simultaneously decreases, and vice versa. Thus, when

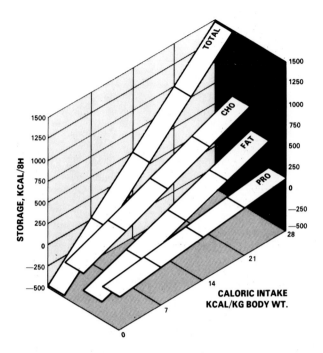

FIGURE 2–11. Fuel storage (kcal/8 hr) as a function of caloric intake (kcal/kg body weight).

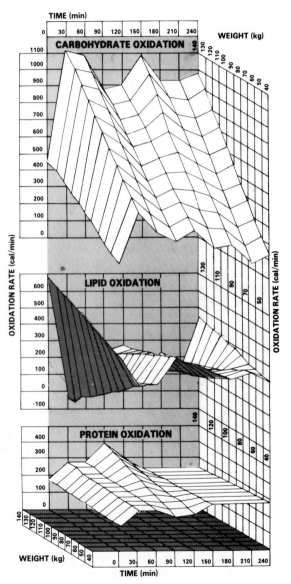

FIGURE 2–10. Three-dimensional response surfaces generated from resistant regression analysis of data from 32 women relating carbohydrate, fat, and protein oxidation with body weight and time before and after breakfast.

macronutrients are ingested as in a common mixed breakfast or other meal, there is preferential oxidation of glucose and amino acids while fat oxidation is suppressed. An exception to this postprandial pecking order occurs when alcohol is also consumed with a meal. Under such circumstances ethanol is preferentially oxidized over glucose, protein, and fat.[59]

A large proportion of ingested macronutrients are disposed of by nonoxidative (storage) pathways. When energy requirements are met and proteins are repleted, direct or indirect storage of excessive macronutrients is the most important route of fuel disposal. The larger the incremental increase in caloric intake over energy expenditure, the greater the quantities of fuels destined for adipose tissue and accompanying fat mass. Figure 2–11 shows the relationship between caloric intake contained in mixed meals and storage of macronutrients.

Food ingestion increases the concentrations of blood glucose, lactate, pyruvate, and amino acids and decreases the concentration of blood free fatty acids, glycerol, and urea nitrogen (Figs. 2–12 and 2–13).[60] Mixed meals cause a fivefold to sevenfold increase in serum insulin concentration.[60] Insulin diminishes hepatic extraction of lactate, pyruvate, and alanine,[60–62] promotes amino acid uptake in muscle,[60,63,64] decreases lipolysis, and therefore limits the availability of FFA and glycerol[11,60] and augments lipogenesis. Insulin also converts the liver from an organ that releases glucose into the blood by glycogenolysis and gluconeogenesis into an organ that extracts glucose from the blood and stores it as gly-

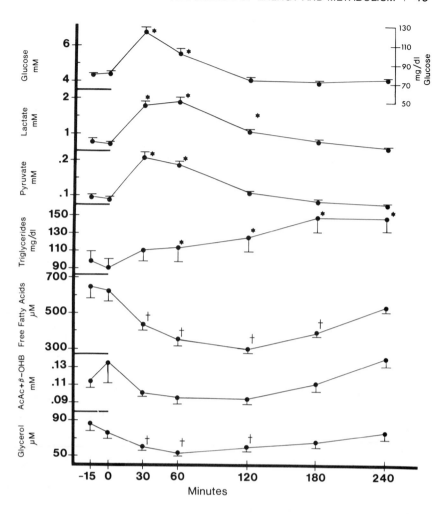

FIGURE 2–12. Substrate (glucose, lactate, pyruvate, triglyceride, free fatty acids [FFA], beta-hydroxybutyrate [β-OHB] plus acetoacetate [AcAc], and glycerol) responses in normal volunteers (six males and six females) to a breakfast. Note the reciprocal relationship between carbohydrate-related (glucose, lactate, and pyruvate) and lipid-related (FFA, β-OHB + AcAc, and glycerol) substrate concentrations. Results are expressed as means ± SE. *Significant increase from basal values, p<0.05. †Significant decrease from basal values, p<0.05. (From Owen OE, Mozzoli MA, Boden G, et al. Metabolism 1980; 29:511–523. Reproduced with permission.)

cogen or converts it into lipids.[65,66] Thus, insulin diminishes not only gluconeogenesis but also ureagenesis[60] and promotes uptake and storage of macronutrients by diverse regulatory mechanisms. For example, insulin modulates gene expressions that control membrane transport systems for glucose and amino acids.[11,67,68] Insulin suppresses gene transcription of gluconeogenic enzymes (phosphoenolpyruvate carboxykinase[69]), augments messenger RNA's of glycolytic enzymes (glyceraldehyde 3-phosphate dehydrogenase[70] and pyruvate kinase[71]) and lipid storage enzymes (fatty acid synthetase[72]), and promotes proteogenic gene transcription (albumin[73]).

Glucagon, in contrast to insulin, is one of the major hormones that promotes release of glucose, amino acid, and fatty acid and catabolism.[12] The postprandial plasma glucagon concentration is more variable than insulin concentration, and it depends upon the nature of the nutrients ingested. Plasma glucagon concentrations increase sharply after a protein meal;[74] promoting hepatic extraction and catabolism of amino acids; decrease after a carbohydrate meal;[74] and remain approximately constant but then increase several hours after a mixed meal.[60] The late rise in circulating glucagon concentration offsets the

postprandial hyperinsulinemia and prevents the development of hypoglycemia.[60]

During fasting, when energy requirements must be met by fuel mobilization, serum insulin concentrations decrease as plasma glucagon concentration increases.[75–77] In contrast to the fed state, during this state of deprivation fat is preferentially oxidized over amino acids and glucose.[77,78]

Several interrelated hormonal systems have regulatory roles in thermogenesis. The iodothyronines play a cardinal role in regulating the basal and resting metabolic rates but do not change the exercise-induced or diet-induced energy expenditure.[79] The central nervous system is integrated with the sympatho-adrenomedullary system, and both interrelate with the iodothyronines. Cortisol promotes the release and thermogenic response of the body to norepinephrine and epinephrine, and the catecholamines augment the thermogenic response of the body to L-triiodothyronine.[66] Special influence has been attributed to the beta-adrenergic activity of norepinephrine in the rise in facultative energy expenditure associated with carbohydrate metabolism.[80,81] Although insulin per se does not exert a thermogenic effect,[82] insulin facilitates extracellular to intracellular translocation, oxidation, and storage

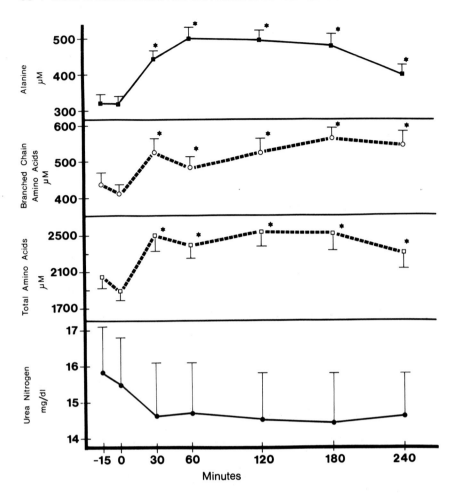

FIGURE 2–13. Plasma amino acid (alanine, branched-chain, and total amino acids) and serum urea nitrogen responses to a breakfast in normal volunteers (six males and six females). Note the reciprocal relationship between amino acid and urea nitrogen concentrations. Results are expressed as means ± SE. *Significant increase from basal values, p<0.05. (From Owen OE, Mozzoli MA, Boden G, et al. Metabolism 1980; 29:511–523. Reproduced with permission.)

of glucose, reduces lipolysis and augments lipogenesis, and promotes amino translocation and protein synthesis. Furthermore, the heightened circulating postprandial insulin concentration can stimulate the ventromedial hypothalamus and enhance norepinephrine secretion.[80,82] The bioactivity of iodothyronine hormones is not influenced by body mass,[14] whereas the bioactivity of catecholamines is controversial in obesity.[30,50,82–84] However, insulin secretion does increase as weight and adiposity increase.[85] Nonetheless, the progressive increase in the RMR and TEF among healthy women and men with weights ranging from 43 to 171 kg discredits any hypothesis suggesting uniformly altered or defective thermogenic mechanisms related to hormonal secretion, Na+, K+ ATPase pumping, substrate recycling, or synthetic processing as causes for more or less energy efficiency among adult humans with vastly different body masses and accompanying leanness or obesity.[16,29]

ORGAN METABOLISM DURING PHYSIOLOGIC CATABOLIC STATES

Humans undergo cyclic periods of feasting and fasting. Whereas eating is associated with macro-

nutrient storage, fasting is associated with FFA, amino acid, and glucose mobilization to furnish the body with fuels needed to maintain normal function.

Under healthy catabolic conditions the liver produces fuels for the other organ systems. It contributes glucose via glycogenolysis, it removes amino acids, glycerol, lactate, pyruvate, and FFA from the blood funneled into it from peripheral tissues, and it releases newly synthesized glucose and ketone bodies into the blood as fuels for brain and peripheral tissues (Fig. 2–14). The liver adds fuels to the blood via glycogenolysis, gluconeogenesis, and ketogenesis.[86] These three processes are inversely related in normal hepatic metabolism. There is a reciprocal relationship between glycogenolysis and gluconeogenesis (both responsible for total hepatic glucose release). In addition, there is a reciprocal relationship between total hepatic glucose release and ketone body release. After an overnight fast normally glucose release is high and ketone body release is low. Conversely, during starvation, when glucose release is low, ketone body release is high. Although the types of substrates contributed to blood from liver vary, the caloric equivalents of these fuels are approximately equal. The total amount of fuel added to the blood from liver that can be terminally oxidized is about one half of the body's caloric needs (Fig. 2–14).

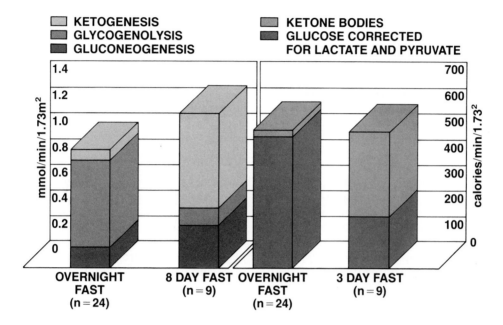

FIGURE 2–14. Relationships among hepatic gluconeogenesis, glycogenolysis, and ketogenesis, and caloric equivalents derived from glucose and ketone bodies in normal subjects who fasted overnight or for 3 days.

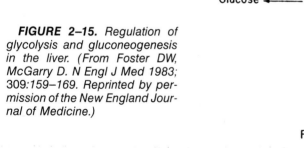

FIGURE 2–15. Regulation of glycolysis and gluconeogenesis in the liver. (From Foster DW, McGarry D. N Engl J Med 1983; 309:159–169. Reprinted by permission of the New England Journal of Medicine.)

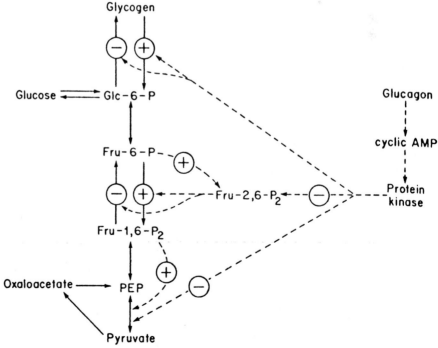

During starvation, hypoinsulinemia coupled with hyperglucagonemia modulates hepatic metabolism. Glucagon regulates hepatic glycolysis and gluconeogenesis by controlling the concentration of fructose 2,6-bisphosphate. Glucagon decreases hepatic fructose-2,6-bisphosphate and thereby inactivates phosphofructokinase, blocking the conversion of fructose-6-phosphate to fructose-1,6-bisphosphate, thus inhibiting glycolysis. Conversely, decreases in hepatic fructose-2,6-bisphosphate allow the conversion of fructose-1,6-bisphosphate to fructose-6-phosphate, thus activating gluconeogenesis (Fig. 2–15).[87]

Glucagon also inhibits glycogen synthesis and effects ketogenesis. Glucagon inhibits acetyl-CoA carboxylase, the enzyme that converts acetyl-CoA to malonyl-CoA. When malonyl-CoA concentrations are lowered by glucagon, fatty acid oxidation and ketogenesis are stimulated (Fig. 2–16). Also, glucagon may increase hepatic carnitine concentrations, which facilitates fatty acylcarnitine translocations across the mitochondria so that FFA undergo beta-oxidation for ketone body synthesis.[87]

The adipose tissue is the other major supplier of body fuel in the form of FFA. In fact, the majority of the differences between total body caloric requirements and hepatic caloric contribution is supplied from mobilized FFA. There is a direct relationship between plasma FFA concentrations and oxidation rates.[88] Although this is true in healthy individuals during fed and starved states, it may not be so in diseased states characterized by abnormal lipid metabolism. Furthermore, all of these integrated, precise mobilization, production, and utilization rates are disturbed in uncontrolled catabolic diseased states.

Normally, there are overlapping hormonal systems that mobilize fuels and prevent fuel-deficient states. During the resting state, alterations occur in insulin and glucagon secretion rates in response to changing blood glucose and ketone body concentrations.[12,89] "Functional" hypoglycemia and hypoketonemia during starvation are accompanied by a decrease in insulin secretion and a rise in glucagon secretion.

During the exercising state, the sympathetic nervous system decreases in muscular utilization of glucose, mobilizes amino acid and FFA, and augments gluconeogenesis and ketogenesis.[12,90]

In more protracted states of starvation, the thyroid hormones play a role in controlling total body energy requirements. The concentration of the most active circulating iodothyronine, triiodothyronine (T_3), falls. Concurrently, reverse triiodothyronine (rT_3) increases and total RMR diminishes. Thus, proteolysis and lipolysis decrease as do gluconeogenesis and ketogenesis.[75] These comments, however, should be cautiously evaluated because the diminution in total body energy requirements and accompanying decreases in organ contributions of fuels after prolonged periods of complete starvation are only about 10 to 15 per cent less than they are after an overnight fast.

The regulation of blood glucose[91] and plasma free fatty acids is discussed in Chapter 8 and will not be detailed here. However, there is a class of substrates that deserves special emphasis during negative energy balance states. The importance of ketone bodies

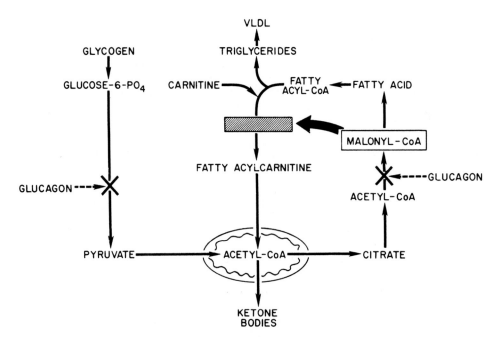

FIGURE 2–16. Relationship between glycolysis and lipid metabolism. (From Foster DW, McGarry D. N Engl J Med 1983; 309:159–169. Reprinted by permission of the New England Journal of Medicine.)

in maintaining fuel homeostasis during physiological catabolic states has been delineated during the last 20 years. The concept that the liver produces ketone bodies to supply alternate fuels to extrahepatic tissue when energy requirements cannot be met by glucose was demonstrated by showing that beta-hydroxybutyrate (β-OHB) and acetoacetate (AcAc) replace glucose as the predominant fuel for the brain during prolonged starvation.[78] This work emanated from George F. Cahill, Jr.'s laboratories housed at the Joslin Research facilities at Harvard University, and launched a new era in the study of metabolism.

During starvation, ketone bodies, AcAc, β-OHB, and acetone, accumulate in the body. AcAc and β-OHB are synthesized in the liver primarily from the partial oxidation of long-chain fatty acids. They are released into the blood as short-chain fatty acids, dissociated to become water-soluble anions, and are distributed at different concentrations in the water components of the body.[57] Acetone, a neutral compound, is probably formed by spontaneous decarboxylation of AcAc and is soluble in both water and lipids. Therefore, it is distributed throughout the body. Unlike AcAc and β-OHB, acetone does not affect blood bicarbonate concentration, arterial blood gases, or pH.[92]

During food deprivation, starvation ketosis is arbitrarily defined as being present when the minimum blood or plasma concentration of AcAc is about 1.0 mmol/L. Concurrent concentrations of β-OHB and acetone are usually about 2.0 to 3.0 and 0.5 mmol/L, respectively. Such values are usually present after 2 to 3 days of total starvation. Maximal blood or plasma concentrations of AcAc (2 to 4 mmol/L), β-OHB (5 to 12 mmol/L), and acetone (3 to 5 mmol/L) develop after several weeks of total fasting.[93]

After an overnight fast the urine of an adult is practically free of ketone bodies. However, as starvation progresses, simultaneously measured ketone body concentrations in urine and blood or plasma show that urine usually has several times greater concentrations than that observed in blood or plasma (Fig. 2–17).[93]

There are several tiers of control regulating ketogenesis, ketonemia, and ketonuria. A major influence regulating ketogenesis and ketonemia is the availability of FFA, the primary precursors of AcAc and β-OHB. Another tier of control is the hormonal milieu. The third factor is the innate energy requirements of tissues: during starvation liver derives most of its energy requirements from beta oxidation of fatty acids in the process of forming ketone bodies. The liver cannot synthesize more ketone bodies than it needs to satisfy its energy needs. On the other hand, peripheral tissues cannot oxidize more ketone bodies than are needed for their fuel requirements. Furthermore, different tissues preferentially select various fuels to meet their energy demands. The fourth factor regulating ketonemia is renal conser-vation of ketone bodies.[93] These substrates have no renal tubular transfer maxima, and renal conservation of ketone bodies during starvation influences the blood concentrations of these valuable fuels. All tiers of regulation have important influences on starvation ketosis. It is illogical to try to isolate and emphasize a single component for governing ketogenesis, ketonemia, and ketonuria.[93]

It has long been held that the liver is the only organ that makes a net contribution of AcAc and β-OHB to the blood. This conclusion was derived from determining net exchange rates of those ketone bodies across the vascular beds of the liver, gut, kidney, muscles, and brain. However, there are discrepancies in the literature between the data collected from catheterization studies and those obtained from kinetic analysis of tracer studies. A possible reason for part, but not all, of these discrepancies resides in the recent observation that under stressful catabolic circumstances the kidney synthesizes and releases ketone bodies into the blood.[86]

Hepatic ketogenesis is accomplished by beta oxidation of FFA to form 3-hydroxy-3-methyl-glutaryl coenzyme A (HMGCoA). HMGCoA undergoes cleavage to form acetyl-CoA and AcAc.[94,95] AcAc equilibrates with β-OHB, and both are released into the blood. Renal ketogenesis is accomplished by direct deacylation of acetoacetyl CoA to form AcAc and β-OHB.[96]

Renal production of ketone bodies is poorly understood and rarely occurs, and for practical purposes, only the liver contributes AcAc and β-OHB to the blood for utilization by virtually all extrahepatic tissues possessing mitochondria.

AcAc plus β-OHB blood concentrations are curvilinearly related to AcAc plus β-OHB production rates. Near-maximum production rates of 0.8 to 1.5 mmol/min/1.73 m² or 70 kg occur after about 4 days of total starvation, when the AcAc plus β-OHB circulating concentration is about 4 or more mmol/L. At higher blood levels there is a dissociation between concentration and production rates of AcAc and β-OHB. In contrast, there is a direct linear relationship between plasma acetone concentrations and production rates.[93,97]

After a few days of starvation, ketone body oxidation can contribute about 30 to 40 per cent of total caloric requirements.[93] However, it is important to recognize that the contribution of ketone bodies as metabolic fuels to specific tissues changes during starvation. Ketone bodies serve only transiently as the major fuels for skeletal muscle in the human during starvation. During the first few days of starvation, AcAc and β-OHB are the predominant fuels for muscle metabolism. Thereafter, net ketone body consumption by muscle paradoxically decreases despite the marked increase in the arterial concentrations of these substrates with progressive starvation. This diminished consumption occurs because muscle extracts AcAc but releases β-OHB during pro-

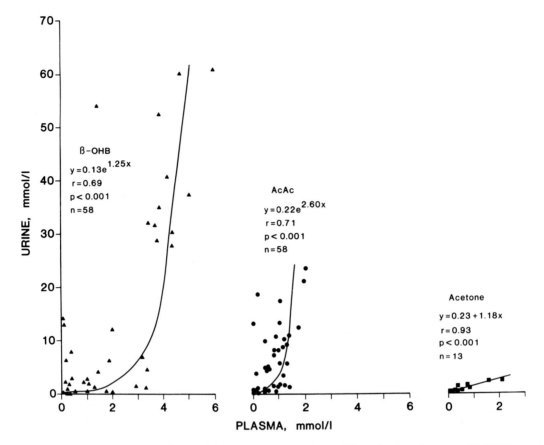

FIGURE 2–17. Correlation between urine and plasma concentrations of beta-hydroxybutyrate (β-OHB), acetoacetate (AcAc), and acetone in obese humans during starvation.

longed starvation.[93] In contradistinction, the kidneys usually, but not always, show increasing ketone body uptake with increasing arterial concentrations of these fuels. Some of the ketone bodies extracted by the kidneys are excreted in the urine, and some are probably oxidized, but the metabolic fate of most of them is unknown. It is possible, however, that ketone bodies along with other substrates are converted into triglycerides and released as lipoproteins by the kidney during starvation.[86,98] Brain consumption of ketone bodies is related to the ambient concentrations of these fuels. The central nervous system is a major organ for oxidizing AcAc and β-OHB after 60 hours of starvation, and during prolonged fasting, ketone bodies are the major fuel for brain functions.[93]

Individual organ metabolism of the third ketone body, acetone, has not been delineated. However, kinetic analysis of ^{14}C acetone showed that the metabolism of this secondarily derived ketone body is different from that of AcAc and β-OHB. Unlike the other two ketone bodies, acetone is excreted in the breath and is also converted into other compounds for subsequent oxidation.[99,100] Studies have identified acetol and propanediol as early intermediates in the pathways of acetone utilization.[97] In addition, methylglyoxal also may be derived from acetone.[101] Methylglyoxal was thought to be the major glucose

precursor at a time when metabolic pathways were virtually unknown,[102] and propanediol is a well-recognized gluconeogenic precursor.[103–105] Thus, a small but significant amount of newly gained glucose can be derived from FFA via acetone. The most likely pathway involves acetone → propanediol → pyruvate → oxaloacetate → phosphoenolpyruvate → glucose.[97] Glucose production from acetone may also occur from methylglyoxal → glucose during catabolic states.[101]

ORGAN METABOLISM DURING NONPHYSIOLOGIC CATABOLIC STATES

The highly regulated and integrated processes of precise mobilization, production, and utilization rates are distorted by a variety of pathological states. Two specific and common disease states with abnormal metabolism, alcoholic cirrhosis and decompensated diabetes mellitus, exemplify opposite extremes of disturbed hepatic production of glucose and ketone bodies (Fig. 2–18). After an overnight fast, hepatic glucose production in patients with cirrhosis is diminished as the result of decreased glycogenolysis.[98] Extensive hepatic fibrosis induces limited space availability to store and release glucose.[98] This deficiency in glycogenolysis is partly compensated by augmented hepatic gluconeogenesis and ketogenesis. Thus, the pattern of hepatic metabolism resembles that in normal humans after more prolonged periods of fasting. However, the caloric delivery of fuels derived from glucose, corrected for recycled lactate and pyruvate plus AcAc and β-OHB, that can be terminally oxidized to CO_2 and H_2O is less in patients with hepatic cirrhosis than in healthy humans after an overnight or more protracted fast (Fig. 2–18).[98] The kidneys in cirrhotic patients usually do not compensate for this diminished delivery of fuels to the blood.[98] Although the kidneys can contribute glucose, ketone bodies, and triglycerides to the blood, the mechanisms controlling the synthesis and release of fuels by the kidneys are not understood.[76,86,98] However, the RMR of patients with alcoholic cirrhosis is maintained at normal (Fig. 2–19) because during fasting periods lipolysis is rapidly augmented and FFA oxidation is heightened (Fig. 2–20).[106] Thus, although maintaining fuel homeostasis during starvation is a struggle for the organs of alcoholic patients with hepatic cirrhosis, it is accomplished.

In contrast to this depressed but compensated state of fuel homeostasis in the cirrhotic patient is the decompensated state of diabetic ketoacidosis. This state is characterized by hyperglycemia, hyperketonemia, and metabolic acidosis.[107] It is a life-threatening metabolic disorder initiated by the lack of a sufficient quantity of circulating insulin to

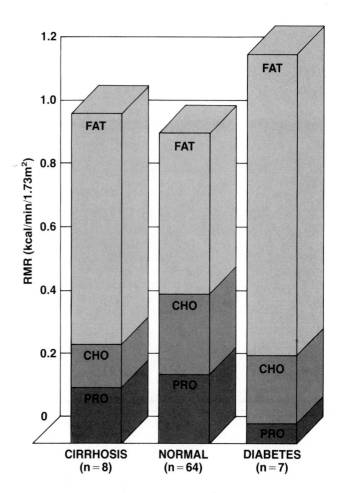

FIGURE 2–19. Nature and quantity of fuels oxidized in overnight fasted cirrhotic and normal subjects and diabetics in ketoacidosis.

restrain unwarranted catabolism. The insulin deficiency is exacerbated by increased glucagon secretion. Hypoinsulinemia coupled with hyperglucagonemia results in the excessive production of glucose from glycogenolysis and gluconeogenesis and of ketone bodies from FFA (Fig. 2–18). The loss of reciprocity among the rates of hepatic glycogenolysis, gluconeogenesis, and ketogenesis results in inappropriately elevated hepatic production rates of glucose and ketone bodies and subsequently hyperglycemia and hyperketonemia.[108] This, coupled with increased FFA mobilization from adipose tissue and concurrent proteolysis, floods the blood stream with an overabundance of fuels (Fig. 2–18) that compete as oxidative substrates (Fig. 2–19).[107,108]

Hyperglycemia produces an osmotic diuresis resulting in volume depletion, which augments catecholamine release. Epinephrine and glucagon synergistically promote the gluconeogenic, glycogenolytic, and ketogenic profile of the liver.[87] In addition, epinephrine diminishes residual insulin

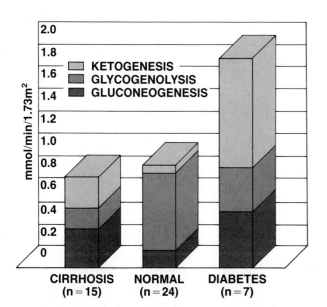

FIGURE 2–18. Relationships among hepatic gluconeogenesis, glycogenolysis, and ketogenesis in cirrhotic, normal, and diabetic human subjects after an overnight fast.

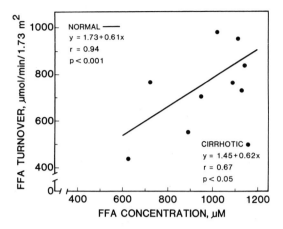

FIGURE 2–20. *Relationships between concentrations and turnover rates of free fatty acids (FFA). The solid line represents results obtained from normal humans undergoing various durations of starvation, and the individual dots represent nine cirrhotic patients who fasted overnight. (Reproduced from The Journal of Clinical Investigation, 1983; 72:1821–1832, by copyright permission of The American Society for Clinical Investigation.)*

secretion, and hypovolemia augments norepinephrine secretion, which stimulates free fatty acid release. Increased ketone body production coupled with diminished ketone body oxidation results in marked hyperketonemia, which induces massive ketonuria, accentuating loss of body water. The release of other stress hormones, cortisol, and growth hormone enhances late developments of diabetic ketoacidosis, since these hormones also exhibit anti-insulin activity. The mechanisms responsible for the maintenance of hyperglycemia and hyperketonemia in established diabetic ketoacidosis may be different from those that initiated the inappropriate and excess hepatic production of glucose and ketone bodies. For example, depressed rates of glucose and ketone body disposal coupled with heightened renal

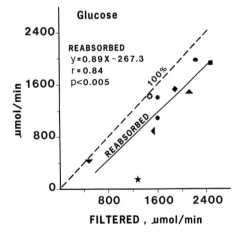

FIGURE 2–21. *Renal reabsorption of glucose. (From Owen OE, Licht JH, Sapir DG. Renal function and effects of partial rehydration during diabetic ketoacidosis. Diabetes 1981; 30:510–518. Reproduced with permission from the American Diabetes Association, Inc.)*

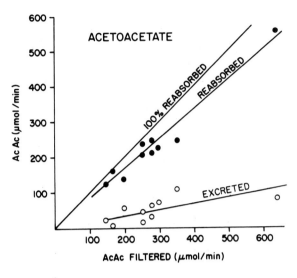

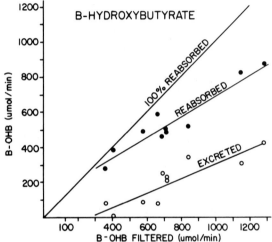

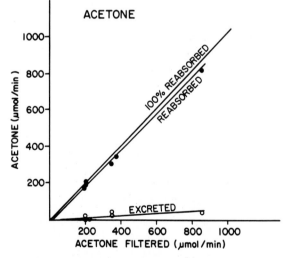

FIGURE 2–22. *Renal reabsorption of acetoacetate (AcAc), beta-hydroxybutyrate (β-OHB), and acetone. (From Owen OE, Licht JH, Sapir DG. Renal function and effects of partial rehydration during diabetic ketoacidosis. Diabetes 1981; 30:510–518. Reproduced with permission from the American Diabetes Association, Inc.)*

retrieval of glucose and ketone bodies during volume depletion may, in part, be responsible for the persistent or progressive hyperglycemia and hyperketonemia. Although glucose (Fig. 2–21) and ketone bodies (Fig. 2–22) have no maximal renal tubular reabsorption rates during diabetic ketoacidosis, glycosuria and ketonuria occur because less than 100 per cent of these filtered compounds are reabsorbed by the renal tubules.[109]

Massive renal glucose and ketone body wastage with induced osmotic diuresis is accompanied by large losses of sodium, potassium, phosphate, ammonium, and other ions in the urine. However, it should be recognized that if glucose and ketone bodies have low renal tubular reabsorption rates, even greater quantities of water and salts would be excreted. Such severe losses of water and electrolytes would further hasten cardiovascular failure and death.

The RQ and nonprotein RQ vary widely during diabetic ketoacidosis, confirming the fact that heterogeneous metabolic states exist in this clinical setting. Thus, it is not surprising to find that the mixture of protein, fat, and glucose oxidized by patients in this state is diverse. In the absence of therapy the RQ ranges from 0.55 to 0.80 and the nonprotein RQ from 0.58 to 0.88.[107] Extremely low RQ values suggest not only fat oxidation but also net gains of glucose from fat with subsequent glycosuria. The caloric requirements during diabetic ketoacidosis are about 25 per cent greater than the RMR of normal humans. Fat contributes about 78 per cent, glucose about 17 per cent, and protein about 5 per cent of the total energy requirements during diabetic ketoacidosis. Not infrequently, however, patients in diabetic ketoacidosis have huge losses of body nitrogen. Such dispossession can have grave effects, since some of these patients are emaciated with depleted lean body tissues. Although the acute metabolic derangements can be corrected in hours, it takes several days of excellent metabolic control to reverse the catabolic aftermath of diabetic ketoacidosis.

Figure 2–19 displays the caloric expenditures and quantities of carbohydrate, fat, and protein oxidized in normal humans and cirrhotic patients in the resting state after an overnight fast and diabetic patients in moderate to severe ketoacidosis.

Acknowledgment

This work was supported in part by a grant, RROO349, General Clinical Research Centers Branch, National Institutes of Health.

REFERENCES

1. White A, Handler P, Smith EL. General metabolism, energy considerations. *In* Principles of Biochemistry. 4th ed. New York, McGraw-Hill, 1968: 291–301.

2. McGilvery RW, Goldstein G. Biochemical energetics. *In* Biochemistry, a Functional Approach. 2nd ed. Philadelphia, WB Saunders, 1979: 337–351, 373–400.

3. Alberts B, Bray D, Lewis J, et al. Energy conversion: mitochondria and chloroplasts. *In* Molecular Biology of the Cell. New York, Garland Publishing, 1983: 483–547.

4. Darnell J, Lodish H, Baltimore D. Molecular Cell Biology. New York, Scientific American Books, 1986: 569–714.

5. Bundgaard M. Vesicular transport in capillary endothelium: does it occur? Fed Proc 1983; *42*:2425–2430.

6. Kaplan J. Patterns in receptor behavior and function. *In* Poste G, Crooke ST (eds). Mechanisms of Receptor Regulation. New York, Plenum, 1985: 13–36.

7. Barnes D. How cells respond to signals. Science 1986; *234*:286–288.

8. Czech MP. The biochemical basis of insulin action. *In* Current Concepts. A Scope Publication. Kalamazoo, MI, Upjohn Co., 1984: 3–40.

9. Petruzelli LM, Stadtmauer L, Herrera R, et al. The insulin receptor as a tyrosine-specific protein kinase. *In* Poste G, Crooke ST (eds). Mechanisms of Receptor Regulation. New York, Plenum Press, 1985: 51–64.

10. Saltiel AR, Fox JA, Sherline P, et al. Insulin-stimulated hydrolysis of a novel glycolipid generates modulators of cAMP phosphodiesterase. Science 1986; *233*:967–972.

11. Cahill GF. Physiology of insulin in man. Diabetes 1971; *20*:785–799.

12. Unger RH. Insulin-glucagon relationships in the defense against hypoglycemia. Diabetes 1983; *32*:575–583.

13. Lehninger AL. Enzymes: kinetics and inhibition. *In* Biochemistry. 2nd ed. New York, Worth Publishers, 1975: 183–216.

14. Ravussin E, Burnand B, Schutz Y, et al. Twenty-four hour energy expenditure and resting metabolic rate in obese, moderately obese, and control subjects. Am J Clin Nutr 1982; *35*:566–573.

15. Jequier E. Long-term measurement of energy expenditure in man: direct or indirect calorimetry. *In* Bjorntorp P, Cairella M (eds). Recent Advances in Obesity Research III. London, John Libbey, 1981: 130–135.

16. Owen OE, Kavle E, Owen RS, et al. A reappraisal of caloric requirements in healthy women. Am J Clin Nutr 1986; *44*:1–19.

17. Bogardus C, Lillioja S, Ravussin E, et al. Familial dependence of the resting metabolic rate. N Engl J Med 1986; *315*:96–100.

18. Jequier E, Schutz Y. Long-term measurements of energy expenditure in humans using a respiration chamber. Am J Clin Nutr 1983; *38*:989–998.

19. Harris JA, Benedict FG. A Biometric Study of Basal Metabolism in Man. Washington, The Carnegie Institute, 1919: 1–266.

20. DuBois BS, DuBois EF. Clinical calorimetry: a formula to estimate the approximate surface area if height and weight be known. Arch Intern Med 1916; *17*:863–871.

21. Boothby WM, Berkson J, Dunn HL. Studies of the energy of metabolism of normal individuals: a standard for basal metabolism, with a nomogram for clinical application. Am J Physiol 1936; *116*:468–484.

22. Boothby WM, Sandiford I. Summary of the basal metabolism data on 8,614 subjects with special reference to the normal standards for the estimation of the basal metabolism rate. J Biochem 1922; *54*:783–803.

23. Robertson JD, Reid DD. Standards for the basal metabolism of normal people in Britain. Lancet 1952; *1*:940–943.

24. DuBois EF. Basal energy metabolism at various ages: man. *In* Altman PL, Dittmer DS (eds). Metabolism. Bethesda, MD, FASEB, 1968: 345.

25. Feurer ID, Crosby LO, Buzby GP, et al. Resting energy expenditure in morbid obesity. Ann Surg 1983; *197*:17–21.

26. Daly JM, Heymsfield SB, Head CA, et al. Human energy requirements: overestimation by widely used prediction equation. Am J Clin Nutr 1985; *42*:1170–1174.

27. Roza AM, Shizgal HM. The Harris-Benedict equation re-evaluated: resting energy requirements and the body cell mass. Am J Clin Nutr 1984; *40*:168–182.

28. Cunningham JJ. A reanalysis of the factors influencing basal metabolic rate in normal adults. Am J Clin Nutr 1980; *33*:2372–2374.

29. Owen OE, Holup JL, D'Alessio DA, et al. A reappraisal of the caloric requirements of men. Am J Clin Nutr, in press.

30. Felig P, Cunningham FP, Levitt M, et al. Energy expenditure in obesity in fasting and postprandial state. Am J Physiol 1983; *244*:E45–51.

31. Miller A, Blyth C. Lean body mass as a metabolic reference standard. J Appl Physiol 1953; *5*:311–316.

32. Behnke AR. Relationship of lean body weight to metabolism and some consequent systematizations. Ann NY Acad Sci 1953; *56*:1095–1142.

33. Keys A, Taylor HL, Grande F. Basal metabolism and age of adult man. Metabolism 1973; *22*:579–587.

34. Tzankoff S, Norris A. Effect of muscle mass decrease on age-related BMR changes. J Appl Physiol 1977; *43*:1001–1006.

35. Tzankoff S, Norris A. Longitudinal changes in basal metabolism in man. J Appl Physiol 1978; *45*:536–539.

36. Bernstein RS, Thornton JC, Yang MU, et al. Prediction of resting metabolic rate in obese patients. Am J Clin Nutr 1983; *37*:595–601.

37. Brozek J, Grande F. Body composition and basal metabolism in man: correlation analysis versus physiological approach. Human Biol 1955; *27*:22–31.

38. Cahill GF, Owen OE. Some observations on carbohydrate metabolism in man. *In* Dickens F, Randle FJ, Whelan WJ (eds). Carbohydrate Metabolism and Its Disorders. Vol. 1. New York, Academic Press, 1968: 497–518.

39. Grande F, Keys A. Body weight, body composition and calorie status. *In* Goodhart RS, Shils ME (eds). Modern Nutrition in Health and Disease. 6th ed. Philadelphia, Lea & Febiger, 1980: 3–34.

40. Garrow GS. Energy Balance and Obesity in Man. 2nd ed. New York, Elsevier/North-Holland Biomedical Press, 1978: 125.

41. Flatt JP. On the maximal possible rate of ketogenesis. Diabetes 1972; *21*:50–53.

42. Trayburn P, James WPT. Thermogenesis: dietary and non-shivering aspects. *In* Cioffi LA, James WPT, Van Itallie TB (eds). The Body Weight Regulatory System: Normal and Disturbed Mechanisms. New York, Raven Press, 1981: 97–105.

43. Himms-Hagen J. Thermogenesis in brown adipose tissue as an energy buffer: implications for obesity. N Engl J Med 1984; *311*:1549–1558.

44. Bray GA, York DA. Hypothalamic and genetic obesity in experimental animals: an autonomic and endocrine hypothesis. Physiol Rev 1979; *59*:719–809.

45. Guernsey DC, Stevens DD. The cell membrane sodium pump as a mechanism for increasing thermogenesis during cold acclimation in rats. Science 1977; *196*:908–910.

46. Miller BG, Otto WR, Grimble RF, et al. The relationship between protein turnover and energy balance in lean and genetically obese (ob/ob) mice. Br J Nutr 1979; *41*:185–199.

47. Newsholme EA, Crabtree B. Substrate cycles in metabolic regulation and in heat generation. Biochem Soc Symp 1976; *41*:61–109.

48. Katz J. Energy balance and futile cycling. *In* Kinney JM, Lense E (eds). Assessment of Energy Metabolism in Health and Disease. Columbus, OH, Ross Laboratories, 1980: 63–66.

49. Kaplan ML, Leveille GA. Calorigenic response in obese and nonobese women. Am J Clin Nutr 1976; *29*:1108–1113.

50. Shetty PS, Jung RT, James WPT, et al. Postprandial thermogenesis in obesity. Clin Sci 1981; *60*:519–525.

51. Schwartz RS, Halter JB, Bierman E. Reduced thermic effect of feeding in obesity: role of norepinephrine. Metabolism 1983; *32*:114–117.

52. Sharief NN, Macdonald I. Difference in dietary-induced thermogenesis with various carbohydrates in normal and overweight man. Am J Clin Nutr 1982; *35*:267–272.

53. Welle SL, Campbell RG. Normal thermic effect of glucose in obese women. Am J Clin Nutr 1983; *37*:87–92.

54. Hill JO, Heymsfield SB, McMannus C III, et al. Meal size and thermic response to food in male subjects as a function of maximum aerobic capacity. Metabolism 1984; *33*:743–749.

55. Pittet PH, Chappius PH, Acheson K, et al. Thermic effect of glucose in obese subjects studied by direct and indirect calorimetry. Br J Nutr 1976; *35*:281–292.

56. Golay A, Schutz Y, Meyer HU, et al. Glucose-induced thermogenesis in nondiabetic and diabetic obese subjects. Diabetes 1982; *31*:1023–1028.

57. Horton ES, Danforth E Jr. Energy metabolism and obesity. *In* Brodoff NB, Bleicher SJ (eds). Diabetes Mellitus and Obesity. Baltimore, Williams & Wilkins, 1982: 261–268.

58. D'Alessio DA, Kavle EC, Mozzoli MA, et al. Oxidative and nonoxidative macronutrient disposal in lean and obese men, in press.

59. Shelmet JJ, Reichard GA, Skutches CL, et al. Ethanol causes acute inhibition of carbohydrate oxidation and insulin resistance, in press.

60. Owen OE, Mozzoli MA, Boden G, et al. Substrate, hormone, and temperature responses in males and females to a common breakfast. Metabolism 1980; *29*:511–523.

61. Felig P, Wahren J, Hendler R. Influence of oral glucose ingestion on splanchnic glucose and gluconeogenic substrate metabolism in man. Diabetes 1975; *24*:468–475.

62. Owen OE, Patel MS, Block BSB, et al. Gluconeogenesis in normal, cirrhotic and diabetic humans. *In* Hanson RW, Mehlman MA (eds). Gluconeogenesis: Its Regulation in Mammalian Species. New York, John Wiley and Sons, 1976: 533–558.

63. Pozefsky T, Felig P, Tobin JD, et al. Amino acid balance across tissues of the forearm in postabsorptive man. Effects of insulin at two dose levels. J Clin Invest 1969; *48*:2273–2282.

64. Wahren J, Felig P, Hagenfeldt L. Effect of protein ingestion on splanchnic and leg metabolism in normal man and in patients with diabetes mellitus. J Clin Invest 1976; *57*:987–999.

65. Madison LL, Mebane D, Lecocq F, et al. Physiological significance of the secretion of endogenous insulin into the portal circulation. V. The quantitative importance of the liver in the disposition of glucose loads. Diabetes 1963; *12*:8–15.

66. Owen OE, Reichard GA Jr, Boden G, et al. Interrelationships among key tissues in the utilization of metabolic substrates. *In* Katzen HM, Mahler RJ (eds). Diabetes, Obesity, and Vascular Disease. Part 2: Metabolic and Molecular Interrelationships. New York, John Wiley and Sons, 1978: 517–550.

67. Kahn CR. The molecular mechanism of insulin action. Ann Rev Med 1985; *36*:429–451.

68. Czech MP. Molecular Basis of Insulin Action. New York, Plenum, 1985.

69. Granner D, Andreone T, Sasaki K, et al. Inhibition of transcription of the phosphoenolpyruvate carboxykinase gene by insulin. Nature (London) 1983; *305*:549–551.

70. Alexander M, Curtis G, Avruch J, et al. Insulin regulation of protein biosynthesis in differentiated 3T3 adipocytes: regulation of glyceraldehyde-3-phosphate dehydrogenase. J Biol Chem 1985; *260*:11978–11985.

71. Naguchi T, Inoue H, Tanaka T. Regulation of rat liver L-type pyruvate kinase mRNA by insulin and by fructose. Eur J Biochem 1982; *128*:583–588.

72. Pry TA, Porter JW. Control of fatty acid synthetase mRNA levels in rat liver by insulin, glucagon and dibutyryl cyclic AMP. Biochem Biophys Res Comm 1981; *100*:1002–1009.

73. Lloyd CE, Jefferson LS. Insulin stimulates transcription of

the albumin gene in primary cultures of rat hepatocyte. Am Diabetes Assoc 45th Ann Meet 1985: Abstract 39.

74. Muller WA, Faloona GR, Aguilar-Parada E, et al. Abnormal alpha-cell function in diabetes. Response to carbohydrate and protein ingestion. N Engl J Med 1970; *283*:109–115.

75. Cahill GF Jr, Herrera MG, Morgan AP, et al. Hormone-fuel interrelationships during fasting. J Clin Invest 1966; *45*:1751–1769.

76. Owen OE, Felig P, Morgan AP, et al. Liver and kidney metabolism during prolonged starvation. J Clin Invest 1969; *48*:574–583.

77. Marliss EB, Aoki TT, Unger RH, et al. Glucagon levels and metabolic effects in fasting man. J Clin Invest 1970; *49*:2256–2270.

78. Owen OE, Morgan AP, Kemp HG, et al. Brain metabolism during fasting. J Clin Invest 1967; *46*:1589–1595.

79. Acheson K, Jequier E, Burger A, et al. Thyroid hormones and thermogenesis: the metabolic cost of food and exercise. Metabolism 1984; *33*:262–265.

80. Anand RK, Chhina GS, Sharma KN, et al. Activity of single neurons in the hypothalamic feeding centers: effects of glucose. Am J Physiol 1964; *207*:1146–1154.

81. Young JB, Landsberg L. Catecholamines and the sympathoadrenal system: the regulation of metabolism. *In* Ingbar SH (ed). Contemporary Endocrinology. Vol 1. New York, Plenum, 1979: 245–303.

82. Acheson KJ, Ravussin E, Wahren J, et al. Thermic effect of glucose in man: obligatory and facultative thermogenesis. J Clin Invest 1984; *74*:1572–1580.

83. Welle S, Campbell RG. Stimulation of thermogenesis by carbohydrate overfeeding: evidence against sympathetic nervous system mediation. J Clin Invest 1983; *71*:916–925.

84. Acheson K, Jequier E, Wahren J. Influence of beta-adrenergic blockage on glucose-induced thermogenesis in man. J Clin Invest 1983; *72*:981–986.

85. Cahill GF. Obesity. *In* Brodoff BN, Bleicher SI (eds). Diabetes Mellitus and Obesity. Baltimore, Williams & Wilkins, 1982: 215–218.

86. Owen OE, Mozzoli MA, Reichle FA, et al. Hepatic and renal metabolism before and after portasystemic shunts in patients with cirrhosis. J Clin Invest 1985; *76*:1209–1217.

87. Foster DW, McGarry D. The metabolic derangements and treatment of diabetic ketoacidosis. N Engl J Med 1983; *309*:159–169.

88. Owen OE, Reichard GA. Fuels consumed by man: the interplay between carbohydrates and fatty acids. Prog Biochem Pharmacol 1971; *6*:177–213.

89. Cryer P. Does central nervous system adaptation to antecedent glycemia occur in patients with insulin-dependent diabetes mellitus? Ann Intern Med 1985; *103*:284–286.

90. Hendler RG, Sherwin RS. Epinephrine-stimulated glucose production is not diminished by starvation: evidence for an effect on gluconeogenesis. J Clin Endocrin Metab 1984; *58*:1014–1021.

91. Felig P, Havel RJ, Smith LH, et al. Metabolism and nutrition. *In* Smith LH, Thier SO (eds). Pathophysiology: the Biological Principles of Disease. Philadelphia, WB Saunders, 1981; *6*:479–652.

92. Sulway MJ, Malins JM. Acetone in diabetic ketoacidosis. Lancet 1970; *1*:736–740.

93. Owen OE, Caprio S, Reichard GA Jr, et al. Ketosis of starvation: a revisit and new perspectives. Clin Endocrinol Metab 1983; *12*:359–379.

94. Robinson AM, Williamson DH. Physiological role of ketone bodies and substrates and signals in mammalian tissues. Physiol Rev 1980; *60*:143–187.

95. Owen OE, Caprio S, Sapir DG, et al. Ketogenesis and metabolic acidosis during diabetic ketoacidosis: new perspectives. *In* Melchionda N (ed). Recent Advances in Obesity and Diabetes. New York, Raven Press, 1984: 309–318.

96. Brady PS, Scofield RF, Ohgaku S, et al. A method for quantitating the contributions of the pathways of acetoacetate formation and its application to diabetic ketosis in vivo. J Biol Chem 1982; *257*:9283–9289.

97. Reichard GA Jr, Skutches CL, Hoeldtke RD, et al. Acetone metabolism in humans during diabetic ketoacidosis. Diabetes 1986; *35*:668–674.

98. Owen OE, Reichle FA, Mozzoli MA, et al. Hepatic, gut and renal substrate flux rates in patients with hepatic cirrhosis. J Clin Invest 1981; *68*:240–252.

99. Reichard GA Jr, Haff AC, Skutches CL, et al. Plasma acetone metabolism in fasting humans. J Clin Invest 1979; *63*:619–626.

100. Owen OE, Trapp VE, Skutches CL, et al. Acetone metabolism during diabetic ketoacidosis. Diabetes 1982; *31*:242–248.

101. Casazza JP, Felver ME, Veech RL. The metabolism of acetone in rat. J Biol Chem 1984; *259*:231–236.

102. Stetten D Jr. High-powered research and the microscopic viewpoint. J Med Educ 1981; *56*:3–7.

103. Rudney H. Propanediol phosphate as a possible intermediate in the metabolism of acetone. J Biol Chem 1954; *210*:361–371.

104. Hanzlik PJ, Lehman AJ, VanWinkle W Jr, et al. General metabolic and glycogenic actions of propylene glycol and other glycols. J Pharmacol Exp Ther 1939; *67*:114–126.

105. Wittman JS, Bawin RR. Stimulation of gluconeogenesis by propylene glycol in the fasting rat. Life Sci 1974; *15*:515–524.

106. Owen OE, Trapp VE, Reichard GA Jr, et al. Nature and quantity of fuels consumed in patients with alcoholic cirrhosis. J Clin Invest 1983; *72*:1821–1832.

107. Owen OE, Trapp VE, Reichard GA Jr, et al. Effects of therapy on the nature and quantity of fuels oxidized during diabetic ketoacidosis. Diabetes 1980; *29*:365–372.

108. Owen OE, Block BSB, Patel M, et al. Human splanchnic metabolism during diabetic ketoacidosis. Metabolism 1977; *26*:381–398.

109. Owen OE, Licht JH, Sapir DG. Renal function and effects of partial rehydration during diabetic ketoacidosis. Diabetes 1981; *30*:510–518.

3

NUTRIENT METABOLISM

K.N. JEEJEEBHOY

MACRONUTRIENTS

Proteins

GENERAL ASPECTS OF PROTEIN METABOLISM

Protein. The word protein is derived from the Greek *protos*, which means "first." Thus, this nutrient is acknowledged as the most important. Indeed, in the animal and plant world proteins make up the basic structure of the body. Of the "average" man's body weight, 2.6 per cent is nitrogen,[1] or nearly 16 per cent is protein. Half of this is intracellular and the rest extracellular.

Chemical Composition. Proteins are composed of amino acids joined by peptide bonds. Amino acids are composed of one or more amino groups (NH_2) associated with one or more carboxyl groups (COOH). The amino groups are in the alpha position to the carboxyl group.

$$
\begin{array}{c}
NH_2 \\
| \\
R\!-\!C\alpha\!-\!COOH \\
| \\
H
\end{array}
$$

The asymmetry about the alpha-carbon renders the molecule optically active except when R = H, as in glycine. It is the L-isomer that is biologically active. This is of importance, for artificial mixtures of DL-amino acids are not completely utilized. Because of the presence of both the NH_2 and COOH groups, these acids behave as amphoteric compounds depending upon the pH.

$$
\begin{array}{c}
NH_3{}^+ \\
| \\
R\!-\!CH\!-\!COO^-
\end{array}
$$

Essential Amino Acids. In proteins any of 22 amino acids can occur. Of these, eight cannot be synthesized endogenously unless the corresponding keto acids are available from exogenous sources. These eight—threonine, lysine, phenylalanine, leucine, isoleucine, valine, methionine, and tryptophan—are called essential amino acids. Since they can be synthesized in vivo when the keto acids are fed, it is really the keto acids that are essential and cannot be synthesized from other substrates. By contrast, the keto acids of the nonessential amino acids are metabolites of carbohydrate metabolism. For example, pyruvate derived from glucose metabolism is transaminated to alanine.

Transformation. Since amino acids are composed of carboxyl and amino groups, they can undergo three main transformations.

The first and most important process is *transamination*. This is a reversible reaction between an amino and a keto acid. The keto acid alpha-ketoglutarate is frequently the recipient of amino groups in this reaction. The donor is often aspartate but can be almost any other alpha-amino acid.

The second transformation is oxidative *deamination*, resulting in the formation of a keto acid and free ammonia:

$$
\begin{array}{c}
NH_2 \\
| \\
R\!-\!C\!-\!COOH + \frac{1}{2}O_2 \rightarrow \\
| \\
H \\
\text{L-Amino acid}
\end{array}
\qquad
\begin{array}{c}
R \\
| \\
C\!=\!O + NH_3 \\
| \\
COOH \\
\text{alpha-Keto acid}
\end{array}
$$

This reaction occurs especially with glutamic acid, resulting in the formation of alpha-ketoglutaric acid (see bottom of page).

The third process is *decarboxylation*. This reaction results in the formation of amines. This reaction is important in the production of biologically active amines.

$$
\begin{array}{c}
R \\
| \\
CH\!-\!NH_2 \\
| \\
COOH
\end{array}
\rightarrow
\begin{array}{c}
R \\
| \\
CH_2\!-\!NH_2 + CO_2
\end{array}
$$

In this way histamine is formed from histidine, pu-

trescine from ornithine, tyramine from tyrosine, and serotonin from tryptophan. Of particular interest is the production of polyamines derived from putrescine, which in turn aid nucleic acid synthesis and promote protein metabolism.

Acidic, Neutral, and Basic Amino Acids. Dicarboxylic acids such as glutamic acid produce excess bicarbonate when deaminated and oxidized to CO_2 and water. In contrast, the basic amino acids histidine, lysine, and arginine donate H^+ when metabolized. Hence their catabolism results in acidosis unless buffered by another bicarbonate-generating anion such as acetate or lactate. The remaining neutral amino acids do not donate or receive H^+, nor do they generate bicarbonate.

Intake and Absorption. Dietary protein is partially digested by pepsin in the stomach to polypeptides. However, gastric digestion is not essential, and the major part of protein digestion occurs in the duodenum and upper jejunum under the influence of pancreatic proteases. It is of interest that intestinal perfusion studies indicate that protein digestion continues up to the proximal ileum.[2] In the small intestine the pancreatic enzymes trypsin, chymotrypsin, and elastase hydrolyze protein to peptides. These are then hydrolyzed by exopeptidases, which remove an amino acid and leave smaller peptides.

$$
\text{Protein} \xrightarrow{\text{endopeptidase}} \text{Peptide} \xrightarrow{\text{exopeptidase}}
$$
$$
\text{Amino acid} + \text{small peptide}
$$

These small peptides are either hydrolyzed by other peptidases at the brush border or transported into the cell and then hydrolyzed by cellular peptidases to amino acids. Peptide absorption by a mucosal cell is more rapid and efficient than amino acid transport into the cell.

Amino Acid Metabolism

General Considerations. Amino acids that are in excess of requirements are not stored but are used as metabolic fuel. The alpha-amino group is removed and the carbon skeleton remaining is transformed into acetyl CoA, acetoacetyl CoA, pyruvate, alpha-ketoglutarate, succinate, fumarate, or oxaloacetate.

$$
\begin{array}{c}
COOH \\
| \\
CH_2 \\
| \\
CH_2 \\
| \\
CO \\
| \\
COOH \\
\text{alpha-Ketoglutaric acid}
\end{array}
+
\begin{array}{c}
COOH \\
| \\
CH_2 \\
| \\
CH\!-\!NH_2 \\
| \\
COOH \\
\text{Aspartic acid}
\end{array}
\rightarrow
\begin{array}{c}
COOH \\
| \\
CH_2 \\
| \\
CH_2 \\
| \\
CH\!-\!NH_2 \\
| \\
COOH \\
\text{Glutamic acid}
\end{array}
+
\begin{array}{c}
COOH \\
| \\
CH_2 \\
| \\
CO \\
| \\
COOH \\
\text{alpha-Keto acid}
\end{array}
$$

Transamination and NH_4^+. Transamination is a process by which the alpha-amino group of an amino acid is transferred to a keto acid.

$$\text{Amino acid (1)} + \text{Keto acid (2)} \xrightarrow{\text{aminotransferase}}$$
$$\text{Keto acid (1)} + \text{Amino acid (2)}$$

Glutamate Transaminase. This catalyzes the transamination by which the nitrogen of excess amino acids is transferred to alpha-ketoglutarate to form glutamate, leaving the keto acid of the amino acid transaminated. In turn, the keto acid is oxidized for energy. Hence this process aids amino acid oxidation. Glutamate is deaminated to alpha-ketoglutarate and NH_4^+. The deamination is catalyzed by glutamate dehydrogenase. The NH_4^+ is converted into urea and excreted. Glutamate dehydrogenase is activated by low ATP and high ADP levels. Hence reduced energy states increase amino acid oxidation.

Alanine Transaminase. This enzyme catalyzes the transfer of nitrogen to pyruvate from other amino acids, alanine, and the keto acid of the amino acid that is transaminated. In turn, alanine can transfer its nitrogen to alpha-ketoglutarate to form glutamate.

Thus these two transaminases funnel the nitrogen from excess amino acids to urea. The remaining carbon skeletons of the transaminated amino acids are used for energy.

Control of Ureagenesis. The ultimate disposal of nitrogen from excess amino acids depends upon urea formation. Hence nitrogen loss is controlled by ureagenesis. It was shown by Rafoth and Onstad[3] that there is a linear relation between urea formation and protein fed. This relationship was subsequently shown to be due to the fact that the activity of carbamoyl phosphate synthetase increased with amino acid feeding. The activation of carbamoyl phosphate synthetase depends on the level of N-acetylglutamate. Amino acid or protein feeding increases the level of N-acetylglutamate, which in turn activates carbamoyl phosphate synthetase.

The enzyme carbamoyl phosphate synthetase catalyzes the condensation of NH_4^+ and CO_2 in the presence of ATP to form carbamoyl phosphate, which is the most important step in the entry of NH_4^+ derived from amino acids into the urea cycle. Carbamoyl phosphate reacts with ornithine to form citrulline.[4]

Hepatic Metabolism of Amino Acids. Amino acids absorbed from the gastrointestinal tract enter the portal circulation and pass through the liver. The passage through the liver results in the removal of most of the amino acids except for the branched-chain amino acids (leucine, isoleucine, and valine).[5] Dietary intake of these amino acids is about 8 per cent of the amino acid content of the diet. In contrast, more than 60 per cent of the amino acids released into the peripheral circulation are of the branched-chain variety.[6] The stimulation of hepatic and plasma protein synthesis is aided by the branched-chain and other amino acids ingested during each meal.[7,8]

In addition to dietary amino acids, the liver receives alanine from muscle. Alanine transfers its nitrogen for urea synthesis to alpha-ketoglutarate, resulting in the formation of glutamate and pyruvate. The glutamate in turn transfers its nitrogen for urea synthesis and the pyruvate is used for gluconeogenesis. In addition, glutamine from muscle is taken up by the intestine and transaminated to alanine, which is again metabolized by the liver as mentioned above. Thus alanine is the major path by which muscle nitrogen is conveyed to the liver and excreted as urea.

Peripheral Metabolism of Amino Acids. The branched-chain amino acids entering the systemic circulation after each meal are taken up by muscles and other peripheral tissues for protein synthesis. On the other hand, there is a release of nitrogen from muscle in the form of alanine and glutamine. Thus, muscle is constantly turning over by the processes of synthesis and catabolism. Muscle proteins that are catabolized release branched-chain amino acids, which are transaminated to alanine and glutamine and the corresponding branched-chain keto acid (BCKA). Alanine and glutamine flow from muscle and are taken up by the viscera. The BCKA is used as a fuel by muscle.

Relationship of Branched-Chain Amino Acids and Other Energy Substrates

Glucose. Branched-chain amino acids inhibit glucose oxidation[9] and glucose restriction reduces utilization of branched-chain amino acids,[10] probably because BCKA's inhibit pyruvate dehydrogenase.

Fat. In contrast to glucose, fat inhibits the utilization of branched-chain amino acids, and isocaloric replacement of carbohydrate by fat increases the levels of branched-chain amino acids.[11]

Interaction of Leucine, Isoleucine, and Valine. Leucine activates the degradation of other branched-chain amino acids. Thus when leucine alone is infused, the levels of valine and isoleucine fall.[12] In contrast, the other two branched-chain amino acids do not influence leucine degradation.

Transformation of Branched-Chain Keto Acids to Amino Acids. The branched-chain amino acids are essential because they are transaminated to BCKA's, which are oxidized for energy by the corresponding dehydrogenase. This irreversible step makes the amino acid essential. However, if BCKA's are provided exogenously, they are transaminated to the corresponding amino acid. Hence BCKA's can be substituted for the corresponding amino acids.[13]

Role of Branched-Chain Amino Acids and Branched-Chain Keto Acids in Promoting Nitrogen Retention. Initial studies seemed to indicate that branched-chain amino acids reduced nitrogen excretion in fasted individuals. The implication was that giving branched-chain amino acids increased nitrogen retention. Since nitrogen excretion falls as fasting progresses, it is necessary to distinguish between a fall in nitrogen excretion during such studies due to fasting and that due to feeding an amino acid. In controlled studies Mitch et al.[14] showed that it was the branched-chain keto and not amino acids that significantly reduced nitrogen loss. A possible explanation resides in the fact that the reaction of transamination between a branched-chain keto acid and pyruvate or alpha-ketoglutarate is an equilibrium reaction and can be driven backward only by the keto acid. In contrast, the amino acid will drive it forward and increase nitrogen output. The above is supported by the fact that leucine augments alanine and glutamine release from muscle,[14,15] whereas the keto acids do not.[13,16]

GENERAL EFFECTS OF PROTEIN INTAKES

The fasting animal and human excrete nitrogen at rates that are proportional to their metabolic rates. Munro[17] has indicated that endogenous nitrogen excretion is 230, 77, and 45 mg/kg/day in rat, dog, and human in relation to the basal metabolic rates of 108, 38, and 23 kcal/kg/day, making the endogenous loss about 2 mg N/kcal/day. This value fits with the finding in several human studies that when normal subjects starve the urine nitrogen falls to about 2 g/day.[17] On the other hand, when a person who has been fasted is refed protein, nitrogen excretion does not rise in proportion to the intake, so that there is a gain of body nitrogen. This gain in early refeeding has been found to be due to a rapid accumulation of nitrogen in the liver, to a lesser extent in kidneys, and very little in muscle.[17] Thus, the early benefit of refeeding protein appears to be a rise in liver protein. However, this early and spectacular nitrogen retention is not sustained, and nitrogen retention slows rapidly within 4 to 7 days. This phenomenon should be considered when interpreting short-term nitrogen balance data. Later it will be shown that whereas nitrogen balance data have suggested marked increases in nitrogen retention during parenteral feeding, this has not been confirmed by long-term studies with whole-body neutron activation analysis.

Protein-Energy Interrelationship. In man it was shown years ago that increasing energy intake either as fat or carbohydrate increased nitrogen retention by 4 and 2 mg N per extra kcal fed respectively.[17] Later Calloway and Spector[18] showed that nitrogen retention increased when either nitrogen or energy intake was increased. However, the effect of each alone was restricted if given in insufficient amounts to meet requirements.

In injured subjects nitrogen excretion rises in proportion to the rise in metabolic rate.[19] Even when insulin infusions are given to maintain euglycemia it can be shown that nitrogen loss and excess energy production from protein oxidation occurs, while glucose oxidation falls.[20] Thus, protein appears to become an important source of energy in injured subjects.

FACTORS AFFECTING PROTEIN UTILIZATION

Protein utilization has been estimated by observing the amount of protein and energy needed to create a positive nitrogen balance. By this we mean the observed difference between intake and measured losses. The tacit assumption is that when losses exceed intake the patient is losing body protein, and vice versa. Recent papers have emphasized the role of nitrogen balance for determining nutrient needs during parenteral nutritional therapy. Hence it is appropriate to analyze the value and interpretation of nitrogen balance data. The human adult has finite cellularity of muscle and viscera, which in turn determines the body nitrogen content. Hence a well-nourished adult cannot go into positive nitrogen balance unless there is hypertrophy of existing muscle and viscera or an increase in tissue that is a part neither of muscle nor of viscera. Such an increase has been shown to occur mainly with deposition of adipose tissue; it is believed that the added nitrogen is required to permit the development of supporting structures such as connective tissue, blood vessels, and the increase in muscle fiber size required to support the additional weight of the adiposity. Experimentally this concept has been supported by the studies of Keys et al.[21] in volunteers and by Elwyn[22] in patients receiving parenteral nutrition.

Munro[17] had noted earlier work showing that the nitrogen excretion in urine is dependent in part upon the preceding nitrogen intake. Hence the amount of nitrogen required to maintain balance in any individual depends to some extent on the previous intake of dietary nitrogen. When an individual receiving a high-protein diet starves or reduces his protein intake, the previously high urinary nitrogen loss continues for a few days despite the reduced intake, resulting in a negative nitrogen balance, the magnitude of which is directly proportional to the previous level of intake. The higher the preceding nitrogen intake, the greater the negative balance upon starvation and vice versa. It is of interest that in experimental animals (rats), Munro[17] showed that the catabolic reaction to injury was greatest in well-nourished animals. The reaction was not clearly seen in malnourished rats. It is also a clinical finding that nitrogen loss following injury is greatest in healthy males and is least in malnourished subjects. However, within a few days of injury the urinary nitrogen excretion falls until it is equal to the level of protein intake or equivalent to at least 2 mg/kcal of metabolic rate. Hence protein catabolism will rise with an increase in metabolic rate. However, the high initial negative nitrogen balance referred to above results in a limited loss of about 50 to 60 g (out of a total of about 1800 to 2000 g of total body nitrogen), after which excretion falls to the low value of about 2 mg/kcal of metabolic rate. Therefore, in order to meet solely ongoing losses, it is necessary to replace about 2 mg/kcal of metabolic rate. Obviously, more is needed in situations in which muscle catabolism is enhanced and to allow for the reduced efficiency of utilization of the currently available amino acid solutions.

Recognition of these principles can aid in reconciling various studies with apparently contradictory results. Calloway and Spector[18] and more recently Richardson et al.[23] showed that in healthy adults it is necessary to give at least 1 g of protein and 45 kcal/kg body weight to maintain nitrogen balance. In contrast, in malnourished and postoperative subjects, apart from the need for energy substrate (glucose or fat), Greenberg et al.[24,25] noticed that the quantity of nitrogen given was an important determinant of nitrogen balance; provided that 2 g/kg of amino acids were given per day to such patients, a positive nitrogen balance was seen, even when total calories were less than metabolic requirements. Similar results have been obtained by Bozzetti[26] in postoperative patients. Recently Hoffer et al.[27] showed that in the obese patient on a protein modified fast, feeding a high nitrogen intake of 1.4 g/kg maintained nitrogen balance, whereas a lower nitrogen intake of 0.8 g/kg was associated with a negative nitrogen balance. Hence, by giving amino acids alone it is possible to induce nitrogen balance in depleted adults. By contrast, the well-nourished adult needs excess energy (to deposit fat) before a positive nitrogen balance is attained.

Experimental proof for this contention is found in the studies of Yeung et al.,[28] who showed that patients receiving total parenteral nutrition gained a lot of weight compared with those on a more modest calorie intake in the form of an elemental diet. However, all this weight gain was shown to be water and/or fat, with nitrogen retention being equivalent in the two groups. Even in patients with burns, who are traditionally regarded as having high caloric needs, Burke et al.[29] have shown that when the protein intake was as high as 2.78 g/kg/day, the effect of adding glucose calories on protein synthesis or catabolism was minimal.

In studies by Collins et al.[30] the total body nitrogen after major surgery was as well maintained with an infusion of amino acids as with amino acids and glucose. Thus, based purely on nitrogen balance it would appear that amino acid infusions by themselves do meet the previously held goal of a positive nitrogen balance. However, in functional terms it is of interest that Young and Hill[31] showed that even though body nitrogen was as well maintained with amino acids alone as with amino acids plus "energy," the group of patients receiving supplemental calories recovered earlier and had fewer complications. This observation underscores the need for altering

our views concerning nitrogen balance and body nitrogen as the best way of measuring the effects of nutritional therapy. As indicated in Chapter 42, the effect of nutrition on muscle function may be rapid and may occur even when there is little or no detectable change in overall body composition.

PROTEIN REQUIREMENTS

From the foregoing discussion of protein metabolism it is clear that the requirement for protein is dependent on a number of metabolic factors such as previous nutritional status, degree of nutritional depletion, provision of nonprotein energy, and the rate of desired repletion. In general it appears that the more protein is given, the less is the effect of nonprotein energy intake and the greater is the degree of nitrogen retention in the depleted patient.

In addition to these purely metabolic factors, the question is often asked whether intravenously given amino acids are as effective in promoting nitrogen retention as oral proteins, and whether all amino acid preparations are comparable in regard to their ability to promote nitrogen retention. To answer this question Patel et al.[32] did a study of the effect on nitrogen balance of casein hydrolysate given in graded amounts and compared the results with those when giving oral casein and oral hydrolysate. This study demonstrated that the amino acid composition of the hydrolysate given intravenously was not optimum and resulted in a lower balance than when the same casein, as intact protein, was administered orally. The finding that the nitrogen balance during the intravenous administration of casein hydrolysate was the same as the one observed when it was given orally, keeping all other parameters constant, indicated that oral and intravenous amino acids were handled identically as far as gross nitrogen economy was concerned. It was surmised in that study that the difference between the hydrolysate and the whole casein was due to a loss of sulfur-containing and aromatic amino acids during the process of hydrolysis.

To prove this point Anderson et al.[33] devised and infused an amino acid mixture enriched in these two groups of amino acids. Using a similar study design they showed that with this more suitable amino acid composition the intravenously administered amino acids were as effective in promoting nitrogen balance as oral protein, and about 1 g/kg ideal body weight was sufficient to promote positive nitrogen balance in patients.

RECOMMENDATIONS FOR INTRAVENOUSLY ADMINISTERED AMINO ACIDS

There are several interacting factors that determine how much protein should be given. The nitrogen requirement for balance in stable adults is only 0.4 g/kg/day, and this was also found to be true for intravenously administered amino acids in the study by Anderson et al.[33] For stable individuals receiving enteral feeding the Recommended Nutrient Intake for Canadians is given in Table 3–1. However, there is increased nitrogen retention with increasing intake, and this gain is linear over a range of 0.25 to 2 g/kg/day.[34] Also, an increase in metabolic rate increases nitrogen loss, raising the basal needs for balance. Finally, the higher the nitrogen intake, the less dependent is the balance on energy intake in depleted patients. On the other hand, poor renal and hepatic function will reduce tolerance to amino acid loads. Taking all these factors into account, it seems desirable to give, as a first approximation, 1 to 1.5 g/kg of ideal body weight/day of a balanced amino acid mixture and to monitor the response of plasma proteins and urea nitrogen excretion.

Energy Metabolism

BIOCHEMISTRY

Energy is derived from all three macronutrients, namely proteins, carbohydrates, and fats. These nutrients act as sources of energy by a three-phase transformation. In the first stage these macromolecules are hydrolyzed to simpler molecules: proteins to amino acids, carbohydrates to monosaccharides, and fats to fatty acids and glycerol. In the second stage these simpler molecules are degraded to two-carbon fragments and linked to coenzyme A (CoA) as acetyl CoA. In the final stage acetyl CoA enters the tricarboxylic acid (Krebs or citric acid) cycle and is oxidized to provide energy, which is then stored as high-energy phosphates.

Under normal circumstances, however, energy in the diet is derived mainly from carbohydrates and fats.

Carbohydrates. The carbohydrate of a normal diet consists of 60 per cent starch, 30 per cent sucrose, and 10 per cent lactose. A total of about 400 g is eaten per day.

Starch is made up of 80 per cent amylopectin and 20 per cent amylose. Amylose is a straight-chain molecule with $\alpha(1\rightarrow4)$ linkages. In contrast amylopectin, in addition to these linkages, has branch points with $\alpha(1\rightarrow6)$ linkages.

Sucrose and lactose are disaccharides composed of glucose and fructose (sucrose) and glucose and galactose (lactose).

TABLE 3–1. Recommended Nutrient Intakes for Canadians

Age	Sex	Weight kg	Protein g/day	Fat Soluble Vitamins A RE*/day	D µg/day	E mg/day	Water Soluble Vitamins C mg/day	Folacin µg/day	B₁₂ µg/day	Minerals Calcium mg/day	Magnesium mg/day	Iron mg/day	Iodine µg/day	Zinc mg/day
Months														
0–2	Both	4.5	11	400	10	3	20	50	0.3	350	30	0.4	25	2
3–5	Both	7.0	14	400	10	3	20	50	0.3	350	40	5	35	3
6–8	Both	8.5	16	400	10	3	20	50	0.3	400	45	7	40	3
9–11	Both	9.5	18	400	10	3	20	55	0.3	400	50	7	45	3
Years														
1	Both	11	18	400	10	3	20	65	0.3	500	55	6	55	4
2–3	Both	14	20	400	5	4	20	80	0.4	500	65	6	65	4
4–6	Both	18	25	500	5	5	25	90	0.5	600	90	6	85	5
7–9	M	25	31	700	2.5	7	35	125	0.8	700	110	7	110	6
	F	25	29	700	2.5	6	30	125	0.8	700	110	7	95	6
10–12	M	34	38	800	2.5	8	40	170	1.0	900	150	10	125	7
	F	36	39	800	2.5	7	40	170	1.0	1000	160	10	110	7
13–15	M	50	49	900	2.5	9	50	160	1.5	1100	220	12	160	9
	F	48	43	800	2.5	7	45	160	1.5	800	190	13	160	8
16–18	M	62	54	1000	2.5	10	55	190	1.9	900	240	10	160	9
	F	53	47	800	2.5	7	45	160	1.9	700	220	14	160	8
19–24	M	71	57	1000	2.5	10	60	210	2.0	800	240	8	160	9
	F	58	41	800	2.5	7	45	165	2.0	700	190	14	160	8
25–49	M	74	57	1000	2.5	9	60	210	2.0	800	240	8	160	9
	F	59	41	800	2.5	6	45	165	2.0	700	190	14	160	8
50–74	M	73	57	1000	2.5	7	60	210	2.0	800	240	8	160	9
	F	63	41	800	2.5	6	45	165	2.0	800	190	7	160	8
75+	M	69	57	1000	2.5	6	60	210	2.0	800	240	8	160	9
	F	64	41	800	2.5	5	45	165	2.0	800	190	7	160	8
Pregnancy (additional)														
1st trimester			15	100	2.5	2	0	305	1.0	500	15	6	25	0
2nd trimester			20	100	2.5	2	20	305	1.0	500	20	6	25	1
3rd trimester			25	100	2.5	2	20	305	1.0	500	25	6	25	2
Lactation			20	400	2.5	3	30	120	0.5	500	80	0	50	6

Published 1983 by The Bureau of Nutritional Sciences, Food Directorate, Health Protection Branch, Dept. of National Health and Welfare, Ottawa, Canada, K1A 0L2.

*RE = Retinol equivalent.

Digestion and Absorption of Carbohydrates.[35]
Digestion mainly occurs in the duodenum and small
bowel. Amylose and amylopectin are hydrolyzed to
oligosaccharides by pancreatic alpha-amylase. These
oligosaccharides are maltose, maltotriose, and alpha-
limit dextrins. The oligosaccharides and disaccharides are hydrolyzed to their constituent monosaccharides by the brush border enzymes glucoamylase, sucrase, and lactase. The monosaccharides
are transported into the mucosal cell by an active
transport process linked to the pumping of sodium.
Fructose is the only monosaccharide that enters by
facilitated diffusion.

Fats. Dietary fat is composed of triglycerides of
mainly four long-chain fatty acids. There are two
saturated fatty acids, palmitic (C_{16}) and stearic (C_{18}),
and two unsaturated fatty acids, oleic (C_{18} with one
double bond) and linoleic (C_{18} with two double
bonds). In addition, smaller amounts of linolenic
acid (C_{18} with three double bonds) and medium-
chain fatty acids (C_6 to C_{10}) are contained in the diet.

Two unsaturated fatty acids, linoleic and linolenic
acids, are called essential fatty acids because they
cannot be synthesized in vivo from nondietary
sources. Both fatty acids have 18 carbon atoms, but
the position of the first double bond, called the omega (ω) number, is between the sixth and seventh
carbons for linoleic acid and between the third and
fourth carbons for linolenic acid. Linoleic acid is converted by chain elongation to arachidonic acid,
which is the precursor of prostaglandins.

Digestion and Absorption of Fats. Triglycerides in
a diet are hydrolyzed to beta-monoglycerides and
free fatty acids by pancreatic lipase and colipase.[36–38]
These products of pancreatic digestion are poorly
soluble in water, but are taken up into an aqueous
medium through the action of bile salts. Bile salts
are composed of both hydrophilic and hydrophobic
molecules. When dissolved in water they form micelles, which are particles composed of a central hydrophobic core surrounded by hydrophilic radicals,
interfacing with the aqueous environment. These
micelles can take up the hydrophobic digestion
products of triglycerides into their hydrophobic core
and thus solubilize them in an aqueous environment.[39] The dispersion of the fatty acids and monoglycerides in micelles enormously increases the surface area of interaction with the mucosa and thus
aids absorption. The micellar contents diffuse
through the unstirred water layer, the intestinal mucus, and the cell wall to enter the cell, where they
are re-esterified to triglyceride and linked to an apoprotein to form a chylomicron.

Medium-chain triglycerides (MCT's), with 6 to 10
carbon atoms, are absorbed to the extent of 30 per
cent as intact triglycerides. The remaining 70 per
cent is hydrolyzed to medium-chain fatty acids,
which are soluble in water and absorbed directly by
the mucosa or via micellar solubilization. In the mucosal cell MCT's are completely hydrolyzed to fatty

acids and transported in the circulation as free fatty
acids.[40]

ENERGY REQUIREMENTS

Energy requirement is dependent on a number of
factors which include the body surface area (derived
from height and weight), age, and sex. Basal requirements are most commonly predicted for normal humans by the Harris-Benedict equation.[41] In
a study done in 21 adults of various heights and
weights the predicted requirement agreed with the
energy consumption obtained by indirect calorimetry with a variation of ±5 per cent.[42] The equations
for calculating the expected basal energy expenditure (EBEE) are given below.[41]

Men

$$kcal/24h = 66.473 + 13.7516 \times wt\ (kg)$$
$$+ 5.0033 \times ht\ (cm) - 6.7550 \times age\ (yr)$$

Women

$$kcal/24h = 655.0955 + 9.5634 \times wt\ (kg)$$
$$+ 1.8496 \times ht\ (cm) - 4.6756 \times age\ (yr)$$

These estimates are for basal energy expenditure
(BEE), and to these values must be added that for
the specific dynamic action of food in order to give
the resting energy expenditure (REE) in the bedridden patient. The REE can be approximated from
the BEE by increasing it by 10 per cent. In contrast,
malnutrition reduces the BEE to an extent exceeding that expected simply on the basis of weight loss.
Injury, sepsis, and especially burns were believed to
increase energy requirements by approximately 30,
60, and 100 per cent, respectively. However, recently
the degree of hypermetabolism in injured and septic
patients has come into question. This matter is not
only of theoretical but of practical importance. If it
is held that such patients lose weight because of hypermetabolism, then the logical treatment is to give
a large excess of calories. Such excess feeding, however, increases the risk of metabolic complications,
as will be shown later.

Three studies, two of them based on controlled
protocols, have failed to find that injured and septic
patients are markedly hypermetabolic. The mean
increase in metabolic rate of injured and septic patients studied by Askanazi et al.[43] exceeded the expected value by only 14 per cent. Similarly Roulet
et al.[44] found an increase of only 12.9 per cent in
critically sick patients in respiratory failure. Baker
et al.[45] in a third study came to the same conclusion.
In any case it should be recognized that an increase
in metabolic rate of 60 per cent in a 70 kg man,
when referred to the BEE (which is about 25 kcal/
kg/day), works out to a requirement of only 40 kcal/

kg/day or 2800 kcal. Hence there is little evidence of a need for 4000 to 6000 kcal as has been claimed in the past. (For further discussion see Chapter 38.)

SOURCES OF ENERGY

Gamble[46] in his classic studies showed that feeding a modest amount (100 g) of glucose reduced the urinary excretion of nitrogen in normal fasting subjects, demonstrating the protein-sparing effect of glucose. Subsquently Kinney et al.[19] showed that in injured and septic patients there was an increase in energy consumption and that nitrogen loss paralleled the metabolic rate. Based on the known protein-sparing effects of glucose and the increased metabolic rate and nitrogen loss observed in such subjects, parenteral nutrition using very large amounts of glucose was advocated for treating patients, in the belief that this therapy would promote nitrogen retention or reduce catabolism, especially in injured and septic patients. This concept received support from the studies of Woolfson et al.[47] and Long et al.,[48] who showed that in burned patients glucose was the only substrate capable of reducing nitrogen excretion and of improving nitrogen balance. However, in injured and septic patients Kinney et al.[19] had shown that the respiratory quotient was in fact low, indicating that in such patients fat was the principal source of energy. This finding was obviously at variance with the above concepts. Recently, for this and other reasons, the paramount importance of glucose has come into question.

Jeejeebhoy et al.[49] showed that in contrast to the observation of Long et al. in burned subjects,[48] patients with gastrointestinal disease utilize glucose and fat equally well, and both promote nitrogen retention to a similar extent. This finding has been confirmed by several other investigators.[50–53] Recently in a controlled trial, MacFie et al.[54] showed that a glucose-lipid mixture promoted nitrogen retention, but glucose alone did not do so. Parallel observations by Wolfe et al.,[55] Burke et al.,[29] and Askanazi et al.[43] have shown that injured and septic patients, including those with burns, have an obligatory need for fat energy and continue to oxidize significant amounts of fat despite being provided with all nonprotein calories as glucose. Furthermore, when a substantial amount of glucose is administered, not all the infused glucose is utilized directly for energy.[55] The excess glucose calories have to be stored. Once liver glycogen is repleted, the excess is converted to fat which is deposited in the liver, resulting in the hepatic steatosis seen by Jeejeebhoy et al.[56] and Messing et al.[57]

This picture, encountered when glucose is used as an exclusive source of nonprotein calories, is not seen when a glucose-lipid mixture is used.[58] Finally, Roulet et al.[44] demonstrated in a controlled trial that acutely sick patients in respiratory failure showed a significant increase in net protein synthesis over ca-

tabolism (as measured by ^{14}C-leucine turnover studies) only when a mixed substrate of fat and carbohydrate was infused. In contrast, infusing equivalent amounts of amino acids without calories, or with glucose calories alone, only maintained balance between synthesis and catabolism—observations in accordance with those of Yeung et al.[28] and MacFie et al.[54] Hence it is now clear that the injured or septic patient needs a mixed substrate of glucose and fat for meeting energy needs.

ESSENTIAL FATTY ACID DEFICIENCY (EFAD)

Holman[59] showed that certain fatty acids, principally linoleic acid, are essential for the human. He also showed that linoleic acid (18 carbon atoms, two double bonds) is converted to a longer chain fatty acid (20 carbon atoms, four double bonds, i.e., a tetraene) called arachidonic acid. It appears that, when linoleate is deficient, the same system that elongates the chain of linoleate will use oleate (18 carbon atoms, one double bond) as a substrate and will elongate it to a 20-carbon fatty acid with three double bonds (i.e., a triene) called eicosatrienoic acid. Since oleate can be synthesized from carbohydrates, there is an alteration in the plasma fatty acid pattern during essential fatty acid deficiency. Linoleic acid and its daughter product arachidonic acid are both reduced and, in place of the latter, eicosatrienoic acid appears in the circulation. Holman[59] compared the amounts of eicosatrienoic and arachidonic acid and expressed them as the triene-tetraene ratio. He found that elevation of this ratio was indicative of essential fatty acid deficiency.

Prior to the advent of parenteral nutrition, a clinical syndrome of skin rash with appropriate alterations in plasma fatty acid pattern had been recognized as indicating essential fatty acid deficiency in infants. Adults did not seem to suffer the syndrome, probably because they have sufficient stores of essential fatty acids in their adipose tissue to prevent this deficiency. However, with the advent of that parenteral nutrition which was based on a system of continuous infusion of a fat-free hypertonic glucose solution, essential fatty acid deficiency was found to occur in adults. Clinically, EFA deficiency in patients receiving TPN is characterized by a skin rash, reduced plasma levels of linoleate, and an elevated triene-tetraene ratio. These changes were corrected by infusing an intravenous lipid emulsion containing linoleate.

More recently Wene et al.[60] showed that the plasma pattern of essential fatty acid deficiency can be observed as early as 10 days after starting fat-free parenteral nutrition, prior to the onset of any clinically observable features. The reason for the early occurrence of EFA deficiency in adults receiving TPN is due to the fact that, when glucose is infused continuously, high insulin levels prevent the release of free fatty acids from adipose tissue stores. Hence plasma fatty acids can originate only from either exogenously infused lipids or, in the case of fat-free parenteral nutrition, from endogenously synthesized lipids derived from carbohydrates. Since the endogenously synthesized lipids do not include linoleate, the pattern of fatty acids alters rapidly to that seen with EFA deficiency. Hence, during continuous glucose infusion the only way to maintain plasma essential fatty acid levels is to infuse continuously lipids containing them. Since intravenous lipid can reverse and prevent EFAD, various regimens have been suggested with variable amounts of lipid given either once a week, twice a week, or three times a week, but none of these regimens has been tested rigorously. However, the more recent indication that lipid would be advantageous as a calorie source has made superfluous the concept of giving lipids only as a source of essential fatty acid.

One remaining question is whether linoleate is the only essential fatty acid in the human or whether linolenate also serves as an essential fatty acid. The latter appears to be necessary for the proper myelination of the central nervous system in newborn animals and therefore may have to be provided when parenteral nutrition is used in the newborn. However, the exact need for, and role of, this fatty acid in the adult human remains to be determined.

RECOMMENDATIONS FOR ENERGY INTAKE

The next question is the magnitude of the optimum caloric intake in the majority of patients. In stable or malnourished individuals receiving either parenteral or enteral diets, the caloric requirements can be roughly computed from the relationships that about 30 kcal/kg (0.13 MJ/kg) maintains body weight and 40 kcal/kg (0.17 MJ/kg) induces weight gain. What about the critically ill patient? Hitherto, based on the concept that these patients are grossly hypercatabolic, 4000 to 5000 kcal was often given to sick patients. In experiments using graded inputs of calories we found that the most striking increase in nitrogen balance, with an increase in caloric intake, occurred when the intake increased from 0 to 40 kcal/kg ideal body weight, and that increasing the intake of calories above this level did not appreciably increase nitrogen balance.[34] This figure corresponds to the theoretical maximum calculated on the basis of a 60 per cent increase in the metabolic rate referred to earlier in this discourse and amounts to an intake of 2800 kcal/day in the 70-kg man. This caloric intake will also comfortably exceed the energy requirements noted for injured and septic patients by Askanazi et al.,[43] Roulet et al.,[44] and Baker et al.[45]

Electrolytes

The importance of fluid and electrolyte replacement for promoting tissue perfusion and ionic equilibrium is self-evident. In addition, the processes of malnutrition and refeeding are both associated with major changes in electrolyte balance. With protein-caloric malnutrition there is loss of the intracellular ions potassium (K^+)[61,62] and magnesium (Mg^{2+}),[63] together with a gain in sodium (Na^+)[64] and water.[65] On refeeding it is necessary to give potassium,[66] magnesium,[67] phosphorus (as monovalent or divalent phosphate),[66] and zinc (Zn^{2+})[68] to ensure optimum nitrogen retention. Initially the sodium balance may become markedly positive and cause water retention during refeeding, particularly with carbohydrate.[69] This rapid gain in weight, seen during the early phases of resumption of food intake, has been noted clinically—the so-called refeeding edema. Diuresis occurs as the nutritional status improves, and the edema disappears. In emaciated patients refeeding has to be undertaken with caution since pulmonary edema may occur if the attempts are too vigorous. Furthermore, these patients may have hyponatremia[70] due to an inability to excrete free water, perhaps as a result of Mg^{2+} and K^+ deficiencies.[71,72]

SODIUM

Source. Milk, cheese, bread, and cereals are rich sources of sodium. Fruits and potatoes are relatively low in sodium. Processing and preserving foods introduce large amounts of sodium.

Absorption. Sodium is actively transported in association with carbohydrate. The absorption of sodium is enhanced by the ingestion of glucose.

Distribution. Sodium is the most abundant extracellular cation and is responsible for maintaining the osmolality of the extracellular fluid. It is distributed widely in many foods. When intake is restricted, sodium is avidly reabsorbed by the kidneys under the influence of aldosterone. Normally the major part of body sodium is in the extracellular fluid, where it is present in a concentration of about 140 mmol/L. Since extracellular fluid amounts to about 20 per cent of body weight, the total amount of sodium in the extracellular fluid is about 1960 mmol. In contrast the sodium concentration in the intracellular fluid is only about 5 mmol/L and intracellular fluid amounts to 50 per cent of body weight, so that total intracellular sodium therefore is only 175 mmol. Thus total body sodium in the adult will average 30 mmol/kg body weight. In malnourished children it has been shown that total body sodium is increased.[64] In surgical patients, the majority of whom were below 85 per cent of ideal body weight, Hill et al.[73] found that total body sodium was 2789 mmol in patients whose average weight was 51.7 kg. This amounts to 53.9 mmol/kg, close to double the expected normal value of 30 mmol/kg. On giving TPN this rose to a mean of 3038 mmol and was accompanied by an average weight gain of 2.6 kg. Thus total body sodium of these surgical patients increased to 56 mmol/kg, although the authors did not find this elevation to be statistically significant. In another study, using oral diets, Veverbrants et al.[69] indicated that carbohydrate feeding induces sodium retention, which is not seen when isocaloric amounts of fat or protein are fed. Hence it is clear that in malnourished patients great care should be taken to prevent salt and water overload, especially in elderly subjects and those with cardiopulmonary disease. The more malnourished the patient, the greater this danger is, especially when large amounts of carbohydrate are being infused. The obvious clinical manifestation of fluid overload is the appearance of "refeeding edema."

Recommendations. The range of normal intake is given in Table 3–1. In the average patient about 100 to 200 mmol/day of sodium can be given. This amount should be supplemented with extra sodium to cover abnormal losses via the gastrointestinal tract. In severely malnourished patients and those with cardiopulmonary disease the sodium intake should be restricted to 50 to 60 mmol/day and the amount infused gradually increased as the patient tolerates the fluid load. In this context it has been shown that potassium[72] and magnesium[71] deficiency may hinder the excretion of free water, resulting in hyponatremia, because even though total body sodium is increased, total body water is increased even more. Under these circumstances replacement of these two ions and the use of diuretics may be necessary.

POTASSIUM

Source. Potassium is present in a variety of foods and is especially abundant in milk, meat, potatoes, and fruits. Traditionally, orange juice and bananas are given as rich sources of potassium.

Absorption. Potassium absorption in the ileum is a passive process and depends upon the concentration gradient. Potassium is secreted by the colon, and in states of diarrhea this loss may be aggravated, as it may be also by the chronic use of laxatives.

Distribution. Potassium is the main intracellular cation, and its concentration in cells amounts to about 140 mmol/L. On the basis of water distribution in different body compartments, it can be calculated that the 70-kg man has 4900 mmol of intracellular potassium. Based on an average extracellular potassium of 4 mmol/L, the extracellular content of potassium amounts to a total of only 56 mmol, giving a total body potassium of 71 mmol/kg. In children with protein-calorie malnutrition the total body potassium is markedly reduced, but this deficiency is not reflected in lower plasma levels.[61,62] In malnourished surgical patients recalculation of the data by Hill et al.[73] for the total body showed that potassium was only 39 mmol/kg and that TPN increased it to 43 mmol/kg without increasing total body nitrogen. Jeejeebhoy et al.[74] and Russel et al.[75] also noted that

body potassium was disproportionately reduced in malnourished patients compared with nitrogen, and was repleted by short-term (30 days) TPN[74] and oral refeeding[75] without altering total body nitrogen. In contrast, it was noted by Jeejeebhoy et al.[74] that long-term TPN increased both nitrogen and potassium. Accordingly, it should be recognized that potassium deficiency is an integral part of malnutrition and needs repletion apart from nitrogen. Rudman et al.[66] showed that a positive nitrogen balance during glucose-based TPN did not occur unless potassium was also given.

Recommendations. The range of normal dietary intake is noted in Table 3–1. The next question is the potassium requirement during parenteral nutrition. To answer this question three facts need to be considered: first, glucose infusions will increase the need for potassium; second, about 3 mEq of K^+ are retained with each gram of nitrogen; and third, based on the data of both Hill[73] and Jeejeebhoy,[74] the total deficit of potassium may amount to between 800 to 900 mmol in the 50 to 70-kg adult. Hence during TPN relatively larger amounts of potassium need to be infused. The infusion of about 80 to 120 mEq/day will aid in replenishing stores and meeting daily needs.

MAGNESIUM

Source. Milk, meat, cheese, and leafy vegetables are rich in magnesium.

Absorption. Only about 30 per cent of oral intake is absorbed. Most of the absorption takes place in the ileum because of slow transit in that area and the fact that uptake is passive. Absorption is linearly related to intake, without obligatory losses.

Distribution. After potassium, magnesium is the next most abundant intracellular cation. Intracellularly it is bound to protein and is necessary for a number of vital cellular functions which include membrane and mitochondrial integrity, enzyme activation including that of ATPase and adenylate cyclase, and also for the synthesis and stability of nuclear DNA. It is also necessary for control of neuromuscular excitability. The average concentration of magnesium in plasma is 1.0 mmol/L or 2.0 mEq/L. Based on a normal extracellular volume, a 70-kg man has about 14 mmol of magnesium extracellularly. This constitutes only about 3 per cent of the total, since intracellular magnesium is about 500 mmol in the average 70-kg adult. In protein-calorie malnutrition magnesium deficiency has been documented,[63] and in surgical patients Freeman[57] has found that increasing the magnesium intake to about 15 mmol per day improved nitrogen balance. In malnourished patients receiving home TPN we have documented markedly positive magnesium balance and noted that 15 to 17 mmol/day was required to maintain balance and normal serum levels over the long term, figures which agree with the finding of

Freeman.[67] Furthermore it should be noted that in patients with a short bowel the needs were especially high owing to losses from diarrhea and stomal drainage.

CALCIUM

Source. The major source is milk and milk products. Calcium in vegetables is less available because of complexing with phytates and oxalates.

Absorption. The luminal contents influence the availability of calcium. Gastric acid converts calcium to an ionized absorbable chloride salt. In contrast high intraluminal phosphate, fatty acids, oxalates, and phytates bind calcium and prevent absorption. Hence most calcium is absorbed proximally. Bile acids, amino acids and mono- and disaccharides enhance absorption. The mucosal cell binds and pumps calcium aided by a vitamin D–dependent system of calcium-binding protein and a Ca^{2+}-Mg^{2+} ATPase complex. The 1,25-dihydroxy derivative of vitamin D is the most potent facilitator of calcium absorption. Details of calcium metabolism are given in Chapter 40.

Recommendations. The recommended intake of calcium in an oral diet is given in Table 3–1. This intake has to be augmented in patients with short bowel because of increased losses. Calcium should always be added to parenteral nutrition regimens. At least 12 to 15 mmol/day should be given, and in addition more should be added to cover losses in gastrointestinal secretions.

PHOSPHORUS

Source. Milk, meat, and cereals are rich sources of phosphorus.

Absorption. The absorption of phosphorus is remarkably efficient, and 70 to 90 per cent of dietary intake is absorbed. Hence dietary hypophosphatemia is rare.

Distribution. Phosphorus is the major intracellular anion. In the cell, among other functions, it is a part of buffer systems, of energy-storing nucleotides (ATP), of membranes (as phospholipids), and of oxygen transfer systems in the form of erythrocyte 2,3-diphosphoglycerate (2,3-DPG). The total body extraskeletal phosphorus amounts to 600 mmol in the 70-kg man.

Since serum levels are only about 1.2 mmol/L, total extracellular phosphorus is only 17 mmol in the 70-kg man. Thus the majority of this element is in bone or intracellular. Data recalculated from Hill et al.[73] show that the total body phosphorus in malnourished surgical patients was only 281 mmol/kg compared with their normal of 374 mmol/kg. If it is assumed that in acute malnutrition skeletal phosphorus is unchanged, the lower total body phosphorus would suggest that intracellular phosphorus is proportionately even more depleted.

The serum phosphorus falls rapidly during TPN, and the literature is full of reports about the serious effects of hypophosphatemia, which in some cases has proved lethal. Silvis[76] showed that during parenteral nutrition in which all nonprotein calories were given as glucose, serum phosphorus may drop precipitously followed by the development of tremors, impaired mentation, paresthesias, muscular weakness, convulsions, and coma. These symptoms usually occur only when glucose is used to provide all caloric needs for a malnourished patient, i.e., in a system of parenteral nutrition not using fat. However, in our experience this syndrome has not been seen in any patient infused with a mixed fuel (glucose-lipid) based nutrient regimen, and hence such a dual substrate system is safer in severely malnourished patients. In addition Rudman et al.[66] showed that a positive nitrogen balance was associated with phosphorus retention, so that this element is of importance in promoting anabolism.

Recommendation. The phosphorus requirements for a normal oral diet are given in Table 3–1. In patients receiving TPN, the total needs for phosphorus amount to about 14 to 16 mmol/day when a glucose-lipid source of nonprotein energy is being given. These requirements are increased when glucose alone is given as a source of energy. This is due partly to the fact that lipid emulsions have phospholipids which of themselves act as an additional source of phosphorus in the dual energy system, and partly to the high insulin level associated with the glucose-only system, which increases cellular uptake of phosphorus.

MICRONUTRIENTS

The major part of our dietary intake, as covered in the foregoing discussion, is composed of water, proteins, carbohydrates, fats, and electrolytes. However, for the utilization of these nutrients it is essential to absorb other substances, called micronutrients, in relatively smaller and in some instances minute amounts. These micronutrients belong to two main groups of substances called trace elements and vitamins. The former are inorganic elements, while the latter are complex organic compounds. Both are essential because they regulate metabolic processes in many elemental constituents of enzyme complexes regulating the utilization of carbohydrates, proteins, and fats.

Trace Elements

Cotzias[77] defined an essential trace element as one that has the following characteristics: (1) present in the healthy tissues of all living things; (2) constant tissue concentration from one animal to the next; (3) withdrawal leads to a reproducible functional and/or structural abnormality; (4) addition of the element prevents the abnormality; (5) the abnormality is associated with a specific biochemical change; and (6) the biochemical change is prevented and/or cured along with the observed clinical abnormality by giving the nutrient.

In animal studies, 15 elements have been found to be essential for health. They are iron, zinc, copper, chromium, selenium, iodine, cobalt, manganese, nickel, molybdenum, fluorine, tin, silicon, vanadium, and arsenic. However, using the strict criteria suggested by Cotzias,[77] only the first seven have been shown to be necessary for health in humans. Of these cobalt is essential only insofar as it is a part of the corrin ring in vitamin B_{12}. The possibility that nutritional edema may be a sign of vanadium deficiency has been raised by Golden and Golden,[78] and a case of molybdenum deficiency has been described.[79]

GENERAL OBSERVATIONS

Trace elements are absorbed as inorganic substances and as organic compounds. In natural foods the latter often predominate. Since the absorption of the two forms may differ, results of studies with inorganic test substances cannot be equated with the availability of the same elements in organic form in food. For example, heme iron is absorbed very efficiently,[80] and the availability of this form of iron cannot be judged from studies with elemental iron. Similarly, chromium as an inorganic salt is poorly absorbed,[81] but the organic form in yeast is well absorbed.

Absorbed trace elements circulate as protein-bound complexes that are not always in free equilibrium with tissue stores. For example, the exchangeable plasma copper is present in very small amounts bound to albumin.[82] In contrast, the major form of circulating copper, ceruloplasmin, is not freely exchangeable.[83] For this and other reasons total circulating levels may not reflect the availability of an element for nutritional needs.

Tissue stores of a trace element may not be available to meet needs during a period of deficient supply because of two factors. First, they may be incorporated in enzyme proteins that do not exchange with the free pool. Second, during anabolism there is net flow of trace elements into cells, so that cellular stores cannot be mobilized; the converse applies as well in catabolism. For example, in hypercatabolic states, even though zinc is being lost and the patient is in negative zinc balance, deficiency does not occur and plasma zinc is normal because of net outflow from tissue stores.[68] When nutritional support is given, resulting in protein synthesis, a positive zinc balance occurs, but plasma levels fall and deficiency will result unless exogenous zinc is given. Because the action of trace elements depends upon other factors such as age, metabolic and nutritional states (anabolic or catabolic), and availability of agonists and antagonists, clinical deficiency cannot be predicted by simple demonstration of a low blood level of the element. As an example of this complexity, it has been found that at least some degree of selenium deficiency can be overcome by giving vitamin E. Also, children with selenium-responsive Keshan disease have levels of plasma selenium no lower than those in children with phenylketonuria receiving artificial diets, and yet the latter do not show a clinical deficiency.[84]

These findings make it imperative to look for subclinical functional changes to enable us to define needs. For example, even in patients who do not have overt clinical deficiency of zinc, Wolman et al.[68] have shown that a negative zinc balance was associated with reduced nitrogen retention and carbohydrate tolerance, thus justifying the need for maintaining balance. Finally, the route of excretion of most trace elements, excepting chromium, is mainly through the gastrointestinal tract. This raises the possibility that abnormal gastrointestinal losses may raise requirements in patients with disease of the gastrointestinal tract. Another consequence of the gastrointestinal route of excretion is that renal disease does not reduce the need for giving these elements.

IRON[80]

Distribution. Iron is an essential constituent of porphyrin-based compounds bound to protein such as hemoglobin and myoglobin (hence the value of red meat as a food source). In addition, smaller amounts of tissue iron associated with enzymes and mitochondria have important metabolic functions. Iron is also found in storage or transport forms bound to protein as ferritin and transferrin. In storage another protein-free form, hemosiderin, also occurs. The proportion of ferritin to hemosiderin in the liver depends upon the iron concentration. At lower concentrations ferritin predominates and at higher concentrations hemosiderin predominates.[85]

Control of Body Iron Stores. There is little physiological excretion of iron. About 0.2 to 0.5 mg/day is excreted in feces,[86] 0.2 mg in urine,[87] and variable amounts in sweat.[88] The last neverthleless may be high in climates where sweating is profuse. Thus in normal men total losses may amount to 0.6 to 1.0 mg/day. However, in women menstrual losses increase iron loss by an additional 0.5 to 0.8 mg/day or more. Hence iron stores are governed by the control of absorption from the gastrointestinal tract. Substantial absorption is said to occur from the duodenum.

The following factors influence iron absorption:
1. Heme iron is absorbed directly, and its absorption is not sensitive to gastric pH and intestinal factors as is that of non-heme iron, which is absorbed less easily.
2. Normal gastric secretion is necessary to release protein-bound iron in food.

3. Ascorbic and organic acids enhance absorption.
4. Trace elements in large amounts reduce iron absorption.
5. Copper deficiency reduces iron absorption.
6. Iron deficiency, hypoxia, and anemia from various causes increase iron absorption.

Abnormal Iron Losses. Blood loss from the gastrointestinal tract and inflamed surfaces, and bile or small bowel drainage enhance iron losses. Venesection for laboratory tests in hospital adds to this load. Thus in seriously sick patients the need for iron can be increased at times from iatrogenic losses.

Assessment of Iron Requirements. The best means of assessing iron needs is to assay the iron content of bone marrow chemically.[89] A less quantitative method is to evaluate the stainable hemosiderin in the marrow. Ferritin levels in plasma do reflect iron stores in general but are unreliably high in patients with inflammation and liver disease.[90] If there is no inflammation, a plasma ferritin concentration of 1 µg/L corresponds to 140 µg/kg body weight of iron stores.[80] Another situation raising circulating ferritin levels is the administration of iron-dextran injections.

Transferrin saturation determines the flow of iron to tissues, and when it falls below 16 per cent then iron supply is suboptimal.[91] Unfortunately this fall can occur as a result both of deficiency and inflammation. Transferrin levels and serum iron are unreliably low when infection and malnutrition reduce protein synthesis and alter the distribution of iron. Iron released from erythrocytes is taken up by macrophages and then transferred to transferrin. With inflammation macrophages do not release iron, thus reducing circulating serum iron levels and saturation. In malnutrition transferrin synthesis falls and thus circulating iron levels are reduced.

Iron Requirements. Normal males require about 1 mg of absorbed iron per day, menstruating females 2 mg/day. In TPN patients the needs may well be enhanced because of abnormal losses. Unfortunately, no carefully controlled study of iron needs has been done. Peters et al.[92] found that up to 25 mg of iron per week given to patients receiving TPN significantly reduced the need for blood transfusion. However, in patients receiving parenteral nutrition, a combination of factors may alter the availability of iron to the tissues. In these patients a deficiency in tissues can result from a reduction of iron stores, reduced macrophage transfer despite normal stores, or reduced transferrin levels decreasing the availability of total circulating iron. Only the first can be treated by giving more iron.

Recommendations for Intravenous Iron. A dilute solution of iron dextran can be used to provide 1 to 2 mg of iron per day to replace physiologic losses.[93] This should be increased by 1 to 2 mg/day in women. Additional needs due to abnormal losses should be met by infusing a calculated amount of iron-dextran to meet the losses. This has been our practice for the last 4 years and has been carried out in over 1200 patients without adverse reactions. In home TPN (HTPN) patients we give 1 to 2 mg/day and monitor the bone marrow at intervals of 1 to 2 years.

ZINC

Zinc is a widely distributed element in foodstuffs (shellfish, liver, milk, and wheat bran) and in the human body. It has been identified as a part of about 120 enzymes.[94] Among them are carbonic anhydrase, carboxypeptidase, alkaline phosphatase, oxidoreductases, transferases, ligases, hydrolases, lyases, and isomerases. While the syndrome of zinc deficiency cannot be identified with the dearth of any one enzyme, zinc deficiency does have a pronounced effect on nucleic acid metabolism, thus influencing protein and amino acid metabolism.

Zinc is an integral constituent of DNA polymerase, reverse transcriptase, RNA polymerase, tRNA synthetase, and the protein chain elongation factor.[94] Thus zinc deficiency can alter protein synthesis at a number of different points, and it is not surprising that in the absence of zinc, growth arrest occurs.[95] Furthermore, zinc deficiency is teratogenic as determined by animal studies and observations in patients with untreated acrodermatitis enteropathica.[96] This finding suggests that zinc deficiency may affect gene expression. In experimental studies in unicellular organisms it has been shown that zinc deficiency changes the nature of RNA polymerase and the base composition of mRNA. The translated peptides contain a preponderance of arginine-rich peptides which can bind to anions such as phosphate groups in nucleic acids and alter their action. Such an alteration could affect the synthesis of histones, proteins which are known to reduce the activity of DNA as a template.[94]

The above-mentioned experimental findings about zinc and nucleic acids are interesting in view of the clinical observation that a number of functions dependent on protein synthesis are suppressed by zinc deficiency. These include growth,[95] cellular immunity[97,98] (see also Chapter 33), fertility,[95] hair growth,[95] wound healing,[99] and plasma protein levels. Thus it is obvious that zinc deficiency leads to profound disturbances of protein synthesis.

Distribution. Zinc is widely distributed in all soft tissues,[100] blood cells, bone, and teeth.[101] However, zinc at these sites is firmly bound to protein, and during deficiency and refeeding the concentrations of zinc in tissues (with the exception of blood, milk, hair, and liver) do not change significantly.[102] Endogenous stores of zinc are mobilized in the fasting state but do not meet metabolic needs during anabolism, because the net movement of zinc is into tissues and there is little free zinc circulating.

Control of Body Zinc. Zinc absorption has a significant effect on body zinc. Zinc is absorbed by a process which involves binding to a surface receptor, followed by uptake into the enterocyte.[103] The process is saturable and the efficiency of absorption decreases at high zinc intakes. From the enterocyte, some zinc is removed by albumin or an alpha-2 macroglobulin and carried to the liver, the remainder being bound to a metallothionein,[104] the proportion bound depending on the metallothionein content of the enterocyte. Since zinc is not transferred to plasma when so bound, this binding action inhibits absorption.[105] Subsequently such bound zinc returns to the bowel lumen when the enterocyte is shed. When body zinc is high there is a stimulation of metallothionein synthesis, thus inhibiting absorption. In addition, absorption is influenced by the following factors:

1. Binding to a ligand secreted by the pancreas enhances absorption.
2. Luminal amino acids bind zinc and prevent its precipitation by substances such as phosphates and phytates.
3. Pregnancy, corticosteroids, endotoxin, and leukocyte endogenous mediator (LEM) all enhance absorption.
4. Phytates, phosphates, iron, copper, lead, and calcium inhibit absorption.

Excretion. Zinc is excreted mainly in the feces, with a smaller amount in the urine.[87] The fecal losses rise with increased intake, as they consist mainly of unabsorbed zinc shed as noted above. In contrast urinary excretion is not influenced by intake. Significant losses may occur in sweat in the tropics, but such losses diminish with deficiency.[106]

Abnormal Losses. Wolman et al.[68] showed that diarrhea and stomal and fistula losses were the major sites of enhanced abnormal losses of zinc from endogenous sources in patients kept NPO. Increased losses also occurred in urine in hypercatabolic individuals. Amino acid infusions also increase urinary zinc losses. In the kidney, zinc infusions enhance distal reabsorption of zinc, while amino acid infusion increases proximal secretion.[107]

Metabolism of Zinc. As already noted, zinc reaching the circulation is bound to albumin and an alpha-2 macroglobulin.[108] From the circulation it is taken up by the liver and other tissues. Infection results in increased uptake of zinc by the liver.[109] This process is stimulated by leukocyte endogenous mediator (LEM). Enhanced uptake of zinc into the liver reduces plasma concentrations, and so circulating zinc concentrations may be reduced by factors other than deficiency.[110–112]

Assessment of Zinc Status and Requirements. While circulating zinc levels fall in the deficient state, there are other causes of low circulating zinc levels (as noted above) that make this measurement unreliable. Hair zinc levels are low when there is low-grade chronic deficiency, but in acute deficiency hair does not grow, and with profound deficiency hair loss occurs and the remaining hair may have normal zinc concentrations.[113] It has recently been shown that leukocyte zinc levels are a reliable indicator of zinc deficiency, but this is not an easy measurement to perform.[114] Currently the best way of assessing zinc status and requirements is through multiple clinical parameters. Abnormal gastrointestinal losses, hypercatabolism, or amino acid infusions raise the need for zinc supplementation. The clinical syndrome of acrodermatitis enteropathica confirms the need for zinc supplementation.

Zinc Requirements. It is recommended that 15 mg/day of zinc be taken in the diet of adults.[95] Based on a mean absorption of 7 per cent, this amounts to about 1 mg of absorbed zinc per day. In patients receiving parenteral nutrition that included intravenous amino acids, Wolman et al.[68] found that about 2.5 mg/day was required for balance in patients without diarrhea. Requirements increased with increased catabolism and gastrointestinal losses by 12 mg/L of small intestinal fluid and 17 mg/L of stool measured in the NPO state.

Requirements in Infants. In addition to replacing losses, infants need zinc for growth. This is especially true of preterm infants, because two thirds of the infant's zinc is transferred from the mother during the last 10 to 12 weeks of normal gestation. It has been estimated that 0.5 to 0.75 mg of zinc is taken up per day during the last 3 weeks of gestation and the first 3 weeks of postnatal life in babies gaining 1.5 kg, making the requirements about 300 to 500 µg/kg/day.[115] James and MacMahon[116] found that infants required 300 µg/kg/day to maintain balance. In older children 50 µg/kg/day maintained normal serum levels and for growth it is recommended that 100 µg/kg/day be given as a safe intake.[117] In addition supplementation will be required for abnormal gastrointestinal losses, but these have not been determined experimentally.

COPPER

Copper is found in many foods, including organ meats, shellfish, legumes, and cocoa. It is widely distributed in human tissues and is a part of enzymes such as cytochrome *c* oxidase, superoxide dismutase, dopamine beta-hydroxylase, monoamine oxidase, and lysyl oxidase.[118] In addition, 90 per cent of the plasma copper is in the form of ceruloplasmin.[119] The major effects of copper deficiency are expressed through the consequences of ceruloplasmin and lysyl oxidase deficiencies,[120,121] although abnormalities in catecholamine metabolism have also been described as a result of its association with dopamine beta-hydroxylase.[122]

Ceruloplasmin is an iron oxidase. Iron released by red cell breakdown is taken up by macrophages. It is then released from macrophages and bound to transferrin for transport to iron-storing and iron-requiring tissues. Similarly, storage iron in the liver is in equilibrium with transferrin. Ceruloplasmin ox-

$$\text{HC}-(CH_2)_2-\overset{H}{\underset{R}{C}}-\overset{H}{\underset{H}{C}}-NH_2+O_2+H_2O \xrightarrow[\text{oxidase}]{\text{lysyl}} \text{HC}-(CH_2)_2-\overset{H}{\underset{R}{C}}-\overset{H}{C}=O+NH_3+H_2O_2$$

lysyl (R = H)
hydroxylysine (R = OH)

allysyl (R = H)
hydroxyallysyl (R = OH)

idizes ferrous iron and aids in transfer of iron from stores to transferrin.[123] It is believed that iron in cells is reduced by riboflavin to the ferrous form to cross the cell membrane, and that after crossing it has to be reoxidized to the ferric form to bind to transferrin.[124] Therefore copper deficiency results in conditioned iron deficiency.

Mature collagen and elastin are characterized by the presence of crosslinks formed from precursor peptides such as alpha-aminoadipic acid delta-semialdehyde or allysine, and delta-hydroxy-alpha-aminoadipic acid delta-semialdehyde or hydroxyallysine.[125] These substances are formed by the oxidative deamination of peptidyl lysine or hydroxylysine residues (see top of page).[126] This process depends on the copper-containing enzyme lysyl oxidase.

In addition to the effects on iron and collagen, another result of copper deficiency is the phenomenon of leukopenia.[127]

Distribution. Copper is mainly concentrated in liver and brain, with smaller amounts in the heart, kidneys, spleen, and skeleton.[128] Of a total of 23 mg of copper in the human body, 16 mg is found in liver and brain. In the blood, copper circulates mainly as ceruloplasmin and a small amount is also bound to albumin.[129] The latter form is the true transport copper which exchanges with tissue.

Control of Body Copper. Body copper is likely to be controlled by absorption and biliary secretion.[130,131] Copper absorption is enhanced by deficiency and is depressed by phytates, ascorbic acid, and cadmium in the diet. Zinc inhibits copper absorption by promoting intestinal metallothionein synthesis. The increased metallothionein binds copper and prevents its transfer to the circulation.[132] The dietary requirement is estimated to be 2 to 5 mg/day, of which about 32 per cent is absorbed (0.6 to 1.6 mg/day).[119] However, in normal humans balance studies have indicated that an intake of about 1.2 mg/day is sufficient.[133,134] The major route of excretion is via bile, in which about 0.5 to 1.3 mg is excreted per day. The copper excreted in bile is not reabsorbed, and there is no enterohepatic circulation of copper.[119] Urinary losses are very small and amount to a mean of about 10 to 60 µg/day.[119] The intravenous infusion of copper does not increase urinary excretion.[134] Loss of copper in sweat is variable and is estimated to be 0.34 ± 0.24 mg/day.[135]

Abnormalities of Copper Excretion. Diarrhea increases copper losses, but the increase is not related to the volume of diarrhea.[134] Abnormalities of liver function reduce copper losses.[134] Adrenocortical deficiency reduces and excess increases urinary copper excretion.[136] In injured patients urinary copper excretion rises to a mean of 256 µg/day.[137]

Copper Metabolism. Copper in the circulation is bound to albumin and also to amino acids such as histidine, threonine, and glutamine, whence it is taken up by the liver and bone marrow among other sites. In the liver copper is incorporated into ceruloplasmin and released into the circulation or excreted into the bile. In the marrow it is incorporated into erythrocuprein and released as red cells. Ceruloplasmin has also been recognized as donating copper for incorporation into enzymes such as superoxide dismutase, lysyl oxidase, and cytochrome oxidase.[138]

Assessment of Copper Status and Requirements. Plasma copper is reduced in copper deficiency and is also affected by a variety of factors that alter the serum concentration of ceruloplasmin. These include deficiency production due to protein-calorie malnutrition and increased loss in patients with nephrosis, both being situations in which reduced levels of copper are found.[139] Infections, inflammatory conditions, leukemia, and Hodgkin's disease all increase the levels of serum copper.[140] Oral contraceptive agents likewise increase plasma copper levels to 300 ± 7 µg/dl from a mean normal of 118 ± 2 µg/dl.[141] For reasons already noted, the copper content of hair is not a reliable index of this element's deficiency.[142]

Copper Requirements. The normal diet supplies 2 to 4 mg/day, and on this intake deficiency has never been observed in adults. In utero a major part of body copper is gained during the last 10 weeks of gestation,[115] and it is estimated that a premature or neonatal infant will retain 100 to 130 µg/kg/day over a 3-week period. In malnourished infants between 40 and 135 µg/kg/day will be required.

In adult patients receiving a parenteral nutrition regimen, Shike et al.[134] found that 0.3 mg/day was sufficient to meet the needs of patients without diarrhea. Requirements rose to 0.5 mg/day in those with diarrhea. In contrast, requirements fell to 0.1 mg/day in patients with abnormal liver function[134] (owing to reduced excretion in bile). These figures compare well with those of Jacobson and Western,[143] who obtained a positive balance with all patients but one by giving 0.24 to 0.29 mg of copper per day. In critically ill patients Phillips and Garnys[144] have recommended 0.5 mg/day. In infants the need, based on balance, is for 50 μg/kg/day. However, the range varies between 10 and 50 μg/kg/day.[116] Hence caution should be exercised in order to avoid overload, and the lower figure of 20 μg/kg/day has been suggested. In older children 20 μg/kg/day has been found sufficient to meet needs.[117]

CHROMIUM

Good dietary sources of chromium are brewer's yeast, corn oil, vegetables, and whole grains. Chromium deficiency in animals has been found to cause a syndrome of glucose intolerance similar to that of clinical diabetes. The abnormalities found were corrected by giving chromium.[145] This element is also important in promoting insulin action in peripheral tissues. In vitro chromium enhances insulin stimulation of glucose oxidation and lipogenesis in adipose tissue.[145] In muscle it also increases insulin-induced glycogenesis. Insulin-stimulated amino acid transport is also positively influenced by chromium.[146]

This set of observations in animals is supported by the finding that the intravenous administration of chromium increased glucose utilization in a patient with chromium deficiency.[147] Chromium administration to this patient also increased the fall in circulating leucine levels in response to a glucose load.[147] Since the insulin response to the glucose load was normal, the above observation suggests that chromium enhances insulin-stimulated tissue uptake of leucine. The respiratory quotient (RQ) was low and the plasma free fatty acid (FFA) levels were high before the administration of chromium. The low RQ and high FFA levels show that fat mobilization and oxidation were continuing despite normal insulin levels. Administration of chromium reduced free fatty acid levels, increased the RQ, and promoted glucose oxidation for energy. Thus chromium is one of the factors that influences insulin sensitivity.

Distribution. Chromium is distributed throughout the human body and its concentration declines with age.[148] Thus it would be expected that glucose intolerance would increase with age, and indeed such an increase is well known. If chromium deficiency were the cause of this increased intolerance, then chromium substitution should improve glucose tolerance. To test this hypothesis Offenbacher and Pi-Sunyer[149] did a controlled trial in older persons, comparing the effect of giving brewer's yeast, a preparation rich in chromium (in a bound form), with giving another yeast (*Torula*) that contains almost no chromium. Those receiving the brewer's yeast improved their glucose tolerance by comparison with those given the *Torula* yeast. Hence a decline in body chromium may contribute to the glucose intolerance of the elderly.

Control of Body Chromium. Chromium is probably absorbed as organic compounds; inorganic chromium is absorbed to an extent that is less than 3 per cent of the dose.[81] In contrast, chromium in yeast is absorbed to the extent of 10 to 25 per cent of the oral dose.[150] Absorption is inhibited by zinc and phytate. However, since these last absorption studies were done with inorganic chromium, the relation of these findings to chromium in food is not clear. In natural foods chromium exists as a dinicotino-glutathionine complex[151] called glucose tolerance factor (GTF).[152] This organic complex appears to be the form in which chromium becomes available from food. As indicated earlier, this form of chromium is absorbed easily, and animal studies have confirmed its ability to enhance the action of insulin upon glucose metabolism.

Excretion occurs in the urine and urinary losses are enhanced by glucose loading in diabetic subjects (degree of "control" not stated).[153] Smaller amounts are lost in stool. Total chromium losses in healthy adults amount to between 5.9 and 10.0 μg/day.[154] This is increased to 19.2 μg/day in diabetics. In one patient receiving parenteral nutrition, losses amounted to about 20 μg/day.[147]

Assessment of Chromium Status and Requirements. This area is as yet not clearly defined. Plasma chromium levels are reduced in deficiency but are also reduced by acute illness[155] and increased by glucose loads in young healthy subjects and in diabetics during periods of improved glucose tolerance (presumably by insulin administration).[156] Hair chromium declines in situations likely to be associated with deficiency.[147] Urinary chromium excretion in response to a glucose challenge has been used as an indirect index of deficiency. At present it appears that the only convincing way of assessing chromium deficiency is to demonstrate abnormal glucose clearance responding to chromium supplementation.

Chromium Requirements. In the adult, oral chromium requirements have not been determined. Deficiency in patients receiving total parenteral nutrition[147,157,157a] may be due to continuous glucose loading resulting in a higher urinary excretion, which in turn increases requirements. It was estimated that in one such patient the needs might have been increased to 10 to 20 μg/day.[147] In infants, balance studies by James et al.[116] indicated a requirement of 0.14 to 0.2 μg/kg/day. However, balance studies in more patients with a spectrum of clinical conditions need to be done to obtain the required information.

SELENIUM AND VITAMIN E

These two substances are interrelated in their actions, and a deficiency of one can be partially corrected by giving the other. To understand the need for these two micronutrients it is necessary to examine the alternative means by which oxygen is reduced in biological systems. Normally the enzyme cytochrome oxidase accepts electrons from cytochrome *c* at the end exposed to the cytosol and discharges them by reacting with $4H^+$ to form water.[158] The alternative path involves the monovalent addition of electrons to form superoxide.[159] The superoxide, if left unaltered, disproportionates to H_2O_2 and oxygen. The H_2O_2 can also react by the Haber-Weiss[160] reaction with superoxide to form hydroxyl ions. Thus in the absence of appropriate controls, a number of reactive peroxide and hydroxyl radicals can form and damage the cell. In well-nourished cells superoxide dismutase (SOD) disproportionates superoxide to H_2O_2, and the peroxide so formed is reduced by glutathione peroxidase (GSHpx) to water.

$$O_2 \xrightarrow{e^-} O_2^- \xrightarrow{e^-} O_2^{2-}$$

$$O_2^- + H_2O_2 \rightarrow O_2 + OH^- + OH\cdot$$

$$O_2^- + H^+ \xrightarrow{SOD} H_2O_2 \xrightarrow{GSHpx} H_2O$$

Glutathione peroxidase is an enzyme made up of four subunits each containing selenocysteine as an integral part of the molecule.[161] In association with superoxide dismutase it controls the levels of superoxide and peroxide in the cell. This in turn affects lipid peroxidation of polyunsaturated fatty acids in cell membranes. Vitamin E is the second line of defense and controls the formation of hydroperoxides in the fatty acid residues of phospholipids, a process which depends on the antioxidant role of the vitamin and also involves its entering into a structural relation with membrane phospholipids.[162] Finally, any lipid hydroperoxides may be reduced by GSHpx to hydroxyacids.

Biological reactions that produce superoxide are (1) enzyme reactions such as those involving xanthine oxidase and galactose oxidase; (2) metabolic pathways such as the hexose monophosphate shunt and oxidative reactions mediated by cytochrome p_{450}; (3) interaction of dioxygen with the electron transport chain in the mitochondria; and (4) phagocytosis, where a burst of oxidative metabolism is associated with generation of NADPH by the hexose monophosphate shunt, which in turn is used by NADPH oxidase to generate superoxide. The excess superoxide is controlled by SOD and GSHpx. Hence it is not surprising that bacterial killing is affected by selenium deficiency. In addition, some antibiotics such as bleomycin produce superoxide.

Thus a number of different pathophysiological situations and metabolic states can increase superoxide evolution and the need for protection by vitamin E and GSHpx.

Distribution. Selenium is present in good concentration in seafood (tuna), meat, and onions, and in all cells of the body. Liver, kidney, and pancreas have the highest concentrations.[163] Cardiac muscle is a close fourth. These levels are responsive to dietary intake. In blood selenium is present in plasma and red cells. In tissues selenium occurs as a part of GSHpx or as seleno-substituted sulfur-containing amino acids.

Control of Body Selenium. Selenium in inorganic and organic form is absorbed in the duodenum and carried in the plasma to tissues. Absorption is very efficient and amounts to between 76 and 100 per cent of an oral dose.[164] It is excreted in the feces, urine, and breath. In human studies with orally ingested selenite, 14 to 20 per cent was excreted during the first week in the urine and 33 to 58 per cent in stool over 3 weeks. The half-life was found to have a slow component of 96 to 144 days.[165]

Metabolism. Absorbed selenium is initially bound to albumin and also, after being processed by red cells, circulates in association with beta-lipoprotein.[166] It is taken up by tissues and incorporated into proteins and GSHpx. Selenium is excreted in both feces and urine. Fecal excretion varies between 57 and 61 per cent and urinary excretion between 29 and 43 per cent of total losses.[167,168]

Assessing Selenium Status and Requirements. Plasma selenium and GSHpx levels are sensitive to selenium intake[166] and can be used to assess the need for this element. However, in functional terms selenium and vitamin E are interrelated, and it has not been determined how much the supply of one conditions the need for the other in humans.

Abnormal Losses. The concentration of selenium in wounds and pus may be as high as 130 μg/L, and in fistula fluids 100 to 380 μg/L, in patients living in a low-selenium diet area (e.g., New Zealand).[169,170] Similar data are not available for other parts of the world.

Selenium Requirements. The dietary intake of selenium varies from a low of 18 to 26 μg/day in New Zealand[87,171] to a high of 150 to 220 μg/day in Canada.[172] Garlic contains substantial amounts of the element. Human metabolic studies would suggest a minimum intake of 20 μg/day,[168] and in studies from China 30 μg/day was considered to constitute a minimal intake.[173] In North American volunteers, the requirements have been estimated to be 54 μg/day.[167]

Patients receiving parenteral nutrition may develop selenium deficiency with associated muscle pains, and in two patients receiving long-term TPN cardiomyopathy has also been described.[174-176] However, the need for selenium will be conditioned by other factors such as vitamin E status, heavy metal intake, abnormal losses, and the presence of oxidants and other antioxidants. These aspects require resolution.

Selenium–Vitamin E Interaction. In animals it has been shown that the myonecrosis induced by a diet deficient in selenium and vitamin E can be corrected by giving either one to the animal.[177] They protect equally well against several experimentally induced cardiomyopathies in animals. In patients receiving TPN the amount of vitamin E required to prevent functional changes appears to be five times as great as the recommended dietary allowances.[178] This could be due to the fact that selenium was not added to the TPN solutions used.

Assessment of Vitamin E Status. Vitamin E status can be estimated from the circulating levels of the vitamin and functionally by observing the red cell hemolysis induced by peroxide[179] and the platelet aggregation response to the addition of ADP.[180] Experimentally it has been shown that with vitamin E deficiency, lipid peroxidation increases and this results in increased ethane and pentane loss in the breath.[181] Monitoring breath ethane and pentane may be a means of assessing lipid peroxidation.

Peroxidation cleaves the polyunsaturated fatty acid molecule at the first double bond from the methyl end. The size of the alkane thus released depends on the omega number of the fatty acid involved.

Peroxy fatty acid

$$CH_3-(CH_2)_3-CH_2-CH-CH=CH-R \dashrightarrow$$
$$| $$
$$\overset{.}{O}$$

$$CH_3-(CH_2)_3-\overset{.}{C}H_2 + \quad \overset{H}{\underset{O}{\overset{\diagdown}{C}}}-CH=CH-R$$

$$+ \cdot H \downarrow$$

$$CH_3-(CH_2)_3-CH_3 \qquad \text{Lipid peroxide}$$
$$\text{Pentane}$$

Requirements for Vitamin E. The RDA of vitamin E is 10 IU of alpha-tocopherol per day. However, in TPN patients Thurlow and Grant found that correction of resistance to peroxide-induced hemolysis and normalization of platelet aggregation with ADP required about 50 IU per day.[178] This requirement has not been studied with different amounts of selenium in the infusion. In home TPN patients, the same amounts were required to maintain normal levels.[182] This area needs further study.

MANGANESE

The role of this trace element is not well defined in the human. It is important for the action of glycosyltransferases.[183] In this role its deficiency leads to abnormality of cartilage growth in young animals. In addition it appears to be necessary for the action of vitamin K in adding the carbohydrate component of prothrombin to the preprothrombin protein. In this regard Doisy[184] described a patient in whom vitamin K could not correct prothrombin levels until the patient was given manganese. Finally, the mitochondria are very rich in manganese, and at that site manganese is an essential component of mitochondrial superoxide dismutase.[185] Rich food sources of this element are whole-grain cereals, dried legumes, and especially tea.

Distribution. The human body contains 12 to 20 mg of manganese, which is mainly distributed in the mitochondria.[186]

Control of Body Manganese. Only 3 to 4 per cent of an oral dose of manganese is absorbed.[187] Manganese is very efficiently excreted by the intestine. Excretion occurs mainly in bile with lesser amounts in pancreatic juice and through the intestinal wall. There is negligible excretion of manganese in the urine. The absorption of manganese is enhanced with low intakes and depressed when intake is high.

Metabolism. Manganese in circulation is bound to a beta-globulin, transferrin. It is taken up rapidly by the mitochondria and at a slower rate by the nuclei. The manganese in cells is in dynamic equilibrium with that in the circulation. Intake in excess of needs increases excretion into the gastrointestinal tract.[188]

Requirements. The dietary intake varies but is between 2 and 3 mg/day.[189] The amount retained varies between 50 and 400 μg/day.[190] Patients receiving home TPN that contained 2.0 mg/day had elevated levels of whole blood manganese.[182] However, requirements have not been determined for human TPN.

MOLYBDENUM

Molybdenum is an essential component of xanthine oxidase,[191] sulfite oxidase,[192] and aldehyde oxidase.[193] Xanthine oxidase catalyzes the conversion of oxypurines to uric acid. In its absence the levels of oxypurines will rise and those of uric acid fall. Sulfite oxidase similarly influences the conversion of sulfite to sulfate. The lack of sulfite oxidase has been shown to be responsible for neurological abnormalities,[194] and it is of interest that Abumrad et al.[195] described a TPN patient who developed coma when infused with amino acid solutions containing sulfite. The coma was reversible by supplementing the TPN solutions with 300 μg of molybdenum per day. The concurrent finding of hyperoxipurinemia, hypouricemia, and low sulfate excretion, also corrected by giving molybdenum, is supportive evidence for molybdenum deficiency as a cause of this syndrome. Legumes, organ meats, and yeast are relatively good food sources of this element.

Distribution of Molybdenum. Human liver and kidney have the highest concentrations of molybdenum.[128]

Control of Body Molybdenum. This element, in the molybdate hexavalent form, is easily absorbed from salts and from herbage.[196] Excretion is mainly in the urine, but urinary excretion rises as sulfate intake or endogenous sulfate production increases. Interestingly, urinary copper excretion rises in humans on a high-molybdenum diet. Hence copper requirements will be influenced by molybdenum intake.

Abnormal Losses. Patients with Crohn's disease have been found to excrete 600 µg of molybdenum in stools per day.[197]

Requirements. These are not known, but preliminary balance studies indicate that individuals may be in equilibrium with as little as 48 to 96 µg/day. However, if patients have abnormal losses then requirements may become much larger. Abumrad et al.[195] gave 300 µg/day to restore the metabolism of the patient referred to earlier with Crohn's disease and short bowel. More studies are required.

All other trace elements, including fluorine, tin, arsenic, silicon, vanadium, cadmium, lead, and mercury, have not been shown to be of dietary importance in the human, and some such as lead, aluminum, cadmium, and mercury, may be toxic. Clearly much more needs to be done to assess the requirements of substances like selenium, molybdenum, and chromium in TPN patients, especially those with gastrointestinal losses and those with acute illness.

Vitamins

Vitamins are essential nutrients which are active in minute quantities. While it seems obvious that these substances have to be included in any regimen of total parenteral nutrition (TPN) in order to avoid deficiency, their optimum dose and frequency of administration have not been studied in detail (with the exception of vitamin D) in patients receiving TPN. The current available studies and the recommendations based on them have been simple observations of plasma or blood levels during a given regimen.[198-200]

FAT-SOLUBLE VITAMINS

Vitamin A. Vitamin A occurs in nature in three forms. All-trans-retinol or A_1 and 3-dehydroretinol or A_2 are the forms found in mammals. In vegetables it occurs as the precursor beta-carotene.

Characteristics. Vitamin A is a reddish-yellow crystalline substance, easily oxidized but stable to acids and alkalies in the absence of oxygen. It is composed of a six-membered carbocyclic ring with an 11-carbon side chain.

Units. One international unit (1 IU) = 1 USP unit = 0.3 µg A_1 alcohol or 0.6 µg beta-carotene. One retinol equivalent (1 RE) corresponds to the biological activity in humans of 1 µg retinol (3.33 IU of A_1) or 6 µg beta-carotene (10 IU).

Sources. Vitamin A: fish liver oils (0.1 to 5 million IU/100 g), liver (2700 to 50,000 IU/100 g), egg yolk (3200 IU/100 g), milk (seasonal variations, 130 to 1000 IU/100 g); carotenoids: palm oil (50,000 to 500,000 IU/100 g), green leaved and yellow root vegetables (8000 to 9000 IU/100 g).

Absorption. Vitamin A is absorbed as the ester; this process is aided by micellar solubilization, which requires bile salts. In the mucosa it is incorporated into chylomicrons and carried through the lymphatics. After an oral dose peak levels are reached in 3 to 4 hours. Carotene is oxidized to two molecules of retinaldehyde and the latter is reduced to retinol,[201] the transport and storage form of the vitamin. The availability of carotene from vegetables is incomplete and is further reduced in infants and in hypothyroid subjects.[202] Conversion is also reduced in diabetes and in intestinal, liver, and renal diseases.[203]

Storage. Retinol is stored mainly in the liver but also in the lungs and the gonads. Total body retinol varies between 300 and 900 mg. From the liver retinol is secreted bound to retinol-binding protein as the free alcohol.

Function. The whole body is affected by vitamin A because it aids the sugar transfer in glycoprotein synthesis. However, its most prominent clinical effect is seen in the eyes. In the retina, in the form of 11-cis-retinal, it is associated with a protein, opsin, to form the light-sensitive pigment rhodopsin. When light strikes rhodopsin the 11-cis-retinal is isomerized to all-trans-retinal with dissociation from the rhodopsin molecule.[204] This process releases Ca^{2+}, which results in a nerve impulse.

Normal Values. Circulating levels of vitamin A and other vitamins are given in Table 3–2.

Deficiency. Reduced intake due to lack of animal and vegetable food items containing vitamin A or carotene, malabsorption, liver disease, and loss of retinol in the urine in the nephrotic syndrome will result in a fall in the circulating retinol levels to below 10 µg/ml with the development of symptoms. Patients receiving TPN may also become deficient if the vitamin is added to the infusion too far in advance of its administration, owing to its moderately rapid degradation. Clinically vitamin A deficiency results in night blindness due to decreased rod function. In addition, because glycoprotein synthesis is reduced there is drying of the conjunctiva (xerophthalmia), hyperkeratosis of the skin, and an increased susceptibility to infection. The xerosis of the eye is manifested as shiny gray foamy triangular areas called Bitot's spots and may cause corneal ulceration and blindness. Regarding the diagnosis of deficiency it should be noted that the plasma concentration may not fall to a deficiency level at the time the first symptoms arise. The reliable diagnostic test is a study of the electroretinogram and of dark adaptation.

Toxicity. Toxicity results from eating polar bear liver, food faddism, and inappropriately high doses as therapy. There is acute abdominal pain, nausea, headache, and dizziness. If intake exceeds 40,000 IU/day a syndrome characterized by bone and joint pains, hair loss, dryness of lips, intracranial hypertension, and hepatomegaly occurs. Although the levels of retinol ester are high, the retinol-binding protein level is normal.

Carotenemia. Upon eating a large excess of caro-

TABLE 3–2. *Assessment of Vitamin Status and Normal Values*

Assay	Normal Range	Deficiency Level
Plasma retinol (μg/dl)	20–80	<10
Plasma alpha-tocopherol (μg/ml)	7–20	<5
Blood thiamine (ng/ml)[222]	25–75	<17
Plasma thiamine (ng/ml)	15–42	<10
Urinary thiamine (μg/g creatinine)	66–129	<27
Erythrocyte transketolase stimulation (%)[223]	0–15	>25
Blood riboflavin (μg/dl)[224]	10–50	<10
Serum riboflavin (μg/dl)[224]	4–24	<4
Urinary riboflavin (μg/g creatinine)	>79	<27
Glutathione reductase stimulation (%)	0–20	>40
Plasma pyridoxal (ng/ml)	$\geq$8	<5
Plasma vitamin B_6 (ng/ml)[225]	>50	<25
Urinary free vitamin B_6 (μg/g creatinine)	$\geq$20	<20
Erythrocyte aminotransferase (formerly oxaloacetic transaminase) stimulation test (EGOT) (%)[225]	<50	>50
Tryptophan load test (xanthurenic acid mg/day)[225,226]	<25	>50
Serum niacin (μg/ml)	3–6	<3
Urinary N^1-methylnicotinamide[227] (mg/24 hr)	5.8 ± 3.6	<0.5
Urinary 2-pyridone/N^1-methylnicotinamide ratio[227]	3.60 ± 1.06	<1.0
Urinary pantothenic acid (mg/g creatinine)	$\geq$2.0	<2.0
Plasma ascorbic acid (mg/dl)	>0.30	<0.20
Platelet ascorbic acid (μmol/10^9)[228]	0.017–0.043	<0.008
Plasma biotin (pg/ml)[229]	520 ± 220	
Urinary biotin (μg/day)[230]	6–50	<6

Data from reference 221 except as noted otherwise.

tene-containing foods such as carrots, or in patients with hypothyroidism who cannot convert beta-carotene to retinol, the plasma carotene levels rise and the patient turns yellow. Retinol levels are normal as there is still regulation of the conversion of carotene to retinol.

Requirements and Treatment of Deficiency. The Recommended Nutrient Intake for Canadians (RNIFC) for this vitamin in patients taking an oral diet is given in Table 3–1. Patients with steatorrhea, short bowel, bile salt deficiency, and jaundice will require larger amounts to offset malabsorption. In such patients doses of 10,000 to 30,000 IU/day may have to be given while the plasma vitamin A levels are monitored. For example, a recent study[205] of patients with pancreatic malabsorption showed subclinical deficiency in a significant number.

In patients receiving TPN the American Medical Association (AMA) recommendations are 3300 IU/day.[200] We have demonstrated normal levels of plasma vitamin A in long-term home TPN patients receiving 2500 IU/day.[182]

When deficiency is noted, and especially if xerosis is seen, then it is a medical emergency requiring 10,000 IU/kg/day of retinol for 5 days followed by 5000 IU/kg/day until the lesion has healed. In others 30,000 IU/day for a week should be given.

Vitamin D. See Chapter 40.

Vitamin E. There are seven forms of vitamin E.

Four of these, alpha-, beta-, gamma-, and delta-tocopherols, have biologic activities in the proportion of 100:30:20:1.

Characteristics. All forms are viscous oils, insoluble in water and stable to the effects of light, heat, and acids under anaerobic conditions. On the other hand, they are easily oxidized and decomposed by ultraviolet light and alkalies.

Units. One international unit (1 IU) = 1.0 mg of racemic alpha-tocopheryl acetate or 0.67 D-alpha tocopherol equivalents.

Sources. The tocopherols are distributed in green plants. Rich sources are wheat germ oil (150 IU/100 g), whole wheat (1 IU/100 g), oils (15 to 60 IU/100 g), and wheat germ (14 IU/100 g).

Absorption. Micellar solubilization by bile salts is necessary for absorption of vitamin E.[206] In addition, although concomitant absorption of fat in general enhances absorption, linolenate inhibits it.

Storage. The absorbed vitamin is stored in adipose tissue (0.1 to 1.1 mg/g of fat).

Function. Vitamin E protects against the action of superoxide (see preceding section on Selenium).

Normal Values. Circulating levels are given in Table 3–2.

Deficiency. Clinically in children vitamin E deficiency has been associated with hemolytic anemia. In patients with severe steatorrhea (as in abetalipoproteinemia and biliary atresia), vitamin E deficiency has been shown to be responsible for neurological syndromes associated with spinocerebellar degeneration and neuropathy. A patient receiving home TPN who developed deficiency showed retinal damage which was partially restored by giving the vitamin.[207] Subclinical deficiency, shown by increased red cell hemolysis and increased platelet aggregation, has been noted in patients receiving TPN.[178]

Requirements. The RNIFC for patients taking an oral diet is given in Table 3–1. In patients receiving TPN the AMA committee has recommended 10 mg/day.[200] However, in home TPN patients we found that about 50 mg/day was required to maintain normal levels.[182] Thurlow and Grant[178] found the same in patients receiving TPN. The question of whether the infusion of polyunsaturated fatty acids (PUFA) in lipid emulsions increases the need for vitamin E is, as yet, not settled, although previous studies suggest that this may be so.

Vitamin K. There are several chemical forms of vitamin K, but all are characterized by a quinone ring connected to a side chain which varies with the compound. Three main forms, K_1 (synthesized by plants), K_2 (of microbial origin), and the synthetic parent compound K_3 or menadione (2-methyl-1,4-naphthoquinone) are important in human nutrition. K_2 is formed in the gut by bacteria through the removal of the side chain from longer-chain analogues.

Characteristics. All forms of vitamin K are soluble in fats and are heat stable, but unstable in alkali and light.

Units. The reference unit is 1 mg of synthetic menadione.

Sources. Green vegetables are the chief source, as the vitamin K content of fruits, milk, and meat is minimal. Endogenous gut bacteria synthesize vitamin K, and therefore dietary deficiency does not occur normally.

Absorption and Storage. Absorption of K_2 in the colon and of menadione in the distal intestine and colon is by a passive process facilitated by bile salts and fatty acids.[208–210] By contrast, absorption of K_1, chiefly in the jejunum, requires an energy-dependent process.[211] The vitamin is absorbed into lymph, but little is stored. Since vitamin K_2 may supply as much as 50 per cent of the total vitamin K required, the need for dietary vitamin K may be modified in the presence of an intact colon with bacteria.

Function. Vitamin K is required for the gamma-carboxylation of glutamic acid in the synthesis of a number of proteins in liver, bone, and kidney, including the clotting factors II (prothrombin), VII, IX, and X.

Deficiency. Deficiency of vitamin K occurs in situations in which there is fat malabsorption, such as celiac disease, obstructive jaundice, and short bowel. In addition the use of antibiotics may reduce endogenous flora, thereby causing deficiency. The main result of deficiency is a bleeding tendency noted at venepuncture sites, spontaneous bruising, hematuria, and gastrointestinal hemorrhage. The prothrombin time is prolonged and can be corrected by giving vitamin K. Warfarin also inhibits gamma-carboxylation and antagonizes the action of vitamin K. Liver disease results in hypoprothrombinemia because of depressed liver protein synthesis.

Requirement. During parenteral nutrition 10 mg of menadione once a week has been sufficient to prevent any abnormalities of prothrombin time. When it is necessary to reverse the action of anticoagulants, K_1 is the most potent preparation and reverses the coagulation abnormality within 6 to 8 hours. The synthetic preparation can then be given for maintenance.

WATER-SOLUBLE VITAMINS

These vitamins are distinguished by the fact that most contain nitrogen (unlike fat-soluble vitamins) and are components of coenzymes catalyzing biochemical reactions. Five of these vitamins are especially concerned with energy metabolism: thiamine, riboflavin, niacin, biotin, and pantothenate.

Thiamine (B_1)

Characteristics. Thiamine contains an amine group and a thiazole residue. The biologically active form has two phosphate groups in thiamine pyrophosphate (formerly known as cocarboxylase). The hydrochloride salt is soluble and resistant to oxidation, but is the most labile in solution. In contrast, the powder is much more stable, but it too is labile when dissolved, especially in alkaline solution. Of note is that the addition of baking soda to vegetables and the SO_2 preservation of fruits destroy this vitamin.

Units. One international unit (1 IU) = 0.003 μg of thiamine hydrochloride.

Sources. In the ordinary diet most thiamine comes from the consumption of cereals and enriched grain products. However, the highest amounts are found in pork, legumes, and wheat germ.

Absorption. Absorption occurs in the upper small intestine and is by active transport when small amounts are taken. Larger amounts may be absorbed by passive diffusion. Barbiturates and ethanol reduce absorption.

Storage. The total body stores of about 30 mg are divided, half being in muscle and the rest in viscera.

Function. This vitamin catalyzes reactions that involve the metabolism of aldehyde groups. One such reaction is decarboxylation of alpha-keto acids, in which thiamine pyrophosphate converts pyruvate to acetyl CoA and CO_2, and alpha-ketoglutarate to succinyl CoA and CO_2. Another reaction is metabolism of alpha-ketols, in which thiamine is present in transketolase.

Normal Values. See Table 3–2.

Clinical Effects of Deficiency. In adults there are two clinical syndromes of deficiency. *Wet beriberi* presents as high-output left ventricular heart failure. Severe physical exertion and a high carbohydrate intake tend to result in wet beriberi. Peripheral vasodilation results in tachycardia and increased central venous pressure. There is also sodium retention and edema. When treated, peripheral vasoconstriction occurs and worsens existing hypertension. If the deficiency is acute, then there is severe dyspnea, intense thirst, and acute cardiac failure. Physical findings include glove-stocking cyanosis, marked cardiomegaly, and hepatomegaly.

Dry beriberi is usually associated with neuropathy and Wernicke-Korsakoff psychosis. There is symmetrical motor and sensory dysfunction affecting all four limbs due to demyelination. With Wernicke's syndrome there is nystagmus followed by ophthalmoplegia and ataxia. After these symptoms the patient develops confusion and coma, and may die. Treatment improves symptoms, but total regression may not occur. Nystagmus and ataxia may remain, but after some late improvement, Korsakoff's psychosis may be a residual phenomenon. The patient will have retrograde amnesia, confabulation, and impaired ability to learn, but is otherwise alert and shows no other behavioral disturbance.

Biochemical Abnormalities in Deficiency. There is a rise in blood lactate, pyruvate, and alpha-ketoglutarate levels. In addition, there is a fall in blood and urinary thiamine. The most reliable means of diagnosing deficiency is by observing an increase in erythrocyte transketolase activity when thiamine pyrophosphate is added to the in vitro assay. A rise of more than 15 per cent occurs in deficiency states.

Requirements. The requirements are proportional to the intake of carbohydrate and average 0.5 mg/1000 kcal ingested per day. There have been three studies of TPN with fixed doses of thiamine that measured transketolase activity. With 1.2 mg/day a few patients developed deficiency.[212] In another study, 5 mg/day was found to be sufficient.[213] The third study[214] used massive doses of thiamine and showed that B$_1$-dependent enzyme activity was not increased by adding vitamin B$_1$ in vitro to red cells, indicating no deficiency either before or after TPN. Thus the recommendation of the nutrition advisory group of the Food and Nutrition Department of the American Medical Association is 3 mg/day in adults and spans the range of 1.2 to 5 mg.[200] However, the optimal value in critically sick patients has not been determined, although 55 mg/day avoids deficiency.[213] In home TPN patients, 50 mg twice weekly avoids deficiency.

Riboflavin (B$_2$)

Characteristics. Riboflavin is a yellow-orange compound, only slightly soluble in water. It is then most stable, and oxidizes slowly. However, it is unstable in alkaline solutions (like thiamine) and in bright light. Hence it should be stored in acid solutions and protected from light, especially ultraviolet. Chemically it is a flavin combined with ribitol.

Sources. Milk, milk products, and vegetables are the main sources of dietary riboflavin. Whole grains and enriched bread are also good sources of this vitamin. Milk should be kept in opaque containers to avoid photodegradation of this vitamin.

Absorption. Riboflavin is absorbed and phosphorylated in the intestine. Absorption is by a specific transporter. It is of interest that fecal riboflavin levels are high because of bacterial synthesis in the bowel. The nutritional significance of bacterial riboflavin is unknown.

Storage. Storage of riboflavin is minimal.

Function. Riboflavin is a component of mono- and dinucleotides with adenine as flavin mononucleotide (FMN) and flavin adenine dinucleotide (FAD). These compounds combine with proteins to form enzymes called flavoproteins. These enzymes are concerned with dehydrogenation and oxidation reactions involving pyruvate, acetyl-CoA, and amino acids. In the process the flavin becomes reduced by accepting hydrogen. The reduced form is reoxidized and again available to accept hydrogen. It also acts as a part of the electron transfer chain (Fig. 3–1).

Normal Values. See Table 3–2.

Clinical Effects of Deficiency. In a deficiency state there may be sore throat, stomatitis, glossitis, and seborrheic dermatitis of the face, trunk, and scrotum. In addition photophia and vascularization of the cornea have been observed. Marrow aplasia and a normocytic normochromic anemia may occur.

Biochemical Abnormalities in Deficiency. Reduced urinary excretion of riboflavin and reduced levels of erythrocyte glutathione reductase activity are observed.

Requirements. The oral intake should be 0.6 mg/1000 kcal. Hence in an average adult intake should be 1.2 to 1.6 mg/day. For TPN the AMA[200] recommends 3.6 mg/day in adults. In other studies 1.8 to 10 mg have been used and shown to be adequate biochemically.[212,214]

Pantothenic Acid

Characteristics. This acid is a yellow liquid but as a salt is a water-soluble powder. It is not stable in acid or alkaline solutions.

Sources. Pantothenic acid is found in all foods except fruit, especially in liver, eggs, mushrooms, milk, and milk products.

Absorption. The mechanism of absorption is not well known but is probably diffusion.

Storage. Small amounts are stored in liver, adrenal glands, brain, kidneys, and heart as coenzyme A.

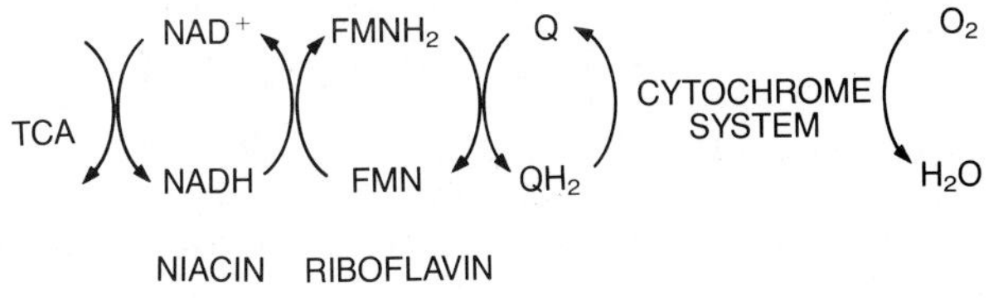

FIGURE 3–1. *Role of water-soluble vitamins in electron transfer.*

Function. Pantothenic acid is a component of the acyl carrier protein required for fatty acid metabolism and as a coenzyme (CoA) becomes a component of acetyl CoA, which is central to the metabolism of carbohydrates, proteins, and fats. It is also the entry point of substrates from these sources into the tricarboxylic acid (Krebs) cycle.

Normal Values. See Table 3–2.

Clinical Effects of Deficiency. Deficiency has been seen only in experimental situations, artificially induced by administering purified diets and antagonists. In such situations insomnia, fatigue, irritability, muscle cramps, and numbness of feet have been described.

Requirements. There is insufficient evidence regarding oral requirements for humans, but 4 to 7 mg/day is suggested. For TPN, the AMA recommends 15 mg/day in adults.[200]

Niacin

Characteristics. Niacin is a white powder stable in the presence of light, oxygen, acid, alkali, and heat.

Sources. Animal sources, meat, milk, and fish contain large amounts of niacin. In addition, the tryptophan content of food adds to the niacin potentially available. The first-class proteins of animal products add more niacin than those of vegetable origin.

Tryptophan and Niacin. In addition to niacin being available from the diet, it should be recognized that tryptophan is converted to niacin in the body. This conversion requires the presence of thiamine, riboflavin, and pyridoxine.

Absorption. Niacin is rapidly absorbed by diffusion.

Function. Niacin is a component of two nucleotides in its active form, nicotinamide. These nucleotides are nicotinamide adenine mono- (NAD) and di- (NADP) nucleotides. They combine with various carrier proteins to form enzymes concerned with electron transfer reactions related to energy metabolism as shown in Figure 3–1.

Normal Values. See Table 3–2.

Clinical Effects of Deficiency. Niacin deficiency is due not only to poor intake of niacin but also to a deficiency or reduced conversion of tryptophan to niacin. Clinical deficiency is the result of a complex disorder involving not only a lack of niacin and tryptophan but also an excessive leucine intake, which inhibits the conversion of tryptophan to niacin. There must also be concurrent deficiencies of riboflavin, thiamine, and pyridoxine, which are needed for this conversion.

Clinically, pellagra presents as a wasting disease with dermatitis of the exposed areas due to photosensitivity. Fatigue, insomnia, and apathy are followed by confusion, hallucinations, disorientation, and finally psychosis. Widespread mucosal inflammation causes glossitis, stomatitis, vaginitis, and diarrhea.

Biochemical Abnormalities in Deficiency. A drop in blood levels of niacin is not a reliable index of deficiency. However, the excretions of urinary N^1-methylnicotinamide and N^1-methyl-2-pyridine-5-carboxyl-amide (2-pyridone) are altered in deficiency, the ratio of the latter to the former normally being at least 1.0. If this ratio is below 1.0, then there is deficiency.

Requirements. The recommended oral intake is 6.6 mg of niacin/1000 kcal. Thus about 13 to 18 mg per day should be taken by adults. In calculating the effect of dietary tryptophan, 60 mg of tryptophan are taken as equivalent to 1 mg of niacin. For TPN the AMA recommends 40 mg/day in adults.[200] In home TPN patients, 100 mg twice weekly avoids deficiency.[215]

Pyridoxine (B₆)

Characteristics. Vitamin B_6 exists with an alcohol (pyridoxine), aldehyde (pyridoxal), or amine (pyridoxamine) side chain, resulting in compounds that are equally active. It is soluble in water, stable in acid but not in alkali, and photodegradable.

Sources. Animal products such as liver, meat, and fish are good sources of pyridoxine. Bananas and avocados are also rich sources, but other fruits do not contain as much. Grains and legumes contain significant amounts of pyridoxine.

Absorption. Pyridoxine is absorbed readily, but the mechanism is not understood. Malabsorption has been described in celiac disease, in alcoholism, and after jejunoileal bypass.

Storage. Pyridoxine is mainly stored attached to muscle phosphorylase.

Function. Pyridoxine is converted in the body to the active form pyridoxal-5-phosphate. This is a cofactor that catalyzes the metabolism of amino acids in the form of (1) a transaminase, (2) a decarboxylase used in synthesis of neurotransmitter amines, and (3) cystathionine-γ-lyase. In addition it is required in the synthesis of delta-aminolevulinic acid, which in turn functions in heme synthesis. Attached to phosphorylase it stabilizes the enzyme. Finally, it catalyzes the conversion of tryptophan to niacin.

Normal Values. See Table 3–2.

Clinical Effects of Deficiency. Muscle weakness, irritability, microcytic anemia, and electroencephalographic changes have been described. The latter may lead to seizures. When experimental deficiency is induced by feeding a vitamin antagonist, then nausea, vomiting, neuropathy, and seborrheic dermatitis occur. The administration of a number of drugs can cause symptoms correctable by giving pyridoxine. Isoniazid-induced neuropathy can be prevented by giving pyridoxine. Similarly, neurological syndromes seen with cycloserine and penicillamine administration are responsive to pyridoxine. Some of the depressions seen in women can also be alleviated by the administration of pyridoxine.

Biochemical Abnormalities in Deficiency. The levels of pyridoxal phosphate in serum and erythrocytes are responsive to intake. Also, urinary excretion of pyridoxine falls when intake is marginal. The effect on transaminase levels in vitro of added pyridoxal phosphate can be an index of deficiency. A rise of the erythrocyte glutamic pyruvic transaminase above 25 per cent of control in response to addition of pyridoxal phosphate is indicative of deficiency.

Requirements. The oral intake in adults should be 2.0 to 2.2 mg/day. During pregnancy and lactation intake should be increased to 2.5 to 2.6 mg/day. Kishi et al.[213] found that 3 mg/day during TPN was adequate based on transaminase activity. By contrast, in home TPN patients 5.5 mg/day was not sufficient in all patients.[182] In such patients, pyridoxine has also been given as 15 mg twice weekly.[215] In acutely sick patients 15 mg caused serum levels to rise.[214] For TPN the AMA recommends 4 mg/day in adults.[200]

Biotin

Characteristics. Biotin is a heat-stable white powder destroyed by oxidation and alkali.

Sources. Liver and oatmeal are rich sources. Eggs, milk, and milk products are also good sources.

Absorption. Biotin is readily absorbed except in the presence of the protein avidin, found in raw egg white. Biotin is also synthesized by intestinal bacteria. Since urinary biotin exceeds intake, bacterial biotin must contribute to the nutritional requirements of the individual.

Function. This vitamin is a cofactor in carboxylation reactions by carrying CO_2 to substrates for the purposes of elongating the carbon chain. For example, pyruvate is carboxylated to oxaloacetate, which enters the tricarboxylic acid cycle. Elongation of acetyl CoA to malonyl CoA aids the synthesis of fatty acids. In addition it is involved in transcarboxylation of amino acids.

Normal Values. See Table 3–2.

Clinical Effects of Deficiency. Without an abnormal intake of egg white, natural deficiency of biotin in adults seems unknown, but it has been described as occurring during TPN in adults[216,217] as well as in children.[218,219] The clinical syndrome consists of lassitude, anorexia, alopecia, scaly skin, dermatitis, and paresthesias.

Biochemical Abnormalities in Deficiency. Blood and especially urine levels of biotin fall with deficiency. In addition there tends to be a metabolic acidosis with the normally negligible urinary excretion of a number of organic acids distinctly increased. These acids are chiefly methylcitrate, 3-methylcrotonylglycine, and 3-hydroxyisovalerate.

Requirements. About 100 to 200 μg/day is the recommended oral intake. However, the dietary intake is only an approximation, especially in the case of TPN, since a significant amount is synthesized in the intestine, though the availability of synthesized biotin has been questioned. For TPN the AMA recommends an intake of 60 μg/day.[200] In the absence of supplementation, low levels of circulating biotin have been observed.[182]

Folacin and Vitamin B$_{12}$. These vitamins are discussed in detail in Chapter 27.

Ascorbic Acid

Characteristics. Ascorbic acid is a white water-soluble powder. In solution it oxidizes readily, especially when heated or in the presence of alkali. The biologically active forms are L-ascorbic acid and L-dehydroascorbic acid. The latter has 80 per cent of the activity of ascorbic acid. Further oxidation to diketogluconic acid makes both forms inactive.

Sources. Citrus fruits, green vegetables, tomatoes, and fruits are rich sources of ascorbic acid. With the exception of liver, animal products have little ascorbic acid.

Absorption. Ascorbic acid is readily absorbed from the small bowel and distributed to all tissues.

Storage. About 1500 mg are stored in the body in various tissues.

Function. While it undergoes reversible oxidation and can act as a reducing agent, the main and unique action of ascorbic acid is in collagen synthesis. In the absence of this vitamin hydroxylation of procollagen does not occur. This hydroxylation occurs at lysine and proline residues, making it possible for collagen to form a triple helix, giving the tissue strength and stability.

Normal Levels. See Table 3–2.

Clinical Effects of Deficiency. The initial manifestation of scurvy is perifollicular hyperkeratosis. Then perifollicular hemorrhages occur, followed by hemorrhages into skin, joints, and nails, and swelling, friability, and bleeding of the gums. There may be terminal icterus, fever, and edema.

In children, metaphyseal fractures below the epiphysis and hemorrhage may occur. Normocytic normochromic anemia is also commonly present. In some cases a macrocytic megaloblastic anemia may develop, perhaps due to a disturbance of folate metabolism caused by the ascorbic acid deficiency.

Deficiency of the vitamin is believed to reduce the synthesis of PGE$_1$ in lymphocytes[220] and thus interfere with their function.

Biochemical Abnormalities in Deficiency. A fall in white cell and platelet ascorbic acid levels is diagnostic of deficiency. Plasma levels are often undetectable even when tissue levels are adequate. In deficiency buffy coat ascorbate falls below 0.2 mg/dl and platelet levels below 25 per cent of normal.

Requirements. In adults an oral intake of 60 mg/day is recommended, with an increase to 80 to 100 mg/day in pregnancy and during lactation. On the other hand, clinical deficiency can be prevented by as little as 10 mg/day. For TPN the AMA recommends 100 mg/day in adults.[200] In critically sick patients 500 mg/day raised white cell ascorbic acids above the normal range.[214]

Requirements for a number of these vitamins are known for the normal state, but the effect of sepsis and trauma on these requirements when the vitamins are introduced by intravenous and commercial enteral feedings is still not well understood.

References

Macronutrients

1. International Commission on Radiological Protection (ICRP). Report of the Task Group on Reference Man, publication 23. Oxford, Pergamon Press, 1975: 281, 327.
2. Chung VC, Young SK, Shadehehr A, et al. Protein digestion and absorption in human small intestine. Gastroenterology 1979; 76:1415–1421.
3. Rafoth RJ, Onstad, GR. Urea synthesis after oral protein ingestion in man. J Clin Invest 1973; 56:1170–1174.
4. Stewart PM, Walser M. Short term regulation of ureagenesis. J Biol Chem 1980; 225:5270–5280.
5. Elwyn DH, Parikh HC, Shoemaker WC. Amino acid movements between gut, liver, and periphery in unanesthetized dogs. Am J Physiol 1968; 215:1260–1275.
6. Wharen J, Felig P, Hagenfeldt L. Effect of protein ingestion on splanchnic and leg metabolism in normal man and in patients with diabetes mellitus. J Clin Invest 1976; 57:987–999.
7. Kirsch RE, Saunders SJ, Frith L, et al. Plasma amino acid concentration and regulation of albumin synthesis. Am J Clin Nutr 1969; 22:1559–1562.
8. Elwyn DH. The role of the liver in regulation of amino acid and protein metabolism. In Munro HN (ed). Mammalian Protein Metabolism. Vol. 4. New York, Academic Press, 1970:523–557.
9. Chang TW, Goldberg AL. Leucine inhibits oxidation of glucose and pyruvate in skeletal muscles during fasting. J Biol Chem 1978; 253:3696–3701.
10. Gelfand RA, Hendler RG, Sherwin RS. Dietary carbohydrate and metabolism of ingested protein. Lancet 1979; 1:65–68.
11. Fery F, Bourdoux P, Christophe J, et al. Hormonal and metabolic changes induced by an isocaloric isoproteinic ketogenic diet in healthy subjects. Diabetes Metab 1982; 8:299–305.
12. Hagenfeldt L, Eriksson S, Wharen J. Influence of leucine on arterial concentrations and regional exchange of amino acids in healthy subjects. Clin Sci 1980; 59:173–181.
13. Mitch WE, Walser M, Sapir DG. Nitrogen sparing induced by leucine compared with that induced by its keto analogue, alpha-ketoisocaproate, in fasting obese man. J Clin Invest 1981; 67:553–562.
14. Snell K. Muscle alanine synthesis and hepatic gluconeogenesis. Biochem Soc Trans 1980; 8:205–213.
15. Elia M, Livesey G. Branched chain amino acid and oxo acid metabolism in human and rat muscle. In Walser M, Williamson JR (eds). Metabolism and Clinical Implications of Branched Chain Amino and Ketoacids. (International symposium, Charleston, SC, 1980.) New York, Elsevier/North-Holland, 1981:257–262.
16. Pozefsky T, Walser M. Effect of intraarterial infusion of the ketoanalogue of leucine on amino acid release by forearm muscle. Metabolism 1977; 26:807–815.
17. Munro HN. General aspects of the regulation of protein metabolism by diet and by hormones. In Munro HN, Allison JB (eds). Mammalian Protein Metabolism. Vol. 1. New York, Academic Press, 1964:381–481.
18. Calloway DH, Spector H. Nitrogen balance as related to calorie and protein intake in active young men. Am J Clin Nutr 1954; 2:405–415.
19. Kinney JM, Long CL, Duke JH. Carbohydrate and nitrogen metabolism after injury. In Porter R, Knight J (eds). Energy Metabolism in Trauma (Ciba Foundation Symposium). London, Churchill, 1970: 103–126.
20. Whittaker JS, Stewart S, Vaughan K, et al. The effect of major abdominal surgery on glucose metabolism. (Abst.) Clin Nutr 1985; 5 (Suppl. 1): No. O.47.
21. Keys A, Brozek J, Hanschel A, et al. The Biology of Human Starvation. Minneapolis, University of Minnesota Press, 1950.
22. Elwyn DH. Nutritional requirements of adult surgical patients. Crit Care Med 1980; 8:9–20.
23. Richardson DP, Wayler AH, Scrimshaw NS, et al. Quantitative effect of an isoenergetic exchange of fat for carbohydrate on dietary protein utilization in healthy young men. Am J Clin Nutr 1979; 32:2217–2226.
24. Greenberg GR, Marliss EB, Anderson GH, et al. Protein-sparing therapy in the postoperative patient: effects of added hypocaloric glucose or lipid. N Engl J Med 1976; 194:1411–1416.
25. Greenberg GR, Jeejeebhoy KN. Intravenous protein-sparing therapy in patients with gastrointestinal disease. JPEN 1979; 3:427–432.
26. Bozzetti F. Parenteral nutrition in surgical patients. Surg Gynecol Obstet 1976; 142:16–20.
27. Hoffer LJ, Bistrian BR, Young VR et al. Metabolic effects of very low calorie weight reduction diets. J Clin Invest 1984; 73:750–758.
28. Yeung CK, Smith RC, Hill GL. Effect of an elemental diet on body composition. Comparison with intravenous nutrition. Gastroenterology 1979; 77:652–657.
29. Burke JF, Wolfe RR, Mullany CJ, et al. Glucose requirements following burn injury. Ann Surg 1979; 190:274–285.
30. Collins JP, Oxby CB, Hill GL. Intravenous amino acids and intravenous hyperalimentation as protein-sparing therapy after major surgery: a controlled clinical trial. Lancet 1978; 1:788–791.
31. Young GA, Hill GL. A controlled study of protein-sparing therapy after excision of the rectum. Ann Surg 1980; 192:183–190.
32. Patel D, Anderson GH, Jeejeebhoy KN. Amino acid adequacy of parenteral casein hydrolysate and oral cottage cheese in patients with gastrointestinal disease as measured by nitrogen balance and blood aminogram. Gastroenterology 1973; 65:427–437.
33. Anderson GH, Patel DG, Jeejeebhoy KN. Design and evaluation by nitrogen balance and blood aminograms of an amino acid mixture for total parenteral nutrition of adults with gastrointestinal disease. J Clin Invest 1974; 53:904–912.
34. Jeejeebhoy KN. Total parenteral nutrition (TPN)—a review. Ann Roy Coll Phys Surg Can 1976; 9:287–300.
35. Gray GM. Carbohydrate digestion and absorption. Role of the small intestine. N Engl J Med 1975; 292:1225–1230.
36. Mattson FH, Volpenhein RA. The digestion and absorption of triglycerides. J Biol Chem 1964; 239:2772–2777.
37. Kayden HJ, Senior JR, Mattson FH. The monoglyceride pathway of fat absorption in man. J Clin Invest 1967; 46:1695–1703.
38. Borgstrom B. On the interactions between pancreatic lipase and colipase and the substrate, and the importance of bile salts. J Lipid Res 1975; 16:411–417.
39. Hofmann AF, Small DM. Detergent properties of bile salts: correlation with physiological function. Ann Rev Med 1967; 18:333–376.
40. Greenberger NJ, Skillman TG. Medium-chain triglycerides. Physiologic considerations and clinical implications. N Engl J Med 1969; 280:1045–1058.
41. Harris JA, Benedict FG. Standard basal metabolism constants for physiologists and clinicians. In A Biometric Study of Basal Metabolism in Man. Publication 279, The Carnegie Institute of Washington. Philadelphia, JB Lippincott, 1919:223–250.
42. Russell DMcR, Shike M, Marliss EB, et al. Effects of total parenteral nutrition and chemotherapy on the metabolic derangements in small cell lung cancer. Cancer Res 1984; 44:1706–1711.
43. Askanazi J, Carpentier YA, Elwyn DH, et al. Influence of total parenteral nutrition on fuel utilization in injury and sepsis. Ann Surg 1980; 191:40–46.
44. Roulet M, Detsky AS, Marliss EB, et al. A controlled trial of the effect of parental nutritional support on patients

with respiratory failure and sepsis. Clin Nutr 1983; 2:97–105.

45. Baker JP, Detsky AS, Stewart S, et al. A randomized trial of total parenteral nutrition in critically ill patients: metabolic effects of varying glucose-lipid ratios as the energy source. Gastroenterology 1984; 87:53–59.

46. Gamble JL. Physiological information gained from studies on the life raft ration. The Harvey Lectures, Ser. 42, 1946–1947:247–273.

47. Woolfson AMJ, Heatley RV, Allison SP. Insulin to inhibit protein catabolism after injury. N Engl J Med 1979; 300:14–17.

48. Long JM, Wilmore DW, Mason AD Jr, et al. Fat-carbohydrate interaction: nitrogen-sparing effect of varying caloric sources for total intravenous feeding. Surg Forum 1974; 25:61–63.

49. Jeejeebhoy KN, Anderson GH, Nakhooda AF, et al. Metabolic studies in total parenteral nutrition with lipid in man: comparison with glucose. J Clin Invest 1976; 57:125–136.

50. Bark S, Holm I, Hakansson I, et al. Nitrogen-sparing effect of fat emulsion compared with glucose in the postoperative period. Acta Chir Scand 1976; 142:423–427.

51. Gazzaniga AB, Bartlett RH, Shobe JB. Nitrogen balance in patients receiving either fat or carbohydrate for total intravenous nutrition. Ann Surg 1975; 182:163–168.

52. Van Way CW III, Buerk CA, Peterson R, et al. Nitrogen balance and electrolyte requirement in Intralipid-based hyperalimentation. JPEN 1979; 3:174–177.

53. Wannemacher RW, Kaminski MV, Dinterman RE, et al. Protein-sparing therapy during pneumococcal infection in rhesus monkeys. JPEN 1978; 2:507–518.

54. MacFie J, Smith RC, Hill GL. Glucose or fat as a non-protein energy source? A controlled clinical trial in gastroenterological patients requiring intravenous nutrition. Gastroenterology 1981; 80:103–107.

55. Wolfe RR, Durkot MJ, Allsop JR, et al. Glucose metabolism in severely burned patients. Metabolism 1979; 28:1031–1039.

56. Jeejeebhoy KN, Zohrab WJ, Langer B, et al. Total parenteral nutrition at home for 23 months without complication and with good rehabilitation. A study of technical and metabolic features. Gastroenterology 1973; 65:811–820.

57. Messing B, Bitoun A, Galian A, et al. La stéatose hépatique au cours de la nutrition parentérale dépend-elle de l'apport calorique glucidique? Gastroenterol Clin Biol 1977; 1:1015–1025.

58. Messing B, Latrive JP, Bitoun A, et al. La stéatose hépatique au cours de la nutrition parentérale totale dépend-elle de l'apport calorique lipidique? Gastroenterol Clin Biol 1979; 3:719–724.

59. Holman RT. Essential fatty acid deficiency. In Holman RT (ed). Progress in the Chemistry of Fats and Other Lipids. Oxford, Pergamon Press, 1968; 9(2):275–348.

60. Wene JD, Connor WE, DenBesten L. The development of essential fatty acid deficiency in healthy men fed fat-free diets intravenously and orally. J Clin Invest 1975; 56:127–134.

61. Mann MD, Bowie MD, Hansen JDL. Total body potassium and serum electrolyte concentrations in protein energy malnutrition. S Afr Med J 1975; 49:76–78.

62. Garrow, JS. Total body potassium in kwashiorkor and marasmus. Lancet 1965; 2:455–458.

63. Montgomery RD. Magnesium metabolism in infantile protein malnutrition. Lancet 1960; 2:74–76.

64. Garrow JS, Smith R, Ward EE. Electrolyte Metabolism in Severe Infantile Malnutrition. Oxford, Pergamon Press, 1968: 56.

65. Brinkman GL, Bowie MD, Friis-Hansen B, et al. Body water composition in kwashiorkor before and after loss of edema. Pediatrics 1965; 36:94–103.

66. Rudman D, Millikan, WJ, Richardson, TJ, et al. Elemental balances during intravenous hyperalimentation of underweight adult subjects. J Clin Invest 1975; 55:94–104.

67. Freeman JB. Magnesium requirements are increased during total parenteral nutrition. Surg Forum 1977; 28:61–62.

68. Wolman SL, Anderson GH, Marliss EB, et al. Zinc in total parenteral nutrition. Requirements and metabolic effects. Gastroenterology 1979; 76:458–467.

69. Veverbrants E, Arky PA. Effects of fasting and refeeding. I. Studies on sodium, potassium and water excretion on a constant electrolyte and fluid intake. J Clin Endocrinol 1969; 29:55–62.

70. Waterlow JC, Golden MHN, Patrick J. Protein-energy malnutrition: treatment. In Dickerson JWT, Lee HA (eds). Nutrition in the Clinical Management of Disease. London, Edward Arnold Ltd., 1978: 49–71.

71. Manitius A, Epstein FH. Some observations on the influence of a magnesium-deficient diet on rats, with special reference to renal concentrating ability. J Clin Invest 1963; 42:208–215.

72. Albrecht PH. Effect of potassium deficiency on renal function in the dog. J Clin Invest 1969; 48:432–442.

73. Hill GL, King RFGJ, Smith RC, et al. Multi-element analysis of the living body by neutron activation analysis—application to critically ill patients receiving intravenous nutrition. Br J Surg 1979; 66:868–872.

74. Jeejeebhoy KN, Baker JP, Wolman SL, et al. Critical evaluation of the role of clinical assessment and body composition studies in patients with malnutrition and after total parenteral nutrition. Am J Clin Nutr 1982; 35:1117–1127.

75. Russell DMcR, Prendergast PJ, Darby PL, et al. A comparison between muscle function and body composition in anorexia nervosa: the effect of refeeding. Am J Clin Nutr 1983; 38:229–237.

76. Silvis SE, Paragas PD. Paresthesias, weakness, seizures and hypophosphatemia in patients receiving hyperalimentation. Gastroenterology 1972; 62:513–520.

Trace Elements

77. Cotzias GC. Role and importance of trace substances in environmental health. In DD Hemphill (ed). Proc First Ann Conf on Trace Subst Environ Health. Columbia, MO, University of Missouri, 1967: 1:5–19.

78. Golden MHN, Golden BE. Trace elements. Br Med Bull 1981; 37:31–36.

79. Abumrad NN, Schneider AJ, Steel D, et al. Amino acid intolerance during prolonged total parenteral nutrition (TPN) reversed by molybdenum. (Abstr.) Am J Clin Nutr 1981; 34:618.

80. Finch CA, Hubers H. Perspectives in iron metabolism. N Engl J Med 1982; 306:1520–1528.

81. Donaldson RM, Barreras RF. Intestinal absorption of trace quantities of chromium. J Lab Clin Med 1966; 68:484–493.

82. Bush JA, Mahoney JP, Gubler CJ, et al. Studies on copper metabolism; transfer of radio-copper between erythrocytes and plasma. J Lab Clin Med 1956; 47:898–906.

83. Sternlieb I, Morell AG, Tucker WD, et al. The incorporation of copper into ceruloplasmin in vivo: studies with copper-64 and copper-67. J Clin Invest 1961; 40:1834–1840.

84. Diplock AT. Metabolic and functional defects in selenium deficiency. Phil Trans R Soc Lond B 1981; 294:105–117.

85. Shoden A, Gabrio BW, Finch CA. The relationship between ferritin and hemosiderin in rabbits and man. J Biol Chem 1953; 204:823–830.

86. Dubach R, Moore CV, Callender S. Studies in iron transportation and metabolism. IX. The excretion of iron as measured by the isotope technique. J Lab Clin Med 1955; 45:599–615.

87. Robinson MF, McKenzie JM, Thomson CD, et al. Metabolic balance of zinc, copper, cadmium, iron, molybdenum and

selenium in young New Zealand women. Br J Nutr 1973; 30:195–205.

88. Foy H, Kondi A. Anaemias of the tropics; relation to iron intake, absorption and losses during growth, pregnancy and lactation. J Trop Med Hyg 1957; 60:105–118.

89. Morgan EH, Walters MNI. Iron storage in human disease. Fractionation of hepatic and splenic iron into ferritin and hemosiderin with histochemical correlations. J Clin Path 1963; 16:101–107.

90. Lipschitz DA, Cook JD, Finch CA. A clinical evaluation of serum ferritin as an index of iron stores. N Engl J Med 1974; 290:1213–1216.

91. Bainton DF, Finch CA. The diagnosis of iron deficiency anemia. Am J Med 1964; 37:62–70.

92. Peters ML, Maher M, Brennan MF. Minimal IV iron requirements in TPN. (Abstract.) JPEN 1980; 4:601.

93. Wan KK, Tsallas G. Dilute iron dextran formulation for addition to parenteral nutrient solutions. Am J Hosp Pharm 1980; 37:206–210.

94. Vallee BL, Falchuk KH. Zinc and gene expression. Phil Trans R Soc Lond B 1981; 294:185–197.

95. Prasad AS. Zinc in Human Nutrition. Boca Raton, FL, CRC Press, 1979: 1–80.

96. Hambidge KM, Neldner KH, Walravens, PA. Zinc, acrodermatitis enteropathica and congenital malformations. Lancet 1975; 1:577–578.

97. Golden MHN, Golden BE, Harland PSEG, et al. Zinc and immunocompetence in protein-energy malnutrition. Lancet 1978; 1:1226–1227.

98. Fernandes G, Nair M, Onoe K, et al. Impairment of cell-mediated immunity functions by dietary zinc deficiency in mice. Proc Natl Acad Sci USA 1979; 76:457–461.

99. Golden MHN, Golden BE, Jackson AA. Skin breakdown in kwashiorkor responds to zinc. (Letter.) Lancet 1980; 1:1256.

100. Tipton IH, Cook MJ. Trace elements in human tissue. II. Adult subjects from the United States. Health Phys 1963; 9:103–145.

101. Underwood EJ. Zinc. In Trace Elements in Human and Animal Nutrition. 4th ed. New York, Academic Press, 1977: 196–242.

102. Kirchgessner M, Roth HP, Weigand E. Biochemical changes in zinc deficiency. In Prasad AS (ed). Trace Elements in Human Health and Disease. Vol. 1: Zinc and Copper. New York, Academic Press, 1976:189–225.

103. Davies NT. Studies on the absorption of zinc by rat intestine. Br J Nutr 1980; 43:189–203.

104. Richards MP, Cousins RJ. Isolation of intestinal zinc: proposed function in zinc absorption. (Abstract.) Fed Proc 1977; 36:1106.

105. Cousins RJ. Regulation of zinc absorption: role of intracellular ligands. Am J Clin Nutr 1979; 32:339–345.

106. Prasad AS, Schulert AR, Sandstead HH, et al. Zinc, iron and nitrogen content of sweat in normal and deficient subjects. J Lab Clin Med 1963; 62:84–89.

107. Abu-Hamdan DK, Migdal SD, Whitehouse AS, et al. Disparate urinary zinc (ZN) handling in response to ZN infusion and amino acids. (Abstract.) Kidney Int 1979; 16:818.

108. Smith KT, Cousins RJ. Quantitative aspects of zinc absorption by isolated, vascularly perfused rat intestine. J Nutr 1980; 110:316–323.

109. Beisel WR, Pekarek RS, Wannemacher RW Jr. The impact of infectious disease on trace-element metabolism of the host. In Hoekstra WG, Suttie JW, Ganther HE, et al. (eds). Trace Element Metabolism in Animals. Vol. 2. Baltimore, University Park Press, 1974:217–240.

110. Talbot TR, Ross JF. The zinc content of plasma erythrocytes of patients with pernicious anemia, sickle cell anemia, polycythemia vera, leukemia and neoplastic disease. Lab Invest 1960; 9:174–184.

111. Vallee BL, Wacker WEC, Bartholmay AF, et al. Zinc metabolism in hepatic dysfunction. Ann Intern Med 1959; 50:1077–1091.

112. Vikbladh I. Studies on zinc in blood. Scand J Clin Lab Invest 1950; 2:143–148.

113. Hambidge KM. Zinc deficiency in man: its origins and effects. Phil Trans R Soc Lond B 1981; 294:129–144.

114. Whitehouse RC, Prasad AS, Rabbani PI, et al. Zinc in plasma, neutrophils, lymphocytes, and erythrocytes as determined by flameless atomic absorption spectrophotometry. Clin Chem 1982; 28:475–480.

115. Widdowson EM, Dauncey J, Shaw JCL. Trace elements in foetal and early postnatal development. Proc Nutr Soc 1974; 33:275–284.

116. James BE, MacMahon RA. Balance studies of 9 elements during complete intravenous feeding of small premature infants. Aust Ped J 1976; 12:154–162.

117. Ricour C, Duhamel J-F, Gros J, et al. Estimates of trace element requirements of children receiving total parenteral nutrition. Arch Fr Pediat 1977; 34(Suppl 7):92–100.

118. Mason KE. A conspectus of research on copper metabolism and requirements in man. J Nutr 1979; 109:1979–2066.

119. Cartwright GE, Wintrobe MM. Copper metabolism in normal subjects. Am J Clin Nutr 1964; 14:224–232.

120. Evans JL, Abraham PA. Anemia, iron storage and ceruloplasmin in copper nutrition in the growing rat. J Nutr 1973; 103:196–201.

121. O'Dell BL. Roles for iron and copper in connective tissue biosynthesis. Phil Trans R Soc Lond B 1981; 294:91–104.

122. Fell BF. Pathological consequences of copper deficiency and cobalt deficiency. Phil Trans R Soc Lond B 1981; 294:153–169.

123. Osaki S, Johnson DA, Freiden E. The possible significance of the ferrous oxidase activity of ceruloplasmin in normal human serum. J Biol Chem 1966; 241:2746–2751.

124. Golden MHN. Trace elements in human nutrition. Hum Nutr Clin Nutr 1982; 36C:185–202.

125. Pinnell SR, Martin GR. The crosslinking of collagen and elastin. Proc Natl Acad Sci USA 1968; 61:708–714.

126. Siegel RC, Pinnell SR, Martin GR. Crosslinking of collagen and elastin. Properties of lysyl oxidase. Biochemistry 1970; 9:4486–4492.

127. Cordano A, Baertl JM, Graham GG. Copper deficiency in infancy. Pediatrics 1964; 34:324–336.

128. Hamilton EI, Minsky MJ, Cleary JJ. The concentration and distribution of some stable elements in healthy human tissues from the United Kingdom. Sci Total Environ 1972; 1:341–374.

129. Gubler CJ, Lahey ME, Cartwright GE, et al. Studies on copper metabolism; transportation of copper in blood. J Clin Invest 1953; 32:405–414.

130. Bremner I. Absorption, transport and storage of copper. In Biological Roles of Copper. Ciba Foundation Symposium. Amsterdam, Excerpta Medica, 1980: 79:23–48.

131. Owen CA. Absorption and excretion of ^{64}Cu-labelled copper by the rat. Am J Physiol 1964; 207:1203–1206.

132. Hall AC, Young BW, Bremner I. Intestinal metallothionein and the mutual antagonism between copper and zinc. J Inorg Biochem 1979; 11:57–66.

133. Sandstead HH. Copper bioavailability and requirements. Am J Clin Nutr 1982; 35:809–814.

134. Shike M, Roulet M, Kurian R, et al. Copper metabolism and requirements in total parenteral nutrition. Gastroenterology 1981; 81:290–297.

135. Jacob RA, Sandstead HH, Munoz JM, et al. Whole body surface loss of trace metals in normal males. Am J Clin Nutr 1981; 34:1379–1383.

136. Henkin RI. On the role of adrenocorticosteroids in the control of zinc and copper metabolism. In Hoekstra WG, Suttie JW, Ganther HE, et al. (eds). Trace Element Metabolism in Animals. Vol. 2. Baltimore, University Park Press, 1974: 647–651.

137. Askari A, Long CL, Murray RRL, et al. Zinc and copper balance in the severely injured patient. (Abstr.) Fed Proc 1979; 38:707.

138. Bremner I, Mills CF. Absorption, transport and tissue stor-

age of essential trace elements. Phil Trans R Soc Lond B 1981; *294*:75–89.

139. Kovalsky VV. The geochemical ecology of organisms under conditions of varying contents of trace elements in the environment. *In* Mills CF (ed). Trace Element Metabolism in Animals. Vol. 1. Edinburgh: Livingstone, 1970: 385–397.

140. Wintrobe MM, Cartwright GE, Gubler CJ. Studies on the function and metabolism of copper. J Nutr 1953; *50*:395–419.

141. Halsted JA, Hackley BM, Smith JC. Plasma zinc and copper in pregnancy and after oral contraceptives. Lancet 1968; *2*:278–279.

142. Hambidge KM. Increase in hair copper concentration with increasing distance from the scalp. Am J Clin Nutr 1973; *26*:1212–1215.

143. Jacobson S, Western P-O. Balance study of twenty trace elements during total parenteral nutrition in man. Br J Nutr 1977; *37*:107–126.

144. Phillips GD, Garnys VP. Parenteral administration of trace elements to critically ill patients. Ann Intens Care 1981; *9*:221–225.

145. Mertz W, Roginski EE, Schwartz K. Effects of trivalent chromium complexes on glucose uptake by epididymal fat tissue of rats. J Biol Chem 1961; *236*:318–322.

146. Roginski EE, Mertz W. Effects of Chromium 3 + supplementation on glucose and amino acid metabolism in rats fed a low protein diet. J Nutr 1969; *97*:525–530.

147. Jeejeebhoy KN, Chu RC, Marliss EB, et al. Chromium deficiency, glucose intolerance and neuropathy reversed by chromium supplementation in a patient receiving long-term total parenteral nutrition. Am J Clin Nutr 1977; *30*:531–538.

148. Schroeder HA, Balassa JJ, Tipton IH. Abnormal trace metals in man—chromium. J Chron Dis 1962; *15*:941–964.

149. Offenbacher EG, Pi-Sunyer FX. Beneficial effects of chromium-rich yeast on glucose tolerance and blood lipids in elderly subjects. Diabetes 1980; *29*:919–925.

150. World Health Organization, WHO Tech Rep Ser 1973; No. 532:20–24.

151. Toepfer WW, Mertz W, Polansky MM, et al. Synthetic organic chromium complexes and glucose tolerance. J Agri Food Chem 1977; *25*:162–165.

152. Anderson RA, Mertz W. Glucose tolerance factor: an essential dietary agent. Trends Biochem Sci 1977; *2*:277–279.

153. Schroeder HA. The role of chromium in mammalian nutrition. Am J Clin Nutr 1968; *21*:230–244.

154. Hambidge KM. Chromium nutrition in the mother and the growing child. *In* Mertz W, Cornatzer WE (eds). Newer Trace Elements in Nutrition. New York, Marcel Dekker Inc., 1971: 169–194.

155. Pekarek RS, Hauer EC, Bayfield EJ, et al. Relationship between serum chromium concentrations and glucose utilization in normal and infected subjects. Diabetes 1975; *24*:350–353.

156. Glinsmann WH, Feldman FJ, Mertz W. Plasma chromium after glucose administration. Science 1966; *152*:1243–1245.

157. Freund H, Atamin S, Fischer JE. Chromium deficiency during total parenteral nutrition. JAMA 1979; *241*:496–498.

157a. Freed BA, Pinchofsky G, Nasr N, et al. Normalization of serum glucose levels and decreasing insulin requirements by the addition of chromium to TPN. (Abstr.) JPEN 1981; *5*:568.

158. Chance B, Sies H, Boveris A. Hydroperoxide metabolism in mammalian organs. Physiol Rev 1979; *59*:527–605.

159. Hill HAO. The superoxide ion and the toxicity of molecular oxygen. *In* Fraustro da Silva JRR, Williams JRP (eds). New Trends in Bioinorganic Chemistry. London, Academic Press, 1978: 173–208.

160. Haber F, Weiss J. The catalytic decomposition of hydrogen peroxide by iron salts. Phil Trans R Soc Lond A 1934; *147*:332–351.

161. Rotruck JT, Pope AL, Ganther HE, et al. Selenium: bio-

162. Diplock AT, Lucy JA. The biochemical modes of action of vitamin E and selenium: a hypothesis. FEBS Lett 1973; *29*:205–210.

163. Dickson RC, Tomlinson RN. Selenium in blood and human tissues. Clin Chim Acta 1967; *16*:311–321.

164. Heinrich HC, Gabbe EE, Bartels H, et al. Bioavailability of food iron-(^{59}Fe), vitamin B_{12}-(^{60}Co) and protein bound selenomethionine-(^{75}Se) in pancreatic exocrine insufficiency due to cystic fibrosis. Klin Wochenschr 1977; *55*:595–601.

165. Thompson CD, Stewart RDH. The metabolism of ^{75}Se-selenite in young women. Br J Nutr 1974; *32*:47–57.

166. Underwood EJ. Selenium. *In* Trace Elements in Human and Animal Nutrition. 4th ed. New York, Academic Press, 1977: 302–246.

167. Levander OA, Sutherland B, Morris VC, et al. Selenium balance in young men during selenium depletion and repletion. Am J Clin Nutr 1981; *34*:2662–2669.

168. Stewart RDH, Griffiths NM, Thomson CD, et al. Quantitative selenium metabolism in normal New Zealand women. Br J Nutr 1978; *40*:45–54.

169. van Rij AM, Thomson CD, McKenzie JM, et al. Selenium deficiency in total parenteral nutrition. Am J Clin Nutr 1979; *32*:2076–2085.

170. van Rij AM, McKenzie JM, Thomson CD, et al. Selenium supplementation in total parenteral nutrition. JPEN 1981; *5*:120–124.

171. Griffith NM. Dietary intake and urinary excretion of selenium in some New Zealand women. Proc Univ Otago Med School 1973; *51*:8.

172. Thompson JN, Erdody P, Smith DC. Selenium content of food consumed by Canadians. J Nutr 1975; *105*:274–277.

173. Chen X, Yang G, Chen J, et al. Studies on the relations of selenium and Keshan disease. Biol Trace Elem Res 1980; *2*:91–107.

174. Lane HW, Dudrick S, Warren DC. Blood selenium levels and glutathione peroxidase activies in university students and chronic intravenous hyperalimentation subjects. Proc Soc Exp Biol Med 1981; *167*:383–390.

175. Fleming CR, Fleming JT, McCall JT, et al. Selenium deficiency and fatal cardiomyopathy in a patient on home parental nutrition. Gastroenterology 1982; *83*:689–693.

176. Johnson RA, Baker SS, Fallon JT, et al. An occidental case of cardiomyopathy and selenium deficiency. N Engl J Med 1981; *304*:1210–1212.

177. Van Vleet JF. An evaluation of protection offered by various dietary supplements against experimentally induced selenium–vitamin E deficiency in ducklings. Am J Vet Res 1977; *38*:1231–1236.

178. Thurlow PM, Grant JP. Vitamin E, essential fatty acids and platelet function during total parenteral nutrition. (Abstr.) JPEN 1981; *4*:586.

179. Losowsky MS, Leonard PJ. Evidence of vitamin E deficiency in patients with malabsorption of alcoholism and the effects of therapy. Gut 1967; *8*:539–543.

180. Ali M, Gudbranson CG, McDonald JWD. Inhibition of human platelet cyclooxygenase by alpha-tocopherol. Prostaglandins Med 1980; *4*:79–85.

181. Hafeman DG, Hoekstra WG. Lipid peroxidation in vivo during vitamin E and selenium deficiency monitored by ethane evolution. J Nutr 1977; *107*:666–672.

182. Jeejeebhoy KN, Langer B, Tsallas G, et al. Total parenteral nutrition at home: studies in patients surviving 4 months to 5 years. Gastroenterology 1976; *71*:943–953.

183. Leach RM, Jr, Muenster AM, Wein EM. Studies on the role of manganese in bone formation. II. Effect upon chondroitin sulfate synthesis in chick epiphyseal cartilage. Arch Biochem Biophys 1969; *133*:22–28.

184. Doisy EA Jr. Micronutrient controls on biosynthesis of clotting proteins and cholesterol. *In* DD Hemphill (ed). Trace

Substances in Environmental Health. Columbia, MO, Curators of the Univ. of Missouri, 1972: 6:193–199.

185. Weisiger RA, Fridovich I. Superoxide dismutase. Organelle specificity. J Biol Chem 1973; 248:3582–3592.

186. Cotzias GC. Manganese in health and disease. Physiol Rev 1958; 38:503–532.

187. Greenberg DM, Copp DH, Cuthbertson EM. Studies in mineral metabolism with the aid of artificial radioactive isotopes. J Biol Chem 1943; 147:749–757.

188. Bertinchamps AJ, Miller ST, Cotzias GC. Interdependence of routes excreting manganese. Am J Physiol 1966; 211:217–224.

189. Wenlock RW, Buss DH, Dixon EJ. Trace nutrients. 2. Manganese in British foods. Br J Nutr 1979; 41:253–261.

190. McLeod BE, Robinson MF. Metabolic balance of manganese in young women. Br J Nutr 1972; 27:221–227.

191. de Renzo EC, Kaleita E, Heytler P, et al. Identification of the xanthine oxidase factor as molybdenum. Arch Biochem Biophys 1953; 45:247–253.

192. Cohen HJ, Fridovich I, Rajagopalan KV. Hepatic sulfite oxidase. A functional role for molybdenum. J Biol Chem 1971; 246:374–382.

193. Mahler HR, Mackler B, Green DE, et al. Studies on metalloflavoproteins. III. Aldehyde oxidase: a molybdoflavoprotein. J Biol Chem 1954; 210:465–480.

194. Cohen HJ, Drew RT, Johnson J, et al. Molecular basis of the biological function of molybdenum: the relationship between sulfite oxidase and the acute toxicity of bisulfite and SO_2. Proc Natl Acad Sci USA 1973; 70:3655–3659.

195. Abumrad NN, Schneider AJ, Steel D, et al. Amino acid intolerance during prolonged total parenteral nutrition reversed by molybdate therapy. Am J Clin Nutr 1981; 34:2551–2559.

196. Underwood EJ. Molybdenum. *In* Trace Elements in Human and Animal Nutrition. 4th Ed. New York, Academic Press, 1977: 109–131.

197. Abumrad NN. Molybdenum—is it an essential trace metal? Bull NY Acad Med 1984; 60:163–171.

Vitamins

198. Lowry SF, Goodgame JT, Maher MM, et al. Parenteral vitamin requirements during feeding. Am J Clin Nutr 1978; 31:2149–2158.

199. Nichoalds GE, Meng HC, Caldwell MD. Vitamin requirements in patients receiving total parenteral nutrition. Arch Surg 1977; 112:1061–1064.

200. Vanamee P, Shils ME, Burke AW, et al. Multivitamin preparations for parenteral use. A statement by the nutrition advisory group. JPEN 1979; 3:258–261.

201. Goodman DS, Olson JA. The conversion of all-trans beta-carotene into retinal. *In* RB Clayton (ed). Methods in Enzymology. Vol 15. Steroids and Terpenoids. New York, Academic Press, 1969: 462–475.

202. Moore T. Vitamin A in the normal individual. *In* Herriott RM (Ed). Symposium on Nutrition. Johns Hopkins University Press, Baltimore, 1953: 28–70.

203. Baker H, Frank O. Vitamin A and carotenes. *In* Clinical Vitaminology. Methods and Interpretation. New York, Interscience Publishers, 1968: 161–168.

204. Wald G. The molecular basis of visual excitation. Nature (London) 1968; 219:800–807.

205. Dutta SK, Bustin MP, Russel RM, et al. Deficiency of fat-soluble vitamins in treated patients with pancreatic insufficiency. Ann Intern Med 1982; 97:549–552.

206. Gallo-Torres HE. Obligatory role of bile for the intestinal absorption of vitamin E. Lipids 1970; 5:379–384.

207. Howard L, Ovesen L, Satya-Murti S, et al. Reversible neurological symptoms caused by vitamin E deficiency in a patient with short bowel syndrome. Am J Clin Nutr 1982; 36:1243–1249.

208. Hollander D, Muralidhara KS, Rim E. Colonic absorption of bacterially synthesized vitamin K_2 in the rat. Am J Physiol 1976; 230:251–255.

209. Hollander D, Truscott TC. Colonic absorption of vitamin K_3. J Lab Clin Med 1974; 83:648–656.

210. Hollander D, Truscott TC. Mechanism and site of vitamin K_3 small intestinal transport. Am J Physiol 1974; 226:1516–1522.

211. Hollander D. Vitamin K_1 absorption by everted intestinal sacs of the rat. Am J Physiol 1973; 225:360–364.

212. Stromberg P, Shenkin A, Campbell RA, et al. Vitamin status during total parenteral nutrition. JPEN 1981; 5:295–299.

213. Kishi H, Nishii, S, Ono T, et al. Thiamin and pyridoxine requirements during intravenous hyperalimentation. Am J Clin Nutr 1979; 32:332–338.

214. Bradley JA, King RFJG, Schorah CJ. Vitamins in intravenous feeding: a study of water-soluble vitamins and folate in critically ill patients receiving intravenous nutrition. Br J Surg 1978; 65:492–494.

215. Howard L, Bigaouette J, Chu R, et al. Water soluble vitamin requirements in home parenteral nutrition patients. Am J Clin Nutr 1983; 37:421–428.

216. McClain CJ, Baker H, Onstad GR. Biotin deficiency in an adult during home parenteral nutrition. JAMA 1982; 247:3116–3117.

217. Khalidi N, Wesley JR, Thoene JG, et al. Biotin deficiency in a patient with short bowel syndrome during home parenteral nutrition. JPEN 1984; 8:311–314.

218. Mock DM, deLorimer AA, Liebman WM, et al. Biotin deficiency: an unusual complication of parenteral alimentation. N Engl J Med 1981; 304:820–823.

219. Kien CL, Goodman SI, Horowitz SP. Biotin–responsive in vivo carboxylase deficiency in two siblings with secretory diarrhea receiving total parenteral nutrition. J Pediatr 1981; 99:546–550.

220. Manku MS, Oka M, Horrobin DF. Differential regulation of the formation of prostaglandins and related substances from arachidonic acid and from dihomogammalinolenic acid. II. Effects of vitamin C. Prostaglandins Med 1979; 3:129–137.

221. Sauberlich HE. Laboratory procedures used in vitamin nutritional assessment. *In* Levenson SM (ed). Nutritional Assessment—Present Status, Future Directions and Prospects. Report of the Second Ross Conference on Medical Research. Columbus, OH, Ross Laboratories, 1981: 65–67.

222. Baker H, Frank O. Thiamine. *In* Clinical Vitaminology. Methods and Interpretation. New York, Interscience Publishers, 1968: 7–21.

223. Brin M. Transketolase (sedoheptulose-7-phosphate: D-glyceraldehyde-phosphate dihydroxyacetonetransferase, EC 2.2.1.1) and the TPP effect in assessing thiamine adequacy. *In* McCormick DB, Wright LD (eds). Methods in Enzymology, Vol. 18. Vitamins and Coenzymes. Part A. New York, Academic Press, 1971: 125–133.

224. Baker H, Frank O, Feingold S, et al. A riboflavin assay suitable for clinical use and nutritional surveys. Am J Clin Nutr 1966; 19:17–26.

225. Sauberlich HE, Canham JE, Baker EM, et al. Biochemical assessment of the nutritional status of vitamin B6 in the human. Am J Clin Nutr 1972; 25:625–642.

226. Baker EM, Canham JE, Nunes WT, et al. Vitamin B6 requirement for adult men. Am J Clin Nutr 1964; 15:59–66.

227. Terry RC, Simon M. Determination of niacin metabolites 1-methyl-5-carboxylamide-2-pyridone and N^1-methylnicotinamide in urine by high-performance liquid chromatography. J Chromatogr 1982; 232:261–274.

228. Evans RM, Currie L, Campbell A. The distribution of ascorbic acid between various cellular components of blood, in normal individuals, and its relation to the plasma concentration. Br J Nutr 1982; 47:473–482.

229. Sanghvi RS, Lemons RM, Baker H, et al. A simple method for determination of plasma and urinary biotin. Clin Chim Acta 1982; 124:85–90.

230. Baker H, Frank O. Biotin. *In* Clinical Vitaminology. Methods and Interpretation. New York, Interscience Publishers, 1968: 22–30.

4

DIMENSIONS OF THE HUMAN BODY AND ITS COMPARTMENTS

GRAHAM L. HILL / ALUN H. BEDDOE

"Nothing is measured with greater error than the human body"

BENEKE, 1878

For a proper understanding of the alterations brought about by nutritional and metabolic imbalances during illness and recovery, detailed information on the morphological changes induced together with their accompanying physiological, biochemical, and psychological effects is required. Although the sciences of anthropometry, nuclear medicine, radiology, medical physics, and anatomy have combined to make it possible to measure the size of the human body and its compartments, there are considerable limitations in applying such measurements to the clinical situation. First, the application of body size measurements to an individual patient may be misleading and inaccurate. This is usually because tables of normal reference values show widespread variation between individuals that are often greater than the changes induced in a patient by his illness. But there is also a problem in that most of the techniques for direct measurement of body composition, which have now reached a high state of sophistication, have not proved to be suitable for use in the daily care of the sick and are at present confined to research institutions. Second, there are the considerable difficulties involved in relating the morphological changes induced by illness to alterations in physiological, biochemical, and psychological function. In spite of these considerable limitations to the use of morphological data, anthropometric and body composition studies have gained a new impetus as the growing awareness of the importance of nutrition in patient care has emerged.

BODY WEIGHT

Body weight is one of the basic anthropometric characteristics. Loss of weight is a universal accompaniment of starvation and is associated with many illnesses. Weight change may serve as a gross index of the disturbed balance between caloric intake and caloric output. If body water is present in normal proportions, gain of body weight over a period of time indicates a positive energy balance; conversely, weight loss over a period of time is an expression of a negative energy balance. Before the physiological importance of body weight in sickness and health can be understood, it is important to know the approximate value of its components. Broadly speaking, the mass of the body consists of fat mass and fat-free body mass, the latter being composed of water, protein, minerals, and glycogen. Values of these components for a typical healthy adult are given in Figure 4–1.[1] The changes in these components that occur in nutritional and metabolic illnesses of different types are discussed below.

Measurement of Body Weight

In the initial assessment and subsequent evaluation of patients with nutritional and metabolic disorders measurements of body weight should always be made. Although it might be expected that this would be a normal part of clinical practice, recent studies suggest that body weight measurements are not always made in sick patients and that many medical staff members do not believe it important to do so.[2] Body weight can be measured on chair-type ward scales to the nearest 0.1 kg. In some cases chair scales cannot be used for acutely ill patients, and

Components of Body Weight

M. Age 40
74.1 kg.

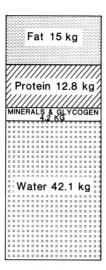

FIGURE 4–1. *The components of body weight in a healthy male subject. An in vivo neutron activation technique and measurements of body water and body weight were used to measure these body compartments.*[1]

bed-type scales onto which the patient is moved can be used. Other scales are available that make it possible to weigh the patient without moving the bed, but here it is important to ensure that the same "patient extras" such as sheets and pillows are included in exactly the same way at each weighing. All scales need to be checked for accuracy and precision and tested to see if different positions of the patient affect the result. It is also important to measure the patient who is being followed according to a strict routine. This should include making the measurement at approximately the same time each day (best first thing in the morning), weighing the patient in approximately the same clothing each day, and ensuring that the bladder has been emptied immediately or a short time before the weighing. The weighings should be always made on the same properly calibrated scales, and if there are any gross or unexpected inconsistencies these should be checked by a second observer.

Determinants of Body Weight

The body weight of an adult is primarily determined by genetic factors. Sex, dietary habits, and exercise determine the relative proportions of the different components of the body. The female body contains a higher percentage of body fat, the male more protein, but in either overeating is associated with an increase in fat and active exercise throws the balance in the other direction with an increase in protein. As a general rule sick patients who have lost weight have an increased hydration of their fat-free body mass due to an increase in extracellular water.[3]

Components of Body Weight

It has already been pointed out that to understand surgical metabolism properly body weight should be broken down into fat mass and fat-free body mass, the latter comprising total body water, total body protein, minerals, and glycogen (Fig. 4–1). It is helpful to further subdivide both the body water (plasma, interstitial water, and intracellular water) and body protein (muscle protein, visceral protein, and structural protein). From Figure 4–1 it can be seen that much of body weight comprises water, and this means in clinical practice that appreciable gains in weight over the short term (anything less than 48 hours) are largely due to increases in body water. The synthesis of new lean tissue, about one fifth of which is protein and four fifths water, proceeds so slowly that it is a cause of weight change that is discernible only over a period of a week or so. The synthesis of lean tissue rarely proceeds at a rate faster than 150 g/day (corresponding to 31 g of protein or 5 g of nitrogen).

Weight loss due to the breakdown of tissue can

occur much more rapidly than its synthesis. Fat and protein can be lost at rates as rapid as 500 g/day, but rapid loss of body water, as from an enterocutaneous fistula, may produce weight loss approximately 10 times as fast. Thus, short-term rapid weight loss generally signifies loss of salt and water. Continuing severe tissue trauma which, for example, accompanies invasive sepsis may account for about 500 g/day. Weight loss over and above this is water loss.

Evaluation of the Normality of Body Weight

Determining the normality of body weight for an individual can be quite difficult. Probably the most commonly used standard is the table produced by the Metropolitan Life Insurance Company in 1959 that relates to a population in the United States. The data for these actuarial standards were obtained from a section of the American population who applied for life insurance, and standards of desirable weights were given for people of a given height and frame, the desirable weights being those found to be associated with the lowest mortality. A new range of desirable weights has recently been published based on the life insurance experience of 4.2 million people between 1959 and 1979,[4] and these may well come to be the most widely used tables of this type. Recently published data compiled from the first and second Health and Nutrition Examination Surveys (HANES I and HANES II) include measurements of height, weight, triceps skinfold, subscapular skinfold, upper arm circumference, and elbow breadth of a cross-sectional multiracial sample of more than 20,000 subjects aged 25 to 74 years.[5] Based on these data, percentages of weight, skinfolds, and bone-free upper arm muscle area by height, sex, and frame size (elbow breadth was used as indicator of frame size) were established for all races combined in two groups: adults aged 25 to 54 years and the elderly aged 55 to 74 years. Using Tables 4–1 to 4–6 and applying age corrections from Table 4–7 these new standards can be used to differentiate those subjects at risk of being obese and undernourished.

A major limitation for the measurement of weight related to height compared with standard values is that they are unable to differentiate between differences in weight due to fat, muscle, water, or bone.[6] In this way superbly fit marathon runners could be classified as being malnourished or equally fit weight lifters could be designated "overweight" or "obese."

Evaluation of Weight Loss

Weight loss is an important index of the presence, severity, and progress of many diseases, as well as nutritional disorders such as protein-energy malnutrition. Body weight can be measured simply and accurately, and therefore weight loss can be determined easily if the patient's weight is measured before and after the occurrence of the loss. Usually, however, patients have already lost weight when they are first seen, and then the size of the loss must be evaluated by comparing measured weight with some estimate of original weight. The accuracy of the result therefore depends on the accuracy with which the original weight can be estimated. It must be borne in mind that, as with many other quantities measured in clinical medicine, clinically significant changes are often smaller than the range of values in healthy people.

Weight is nearly unique in that it is a measurement that many people make on themselves. Therefore, many patients can give some estimate of their weight when they are well, and there is good evidence that this estimate is reliable and accurate.[7] Generally speaking, though, tall and heavy persons tend to underestimate their height and weight and short, light persons overestimate theirs.[8] There are fewer data on the accuracy of recollection of weight before a period of illness, but a recent study suggests that "well weight" is not as reliably recalled in patients as in normal subjects.[9]

An alternative to recalled weight is predicted or standard weight. This is the mean weight of a group of healthy persons of the same age, sex, and height as the patient and usually taken from published tables. It is the only possible estimate of healthy weight when the patient is unable to remember his well weight and has been widely used in studies of hospital patients. However, for the individual patient it is important to realize that it is subject to large errors since it makes no allowance for the wide variation of individual weights about the mean. It has now been clearly shown that it is more reliable to estimate weight loss by using the patient's recalled well weight than by using published tables.[9]

Since the procedure of estimating weight loss by either method may be quite misleading, in individual cases it is important to relate this to the physical examination of the patient. There are marked changes in the physique characteristically associated with severe weight loss, and these should be carefully looked for. For example, Keys and colleagues[10] showed that after 6 months of semistarvation that resulted in weight loss of around 24 per cent there were decreases in muscle tissues and subcutaneous fat that made the subjects who were studied haggard and emaciated in appearance. They wrote, "Their faces were thin and their cheek bones prominent. The padding around the shoulder girdle was greatly reduced with marked decrease in the breadth of the shoulders. The ribs had become prominent and there were winged scapulae. The patients' waists were narrow and pinched and the iliac crests were prominent. The wasting of soft tissues was particularly marked in the region of the buttocks which had become thin and flat. The arms and legs were spindly." It is important to remember that these char-

TABLE 4–1. Selected Percentiles of Weight, Triceps and Subscapular Skinfolds, and Bone-Free Upper Arm Muscle Area for U.S. Males and Females with Small Frames, 25 to 54 Years Old, Derived from the Combined HANES I and II Data Sets

Ht (in)	Ht (cm)	n	Wt (kg) 5	10	15	50	85	90	95	Triceps (mm) 5	10	15	50	85	90	95	Subscapular (mm) 5	10	15	50	85	90	95	Bone-free AMA (cm²) 5	10	15	50	85	90	95
Males																														
62	157	23	46*	50*	52*	64	71*	74*	77*				11	17						16							52			
63	160	43	48*	51*	53	61	70	75*	79*			6	10	16	18			7	8	12	20					32	48	54		
64	163	73	49*	53	55	66	76	76	80*		5	6	10	17	18	21		8	8	15	25	29	35			38	49	58	63	
65	165	112	52	53	58	66	77	81	84	4	5	6	11	17	18	20		8	9	14	25	28	32		37	37	47	60	63	71
66	168	129	56	57	59	67	78	83	84	5	5	6	11	18	20	22		8	8	14	26	25	30		35	38	49	58	62	71
67	170	132	56	60	62	71	82	83	88	5	6	6	10	15	16	20		7	9	15	23	25	40		36	41	49	58	60	62
68	173	107	56	59	62	71	79	82	88	5	6	6	11	17				8	7	13	24	30	26		39	40	49	59	62	69
69	175	97	57*	62*	65	74	84	87	88*	5	6	6	10	17	20			7	9	13	24				37	40	58	61	63	
70	178	46	59*	62*	67	75	87	86*	90*		6	7	10	16				8	8	13	23				36	35	48	57		
71	180	49	60*	64*	70	76	79	88*	91*			7	10		20					14	22					39	47	52		
72	183	21	62*	65*	67*	74	87*	89*	93*	7										14							45			
73	185	9	63*	67*	69*	79*	89*	91*	94*	7																				
74	188	6	65*	68*	71*	80*	90*	92*	96*	6																				
Females																														
58	147	53	37*	43	43	52	58	62	66*			13	24	30	33		8	10	12	23	34	38			22	24	29	36	44	
59	150	108	42	43	44	53	63	69	72	6	12	14	21	29	36	37	6	9	10	17	29	32	34	17	20	22	28	38	39	43
60	152	142	42	44	45	53	63	65	70	8	11	12	21	28	29	33	7	7	8	18	27	32	39	19	21	22	28	36	40	44
61	155	218	44	46	47	54	64	66	72	8	11	14	21	28	31	34	7	8	8	16	28	32	36	20	21	23	28	38	39	42
62	157	255	44	47	48	55	63	64	70	7	12	14	20	28	31	36	6	7	7	14	22	27	32	20	21	21	27	33	35	37
63	160	239	46	48	49	55	65	68	79	6	11	13	20	27	30	34	6	7	8	14	27	29	31	21	22	23	27	33	35	38
64	163	146	49	50	51	57	67	68	74	6	13	14	20	28	31	34	6	7	8	13	24	30	34	22	23	23	28	34	38	42
65	165	113	50	52	53	60	70	72	80	7	13	12	22	29		33	7	8	8	15	26	30	33	21	22	23	28	37	39	47
66	168	47	46*	49*	54	58	65	71*	74*			12	19	30					9	12	25					23	27	35		
67	170	18	47*	50*	52*	59	70*	72*	76*	6			18							13							26			
68	173	18	48*	51*	53*	62	71*	73*	77*				20							15							25			
69	175	5	49*	52*	54*	63*	72*	74*	78*																					
70	178	1	50*	53*	55*	64*	73*	75*	79*																					

*Value estimated through linear regression equation.
From Frisancho AR. Am J Clin Nutr 1984; *40*:808–819. ©Am J Clin Nutr, American Society for Clinical Nutrition. Reproduced with permission.

TABLE 4–2. Selected Percentiles of Weight, Triceps and Subscapular Skinfolds, and Bone-Free Upper Arm Muscle Area for U.S. Males and Females with Medium Frames, 25 to 54 Years Old, Derived from the Combined HANES I and II Data Sets

Ht (in)	Ht (cm)	n	Wt (kg) 5	10	15	50	85	90	95	Triceps (mm) 5	10	15	50	85	90	95	Subscapular (mm) 5	10	15	50	85	90	95	Bone-free AMA (cm²) 5	10	15	50	85	90	95
Males																														
62	157	10	51*	55*	58*	68	81*	83*	87*				15	18	20					13	30	32					58			
63	160	30	52*	56*	59*	71	82*	85*	89*				11	20	22	25				18	26	29					55			
64	163	71	54*	60	61	71	83	84	90*	6	6	6	12	16	18	22		7	9	17	30	32			43	47	56	67	71	
65	165	154	59	62	65	74	87	90	94	8	7	8	12	21	23	28	8	9	10	16	26	29	32	40	43	45	55	67	69	70
66	168	212	58	61	65	75	85	87	93	7	6	7	11	18	20	24	7	7	9	16	25	27	33	38	42	44	53	66	72	78
67	170	409	62	66	68	77	89	93	100	8	7	7	13	18	20	24	8	9	10	18	26	30	33	39	42	44	55	67	69	73
68	173	478	60	64	66	78	89	92	97	7	5	7	11	18	20	23	7	8	9	16	25	28	31	41	44	45	55	67	71	76
69	175	464	63	66	68	78	90	93	97	7	6	7	12	18	20	25	7	8	9	16	25	27	31	38	41	44	54	66	69	73
70	178	419	64	66	70	81	90	93	97	4	5	7	12	19	21	25	7	8	9	15	24	27	30	39	42	43	55	65	68	72
71	180	282	62	68	70	81	92	96	100	5	7	7	12	20	22	26	7	8	9	14	24	27	30	37	41	44	54	67	67	73
72	183	231	68	71	74	84	97	100	104	6	7	8	12	20	24	27	7	9	9	15	26	30	32	40	42	44	56	65	69	74
73	185	106	70	72	75	85	100	101	104		7	8	12	20	24		8	9	9	15	25	29	32	39	42	43	55	67	69	73
74	188	50	68*	76	77	88	100	100	104*		6	9	13	21	23	27		7	9	14	25	30			43	43	55	62	63	
Females																														
58	147	40	41*	46*	50	63	77	75*	79*	15	19	20	25	40	40	40	10	12	15	23	38	39	43	23	24	24	35	42	45	49
59	150	104	47	50	52	66	76	79	85	14	15	21	30	37	37	41	8	10	13	29	38	37	41	22	25	26	33	43	45	49
60	152	208	47	50	52	60	77	79	85	11	15	17	26	35	36	42	7	9	11	22	35	36	42	21	24	25	32	42	45	51
61	155	465	49	49	51	61	73	78	86	12	14	15	25	34	36	40	7	9	10	19	32	36	42	21	23	25	31	42	43	48
62	157	644	50	51	53	61	73	77	83	12	13	16	24	34	36	40	7	8	10	18	33	37	40	21	23	25	31	40	43	50
63	160	685	50	52	54	62	77	80	88	11	14	15	23	33	35	38	7	8	10	18	31	35	38	21	22	24	31	41	43	48
64	163	722	52	52	55	62	76	82	87	12	14	15	24	33	36	38	7	7	8	16	31	33	38	21	23	24	31	40	43	49
65	165	628	52	54	55	63	75	80	89	11	14	15	22	31	34	38	7	8	8	15	29	30	35	21	23	24	30	39	41	44
66	168	428	52	54	55	63	75	78	83	11	13	14	22	31	33	37	7	8	8	14	28	30	37	22	23	24	30	40	43	48
67	170	257	54	56	57	65	79	82	88	12	13	15	21	29	30	35	7	8	9	15	28	32	37	22	24	25	30	40	41	48
68	173	119	58	59	60	67	77	85	87	10	14	15	22	31	32	36	8	8	9	15	29	33	35		24	25	30	37	38	39
69	175	59	49*	58	60	68	79	82	87*		11	12	19	29	31	36		8	8	12	25	29			23	24	30	36	39	
70	178	15	50*	54*	57*	70	80*	83*	87*				19							20							32			

*Value estimated through linear regression equation.
From Frisancho AR. Am J Clin Nutr 1984; *40*:808–819. ©Am J Clin Nutr, American Society for Clinical Nutrition. Reproduced with permission.

TABLE 4–3. Selected Percentiles of Weight, Triceps and Subscapular Skinfolds, and Bone-Free Upper Arm Muscle Area for U.S. Males and Females with Large Frames, 25 to 54 Years Old, Derived from the Combined HANES I and II Data Sets

Ht (in)	Ht (cm)	n	Wt (kg)							Triceps (mm)							Subscapular (mm)							Bone-free AMA (cm²)						
			5	10	15	50	85	90	95	5	10	15	50	85	90	95	5	10	15	50	85	90	95	5	10	15	50	85	90	95
Males																														
62	157	1	57*	62*	66*	82*	99*	103*	108*																					
63	160	1	58*	63*	67*	83*	100*	104*	109*																					
64	163	5	59*	64*	68*	84*	101*	105*	110*																					
65	165	15	60*	65*	69*	79	102*	106*	111*																					
66	168	37	60*	65*	75	84	103	106*	112*				14	30					13	21	36						62			
67	170	54	62*	70	71	84	102	111	113*			9	14	23	27				11	20	36					48	58	76		
68	173	84	63*	74	76	86	101	104	114*		7	7	11	22	23			8	14	20	31	40			50	52	61	73	78	
69	175	126	68	71	74	89	103	105	114	9	9	10	14	25	29	31	9	12	11	18	31	35	38	46	51	53	65	78	86	83
70	178	150	68	72	74	87	106	112	114	7	7	8	15	23	25	30	7	10	11	17	31	32	38	43	48	49	61	73	78	86
71	180	123	73	78	82	91	113	116	123	6	7	10	14	25	27	31	9	10	11	20	35	35	46	47	47	50	61	75	77	83
72	183	114	73	76	78	91	109	112	121	7	8	7	15	20	25	25	8	11	9	19	28	40	48	45	48	50	62	75	81	86
73	185	109	72	77	79	93	106	107	116	5	6	8	12	19	22	31	7	9	9	18	27	36	30	47	48	51	66	79	80	86
74	188	37	69*	74*	82	92	105	115*	120*	5	6		13	19	22			9	9	18	32	28			49	53	66	78	83	
Females																														
58	147	6	56*	63*	67*	86*	105*	110*	117*																				
59	150	19	56*	62*	67*	78	105*	109*	116*				36														45		
60	152	32	55*	62*	66*	87	104*	109*	116*				38							35							44		
61	155	92	54*	64	66	81	105	117	115*		25		36	48	50	50		17		42	48	53	55		29		41	62	74	72
62	157	135	59	61	65	81	103	107	113	16	19	26	34	48	48	51	13	16	17	35	48	51	50	26	28	33	44	56	63	77
63	160	162	58	63	67	83	105	109	119	18	20	22	34	46	48	49	11	14	18	32	44	48	50	27	30	31	43	60	65	63
64	163	196	58	62	63	79	102	104	112	16	20	22	32	43	46	48	9	12	16	32	42	46	50	26	28	32	39	50	55	67
65	165	242	59	61	63	81	103	109	114	17	17	21	31	40	43	45	10	12	15	28	42	48	52	27	28	29	39	50	59	69
66	168	166	55	58	62	75	95	100	107	13	16	18	27	41	43	49	8	9	14	25	36	40	45	23	24	27	35	49	53	55
67	170	144	58	60	65	80	100	108	114	13	16	17	30	37	40		7	10	11	25	41	46	55	25	28	30	37	50	53	
68	173	81	51*	58	66	76	104	105	111*			20	29	42				10	11	21	45	48			28	30	38	51	54	
69	175	39	50*	57*	68	79	105	104*	111*			21	30						12	20	43					30	35	49		
70	178	17	50*	56*	61*	76	99*	104*	110*				20						11	16						27	37		

*Value estimated through linear regression equation.

From Frisancho AR. Am J Clin Nutr 1984; *40*:808–819. ©Am J Clin Nutr, American Society for Clinical Nutrition. Reproduced with permission.

TABLE 4-4. Selected Percentiles of Weight, Triceps and Subscapular Skinfolds, and Bone-Free Upper Arm Muscle Area for U.S. Males and Females with Small Frames, 55 to 74 Years Old, Derived from the Combined HANES I and II Data Sets

Ht		n	Wt (kg)							Triceps (mm)							Subscapular (mm)							Bone-free AMA (cm²)						
in	cm		5	10	15	50	85	90	95	5	10	15	50	85	90	95	5	10	15	50	85	90	95	5	10	15	50	85	90	95
Males																														
62	157	47	45*	49*	56	61	68	73*	77*			6	9	12					11	16	23					38	46	52		
63	160	78	47*	49	51	62	71	71	79*		5	5	10	16	17			6	6	12	21	22			34	35	43	54	55	
64	163	107	47	50	54	63	72	74	80		4	4	9	20	21	22		7	8	14	24	25	29		30	31	44	53	54	56
65	165	132	48	54	59	70	80	90	90	4	6	7	11	16	19	24	6	8	8	16	28	28	29	26	30	34	48	57	60	62
66	168	112	51	55	59	68	77	80	84	5	6	7	11	16	20	20	6	7	8	15	25	26	30	26	31	35	45	54	58	64
67	170	128	55	60	61	69	79	81	88	5	6	6	10	15	17	25	7	8	9	13	22	25	31	25	36	37	45	53	55	59
68	173	95	54*	54	58	70	79	81	86*		5	5	10	15	17		7	7	7	13	21	22		30	35	35	43	55	60	
69	175	47	56*	59*	63	75	81	84*	88*			8	10	15					10	16	27					38	47	62		
70	178	29	57*	61*	63*	76	83*	86*	89*				11							13							48			
71	180	14	59*	62*	65*	69	85*	87*	91*				9							10							43			
72	183	6	60*	64*	66*	76*	86*	89*	92*																				
73	185	1	62*	65*	68*	78*	88*	90*	94*																				
74	188	1	63*	67*	69*	77*	89*	92*	95*																				
Females																														
58	147	85	39*	46	48	54	63	65	71*	11	14	16	21	31	34	33	6	8	9	18	32	33	33	22	22	23	29	40	42	44
59	150	122	41	45	48	55	66	68	74	10	13	15	21	30	31	35	5	7	9	19	29	30	36	20	23	24	30	39	40	44
60	152	157	43	45	47	54	67	70	73	10	11	13	20	29	31	32	6	7	8	15	27	32	34	18	22	23	30	37	41	42
61	155	145	43	43	45	56	65	70	71	11	12	14	22	29	29	32	7	7	8	17	29	31	30	20	21	23	28	36	40	43
62	157	158	47	49	52	58	67	69	73		11	12	21	29	30			8	7	17	25	26			23	24	30	37	40	
63	160	89	42*	45	49	58	67	68	74*		12	13	20	29	30			6	6	14	25	27			19	20	27	35	36	
64	163	50	43*	47*	49*	60	68	70	75*		12	13	21	27	29			6	7	18	24	25			21	21	28	37	42	
65	165	26	43*	47*	49*	60	69*	72*	75*				18							13							28			
66	168	12	44*	48*	50*	68	70*	72*	76*				23							13							33			
67	170	1	45*	48*	51*	61*	71*	73*	77*																				
68	173	0	45*	49*	51*	61*	71*	74*	77*																				
69	175	0	46*	49*	52*	62*	72*	74*	78*																				
70	178	0	47*	50*	52*	63*	73*	75*	79*																				

*Value estimated through linear regression equation.

From Frisancho AR. Am J Clin Nutr 1984; 40:808–819. ©Am J Clin Nutr, American Society for Clinical Nutrition. Reproduced with permission.

TABLE 4–5. Selected Percentiles of Weight, Triceps and Subscapular Skinfolds, and Bone-Free Upper Arm Muscle Area for U.S. Males and Females with Medium Frames, 55 to 74 Years Old, Derived from the Combined HANES I and II Data Sets

Ht (in)	Ht (cm)	n	Wt 5	Wt 10	Wt 15	Wt 50	Wt 85	Wt 90	Wt 95	Tri 5	Tri 10	Tri 15	Tri 50	Tri 85	Tri 90	Tri 95	Sub 5	Sub 10	Sub 15	Sub 50	Sub 85	Sub 90	Sub 95	AMA 5	AMA 10	AMA 15	AMA 50	AMA 85	AMA 90	AMA 95
Males																													
62	157	49	50*	54*	59	68	77	81*	85*			5	12	25					11	19	27	28				39	48	61		
63	160	89	51*	57	60	70	80	82	87*		7	7	11	20	23			8	10	15	26	27				38	50	60	63	
64	163	210	55	59	62	71	82	83	91	5	6	6	10	17	20	26	7	7	9	15	25	29	35	35	36	40	51	64	66	71
65	165	335	56	60	64	72	83	86	89	5	6	7	11	17	19	24	7	9	10	16	25	28	31	35	39	41	52	63	65	72
66	168	405	57	62	66	74	83	84	89	6	6	7	12	18	19	22	9	9	10	17	26	29	34	34	38	42	51	60	62	67
67	170	509	59	64	66	78	87	89	94	5	6	8	12	18	20	23	9	9	10	17	26	28	32	35	39	42	52	65	67	70
68	173	413	62	66	68	78	89	95	101	5	7	7	12	18	21	23	8	8	9	16	25	27	30	37	40	40	52	65	65	70
69	175	366	62	66	68	77	90	93	99	6	6	7	11	19	22	25	9	9	10	16	25	26	31	31	36	44	51	62	65	72
70	178	248	68	68	71	80	90	95	101	5	7	6	11	18	19	21	9	9	10	15	25	27	—	36	41	44	53	63	65	68
71	180	146	68	72	72	84	96	97	101	5	6	8	13	16	17	20	8	8	10	16	28	26	—	36	42	39	56	65	67	71
72	183	81	66*	65	69	81	93	97	101*		6	8	11	19	20				10	15	26	30				43	50	58	59	
73	185	35	68*	72*	79	88	98*	99*	103*				13	16					10	18					27		56	67		
74	188	11	69*	73*	76*	95	98*	101*	104*				11														56			
Females																													
58	147	105	40	44	49	57	72	82	85	5	13	17	28	40	40	41	3	7	10	25	37	43	48	21		25	32	46	47	51
59	150	198	47	49	52	62	74	78	86	12	15	18	26	34	38	41	8	9	11	23	32	36	43	24	23	27	35	44	48	48
60	152	358	47	50	52	65	76	79	86	13	17	18	25	33	34	38	8	10	12	22	34	36	40	21	26	26	35	45	49	57
61	155	543	49	51	54	64	78	81	86	13	16	18	25	35	37	42	8	10	10	20	33	36	42	22	24	26	34	44	49	52
62	157	576	49	53	54	64	78	82	88	13	15	16	24	33	36	39	8	8	10	20	33	36	38	24	25	26	35	45	47	54
63	160	551	52	54	55	65	78	83	89	12	14	16	24	32	35	38	7	9	10	18	32	37	41	24	26	27	35	44	45	51
64	163	406	54	56	57	66	78	81	87	14	14	17	25	33	35	37	7	8	9	17	30	33	37	21	25	26	33	44	46	49
65	165	307	54	57	59	67	78	84	88	12	16	16	24	33	33	39	6	7	8	17	30	35	37	24	26	27	34	44	45	50
66	168	119	54	57	57	66	79	85	88	12	13	17	24	35	35	36	8	9	10	16	35	31	34	24	25	27	33	41	43	49
67	170	63	51*	59	61	72	82	85	89*		17	17	27					9		19	35	35			27	28	32	41	43	
68	173	28	52*	56*	59*	70	83*	86*	90*				25							16							36			
69	175	5	53*	57*	60*	72*	84*	87*	91*																					
70	178	1	54*	58*	61*	73*	85*	88*	92*																					

*Value estimated through linear regression equation.

From Frisancho AR. Am J Clin Nutr 1984; 40:808–819. ©Am J Clin Nutr, American Society for Clinical Nutrition. Reproduced with permission.

TABLE 4–6. Selected Percentiles of Weight, Triceps and Subscapular Skinfolds, and Bone-Free Upper Arm Muscle Area for U.S. Males and Females with Large Frames, 55 to 74 Years Old, Derived from the Combined HANES I and II Data Sets

Ht			Wt (kg)							Triceps (mm)							Subscapular (mm)							Bone-free AMA (cm²)						
in	cm	n	5	10	15	50	85	90	95	5	10	15	50	85	90	95	5	10	15	50	85	90	95	5	10	15	50	85	90	95
Males																														
62	157	7	54*	59*	63*	77*	91*	95*	100*				15							20										
63	160	12	55*	60*	64*	80	92*	96*	101*				21							31							57			
64	163	20	57*	62*	65*	77	94*	97*	102*			11	14	22					14	19	27						44			
65	165	36	58*	63*	73	79	89	98*	103*		7	8	13	21	25			9	11	20	31					44	59			
66	168	58	59*	67	73	80	101	102	105*		8	9	16	21	25	27	8	11	12	20	35	35			43	47	56	66	72	
67	170	114	65	71	73	85	103	108	112	6	7	8	13	20	21	23	8	10	11	18	27	35	38	41	43	44	56	67	73	79
68	173	128	67	71	73	83	95	98	111	6	7	8	12	18	20	23	7	11	11	19	27	30	32	41	43	46	57	69	70	74
69	175	131	65	70	74	84	96	98	105	6	6	8	14	22	25	31	9	11	13	20	30	30	33	40	45	45	58	70	72	79
70	178	144	68	73	77	87	102	104	117	5	6	6	13	18	22			8	9	15	30	33	37	43	48	50	59	70	71	87
71	180	95	65*	70	70	84	102	109	111*		8	8	13	23	26			8	9	20	28	30			46	47	54	70	75	
72	183	72	67*	76	81	90	108	112	112*				11							19	31	31			47	48	59	73	78	
73	185	23	68*	73*	76*	88	105*	108*	113*				12							15							59			
74	188	15	69*	74*	78*	89	106*	109*	114*																		54			
Females																														
58	147	14	53*	59*	63*	92	95*	99*	104*				45							44							50			
59	150	26	54*	59*	63*	78	95*	99*	105*				36							31							49			
60	152	72	54*	65	69	78	87	88	106	18	25	26	35	44	45	46	13	19	21	31	42	45	48		28	33	41	58	60	71
61	155	117	64	68	69	79	94	101	111	19	22	24	33	40	44	50	13	16	19	29	40	43	53	31	32	34	44	59	61	76
62	157	126	59	61	63	82	93	101	118	20	24	24	32	40	43	45	13	19	22	30	39	48	51	28	29	34	43	59	63	67
63	160	154	61	65	67	80	100	102	119	18	24	25	33	41	43	50	10	15	16	33	40	45	55	27	32	33	41	56	62	78
64	163	147	60	65	69	77	97	102	111	15	22	23	29	42	46	46	8	12	16	29	41	46	48	28	29	32	41	54	60	65
65	165	117	60	66	69	80	98	102	111		17	23	30	43	44			9	12	24	42	46		29	32	32	42	53	57	
66	168	64	57*	60	63	82	98	105	109*		18	18	27	35	40				12	26	34	36			31	31	40	58	58	
67	170	40	58*	64*	68	80	105	104*	109*			22	32	44					14	25	46					30	40			
68	173	17	58*	64*	68*	79	100*	104*	110*				26							21							48			
69	175	7	59*	65*	69*	85*	101*	105*	110*																					
70	178	2	60*	65*	69*	85*	101*	105*	111*																					

*Value estimated through linear regression equation.

From Frisancho AR. Am J Clin Nutr 1984; *40*:808–819. ©Am J Clin Nutr, American Society for Clinical Nutrition. Reproduced with permission.

TABLE 4–7. Age Correction for Estimates of Weight, Triceps and Subscapular Skinfold Thicknesses, and Bone-Free Upper Arm Muscle Area

Age Group: Frame Size	Median Age	Weight	Triceps Skinfold	Subscapular Skinfold	Arm Muscle Area
Males					
25–54					
Small	39	0.074	0.016	0.080	0.030
Medium	39	0.080	0.005	0.083	0.055
Large	40	0.000	−0.024	0.049	0.026
55–74					
Small	66	−0.329	−0.036	−0.115	−0.407
Medium	67	−0.435	−0.040	−0.125	−0.521
Large	67	−0.562	−0.054	−0.185	−0.644
Females					
25–54					
Small	37	0.165	0.166	0.142	0.087
Medium	37	0.234	0.189	0.214	0.191
Large	37	0.284	0.191	0.233	0.270
55–74					
Small	67	−0.027	−0.072	−0.013	0.036
Medium	66	−0.196	−0.210	−0.221	−0.033
Large	67	−0.466	−0.370	−0.515	−0.378

These age correction coefficient factors are used as in the following example:

Given a 57-year-old, large-framed male who is 170 cm (67 in) tall, we wish to determine whether he is above or below the United States median, if he weighs 90 kg. The general equation used to determine the age-adjusted median weight for such an individual would be:

Adjusted weight standard
= unadjusted weight standard
+ (age-correction factor)
× (deviation from median age)

Where:

Unadjusted weight standard = 85 kg (see Table 4–6)
Age-correction factor = −0.562 (see above)
Median age = 67 years
Actual age = 57 years

From this information:

Adjusted weight standard
= 85 + (−0.562) (57−67)
= 85 + (−0.562) (−10)
= 90.62 kg

Therefore, the age-adjusted weight standard indicates that this individual is actually *below* the United States median (90 vs 91 kg), whereas without the age correction, he would have appeared to be about 5 kg *above* the median weight for his height and frame size.

From Frisancho AR. Am J Clin Nutr 1984; *40*:808–819. ©Am J Clin Nutr, American Society for Clinical Nutrition. Reproduced with permission.

acteristics and changes take place gradually, and close relatives and the patient himself tend to forget the original appearance. Photographs taken when the patient was well can be useful and can quite vividly be used to bring out the degree of emaciation in starvation.

Functional Effects of Weight Loss and Weight Gain

In the Minnesota experiment, mentioned above, Keys and colleagues studied 32 previously healthy men who were subjected to a 6-month period of semistarvation.[10] This regimen resulted in a 24 per cent weight loss. Observations of fitness were made at 3 months and at 6 months during the period of diet restriction. After 3 months of semistarvation the men lost an average of 17.5 per cent of their body weight. Marked deterioration in maximal oxygen intake, Harvard Fitness Test score, and strength had occurred. Once normal diet was resumed it was a

further 3 to 6 months before the subjects recovered and returned to normal.

The importance of weight loss in surgical patients presenting for major surgery was shown by the classic study of Studley,[11] who, over 50 years ago, found an increase in mortality among patients undergoing surgery for peptic ulceration who had lost 20 per cent or more of their body weight. Although recent studies have failed to show such a clear-cut association between weight loss and capacity to withstand a surgical procedure, an association is still apparent, particularly in those with massive weight loss, in spite of modern surgical techniques, anesthesia, and antibiotics.[12] The significance of lesser degrees of weight loss is not quite so clear. Most studies indicate that normal subjects evaluated in semistarvation for 10 days with weight loss less than 10 per cent demonstrate no impairment of physical performance,[13] but some authors suggest that physical performance is affected more by the rate of weight loss than by the absolute extent of it.

Although it is difficult to quantify the precise functional effects of being overweight, very fat people tend to be relatively inactive and have been shown to make fewer movements than persons of average weight. When a fat person has to move quickly there is an excessive demand on the whole organism, and this may mean a strain on one or more of the vulnerable organs or functions. Insurance companies report an excessive death rate in overweight persons from a variety of causes, including accidents.

Changes in Body Weight in Health

The body weight of normal subjects fluctuates throughout the day as a function of ingestion and excretion of food and water. Weight is at its peak in the late afternoon or early evening. Throughout the night 1 to 2 kg disappear by the insensible loss of water through the lungs and, as food is oxidized, by the exhalation of the resultant carbon dioxide and urinary excretion of water of oxidation. The fluctuations from day to day can be quite large.

Studies of normal subjects carried out under very controlled conditions have shown that there are body weight changes as high as 1 kg from one day to the next. In an important study Khosla and Billewicz[14] showed that the daily variation of body weight is a function of body weight itself; that the standard deviation of weight about its trend is close to 0.5 per cent of the body weight; and that the maximum change from one day to the next rarely exceeds 1.5 per cent of body weight, regardless of body size, age, or sex.

It is important to understand the changes that occur as part of the normal aging process. Although body weight may remain quite constant from year to year and into old age, there is a higher proportion of fat and a reduction of fat-free body mass as age advances.[15, 16]

Body Weight Changes in Disease and Recovery

Starvation. In a classic work published in 1915, Benedict[17] gathered together the records of body weight obtained during a considerable number of closely controlled fasting experiments. The data are summarized in Figure 4–2, where it can be seen that, on average, total starvation results in a weight loss of about 15 per cent (10 kg) over a 3-week period. In the clinical setting it is not uncommon for periods of total starvation to go untreated for as long as 3 weeks, and periods of semistarvation are more frequently encountered. It is important, therefore, to have an idea of the degree of weight loss that is associated with different aspects of semistarvation. In this context Table 4–8, adapted from Keys' book,[10] gives data that can be of direct clinical use. It can be seen from this table that the general mag-

nitude of weight loss (expressed as a percentage of original body weight) in patients who are consuming only 50 per cent of their normal diet is 15 per cent at 3 months, 25 per cent at 6 months, and 30 per cent at 12 months or more.

Weight Loss after Operation. When body weight changes following operation are plotted in graphical form it can be seen that an initial phase during which the curve declines is followed by a second phase in which the curve is more nearly level or tending in a positive direction (Fig. 4–2). The minimal weight is frequently found at the point of transition from one to the other phase. From the figure it can be seen that weight loss after surgery is less than that which occurs with total starvation and reflects known data about energy balance in these circumstances.[18] It has been shown that over the 2 weeks following abdominoperineal excision of the rectum an average of about 7 to 8 per cent of body weight is lost, this being less than that which would have been expected in total starvation, when about 13 per cent would be expected to be lost. Energy balance studies show that such patients consume about half the energy intake required over the first 2 weeks after operation, thereby accounting for a lesser weight loss than that which occurs in total starvation. As might be expected, it has been found that the duration of postoperative weight loss is generally proportional to the degree of trauma; furthermore, when intensity of surgical trauma is nearly uniform, postoperative weight loss continues longer for heavier than for lighter patients.[19]

Weight Loss Associated with Trauma and Sepsis. It has been seen that patients recovering from major elective surgical procedures will usually lose 4 to 8 per cent of their body weight in the early postoperative period. There seems to be general acceptance among physicians of the idea that a loss of up to 10 per cent of body weight can be sustained without jeopardizing convalescence, and hence normal postoperative recovery is thought not to be influenced by this degree of weight loss. However, the situation is more complicated after trauma and sepsis. Kinney[20] showed that severely traumatized patients who receive about 50 per cent of the normal intake of calories and nitrogen during a 3-week period following injury sustained weight losses equivalent to those observed in subjects undergoing total starvation (Fig. 4–2). Further studies of this type are complicated by the fact that such patients, particularly when septic, are now treated vigorously with fluid replacement together with intravenous nutrition. Thus, as Figure 4–2 shows, many septic patients have rapidly increasing body weight owing to fluid retention, and it is only during recovery, when water and sodium are lost, that weight loss becomes apparent.[21] In spite of this apparent weight gain there are profound falls in body protein in spite of aggressive intravenous nutrition, although evidence

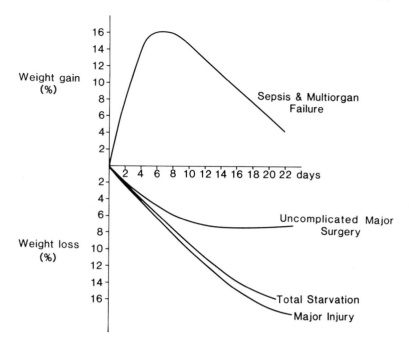

FIGURE 4–2. Changes in body weight that occur in serious sepsis, after uncomplicated surgery, in total starvation, and after major injury.

now suggests that body fat may be gained in these circumstances.

Body Weight Changes Associated with Cancer. Weight loss is recognized as a common accompaniment of cancer and it almost always occurs when the disease is far advanced. It has been shown to influence the response to chemotherapy[22] and the duration of survival.[23] It is seen particularly in patients with gastrointestinal cancer. In a massive study[24] of over 3000 patients, those with favorable subtypes of non-Hodgkin's lymphoma, breast cancer, acute non-lymphocytic leukemia, and sarcomas had the lowest frequency of weight loss, with 60 to 70 per cent of the patients having no weight loss at all. On the other hand, patients with pancreatic or gastric cancer had a higher frequency of weight loss (83 to 87 per cent) and about a third of these patients had lost more than 10 per cent of their body weight. Generally speaking, the cause of the weight loss in patients with gastrointestinal cancer is impaired dietary intake rather than increased metabolic expenditure.[25, 26]

Anabolic Recovery. Long-term studies of patients recovering from major surgery are few and far between. One study looking at weight and body com-

positional changes in ten patients recovering after panproctocolectomy and ileostomy showed that 6 months after surgery only four had returned to what was considered to be their well weight. Nevertheless, the group as a whole, over the 6-month period, had a mean weight gain of 13.7 per cent.[27] Even though it may take some months to return to normality following very major surgery, it is worth noting that some patients ultimately become heavier than they were before the surgical procedure. In some situations, though, body weight never returns to normal; a classic example is subtotal gastrectomy, after which permanent weight loss occurs in nearly half the patients.[28]

Intravenous Nutrition. Although weight gain is seen regularly in patients being treated with adequate intravenous nutrition, this weight gain does not always represent tissue gain. During short periods of intravenous nutrition it is more likely to be due to water gain associated with glycogen deposition in muscle tissue than to a true gain in cellular protein (Fig. 4–3). Fat is quite frequently gained during intravenous feeding and represents a small part of the weight gain observed.[29]

Changes in Physical Appearance Associated with Weight Loss. Chronically starved patients can be recognized easily by their haggard faces: they are lean and bony. Generally speaking, they have profound wasting of both subcutaneous fat and muscle, and since the body framework remains the same the skeleton becomes prominent and the appearance angular. Sheldon[30] proposed a scheme of somatotypes which he suggested represent the basic body characteristic and are relatively independent of body fat. Soft roundness (*endomorphy*), muscular solidity (*mesomorphy*), and linearity-delicacy (*ectomorphy*) have been described as basic somatotypes. Sheldon be-

TABLE 4–8. Weight Loss in Patients on Reduced-Energy Diets

Duration of Reduced Intake (Months)	Energy Intake as Percentage of Intake Needed to Maintain Normal Weight				
	80	*70*	*50*	*30*	*20*
3	8%	10%	15%	25%	30%
6	12%	15%	25%	35%	45%
12 or more	15%	20%	30%	40%	

Weight loss expressed as a percentage of original body weight. After Keys A, Brozek J, Henschel A, et al. The Biology of Human Starvation. Minneapolis, University of Minnesota Press, 1950.

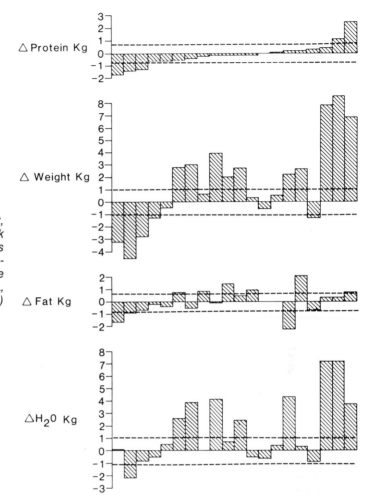

FIGURE 4–3. Changes in body protein, weight, fat, and water that occurred in 20 patients during a 2-week course of total parenteral nutrition. The broken lines indicate the maximum difference between the measurements, which can with 95 per cent probability be attributed to measurement error alone. (After Hill GL, Bradley JA, Smith RC, et al. JPEN 1979; 3:215–218.)

lieved that the basic somatotype did not change even with severe weight loss, but other workers have shown this not to be so, pointing out that when starved the endomorph is so changed that he appears more like an ectomorph.

In the first few months of rehabilitation after nutritional depletion the patient does not simply return to normal body composition. Keys[10] showed that fat is laid down more rapidly than muscle tissue and "soft roundness" becomes the dominant characteristic, reflecting a tendency to a relative obesity. Mention has already been made of the fact that in later rehabilitation, even after body composition has been restored to normal levels and anabolism ceases, the patient may continue to gain weight and become fatter than normal.

There is a small decrease in height in patients who have been starved, and this is not always corrected after rehabilitation. It is thought that the decrease in height is due to a decrease in the thickness of the intervertebral discs and that these changes may be irreversible, essentially paralleling the process of aging, in which a decrease in stature has also been observed.

Organ Changes Associated with Weight Loss

The degree of wasting of various organs of the body that accompanies body weight loss has been computed by comparing weights of different organs in emaciated patients subjected to necropsy with normal standards. Unfortunately many of the standards are unsatisfactory and proper longitudinal studies are lacking. Nevertheless, available data are instructive. Results of the autopsy studies of Krieger[31] are given in Table 4–9 and show the striking fact that most organs have a percentage mass loss roughly similar to that of the total body, the exception being the brain. Generally speaking, skin, muscle, and particularly liver waste more than the heart, although it must be said that there is great variability among individuals.

The Concept of Lethal Weight Loss

Although weight loss after uncomplicated surgery is usually small and perhaps unimportant physio-

TABLE 4–9. Percentage Losses of Weight of the Body and Various Organs in Autopsies on Emaciated Bodies

	Cachexia (% Loss)	Tumor (% Loss)	Sepsis (% Loss)	Old Age (% Loss)
Body weight	39	38	44	36
Heart	35	33	31	30
Liver	42	33	28	26
Kidney	36	28	16	20
Spleen	47	28	—	36
Brain	5	3	3	3
Pancreas	—	33	31	—
Endocrine glands	—	22	30	—

After Krieger M. Anat Konstitutionsl 1921; 7:87–134.

logically, some patients with septic complications may sustain considerable losses of weight. Before death from tissue depletion occurs, complications such as pulmonary infection, hepatic failure, or upper gastrointestinal hemorrhage generally occur. In anorexia nervosa even greater weight losses occur, and patients with this disorder may die from tissue depletion without other complications. In this condition three factors are thought to contribute to the extreme degree of weight loss, which may reach 45 to 55 per cent of normal body weight. The reduction in food intake is gradual, there is no major catabolic stimulus limiting the adaptation to starvation, and the limitation of water intake as well as food intake restricts the development of nutritional edema. Thus, weight loss can be serious both because of its ultimate extent and because of the rapid rate of development such as occurs in major surgical catabolic states. The extent of weight loss that can be tolerated in major metabolic illness is less than that which can be tolerated in partial starvation without injury or sepsis. Loss of 30 to 40 per cent of body weight may be considered as cachexia. This degree of weight loss in a concentration camp has been shown to be followed by increasing trouble from weakness, decubitus ulcers, and joint contractures. An equivalent degree of protein and fat depletion may occur in hospital patients without recognition of the severity of the problem because of the extracellular water retention that accompanies prolonged clinical care.[32]

It is sometimes said that there is a definite level of loss of body weight that is lethal. Krieger[31] set the lethal level of loss of original body weight at 20 per cent for the young, 40 per cent for adults exposed to acute starvation, and up to 50 per cent in cases of semistarvation. Although these are broad guidelines, it is important from a clinical point of view to realize that there is no state except final coma when the disease and starvation can be said to be irreversible. Many clinicians have reported recovery in some patients who have suffered a striking loss of body weight and exhibited profound cachexia.

BODY FAT

The layman often considers that the difference between undernourished and well-fed persons is their degree of "fatness." While this is clearly wrong, the fact remains that changes in the relative amount of fat at different levels of nutrition are nearly always greater than changes in the fat-free tissues of the body. For the intelligent interpretation of body weight and its changes in different physiological conditions we need to know the components of the body and its parts. Traditionally body composition studies have broken down the living body in terms of fat and fat-free tissues, and it is because of this and the fact that the relationship of the fat content of the body to health and illness is an important problem that "body fat" and its measurement will be dealt with in some depth.

Techniques for Measuring Body Fat

Of the major body compartments the most elusive to measure in the living subject is undoubtedly fat, especially since it has not yet been possible to measure this substance by a direct means. Nevertheless many methods have been used and these can be grouped together into five general approaches including *densitometry* (usually by underwater weighing), *skinfold anthropometry*, *imaging techniques* (x-ray radiometry, computer scanning, or ultrasonography), *electrical conductivity* or *impedance measurement*, and, finally, measurement of other major compartments and subtraction of these from measured body weight (the so-called difference methods). This list is by no means exhaustive.

In the absence of any absolute method, research workers have always been in the position of having to compare results of any new technique with those of an earlier technique. Since densitometry was the technique first developed,[33] it has generally been the practice to compare new techniques with densitometry, thereby, quite arbitrarily, investing the latter technique with the status of a "gold standard." This has been unfortunate, since densitometry is an indirect technique that critically depends on a priori assumptions about the density of the fat-free component of the body, assumptions that are unsubstantiated in normal humans and that certainly cannot be expected to apply in the clinical situation. Before describing some of the methods of measuring body fat it is pertinent to briefly examine some of the factors that affect the precision and accuracy of estimates of one entity from measurements of another.

Statistical Considerations. The development of predictor relationships to predict a quantity y from a measured quantity x depends on first being able to measure both x and y in a representative sample of a patient population and then on imposing a relationship between the two quantities. Assuming for the sake of argument that the imposed relationship is linear, then the residual error (sometimes called the standard error of the estimate) of y upon x, σ_R, is made up of two components, namely a measured or technical component, σ_M, and a biological component, σ_B, such that

$$\sigma_R^2 = \sigma_M^2 + \sigma_B^2$$

The biological component arises from the fact that, discounting measurement error, the relationship between x and y is not perfectly linear. Put another way, σ_B^2 represents the refusal of nature to conform to the imposed relationship. In many clinical situations $\sigma_B^2 > \sigma_M^2$. Furthermore, if we subsequently measure a value of x, then the propagated error in the estimate of the true value of y can be shown to depend only on the biological component of the residual error in the original regression.* This biological component is clearly subject-specific, and one can have no a priori knowledge of its magnitude in an individual. It affects not only the accuracy of each individual estimate but also the precision of an estimate of the mean value of y from a number of different measured values of x, despite the fact that it arises from systematic sources that do not affect the precision of an individual estimate; because of this it is frequently missed or ignored.

However, when groups of patients are to be studied, further problems arise. The regression equations to be used on patient studies are usually derived from studies of normal populations, and two effects result from the inevitable heterogeneity of patient groups. The first is an increase in the biological component of the residual error, which clearly leads to reduced accuracy for individual estimates and poorer precision for group means than is obtainable with studies of normals. The second result is the generation of a systematic error on the group mean, arising because the true regression relationship between x and y for the patient group is systematically different from that derived from normal studies; it is frequently not possible to derive the true relationship for a patient group for logistic reasons, so that regressions derived from normal studies have to be used instead.

The implication is that the use of indirect estimates of an entity (such as body fat) should be treated with extreme caution, especially if estimates are to be made for individual patients or small groups ($n < 50$) of patients. The problem is also important with longitudinal studies, in which the biological component of the residual error may systematically change with time as the result of changes in the patient's condition. Thus apparent changes in an entity derived via an indirect means may in fact reflect only changes in the biological error.

---

*It should be noted that if x is also measured with random error, as it usually is, then strictly speaking regression analysis is inappropriate and one should resort to factor analysis to get unbiased estimates of the relationship between *true* values of measured quantities.[34, 35] The present argument ignores such considerations because the biological errors associated with indirect body composition techniques are generally large compared with the measurement errors.

Finally, mention should be made of the effects of measurement error. These errors are either systematic in character, not affecting the precision but clearly affecting the accuracy of both individual and grouped data, or they are random, clearly affecting the precision for both individuals and groups. However, technical errors are generally readily measured and their effects well appreciated, so that further discussion is not necessary here.

Densitometry. Measurements of the density of the human body have been undertaken since the beginning of this century,[36] but it is probably not unfair to state that the originators of this body composition technique were Behnke and colleagues in the early 1940's.[33, 37] These workers were the first to recognize the importance of measuring residual lung volume, thereby correcting the measured densities, and used their results to classify individuals as to degree of obesity. Indeed, by suggesting body density as an index of obesity (and body fitness), Behnke and colleagues were able to classify athletes and well-developed individuals as normal where age-height-weight tables tended to categorize them as overweight. Conversely, some apparently normal people could be classified as obese with density measurement, as indeed they were. Accurate densitometry therefore represented a major step forward in body composition assessment.

The use of densitometry to estimate body fat depends first on the fact that body fat is much less dense than the other compartments of the body, but more importantly on the assumption that variations in body density are the result of variations in body fat content. This implies that the density (D) of the fat-free body is assumed to be constant and therefore that

$$\frac{m_f}{M} \propto \frac{1}{D}$$

where m_f and M are the mass of fat and body mass, respectively. Various equations have been suggested, but the most commonly used is probably that proposed by Siri,[38] namely

$$\frac{m_f}{M} = \frac{4.95}{D} - 4.50$$

which assumes densities of 0.90 and 1.100 g/cc for fat and fat-free mass, respectively.

Since this is an indirect method of measuring body fat, there are biological as well as technical sources of error that affect the precision and accuracy of the calculated body fat. Siri[39] calculated that the variation in density of fat and the lean body mass (LBM) would give rise to a precision standard deviation in the estimate of fat in normal man of the order of 3.8 per cent of body fat, equivalent to 0.006 g/cc in density units. Measurement error of 0.002 g/cc[40] will add in quadrature to produce a total precision of

0.0063 g/cc. Finally, the possibility of important systematic errors arising from the underwater technique should not be underestimated, and the problem of estimation of residual lung volume is particularly important.[41]

Clearly, densitometry based on underwater weighing is not a satisfactory method for measuring most patients purely for logistical reasons. Other methods of measuring body density have been used, such as that reported by Siri[42] in which body volume is measured in a sealed chamber by helium dilution; this method and other plethysmographic methods could also be applied to some moderately sick patient groups but not to many of the patients in our surgical wards or intensive care units. Furthermore, the variability of density in the LBM could be expected to be much greater in patients than in normal individuals, so that poorer precision would result; also, systematic errors would be highly probable, especially in those patients who have undergone profound weight changes as the result of their illness or treatment.

Skinfold Anthropometry. Since one of the major sites of fat deposition in the human body is subcutaneously located, measurement of skinfold thickness could be expected to correlate with total body fat, provided that the ratio of subcutaneous to total body fat is reasonably constant for a given sex and age range. As shown in Table 4–10, subcutaneous fat represents about 30 and 33 per cent of total body fat in men and women, respectively, though according to Lohman[43] estimates by various investigators range from 20 to 70 per cent depending on factors such as age, sex, obesity, and measurement technique. Furthermore, the accuracy of an estimate of subcutaneous fat is very much dependent on the number of sites measured and on the degree to which those sites correlate with total subcutaneous fat. In clinical practice, especially in dealing with the very sick nonambulatory patient, measurements can be reliably made only in two or three sites, and these usually include biceps and triceps skinfolds with or without subscapular skinfold.

Body fat assessment by skinfold anthropometry is perhaps one of the most widely investigated fields in the biological sciences, and a plethora of studies, certainly far too numerous to mention in detail in the present context, have been reported for specific population groups of interest to nutritionists and to those workers involved in exercise or sports medicine. These investigators have generally derived regression equations relating body density to functions involving skinfold thickness at one or more sites. The derived body density is then used to determine the percentage of body fat by Siri's equation[38] or a similar such relationship.

Perhaps one of the more widely used sets of regression relationships is that reported by Durnin and Womersley;[45] Table 4–11 has been adapted from their published regression equation for normal males and females ranging in age from 17 to above 50 years in which the general form of the relationship is

$$D = C - m \log_{10} \left(\sum_i s_i \right)$$

where s_i is the mean measured skinfold thickness at a specified site and where C and m are the tabulated linear regression constants. Residual errors (standard errors of the estimates) for the sum of three skinfolds range between 0.0080 and 0.0121 g/cc for females, with no obvious trend with age, and between 0.0059 and 0.0100 g/cc for males, with a clear trend towards increased residual error with age. It is possible to calculate the effect of such residual errors on estimates of total body fat by assuming that the only error variance is that observed for the above empirical relationships. For example, taking the residual error for 20- to 29-year-old men (0.0087 g/cc) together with the mean measured density for this group (1.064 g/cc), one can compute the error on the estimate of body fat for a typical individual to be 24 per cent, implying that approximately two thirds of a subpopulation of males in the 20 to 29 year age range will have fat estimates up to 24 per cent in error and one third will have errors greater

TABLE 4–10. Fat Distribution in Reference Man and Woman

Fat Location	Reference Man		Reference Woman	
Essential fat (lipids of the bone marrow, central nervous system, mammary glands and other organs)	2.1		4.9	
Storage fat (depot)	8.2		10.4	
Subcutaneous		3.1		5.1
Intermuscular		3.3		3.5
Intramuscular		0.8		0.6
Others (fat of thoracic and abdominal cavity)		1.0		1.2
Total fat, kg	10.3		15.3	
Body weight, kg	70.0		56.8	
% fat	14.7		26.9	

From Lohman TG. Hum Biol 1981; 53:181–225. Data from Behnke AR. In Wilson NL (ed). Obesity. Philadelphia, FA Davis, 1969:25–53.

TABLE 4–11. Linear Regression Equations for the Estimation of Body Density (g/cc) from the Logarithm of the Sum of Skinfold Thicknesses (mm)

Skinfold Site	Males	Age (Years) 17–19	20–29	30–39	40–49	50+	17–72
Biceps	C	1.1066	1.1015	1.0781	1.0829	1.0833	1.0997
	M	0.0686	0.0616	0.0396	0.0508	0.0617	0.0659
Triceps	C	1.1252	1.1131	1.0834	1.1041	1.1027	1.1143
	M	0.0625	0.0530	0.0361	0.0609	0.0662	0.0618
Subscapular	C	1.1312	1.1360	1.0978	1.1246	1.1334	1.1369
	M	0.0670	0.0700	0.0416	0.0686	0.0760	0.0741
Biceps & triceps	C	1.1423	1.1307	1.0995	1.1174	1.1185	1.1356
	M	0.0687	0.0603	0.0431	0.0614	0.0683	0.0700
Biceps & triceps & subscapular	C	1.1643	1.1593	1.1213	1.1530	1.1569	1.1689
	M	0.0727	0.0694	0.0487	0.0730	0.0780	0.0793

Skinfold Site	Females	Age (Years) 16–19	20–29	30–39	40–49	50+	16–68
Biceps	C	1.0889	1.0903	1.0794	1.0736	1.0682	1.0871
	M	0.0553	0.0601	0.0511	0.0492	0.0510	0.0593
Triceps	C	1.1159	1.1319	1.1176	1.1121	1.1160	1.1278
	M	0.0648	0.0776	0.0686	0.0691	0.0762	0.0775
Subscapular	C	1.1081	1.1184	1.0979	1.0860	1.0899	1.1100
	M	0.0621	0.0716	0.0567	0.0505	0.0590	0.0669
Biceps & triceps	C	1.1290	1.1398	1.1243	1.1230	1.1226	1.1362
	M	0.0657	0.0738	0.0646	0.0672	0.0710	0.0740
Biceps & triceps & subscapular	C	1.1509	1.1605	1.1385	1.1303	1.1372	1.1543
	M	0.0715	0.0777	0.0654	0.0635	0.0710	0.0756

Adapted from Durnin JVGA, Womersley J. Br J Nutr 1974; 32:77–97.

than 24 per cent; the corresponding value for 40- to 49-year-old women is 14.3 per cent, corresponding to a residual error of 0.0107 g/cc and a mean density of 1.020 g/cc. Clearly the measurement of total body fat is more precise for people with higher percentages of body fat, a fact that is not always appreciated.

Furthermore, it should be emphasized that the above computations assume that the relationship between density and total body fat is free from biological imprecision, which is not the case, since the density of the lean body varies considerably owing to variations in hydration, minerals, and protein between individuals. Siri[39] has calculated the biological residual error in this relationship to be approximately 0.006 g/cc, expressed in units of density. It is difficult to assess the effects of the combined variances because one cannot assume the two sources of biological error to be independent; that is, there is probably considerable covariance present. One point, however, is clear, and this is that the derivation of body density as an intermediary step in the estimate of body fat from skinfold anthropometry is counterproductive. Until more direct ways of deriving body fat are demonstrated, it is difficult to see how this can be avoided. This point will be further addressed a little later in this chapter.

At the present state of the art the authors feel that is would be unwise to place too much emphasis on the value of skinfold anthropometry in body composition assessment. For the reasons outlined earlier skinfold anthropometry is unsuitable for measurement of body fat in individuals or small groups. This is especially true of patient studies in which major changes in body composition are suspected. Such changes will in principle affect the density of the fat-free mass as well as the relationship between subcutaneous and total body fat. The heterogeneity of many patient populations will result in increased (but not quantifiable) residual error as well as significant systematic errors, especially as the only available relationships between skinfold thickness and body density have been derived from studies of normal individuals. If such studies are unavoidable it is suggested that the minimum number of patients in any group studied (or arm of a clinical trial) be at least 50 to minimize the effects of the heterogeneity on the precision of estimated group means.

Imaging Techniques. X-ray imaging allows the volume of fat over a given site to be determined from surface area measurements. As far as conventional radiography is concerned, measurements are generally obtained for subcutaneous sites, those over the biceps and triceps being typical; in this case radiography or x-ray radiometry, as it is more generally known, replaces skinfold calipers. The method enables detailed evaluation to be made of changes in skinfold thickness with position along the humerus, and is useful to evaluate the accuracy of conventional skinfold anthropometry.

On the other hand, computerized tomography (CT) enables transverse cross-sectional radiographs to be obtained at any site in the human body. The CT image allows calculation of total fat area in a given cut, and sequential cuts at known separations enable fat volume to be estimated. The method is particularly suited to the differentiation of subcutaneous from intra-abdominal fat[46] and evaluation of changes in distribution with aging,[47] but has limited application as a means of determining total body fat because of both cost and radiation dose considerations. Nevertheless, in principle the method could be most useful as a nearly absolute means of determining total adipose tissue, provided sufficient numbers of scans were made on the subject. One of the problems with the technique is the differentiation of fat and other tissues at the interfaces between these components.

Electrical Conductivity. The measurement of electrical conductivity provides another method of estimating total body fat. In this technique[48, 49] the differential conductivity of fat and lean tissue is exploited, with the latter displaying better conductivity owing to its greater electrolyte concentration. Measurement of total body electrical conductivity (TOBEC) can be achieved, for example, by placing the subject in a large solenoidal coil driven by a 5 MHz oscillating radiofrequency current; impedence measurement can be used to derive conductivity, which is a function of lean body mass.

To date validation of the TOBEC method in human studies has been against densitometric estimates of lean body mass;[49] consequently the method suffers from the same validation problem as other indirect techniques calibrated via densitometry, namely that the greater contribution to biological variance probably arises from the assumption of a constant density for the fat-free component of the body. The advantages of the method are that it is rapid, reproducible, safe, noninvasive, and applicable to most groups of hospitalized patients.

Difference Methods. Undoubtedly the most simple form of the difference method is the use of measured total body water (TBW) to determine the fat-free mass (FFM) by the relation

$$FFM = TBW/f$$

where f is the assumed fraction of the FFM that consists of water; f is usually taken to be 0.73 for normal man based upon the studies of Pace and Rathburn.[50] However, recent work by Streat and colleagues[41] has shown that this ratio varies from 0.685 to 0.754 in normal subjects, with a mean value of 0.729, so that the assumption of constancy will lead to errors in individual estimates of FFM (and hence of total body fat [TBF]) by the relation

$$TBF = M - FFM$$

Furthermore, the hydration ratio has been shown to vary from 0.67 to 0.83 (mean = 0.74) in a group of surgical patients presenting for nutritional support,[41] implying that application of 0.73 will lead to gross errors in individual values of FFM or TBF, and large systematic errors in the mean values of these entities. Unless appropriate values of f can be experimentally determined, this method of determining TBF is not recommended for studies of groups of patients. Nevertheless it continues to be a very popular method.[51–53]

Perhaps the original difference method was proposed by McCance and Widdowson in 1951.[54] These authors considered the living body in terms of extracellular fluid and body cell mass, with fat being obtained by subtraction of those compartments from body weight after making allowance for minerals. The method was further extended by Cohn and colleagues some 30 years later[55] using the technique of in vivo neutron activation analysis (IVNAA). These authors considered several variables, including a model in which TBW was determined by tritium dilution, total body protein (TBProt) by the measurement of nitrogen using IVNAA, and bone mineral mass (BMM) by IVNAA. The FFM was considered to be the sum of these three entities, so that TBF is again obtained by the relationship TBF = M − FFM. It is important to note that in a large series of normal volunteers Cohn and colleagues[55] found that skinfold anthropometry consistently underestimated TBF relative to both difference methods outlined above as well as relative to methods based on the measurement of total body potassium.

A similar difference method has also been developed by Beddoe and co-workers[1] using IVNAA and tritium dilution, and results confirming the findings of Cohn and colleagues[55] have also been reported.[41] Indeed, this work showed that underestimation of TBF is even greater in a group of patients presenting for nutritional support than in normal subjects. To illustrate the above contention and to emphasize the inherent problem of applying skinfold anthropometry to patient populations (via calculations of body density), Table 4–12 summarizes regressions of measurements of TBF by two techniques in 68 normal volunteers and 94 patients presenting for nutritional support. The patients were predominantly ambulant and included 30 preoperative and 64 postoperative subjects, with a wide variety of gastrointestinal and surgical diseases. While in both groups the mean TBF was underestimated by skinfold anthropometry, the error was more marked in the patient group. The residual error (expressed as a coefficient of variation) is also much greater for the patient group, reflecting the heterogeneity of the patients, some of whom have a normal relationship between skinfold thickness and TBF whereas others do not. However, the reader may not be convinced that the observed residual errors are largely due to imprecision in the estimate of fat by anthropometry rather than by the difference method. To demon-

TABLE 4–12. *Total Body Fat (TBF) by Difference Method and Skinfold Anthropometry in Normal Individuals and Surgical Patients Presenting for Nutritional Support*

| Subjects | Mean TBF (sd) kg | | Δ | p | r | CV (%) |
	Difference Method	Anthropometry				
68 volunteers	16.9 (5.1)	15.7 (5.8)	1.26	2.5×10^{-4}	0.91	14.3
94 patients	16.4 (8.3)	14.2 (6.6)	2.2	1.3×10^{-5}	0.90	22.5

Δ, difference between means; p, probability based on paired t-test; r, correlation coefficient of regression of TBF (difference) against TBF (anthropometry); CV, residual error divided by mean value of TBF (difference) expressed as a percentage.

Means and ranges of ages in the normal and patient groups were 30 years (19–59) and 57 years (20–92), respectively.

strate this it is necessary to examine the frequency histogram of the ratio of total body water to fat-free mass (TBW:FFM) for the same groups of subjects; these are plotted in Figures 4–4 and 4–5. In both figures FFM has been calculated by an IVNAA/tritium dilution method[1] as well as by skinfold anthropometry. Clearly anthropometry yields values of TBW:FFM that are outside accepted biological limits, reflecting the inherent dangers of using current skinfold methods, especially on patient groups. In fairness to proponents of skinfold anthropometry it should be noted that this technique might well prove to be more useful if it were to be calibrated against techniques that would provide more accurate estimates of body fat than densitometry is capable of doing.

This subsection has discussed the use of IVNAA as a useful method for deriving TBF, but has not discussed the technique itself. Such a discussion will appear later in this chapter.

Normal Body Fatness

Setting the range of body fatness in normal humans is difficult since adipose tissue has no normal functional role (disregarding the importance of essential lipids). The problem is not enhanced by the fact that there is no direct way of measuring total adipose tissue. There have, of course, been multitudinous studies of total body fat in various popu-

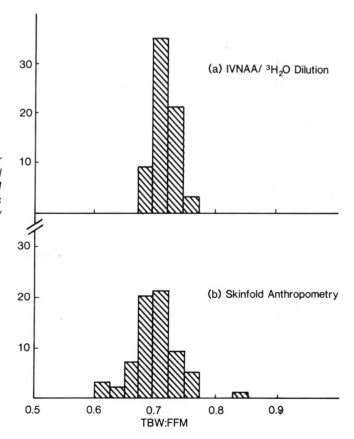

TBW:FFM RATIOS IN 68 NORMAL VOLUNTEERS

FIGURE 4–4. *Histograms of the ratio of total body water (TBW) to the fat-free body mass (FFM) for 68 normal volunteers. (a) TBW measured by tritium dilution and FFM measured by the in vivo neutron activation analysis (IVNAA)/tritium dilution method. (b) TBW measured by tritium dilution and FFM via skinfold anthropometry.*

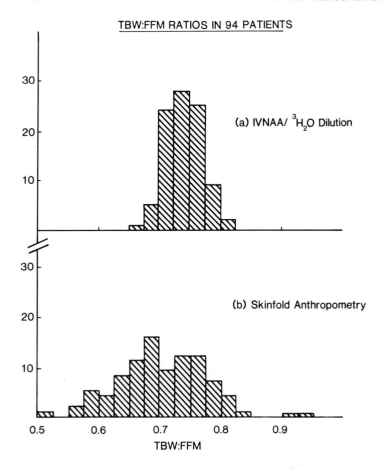

FIGURE 4–5. Histograms of the TBW:FFM ratio for 94 patients presenting for nutritional support. (a) TBW measured by tritium dilution and FFM measured by the IVNAA/tritium dilution method. (b) TBW measured by tritium dilution and FFM via skinfold anthropometry.

lations, usually in college-age males and females, and most of these studies have been performed using either densitometry or skinfold anthropometry or both. Perhaps the most general study is that reported by Durnin and Womersley in the mid-1970's,[45] and Table 4–13 shows data extracted from this paper on mean percentage body fat together with standard deviations and ranges for groups of normal subjects ranging in age from 17 to 72; these values are based on densitometric studies using the underwater weighing method of Durnin and Rahaman.[56]

Clearly the mean percentage of fat increases steadily with age, varying from 15 to 28 per cent in males and 26 to 39 per cent in females. Individual values vary tremendously, ranging from 7 to 30 per cent in young men (17 to 19 years old) and from 24 to 61 per cent in middle-aged women (40 to 49 years old).

TABLE 4–13. Percentage Body Fat As Determined by Densitometry in Normal Humans

Age Range	Number of Subjects	Percentage Body Fat (% of Body Mass)		
		Mean	*sd*	*Range*
Males				
17–19	24	15	7.0	7–30
20–29	92	15	7.0	5–38
30–39	34	23	5.4	13–38
40–49	35	25	6.7	11–37
50–72	24	28	8.5	11–50
Females				
16–19	29	26	7.8	14–43
20–29	100	29	10	10–54
30–39	58	33	9.5	19–53
40–49	48	35	7.5	24–61
50–68	37	39	7.6	26–52

From Durnin JVGA, Womersley J. Br J Nutr 1974; *32*:77–97. Reproduced with permission.

TABLE 4–14. Percentage Body Fat in Normal Humans As Determined by an IVNAA Difference Method and by Skinfold Anthropometry

Age Range	Number of Subjects	Percentage Body Fat (% of Body Mass)	
		Difference Method	*Skinfold Method*
Males			
20–29	22	17.2	19.8
30–39	13	20.1	17.7
40–49	10	22.6	18.5
50–59	10	23.8	18.3
60–69	9	28.1	18.8
70–79	10	29.1	20.1
Females			
20–29	10	24.6	29.1
30–39	10	30.0	29.1
40–49	10	31.0	31.6
50–59	8	40.0	34.1
60–69	13	36.1	29.1
70–79	10	35.9	29.3

Data from Cohn SH, Ellis KJ, Vartsky D, et al. Am J Clin Nutr 1981; *34*:2839–2847.

To underline the problem of characterizing fat, even in normal subjects, Table 4–14 lists mean percentage of body fat over a similar age range as calculated by a difference method and a skinfold anthropometric method. Clearly the results generally show rather poor agreement between methods, though it should be noted that part of the mean difference between methods can be attributed to systematic error in either technique and part (probably the larger part) is due to the biological component of the residual error discussed in the previous section; the latter affects the precision of each group mean based on the skinfold method in a nonquantifiable manner. Larger numbers of subjects in each age cohort may have resulted in better average agreement. It is also interesting to note that the results by the difference method agree quite well, on average, with the means quoted in Table 4–13 (the latter study being based on much larger groups), allowing for the fact that the two studies were on different populations. Discounting serendipitous agreement, this concurrence suggests that the average systematic errors in both densitometric and difference methods are small, at least as applied to studies of normal people.

Body Fatness in Wasting Disease and Obesity

Mean values of percentage body fat for 137 ward patients presenting for total parenteral nutrition are shown in Table 4–15. These values are based on a difference method recently reported.[1] Clearly, as one would expect, there is again a wide variation of fatness in patients, though mean values tend to be less than the equivalent values quoted in Table 4–13 and enclosed in parentheses in Table 4–15. In point of fact the men had an average reduction of 24 per cent in body fat, whereas the women lost 16 per cent

of body fat. This difference reflects the higher percentage of body mass represented by fat in females and also the lower energy expenditure per unit mass of females. It should be stressed that the data presented are tentative, and that greater numbers of patients need to be studied before definitive conclusions about typical fat depletion in patients presenting for nutritional support can be determined.

The difficulty of measuring fat by anthropometric techniques in persons with morbid obesity is well known.[57] This difficulty relates partly to the poor reproducibility inherent in measuring skinfold thicknesses in the obese and partly to the biological problems discussed above. However, more recently several studies of morbid obesity have been performed using alternative methods of measuring fat, including the analysis of the composition of weight loss in patients undergoing rigid dietary control via IVNAA and TBK measurement[58] and a major study of body composition changes following gastric operations for morbid obesity by MacLean and co-workers.[59] Shizgal[60] described body composition measurements in 42 morbidly obese patients just prior to weight-reducing surgery. Body fat accounted for more than 50 per cent of the measured body weight. Although the lean body mass in most of these patients was greater than in a group of normal individuals, in a few patients it was abnormally decreased in size. In the same article Shizgal described a group of fat subjects with a mean body weight of about 74 kg in whom measured body cell mass was only two thirds that of a group of normal persons of similar weight. He states that this "body cell mass depletion" was not suspected clinically because the patients' excessive body fat obscured the presence of muscle wasting.

Relation of Body Fat to Mortality

The ratio of body weight to height squared (W/H^2) is variously termed Quetelet's index or the Body Mass Index. Although a number of workers have sought to derive a precise relationship between the percentage of body fat and W/H^2, Garrow[57] has pointed out that it is curvilinear and that the nature of the curve depends on the proportion of lean to fat involved in changes in body weight. Nevertheless W/H^2 is used as a measure of obesity and in the experience of life insurance companies a range of W/H^2 between 20 and 25 is associated with minimum mortality.

Relation of Body Fat to Starvation Resistance

Clinically, it can be observed that fat patients withstand starvation better than thin patients. It has long been known that women withstand semistarvation

TABLE 4–15. Percentage Body Fat As Determined by a Difference Technique in 137 Patients Presenting for Nutritional Support

Age Range	Number of Subjects	Percentage Body Fat (% of Body Mass)		
		Mean	*sd*	*Range*
Males				
18–29	8	11.1 (15)	9.8	2–32
30–39	8	15.2 (23)	6.7	5–22
40–49	9	19.6 (25)	4.5	11–24
50–59	24	22.3 (28)	6.8	5–34
60–69	17	21.3 (28)	8.3	4–34
70+	13	23.5 (28)	9.6	5–45
Females				
20–29	7	28.0 (29)	5.2	20–34
30–39	6	29.0 (33)	11.0	14–40
40–49	4	23.5 (35)	9.1	14–31
50–59	12	28.9 (39)	9.5	14–44
60–69	10	36.1 (39)	7.3	23–45
70+	19	32.7 (—)	6.7	21–44

Data from Beddoe AH, Streat SJ, and Hill GL (unpublished).

better than men, and in famines the mortality among men is often twice that of women.[10] One of the factors contributing to the better resistance of women to starvation may be their larger stores of body fat.[10]

COMPARTMENTS OF THE BODY

In general the body is made up of the living cells and, in contrast, the less immediately vital materials such as interstitial fluid, fat, and bone. Blood, with its two divisions of plasma and cells, needs consideration also. Here we will consider first the living body as comprising total body fat and the fat-free body mass. The methods of measuring the components of the fat-free body will be discussed before the changes that occur in these components during disease and recovery are described.

Fat-Free Mass and Lean Body Mass

In the previous section we have discussed two terms that are often used synonymously but that are conceptually slightly different. The concept of the lean body mass (LBM) was originally used by Behnke and colleagues[33] in the early 1940's; these workers visualized the LBM as a compositional entity of the human body with specific gravity of 1.1 that was totally devoid of fat except for a small amount of essential lipid. On the other hand the concept of the fat-free mass (FFM) is more straightforward, being simply the mass of the body minus the total mass of fat (essential and nonessential).

There the discussion should rest. Unfortunately there still seems to be ample confusion in the literature over the two terms, and, at the risk of compounding the problem, it is of interest to illustrate this. Moore[61] in 1980 claimed that LBM and FFM are "compositionally synonymous, while methodologically very different." He defined both terms as being the weight of the entire human body minus the weight of neutral fat and used the terms interchangeably. On the other hand, Garrow[62] more recently defined LBM as the difference between body mass and adipose tissue, with the latter comprising 83 per cent fat, 2 per cent protein, and 15 per cent water. Nevertheless, he claimed that in "fairly lean people the contribution of non fat components in adipose tissue is fairly small, so it is not very important to distinguish between LBM and FFM" provided the people are lean. According to Grande and Keys,[63] Behnke originally conceived the LBM as containing essential fat amounting to 10 per cent of its mass, but later revised the percentage to 2 per cent. Since it is impossible to decide how much fat is essential, there being no way of absolutely distinguishing essential from nonessential fat, it is perhaps best to avoid the term altogether. Furthermore, we can tighten our definition of the FFM by defining fat as the ether-extractable substances in the body. This at least has the advantage of allowing us to define the FFM as something that actually can be measured.

Metabolic Body Size

An undoubted aim of body composition research is the characterization of the size of the metabolically active tissues of the human body. Behnke and colleagues,[33] through their concept of the lean body mass as measured by densitometry, were the first workers to suggest that "the presence of an indeterminate amount of excess adipose tissue renders difficult any precise computation, for example, of metabolic rate or dosage of drugs in terms of total body weight." Certainly the lean body mass provided an entity that was related to the size of the "metabolic machinery," at least in normal man. McCance and Widdowson's concept of the human body comprising fat, cellular tissues, and extracellular supporting tissues[54] came close to the concept of the body cell mass (BCM) elaborated later so elegantly by Moore and co-workers.[64] The BCM was defined by Moore "as that component of body composition containing the oxygen-exchanging, potassium-rich, glucose-oxidizing, work-performing tissue." By definition it is the sum of all cellular components of the body including those of muscle, viscera, central nervous system, and hematopoietic system as well as the cells in cartilage, tendon, bone, and adipose tissue. Furthermore, because potassium is almost entirely intracellular, Moore considered that measurement of this element would serve as an index of BCM. Kinney and associates[65] appeared to complete the scenario by showing that total body potassium (TBK) was closely related to resting metabolic expenditure, although the curvilinear relationship between oxygen consumption and TBK demonstrated clearly the existence of populations of cells with differing levels of oxidative metabolism.

However, in many diseases characterized by protein depletion, including critical illness, changes in TBK are accompanied by changes in cellular hydration which may or may not be associated with changes in the metabolically active component of the BCM, namely the intracellular protein. Clearly in the hospital patient the BCM is probably most independent (at least in the short term) of changes in intracellular water mass, and oxidative metabolism is more likely to be related to intracellular protein than to BCM. Research efforts should therefore be aiming to develop the methodology capable of measuring or deriving intracellular protein.

Historically the first step toward the goal was the measurement of total body nitrogen and the derivation of total body protein by the application of the universally used multiplicative factor 6.25. This factor, however, is as yet unsupported by cadaver analysis apart from the single cadaver studied by Moore and co-workers,[66] and much work needs to be done to examine the ranges of this factor in both normality and wasting disease. The next step taken by Burkinshaw and colleagues used total body protein and TBK to derive muscle and non-muscle mass.[67] Cohn and associates[68] recognized the difficulty with this two-compartment model; they argued that, since the non-muscle compartment necessarily includes both the metabolically active viscera and the noncellular structural proteins in cartilage, fibrous tissues, and skeletal tissues, it is metabolically more reasonable to separate the proteinogenous compartments into the actively metabolizing body cell mass and the slowly metabolizing structural components. The final step, which has yet to be undertaken experimentally, is to consider only the protein components of the respective tissues and derive muscle protein (MP) and intracellular protein (ICP) in terms of measurable entities thus:

$$MP = \frac{TBK - ECK - r_{NM}\, TBN}{r_M - r_{NM}} \psi_{MP}$$

$$ICP = \frac{TBK - ECK}{r_C} \psi_{ICP}$$

where ECK is the total extracellular potassium (< 5 per cent of TBK), r_{NM}, r_M, and r_C are the respective mean ratios of K/N in non-muscle, muscle, and the BCM, and where ψ_{MP} and ψ_{ICP} are the weighted mean nitrogen conversion factors in muscle protein and total intracellular protein respectively. Clearly the r and ψ factors will require extensive experimental work via tissue biopsy and cadaver analysis through a range of diseases and nutritional states before much use can be made of the model in clinical medicine.

Measurement of Whole Body Compartments

We have already considered the methodologies used to measure the fat and fat-free compartments of the human body. In this section we consider the further partition of the FFM into its components, water, protein, and minerals, not to mention glycogen. In addition, we examine the partitioning of the water space into its intra- and extracellular components and discuss the more recent techniques that have previously been granted only brief mention. We finish the section by reviewing the findings of the few cadaver analyses that have been reported.

Dilution Methods. The dilution principle is remarkable for its simplicity. If a solute of volume v_i is tagged with a label (radioactive or chemical) of concentration C_i and injected into a given compartment within a patient, then the size of that compartment V_i can be determined by measuring the concentration of the label in the compartment such that

$$V = \frac{C_i}{C_m} v_i$$

Dilution of course is never instantaneous, and measurement of the concentration must be carried out after equilibration has been achieved if underestimates of the compartment size are to be avoided. Several simple rules apply. For example, v_i must be small compared with V so that its presence does not upset the homeostatic mechanisms regulating the size of V. Clearly true V should remain constant over the equilibration period, although the effects of changing compartment size during the measurement period can be accounted for in certain circumstances. Furthermore, any excretion of the labeled solute from the compartment being measured should be minimal, otherwise overestimation of compartment size will result. It is also important that the solute is not metabolized significantly during the equilibration period. Careful choice of tracer can usually avoid any of the above problems. Finally, and most importantly, the tracer must not distribute to any pool other than V; this is usually the most difficult part of the exercise to establish, as the following discussion will show.

Undoubtedly the most important dilution method is that involved in the measurement of total body water (TBW), which can be achieved by tritium-labeled or deuterium-labeled water, by ^{18}O-labeled water,[69] or indeed by ethanol[70] or urea[54] dilution. The most popular technique uses the ^{3}H label (with a precision of the order of 1 per cent), which in effect measures the total exchangeable hydrogen including any hydrogen atoms in protein, glycogen, and fat. The nonaqueous exchangeable hydrogen has been calculated by Culebras and colleagues[71] to be approximately 5.2 per cent of the aqueous hydrogen, but these authors considered that much of this is "hard to exchange" in the short equilibration times usually employed (2½ hours). Experimental work from the same laboratories[72] suggested 2 per cent maximum overestimation of the water space, though more recent data[69] suggest that the use of the tritium or deuterium label gives rise to a 2.3 per cent (sem = 0.6 per cent) overestimate of TBW relative to that obtained by the $H_2{}^{18}O$ dilution technique, which itself may overestimate TBW by 0.7 per cent. The true systematic error in using [2]H- or ^{3}H-labeled water is as yet unknown, but clearly depends on factors such as equilibration time, the relative proportions of protein, water, and fat, and the nutritional status of the subject being measured. For most practical purposes the tritium (or deuterium) space can be considered to be synonymous with TBW.

Partitioning the water space into intra- and extracellular water represents the next step in the unfolding of the composition of the human body. As far as isotope dilution is concerned, ^{82}Br dilution has been most commonly used to determine ECW, yielding a precision of typically around 4 per cent (sd).[73] Measurement of ECW and TBW allows ICW to be inferred by difference. Moore[61] points out that the bromide dilution volume is larger than the thiosulfate and inulin dilution volumes but yields a very satisfactory equilibration plateau. Bromide ions of course follow chloride ions into red cells, so that some estimate of the fraction of bromide that is taken up by red cells is necessary if an overestimation of the ECW is to be avoided. Red cell volume can normally be achieved via ^{51}Cr-tagged red cells and dilution of ^{125}I-labeled human serum albumin.

Estimation of the BCM has usually been achieved by measurement of total body potassium (TBK), since potassium is the most abundant intracellular cation and because almost all ($\sim$ 98 per cent) of the body's potassium is located within cells. Furthermore, the total exchangeable potassium (TBK$_e$) is approximately equal to TBK. Moore and colleagues[64] have in fact shown that potassium is linearly related to both ICW and BCM. The potassium isotope used is ^{42}K, which has a half-life of only $12\frac{1}{2}$ hours, which limits its usefulness. Shizgal and colleagues[74] have shown that an indirect estimate of TBK can be obtained by measurement of exchangeable sodium (TBNa$_e$). This method is based on the observation that the ratio of sodium plus potassium to water content in all tissues (except bone) is approximately constant. Therefore

$$\frac{TBNa_e + TBK_e}{TBW} = \frac{Na + K}{H_2O} = \alpha$$

so that

$$TBK_e = \alpha\, TBW - TBNa_e$$

TBNa$_e$ is measured via the dilution of ^{22}Na and TBW by ^{3}H$_2$O dilution. Assessment of the "constant" α is achieved by measuring the sodium, potassium, and water contents of whole blood.

A summary of the uses of two well-known multiple isotope dilution methods[60, 64] for determining body composition is shown in Table 4–16. The two techniques are similar except for the measurement of ECW and TBK$_e$.

Isotopic dilution techniques do present a problem in situations in which the patient's clinical condition and treatment can interfere with the measurement process, especially where extended equilibration times are necessary. For example, the patient may be receiving intravenous fluid and nutrients, may not be hemodynamically stable, or may be gaining or losing water at a prodigious rate (10 L per day is not uncommon). In these situations the measurement of TBK by whole body counting may offer some advantage.

Measurement of Total Body Potassium Using a

TABLE 4–16. Body Composition As Determined by Isotope Dilution

Compositional Entity	Moore et al.[64]	Shizgal et al.[60]
Red cell volume (RCV)	^{51}Cr–red cells	^{51}Cr–red cells
Plasma volume (PV)	^{125}I-HSA	^{125}I-HSA
Blood volume	RCV + PV	RCV + PV
TBW	^{3}H$_2$O dilution	^{3}H$_2$O dilution
ECW	^{82}Br dilution	^{22}Na (early distribution volume)
TBNa$_e$	^{22}Na dilution	^{22}Na (24-hour distribution volume)
ICW	TBW − ECW	TBW − ECW
TBK$_e$	^{42}K dilution	α TBW − TBNa$_e$
LBM (FFM)	TBW/0.732	TBW/0.73
TBFat	M − LBM	M − LBM
BCM	0.0833 TBK$_e$	0.0833 TBK$_e$

Whole Body Counter. The radioisotope ^{40}K occurs naturally in the human body in a known fixed ratio (0.01 per cent) to its stable sisters ^{39}K and ^{41}K. Therefore a measure of ^{40}K affords a measure of TBK. It decays with a half-life of 1.3×10^9 years, emitting beta and gamma particles of energy 1.46 MeV, which can readily be monitored by arrays of sodium iodide detectors placed above and below the patient. Such an array needs to be enclosed in a lead- and/or steel-lined room to prevent gamma rays from extracorporeal sources, such as ^{40}K, ^{238}U, and ^{232}Th in building materials, from striking the detectors. ^{40}K can also be measured using a shadow shield counter, which is much lighter than the whole body counter relying as it does on appropriate placement of lead shields to prevent radiation from reaching the detectors.[75]

The advantages of measuring TBK by monitoring ^{40}K levels are as follows. First, it is a totally noninvasive technique involving minimal discomfort to the patient and requiring no administered radionuclides. Second, the whole body counting technique provides a rapid (10 to 30 minutes) estimate of TBK, with a precision of the order of 2 per cent (sd). Furthermore, it does not depend on isotopic equilibration as do the isotope dilution methods, in which times vary from 24 to 48 hours; this can be especially important if major fluid shifts are occurring over the measurement period. However, this situation can itself lead to interpretive problems with whole body counting, since changing body habitus leads to variation in internal self-absorption of the emitted gamma rays and to variation in background absorption. Careful calibration is therefore required. In practice known amounts of ^{42}K can be given to volunteers with a range of body shapes and sizes; this technique exploits the close similarity between the gamma energies emitted (1.46 MeV for ^{40}K and 1.52 MeV for ^{42}K), which results in almost identical internal absorption characteristics.[76] Once the calibration study has been carefully performed, relationships to habitus (including weight, height, and skeletal parameters) can be ascertained and used in patient studies.

In Vivo Neutron Activation Analysis. The unique association of the element nitrogen with protein in the human body suggests that a measure of total body nitrogen (TBN) would furnish an estimate of total body protein (TBProt) via the relationship

$$TBProt = 6.25 \, TBN$$

Anderson and colleagues[77] pointed out in 1964 that measurement of TBN would allow assessment of muscle wasting and malnutrition. Measurement of N was first reported by Palmer and co-workers in 1968,[78] but it was not until the latter half of the 1970's that application of the method to nutritional and metabolic studies was reported.[79, 80]

TBN can be measured by two IVNAA methods, namely the delayed gamma method and the prompt gamma method. *Delayed gamma* IVNAA depends on the $^{14}N(n,2n)^{13}N$ reaction, which requires exposure to neutrons of very high energy (greater than 11.3 MeV). Monitoring the reaction is achieved by measuring the 0.15 MeV gamma rays from subsequent positron annihilation. On the other hand, the *prompt gamma* method depends on the $^{14}N(n,\gamma)^{15}N^*$ reaction; $^{15}N^*$ de-excites very quickly (10^{-15} second lifetime) to stable ^{15}N, emitting a range of gamma rays of which the 10.8 MeV gamma is the one monitored. For reviews of the advantages and disadvantages of these two techniques the reader is referred to Cohn[81]

and Beddoe and Hill.[82] The last authors have developed a clinical facility provided with an intensive care environment, in which patients with serious sepsis and multiorgan failure can have measurements of body composition taken (Fig. 4–6).

The value of either IVNAA technique over conventional nitrogen balance is primarily that it affords an estimate of total body protein at any given time, where balance techniques can only provide net changes in total body protein. Moreover, IVNAA is logistically more suitable over long study periods and does not in principle suffer from the cumulative systematic errors that almost inevitably occur with the nitrogen balance technique.

Various combinations including IVNAA, TBK measurement, or tritium dilution have been used by several groups as a means of determining the major nutritionally important compartments of the body, and several models have been proposed. Burkinshaw and co-workers[67] used measurements of TBK, TBN, and bone mineral mass as the primary data in a model of the human body consisting of fat, muscle, non-muscle, and bone mineral mass; this model makes use of the fact that potassium:nitrogen ratios differ in muscle and non-muscle, but does assume that the ratios are constant for both components. A second model developed by Cohn and colleagues[55] used tritium dilution, TBN, and total body calcium measurements to determine a model consisting of protein, water, fat, and minerals. A third method[1] uses just TBN measurement in combination with tritium dilution to determine the same compartments on the assumption that body minerals, largely calcium hydroxyapatite, are relatively unaffected by wasting.

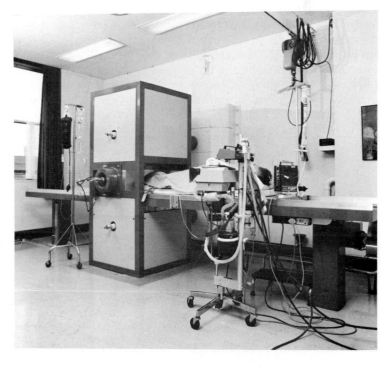

FIGURE 4–6. A "prompt gamma" neutron activation facility designed for clinical use. Here, an intensive care patient is being scanned. On the top right hand side of the photograph is a hoist/weighing system consisting of a simple two-speed electrically operated block and tackle attached via a load cell to a frame that supports a canvas sheet on which the patient lies. The system transfers the patient from his bed to the IVNAA facility couch, weighing him during transfer. The patient enters the scanner "feet first" with all lines (TPN, catheter, drains, EKG leads, etc.) following, with monitors placed at the head of the couch, and with the respective trolley following alongside. The scan takes a total of 35 minutes. (From Beddoe AH, Zuidmeer H, Hill GL. Phys Med Biol 1984; 29:371–383. Reproduced with permission.)

In each case body fat can be determined by subtracting the sum of the measured and estimated non-fat compartments from body mass, as has been described already. The advantages of the latter two models and methods for the measurement of fat are that no a priori assumptions are made about the ratio of the major compartments; that is, it is not necessary to assume that the hydration of fat-free mass is a constant nor that protein or minerals bear constant relations to the FFM. Nevertheless, there are still assumptions that have a small bearing on the results, for example, that the body protein:TBN ratio is a constant (6.25) and that the proportions of hydrogen in protein, water, and fat are constant at 7.0, 11.1, and 12.0 per cent, respectively.[84]

Cadaver Analysis and Its Contribution to Knowledge of Body Composition. The gross chemical analysis of the human body provides in principle the absolute yardstick by which to compare the various in vivo techniques. Nevertheless, the sheer bulk of a human body renders gross chemical analysis a very difficult and time-consuming business. Perhaps this is the reason that so few cadavers have been analyzed. In fact, to the authors' knowledge only ten such analyses have been reported in this century, and these are summarized in Table 4–17. Of these only the three cadavers listed at the top of the table could be considered to have exhibited normal body composition at the time of death. The other seven all suffered from diseases that are known to be associated with protein wasting and/or expansion of the extracellular fluid space.

The data from chemical analysis of cadavers provide baseline composition of human beings in both normal and diseases states. They also provide qualitative assurance that the in vivo body composition methods yield compositional information of similar magnitude. However, the range of values of body compartments in both health and disease is such that for accurate quantitative comparison it is necessary to analyze cadavers by the other in vivo methods prior to undertaking chemical analyses. Such a procedure has been carried out by an IVNAA

technique[1] on the last two cadavers listed in Table 4–17, and the comparative data on one of these are shown in Table 4–18.[88] Clearly the agreement between techniques is encouraging, though many such cadavers should be analyzed before definitive claims about the accuracy of the IVNAA technique can be made.

Compartmental Changes in Disease

Figure 4–1 illustrates the body composition of the typical normal male in terms of fat, water, protein, minerals, and glycogen. Before discussing changes in body composition that occur in nutritional metabolic illness, we will first examine the ranges of components in the major compartments in normal humans, excluding fat, which has already been discussed.

Normative Data on Body Compartments. Table 4–19 shows data derived from work published by Cohn and colleagues[89] on the total body contents of water, protein, and minerals in 135 normal subjects ranging in age from 20 to 79 years, and arranged in 10-year cohorts; the weights and heights of each cohort are also tabulated, together with standard deviations on each compositional entity. The data were derived from measurements of TBN and TBCa using IVNAA and total body water from tritium dilution. These data represent the largest body of data on normal humans yet compiled by one center and as such can be regarded as the normative data with which any other data set on non-normals should be compared.

Body Composition of Hospital Patients Requiring Total Parenteral Nutrition. To illustrate the effects of severe illness on body composition, Table 4–20 presents data from 137 surgical patients presenting for intravenous nutrition. These were predominantly ambulant ward patients with a wide variety of gastrointestinal surgical diseases. Their body composition was studied immediately prior to a course of intravenous nutrition. Body water was

TABLE 4–17. Gross Body Composition of Ten Adult Human Cadavers Analyzed by Chemical Methods

Reference	Sex/Age	Cause of Death	Height (cm)	Weight (kg)	Water (kg)	Protein (kg)	Fat (kg)	Minerals (kg)
Forbes et al.[84]	M46	Skull fracture	168.5	53.8	29.7	10.0	10.5	2.9
Forbes et al.[85]	M60	"Heart attack"	172	73.5	37.2	12.6	20.5	3.6
Widdowson et al.[86]	F42	Drowning	169	45.1	25.3	8.7	10.6	—
Mitchell et al.[87]	M35	"Acute heart attack" (mitral insufficiency)	183	70.6	47.9	10.2	8.8	3.4
Forbes et al.[85]	M48	Infective endocarditis	169	62.0	43.9	12.2	2.7	3.6
Widdowson et al.[86]	M25	Uremia	179	71.8	44.4	11.9	10.7	4.6
Widdowson et al.[86]	M48	Infective endocarditis	—	63.8	52.0	8.2	0.7	3.1
Moore et al.[66]	F67	Advanced malignancy	—	43.4	32.0	5.5	3.8	2.1
Knight et al.[88]	M63	Exsanguination (esophageal cancer)	174	58.6	35.0	9.6	10.5	3.3
Knight et al.[88]	F59	Extreme cachexia	154	25.9	13.3	3.7	7.7	1.2

TABLE 4–18. Gross Composition of a Human Cadaver Analyzed by Neutron Activation Analysis and a Chemical Method

Technique		Water	Protein	Fat	Minerals
Chemical analysis	Mean	35.00	9.56	10.48	3.33
	Sem	0.33	0.21	0.15	0.04
Neutron activation	Mean	—	9.21	10.71	3.31
analysis	Sem	—	0.13	0.13	—

From Knight GS, Beddoe AH, Streat SJ, et al. Body composition of two human cadavers by neutron activation and chemical analysis. Am J Physiol 1986; *250*:E179–185.

TABLE 4–19. Composition of the Fat-Free Mass in 135 Normal Subjects

Age	(Number of Subjects)	Weight		Height		TBW		TBProt		TBMin	
Males		(kg)		(cm)		(kg)		(kg)		(kg)	
20–29	(24)	79.5	(9.1)	178.1	(3.7)	46.9	(5.9)	12.9	(1.4)	5.87	(0.46)
30–39	(10)	72.8	(11.6)	175.2	(6.7)	41.0	(5.9)	11.8	(1.1)	5.56	(0.62)
40–49	(10)	80.5	(11.7)	178.1	(5.2)	44.7	(3.8)	12.0	(0.9)	5.58	(0.56)
50–59	(10)	82.4	(17.3)	178.2	(7.8)	45.2	(8.0)	11.9	(1.6)	5.65	(0.56)
60–69	(10)	78.7	(10.1)	177.0	(4.2)	41.0	(5.4)	11.3	(1.5)	5.44	(0.93)
70–79	(9)	79.8	(11.7)	169.9	(6.5)	40.3	(4.2)	11.1	(1.0)	5.30	(0.76)
Females											
20–29	(10)	60.1	(4.7)	164.6	(4.4)	32.2	(2.4)	9.1	(1.1)	4.44	(0.46)
30–39	(10)	66.4	(6.0)	165.0	(5.0)	33.1	(2.4)	8.9	(1.0)	4.37	(0.38)
40–49	(10)	64.3	(8.4)	162.5	(4.4)	31.5	(3.5)	8.5	(1.0)	4.29	(0.50)
50–59	(10)	73.2	(9.1)	163.9	(7.7)	32.0	(3.2)	7.9	(0.7)	3.87	(0.27)
60–69	(14)	63.0	(9.2)	158.3	(7.9)	28.5	(3.4)	7.5	(1.0)	3.50	(0.64)
70–79	(8)	59.3	(5.2)	154.8	(4.5)	26.6	(3.1)	7.3	(0.7)	3.20	(0.57)

The numbers in parentheses are standard deviations.
From Cohn SH, Vartsky D, Yasumura S, et al. Am J Physiol 1980; *239*:E524–E530. Reproduced with permission.

TABLE 4–20. Composition of Fat-Free Mass in 137 Patients Presenting for Intravenous Nutrition

Age	(Number of Subjects)	Weight		TBW		TBProt		TBMin
Males		(kg)		(kg)		(kg)		(kg)
18–29	(8)	64.5	(9.3)	42.2	(5.6)	10.8	(2.0)	3.8
30–39	(8)	61.3	(11.6)	38.2	(7.2)	9.6	(2.1)	3.6
40–49	(9)	64.2	(10.7)	37.8	(6.8)	9.7	(2.0)	3.6
50–59	(24)	66.7	(11.6)	37.7	(4.6)	9.5	(1.9)	4.0
60–69	(17)	64.3	(9.3)	37.0	(4.6)	9.4	(1.8)	3.7
70+	(13)	64.2	(14.0)	35.8	(7.4)	8.8	(2.5)	3.9
Females								
20–29	(7)	47.0	(3.9)	25.1	(1.9)	5.7	(1.1)	2.7
30–39	(6)	57.4	(7.2)	29.8	(6.3)	7.2	(2.3)	3.3
40–49	(4)	48.7	(8.1)	28.5	(4.9)	5.8	(1.7)	2.6
50–59	(12)	56.4	(9.8)	30.4	(7.7)	6.8	(2.1)	2.5
60–69	(10)	61.0	(15.7)	28.5	(3.5)	6.2	(2.5)	3.7
70+	(19)	54.6	(11.2)	27.6	(4.6)	5.7	(1.5)	3.0

Data from Beddoe AH, Streat SJ, and Hill GL (unpublished).

measured by tritium dilution and body protein by prompt gamma IVNAA. The total body minerals (TBMin) component was determined via a regression equation derived from studies of normal volunteers relating TBMin to the product of height, mediastinal thickness, and biacromial diameter.[1] Clearly in comparing results with those given in Table 4–19 it is apparent that weight is typically about 20 per cent lower in all groups in the case of males and varies from 3 to 24 per cent lower in the females. For example, in males TBW ranges from 7 to 17 per cent below the TBW in the corresponding normal group in Table 4–19, whereas for females the difference in TBW ranged from −22 to +4 per

cent, with the changes in water largely reflecting the changes in weight. On the other hand, differences in mean protein ranged from 16 to 21 per cent reduction in all age groups for males but from 14 to 27 per cent in females. It should be stressed that this approach takes no account of the nature of the predominant disease category in the various groups; for example, at the younger end of the age spectrum the patients tend to have a high concentration of Crohn's disease (females) and ulcerative colitis (males). In particular Crohn's disease is often associated with gross wasting, which undoubtedly explains the large deficits observed in females in the 20 to 49 year age range. In addition, patient numbers are small in the lower age ranges, so that statistical bias will probably be present, especially in the female group.

Changes in Body Composition after Major Surgery. Using in vivo neutron activation analysis Hill and colleagues[79] measured the tissue composition of the weight lost by 16 patients over the 2 weeks following abdominoperineal excision of the rectum. For the group there was an average weight loss of 4.1 kg. This was composed of 1 kg protein, 1.3 kg fat, and 1.8 kg water. These are the only data available that describe direct measurements of body composition in such patients.

Effect of Intravenous Nutrition on Body Composition of Surgical Patients and Patients with Serious Sepsis. In Figure 4–3 the changes in body protein, weight, fat, and water that occurred in 20 ward surgical patients with gastrointestinal dysfunction over a 2-week period are shown. It can be seen that only two patients gained protein over this time period, and most of the weight gain could be accounted for in terms of water and to a lesser extent fat. The water accumulation occurring during short-term intravenous nutrition is a consequence of glycogen storage, with 1 g of glycogen obligating about 3 g of water.[90] Although the changes seen in Figure 4–3 are typical of those which occur during routine administration of intravenous nutrition in the hospital setting, when high intakes of energy and protein are administered, depleted patients will gain both fat and protein during short courses of intravenous nutrition.[91] Serious sepsis is another matter. Recently it was shown[92] that a group of septic patients with multiorgan failure who received maximum intravenous nutritional intakes lost an average of 12 per cent of their body protein over a 10-day period even though they were in positive energy balance.

References

1. Beddoe AH, Streat SJ, Hill GL. Evaluation of an in vivo prompt gamma neutron activation facility for body composition studies in critically ill intensive care patients: results on 41 normals. Metabolism 1984; *33*:270–280.
2. Guenter PA, Moore K, Crosby LO, et al. Body weight measurement of patients receiving nutritional support. JPEN 1982; *6*:441-443.
3. Moore FD, Boyden CM. Body cell mass and limits of hydration of the fat free body: their relation to estimated skeletal weight. Ann NY Acad Sci 1963; *110*:62–71.
4. Society of Actuaries. Build Study 1979. Association of Life Insurance Medical Directors of America.
5. Frisancho AR. New standards of weight and body composition by frame sizes and height for assessment of nutritional status of adults and the elderly. Am J Clin Nutr 1984; *40*:808–819.
6. Keys A, Fidanza F, Karvonen MJ, et al. Indices of relative weight and obesity. J Chron Dis 1972; *25*:329–343.
7. Stewart AL. The reliability and validity of self reported weight and height. J Chron Dis 1982; *35*:295–309.
8. Schlichting P, Hoilund-Carlsen PF, Quade F. Comparison of self reported height and weight with controlled height and weight in women and men. Int J Obesity 1981; *5*:67–76.
9. Morgan DB, Hill GL, Burkinshaw L. The assessment of weight loss from a single measurement of body weight: the problems and limitations. Am J Clin Nutr 1980; *33*:2110–2105.
10. Keys A, Brozek J, Henschel A, et al. The Biology of Human Starvation. Minneapolis, University of Minnesota Press, 1950.
11. Studley HO. Percentage of weight loss. A basic indicator of surgical risk in patients with chronic peptic ulcer. JAMA 1936; *106*:458–460.
12. Pettigrew RA, Hill GL. Indicators of surgical risk and clinical judgement. A prospective comparative study. Br J Surg 1986; *73*:47–51.
13. Daws TA, Consolazio CF, Hilty SL, et al. Evaluation of cardiopulmonary function and work performance in man during caloric restriction. J Appl Physiol 1972; *33*:211-217.
14. Khosla T, Billewicz WZ. Measurement of change in body weight. Br J Nutr 1964; *18*:227–239.
15. Forbes GB. The adult decline in lean body mass. Hum Biol 1976; *48*:161–173.
16. Lesser GT, Deutsch S, Markofsky J. Use of independent measurement of body fat to evaluate overweight and underweight. Metabolism 1971; *20*:792–804.
17. Benedict FG. A Study of Prolonged Fasting. Washington, DC, Carnegie Institute of Washington, 1915: 69–87.
18. Hackett AF, Yeung CK, Hill GL. Eating patterns in patients recovering from major surgery—a study of voluntary food intake and energy balance. Br J Surg 1979; *66*:415–418.
19. Paquin AJ, Lange J. Studies of postoperative body weight loss. Ann Surg 1956; *144*:809–815.
20. Kinney JM. Surgical diagnosis, patterns of energy, exchange, weight and tissue change. *In* Wilkinson AW, Cuthbertson D (eds). Metabolism in Response to Injury. Tunbridge Wells, England, Medical Publish Co Ltd, 1976: 121–134.
21. Streat SJ, Beddoe AH, Hill GL. Unpublished data.
22. Copeland EM, Daly JM, Dudrick SJ. Nutrition as an adjunct to cancer treatment in the adult. Cancer Res 1977; *37*:2451–2456.
23. Byar D, Kenis Y, Van Andel JG, et al. Results of a E.O.R.T.C. randomised trial of cyclophosphamide and radiotherapy in inoperable lung cancer: prognostic factors and treatment results. Europ J Cancer 1978; *14*:919–930.
24. De Wy S. Nutritional abnormalities in cancer: weight loss in cancer patients: prognostic and pathophysiologic considerations. *In* Kluthe R, Löhr G-W (eds). Nutrition and Metabolism in Cancer. Stuttgart, Theime Verlag, 1981: 8–16.
25. Clarke RG. Cancer. *In* Hill GL (ed). Nutrition and the Surgical Patient. Edinburgh, Churchill Livingstone, 1981: 297–308.
26. Macfie J, Burkinshaw L, Oxby C, et al. The effect of gastrointestinal malignancy on resting and metabolic expenditure. Br J Surg 1982; *69*:443–446.
27. Hill GL, Goligher J, Smith AH, et al. Long term changes in total body water, total exchangeable sodium and total body potassium before and after ileostomy. Br J Surg 1975; *62*:524–527.
28. Ivy AC, Grossman MI, Bachrach WN. Peptic Ulcer. New York, McGraw-Hill, 1950.
29. Hill GL, Bradley JA, Smith RC, et al. Changes in body weight and body protein with intravenous nutrition. JPEN 1979; *3*:215–218.
30. Sheldon WH, Stevens SS, Tucker WB. The varieties of human physique. New York, Harper, 1940.
31. Krieger M. Ueber die Atrophie der menschlichen Organe bie Inanition. Anat Konstitutionsl 1921; *7*:87–134.
32. Hill GL, Pickford I, Young GA, et al. Malnutrition in surgical patients—an unrecognised problem. Lancet 1977; *1*:689–692.
33. Behnke AR, Feen OG, Welham WC. The specific gravity of healthy men. JAMA 1942; *118*:495–498.
34. Burkinshaw L. Measurement of body potassium. Calibrations and intercomparison of two whole body radiation counters. Phys Med Biol 1967; *12*:477–488.
35. Morgan DB, Burkinshaw L. Estimation of non-fat body tis-

sues from measurements of skinfold thickness, total body potassium and total body nitrogen. Clin Sci 1983; 65:407–414.

36. Stern H. Investigations on corporal specific gravity and on the value of this factor in physical diagnosis. Med Rec 1901; 59:204–207.

37. Welham WC, Behnke AR. The specific gravity of healthy men. JAMA 1941; 118:498–501.

38. Siri WE. University of California Radiation Laboratory Publication No. 3349; 1956.

39. Siri WE. Body composition from fluid spaces and density: analysis of methods. In Bozek J, Henschel A (eds). Techniques for Measuring Body Composition. Washington, DC, National Academy of Sciences—National Research Council, 1961: 223–244.

40. Buskirk ER. Underwater weighing and body density: a review of procedures. In Brozek J, Henschel A (eds). Techniques for Measuring Body Composition. Washington, DC, National Academy of Sciences—National Research Council, 1961: 90–106.

41. Streat SJ, Beddoe AH, Hill GL. Measurement of body fat and hydration of the fat free body in health and disease. Metabolism, 1985; 34:509–518.

42. Siri WE. The gross composition of the body. Avd Biol Med Phys 1956; 4:239–280.

43. Lohman TG. Skinfolds and body density and their relation to body fatness: a review. Hum Biol 1981; 25:181–225.

44. Behnke AR. New concepts of height-weight relationships. In Wilson NL (ed). Obesity. Philadelphia, FA Davis Co, 1969: 25–53.

45. Durnin JVGA, Womersley J. Body fat assessed from total body density and its estimation from skinfold thickness: measurements on 481 men and women aged from 16–72 years. Br J Nutr 1974; 32:77–97.

46. Borkan AG, Gerzof SG, Robbins AH, et al. Assessment of abdominal fat content by computed tomography. Am J Clin Nutr 1982; 36:172–177.

47. Borkan GA, Hults DE. Change in fat content and distribution with ageing. Am J Phys Anthropol 1983; 60:175.

48. Harrison GG, Van Italie TB. Estimation of body composition: a new approach based on electromagnetic principles. Am J Clin Nutr 1982; 32:524–526.

49. Presta E, Segal KR, Gutin B, et al. Comparison in man of total electrical conductivity and lean body mass derived from body density: validation of a new body composition method. Metabolism 1983; 32:524–526.

50. Pace N, Rathbun EN. Studies on body composition. III. The body water and chemically combined nitrogen content in relation to fat content. J Biol Chem 1945; 158:685–691.

51. Archibald EH, Harrison JE, Pencharz PB. Effect of weight reducing high-protein diet on the body composition of obese adolescents. Am J Dis Child 1983; 137:658–662.

52. Shike M, Russell DM, Detsky AS, et al. Changes in body composition in patients with small-cell lung cancer. Ann Int Med 1984; 101:303–309.

53. Almond DJ, King RFGJ, Burkinshaw L, et al. Measurement of short-term changes in the fat content of the body: a comparison of three methods in patients receiving intravenous nutrition. Br J Nutr 1984; 52:215–225.

54. McCance RA, Widdowson EM. A method of breaking down the body weights of living persons into terms of extracellular fluid, cell mass and fat, and some applications of it to physiology and medicine. Proc Roy Soc B 1951; 138:115–130.

55. Cohn SH, Ellis KJ, Vartsky D, et al. Comparison of methods of estimating body fat in normal subjects and cancer patients. Am J Clin Nutr 1981; 34:2839–2847.

56. Durnin JVGA, Rahaman MM. The assessment of the amount of fat in the human body from measurements of skinfold thickness. Br J Nutr 1967; 21:681–689.

57. Garrow JS. Indices of adiposity. Nut Abst Rev Clin Nutr Series A 1983; 53:697–707.

58. Vaswani AN, Vartsky D, Ellis K, et al. Effect of caloric restriction on body composition and total nitrogen as measured by neutron activation. Metabolism 1983; 32:185–188.

59. MacLean LD, Rhode BM, Shizgal HM. Nutrition following gastric operations for morbid obesity. Ann Surg 1983; 198:347–355.

60. Shizgal HM. Body composition. In Fischer JE (ed). Surgical Nutrition. Boston, Little, Brown & Co, 1983: 3–17.

61. Moore FD. Energy and the maintenance of the body cell mass. JPEN 1980; 4:228–260.

62. Garrow JS. New approaches to body composition. Am J Clin Nutr 1982; 35:1152–1158.

63. Grande F, Keys A. Body weight, body composition and calorie status. In Goodhart RS, Shils ME (eds). Modern Nutrition in Health and Disease. Philadelphia, Lea & Febiger, 1980: 3–34.

64. Moore FD, Olesen KH, McMurrey JD, et al. The Body Cell Mass and Its Supporting Environment: Body Composition in Health and Disease. Philadelphia, WB Saunders, 1963.

65. Kinney, JM, Lister J, Moore FD. Relationship of energy expenditure to total exchangeable potassium. Ann NY Acad Sci 1963; 110:711–722.

66. Moore FD, Lister J, Boyden CM, et al. The skeleton as a feature of body composition. Hum Biol 1968; 40:135–188.

67. Burkinshaw L, Hill GL, Morgan DB. Assessment of the distribution of protein in the human body by in vivo neutron activation analysis. IAEA-SM 1979; 227/39:787–798.

68. Cohn SH, Vaswani AN, Yasumura S, et al. Improved models for determination of body fat by in vivo neutron activation. Am J Clin Nutr 1984; 40:255–259.

69. Schoeller DA, Von Senten E, Peterson DW, et al. Total body water measurements in humans with ^{18}O and ^{2}H labelled water. Am J Clin Nutr 1980; 33:2686–2693.

70. Leoppky JA, Myhre LG, Venters MD, et al. Total body water and lean body mass estimated by ethanol dilution. J Appl Physiol 1977; 42:803–808.

71. Culebras JM, Moore FD. Total body water and the exchangeable hydrogen. I. Theoretical calculations of nonaqueous exchangeable hydrogen in man. Am J Physiol 1977; 232:R54–59.

72. Culebras JM, Fitzpatrick HF, Brennan CM, et al. Total body water and the exchangeable hydrogen. II. A review of comparative data from animals based on isotope dilution and desiccation, with a report of new data from the rat. Am J Physiol 1977; 232:R60–65.

73. McMurrey JD, Boling EA, Davis JM, et al. Body composition: simultaneous determination of several aspects by the dilution principle. Metabolism 1958; 7:651–667.

74. Shizgal HM, Spanier AH, Humes J, et al. Indirect measurement of total exchangeable potassium. Am J Physiol 1977; 233:F253–F259.

75. Palmer HE, Roesch WC. A shadow shield whole-body counter. Health Phys 1965; 11:1213–1219.

76. Burkinshaw L. Measurement of body potassium. Calibration and intercomparison of two whole-body radiation counters. Phys Med Biol 1967; 12:477–488.

77. Anderson J, Osborn SB, Tomlinson RWS, et al. Neutron activation analysis in man in vivo: a new technique in medical investigation. Lancet 1964; 2:1201–1205.

78. Palmer HE, Nelp WB, Murano R, et al. The feasibility of in vivo neutron activation analysis of total body calcium and other elements of body composition. Phys Med Biol 1968; 13:269–279.

79. Hill GL, McCarthy ID, Collins JP, et al. A new method for the rapid measurement of body composition in critically ill surgical patients. Br J Surg 1978; 65:732–735.

80. McNeill KG, Mernagh JR, Jeejeebhoy KN, et al. In vivo measurements of body protein based on the determination of nitrogen by prompt gamma analysis. Am J Clin Nutr 1979; 32:1955–1961.

81. Cohn SH. The present status of in vivo neutron activation analysis in clinical diagnosis and therapy. Atomic Energy Review (Vienna) 1981; 18(3):599–990.

82. Beddoe AH, Hill GL. Clinical measurement of body com-

position using in vivo neutron activation analysis. JPEN 1985; 9:504–520.

83. Report of the Task Group on Reference Man. Int Comm Radiol Protection Report No 23. Oxford, Pergamon Press, 1975.

84. Forbes RM, Cooper AR, Mitchell HH. The composition of adult human body as determined by chemical analysis. J Biol Chem 1953; 203:359–366.

85. Forbes RM, Mitchell HH, Cooper AR. Further studies on the gross composition and mineral elements of the human body. J Biol Chem 1956; 223:969–975.

86. Widdowson EM, McCance RA, Spray CM. The chemical composition of the human body. Clin Sci 1951; 10:113–125.

87. Mitchell HH, Hamilton TS, Steggerda FR, et al. The chemical composition of the adult human body and its bearing on the biochemistry of growth. J Biol Chem 1945; 158:625.

88. Knight GS, Beddoe AH, Streat SJ, et al. Body composition of two human cadavers by neutron activation and chemical analysis. Am J Physiol 1986; 250:E179–185.

89. Cohn SH, Vartsky D, Yasumura S, et al. Compartmental body composition based on total body nitrogen, potassium and calcium. Am J Physiol 1980; 239:E524–530.

90. Chan STF, Johnson AW, Moore MH, et al. Early weight gain and glycogen-obligated work during nutritional rehabilitation. Hum Nutr Clin Nutr 1982; 36:223–232.

91. Hill GL, Church J. Energy and protein requirements of general surgical patients requiring intravenous nutrition. Br J Surg 1984; 71:1–9.

92. Streat SJ, Hill GL. Nutritional support in the management of critically ill surgical intensive care patients. World J Surg 1987; 11:127.

5

PHOSPHORUS MAGNETIC RESONANCE SPECTROSCOPY AS A PROBE OF NUTRITIONAL STATE

BRITTON CHANCE / RICHARD L. VEECH

The use of magnetic resonance spectroscopy for the detection of muscle work performance and for the detection of tissue hypoxia is now well established through a number of examples in which it is clearly the method of choice as a noninvasive, nondestructive approach to the understanding of oxidative metabolism in work and in hypoxic-ischemic distress. Few studies, if any, have been made on the response of oxidative metabolism to substrate delivery under conditions of quantified tissue function.

This chapter describes how phosphorus magnetic resonance spectroscopy (P-MRS) can be used as a quantitative indicator of the nutritional state in general and of the delivery of substrate for oxidative metabolism to body organs in health and disease.

Nutrition here is identified as the process by which electrons are delivered to the respiratory chain to promote the synthesis of ATP in a process that is not usually rate-limiting, but may be in disease in general and in metabolic defects in particular. Defects of oxidative metabolism may cause ATP synthesis to become rate-limiting and activate high levels of glycolytic activity with consequent tissue acidosis. For example, mitochondrial diseases or diseases leading to flooding of the tissue with glycolysis products, especially lactic acid from excessive glycolysis and glycogenic breakdown, on the one hand, or fatty acids on the other, may fail to deliver adequate substrate or substrates at an abnormal potential to the mitochondrial system. In both cases this may lead to inadequate ATP production or to an inadequate phosphorylation potential.

THEORETICAL BACKGROUND

The prescription of oral and parenteral nutrients is so routine and the reliance upon pharmacological or surgical interventions so dominant in the current practice of clinical medicine that the therapeutic opportunities and power of nutritional and fluid therapy are little considered or optimally utilized. Phosphorus magnetic resonance spectroscopy presents to the clinician for the first time a powerful, noninvasive method for quantitatively determining the central energy parameter of the living cell, the phosphorylation potential or $[\Sigma ATP]/[\Sigma ADP][\Sigma P_i]$ ratio. Critically related to phosphorylation potential are such vital characteristics of the living animal as: (1) the efficiency of cardiac work per mole of coronary O_2 delivered; (2) the oxidation-reduction state of cellular cofactors; (3) whether dietary or tissue amino acids will be synthesized into tissue protein or broken down into glucose; (4) to what extent a hormone or drug will act in a given situation; (5) the extent of the plasma membrane gradients of the essential electrolytes of the cellular fluids; (6) the intracellular pH; and (7) the distribution of water between the various cellular compartments.

By the thoughtful understanding of the fundamental biochemical architecture of the cell, the clinician may now use nutritional therapy to manipulate and alter this fundamental energy parameter of the living cell so as to achieve therapeutic aims for particular patients. In that endeavor, phosphorus magnetic resonance spectroscopy becomes a powerful new tool to aid in the diagnosis of the defect present and to monitor the effectiveness of the therapeutic modalities applied.

What is generally meant by nutrition is the provision to the living organism of the substrates, inorganic ions, and essential vitamins or cofactors required to provide the small amount of structural constituents and the large amount of metabolic energy to sustain life and tissue growth and repair in a maximally efficient or healthy state. The precise pathways by which nutrients are metabolized are discussed elsewhere[1] (see Chapter 3). The dominant portion of foodstuffs eaten is not incorporated into constituents of tissue but rather converted into metabolic energy. Carbohydrates, fats, and the carbon chains of amino acids are converted into CO_2 and water, while the nitrogen of amino acids is converted predominantly into urea or uric acid. This is apparent from studies showing that the heat produced by the burning of glucose in a calorimeter is essentially equivalent to the heat released if the glucose is administered to a living animal. Clearly, therefore, the primary role of nutrition is the provision of metabolic energy. Recent rapid advances in phosphorus magnetic resonance spectroscopy (^{31}P-MRS) provide a new and powerful tool for evaluating the central energy parameter of the cells of living animals in different nutritional conditions or with differing nutrient compositions, thus providing information on the effects of various nutrient mixtures and hormones or pharmacological agents upon the primary resultant of nutrients, metabolic energy.

Pathways of Metabolic Energy Production

Nutrients are substances such as fats, carbohydrates, and proteins that become substrates for diverse metabolic reactions of the cell that all remove H atoms and their two attendant electrons in stereotyped dehydrogenase reactions[2] of the type:

Reduced foodstuff

$$+ NAD^+ \leftrightarrow \text{Oxidized foodstuff} + NADH + H^+ \quad (Eq. 1)$$

High-energy electrons from the foodstuffs, now carried on reduced pyridine nucleotide cofactors (NADH), are transferred into the mitochondria in a series of enzymatic shuttles in which NADH becomes the substrate of the electron transport system. These electrons, at a very negative potential, are passed up the electron transport system of the mitochondria to reduce molecular O_2, at a very positive potential, to form H_2O, while at the same time the process of oxidative phosphorylation conserves the bulk of the energy possessed by these electrons by formation of the anhydride bond of ATP from ADP and P_i in the reaction:[3]

$$NADH_m + H^+_m + 3\ ADP^{3-}_c + 3\ P_i^{2-}_c + 3\ H^+_c$$
$$+ \tfrac{1}{2}\ O_2 \rightarrow NAD^+_m + 3\ ATP^{4-}_c + 4\ H_2O + \text{heat} \quad (Eq. 2)$$

Most of the roughly 1.1 electron volts of energy these electrons carried from foodstuffs by NADH is then used, in their passage up the electron transport system, to form the high-energy anhydride bond of ATP. Only a small but kinetically important portion of that energy is given off as the heat characteristic of living animal cells.

In the most basic sense, then, the living organism may be considered as the most efficient of fuel cells. Instead of storing energy in a battery, however, the living cell stores it as chemical bond energy in anhydrides of phosphate, principally ATP and secondarily in its isomeric partner in muscle and brain, creatine phosphate. ATP is the form of cellular energy generally used for muscle contraction, ion pumping, and a host of synthetic reactions. The energy is released from ATP during its hydrolysis in an ATPase reaction of the type:

$$H_2O + ATP \rightarrow ADP + P_i + H^+ + \Delta G \quad (Eq. 3)$$

The extent and direction of the reaction given in Equation 3, or in other words the energy that can be released to drive other reactions, the ΔG, is independent of the pathway by which this release is achieved, and is determined solely by two factors:

1. The standard free energy, ΔG^0, of ATP's anhydride bond, which is invariant under physiological conditions and has a value of -7.6 kcal/mole at 38°C,

pH 7.0, 1 mmol free $[Mg^{2+}]$, and 0.25 ionic strength.[4]

2. The activity or concentration of the reactants listed in Equation 3, or in other words the value of the $[\Sigma ATP]/[\Sigma ADP][\Sigma P_i]$ ratio, or the phosphorylation potential, which varies widely under normal and pathological conditions, is the quantity which can now be determined in vivo using P-MRS. Within the living mammalian cell, the value of ΔG released under normal intracellular conditions is between -13.6 and -13.9 kcal/mole of ATP hydrolyzed.[5]

The relationship between chemical reactions and energy[6] may be written formally for the case of ATP hydrolysis as:

$$\Delta G = \Delta G^0 + RT \ln (\Sigma ADP)(\Sigma P_i)/(\Sigma ATP) \quad (Eq.\,4)$$

where:

ΔG = the free energy of ATP hydrolysis in the cytosol of the mammalian cells, which is between -13.6 and -13.9 kcal/mole of ATP hydrolyzed

ΔG^0 = standard free energy of ATP hydrolysis or -7.6 kcal/mole

R = the gas constant: 1.987 calories/°K/mole

T = temperature in degrees Kelvin: 38°C = 311°K

$\ln$ = the natural log: $2.303 \times \log_{10}$

Relationship of the Redox State to Phosphorylation Potential

While the biochemical reactions converting the electrons of foodstuffs into energy are basically the same, not all foodstuffs yield protons (H^+) and electrons (e^-) of the same energy. Consequently protons and electrons from different foodstuffs cannot all yield the same amount of ATP. The protons and electrons generated during the metabolism of lactate yield 3 ATP per mole of lactate consumed, while those obtained from the oxidation of succinate yield only 2.[7] This difference in the energy of protons and their attendant electrons between a reduced substrate and its oxidized product is called the "redox state" of a reaction.[8]

In the basic dehydrogenase reaction (Eq. 1) providing NADH, the substrate for oxidative phosphorylation, one pair of substrates, NAD^+, gains 2 electrons (2 e^-), or is reduced, while the other set of substrates, in this case l-lactate$^-$ converting to pyruvate$^-$, loses 2 electrons and 2 protons (H^+) or is oxidized. These pairs of substrates in an oxidation-reduction reaction are called redox couples and take part in half reactions that may be written:[2]

The inherent ease with which a substrate donates its electrons and protons to NAD^+ is called its redox potential, which in turn is an inherent function of the equilibrium constant (K_{eq}) of the reaction involved. The potential of a reduced substrate and its oxidized product is given by the half reaction:[8]

$$E_h = E^0 + \frac{RT}{nF} \ln \frac{[\text{oxidized substrate}]}{[\text{reduced substrate}]} \quad (Eq.\,6)$$

where:

E_h = the redox potential of the couple in volts

E^0 = the standard potential of the couple in volts

n = the number of electrons involved in the reaction

F = the Faraday constant, or 23.085 kcal/V/mole

The standard potential of the normal monoanionic redox pairs that serve as blood-borne nutrients between the various organs are quite different. Thus the standard potential at pH 7 of the l-lactate$^-$/pyruvate couple is about -0.19 V, while that of the ketone body couple, d-beta hydroxybutyrate/acetoacetate, is -0.29 V.[8] The commonly referred to "reducing agent" ascorbic acid has a more oxidized standard potential of -0.06 V. The intracellular carrier of elecrons from foodstuffs to the electron transport system, NAD/NADH, has a standard potential at pH 7 of -0.32 V, while that of the ultimate electron acceptor couple of the electron transport system, $\frac{1}{2} O_2/H_2O$, has a standard potential of $+0.8$ V for a difference of about 1.1 V between NADH and $\frac{1}{2} O_2$.[8]

Within the cell, variable redox states of the pyridine nucleotides exist at widely differing redox potentials.[9] Thus the redox state of the free cytosolic $[NAD^+]/[NADH]$ couple is normally about -0.19 electron volts, and that of the free cytosolic $[NADP^+]/[NADPH]$ used for reductive biosynthesis is a more negative -0.41 V, while the redox state of the free mitochondrial $[NAD^+]/[NADH]$, which serves as the initial substrate for oxidative phosphorylation, is normally at an intermediate value of -0.28 V.[9] It is the difference in voltage between the redox state of the variable free mitochondrial $[NAD^+]/[NADH]$ and the relatively concentration insensitive $[\frac{1}{2} O_2]/[H_2O]$ couple at $+0.8$ V that is the final determinant of the maximum energy in the phosphorylation potential given the stoichiometry of 3 ATP formed for each 2 electrons passed up the chain from NADH to O_2. Thus oxidation of the mitochondrial free $[NAD^+]/[NADH]$, as occurs during substrate depletion, uncoupled electron transport, or inappropriate nutrient loading, must inevitably

$$\text{Sum:} \quad \frac{\begin{array}{l} NAD^+ + 2e^- + H^+ \rightarrow NADH \\ CH_3CH_2COO^- \rightarrow CH_3COCOO^- + 2e^- + 2H^+ \end{array}}{CH_3CH_2COO^- + NAD^+ \rightarrow CH_3CH_2COO^- + NADH + H^+} \quad (Eq.\,5)$$

be accompanied by a decrease in the phosphorylation potential or a decrease in the efficiency of ATP production per each $\frac{1}{2}$ O_2 consumed. In general, however, because of common metabolites that link the various cellular redox states in a network of near equilibrium, reduction of one pyridine nucleotide pool is accompanied by reduction of the other pools as well.[9]

It has long been recognized that the nutritional state of the patient played a major part in the outcome of his or her disease. It has also long been recognized that nutritional formulations currently used have more to do with the historical development of nutrients than with detailed intracellular studies of their effects. Recently it has become apparent that the phosphorylation potential of cells within the living animal may be manipulated and controlled by controlling the redox state of the permeant, monoanionic nutrients supplied to the patient.[10] This is so because the cytosolic redox state can be manipulated by controlling the redox state of the monoanionic nutrients supplied to the organs in the blood.

Relationship of the Cytosolic Redox State to Phosphorylation Potential

The redox state of the free cytosolic [NAD+]/[NADH] couple is in near equilibrium with the [l-lactate]/[pyruvate] ratio. This [NAD+]/[NADH] couple in turn is in near equilibrium with the cytosolic phosphorylation potential through a series of powerful enzymes of the glycolytic pathway, which are present in high activity in all cells.[5] The reaction may be written:

$$K_{G+G} = \frac{[3PG]}{[DHAP]} \times \frac{[\Sigma ATP]}{[\Sigma ADP][\Sigma P_i]}$$
$$\times \frac{[NADH][H^+]}{[NAD^+]} \quad \text{(Eq. 7)}$$

It is obvious that nutrients that cause a decrease in the cytosolic phosphorylation potential will, assuming constancy of the metabolites of glycolysis, result in a lowering of the cellular phosphorylation potential. The energy derived from the hydrolysis of ATP will be proportionately lowered according to the relationship given in Equation 4. Since patients with severe illnesses are characterized almost universally by having an elevated blood [lactate]/[pyruvate] ratio, administration of nutritional regimens that cause further reduction of the cytosolic [NAD+]/[NADH] ratio must exacerbate the problem further. Of particular concern in nutritional therapy are the recent observations[11] that the rate of steroid-induced hepatic conversion of tissue amino acids to glucose is a function of the [l-lactate]/[pyruvate] ratio bathing the hepatic cells. The "catabolic" state of accelerated

tissue breakdown following either surgery or most severe illness, in which blood steroids are generally elevated, may potentially be alleviated by careful control of the effects administered nutrients have upon the redox state of the patient.

Relationship between Phosphorylation Potential and Electrolyte and Water Distribution

One of the primary purposes of nutritional therapy is to provide, in addition to nutrients, the water and electrolytes required to sustain life. It has long been known that severe injury of tissue from any cause leads to a loss of tissue K^+ into the blood and extracellular fluid, and an increase in tissue Na^+ and water.[12] Maintenance of the ion gradients characteristic of living tissue is critically dependent upon the provision of metabolic energy in the form of ATP.[13]

Recently it has been hypothesized that the distribution of the common electrolytes Na^+, K^+, Cl^-, and Ca^{2+} and the distribution of water between intracellular and extracellular space are in a state of near equilibrium with the cytosolic phosphorylation potential in an electroneutral, osmoneutral sum of several plasma membrane transport reactions, which may be written:

$$0 = 3\,\Delta G_{ATPase} + 3\,\Delta G^0_{ion}$$
$$+ 3\,RT \ln \frac{[\Sigma ADP]}{[\Sigma ATP]}[\Sigma P_i] \quad \text{(Eq. 8)}$$
$$+ RT \ln \frac{[Na^+]_o^3[K^+]_i^6[Cl^-]_o[Ca^{2+}]_o^2}{[Na^+]_i^3[K^+]_o^6[Cl^-]_i[Ca^{2+}]_i^2}$$

This equation, which has been discussed elsewhere,[10] attempts to relate such parameters as the resting membrane potential, the distribution of the major tissue electrolytes, and the distribution of water between intracellular and extracellular space to the central phosphorylation potential. It may be thought of as approaching an equation of state for the cell. Because nutritional status can materially affect the redox state of most cells, Equation 8 should be considered in prescribing nutritional regimens. The essential point that the phosphorylation potential is critically related to the essential properties of living cells is certainly likely to be true. It is this central parameter of cellular function that should be considered during any nutritional prescription and that can be manipulated within limits by dietary means. Furthermore, the effect of these manipulations is now quantitatively determinable within the critical organs of the living patient such as brain[14] and heart,[15] using the new technique of phosphorus magnetic resonance spectroscopy.

ROLE OF P-MRS IN MONITORING INTRACELLULAR pH AND PHOSPHORYLATION POTENTIAL IN NUTRITIONAL THERAPY

In a healthy patient in a nonstressful state, the process of ATP synthesis is not self-limiting. However, in most disease states, such as fever, tissue anoxia secondary to circulatory occlusion or pulmonary disease, or certain genetic diseases, or during extreme muscular work, the rate of mitochondrial ATP synthesis becomes rate-limiting and falls below the rate of ATP utilization. When that happens, a second, less efficient form of ATP production is brought into play, namely glycolysis. In that process, glucose is broken down in the cytoplasm to lactic acid with the consequent production of only 2 ATP per mole of glucose consumed, whereas the complete metabolism of lactate through the Krebs cycle[16] to CO_2 and H_2O within the mitochondria and the subsequent oxidation by the electron transport system of the NADH released by the complete metabolism of lactate would have led to the production of 36 ATP. Exuberant anaerobic production of highly ionized lactic acid, rather than neutral H_2O, and rapidly permeant gaseous CO_2, which is efficiently removed by the circulation and ultimately by the lungs, leads to intracellular acidosis. This change in intracellular pH can be monitored using P-MRS by observing the chemical shift of the inorganic phosphate (P_i) peak,[17] whose pK_a is about 6.6,[18] thus existing 20 per cent in the $H_2PO_4^-$ and 80 per cent in the HPO_4^{2-} form at normal intracellular pH.

In monitoring the cellular phosphorylation potential, the concentration of free cytosolic [ΣADP] of 20 to 50 μmol is below the sensitivity of P-MRS to detect. However, the phosphorylation potential in heart, brain, and muscle can be effectively monitored by P-MRS, taking advantage of the strong creatine phosphate signal that is prominent in the spectra of brain and muscle tissue. The reactants of the creatine kinase reaction are in near equilbrium in these tissues.[5] With knowledge of the intracellular pH and of free cytosolic [ΣP_i] and [ΣPCr] derived from P-MRS and on the assumption that the change in [ΣP_i] in equivalent to change in [creatine], the cytosolic phosphorylation potential may be estimated in the living patient by:[19,20]

Free cytosolic [ΣADP]

$$= \frac{[\Sigma ATP]}{K_{CK}} \times \frac{[creatine]}{[\Sigma PCr][H^+]} \quad (Eq.\ 9)$$

where $K_{CK} = 1.66 \times 10^9\ M^{-1}$

From the above equation, the free cytosolic [ΣADP] may be calculated, and the phosphorylation potential estimated as previously described.[19] The MRS-measurable [ΣPCr]/[ΣP_i] ratio becomes equivalent to the [ΣATP]/[ΣADP][ΣP_i] ratio.

ADEQUACY OF ENERGY PRODUCTION RELATIVE TO ENERGY UTILIZATION

We have argued that a major function of nutrients is the provision of adequate metabolic energy to meet the metabolic demands required to sustain living cells in a healthy state. The steady state that characterizes the living organism is a balance between energy production and energy utilization. The central measure of that state is the phosphorylation potential of the cells. The sustenance of that steady state of phosphorylation thus becomes a question of the control of the major pathways of cellular energy production, oxidative phosphorylation and glycolysis, and the rates of the diverse cellular ATPase reactions.

In the normal patient, the rate of O_2 consumption in the reaction of oxidative phosphorylation (Eq. 2) is determined by the rate of ATP hydrolysis (Eq. 3) required to meet metabolic demands at the time in question. From a kinetic point of view[19] the rate-controlling substrate in this process could be given by any of the reactants listed in Equation 2 according to a kinetic statement of the form:[21]

$$\frac{V}{V_{max}} = \frac{1}{1 + \dfrac{Km}{[ADP]} + \dfrac{Km'}{[P_i]} + \dfrac{Km''}{[NADH]} + \dfrac{Km'''}{[O_2]}}$$

$$(Eq.\ 10)$$

where

V = the rate of O_2 consumption

V_{max} = the rate of maximal O_2 consumption

K_m, Km', etc. = the Km of the substrate appearing below

Thus under normal conditions the steady state concentrations of [P_i], [NADH], and [O_2] are such that the concentration of free cytosolic [ADP] of 20 to 50 μmol is rate-limiting for O_2 consumption.[2] Under pathological conditions, or under conditions of abnormal nutrition, either enteral or parenteral, the rate of O_2 consumption may become limited by one or another of the parameters listed in Equation 4. In particular, the administration of conventional parenteral nutrition solutions may impose kinetic limitations upon the rates of O_2 consumption in conformity with the general equation for the process (Eq. 10). This is particularly the case during abnormal redox states of the free [NAD^+]/[NADH] couple, or during abnormalities of [P_i] concentration induced during administration of parenteral nutrients such as those currently used.

EQUATIONS FOR METABOLIC CONTROL BY THE NUTRITIONAL STATE

One of the unexpected fruits of P-MRS study is the ability to detect not only the phosphate potential of the system,

$$\frac{ATP}{ADP} \times P_i \qquad (Eq. 11)$$

which when translated into P-MRS terms by Equation 8 is (PCr/P_i^2), but especially the velocity of oxidative metabolism as indicated by the Michaelis-Menten expression of

$$\frac{V}{V_{max}} = \frac{1}{1 + \dfrac{K_s}{S}} \qquad (Eq. 12)$$

$$\frac{V}{V_{max}} = \frac{1}{1 + \dfrac{0.6}{P_i/PCr}} \qquad (Eq. 13)$$

Thus, for the first time, it is possible to determine the relative velocity of intracellular metabolism by a noninvasive method.

The enzyme indicated in the Michaelis-Menten expression (Eq. 12 and 13) is the oxidative metabolism system that governs the rate of ATP synthesis (see Eq. 3). In Equations 12 and 13, the assumption—justified by experimental studies—was made that the rate-limiting step of oxidative metabolism is the ADP concentration in the cytosol, which is then translocated into the mitochondral matrix to be phosphorylated to ATP. However, it is clear from Equations 2 and 10 that substrate concentration may also govern the rate of ATP synthesis. Most important from the standpoint of nutrition, the NADH concentration, as delivered to the mitochondrial matrix, passes through the citric acid cycle, the Embden-Meyerhof glycolytic pathway, or indeed the fatty acid oxidation pathway. In order to incorporate substrate concentration as a controlling factor in the velocity of oxidative metabolism, we add to Equation 13 the appropriate term.

$$\frac{V}{V_{max}} = \frac{1}{1 + \dfrac{0.6}{P_i/PCr} + \dfrac{K_1}{NADH}} \qquad (Eq. 14)$$

Thus, the substrate level can be a governing factor in the rate of oxidative metabolism. However, certain important homeostatic regulations occur that are even more useful in the study of tissue nutrition. For a constant velocity of metabolism, which is necessary for steady-state life in the brain, heart, and kidney, the denominator is a constant.

$$\frac{V}{V_{max}} = \frac{1}{1 + \dfrac{0.6}{P_i/PCr} + \dfrac{K_1}{NADH}} = const \qquad (Eq. 15)$$

Thus, P_i/PCr directly indicates the NADH and substrate levels. As substrate (NADH) is depleted, P_i/PCr increases in inverse proportion.

Phosphofructokinase Deficiency

An example of the use of these equations is provided by a patient with genetic deficiency of phosphofructokinase (PFK), an enzyme providing NADH to the mitochondria.[22] Oxidative metabolism in this 29-year-old patient depended upon fatty acid metabolism. While this defect had no detectable consequences for resting metabolism of the skeletal tissue ($V < < V_{max}$), the exercise performance ($V/V_{max}/3$) was significantly handicapped. In order to demonstrate this defect P-MRS was employed to observe the work accomplished in exercise and the corresponding P_i/PCr value. It would be expected that the substrate-deficient subject would have a larger P_i/PCr value with a given work load than was normal. Figure 5–1 plots the P_i/PCr value against the work load for a normal subject and for the PFK-deficient subject. The experimental results are in accord with expectations. In the initial portion of the work, fatty

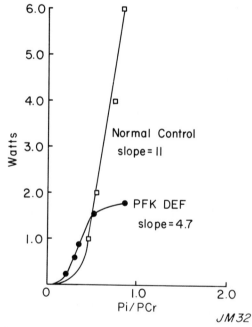

FIGURE 5–1. Graph showing the small fraction of V_{max} available to a substrate-deficient human as compared with a normal control. (From Chance B, Eleff S, Bank W, et al. Proc Natl Acad Sci USA 1982; 79:7714–7718. Reproduced with permission.)

acids allowed the subject to maintain performance similar to that of a normal subject. But when the capacity for substrate delivery of the fatty acid system was exceeded, then, indeed, the P_i/PCr value abruptly increased with work load, while that of the normal subject was maintained under homeostatic control because of the availability of pyruvate through the Embden-Meyerhof pathway. A typical effect of nutritional deficiency was also observed in this case: The trapping of P_i in the sugar phosphate pool was extreme and a severe hypophosphatemia resulted, which exerted an additional control:

$$\frac{V}{V_{max}} = \frac{1}{1 + \dfrac{0.6}{P_i/PCr} + \dfrac{1.0}{P_i} + \dfrac{K_1}{NADH}} \quad \text{(Eq. 16)}$$

where 1.0 mmol is the K_m of mitochondria for P_i.

Muscle Nutrition

While P-MRS is highly responsive to substrate limitation to the muscle, homeostatic mechanisms are called into play to counter gross effects of dietary deficiencies in normal feeding and fasting cycles. One of the key problems in measuring muscle nutrition is the difficulty of depletion of the glycogen stores. Thus, results of voluntary starvation in human subjects for various periods have not yielded striking data. On the other hand, Koruda et al. have employed P-MRS to evaluate substrate deficiencies in rodents.[23]

The use of P-MRS to assess the effectiveness of corticosteroid therapy in hypothyroidism and polymyositis has also been reported.[24]

Vitamin Deficiency

Because P-MRS detects enzyme activities in the metabolic sequence that supplies substrates of oxidative metabolism, and vitamins are frequently components of the active site of enzymes, i.e., coenzymes, vitamin deficiencies might well be studied by P-MRS.

A example of the apparent effect of flavin supplementation upon the diet of a patient with an organic aciduria consistent with glutaric aciduria Type II has been afforded by studies of neonate twins, one of whom had the disease[25] and the other was asymptomatic (R. Kelley, personal communication). As shown by Figure 5–2, gluteus muscle and cardiac tissue both showed elevated inorganic phosphate levels, at rest for the muscle and under resting cardiac activity for the heart. A control for the cardiac tissue is provided by Figure 5–3, which illustrates relative values of phosphocreatine and inorganic phosphate in the hearts of the deficient and normal twins. Figure 5–4 indicates the improvement of phosphocreatine/phosphate ratio coincident with dietary

supplements of riboflavin, which possibly increased activities of the deficient dehydrogenases. As is characteristic of P-MRS studies, which can be made repetitively and noninvasively, this patient has been followed for over 18 months in order to ensure that the therapy was effective, and indeed it was over this interval.

Cytochrome b Deficiency

The effect of vitamins C and K_3 to ameliorate a deficiency of cytochrome b in the skeletal tissues has been reported elsewhere.[26,27] For the purposes of this presentation, it suffices to say that the deficiency of cytochrome b resulted in a very low rate of oxidative metabolism (3 per cent of normal), a high lactic acidosis, and a significantly elevated P_i/PCr even at rest (0.7). Since it was known from in vitro studies that antimycin A–inhibited mitochondrial respiration could be reactivated by a combination of vitamins K and C, we attempted therapy of the P-MRS–diagnosed deficiency of oxidative metabolism. The dose-response curve is shown in Figure 5–5, where the abscissa is dose of K_3 + C over a period of 2 years and the ordinate is the PCr/P_i value at rest. It is seen that significant improvement was obtained through the use of vitamins K_3 and C as electron transfer components bypassing the missing cytochrome.

PROSPECTS FOR FUTURE STUDY

P-MRS monitoring of the nutritional state of tissues is in its infancy. Only proposals for its efficacy can be presented for which detailed human subject studies are not yet available. However, it is clear that merging of the equations for nutritional state developed in the first part of this paper with the significant sensitivity of the PCr/P_i ratio to NADH delivery and to the phosphorylation potential will lead to significant applications of the method to studies in which phosphate potential, redox state, and water and ion balances are optimized. These parameters can be continuously monitored by P-MRS in an organ for which the parenteral fluids are inappropriate. This can be especially important in parenteral fluid therapy, hemodialysis, and many other applications in which an artificial fluid is equilibrated with the plasma, which in turn equilibrates with the body cells.

Acknowledgments

Portions of this work have been supported by NIH Grants HL 31934, RR 02305, AM 37767; the James S. McDonnell Foundation; The Ben Franklin Part-

GLUTARIC ACIDURIA TYPE II:
QUADRICEPS vs CARDIAC REGION

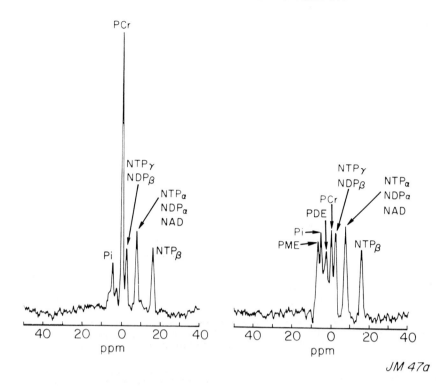

FIGURE 5–2. Elevated P_i in resting quadriceps muscles and low PCr/P_i in hypertrophic heart of neonate having a genetic deficit in glutaric acid metabolism. (From Chance B, Leigh JS Jr, Smith D, et al. Phosphorus magnetic resonance spectroscopy [P MRS] studies of the role of mitochondria in the disease process. New York Academy of Sciences Conference on Biological Membrane Pathology, 1986. Reproduced with permission.)

JM 47a

GLUTARIC ACIDURIA TYPE II : CARDIAC REGION

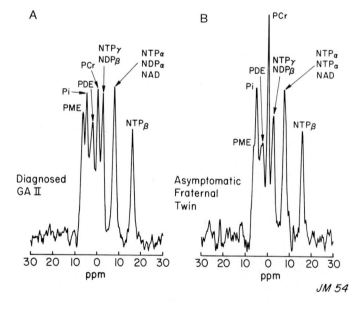

FIGURE 5–3. Heart region of the subject in Figure 5–2 compared with asymptomatic twin. Note higher PCr/P_i in the latter child. (From Chance B, Leigh JS Jr, Smith D, et al. Phosphorus magnetic resonance spectroscopy [P MRS] studies of the role of mitochondria in the disease process. New York Academy of Sciences Conference on Biological Membrane Pathology, 1986. Reproduced with permission.)

JM 54

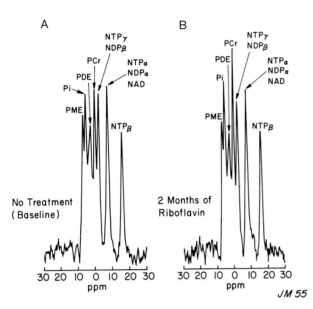

GLUTARIC ACIDURIA TYPE II: CARDIAC REGION

FIGURE 5–4. *Effect of riboflavin therapy upon the subject of Figure 5–2. Note the increase of PCr/P$_i$. (From Chance B, Leigh JS Jr, Smith D, et al. Phosphorus magnetic resonance spectroscopy [P MRS] studies of the role of mitochondria in the disease process. New York Academy of Sciences Conference on Biological Membrane Pathology, 1986. Reproduced with permission.)*

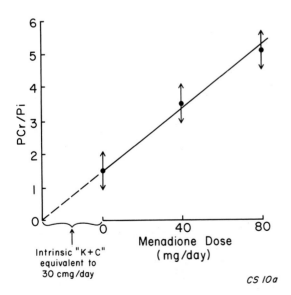

FIGURE 5–5. *Dose-response evaluation of a cytochrome b-deficient young woman. (From Eleff S, Kennaway NG, Buist NRM, et al. Proc Natl Acad Sci USA 1984; 81:3529–3533. Reproduced with permission.)*

nership's Advanced Technology Center of Southeastern Pennsylvania; and the Muscular Dystrophy Association, and aided by Clinical Research Grant 6–482 from the March of Dimes Birth Defects Foundation.

References

1. Krebs HA, Kornberg HL, Burton K. Energy transformations in living matter. Berlin, Springer Verlag, 1957.
2. Theorell H, Chance B. Studies on liver alcohol dehydrogenase. Acta Chem Scand 1951; 5:1127–1144.
3. Chance B, Williams GR. The respiratory chain and oxidative phosphorylation. Adv Enz Reg 1956; 17:65–134.
4. Guynn RW, Veech RL. The equilibrium constants of the adenosine triphosphate hydrolysis and adenosine triphosphate–citrate lyase reactions. J Biol Chem 1973; 248:6966–6972.
5. Veech RL, Lawson JWR, Cornell NW, et al. Cytosolic phosphorylation potential. J Biol Chem 1979; 254:6538–6547.
6. Gibbs JW. On the equilibrium of heterogeneous substances. Trans Conn Acad 1875–1878; 3:108–248, 343–524.
7. Ochoa S. Nature of oxidative phosphorylation. Nature 1940; 146:267.
8. Clark WM. The Oxidation Reduction Potential of Organic Systems. Baltimore, Williams & Wilkins, 1960.
9. Krebs HA, Veech RL. Pyridine nucleotide interrelations. In Papa S, Tager JM, Quagliariello E, et al (eds). The energy level and metabolic control in mitochondria. Bari, Adriatica Editrice, 1969: 329–384.
10. Veech RL. The toxic impact of parenteral solutions on the metabolism of cells: a hypothesis for physiological parenteral therapy. Am J Clin Nutr 1986; 44:519–551.
11. Sistare FD, Haynes RC. Acute stimulation by glucocorticoids of gluconeogenesis from lactate/pyruvate in isolated hepatocytes from normal and adrenalectomized rats. J Biol Chem 1985; 23:12754–12760.
12. Tabor H, Rosenthal SM. Effects of potassium administration, sodium loss, and fluid loss in tourniquet shock. Publ Health Rep 1945; 60:401–419.
13. Stern JR, Eggleston LV, Hems R, et al. Accumulation of glutamic acid in isolated brain tissue. Biochem J 1949; 44:410–418.
14. Nioka S, Chance B, Hilberman M, et al. The relationship between intracellular pH and energy metabolism in dog brain as measured by ^{31}P NMR. Am J Physiol 1986; in press.
15. Chance B, Clark BJ, Nioka S, et al. Phosphorus nuclear magnetic resonance spectroscopy in vivo. Circulation 1985; 72(Suppl IV):103–110.
16. Krebs HA, Johnson WA. The role of citric acid in intermediate metabolism in animal tissues. Enzymologia 1937; 4:148–156.
17. Gadian DG, Radda GK, Richards RE, et al. ^{31}P NMR in living tissue. The road from a promising to an important tool in biology. In Shulman RG (ed). Biological Applications of Magnetic Resonance. New York, Academic Press, 1979: 463–535.
18. Sorensen SPL. Biochem Z. 1909; 22:352–357.
19. Chance B, Eleff S, Leigh JS, et al. Mitochondrial regulation of phosphocreatine/inorganic phosphate in exercising human muscle: a gated ^{31}P NMR study. Proc Natl Acad Sci 1981; 78:6714–6718.
20. Lawson JWR, Veech RL. The effects of pH and free Mg^{2+} on the K$_{eq}$ of the creatine kinase reaction and other phosphate transfer reactions. J Biol Chem 1979; 254:6528–6537.
21. Chance B, Leigh JS Jr, Kent J, et al. Multiple controls of oxidative metabolism of living tissues as studied by ^{31}P MRS. Proc Natl Acad Sci USA 1986; 83:9458–9462.
22. Chance B, Eleff S, Bank W, et al. ^{31}P NMR studies of control

of mitochondrial function in phosphofructokinase-deficient human skeletal muscle. Proc Natl Acad Sci USA 1982; 79:7714–7718.

23. Koruda M, Argov Z, Maris J, et al. Phosphorus-31 magnetic resonance spectroscopy (P-MRS) of stimulated muscle during starvation. Surg Forum. 1985; 36:61–63.

24. McCully KK, Argov Z, Boden BP, et al. Detection of muscle injury in humans with 31-P magnetic resonance spectroscopy. Muscle and Nerve, in press.

25. Chance B, Leigh JS Jr, Smith D, et al. Phosphorus magnetic resonance spectroscopy studies of the role of mitochondria

in the disease process. Ann NY Acad Sci 1986; 488:140–153.

26. Eleff S, Kennaway NG, Buist NRM, et al. ^{31}P NMR study of improvement in oxidative phosphorylation by vitamins K₃ and C in a patient with a defect in electron transport at complex III in skeletal muscle. Proc Natl Acad Sci USA 1984; 81:3529–3533.

27. Argov Z, Bank WJ, Maris J, et al. Treatment of mitochondrial myopathy due to complex III deficiency with vitamins K₃ and C: A ^{31}P NMR follow-up study. Ann Neurol 1986; 19:598–602.

ALTERED NUTRITIONAL STATES

6

PREGNANCY AND LACTATION

MYRON WINICK / PEDRO ROSSO
SALLY A. LEDERMAN

METABOLIC CHANGES IN PREGNANCY AND THEIR NUTRITIONAL IMPLICATIONS

A series of profound metabolic changes occur during pregnancy that affect the way the mother utilizes practically all types of nutrients. Teleologically, the metabolic changes of pregnancy seemed aimed at ensuring efficient and mutually convenient metabolic utilization of fuels and substrates by both the mother and the fetus. However, the biological implications of some of these changes are not always clear.

There are similarities between the metabolic profile of a pregnant woman and the profiles in starvation and diabetes mellitus. For example, tissue glucose utilization is decreased and fat utilization is enhanced in all of these conditions. However, in contrast to either starvation or diabetes, during pregnancy basal insulin secretion is significantly increased relative to plasma glucose values, and anabolism prevails.

In the nonpregnant state the need to maintain blood glucose levels within ranges compatible with normal brain function greatly influences the rates at which the various metabolic fuels are utilized. Glucose is continuously released from the liver at rates of 2 to 3 mg/kg/min.[1] In the postabsorptive state, the transiently increased load of carbohydrate, fat, and protein results in an increased blood glucose level, which in turn stimulates insulin release. During this period plasma insulin levels may increase two- to tenfold. Insulin increases glucose uptake by the liver, where the glucose is converted to glycogen and stored, or into fatty acids and exported. Insulin also promotes the incorporation of amino acids into protein and of lipids into adipose tissue. Thus, the postprandial period is an anabolic phase in which glucose is used as the main metabolic fuel and adipose tissue and muscle have net gains in metabolic substrates.

Between meals the majority of the glucose released from liver (75 per cent) is the product of glycogenolysis. The rest is derived from gluconeogenesis using lactate and alanine and, to a lesser extent, glycerol, as substrates.[1] If the intermeal period is prolonged by several hours, such as during an overnight fast, glycogen continues to be the main source of glucose until blood glucose levels fall by 10 to 50 mg/dl. This small decline signals the pancreas to decrease insulin release and to increase glucagon secretion.[2] As a result of the fall in plasma insulin, free fatty acids are released by lipolysis and utilized as an alternative metabolic fuel. In addition, the reduction in insulin levels results in a decreased uptake of amino acids into muscle and a reduction in the rate of muscle protein synthesis. Thus, the muscle enters a catabolic phase, making more alanine available for gluconeogenesis.[1] During pregnancy the sequence of events described above undergoes drastic modification.

Carbohydrate Metabolism

Carbohydrate metabolism changes markedly during pregnancy: Plasma glucose levels decline, both basal and stimulated insulin secretion increase, and tissues become less sensitive to insulin action.

The reduction in fasting plasma glucose level is gradual and it reaches a nadir during the third trimester, when the average concentration is 5 to 15 mg/dl lower than the prepregnancy levels of 65 to 78 mg/dl.[3–5] A variety of factors may be implicated in lowering plasma glucose, and their relative importance changes with advanced gestation. For example, early in pregnancy as plasma volume expands, the circulating glucose pool may be slightly diluted. The decline in plasma levels due to such dilution, however, would be too small to elicit feedback compensatory mechanisms. Later in gestation the lower glucose levels have been attributed in part to an increased glucose drain by the fetus.[6–8] A term fetus of average weight requires approximately 40 g/day of glucose.[9] Although values of 28 to 30 g/day have been calculated by others, these values are based on the assumption that glucose constitutes the only metabolic fuel of the fetus, but the glucose contribution to the fat stores of the fetus apparently was not considered.[10, 11] In addition to the fetus, the mother expands her red cell mass by about 18 per cent. Since the red cells consume glucose, the increase in red cell mass increases glucose consumption proportionally. In an adult 70-kg male, the daily glucose consumption of the red cell mass would be 50 g.[1] In an average nonpregnant female, because of a smaller red cell mass, it would be approximately 35 g/day. During pregnancy, the red cell mass increase would elevate daily glucose consumption to 43 g/day. In addition, 10 g/day of extra glucose consumption would be required by the placenta, heart, respiratory muscles, and the enlarged uterus and breasts.[12] Thus, the total maternal extra need for glucose would amount to 53 g of glucose per day.

Using a stable tracer, glucose production rates in mothers undergoing elective cesarean sections were estimated to be 2.42 mg/kg/min.[13] In an average pregnant woman near term this would be approximately 238 g/day. The same study revealed production rates in nonpregnant women of approximately 205 g/day. The difference, 33 g, represents approximately 50 per cent of the extra glucose needs estimated above. Therefore, to meet the extra needs the mother must decrease glucose utilization by her own tissues. This is apparently achieved by increased insulin resistance.

A progressive reduction in the sensitivity of the maternal tissues to insulin, reflected by an increasing insulin/glucose ratio, is established by the 25th week of gestation.[14] Tissue sensitivity to insulin in normal pregnant women has been measured using a "glucose clamp" technique in which plasma insulin is determined in response to a fixed degree of hyperglycemia maintained by intravenous infusion.[15] By this technique, tissue sensitivity has been found to decline by as much as 80 per cent. The reduced sensitivity to insulin results in an additional saving of glucose since other metabolic fuels, mostly fatty acids and their derivatives, are used instead. This is reflected by a lower respiratory quotient after an overnight fast in late pregnancy.[16]

Antagonism of insulin action by human chorionic somatomammotropin (hCS, hPL) has been considered to be one of the major causes of gestational insulin resistance. The role of this hormone as a diabetogenic agent in nonpregnant subjects is well established.[17] However, recent studies in women with twin pregnancy have shown that despite much higher plasma levels of hCS than in singleton pregnancies, the rate of glucose disappearance after intravenous injection was similar.[18] Glucagon does not seem to contribute to gestational insulin resistance. Fasting plasma glucagon levels are slightly higher during pregnancy than in nonpregnancy, but after an oral or intravenous glucose load the fall in glucagon levels is more pronounced in pregnancy.[19, 20]

Prolactin is another potential antagonist to insulin action. Women with hyperprolactinemia associated with amenorrhea-galactorrhea syndrome have a decreased carbohydrate tolerance despite a concomitant hyperinsulinemia.[21, 22]

As mentioned above, the increased insulin resistance of pregnancy develops while the basal levels of insulin and the insulin response following a glucose challenge are increased above nonpregnant values. Fasting plasma insulin levels are increased only during the last half of gestation.[23–25] In contrast, the enhanced insulin response following glucose administration can be demonstrated during the first half of gestation.[14] The increased rates of insulin secretion may reflect the influence of estrogen and progesterone on the maternal pancreas. In the rat, estrogen alone or in combination with progesterone increases pancreatic islet size and insulin secretion,[26] while progesterone administration enhances insulin response to glucose in the rhesus monkey.[27]

It has been proposed that the increased rate of insulin secretion during pregnancy could compensate for an increased binding or sequestration of insulin by the placenta.[28] Active systems for insulin cleavage and insulin binding have been described in human placenta.[29–31] However, in vivo measurements of insulin removal in pregnant women have not confirmed the possibility of accelerated insulin catabolism.[32, 33]

The increased insulin resistance may also reflect changes in the insulin receptors of various tissues. The number of insulin receptors in monocytes of pregnant women was found to be reduced by 35 per cent while the affinity of the receptors remained unchanged.[34] Thus, it was concluded that gestational insulin resistance was due to a reduced number of receptors. By contrast, studies in adipocyte cells came to opposite conclusions, finding no change in insulin receptor number during pregnancy but a 50 per cent decrease in affinity.[35] The discrepancy may reflect the characteristics of two markedly different cells.

In the rat the number of insulin receptors increased both in adipocytes and in isolated liver cells[36, 37] during the first half of gestation and then remained unchanged. The increase was attributed to a compensatory mechanism to offset the increased resistance.

Although the hyperinsulinemia and the increased glucose demands of insulin in sensitive compartments, such as the conceptus and the expanded maternal red cell mass, is well accepted, the rate of disappearance of glucose from maternal blood remains unclear. Some authors have found that in pregnant women glucose disappearance rates are considerably higher,[38] slightly increased,[4] or unchanged.[39]

Although glucose production and utilization are greater during pregnancy, animal studies suggest glucose turnover rates similar to rates in nonpregnant animals.[40] For example, in pregnant rats the rates of glycogen synthesis and degradation and the liver glycogen stores are similar to those in nonpregnant rats. Other studies have revealed a similar rate of gluconeogenesis in both groups.[41] These studies in small rodents are highly significant because the fetal mass carried during pregnancy is proportionally five times greater than in humans. The animal studies and the metabolic studies in humans indicate that the reduced glucose plasma levels of late pregnancy are caused not by an excessive glucose drain but simply by hemodilution.

Oral glucose tolerance tests (OGTT) performed serially during gestation suggest a very small, although progressive, decrease in glucose tolerance, but values remain within the normal range.[14] The most significant changes observed in OGTT include a delay in attainment of peak plasma glucose values and, in general, higher peak values than in the nonpregnant state.[14] The differences may reflect a slower rate of intestinal absorption combined with a slower rate of glucose uptake by the liver due to the increased insulin resistance. Studies in nonpregnant subjects have shown that the magnitude of elevation in blood glucose after a high-carbohydrate meal is inversely proportional to liver uptake.[42]

An indication of the efficiency with which a pregnant woman can maintain glucose homeostasis despite some of the changes described above is revealed by the stability of plasma values of glucose during a 24-hour period. After average meals glucose levels do not increase more than 30 to 35 mg/dl over the mean values for the entire period.[43] Similarly, increments in insulin levels average only 30 per cent of average daily values.[43, 44] Although higher increments have been observed,[45] free fatty acids and triglyceride tend to remain high, with high postprandial peaks in free fatty acid concentration.[45]

Lipid Metabolism

Almost every aspect of lipid metabolism is influenced by pregnancy.[46, 47] Plasma levels of most lipid fractions, including free fatty acids, triglycerides, cholesterol, and phospholipids increase during pregnancy. The increase reflects still undefined changes in hepatic and adipose tissue metabolism as well as changes in transport kinetics.

During the first half of gestation, increased food intake and the resulting greater influx of exogenous carbohydrates and fat, together with a moderate postprandial hyperinsulinism, create optimal conditions for lipid synthesis and storage. By contrast, during the second half of gestation, food intake declines and insulin resistance is established. In addition, levels of hCS, which has lipolytic properties, become substantially elevated. The net result of the interaction of these factors is a relative reduction in the rate of lipid accumulation with apparently a small net loss of body fat. The earliest change in the plasma concentration of lipids is an increase in triglycerides at the end of the first trimester.[48, 49] Since plasma triglycerides are a component of lipoprotein complexes, their elevation reflects increases of the various lipoprotein fractions that serve as vehicles for the transport of triglycerides. The hypertriglyceridemia of pregnancy is reflected primarily by an increase in VLDL concentration. However, the composition of the lipid fraction of VLDL remains unchanged. By contrast, the LDL and HDL fractions, which are also elevated, contain a greater proportion of triglycerides relative to cholesterol and phospholipid.[50, 51]

The apoprotein constituents of lipoproteins are also different in pregnancy. Apolipoprotein B (apo B) in VLDL increases while apo C-II decreases in relation to C-III content. An increase in apo A-I in HDL has also been documented.[50, 51]

The lipids present in VLDL are derived from two sources: (1) fatty acids and glycerol synthesized de novo by the liver from carbohydrate and amino acid, and (2) endogenous and exogenous fatty acid sources. In subjects consuming a balanced diet, most of the VLDL triglycerides derive from endogenous circulating FFA. In those consuming a high-carbohydrate diet, de novo synthesis accounts for the larger proportion.[52, 53] The VLDL of pregnant women contain a high proportion of saturated fatty acids. This suggests active de novo synthesis in liver.[54] However, there is no clear experimental evidence demonstrating de novo synthesis. Studies of triglyceride synthesis and removal have produced contradictory results. Some have found no evidence of increased synthesis and, therefore, they have concluded that the rise reflects a slower removal from blood.[55] Others have found that the rate of removal is similar to the rate that occurs in the nonpregnant state and, therefore, they have attributed the change to an increased rate of synthesis.[56] The idea of a gestational increase in triglyceride synthesis is also supported by earlier studies in which plasma removal of triglycerides was blocked by a drug.[57] However, enzyme changes that have been described are more consistent with the possibility of a reduced removal rate. For example, both adipose tissue lipoprotein lipase and postheparin lipase activities decrease in late gestation.[57–59]

Additional indirect evidence also supports the possibility of an increased rate of triglyceride synthesis. Estrogens alone or as part of oral contraceptives increase the endogenous production of VLDL triglycerides.[60, 61] In vitro studies in rat liver slices have shown that corticosterone has a permissive role in the estrogen stimulation of acetyl CoA carboxylase and fatty acid synthetase, rate-limiting enzymes for lipogenesis.[62] Levels of cortisol are maximal during late gestation. Estrogen has also been found to reduce adipose tissue lipoprotein lipase activity drastically in ovariectomized rats.[63] Thus, the estrogenic influence over triglyceride metabolism is one of increased synthesis and reduced removal.

The role of progesterone in the gestational changes in triglyceride metabolism is uncertain. Progesterone administered to premenopausal women increases the rate of plasma triglyceride removal.[64] Studies in rats, however, have shown only a slight or nonsignificant change in plasma triglyceride removal after progesterone administration.[61, 63] Nevertheless, suppression of progesterone secretion is believed to mediate the profound influence of prostaglandins on the triglyceride metabolism of the pregnant rat near term. Injections of prostaglandin $F_{2\alpha}$ near term increased the activity of lipoprotein lipase in the mammary gland fourfold, reduced the activity in adipose tissue by 60 per cent and decreased serum concentration of triglycerides by about 50 per cent.[65] In addition, prostaglandin $F_{2\alpha}$ caused a fivefold increase in prolactin levels and reduced serum progesterone levels by 90 per cent. Prolactin administration to lactating rats mimics the effect of prostaglandin $F_{2\alpha}$ on adipose tissue and mammary gland in late gestation.[66] However, prolactin has no effect on lipoprotein lipase activity in either tissue when injected late in gestation.[65] Therefore, the prostaglandin effect seems to be mediated only by the reduction in plasma progesterone levels. In support of this possibility, progesterone injections block the prostaglandin effect. No effect of prostaglandin $F_{2\alpha}$ on either insulin or 17-estradiol levels was observed.[65]

If prostaglandin $F_{2\alpha}$ is injected in rats on day 16 of gestation (length of gestation in the rat is 21 days), plasma progesterone levels decrease about 80 per cent, but lipoprotein lipase activity remains unchanged. At this time, however, progesterone levels are considerably higher than at day 20. Thus, although the percentage decrease in plasma levels caused by prostaglandin was similar on both days, levels in the rats injected on day 16 were four times higher than on day 20. The results of this study suggest that the prostaglandin effect may be mediated by the suppression of progesterone antagonism for a substance that inhibits lipoprotein lipase activity in the adipose tissue but stimulates this activity in the mammary gland. The most likely candidate for this unknown substance is estrogen. In the pregnant rat, plasma estrogen concentration increases markedly after day 18 of gestation.[67]

The decreased adipose tissue lipoprotein lipase activity presumably caused by the increased estrogen/progesterone ratio of late gestation may enhance free fatty acid utilization by other tissues in place of deposition in fat stores. The simultaneous increase of mammary gland lipoprotein lipase[58] is consistent with this possibility, but no similar increases of this enzyme's activity have been described in other tissues. Furthermore, although as previously mentioned, estrogen decreases lipoprotein lipase in adipose tissue, there is no concomitant change in lipoprotein lipase activity of heart or lung.[63]

Plasma free fatty acid levels decrease until week 30 of gestation and then increase until a few days before delivery.[68] Plasma glycerol concentration changes in a similar fashion. The late gestational increase in FFA and glycerol is compatible with an increased rate of lipid mobilization from adipose tissue. In support of this conclusion, in vitro rates of lipolysis from adipose tissue obtained during surgery at various gestational ages show an increase in both spontaneous and stimulated rates of lipolysis over the rates in nonpregnant women.[69] The results were obtained under conditions in which the production of cAMP was not rate-limiting to the activation of lipolysis, and it is likely that the data reflect increased levels of hormone-sensitive lipase and the lipase activating system. Earlier in vitro studies in pregnant rats also revealed an increased rate of lipolysis with advanced gestation.[70] The studies in human adipose tissue also demonstrate a lack of stimulatory effect of hCS on in vitro lipolysis,[69] but this has been contradicted by more recent findings.[71] Since insulin has an inhibitory effect on hormone-sensitive lipase activity, the progressive insulin resistance of late pregnancy could have a stimulatory effect on the activity of this enzyme.[72] The high levels of plasma cortisol present at this period may also result in enhancement of hormone-sensitive lipase activity. The increase in the circulating pool of FFA may have an important effect on maternal metabolism because it provides an alternative source of metabolic fuel during a time of gestation in which glucose needs are maximal.

Plasma levels of cholesterol are also increased during gestation, but the elevation is proportionally smaller than that of either FFA or triglycerides.[73] The elevated plasma cholesterol concentration probably reflects both increased synthesis and decreased catabolism. In addition, the increased sluggishness of the intestine seems to contribute to a greater degree of cholesterol reabsorption. The increased rate of synthesis is probably related to changes in lipoprotein metabolism, although the nature of these changes is unknown. Experiments with pregnant rats have shown a moderate decrease in the quantity of cholesterol eliminated in bile after injection of ^{14}C-cholesterol.[74] Cholesterol balance studies[75] and studies performed in pregnant guinea pigs have also been inconclusive.[76]

Plasma phospholipid levels increase moderately during gestation.[73] The elevation probably reflects the increased VLDL concentration as well as that of the other lipoproteins. Pregnancy also causes marked changes in phospholipid composition.[73] During the last month of gestation, lysolecithin concentration decreased while other phospholipids, including sphingomyelin, lecithin, and phosphatidyl ethanolamine, tended to increase in varying amounts. The mechanisms responsible for these changes are unknown. Equally unknown are the implications of the changes. Lecithin and lysolecithin are important components of lipoprotein and participate in the conversion of free cholesterol to its ester form. This step is important for the reversed transport of cholesterol from peripheral tissues to the liver for its conversion to bile acids and subsequent excretion. Thus, alterations of these fractions may affect the body's handling of cholesterol.

Protein and Amino Acid Metabolism

Even less is known about protein and amino acid metabolism in the healthy gravida than is known about carbohydrate and lipid metabolism. Most of the available data consist of descriptions of changes in plasma protein concentrations and of urinary excretion of nitrogenous compounds and nitrogen.

Furthermore, only a limited number of studies on protein and amino acid metabolism have been carried out in pregnant animals. Therefore, it is difficult to draw general conclusions regarding the nature of the major metabolic adjustments and their mechanisms.

In the nonpregnant state a woman consuming an average Western diet has a daily protein intake of approximately 80 g. In the intestine this protein combines with 55 to 70 g of endogenous protein derived from desquamated intestinal cells and various intestinal secretions.[77] Both types of protein are digested to small peptides and free amino acids, which are then transported into the mucosal cells. The small peptides, mostly dipeptides, are further hydrolyzed in the mucosal cells to free amino acids. Nitrogen balance studies suggest that the proportion of nitrogen lost in the feces, about 10 per cent of the ingested nitrogen, is similar in pregnant and nonpregnant women.[78]

The liver "retains" a substantial quantity of the absorbed amino acids. Studies carried out in dogs fed a meat diet have shown that much of the incoming amino acid is immediately degraded to urea and eventually excreted in the urine; a small proportion is retained as liver protein, another small proportion is secreted as plasma protein, and the rest, about 25 per cent, passes into the general circulation.[79] In humans, ingestion of 55 to 60 g of protein as eggnog resulted in a 20 per cent elevation in plasma α-amino nitrogen 4 hours after the meal. The branched-chain amino acids (valine, leucine, isoleucine) remained elevated for 8 hours, whereas alanine failed to rise and decreased below basal levels 5 to 8 hours after the meal. Similar changes in plasma branched-chain amino acids have been observed following milk intake.[80]

Studies in pregnant women receiving "mixed meals" during late gestation indicate elevations in the plasma concentration of serine and isoleucine following the meals.[81] Compared with the nonpregnant state, however, the peaks are of a lesser amplitude. The results suggest that branched-chain amino acids preferentially "escape" from the splanchnic bed after a meal whereas others, such as alanine, are mostly retained.

Kinetic studies on the fate of plasma amino acids during gestation are lacking both in humans and in animals. In nonpregnant subjects part of the free amino acid pool is incorporated into tissue protein. These amino acids return to the free amino acid pool after a variable length of time, depending on the catabolic rate of the specific tissue.[82] An exception to this is histidine, which, after being incorporated into muscle protein, is converted to 3-methylhistidine, a nonmetabolizable substance.[77] Another portion of the free amino acids is deaminated and the carbon skeleton is used as a metabolic fuel, that is, converted into CO_2 and H_2O, or used in the synthesis of fatty acids, glucose, or glycogen.

The daily flux of amino acids in the various compartments of the body has been estimated mostly in young male volunteers using a combination of techniques such as disappearance and interconversion rates of stable and radioactive isotopes and balance studies.[83-86]

As previously mentioned, approximately 95 per cent of the exogenous and endogenous protein present in the human intestine will be absorbed. Thus, a total of 130 to 160 g of amino acids will enter the splanchnic veins and after passing through the liver will be transported into the blood and join the free amino acid pool. For an average 70-kg man the quantity of amino acids present in the free pool has been estimated as 70 g, of which 60 g is nonessential amino acids and 10 g is essential.[77] The extremely rapid flux of the amino acids between various tissues and body compartments is reflected by the fact that approximately 300 g of protein, more than four times the size of the free amino acid pool, are synthesized daily by an average 70-kg man.

During the postprandial period, amino acids are actively incorporated into various tissues. Because of its large mass, skeletal muscle is the most important of these tissues. The incorporation of amino acids into muscle is maximal following a meal and is greatly influenced by insulin, as indicated by the decreased amino acid uptake of diabetic subjects.[87] Branched-chain amino acids account for 60 to 90 per cent of all the amino acids taken up by muscle during the absorptive phase.[87] Since this high proportion far exceeds the contribution of branched-chain amino acids to muscle protein synthesis, it has been proposed that the major fate of these amino acids is oxidation in muscle; thus, their amino groups would become available for alanine synthesis from pyruvate.[1]

Alanine and glutamine represent the two major "catabolic" amino acids of skeletal muscle. Except for a brief period following a meal, these two amino acids are being constantly released from muscle. In the postabsorptive state (after a 12- to 14-hour fast) output of alanine and glutamine accounts for over 50 per cent of all the α-amino nitrogen released from muscle.[88, 89] The released alanine is taken up mostly by the liver, where it is used as substrate for gluconeogenesis,[1] while glutamine is taken up largely by the kidney and gut, where it serves as a substrate for ammonia and alanine synthesis, respectively.[42] In the overnight fasted individual, alanine provides about 50 per cent of the glucose not derived from glycogenolysis.[1] Hence, in conditions in which glucose demands are increased, such as pregnancy, the availability of alanine would assume considerable importance. The plasma concentration of alanine is lower after an overnight fast in pregnancy than in the nonpregnant state. This change has been attributed to increased urinary excretion combined with increased fetal uptake,[7] implying an effective reduction in the circulating alanine pool. Nevertheless,

recalculation of the data suggests that the reduced plasma concentration of alanine is apparently caused by dilution of the circulating pool and not by reduced availability. Alanine concentration in plasma increases during gestation, although fasting levels remain below nonpregnant levels. When total circulating alanine is computed, the plasma alanine pool near term is approximately 1452 μmol, compared with 1070 μmol in nonpregnant subjects, or a 35 per cent expansion.

The plasma levels of various amino acids are moderately decreased during gestation.[90, 91] However, when total α-amino nitrogen[92] present in blood is calculated, values in late pregnancy are 144 mg, and in nonpregnant subjects, 113 mg. Therefore, the reduced concentration of plasma amino acids of pregnancy is solely a dilution phenomenon; the availability of free amino acids is increased rather than reduced.

The enlargement of the uterus, the expansion of the red cell mass, and the growth of the placenta and the fetus determine a greater need for body protein. Throughout the entire period of gestation the total amount of extra protein accumulated during pregnancy is 925 g, of which 382 g remains in the maternal body and 543 g is deposited in the conceptus. This represents an average extra need of protein of approximately 4.7 g/day during the last 28 weeks of gestation. The quantity seems very small in relation to the size of the free amino acid pool and one that can be easily met by the greater maternal food consumption. Even during its period of maximal daily growth the fetus would not require more than 7 to 8 g/day of amino acids.[9] Based on these considerations, it seems safe to predict that the pregnant mother does not undergo any drastic changes in protein turnover or, in general, that she does not suffer a net loss in body protein. However, the drastic hormonal changes of pregnancy may affect protein metabolism independently of fetal events. The constant hyperinsulinemia, the high levels of hCS, a hormone that has growth hormone–like properties, are compatible with a state of enhanced anabolism of the skeletal muscles, the greatest of the body's protein "reservoirs." On the other hand, the very high levels of free cortisol present in late gestation[93] would have the opposite effect. Glucocorticosteroids are powerful catabolic hormones for muscle protein. The net result of these interactions could be an increased rate of whole-body protein turnover.

Whole-body protein metabolism has not been studied yet in the pregnant woman. However, there is indirect evidence that the rate of protein catabolism is increased, as indicated by an increased urinary excretion of 3-methylhistidine (3-MH).[94, 95] In normal pregnant rats 3-MH increases shortly after conception and continues to increase linearly until delivery.[95] A similar pattern has been described in pregnant woman.[94] However, the late gestation rise in 3-MH excretion described in humans seems proportionally greater than in the rat. Since 3-MH cannot be reincorporated into protein, its rate of excretion has been used as a marker of protein catabolism.[96]

A decreased tubular reabsorption of 3-MH, as part of the general decrease in amino acid reabsorption of pregnancy, may contribute to the increased urinary excretion of this amino acid; nevertheless, the magnitude of the change suggests a real increase in protein catabolism. In a situation of net protein retention such as pregnancy, an indication of greater protein catabolism can reflect only an increased whole-body protein turnover.

Changes in plasma albumin concentration during pregnancy have been reported by several authors; these data have been recently reviewed.[97] In nonpregnant women serum albumin concentration ranges between 3.33 and 4.63 g/dl, with an average value of 4.12 g/dl. During gestation values decline until the 20th to 25th week and remain rather constant thereafter. At term mean albumin concentration is 2.95 g/dl, with values ranging from 2.38 to 3.33 g/dl. Using estimates of plasma volume reported in the literature, the intravascular albumin pool can be estimated to be approximately 112 g. This value agrees with available direct estimates.[98]

One of the consequences of the reduced albumin concentration is a proportional decrease in the colloid-osmotic pressure of the plasma, a factor that may contribute to the moderate expansion in interstitial fluid of late gestation.[99] It is significant that during late gestation, the ratio of intravascular to extravascular albumin is 1.08, while in nonpregnant subjects it is 0.85.[98] The shift in the distribution of albumin probably contributes to a decrease in the magnitude of water tension in the interstitial space. Studies using ^{131}I-labeled albumin indicate that albumin synthesis and catabolism remain constant at approximately 9 g/day during gestation.[98]

Plasma concentration of globulins increases during gestation.[97] The extent of the change varies from study to study, but, with few exceptions, most authors have confirmed this finding. When total circulating pools for the various globulin fractions are calculated it becomes apparent that all the globulin fractions nearly double their intravascular pool size during gestation. A greater number of the proteins present in these fractions are carrier proteins or binding proteins for a variety of nutrients, hormones and other substances. The specific changes of a few of these proteins have been studied in some detail, including ceruloplasmin,[100, 101] thyroxine binding globulin[102, 103] and transcortin.[104, 105] The increased production of these proteins is probably the result of estrogenic stimulation, since it can be reproduced in nonpregnant subjects by the administration of estrogens.[106, 107]

During pregnancy the excretion of urinary nitrogen remains unchanged and continues to be closely related to total nitrogen intake.[78, 108, 109] For this reason it has been used by some to assess the adequacy of maternal protein intake during pregnancy.

The net gain of body protein during pregnancy has been explored using nitrogen balance techniques. The results of these studies vary widely, although, in general, studies carried out during the last 15 years are in better agreement than earlier studies. The discrepancy probably reflects the limitations of the previous methods. In general, nitrogen balance studies tend to overestimate the input and to underestimate the losses. Most studies measure only fecal and urinary nitrogen excretion and estimate the rest of the losses of skin, hair, and various body secretions. A review of studies[110] in which protein intake was not considered a limiting variable provides 273 metabolic balances, most of which were obtained from women at or beyond the 30th week of gestation. Mean nitrogen retention in these studies was 1.37 ± 1.25 g/day. This figure would reflect a protein retention considerably higher than the theoretical estimates of 925 g (or 148 g of nitrogen). Since the quantity present in the conceptus has been measured directly, the extra protein would be retained in the maternal body. The concept of maternal protein retention has been dismissed as a methodological error.[12] In contrast to fat depots, the body does not have protein depots; hence the extra maternal protein should be distributed either as circulating protein or in the cytoplasm of the various tissues. However, cellular protein accumulation implies a proportional retention of body water. A protein deposition of the magnitude reported by the various balance studies (1500 to 2000 g) would require an extra water retention of several liters. The most recent nitrogen balance studies[78, 111] have found daily nitrogen more similar to the theoretical values.

METABOLIC CHANGES IN LACTATION AND THEIR NUTRITIONAL IMPLICATIONS

Lactation is a difficult period to study in the human mother, as is breast-feeding in the infant. Some difficulties are due in part to changes occurring during the different stages of lactation (colostrum production, milk production, introduction of supplementary food, and gradual weaning). Other difficulties relate to the variation in the quantity and composition of milk over time, during each feed, and from one woman to another. Problems also arise from the interference in the natural process of lactation caused by many measurement procedures. Furthermore, the individual infant, with its unique suckling pattern and growth demands, may also influence the lactation process. Although many studies have been reported, some variables cannot be measured in humans, or at times not with sufficient accuracy to yield unequivocal results, and others cannot be adequately controlled; therefore some basic data derived from animals must be considered despite the fact that their relevance for humans may be questioned.

Physiological changes that are important because they influence the nutritional demands of lactation include changes in body composition, hormone levels, enzyme activities, and substrate utilization. If lactation is to begin, one of the crucial changes that must occur in the maternal body is breast development. This process normally starts long before pregnancy but completes some of its stages only during pregnancy and lactation. Development and differentiation of the various mammary tissues make it possible for the breast to increase blood flow, obtain appropriate blood-borne nutrients, and synthesize and release milk in response to the hormonal changes accompanying parturition. Suckling itself serves to enhance these processes by affecting the secretion of prolactin and oxytocin, the hormones most directly controlling milk production and ejection.

Intestinal hypertrophy is also likely to occur during pregnancy, and possibly even more during lactation, at least if observations in animals apply to humans. It must be recognized, however, that the extreme hypertrophy of the intestine noted in small, lactating mammals may not be necessary in the human. Rats increase their food intake by about 60 per cent during lactation, whereas humans may need to increase intake by only 15 to 20 per cent or less. We do not have the requisite data to permit a definitive conclusion regarding changes in the viscera in lactating humans. Nevertheless, function may be altered even without hypertrophy. In the lactating cow, for example, blood flow through the portal vein and hepatic artery are 56 per cent higher than in nonlactating cows. This flow change may aid in the observed increase in hepatic uptake of the bovine gluconeogenic precursors propionate and lactate.

Probably the maternal biological change most widely believed to be related to lactation is maternal storage of body fat during gestation. It is thought that the nonobese woman will store 3 to 4 kg of fat during pregnancy if permitted to eat to appetite.[12] Most of the fat is stored during the first three fourths of gestation,[112] but women with low weight gains early in pregnancy[112] or marginally nourished women offered food supplements late in pregnancy can store additional fat in the last quarter. Similar observations have been made in rats, where body composition may be measured directly.[113]

By the time parturition occurs, the mother is probably prepared to consume and absorb more nutrients, extract them for milk synthesis, and rely to some extent on fat stores to buffer intermeal intervals. Parturition induces changes to create the essential hormonal milieu to complete these adjustments. The orchestration of these changes is a complex process, not yet fully understood. For example, although many hormones have been shown to play some role in breast preparation and milk production, a complete discussion of hormonal controls is not yet possible. It is widely recognized that oxytocin is crucial to lactation, acting on the myoepithelial cells of the breast to induce contraction. This action causes "let down," the movement of milk from the acini into the milk ducts, where it is accessible to the suckling infant. Although important for successful lactation, oxytocin has not been ascribed any direct influence on maternal metabolic and nutritional changes.

From a nutritional viewpoint, other hormones are of major interest. To understand their role it is necessary to recognize that several synthetic processes are occurring in the lactating breast. Casein, fat, and lactose production are quantitatively the most important. Although some fat is derived from fat or fatty acids taken up from blood,[114] a very large amount is synthesized de novo from glucose, lactate, and pyruvate, at least in the rat.[114] Only about 10 per cent of the glucose taken up by the mammary gland is completely oxidized.[115]

Since glucose is so central to the functioning of the mammary gland, being used as a major substrate for both fat and lactose synthesis, it is not surprising that this gland has been shown to be insulin-sensitive in the rat.[115] Insulin probably acts by enhancing glucose transport as well as by influencing regulatory enzymes that facilitate lipogenesis. Nevertheless, in the rat, lactose synthesis itself does not seem to be regulated by insulin.[115, 116]

Prolactin deficiency also decreases lipogenesis, and isolated acini from prolactin-deficient lactating rats show a reduction in glucose utilization, possibly owing to inactivation of pyruvate dehydrogenase.[115] Glucose uptake, however, does not seem to be affected. Casein synthesis, on the other hand, has been reported to be reduced by 40 per cent when a 24-hour prolactin deficiency was induced by bromocryptine.[114] Aside from these small metabolic effects, which are less dramatic than those of insulin, prolactin has an important role in the development and differentiation of the gland preparatory to milk production. In this capacity it is also essential for the maintenance of lactation. Prolactin plays an important indirect role as well, since it is necessary for the maintenance of insulin receptor number in the gland.[117] Beyond this, little information is available for defining the direct effects of prolactin on mammary metabolism.

Nevertheless, prolactin plays a major role in controlling substrate flow from other tissues. In the presence of prolactin, lipogenesis is depressed in both adipose tissue and liver. Decreased activity in these tissues spares both glucose and lactate for uptake by the mammary gland, whose uptake is increased during lactation.

Fat synthesis in adipose tissue is reduced during lactation, even in rats fed a low-fat diet,[118] and adipocyte uptake of fat is also depressed. These changes are partly a result of decreased activity of adipose tissue lipoprotein lipase; thus, circulating triglycerides as well as glucose can be preferentially used by the mammary gland. While these changes permit a reduction of the use of glucose and fat by adipose tissue, reciprocal changes in enzyme concentration enhance their use by the mammary gland during lactation. The activities of lipogenic enzymes, including fatty acid synthase, glucose-6-phosphate dehydrogenase, and "malic" enzyme, increase in the rat gland during the first 10 days of lactation.[119] The activity of lipoprotein lipase also rises. These changes would aid in glucose and fat use by the mammary gland. Since both lipogenesis and fat uptake are concurrently depressed in adipose tissue, fat stores may be gradually reduced while milk production is maintained. Although other hormonal changes may be responsible for the initiation of these changes in lipoprotein lipase activity, prolactin is important for maintaining the established pattern. In sheep, in which acetate utilization by the udder is substantial, extraction of acetate by muscle is depressed during lactation.[120]

The information discussed so far presents a picture describing lactation in well-nourished animals. During pregnancy the body is prepared for lactation by fat storage and mammary gland development. At parturition and later, with suckling, hormonal changes stimulate transfer of glucose and fat into the mammary gland and depress utilization by the liver and adipose tissue. This picture suggests that fat stored during pregnancy may function to spare substrates (particularly glucose) obtained at meals. That is, maternal tissues capable of using fat between meals will have an adequate supply and will not need to use glucose or its precursors to a great extent. Lower levels of insulin and glucose, which have been observed during lactation by some workers[36] but not by others,[121] would also help to reduce utilization by other tissues, if mammary tissues operate effectively at lower insulin and glucose levels.

The controls may be more complex than this, however. It appears that during pregnancy high insulin levels do not down-regulate adipose tissue receptors for insulin, possibly because of the rising progesterone levels, which probably act with estrogens to simultaneously block the effect of placental lactogen on the breast.[122] At parturition, adipose tissue insulin receptors decline as progesterone declines, and at the same time the mammary gland becomes more responsive to the effects of prolactin.[117] Prolactin then acts to decrease lipoprotein lipase activity in adipose tissue while raising its activity in the mammary gland.[123]

It is often assumed that these adaptations will maintain milk production even if maternal food intake is reduced, just as they may act to support metabolism between meals. Several lines of evidence in animals and humans indicate that this is not so.

When the intermeal fasting interval is prolonged beyond normal, other changes supervene and the mammary gland is no longer so strongly favored metabolically. For example, when lactating goats are starved for 48 hours, milk production decreases 70 per cent.[124] Although plasma glucose is not decreased by this fast, glucose infusion increases plasma glucose more in starved than in fed goats and increases milk production only in the infused starved goats.[125]

In the lactating cow, fasting reduces hepatic blood flow and the hepatic uptake of gluconeogenic substrates. Milk output, which is linearly related to hepatic glucose output, also declines in fasted cows.[126] In rats, 50 per cent food restriction during lactation reduces pup growth, whereas if the restriction occurs during pregnancy (preventing an increase in body fat) but the rats are fed ad libitum during lactation, pup growth is normal.[127] In rats that are food-restricted only 25 per cent for days 4 to 14 of lactation, total milk yield on day 14 is reduced nearly 50 per cent and pup weight is only 80 per cent of the weight of controls.[128] In fact, even in obese rats, if food intake is reduced during lactation, pup growth (and presumably milk quantity and/or quality) is depressed.[129] If intake is raised above normal during lactation by feeding a highly palatable diet, pup growth is enhanced.[129]

The quality of maternal dietary protein can also affect pup growth in the rat. On day 15 of lactation pups of dams fed wheat gluten as the protein weighed only 19 g, whereas dams pair-fed a casein diet had pups weighing 27 g. This effect on pup growth occurred even though dam weight was not different in the two diet groups.[130] Preliminary studies indicate that casein synthesis, though not very sensitive to a 6-hour fast in the rat, is decreased by 80 per cent after 24-hour starvation.[114]

The effect of malnutrition on the mammary gland of the lactating rat has been studied directly. When rats are restricted to 75 per cent of ad libitum intake, synthesis of lactose by the mammary gland decreases. This effect appears to be independent of insulin concentration.[116] Starvation also decreases glucose removal by the mammary gland and more of the extracted glucose is released as lactate.[131] In the mouse, fasting for one day early in lactation also decreases total DNA in the mammary gland (an indication that cell number has not increased normally). Nevertheless, subsequent milk production becomes normal.[132]

Despite the value of these animal studies for clarifying the complex interrelations among various hormonal controls and substrate utilization, their use for studying the consequences of human undernutrition is limited. The calorie demand of lactation in humans is proportionally less than in small mammals. Furthermore, an in vitro study indicates that thermogenesis of brown adipose tissue is suppressed during lactation in mice. A rough estimate indicated that as much as 40 per cent of the maintenance energy requirement of the nonlactating mouse might be conserved in this way.[133] This adaptation may be essential in the small rodent, since lactation demands may raise food intake to maximal levels. In addition, lactating rats may have an increase in basal energy requirement partly caused by an increased relative weight of the vital organs, which have a high expenditure per unit mass[134] and undergo marked hypertrophy. In humans such an adjustment in brown adipose tissue metabolism may not normally be needed for lactation, since lactation demands are lower and the vital organs may not grow very much. Such an adjustment could permit normal or nearly normal lactation, however, when food intake is reduced.

Whether in fact such an adaptation to low intake levels occurs in humans is speculative. The data regarding the effect of malnutrition during lactation on maternal calorie stores and on infant growth are not as easily interpreted, nor as consistent, as the animal data. Many studies suggest that undernourished women produce less milk[135, 136] but very large differences in maternal calorie intake result in relatively small differences in milk output. There is disagreement as to whether milk quality is impaired, since some studies find significant changes in composition[135] but many others do not.[136] It is likely that details of the mother's diet and prior nutritional status determine how well she can maintain milk quality and quantity on low intake. Moreover, reduced energy output has been observed in lactating mothers compared with mothers who were not lactating. This form of conservation may not be available to all women, but may be important to some.

It cannot, however, be assumed that lactation can be maintained by increased use of maternal tissues even when intake is inadequate, because low intake is not associated with excessive weight loss. Weight loss occurs slowly during lactation in many well-nourished women,[137] but they have presumably stored fat during pregnancy. Among chronically undernourished women, lactational weight changes are small and some reports indicate that weight and skinfold may increase during lactation in previously undernourished women, even while milk output is suboptimal.

A study of supplementation during lactation indicated, on the other hand, that effects on maternal weight and on milk volume and composition were small, much less than expected on the basis of the calorie increment. Health and work capacity were apparently improved.[138, 139] These findings may suggest that after delivery the capacity of the breast of malnourished women to increase output is limited as a result of inadequate development during pregnancy. In rats, mammary development is reduced by food restriction during pregnancy.[132] Alternatively, the lack of a marked effect of supplementation may indicate that during undernutrition in lactating women energy is conserved either by reduction in energy-demanding activities or perhaps by adaptations in brown adipose tissue similar to those observed in normally fed, lactating mice. We cannot yet completely describe the energy partitioning or calorie needs of lactating women because of these unresolved issues.

Despite these considerations regarding milk output and composition and maternal energy requirements, we can securely state that maternal nutrition affects infant growth. In general the reported data are confusing because undernourished women tend to have smaller newborns with smaller maintenance energy needs. Therefore, initially even low milk output may suffice to maintain the growth of their smaller infants.[135] This may not be true for dieting women feeding large babies. In addition, since lethargy and reduced activity are frequent adaptations to undernutrition, the newborn may be able to participate in conserving the energy resources of the maternal-infant dyad by reducing random activity and by sleeping more. Whether this occurs, or is innocuous for infant development, has not been examined.

It is clear, however, that undernourished women cannot supply adequate milk after a few months and infant growth falters sufficiently to be statistically detected by 3 or 4 months.[135] In contrast, well-nourished mothers appear to be able to provide for normal infant growth for at least 9 months and perhaps for a year.[140] Studies of well-nourished women breast-feeding twins indicate that milk yield can be maintained at double the value observed in women nursing one infant.[140]

How milk output and maternal calorie intake are related is clearly complex. Even in well-nourished groups, women who have lower intakes generally have lower milk output.[137, 141] Some authors indicate that reduced intake causes lactation failure[137] or accelerates the need for infant supplementation; others conclude that supplementation of the infant begins first, and output falls because infant demand is decreased. No doubt both patterns are followed to some extent.

An important conclusion to be drawn from the array of available data is that lactation is not a time to crash diet to reduce obesity existing from before pregnancy. There are several reasons why this is contraindicated. In the United States dieting often means reduction of carbohydrate intake. Carbohydrate is important for maintaining insulin secretion and lactose synthesis, even if blood glucose is not altered. Lactose probably also is necessary for maintaining milk volume.[142] Development of ketoacidosis and dehydration has been reported in a woman consuming a high-protein, carbohydrate-free reducing diet for one week during her 13th week of lactation.[143] Blood glucose was high; insulin and saline infusions were used to normalize hydration and blood glucose. Whether small amounts of carbohydrate would have eliminated this problem is not known.

Although most research, and our discussion so far, have focused on the effect of maternal nutrition on caloric conditioning, stringent dieting is also likely to result in inadequate intake of other nutrients. Since calcium needs peak during lactation, several studies have examined lactational calcium homeostasis. Women consuming over 1 g/day of calcium have been reported to maintain serum calcium in late lactation, after an initial decrease.[144] Nevertheless, women who have lactated have been reported to have lower bone density which, however, rises with age and exceeds that of nonlactators after menopause.[145] Other workers[146] also observed lower values for bone mineral content in postpartum women over 19 years of age, compared with those under 19. As lactation proceeded, bone demineralization occurred in the younger group concomitant with a lower calcium intake and, presumably, a higher calcium requirement than in the older group. No such demineralization was observed in the over 19 group, which maintained a calcium intake of 1 g/day.[146] It is doubtful that adequate intake of calcium and vitamin D could be maintained if a lactating woman tried to lose weight rapidly. Furthermore, relationships among calcium, magnesium, and phosphorus are unlikely to be optimized by calcium supplements. Reducing diets may also be deficient in other essential nutrients. For example, zinc deficits (unrelated to dietary protein level) have been documented in some low-calorie diets.[147]

The supply of other nutrients may also be compromised if a lactating woman diets. In a study of women of low socioeconomic level, intakes of vitamin B_6 and folate were well below the RDA for lactation. Supplementation increased the milk concentration of these two vitamins. Milk concentration of vitamin B_{12} was also increased by supplementation, although intake was above the RDA levels even without supplementation. Supplementation with ascorbic acid, which raised an already adequate intake, did not affect milk ascorbate.[148] In an African study, however, where ascorbate intake was initially low (34 mg/day), supplementation (103 mg/day) significantly raised milk content, though milk levels approached a plateau at higher intakes.[149] In addition, maternal nutrition may affect the immunologic characteristics of milk. Reduced cell counts (lymphocytes and macrophages) have been observed in milk of undernourished women.[150]

The significance of lower levels of vitamins in breast milk is not clear. We would expect that the protective functions of these substances might be impaired in infants breast-fed by women with marginal vitamin or mineral status, but data are lacking. There have been individual case reports of deficiency diseases of infants, for example, hypocalcemia,[151] thiamine deficiency,[152] and vitamin B_{12} deficiency.[153] Whether these deficits are determined by the mother's deficit during gestation, or whether they can be precipitated from inadequate lactational food patterns alone, is not known.

The conclusion to be drawn from the information discussed above is that too little is known for us to be careless about our dietary recommendations for lactation. Although there may well be adaptations that permit lactation even on low intakes, evidence suggests that the infant will also be deprived if the mother's daily intake is too low. The significance for the child remains even less explored than the significance for the mother. Nevertheless, growth failure, decreased disease resistance, and vitamin and mineral deficiencies are possibilities that are suggested in the literature. Therefore, even more than at other times of life, lactation is a period when good nutrition should be ensured.

References

1. Felig P. The glucose-alanine cycle. Metabolism 1973; 22:179–207.
2. Marliss EB, Aoki TT, Cahill GF Jr. Glucagon levels and metabolic effects in fasting man. J Clin Invest 1970; 49:2256–2270.
3. Lind T, Billewicz WC, Brown G. A serial study of changes occurring in oral glucose tolerance test in pregnancy. J Obstet Gyneacol Br Commonw 1973; 80:1033–1039.
4. Fischer PM, Hamilton PM, Sutherland HW, et al. The effect of gestation on intravenous glucose tolerance in women. J Obstet Gynaecol Br Commonw 1974; 81:285–290
5. Victor A. Normal blood sugar variation during pregnancy. Acta Obstet Gynecol Scand 1974; 53:37–40.
6. Spellacy WN. Maternal and fetal metabolic interrelationships. In Sutherland HW, Stowers JM (eds). Carbohydrate Metabolism in Pregnancy and the Newborn. Edinburgh, Churchill Livingstone, 1975: 42.
7. Adam PAJ, Felig P. Carbohydrate, fat and amino acid metabolism in the pregnant woman and fetus. In Flakner F, Tanner JM (eds). Human Growth. Vol. I. Principles and Prenatal Growth. New York, Plenum Press, 1978: 461.
8. Kalkhoff RK, Kissebah A, Kim HJ. Carbohydrate and lipid metabolism during normal pregnancy: relationship to gestational hormone action. In Merkats I, Adam PAJ (eds). The Diabetic Pregnancy. New York, Grune and Stratton, 1979: 3.
9. Rosso P, Lederman SA. Nutrition and fetal growth. In Milunsky A, Friedman EA, Gluck L (eds). Advances in Perinatal Medicine. Vol. I. New York, Plenum Medical Books, 1985: 1–61.
10. Page EW. Human fetal nutrition and growth. Am J Obstet Gynecol 1969; 104:378–387.
11. Hytten FE. Placental handling of glucose. In Sutherland CW, Stowers JM (eds). Carbohydrate Metabolism in Pregnancy and the Newborn. Berlin, Springer-Verlag, 1979: 76.
12. Hytten FE, Leitch I. The Physiology of Human Pregnancy. Oxford, Blackwell Scientific Publications, 1971.
13. Kalham SC, D'Angelo LJ, Savin SS, et al. Glucose production in pregnant women at term gestation. Source of glucose for human fetus. J Clin Invest 1979; 63:388–394.
14. Kuhl C. Glucose metabolism during and after pregnancy in normal and gestational diabetic women. I. Influence of normal pregnancy on serum glucose and insulin concentration during basal fasting conditions and after a challenge with glucose. Acta Endocrinol 1975; 75:709–719.
15. Sutherland HW, Fisher PM, Stowers JM. Evaluation of maternal carbohydrate metabolism by the intravenous glucose tolerance test in early diabetes in early life. In Camerini-Davalos RA, Cole HS (eds). New York, Academic Press, 1975.

16. Plass ED, Oberst FW. Respiration and pulmonary ventilation in normal, non-pregnant, pregnant and puerperal women, with interpretation of acid-base balance during normal pregnancy. Am J Obstet Gynecol 1938; 35:441–452.

17. Beck P, Daughaday WH. Human placental lactogen: studies of its acute metabolic effects and disposition in normal man. J Clin Invest 1967; 46:103–111.

18. Spellacy WN, Buhi WC, Birk SA. Carbohydrate metabolism in women with a twin pregnancy. Obstet Gynecol 1980; 55:688–691.

19. Daniel RR, Metzger BE, Freinkel N, et al. Carbohydrate metabolism in pregnancy. XI. Response of plasma glucagon to overnight fast and oral glucose during normal pregnancy and in gestational diabetes. Diabetes 1974; 23:771-776.

20. Kuhl C, Holst JJ. Plasma glucagon and insulin: glucagon ratio in gestational diabetes. Diabetes 1976; 25:16–23.

21. Tourneire J. Diminution de la tolerance glucidique et hyperinsulinisme dans l'adenoma a prolactine. Nouv Pr Med 1974; 3:1705–1707.

22. Landgraf R. Prolactin: a diabetogenic hormone. Diabetologia 1977; 13:99–104.

23. Spellacy WN, Goetz FC, Greenberg BZ. Plasma insulin in normal "early" pregnancy. Obstet Gynecol 1965; 25:862–865.

24. Tyson JE, Rabinowitz D, Merimee TJ. Response of plasma insulin and human growth hormone to arginine in pregnancy and postpartum females. Am J Obstet Gynecol 1969; 103:313–319.

25. Felig P, Lynch V. Starvation in human pregnancy: hypoglycemia, hypoinsulinemia and hyperketonemia. Science 1970; 170:990–992.

26. Costrini NV, Kalkhoff RK. Relative effects of pregnancy, estradiol and progesterone on plasma insulin and pancreatic islet insulin secretion. J Clin Invest 1971; 50:992–999.

27. Beck P. Progestin enhancement of the plasma insulin response to glucose in rhesus monkeys. Diabetes 1969; 18:146–152.

28. Freinkel N, Goodner CJ. Carbohydrate metabolism in pregnancy. I. The metabolism of insulin by human placental tissue. J Clin Invest 1960; 39:116–131.

29. Posner BI. Insulin metabolizing enzymes activities in human placental tissue. Diabetes 1973; 22:552–563.

30. Marshall RN, Underwood LE, Voina SJ, et al. Characterization of the insulin and somatomedin-C receptors in human placenta cell membranes. J Clin Endocr Metab 1974; 39:283–292.

31. Posner, BI. Insulin receptor in human and animal placental tissue. Diabetes 1974; 23:209–217.

32. Bellmann O, Hartmann E. Influence of pregnancy on the kinetics of insulin. Am J Obstet Gynecol 1975; 122:829–833.

33. Lind T, Bell S, Gilmore E, et al. Insulin disappearance rate in pregnant and non-pregnant women, and in non-pregnant women given GHRIH. Eur J Clin Invest 1977; 7:47–51.

34. Beck-Nielsen H, Kuhl C, Pedersen O, et al. Decreased insulin binding to monocytes from normal pregnant women. J Clin Endocrinol Metab 1979; 49:810–814.

35. Pagano G, Cassader M, Massobrio M, et al. Insulin binding to human adipocytes during late pregnancy in healthy, obese and diabetic state. Horm Metab Res 1980; 12:177–181.

36. Flint DJ, Sinnett-Smith PA, Clegg RA, et al. Role of insulin receptors in the changing metabolism of adipose tissue during pregnancy and lactation in the rat. Biochem J 1979; 182:421–427.

37. Flint DJ. Changes in the number of insulin receptors of isolated rat hepatocytes during pregnancy and lactation. Biochim Biophys Acta 1980; 628:322–327.

38. Silverstone FA, Solomon E, Rubricius J. The rapid intravenous glucose tolerance test in pregnancy. J Clin Invest 1961; 40:2180–2189.

39. Burt RL. Peripheral utilization of glucose in pregnancy and the puerperium. Obstet Gynecol 1954; 4:58.

40. Sekiba D, Takeda Y, Kudo T, et al. A study of carbohydrate metabolism in pregnancy. A glucose turnover following one shot intravenous injection. Acta Obstet Gynaecol Jpn 1976; 23:195–200.

41. Herrera E, Knopp RH, Freinkel N. Carbohydrate metabolism in pregnancy, VI. Plasma fuels, insulin, liver composition, gluconeogenesis and nitrogen metabolism in the fed and fasted rat. J Clin Invest 1969; 48:2260–2272.

42. Felig P, Wahrer J, Handler R. Influence of oral glucose ingestion on splanchnic glucose and gluconeogenic substrate metabolism in man. Diabetes 1975; 24:468–475.

43. Cousins L, Rigg L, Hollingsworth D, et al. The 24-hr excursion and diurnal rhythm of glucose, insulin and C-peptide in normal pregnancy. Am J Obstet Gynecol 1980; 136:483–488.

44. Lewis SB, Wallin JD, Kuzuya H, et al. Circadian variation of serum glucose, C-peptide immunoreactivity and free insulin normal and insulin-treated diabetic subjects. Diabetologia 1976; 12:343–350.

45. Phelps RL, Metzger BE, Freinkel N. Carbohydrate metabolism in pregnancy. XVII. Diurnal profiles of plasma glucose, insulin, free fatty acids, triglycerides, cholesterol and individual amino acids in normal pregnancy. Am J Obstet Gynecol 1981; 140:730–736.

46. Biezenski JJ. Maternal lipid metabolism. Obstet Gynecol Ann 1974; 3:203–233.

47. Kalkhoff RK, Kissebah AH, Kim H. Carbohydrate and lipid metabolism during normal pregnancy: relationship to gestational hormone action. Semin Perinatol 1978; 2:291–307.

48. Knopp RH, Warth MR, Carroll CJ. Lipid metabolism in pregnancy. I. Changes in lipoprotein triglyceride and cholesterol in normal pregnancy and the effects of diabetes mellitus. J Reprod Med 1973; 10:95–101.

49. Darmody JM, Postle AD. Lipid metabolism in pregnancy. Br J Obstet Gynaecol 1982; 89:211–215.

50. Warth MR, Arky RA, Knopp RH. Lipid metabolism in pregnancy. III. Altered lipid composition in intermediate, very low, low and high density lipoprotein fractions. J Clin Endocr Metab 1975; 41:649–655.

51. Hillman L, Schonfeld G, Miller JP, et al. Apolipoproteins in human pregnancy. Metabolism 1975; 24:943–952.

52. Barter PJ, Nestel PJ. Plasma free fatty acid transport during prolonged glucose consumption and its relationship to plasma triglyceride fatty acids in man. J Lip Res 1972; 13:483–491.

53. Barter PJ, Nestel PJ, Carroll KF. Precursors of plasma triglyceride fatty acid in humans. Effect of glucose consumption, clofibrate administration and alcoholic fatty liver. Metabolism 1972; 21:117–124.

54. De Alvarez RR, Goodwell BW, Zighelboim I. Fatty acid composition of serum lipids in pregnancy and gynecologic cancer. Am J Obstet Gynecol 1967; 97:419–442.

55. Hummel L, Zimmerman T, Schenk H, et al. Studies on the hypertriglyceridemia in the pregnant rat. Acta Biol Med Ger 1978; 37:259–266.

56. Humphrey JL, Tobert-Childs M, Monter A, et al. Lipid metabolism in pregnancy. VII. Kinetics of chylomicron triglyceride removal in fed pregnant rats. Am J Physiol 1980; 239:E81–87.

57. Otway S, Robinson DS. The significance of changes in tissue clearing-factor lipase activity in relation to the lipemia of pregnancy. Biochem J 1968; 106:677–682.

58. Hamosh M, Clary TR, Chernick SS. Lipoprotein lipase activity of adipose tissue and mammary tissue and plasma triglyceride in pregnancy and lactating rats. Biochim Biophys Acta 1970; 210:473–482.

59. Knopp RH, Boroush MA, O'Sullivan JB. Lipid metabolism in pregnancy. II. Postheparin lipocytic activity and hypertriglyceridemia in the pregnant rat. Metabolism 1975; 24:481–493.

60. Glueck CH, Fallat RW, Scheel D. Effects of estrogenic compounds on triglyceride kinetics. Metabolism 1975; 24:537–545.

61. Kim HJ, Kalkhoff RK. Sex steroid influence on triglyceride metabolism. J Clin Invest 1975; 56:888–896.

62. Afolabi S, Tulloch B, Kissebah AH. Mechanism of estrogen-induced hypertriglyceridemia: a role of adrenal cortex. Clin Endocrinol (Oxf) 1976; 5(3):203–208.

63. Hamosh M, Hamosh P. The effect of estrogen on the lipoprotein lipase activity of rat adipose tissue. J Clin Invest 1975; *55*:1132–1135.

64. Kissebah AH, Harrigan P, Wynn V. Mechanisms of hypertriglyceridemia associated with contraceptive steroids. Horm Metab Res 1973; *5*:184–192.

65. Spooner PM, Garrison M, Scow RO. Regulation of mammary and adipose tissue lipoprotein lipase and blood triglyceride in rats during late pregnancy. Effect of prostaglandins. J Clin Invest 1977; *60*:702–708.

66. Zinder O, Hamosh M, Fleck TR, et al. Effects of prolactin on lipoprotein lipase in mammary gland and adipose tissue of rats. Am J Physiol 1974; *226*:744–748.

67. Lahbsetwar AP, Watson DJ. Temporal relationship between secretory patterns of gonadotropins, estrogens, progestins and prostaglandin F in preparturient rats. Biol Reprod 1974; *10*:103–110.

68. McDonald-Gibson RG, Young M, Hytten FE. Changes in plasma non esterified fatty acids and serum glycerol in pregnancy. Br J Obstet Gynaecol 1975; *82*:460–466.

69. Elliott JA. The effect of pregnancy on the control of lipolysis in fat cells isolated from adipose tissue. Eur J Clin Invest 1975; *5*:159–163.

70. Knopp RH, Herrera E, Freinkel N. Carbohydrate metabolism in pregnancy from fed and fasted pregnant rats during late gestation. J Clin Invest 1970; *49*:1438–1446.

71. Williams C, Coltart TM. Adipose tissue metabolism in pregnancy: the lipolytic effect of human placental lactogen. Br J Obstet Gynaecol 1978; *85*:43–46.

72. Coltart TM, Williams C. Effect of insulin on adipose tissue lipolysis in human pregnancy. Br J Obstet Gynaecol 1976; *83*:241–244.

73. Svanborg A, Vikrot O. Plasma lipid fractions, including individual phospholipids at various stages of pregnancy. Acta Med Scand 1975; *178*:615–630.

74. Subbiah MT, Buscaglia MD. Studies concerning the hypercholesterolemia of pregnancy: cholesterol metabolism and excretion during late pregnancy in the rat. Res Comm Chem Pathol Pharmacol 1976; *13*:529–539.

75. Potter J, Nestel PJ. Cholesterol balance during pregnancy. Clin Chim Acta 1978; *87*:57–61.

76. Li JR, Bale LK, Subbiah MTR. Bile acids and cholesterol excretion in the pregnant guinea pig: studies on the hypercholesterolemia of pregnancy. Steroids 1978; *31*:799–807.

77. Munro HN, Grim MC. The proteins and amino acids. *In* Goodhart RS, Shils M (eds). Modern Nutrition in Health and Disease. 6th ed. Philadelphia, Lea & Febiger, 1980: 51.

78. Johnstone FD, McGillivray I, Dennis KJ. Nitrogen retention in pregnancy. J Obstet Gynaecol Brit Comm 1972; *79*:777–781.

79. Elwyn D. The role of the liver in regulation of amino acid and protein metabolism. *In* Munro HN (ed). Mammalian Protein Metabolism. Vol. 4. New York, Academic Press, 1970: 523.

80. Armstrong MD, Stave U. A study of plasma free amino acid levels. I. Study of factors affecting validity of amino acid analyses. Metabolism 1973; *22*:549–560.

81. Freinkel N, Phelps RL, Metzger BE. Intermediary metabolism during pregnancy. *In* Sutherland HW, Stowers JM (eds). Carbohydrate Metabolism in Pregnancy and the Newborn. Berlin, Springer-Verlag, 1979: 1.

82. Felig P. Amino acid metabolism in man. Ann Rev Biochem 1975; *44*:933–955.

83. Fern EB, Garlick PJ, McNurlan MA, et al. The excretion of isotope in urea and ammonia for estimating protein turnover in man with (^{15}N) glycine. Clin Sci 1981; *61*:217–228.

84. Bier DM, Christopherson HL. Rapid micromethod for determination of ^{15}N enrichment in plasma lysine: application to measurement of whole body protein turnover. Analyt Biochem 1979; *94*:242–248.

85. Waterlow JC, Golden MHN, Garlick PJ. Protein turnover in man measured with ^{15}N: comparison of end products and dose regimens. Am J Physiol 1978; *235*:E165–E174.

86. Steffee WP, Goldsmith RS, Pencharz PB, et al. Dietary protein intake and dynamic aspects of whole body nitrogen metabolism in adult humans. Metabolism 1976; *25*:281–297.

87. Wahren J, Felig P, Hagenfeldt L. Effect of protein ingestion on splanchnic and leg metabolism in normal man and patients with diabetes mellitus. J Clin Invest 1976; *57*:987–999.

88. Felig P, Pozefsky T, Marliss E, et al. Alanine: key role in gluconeogenesis. Science 1970; *167*:1003–1004.

89. Marliss EB, Aoki TT, Pozefsky T, et al. Muscle and splanchnic glutamine and glutamate metabolism in postabsorptive and starved man. J Clin Invest 1971; *50*:814–817.

90. Hytten FE, Cheyne GA. The aminoaciduria of pregnancy. J Obstet Gynaecol Brit Comm 1972; *79*:424–432.

91. Schoengold DM, de Fiore RH, Parlett RC. Free amino acids in plasma throughout pregnancy. Am J Obstet Gynecol 1978; *131*:490–499.

92. MacDonald HN, Good W. Changes in plasma total proteins, albumin, urea and alpha-amino nitrogen concentrations in pregnancy and the puerperium. J Obstet Gynaecol Brit Commonw 1971; *78*:912–917.

93. Rosenthal HE, Slaunwhite WR Jr, Sandberg AA. Transcortin: a corticosteroid-binding protein of plasma. X. Cortisol and progesterone interplay and unbound levels of these steroids in pregnancy. J Clin Endocrinol Metab 1969; *29*:352–367.

94. Naismith DJ. Personal communication.

95. Rosso P, Kava R. Effects of food restriction on cardiac output and blood flow to the uterus and placenta in the pregnant rat. J Nutr 1980; *110*:2350–2354.

96. Young VR, Alexis SD, Baliga BS, et al. Metabolism of administered 3-methylhistidine: Lack of muscle transfer ribonucleic acid charging and quantitative excretion as 3-methylhistidine and its N-acetyl derivative. J Biol Chem 1972; *247*:3592–3600.

97. Joseph JC, Baker C, Sprang ML, et al. Changes in plasma protein during pregnancy. Ann Clin Lab Sci 1978; *8*:130–142.

98. Honger PW. Albumin metabolism in normal pregnancy. Scand J Clin Lab Invest 1968; *21*:3–9.

99. Robertson EG. Oedema in normal pregnancy. J Reprod Fert 1969; *9*(Suppl):27–36.

100. De Jorge FB, Delascio D, Antunes ML. Copper and copper oxidase concentrations in the blood serum of normal pregnant women. Obstet Gynecol 1965; *26*:225–227.

101. Markowitz H, Gubler CJ, Mahoney JP, et al. Studies on copper metabolism. XIV. Copper, ceruloplasmin and oxidase activity in sera of normal human subjects, pregnant women, and patients with infection, hepatolenticular degeneration and the nephrotic syndrome. J Clin Invest 1955; *34*:1498–1508.

102. Oppenheimer JH, Squef R, Surks MI, et al. Binding of thyroxine by serum proteins evaluated by equilibrium dialysis and electrophoretic techniques. Alterations in nonthyroidal illness. J Clin Invest 1963; *42*:1769–1782.

103. Robin NI, Refetoff S, Fang V, et al. Parameters of thyroid function in material and cord serum at term pregnancy. J Clin Endocrinol Metab 1969; *29*:1276–1280.

104. Doe RP, Fernandez R, Seal US. Measurement of corticosteroid binding globulin in man. J Clin Endocrinol Metab 1964; *24*:1029–1039.

105. De Moor P, Heyns W. Cortisol binding affinity of plasma transcortin (CBA) as studied by competitive absorption. J Clin Endocrinol Metab 1968; *28*:1281–1286.

106. Mills IH, Schedl HP, Chen PS Jr, et al. The effect of estrogen administration on the metabolism and protein binding of hydrocortisone. J Clin Endocrinol Metab 1960; *20*:515–528.

107. Finucane JF, Griffiths RS, Black EG. Altered patterns of thyroid hormones in serum and urine in pregnancy and during oral contraceptive therapy. Br J Obstet Gynaecol 1976; *83*:733–737.

108. Beydoun S, Cuenca VG, Evans LP, et al. Maternal nutrition. I. The urinary urea nitrogen/total nitrogen ratio as an index of protein nutrition. Am J Obstet Gynecol 1972; *114*:198.

109. Zlatnik FJ. Urinary nitrogen excretion as related to dietary protein in pregnant women. J Reprod Med 1979; *22*:128–132.

110. Calloway DH. Nitrogen balance during pregnancy. *In* Winick M (ed). Nutrition and Fetal Development. New York, John Wiley & Sons, 1974: 79–94.

111. Zuspan FP, Goodrich S. Metabolic studies in normal pregnancy. I. Nitrogen metabolism. Am J Obstet Gynecol 1968; *100*:7–14.

112. Pipe NGJ, Smith T, Halliday D, et al. Changes in fat, fat-free mass and body water in human normal pregnancy. Br J Obstet Gynaecol 1979; *86*:929–940.

113. Lederman SA, Rosso P. Effects of protein and carbohydrate supplements on fetal and maternal weight and on body composition in food restricted rats. Am J Clin Nutr 1980; *33*:1912–1916.

114. Williamson DH, Munday MR, Jones RG. Biochemical basis of dietary influences on the synthesis of the macronutrients of rat milk. Fed Proc 1984; *43*:2443–2447.

115. Williamson DH. Integration of metabolism in tissues of the lactating rat. FEBS Letters 1980; *117*(Suppl):K93–K105.

116. Wilde CJ, Kuhn NJ. Lactose synthesis in the rat, and the effects of litter size and malnutrition. Biochem J 1979; *182*:287–294.

117. Flint DJ. Regulation of insulin receptors by prolactin in lactating rat mammary gland. J Endocrinol 1982; *93*:279–285.

118. Farid M, Baldwin RL, Yang YT, et al. Effects of age, diet and lactation on lipogenesis in rat adipose, liver and mammary tissue. J Nutr 1978; *108*:514–524.

119. Grigor MR, Geursen A, Sneyd MJ. Regulation of lipogenic capacity in lactating rats. Biochem J 1982; *208*:611–618.

120. Pethick DW, Lindsay DB. Acetate metabolism in lactating sheep. Br J Nutr 1982; *48*:319–328.

121. Grimble EF. The effect of dietary protein concentration and quality on the hormonal status, protein metabolism and milk protein concentrations of rats. Ann Nutr Metab 1981; *25*:221–227.

122. Liu J, Rebar RW, Yen SSC. Neuroendocrine control of the postpartum period. Clin Perinatol 1983; *10*:723–736.

123. Steingrimsdottir L, Brasel AJ, Greenwood ERM. Diet, pregnancy and lactation: effects on adipose tissue, lipoprotein lipase and fat cell size. Metabolism 1980; *29*:837–841.

124. Chaiyabutr N, Faulkner A, Peaker M. Glucose metabolism in vivo in fed and 48 h starved goats during pregnancy and lactation. Br J Nutr 1982; *47*:87–94.

125. Chaiyabutr N, Faulkner A, Peaker M. Effects of exogenous glucose metabolism in the lactating goat in vivo. Br J Nutr 1983; *49*:159–165.

126. Lomax MA, Baird GD. Blood flow and nutrient exchange across the liver and gut of the dairy cow. Br J Nutr 1983; *49*:481–496.

127. Rasmussen K, Warman NL. Effect of maternal malnutrition during the reproductive cycle on growth and nutritional status of suckling rat pups. Am J Clin Nutr 1983; *38*:77–83.

128. Grosvenor CE, Mena F. Effect of underfeeding upon the rate of milk ejection in the lactating rat. J Endocrinol 1983; *96*:215–222.

129. Rolls BJ, van Duijvenvoorde PM, Rowe EA. Effects of diet and obesity on body weight regulation during pregnancy and lactation in the rat. Physiol Behav 1984; *32*:161–168.

130. Sampson DA, Jansen GR. Protein synthesis during lactation: no circadian variation in mammary gland and liver of rats fed diets varying in protein quality and level of intake. J Nutr 1984; *114*:1470–1478.

131. Robinson AM, Williamson DH. Comparison of glucose metabolism in the lactating mammary gland of the rat in vivo and in vitro. Biochem J 1977; *164*:153–159.

132. Knight CH, Peaker M. Effects of fasting during mid pregnancy or early lactation on mammary development and milk yield in mice. J Dairy Res 1982; *49*:567–575.

133. Trayhurn P, Douglas JB, McGuckin MM. Brown adipose tissue thermogenesis is "suppressed" during lactation in mice. Nature 1982; *298*:59–60.

134. Canas R, Romero JJ, Baldwin RL. Maintenance energy requirements during lactation in rats. J Nutr 1982; *112*:1876–1880.

135. Hanafy MM, Seddick Y, Habib YA, et al. Maternal nutrition and lactation performance. J Trop Ped Environ Child Health 1972; *18*:187–191.

136. Khin-Maving-Naing, Tin-Tin-Oo KT, Kywe-Thien MS, et al. Study on lactation performance in Burmese mothers. Am J Clin Nutr 1980; *33*:2665–2668.

137. Whichelow MJ. Succeess and failure of breast feeding in relation to energy intake. Proc Nutr Soc 1976; *35*:62A–63A.

138. Prentice AM, Roberts SB, Prentice AA, et al. Dietary supplementation of lactating Gambian women. I. Effect on breast milk volume and quality. Hum Nutr Clin Nutr 1983; *37C*:53–64.

139. Prentice AM, Lunn PG, Watkinson M, et al. Dietary supplementation of lactating Gambian women. II. Effect on maternal health, nutritional status and biochemistry. Hum Nutr Clin Nutr 1983; *37C*:65–74.

140. Hartmann PE, Prosser CG. Physiological basis of longitudinal changes in human milk yield and composition. Fed Proc 1984; *43*:2448–2453.

141. Manning-Dalton C, Allen LH. The effects of lactation on energy and protein consumption, postpartum weight change and body composition of well nourished North American women. Nutr Res 1983; *3*:293–308.

142. Linzell JL, Peaker M. Mechanism of milk secretion. Physiol Rev 1971; *51*:564–597.

143. Altus P, Hickman JW. Severe spontaneous "bovine" ketoacidosis in a lactating woman. J Indiana State Med Assoc 1983; *76*:392–393.

144. Greer FR, Tsang RC, Searcy JE, et al. Mineral homeostasis during lactation—relationship to serum 1,25-dihydroxyvitamin D, 25-hydroxyvitamin D, parathyroid hormone, and calcitonin. Am J Clin Nutr 1982; *36*:431–437.

145. Goldsmith NF, Johnston JO. Bone mineral: effects of oral contraceptives, pregnancy and lactation. J Bone Joint Surg 1975; *57A*:657–668.

146. Chan GM, Slater P, Nonie R, et al. Bone mineral status of lactating mothers of different ages. Am J Obstet Gynecol 1982; *144*:438–441.

147. Kramer L, Spencer H, Osis D. Zinc and mineral content of weight reducing diets. Am J Clin Nutr 1981; *34*:1372–1378.

148. Sneed SM, Zane C, Thomas MR. The effects of ascorbic acid, vitamin B_6, vitamin B_{12} and folic acid supplementation on the breast milk and maternal nutritional status of low socioeconomic lactating women. Am J Clin Nutr 1981; *34*:1338–1346.

149. Bates CJ, Prentice AM, Prentice A, et al. The effect of vitamin C supplementation of lactating women in Keneba, a West African rural community. Int J Vit Nutr Res 1982; *53*:68–76.

150. Narula P, Mettal SK, Gupta S. Cellular and humoral factors of human milk in relation to nutritional status in lactating mothers. Ind J Med Res 1982; *76*:415–423.

151. Rosen JF, Roginsky M, Natheson G, et al. 25-Hydroxyvitamin D. Plasma levels in mothers and their premature infants with neonatal hypocalcemia. Am J Dis Child 1974; *127*:220–223.

152. Van Gelder DW, Darby FU. Congenital and infantile beriberi. J Pediatr 1944; *25*:226–235.

153. Lampkin BC, Saunders EF. Nutritional vitamin B_{12} deficiency in an infant. J Pediatr 1969; *75*:1053–1055.

7

AGING

HAMISH N. MUNRO

The proportion of people over 65 years of age varies in different parts of the world. In many underdeveloped countries their frequency is less than 5 per cent, but in North America the proportion is currently 11 per cent, while in Western Europe this group represents some 16 per cent of the population. This elderly segment, which continues to grow, makes disproportionate demands on health care. Rowe[1] provides a thoughtful account of the health care problems of the elderly in which he emphasizes that the elderly are more than simply old adults, and their care requires an understanding of the physiological, psychosociological, and pathological impacts of aging. Thus we have an elderly population who are more liable to come under medical or surgical care and whose bodily functions have generally diminished as compared with those of younger adults. The impact of age-related degenerative changes in body function is dramatically illustrated by a recent publication analyzing the years of functional integrity remaining to Massachusetts residents after the age of 65 years. Using life-table techniques, Katz et al.[2] have computed the remaining life span in two phases, first for independent living, followed by assisted living. The latter involves help in rising from bed, bathing, dressing, or eating. According to these criteria, men aged 65 to 69 years have an average of 9.3 years during which they can enjoy independent living, followed by 3.8 years of dependence on others. For women of the same age, further independent living averages 10.6 years, followed by a much longer period (8.9 years) of assisted existence.

Here, we examine the relationship between nutrition and the aging process, and try to evaluate the nutritional status of old people. Nutrition can be considered to be related to aging in three ways. First, many bodily functions and metabolic parameters decline progressively throughout adult life. Since nutrient intake usually decreases as adult age advances, it is legitimate to ask whether the reduced intake of nutrients contributes to the age-related loss of tissue functions. For example, do nutritional factors affect bone loss in osteoporosis? Second, many chronic diseases increase in incidence as people grow older. The role of long-term nutritional habits in the etiology of diseases such as cancer, heart disease, and hypertension has long been an area of intensive research. Third, the nutrient intakes of adults become progressively less as age advances, and over the age of 65 years can indeed fall below the intakes recommended for young adults. However, we do not know whether such low intakes contribute to the impairment of bodily functions in the elderly and whether better nutrition would retard the continued loss of functional capacity associated with aging.

In this chapter, we shall deal with the nutrient needs and nutritional status of people of middle age as they merge into the group 65 years and older. This approach emphasizes that old age is part of a continuum of change. The first section is arranged to deal with changes in body composition, in metabolism, and in tissue function occurring during aging. This is followed by a section summarizing the evidence on the role of nutrition in the aging process provided by animal models of aging. Then a major section follows on the nutrient needs of the elderly. The chapter closes with a commentary on the socioeconomic circumstances under which malnutrition is most likely to occur among the elderly and how it can be evaluated. In this way, we shall cover the first and third of the categories of the relationship of nutrition to aging identified in the preceding paragraph. More extensive information on a number of the topics can be found in the proceedings of a recent symposium.[3]

CHANGES IN BODY COMPOSITION, METABOLISM, AND TISSUE AND ORGAN FUNCTION

Body Composition

There is continuous change in body composition during adult life. This has been grossly demonstrated by both longitudinal and cross-sectional studies of populations at different ages using the whole body counter to assess lean body mass from the amount of ^{40}K radiation. In this way, Forbes[4, 5] has demonstrated a continuous decline in the lean body mass of adults of both sexes throughout adult life which is compensated by increasing body fat, so that total body weight tends to increase. Forbes detects some acceleration in loss of lean body mass in later life, and Steen[6] has observed that Swedish people lose an average of 1 kg lean body mass between the ages of 70 and 75 years. Cohn et al.[7] have extended these observations by comparing the age-related reduction in ^{40}K with changes in total body N measured by neutron activation. The latter provides a measure of total body protein, whereas ^{40}K is richer in muscle. Using differential equations, it was thus possible to parcel out muscle and nonmuscle components of the

lean body mass of men of different ages and to demonstrate that aging preferentially reduces muscle by nearly 50 per cent between the ages of 20 and 80 years of age, whereas the remainder of lean body mass is essentially unaffected by age (Table 7–1). This is supported by the output at different ages of creatinine which is derived from muscle creatine, and of 3-methylhistidine which represents muscle protein breakdown.[8] Table 7–2 shows that the output of both these muscle metabolites declines extensively and in parallel. This picture is amplified by autopsy data[10] showing that human subjects dying after the age of 70 years have lost 40 per cent of the muscle mass of a young adult, whereas the loss of visceral mass ranges from 9 to 18 per cent for different organs, some of this loss possibly associated with terminal disease. The actual loss of contractile muscle tissue may well be greater than the diminished mass suggests. Thus computerized tomography (CAT scan) shows that the bundles of contractile muscle within a muscle become separated, probably by intramuscular accumulation of fat.[11] The decrease in muscle mass with age is due to a loss of muscle fibers, which Lexell et al.[12] found to diminish in number by about 25 per cent in the vastus lateralis muscle between early manhood and age 70 and over. Stalberg and Fawcett[13] have provided evidence that this loss is due to a steady loss of motor units within the spinal cord. The loss of muscle results in a parallel reduction in strength. Thus between ages 30 and 80 years the leg and back muscles decrease in strength by some 30 to 40 per cent.[14] The effect of aging on hand grip is illustrated in a later section (see Fig. 7–6). Despite this loss of muscle strength, training can still improve performance to a limited extent among the elderly.[15]

Metabolism

Many authors have contributed to the profile of metabolism in the aging individual. In general, the emerging picture is one of continuous reduction in adaptation to nutrient supply as aging progresses. Basal energy metabolism, measured as oxygen consumption per unit of surface area, declines by about 20 per cent between the ages of 30 and 90 years (Fig. 7–1), but this decline is eliminated if oxygen con-

TABLE 7–1. Age-Related Changes in Body Composition of Adult Men

Age Group (yr)	Body Weight (kg)	Body Fat (kg)	Non-muscle Mass (kg)	Muscle Mass (kg)	Creatine Output (mg/kg/day)
20–29	80	15	37	24	26
40–49	81	19	38	20	—
60–69	79	23	37	17	—
70–79	80	24	38	13	16

Data adapted from Cohn et al.[7] and Uauy et al.[9]

TABLE 7–2. Whole-Body Protein Breakdown and Muscle Protein Breakdown in Young and Old Adults

Group	Mean Age (yr)	Whole Body Protein Breakdown (g/day)		Creatinine Output (mg/kg body weight)	Muscle Protein Breakdown (g/day)	
		per kg body weight	*per kg body cell mass*		*per kg body weight*	*per g creatinine*
Males						
Young	22	2.94	6.7	26	0.76	30
Old	70	2.64	7.5	16	0.53	32
Females						
Young	20	2.35	6.1	23	0.64	28
Old	76	1.94	6.6	13	0.31	26

Adapted from Uauy R, et al. J Gerontol 1978; *33*:663–671.

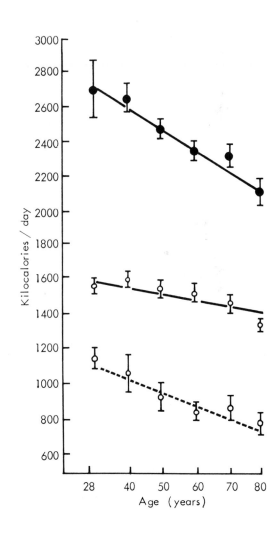

FIGURE 7–1. *Daily intake and expenditure of energy in men of different ages. (From Shock NW. Energy metabolism, caloric intake, and physical activity of the aging. In Carlson LA [ed]. Nutrition in Old Age [10th Symposium of the Swedish Nutrition Foundation]. Uppsala, Almqvist & Wiksell, 1972. Reproduced with permission.)*

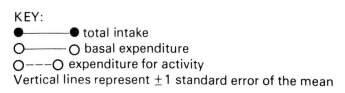

KEY:
●————● total intake
○————○ basal expenditure
○– – –○ expenditure for activity
Vertical lines represent ±1 standard error of the mean

sumption is expressed per unit of lean body mass.[16] This decline in basal metabolism and in lean body mass probably accelerates after 70 years. The decline thus arises from having less active cell mass as one becomes old. As pointed out by Silverberg[17] in an excellent review of carbohydrate metabolism in aging, it is generally accepted that tolerance for carbohydrate diminishes as the person gets older, so that the blood sugar level at 1 hour after a standard dose of glucose given to an individual over 50 years of age rises to a level about 10 mg higher than in a young subject (Fig. 7–2). Using the euglycemic insulin clamp procedure, Rowe et al.[19] have confirmed the reduced sensitivity of the peripheral tissues to insulin (Fig. 7–3). Regarding lipid metabolism, Kritchevsky[20] has reviewed the evidence and has concluded that aging reduces the ability of the subject to degrade and excrete lipids, thus contributing to their accumulation in the tissues. The age-related changes in different classes of blood lipoproteins are shown in Figure 7–4.

The metabolism of protein also shows age-related changes, some of which are probably attributable to the reduced muscle mass of the elderly. Studies by us[22] using ^{13}C-leucine as the precursor of protein synthesis showed that elderly males in the fasting state undergo a reduction in synthesis per kilogram of body weight of about 10 per cent, and a larger reduction of 30 per cent for elderly females, when compared with young adults of the same sex. Since these experiments represent only the fasting state, ^{13}C-glycine was applied to studying protein turnover, since the procedure using this labeled amino acid integrates turnover throughout the whole day (Table 7–2). This confirms that rates of breakdown of

body protein expressed per kilogram of body weight are less in older men and women,[17] which is also in agreement with the findings of Golden and Waterlow.[23] This age-related reduction can be accounted for by the smaller mass of active cells (lean body mass) in the bodies of elderly people. Thus when expressed in relation to lean body mass, turnover of body protein does not appear to be affected by aging.[9] Finally, we[24] have examined the effects of aging and of dietary protein intake on albumin synthesis by the liver. This involved a modified technique using ^{5}N-glycine to label the liver free arginine pool from which albumin is synthesized. When young adults were fed a diet low in protein, they synthesized less albumin than when they were allowed adequate dietary protein, whereas the elderly failed to show this response to the higher level of protein (Table 7–3). We have hypothesized that there is an upper set-point for albumin synthesis beyond which amino acid supply ceases to stimulate, and that this set-point is lowered as age advances.

Finally, continued loss of bone minerals throughout most of adult life (osteoporosis and osteomalacia) is a clinically important phenomenon because of the resultant bone fractures in many adults. Importantly, there is evidence discussed later that indicates a role for dietary factors in reducing the magnitude of this age-related loss.

Tissue Function

The effects of aging on tissue function have been documented by many studies, of which the Baltimore Longitudinal Study of Aging, initiated in 1958 as a continuing study of more than 1000 male volunteers, and summarized in a recent volume,[25] provides the most comprehensive survey available of normal aging. The data have been used both for cross-sectional studies of aging-related changes and also longitudinal evidence of change incurred by the aging process.

Nathan Shock, who established the Gerontology Center at Baltimore, has assembled data on some of the major changes in organ function as a result of aging (Fig. 7–5). This diagram shows that, between the ages of 30 and 80 years, cellular enzymes in general, and also nerve conductance, decline by 15 per cent, cardiac output by 30 per cent, renal blood flow by 50 per cent, maximum breathing capacity by 60 per cent, and so on. In addition to these effects, muscle strength measured by hand-grip strength declines progressively with age (Fig. 7–6). The consequent decline in capacity for sustained effort as one gets older is well known to professional sportsmen and has been studied in specific sporting events; for example, in a Swedish ski race, the *Vasalopet*, the time taken by different competitors for the course increased progressively from those of 30 through those of 65 years of age.[27]

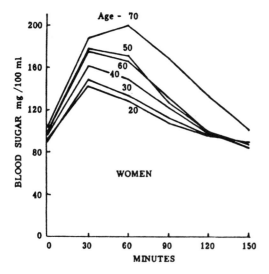

FIGURE 7–2. Effect of age on mean blood sugar levels fasting (0) and at 30, 60, 90, 120, and 150 minutes after oral intake of 50 g of glucose. (From Keen H, Fuller JH. The epidemiology of diabetes. In Exton-Smith A, Caird FC [eds]. Metabolic and Nutritional Disorders in the Elderly. Bristol, John Wright & Sons, 1980. Reproduced with permission.)

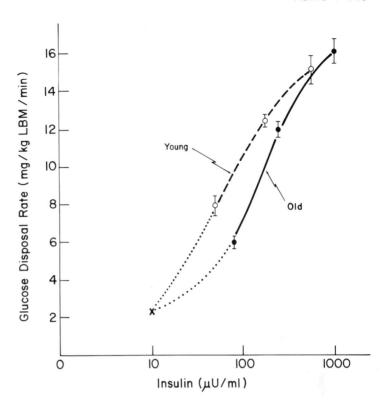

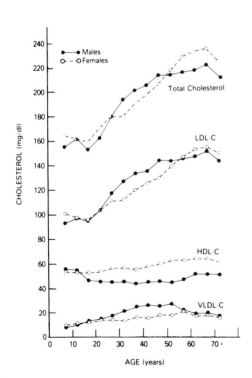

FIGURE 7–3. Dose-response curves for insulin-mediated whole-body glucose disposal. Rates in young (----) and old (——) subjects, expressed as mg glucose per kg body weight disposed of by young and old subjects at different levels of insulin infusion. (From Rowe JW, Minaker KL, Pallotta JA, et al. J Clin Invest 1983; 71:1581–1587. Reproduced with permission.)

FIGURE 7–4. Age-related changes in the concentrations of cholesterol in different classes of plasma lipoproteins in the blood of men and women in the United States. (Drawn by Dr. E.A. Schafer; data from reference 21.)

The endocrine system can also be affected by aging. A review of this field[28] shows that intracellular receptor abundance for androgens, estrogens, and corticosteroids declines with age. These changes suggest that hormone-mediated adaptation must decrease with age. Adelman[29] illustrates the effects of hormonal treatment on liver enzyme response in the rat. As aging progresses, the latent time of response increases. However, analysis of this response has led Adelman to conclude that aging results in this decline in responsiveness through a complex series of changes in endocrine and cellular function. Animal models of aging, discussed in detail below, indicate that food restriction can preserve receptors for at least some hormones against aging.

A major system of importance in aging is that of immunity.[30, 31] With advancing age, both cellular and humoral immunity decrease extensively. This senescence of the immune system can be related to thymic involution with advancing age and to changes in T-lymphocyte populations, possibly due to lack of capacity of the aging thymus to induce differentiation of prethymic lymphocytes.[31] Recent advances in our knowledge of factors controlling lymphocyte function, notably the interleukins, are impacting on the field of immunosenescence. It has long been recognized that immunodeficiency in infants can result from inadequate nutrition, and the time has now arrived for similar exploration of nutritional factors affecting immunosenescence for which there is already some evidence.[32] Recent studies of this kind on the elderly are well summarized by James and Makinodan,[31] who evaluate the alleged adverse im-

TABLE 7–3. Effect of Dietary Protein on Albumin Metabolism in Men

Group	Measurement	Diet		Statistical Significance (P Value)
		Low Protein	Adequate Protein	
Young	Serum albumin (g/L)	46	45	NS*
	Albumin synthesis (mg/kg/day)	140	190	<0.025
Elderly	Serum albumin (g/L)	41	42	NS
	Albumin synthesis (mg/kg/day)	147	149	NS

Adapted from Gersovitz M, et al. Metabolism 1980; 29:1075–1086.

The subjects were fed the adequate level of protein (1.5 g/kg body weight) for 7 days before measurements were taken. They were then fed the low-protein diet (0.4 g/kg body weight) for 14 days preceding repeat measurements. Albumin metabolism was measured with ^{15}N-glycine as the precursor of liver arginine.

*NS, not significant.

pact of caloric restriction, of high fat intakes (notably polyunsaturated fatty acids), and of inadequate dietary intakes of micronutrients, especially zinc. They comment that "recent knowledge of the cellular and subcellular events which comprise intact immune response now permits a more sophisticated approach to assessing the effects of dietary manipulation at the cellular-molecular level." Thus immunosenescence promises to be an important future area for delineating the relationship of nutrition to the aging process. The more extensive evidence of such a relationship provided by studies of aging with animal models is discussed below.

Another major area of functional changes with aging is the nervous system. A new edition of the *Handbook of the Biology of Aging*[33] summarizes recent studies on the impact of aging on neuroendocrine and autonomic functions,[34] on brain structure and energy metabolism,[35] on synaptic structure,[36] on neurotransmitter metabolism and function,[37] and on sleep patterns.[38] This extensive literature contains many contradictory findings, in part due to the complexity of brain structure. From the point of view of nutrition, neurotransmitters are compounds derived from nutrients, mostly amino acids, and Wurtman[39] has made a case for regarding the supply of some nutrients to the brain as being rate-limiting for neurotransmitter synthesis. Cherkin[40] has provided a thoughtful review of the role of these and other nutritional factors in memory function in which he deals with the contributions of vitamin deficiencies, intakes of specific amino acids, and mineral deficiencies to impairment of memory in the elderly, notably in Alzheimer's disease, and provides a review of the contradictory literature on the effects of administered choline. At present, it seems likely that more exploration should be undertaken on the uses of dietary precursors of neurotransmitters as therapeutic adjuvants for elderly subjects with diseases involving nervous system function for which drugs are also being prescribed.

Animal Models of Nutrition and Aging

Although human studies provide some evidence of the role of nutrition in the aging process, there is an extensive literature[41] describing the efficiency of nutritional intervention on the aging process in animals. It is now over 50 years since McCay[42] demonstrated that rats growth-retarded by caloric restriction from an early age live longer. This obser-

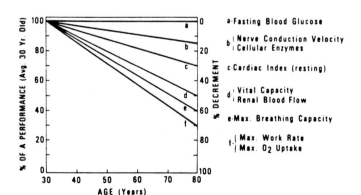

AGE DECREMENTS IN PHYSIOLOGICAL PERFORMANCE

a—Fasting Blood Glucose
b—Nerve Conduction Velocity / Cellular Enzymes
c—Cardiac Index (resting)
d—Vital Capacity / Renal Blood Flow
e—Max. Breathing Capacity
f—Max. Work Rate / Max. O₂ Uptake

FIGURE 7–5. Age-related decrements in physiological functions of men, expressed as percentage of function remaining at different ages. a, Fasting blood glucose; b, nerve conduction velocity; c, resting cardiac index; d, vital capacity, renal blood flow; e, maximum breathing capacity; f, maximum work rate, maximum oxygen uptake. (From Shock NW. Energy metabolism, caloric intake, and physical activity of the aging. In Carlson LA [ed]. Nutrition in Old Age [10th Symposium of the Swedish Nutrition Foundation]. Uppsala, Almqvist & Wiksell, 1972. Reproduced with permission.)

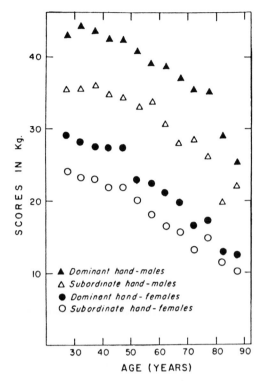

FIGURE 7–6. Age-related decrement in muscle strength for dominant and subordinate hands of men and women. (Reproduced with permission from Miles WR. In Gerard RN [ed]. Methods in Medical Research. Copyright © 1950 by Year Book Medical Publishers, Inc., Chicago.)

vation has been repeatedly confirmed (Fig. 7–7), and it has been shown that caloric restriction need not be instituted at weaning but is still effective if started in rodents that are young adults[43] or even middle aged.[44] This is clearly more relevant to the human situation than restriction beginning in childhood. However, it should be pointed out that the life of the caged rat can also be extended by exercise,[44] and we may regard the ad libitum–fed rat as the equivalent of the overfed, sedentary businessman, whose life expectancy has been reduced by this life-style. The analogy is further extended by examining the patterns of rodent disease associated with ad libitum compared with restricted feeding. If the caloric intake is restricted from an early age, the incidence and severity of chronic nephrosis, periarteritis, myocardial degeneration, and muscular dystrophy is greatly reduced[46] and the frequency of certain tumors is diminished.[47]

Despite these ambiguities about the relevance of the animal model to the role of nutrition in normal human aging, it does provide strong evidence that aging of physiological functions can be influenced by nutritional history. Thus chronic restriction of caloric intake results in better preservation of skeletal muscle into old age,[48] in less accumulation of body fat[49] and of plasma cholesterol,[50] and in better retention of the responsiveness of adipocytes to hormones.[51, 52] Dietary restriction of rodents also re-

duces the age-related impairment of endocrine functions, including the increase in plasma insulin,[53] the decrease in brain serotonin levels,[54] and the loss of brain dopamine receptors[55] that accompany aging in the ad libitum–fed rodent. A detailed account of other endocrine changes in the dietary-restricted rat is provided by Merry and Holehan.[56] The immunological system also undergoes extensive functional alterations as the age of the rodent advances; furthermore, such losses in immunocompetence can mostly be reduced or prevented by dietary restriction of rats or mice. Thus T-cell–dependent immunological responses are better maintained in calorie-restricted animals,[57] and their thymus morphology resembles that of younger animals.[58] Using autoimmune disease–prone mice, Good[59] found that dietary restriction delayed the time of onset of these various autoimmune diseases and reduced their severity. Liv et al.[60] have recently made the significant observation that weekly injection of an antibody to T-suppressor cells into mice eating an ad libitum diet prolonged their survival, thus suggesting that the immune system may be the primary mechanism through which caloric restriction extends life.

It is obvious that dietary restriction as a technique for extending life span and tissue function does not distinguish individual dietary constituents, though the benefits are often attributed to the reduced caloric intake. Restriction of protein intake at an early age prolongs the life of the rat,[61] but this may be related to lower caloric intake that had been caused by reduced growth rate. The same explanation may apply to prolongation of the life of rats given diets restricted in vitamins,[62] essential fatty acids,[63] or zinc.[64]

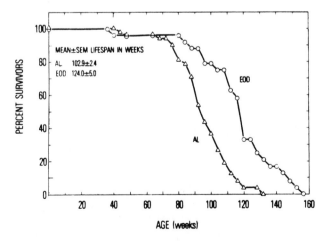

FIGURE 7–7. Survival of male Wistar rats housed in wheel-activity cages and fed ad libitum (AL) or every other day (EOD). (From Goodrick CI, Ingram DK, Reynolds MA, et al. Exp Aging Res 1983; 9:203–209. Reproduced with permission.)

NUTRIENT NEEDS AND INTAKES OF THE ELDERLY

Our knowledge of the needs of older adults is largely based on extrapolations from the better-determined needs of young adults, supplemented by an increasing amount of direct experimentation. The requirements of the elderly nevertheless demand extensive attention, and this is now beginning to be undertaken. The determination of the appropriate intakes of nutrients for all groups in the population is the business of international committees such as those of the Food and Agricultural Organization (FAO) and the World Health Organization (WHO) and is also performed for individual countries by national committees such as the U.S. Committee on Dietary Allowances. The former group issue joint reports on protein and energy needs, of which the most recent has just appeared.[65] The latter committee issues Recommended Dietary Allowances (RDA) for each essential nutrient based on the estimated *mean* requirement of a given age and sex category (e.g., 23- to 50-year-old men) to which is added an additional amount of the nutrient to cover individual variability within the population group. This involves estimating variability as the standard deviation (S.D.) and raising the RDA to two S.D.'s above the mean, thus covering the needs of all the population except the highest 2 per cent. An exception is the requirement for energy, for which the RDA's provide *average* needs with a range. In the case of the 9th edition of the RDA,[66] the elderly were aggregated into an age category called "51 years and over," as if people of 51 and 91 years had the same requirements. In the ensuing section, we shall examine requirements for selected major nutrients by the elderly. Since intakes of nutrients mostly diminish progressively throughout adult life, we shall deal with middle as well as old age as a continuum.

Energy Intakes and Requirements

Several studies performed in different countries agree in showing that the energy intake of the adult diminishes with age. The Baltimore Longitudinal Study of Aging[25] of male executives and civil servants initially provided cross-sectional data on the energy intake of this group.[67] The findings are illustrated in Figure 7–1, which shows a linear reduction in *total* energy intake between 30 and 80 years of age, from 2700 kcal at the younger age to 2100 kcal at the older age. This reduction of 600 kcal can be assigned to two causes. First, 200 kcal represents the reduction in basal metabolism consequent on the progressive age-related loss of active tissue (lean body mass). Second, the decline in physical activity with age accounts for the remaining reduction of 400 kcal between these ages. Since this first cross-sectional study, two subsequent nutrient intake studies on 180

of the same men have been carried out over a 15-year period.[68] These longitudinal studies have shown changes in nutrient consumption patterns due to aging and also those due to changes in food preferences common to the general population. Using multiple analysis for aging, for cohort, and for elapsed time, it was possible to show that different nutrients are affected by various factors as time passes. Advancing age was the main factor causing a reduction in caloric intake and in total intake of fats. On the other hand, intake of polyunsaturated fats and the ratio of polyunsaturated to saturated dietary fats showed an upward trend unrelated to age, but common to all groups. This means that an aging population can share in the general awareness of nutritional trends, such as the benefits claimed for more unsaturated fat in the diet.

These data from the Baltimore Longitudinal Study of Aging provide an excellent basis for observing age-related alterations in nutritional parameters, but the selection and nature of the group raises questions about the general applicability of the findings. It is therefore gratifying to note that other data support and amplify the picture presented by the Baltimore study. The Health and Nutrition Examination Surveys (HANES I and II) represent continuing studies of the food intakes, nutritional status, and health of a large sample balanced to represent all sectors of the U.S. population. Mean energy intakes from HANES II are presented in Table 7–9 and show that, in fair agreement with the Baltimore findings, men reduced their caloric intake from 2700 kcal at 23 to 34 years to 1800 kcal at 65 to 74 years, and women consumed 1600 kcal daily at 25 to 34 years but had reduced their intakes to 1300 kcal by 65 to 74 years. The caloric intakes estimated for elderly people by the National Food Consumption Survey summarized in Table 7–10 provide slightly higher values for men and women over 65 years, while the recorded intakes of elderly nursing-home patients[69] in Colorado showed slightly lower values, 1720 kcal daily for men and 1330 kcal for women. A cross-sectional survey by Exton-Smith and Stanton[70] of elderly women living alone in London showed a reduction of 19 per cent in caloric intake between the ages of 70 and 80 years, which the authors attribute to limitation of physical activity through disability.

The influence of activity is illustrated in two studies. First, it was shown in a French study[71] that the mean daily caloric intake of elderly townswomen averaged 1710 kcal, whereas women living in the country, presumably more active, consumed 2170 kcal/day. Time and geographic location do not seem to alter the picture of the decline with age and the role of exercise. Table 7–4 illustrates a study made 30 years ago of nutrient intakes by young and old men and women in different occupations in Scotland.[72] Young clerks consumed 3000 kcal per day, older clerks averaging 50 years took 2400 kcal, and retired

TABLE 7-4. Protein Intakes of Groups of Adults in Scotland

Group	Number in Group	Mean Age (yr)	Mean Energy Intake per Day (kcal)	Mean Protein Intake per Day		
				Total (g)	As % of Total Energy Intake	Intake per kg Body Weight (with range) (g/kg)
Younger men						
Students	9	22	3060	91	11.9	1.28 (1.05–1.46)
Clerks	10	28	3040	96	12.6	1.49 —
Coal miners	19	36	4030	121	12.0	1.84 —
Older men						
Older clerks	8	56	2440	83	13.6	1.24 (1.04–1.52)
Older workers (heavy work)	26	60	3430	113	13.2	1.48 (1.24–1.86)
Older workers (moderate work)	24	61	2910	90	12.4	1.31 (0.85–1.80)
Retired men (living alone)	9	73	2050	72	14.0	1.03 (0.78–1.24)
Younger women						
Technicians	18	19	2200	64	11.6	1.18 (0.89–1.65)
Young shop assistants	12	21	2220	70	12.3	1.21 (0.99–1.63)
Pregnant women (first child)	489	—	2450	75	12.4	1.20 —
Older women						
Older housewives	21	60	1940	62	12.7	1.02 (0.69–1.39)
Elderly women (living alone)	17	66	1890	62	13.2	1.03 (0.69–1.59)

From Munro HN. An introduction to nutritional aspects of protein metabolism. *In* Munro HN, Alison JB (eds). Mammalian Protein Metabolism. Vol. 2. New York, Academic Press, 1964: 3–39. Reproduced with permission.)

men aged 73 were satisfied with 2050 kcal; these values are parallel to those of the HANES survey data (Table 7–8) but some 200 kcal higher at all points. As expected, occupational differences are seen in Table 7–4. The Scottish data for women (Table 7–4) show a similar picture also bearing a parallelism to the HANES data for American women, but with a larger gap (500 kcal) between the Scottish and U.S. data (compare Tables 7–4 and 7–8). Finally, these low caloric intakes by women examined in recent surveys are often challenged as being erroneous through omission of some sources of energy. However, a recent study[73] of the energy expenditures of English women aged 20 to 40 years using dissociation of $D_2{}^{18}O$ as a new integrating measure of energy expenditure over 2 to 3 weeks, shows low energy expenditures compatible with the estimated caloric intakes of women from dietary surveys. Consequently, the average English woman of today has an energy expenditure of 1.4 times her basal metabolism, and we must accept that modern women are either combating obesity or limiting their work output.

With the reduced caloric intake with aging goes a reduction in the consumption of the nutrients contained in the caloric sources. In the Baltimore Longitudinal Study of Aging, the first cross-sectional dietary survey[67] included evaluation of vitamin and mineral intakes at various ages. These data showed that age caused a decline in intakes of iron, thiamine, riboflavin, and niacin, but no established trend emerged for calcium, vitamin A, or vitamin C. As

pointed out above, this study is not based on a representative population, and it is therefore significant to find that, in the Colorado nursing home study,[69] intakes of thiamine, calcium, and iron averaged less than the recommended dietary allowances. Similarly, the intakes of the elderly poor surveyed in the Ten-State Survey[74] often showed marginal or lower intakes of several nutrients. In England, Exton-Smith[70] found that women 80 years of age and living alone consumed about 20 to 30 per cent less of most nutrients when compared with 70-year-old women living alone. While it is thus apparent that aging reduces intake of many nutrients, the important question is whether these reduced intakes put a proportion of the elderly in jeopardy of subclinical and even florid deficiency. The English elderly have, in fact, been surveyed by biochemical tests for malnutrition as well as by clinical evaluation and food intake recall, and the British Department of Health and Social Security[75] has concluded that 6 per cent of men and 5 per cent of women between 70 and 80 years of age and twice this frequency of men and women over 80 years were suffering from one or more forms of malnutrition.

Protein Requirements and Nutriture

The protein intakes of adults of different ages and work habits are related to their caloric intakes, so that protein contributes a fairly constant 12 to 14 per cent of total calories (Table 7–4). In consequence, elderly people consume less protein as well as less energy-yielding foods. This lands us in a dilemma because it has been well established that caloric intake affects protein utilization (see below). Here we try to establish allowances of protein that will best preserve the diminishing functions of elderly. A more detailed discussion of the evidence is provided elsewhere.[76]

For more than a century, estimates of protein requirements of adults have customarily been based on nitrogen intake versus output (nitrogen balance).[77] The amount of dietary protein needed to prevent loss of body protein has been estimated by either of two methods. In the "factorial" procedure, losses of body protein measured as nitrogen via various routes (urine, feces, skin, etc.) by subjects on a protein-free diet are taken to represent the need for dietary protein to replace these losses. In the other method, subjects are fed dietary protein at several levels of intake below and above the amount needed to achieve N equilibrium; from the resulting negative and positive balances, zero balance is obtained by interpolation. The second of these procedures is now generally regarded as a more accurate reflection of the requirements. Early estimates of the needs of the elderly by this approach are summarized elsewhere.[76] Only more recent studies recognizing newer refinements and considerations in balance techniques[68] will be discussed here. The problems now recognized to be important include (1) estimates of minor routes of nitrogen excretion (cutaneous, etc.), (2) the previous nutritional status of the subject (subjects who are protein-depleted respond to increments in protein intake with a larger nitrogen retention than do repleted subjects), (3) the absence of stress (which promotes loss of body protein), and importantly (4) energy intakes as a significant and persisting factor in setting the amount of dietary protein needed to achieve nitrogen equilibrium (zero nitrogen balance). The continuing relation of energy intake to nitrogen balance has been emphasized before,[79, 80] and Kishi et al.[81] have provided a series of studies on Japanese adults that show the considerable impact of varying energy intake on their apparent protein requirements (Table 7–5).

Four recent studies provide a basis on which to judge the allowance of protein appropriate for achieving nitrogen equilibrium for adults over 60 years of age. Cheng et al.[82] used young and old Chilean subjects who received three protein levels (0.4, 0.8, and 1.6 g/kg) from a wheat-soy-milk mixture for 11 days, and achieved zero N balance in both groups at 0.8 g protein/kg. Unfortunately, they chose to provide 40 kcal/kg to both young and old subjects, although energy needs discussed above show that the elderly have lower energy requirements. Consequently, providing the elderly with the same energy intake as for the young would allow them to retain dietary protein more effectively and would thus obscure a greater need of the elderly for protein. The second study, by Zanni et al.,[85] involved feeding old men on a protein-free diet followed by egg protein at two levels and extrapolating the data to zero nitrogen balance, which showed that 0.59 gm protein/kg body weight prevented loss of body protein. However, the experiment was preceded by a period of feeding the subjects on a protein-free diet, which could have depleted them sufficiently to give more favorable utilization of the dietary protein.

Two subsequent experiments suggest a higher requirement for protein by older people. Uauy et al.[84] barely achieved zero nitrogen balance at a protein intake of 0.8 gm/kg body weight, which is the level recommended for young adults.[85] Similarly, Gersovitz et al.[85] report a study on elderly men and women who receive 0.8 g egg protein/kg and about 30 kcal/kg for 30 days, at the end of which three of the seven men and four of the eight women were still losing body protein (negative nitrogen balance) (Table 7–6). This raises the question of whether the lower caloric intake of the elderly is a factor in the increased amount of dietary protein needed to achieve zero nitrogen balance.

It should be recognized that nitrogen balance procedures are insensitive to small changes in body protein gain or loss, since they have a daily variability of about ± 500 mg N (± 3 g body protein). In contrast, the loss of lean body mass reported by Steen[6] in people over 70 years of age, namely 1 kg over a 5-year period, is equivalent to 20 mg of nitrogen daily, an amount far below the sensitivity of the balance technique to detect. It is therefore not possible to use nitrogen balance to measure sufficiently sensitively the effect of protein or energy intake on rate of loss of lean body mass. All we can conclude is that actual protein consumption in the Western world runs around twice the allowance of 0.8 g/kg body weight, but the people of these countries continue to lose lean body mass as aging progresses.

Finally, there is little information about the requirements of the elderly to satisfy their needs for essential amino acids. Studies based on nitrogen balance have been claimed[86] to show that requirements for methionine and lysine are higher in the elderly, whereas another study[87] shows less of a need for the sulfur-containing amino acids by old people compared with younger adults. Studies using the response of plasma amino acids to various intakes of tryptophan[88] and of threonine[89] suggest that the needs for these two essential amino acids are met by similar or lower intakes per kilogram of body weight compared with the requirements of young adults. In view of the use of amino acid mixtures in formulas for parenteral and enteral administration, which are often given to patients who are old, it would seem desirable to have definitive information about the essential amino acid needs of the elderly.

TABLE 7–5. Effect of Energy Intake on Dietary Protein Requirements in Men

Energy (kcal/kg body weight)	Mean Requirement of Dietary Protein for Zero N Balance (g protein/kg body weight)	Safe Allowance of Protein (Mean Requirement + 2 Standard Deviations)	
		g protein/kg body weight	g protein/ 70-kg man
40	0.78	1.02	72
45	0.56	0.74	52
48	0.51	0.62	44
57	0.42	0.52	37
Recommended dietary allowance (1980)		0.80	56

Calculated from Kishi K, et al. J Nutr 1978; *108*:658–669.

In conclusion, nitrogen balance is too crude a tool to tell us the level of protein intake that preserves tissue mass most effectively during aging. Nevertheless, there is some evidence that some elderly people continue to lose substantial amounts of body protein when receiving 0.8 g protein/kg body weight, which is the basis of the RDA for protein in this age group.[65] This may be because energy intake, which is known to affect protein utilization, diminishes progressively with aging (Fig. 7–1). In addition, the elderly are more liable to chronic diseases that result in periodic losses of body protein through fever and loss of appetite. This suggests the need for a small repletion allowance as part of their protein allowance. As a consequence of these various considerations, it is recommended that people over 60 years old should not consume less than 12 to 14 per cent of their diminishing caloric intake as protein. Finally, the question of toxic effects of excessive protein intake has been occasionally raised. Brenner et al.[90] provide evidence suggesting that high protein intakes may accelerate loss of kidney function. As authenticated adverse effect of high protein intake is to increase loss of bone calcium and thus may contribute to osteoporosis. This is discussed in the section immediately following.

TABLE 7–6. Nitrogen Balances of Elderly Men and Women Receiving 0.8 g Egg Protein per kg Body Weight Over a 30-Day Period

Group of Elderly	10-Day Period on Diet	Average Nitrogen Balance (mg N/kg/day)	Number in Negative Balance
Men	0–10	−7.4	7 of 7
	11–20	+1.6	4 of 7
	21–30	+0.4	3 of 7
	Mean	−1.8	
Women	0–10	−0.8	4 of 7
	11–20	−7.8	7 of 8
	21–30	−2.3	4 of 8
	Mean	−3.6	

Balances are for last 5 days of each 10-day period and represent directly measured N output in urine and feces with an allowance of 5 mg N for skin and other minor routes of N output.

Adapted from Gersovitz M, et al. Am J Clin Nutr 1982; *35*:6–14.

Calcium, Vitamin D, and the Multifaceted Bone Loss Problem

Attempts to modify the loss of bone density with age provide the most persuasive evidence that dietary factors can affect age-related changes in body composition. The onset of perceptible loss of bone density has been variously set at 20 years[91] or 40 years of age.[92] It is agreed that some women show an accelerated rate of loss during the first 20 years following the menopause, eventually leading for many to fractures of the wrist, long bones, or spine. By age 80 years, American women show an average reduction in bone density of 25 per cent, while men have undergone 12 per cent loss.[93] Nordin[94] estimates that, by the age of 80 years, women show a cumulative prevalence of wrist fracture of 14 per cent, with 8 per cent vertebral compression fractures and 5 per cent femoral neck fractures; the frequencies of these fractures in men are computed to be 4 per cent, 4 per cent, and 1.5 per cent, respectively. This emphasizes how processes starting in early middle life can become problems of old age.

Nutritional factors that have been implicated in this process of bone loss include too little calcium, phosphorus, and vitamin D and too much protein, phytate and fiber; exercise is another component of the picture. The significance of calcium intake in the maintenance of bone density has been carefully evaluated by a panel of experts.[93] From the extensive data of the HANES I and II surveys of the nutrient intakes of the American population, they concluded that, compared with adolescents, intakes of calcium were much lower in adults, especially women. During the age range of 18 to 30 years, when deposition of bone is maximal, the survey showed that two thirds of women and one third of men were receiving less than the recommended dietary allowance of calcium. After the age of 35 years, more than 75 per cent of women were consuming less than the adult RDA of 800 mg; this group is especially at risk for osteoporotic fractures.

A question that arises is, at what time of life are adequate calcium intakes most effective? The period between late adolescence and 30 years of age is associated with significant continued deposition of bone calcium. Markovic et al.[95] examined bone density of populations in two regions of Yugoslavia. One provided a low calcium intake (500 mg daily at age 40 to 42 years) and the other a high intake (1100 mg daily). Already at 30 years of age, bone density was greater for men and women in the region receiving the higher intake of calcium (Fig. 7–8). Although bone density decreased thereafter at similar rates in both districts, the population in the low-calcium region had more fractures because they began with less dense bones and thus reached a critical stage of fragility sooner. These observations would point to the period of adolescence and early adult life as a time when a high intake of calcium confers benefits for skeletal integrity in later life. Garn[92] draws attention to the same phenomenon among American blacks, who have thicker bones than the rest of the U.S. population as young adults. Although they lose bone in parallel with those of other racial groups, American blacks rarely reach the level of osteoporotic fracture.

This observation should not imply that intake of calcium has no significance in later adult life. High calcium intakes have beneficial actions. Two independent studies[96, 97] show that an intake of 1.5 g calcium daily over a period of years can reduce or prevent bone calcium loss in postmenopausal women. An interaction between intake of calcium and estrogens has also been documented in menopausal women. Heaney et al.[98] have shown that a dietary level of 1 g calcium per day can maintain zero calcium balance in premenopausal women and in estrogen-treated postmenopausal women, compared with 1.5 g calcium needed by postmenopausal women without estrogen treatment. Horsman et al.[99] have found that less estrogen has to be given in the treatment of postmenopausal osteoporosis if calcium intake is raised, thus reducing the risks of high levels of estrogen administration. These conclusions are based on long-term observations. Heaney et al.[93] comment, "The balance method and bone mass measurement can yield reliable results in only two circumstances: (1) when the duration of observations on a supplement extends to more than 2 years (and preferably more than 3 years), or (2) when the subjects are studied on their own self-selected home intakes."

The prevention of osteoporosis involves other nutritional factors affecting bone integrity. Using formula diets in which the amounts of single nutrients were varied, Anand and Linksweiler[100] showed that raising protein intake increases urinary output of calcium and impairs calcium balance. This effect has been confirmed by others, including Bengoa et al.,[101] who observed increased calciuria and negative calcium balances during intravenous infusions of increasing levels of amino acids, an important observation for parenteral nutrition. Spencer et al.,[102] however, observed only a transient effect on calcium balance following raising protein intake when the supplementary protein consisted of meat. They attributed this to the beneficial effect of the phosphorus contained in the meat, but Heaney and Recker[103] conclude from studying the calcium balances of women on self-selected diets that the action of phosphorus is not sufficient to counteract fully the adverse effect of dietary protein.

The role of vitamin D in the causation of metabolic bone loss in the elderly is complex, as summarized in a consensus reported by a group of experts.[104] Osteomalacia, the metabolic bone disease caused in adults by vitamin D deficiency, gives rise to accumulation of osteoid tissue that can be confirmed by biopsy of iliac crest bone.[94] Osteomalacia is commoner in Europe than in the United States, where milk and margarine are fortified with vitamin D. In addition, greater exposure to sunshine in the U.S. provides more vitamin D from its synthesis in the irradiated skin. It is thus not surprising that osteomalacia is also present in about 25 per cent of cases of osteoporosis in Britain;[94] in addition to preventing osteoid from being laid down, part of the action of vitamin D may be to ensure adequate absorption of calcium by the aging intestine through induction of calcium carrier proteins by stimulation with 1,25-dihydroxyvitamin D.[105] The role of vitamin D and its metabolites in regulating bone metabolism is, however, complex, involving the diminishing efficiency of the aging kidney to convert 25-hydroxyvitamin D to the dihydroxy derivative and the reduced response of this reaction to administration of parathyroid hormone to man[106] or rats.[107] The sig-

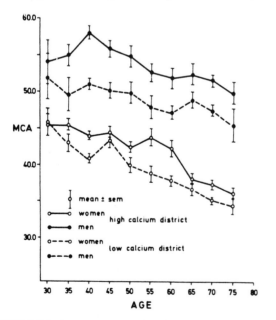

FIGURE 7–8. Age-related changes in metacarpal bone density in men and women in two districts in Yugoslavia, one providing a high calcium intake, the other a low intake. (From Markovic V, Kostial K, Simonvic I, et al. Am J Clin Nutr 1979; 32:540–549. © Am J Clin Nutr. American Society for Clinical Nutrition. Reproduced with permission.)

nificance of vitamin D metabolic bone disease is discussed in detail by Parfitt et al.[104]

Other factors affecting calcium absorption include fiber and phytate. For this reason, consumption of large amounts of unrefined cereals can reduce available calcium and other minerals.[93] In addition, prolonged exercise has been shown to result in denser bones. Using neutron activation to measure skeletal calcium in 30 male marathon runners about 42 years of age, Aloia et al.[108] found that they had 11 per cent more body calcium as compared with sedentary individuals of the same age. The same investigators[109] also showed that bone loss by postmenopausal women can be prevented by exercise. This has been confirmed in Denmark,[110] where women aged 50 to 73 years with a previous forearm fracture were given exercise for 1 hour twice weekly over an 8-month period. They showed a 3.5 per cent gain in lumbar spine density, compared with a loss of 2.7 per cent by an unexercised control group. Finally, Smith et al.[111] studied a series of women aged 69 to 95 years who exercised and/or were given calcium and vitamin D. Over a 3-year period, a control group showed a bone loss of 3.3 per cent, physical activity caused a gain of 2.3 per cent, and the calcium–vitamin D group gained 1.4 per cent; surprisingly, however, those who exercised and received supplemental nutrients showed no gain, though they did not lose bone density like the untreated controls.

Trace Element Nutriture

Iron deficiency anemia is widespread in the developing world and also occurs in some groups in industrialized countries. The iron status of elderly Americans has recently been the subject of a consensus report chaired by Lynch.[112] In order to determine iron status, it is not sufficient to measure hemoglobin levels. Adequate assessment of a population requires additional criteria, which include the level of saturation of serum transferrin, the serum ferritin concentration, and the level of free protoporphyrin in the erythrocytes. These combined estimations provide indices of deficiency of stored iron as well as anemia due to iron deficiency. When these criteria were applied to an inner city population (Table 7–7), stored iron was found to be low among 20 per cent of menstruating women, but in only 6 per cent of older women and 3 to 4 per cent in men of all ages.[113] Indeed, serum ferritin, an index of iron stores, rose steadily throughout the adult life of men but only after the menopause in women (Fig. 7–9). Half of the subjects who had low iron stores were anemic (Table 7–7). However, this table does not differentiate those over 65 from those over 45 years, so that the incidence of anemia among the elderly is not reported.

Fortunately, some indication of the frequency of low hemoglobin values is available for men and women of 65 to 74 years from the HANES survey, which provides a sample representative of the U.S. population. A careful analysis of the HANES data has been made by Dallman et al.,[114] who used hemoglobin levels, serum iron and iron-binding capacity, erythrocyte protoporphyrin content of red cells, and in some cases serum ferritin values to assess the iron status of elderly people. These authors conclude that the 4.4 per cent frequency of anemia found among elderly men is mostly due to infections, whereas the small incidence of anemia in elderly women is indeed due to iron deficiency. This low incidence is confirmed for an inner city group by Gershoff et al.,[115] who found low hemoglobin values to be infrequent and to revert to normal on repeat testing whether iron was given or not. Lipschitz et al.[116] conclude from studies of the abundance of white and red cell precursors that the mild anemia found in some el-

TABLE 7–7. Evaluation of Iron Status of an Inner City Population

	15–45 years		46+ years	
	Men	*Women*	*Men*	*Women*
Serum ferritin	1.7	21.1	3.6	3.7
Transferrin saturation	5.0	24.7	7.3	8.8
RBC protoporphyrin	3.3	16.0	12.1	14.3
Hemoglobin	4.2	14.1	9.1	8.3
Iron deficiency	3.3	20.0	4.2	5.6
Iron-deficiency anemia	1.2	8.4	2.4	2.3

Figures represent percentages of subjects found to have abnormal values for each criterion, or to have iron deficiency or iron deficiency anemia.

Adapted from Cooke JD, et al. Blood 1976; 48:449–455.

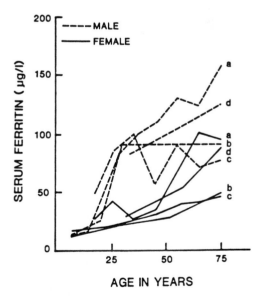

FIGURE 7–9. Effect of age on serum ferritin concentration measured in men (----) and women (——) in (a) the United States, (b) Canada, (c) Britain, and (d) Italy. (From Lynch SR, Finch CA, Monsen ER, et al. Am J Clin Nutr 1982; 36:1032–1045. © Am J Clin Nutr. American Society for Clinical Nutrition. Reproduced with permission.)

derly people can be due to a reduction in reserves of hematopoietic stem cells.

These observations lead to the conclusion that iron deficiency anemia is not likely to be significant among the elderly in most Western countries, which is compatible with the tendency of iron stores to increase with age. This is in agreement with the evidence of the HANES surveys (Table 7–8) that the daily iron intake of elderly people averages 10 mg or more. Since caloric intake decreases with age, the adequacy of iron intake is maintained by the increase in the proportion of iron-rich foods in the diet selected by older people. The adequacy of the iron intake of elderly people is also supported by the extensive population study of Garry et al.[117] In their survey of healthy old people in New Mexico, only 6 per cent of men and one third of women were not consuming the Recommended Dietary Allowance of 10 mg iron daily. This should not be construed as meaning that some inner city populations are also immune from iron deficiency anemia. Thus the Ten-State Survey[74] showed inadequate intakes of iron by some low-income white and black women 60 years and older, and this was also found to be true for some members of inner city groups in Syracuse.[118]

The other trace metal to be discussed here is zinc. Like iron, zinc has been the subject of a consensus report.[119] An extensive review of the literature is also provided by Golden.[120] The consensus report[119] is the source of the data in Table 7–9, representing a digest of the energy and zinc intakes of older people obtained from two U.S. surveys, the HANES II Survey and the National Food Consumption Survey. In contrast to iron nutriture, few elderly people met the RDA of 15 mg zinc daily, the average intake being about 10 mg for men and 7 to 8 mg for women (Table 7–9). Again, in contrast to iron, the intake of zinc falls steadily with age as energy intake diminishes. In a survey of healthy, noninstitutionalized elderly people in New Mexico, Garry et al.[117] found that 98 per cent received less than the RDA from their diet, though supplements changed this picture to one of adequacy for the majority of elderly. The significance of these low values depends on the level of absorption provided by the dietary constituents. Some 30 per cent of dietary zinc is regarded as available through absorption, but this proportion is reduced by high intakes of some other dietary constituents, especially phytate, some types of fiber, phosphate, and protein.[119] The consensus report has also evaluated seven studies of plasma or serum zinc levels made in older subjects.[119] Most of these studies failed to demonstrate a relationship between age and the plasma zinc levels; the zinc content of hair from older people was no more indicative of significant deficiency in the elderly population. It is equally difficult to find evidence of functional defects in older people attributable to lack of zinc. Loss of taste acuity (hypogeusia) can be induced in animals and in young human subjects by experimental zinc deficiency and by diseases causing malabsorption.[119] However, five studies of taste threshold of older people failed to show a relationship to zinc nutriture, nor did hypogeusic elderly subjects respond to zinc.[119]

Of more interest in a surgical setting is the relationship of zinc to wound healing. Some subjects who have delayed wound healing respond to zinc administration and may be zinc-deficient,[121] which can be compounded by loss of body zinc accompanying the catabolic response to injury.[122] The role of zinc in wound healing also emerges in two studies on elderly people with varicose ulcers.[123, 124] Those with relatively low plasma levels of zinc responded to zinc administration. Finally, the consensus review of zinc nutriture in the elderly[119] identifies a series of publications demonstrating a relationship between zinc status and immune function both in animal studies and in diseases associated with severe zinc deficiency. These studies on older people suggest that adequacy of zinc nutriture may play a part in the response to immunization and the delayed hypersensitivity to antigens and may affect the population of T-lymphocytes in circulation.[119] Thus, the observations of a relationship of zinc nutriture to the function of the immune system, on the role of zinc in the healing of wounds, and on the loss of zinc during the metabolic response to injury all suggest that zinc status of elderly patients may be an important area for evaluation in a surgical setting. In this context, it should be remembered that older people have less skeletal muscle, a tissue containing most of the available zinc in the body. They may thus be less able to bear the loss of zinc accompanying the metabolic response to injury or infection.

TABLE 7–8. Mean Daily Energy and Iron Intakes of Adults in the United States (HANES II, as condensed from Lynch, et al.[112])

Age (yr)	Males			Females		
	Energy (kcal)	Iron (mg)	Iron/Energy (mg/1000 kcal)	Energy (kcal)	Iron (mg)	Iron/Energy (mg/1000 kcal)
25–34	2734	17.3	6.3	1643	10.9	6.6
35–44	2924	16.1	6.6	1579	11.2	7.1
45–54	2361	16.2	6.9	1439	10.4	7.3
55–64	2071	14.8	7.1	1401	10.7	7.6
65–74	1828	14.1	7.7	1295	10.2	7.9

Adapted from Lynch SR, et al. Am J Clin Nutr 1982; 36:1032–1045.

TABLE 7-9. Effect of Age on Daily Energy and Dietary Zinc Consumption in the United States

Sex and Age Group (yr)	Energy (kcal)		Zinc (mg)	
	HANES II	*NFCS*	*HANES II*	*NFCS*
Males: 55–64	2071	—	12.6	—
65–74	1828	1970	10.6	10.5
75+	—	1808	—	9.3
Females: 55–64	1401	—	8.2	—
65–74	1295	1444	7.2	7.6
75+	—	1367	—	7.0

Adapted from Sandstead HH, et al. Am J Clin Nutr 1982; *36*:1046–1059. Data from HANES II and National Food Consumption Survey.

Water-Soluble Vitamin Needs

In a review of vitamin insufficiency among the elderly, Exton-Smith[125] points out that deficiency is nowadays commoner among old people than among the young and attributes this to a combination of marginal intakes and endogenous factors impairing absorption, metabolism, and utilization. In this section, we deal with the needs of the elderly for thiamine, folic acid, and ascorbic acid.

The metabolic role of thiamine (vitamin B_1) in energy metabolism suggests that the requirement for this vitamin may diminish as caloric intake falls with aging. The 9th edition of the RDA handbook[66] advises 0.5 mg thiamine/1000 kcal but, on the basis of two reports that the elderly use thiamine less efficiently, it is recommended in the handbook that thiamine intake by the elderly should not fall below 1.0 mg daily even though caloric consumption is less than 2000 kcal. The recommended intake over age 50 years is 1.2 mg for men and 1.0 mg for women; for caloric intakes of people over 75 years given in the same handbook, this would represent about 0.6 mg/1000 kcal.

In a consensus report, Iber et al.[126] have recently reviewed the evidence relating to thiamine needs and deficiencies in the elderly. They have used HANES I and HANES II surveys of U.S. nutrient intakes to show that the average American consumes thiamine in proportion to his or her caloric intake (Table 7–10). In the oldest group surveyed in HANES II (65 to 74 years), men had an average daily intake of 1.35 mg thiamine and women consumed 0.99 mg daily. This provided a somewhat higher ratio (0.75 mg/1000 kcal) than did young con-

sumers. In their review, Iber et al.[126] imply that the recommended intakes for older Americans (51 years upwards) in the 9th edition of the Recommended Dietary Allowances,[66] namely 1.2 mg daily for men and 1.0 mg for women, are unnecessarily generous, since they exceed 0.5 mg/1000 kcal. In defense of this view, they cite among other studies that of Sauberlich et al.,[127] who were unable to induce biochemical evidence of thiamine deficiency in young men receiving only 0.3 mg/100 kcal. However, there is no discrepancy. The 9th edition of the RDA[66] for the elderly assumes an average calorie intake of 2400 and 1800 kcal, respectively, for men and women between 51 and 75 years of age (giving about 0.55 mg thiamine/1000 kcal), compared with an average of 1950 kcal and 1350 kcal, respectively, for men and women aged 55 to 74 years surveyed in HANES II (Table 7–10). Furthermore, free-living communities of middle-class elderly in the U.S. can more than satisfy the Recommended Dietary Allowances.[66] Thus in New Mexico, middle-income elderly men and women were mostly consuming more than the RDA from the diet alone, to which about half added a supplement of thiamine averaging some five times the RDA.[117] A recent survey in Boston of the nutrient intakes of free-living elderly[129] demonstrated that only about 5 per cent of men and women within the age groups 60 to 69, 70 to 79, and 80+ years were receiving less than two thirds of the RDA for thiamine from the diet.

What is the evidence regarding the thiamine intake of specific target groups of elderly, and what is the incidence of thiamine deficiency in such groups? The latter is usually measured by biochemical tests, since no constellation of clinical changes is distinctive

TABLE 7-10. Dietary Intakes of Thiamine and Calories by Adults

Age (yr)	Males			Females		
	Energy (kcal)	*Thiamine (mg)*	*Thiamine/Energy (mg/1000 kcal)*	*Energy (kcal)*	*Thiamine (mg)*	*Thiamine/Energy (mg/1000 kcal)*
25–34	2734	1.69	0.62	1643	1.08	0.66
35–44	2424	1.55	0.64	1579	1.05	0.66
45–54	2361	1.51	0.64	1439	0.98	0.68
55–64	2071	1.40	0.68	1401	1.00	0.71
65–74	1828	1.33	0.73	1295	0.99	0.76

Adapted from Iber FL, et al. Am J Clin Nutr 1982; *36*:1067–1082. Data from HANES II.

enough for screening deficiency.[126] Measurement of the thiamine intakes of a nursing home population in Colorado[69] provided mean values of 0.5 to 0.6 mg/1000 kcal, while biochemical tests suggested marginal deficiency in 19 per cent of these. A study in Belfast, Northern Ireland[128] showed intakes by free-living subjects and hospital and nursing home patients to be about 0.4 mg/1000 kcal, but the frequency of unacceptably low biochemical values by the transketolase test varied considerably from one group to another. From an extensive in-depth survey of the literature on thiamine intakes and incidence of deficiency among the elderly within the U.S. and in Europe, Iber et al.[126] conclude that

Deficiency of thiamin and its phospate ester coenzyme forms is not common in free-living older people in the U.S.A. However, when one considers data from Ireland, the Netherlands or England, where the thiamin intakes are comparable to the lowest in America, one finds an increasing incidence of marginal or severe deficiency. If one considers the infirm in North America, there is an increase in the fraction of the subjects showing marginal or severe deficiency. Thus disease seems clearly to increase the frequency and severity of deficiency.

The same consensus group[126] concluded that about 10 per cent of persons in some selected U.S. subgroups are thiamine-deficient, and are usually from poor or diseased populations. Alcohol is a major cause of deficiency, since it interferes with absorption of thiamine, diminishes dietary intake, and increases requirements. The sites of action of alcohol are discussed in detail elsewhere.[126, 130]

The RDA for folic acid by the elderly is 400 µg daily.[66] A consensus report[131] on folic acid status among the elderly suggests that this it too high an allowance. Unlike thiamine intake, folate intake could not be included in the HANES surveys because of incomplete analytical data on the constituent foods at the time these surveys were undertaken. However, a survey of food consumption patterns in Canada[132] showed that the average adult male over 65 years of age consumed 151 µg folate daily, while older Canadian women consumed 130 µg. A Swedish survey[133] gave average intakes of 157 and 129 µg, respectively, in older men and women. In the latter survey, blood folate levels were within normal limits and no cases of megaloblastic anemia were encountered. The American experience is similar for selected groups of elderly. The survey of middle-income elderly in New Mexico[117] showed that 40 per cent of subjects were consuming less than 50 per cent of the RDA value of 400 µg folate per day from their diets. A similar study in Florida, reported in the consensus statement on the folate status of the elderly,[131] showed that about 90 per cent were receiving less than 400 µg folate, while 37 to 65 per cent of individuals in different communities were consuming less than 200 µg folate, the magnitude of the deficit being highest for those with the lowest incomes. In the Boston survey,[129] mean intakes at

each decade after 60 years were about 275 µg daily for men and 240 µg for women, and the proportions receiving less than two thirds of the RDA of 400 µg folate were about 60 per cent of elderly men of all ages after 60 years and 70 per cent of women of similar ages. From these various observations, it is clear that few old people consume the U.S. recommended intake of 400 µg folacin daily.

These surveys thus show much lower folate intakes by the elderly than those recommended by the U.S. Dietary Allowances Committee. In their consensus report on folate nutrition in the elderly, Rosenberg et al.[131] accept serum folate levels of 3 ng/ml and red cell folate levels of 140 ng/ml as the dividing lines for deficiency. They point out that the Ten-State Survey and the HANES I study identified few elderly who failed to meet this criterion for serum folate levels. However, erythrocyte folate concentrations seem to be more sensitive. A series of four studies in Florida showed few low serum values, whereas the proportion of red cell folate levels below the critical level of 140 ng/ml varied from 6 per cent in a higher socioeconomic status retirement community to 60 per cent in a low-income urban population.[131] Reports from various countries show that the frequency of low serum and erythrocyte folate values among the elderly is about 18 per cent for nursing home and hospitalized subjects, compared with 9 per cent of the elderly living at home.[131]

In conclusion, the data on the folate needs of the elderly suggest that some 200 to 300 µg folate daily should be adequate. Thus, the mean folate intakes by the elderly in four areas of Florida are reported to be 250, 217, 192, and 184 µg and the frequency of unacceptably low erythrocyte folate levels in these four studies were 13, 6, 60, and 31 per cent, respectively[131] (the latter two surveys were made on low-income elderly). This variability in the degree of deficiency of different elderly populations on low folate intakes may arise from factors impairing absorption. These include alcohol, which alters the kinetics of folate metabolism and increases its excretion in the urine.[134] Chronic alcoholism can thus be a cause of folate-dependent megaloblastic anemia.[131] In addition to alcohol, decreased or absent secretion of gastric acid in old people is associated with diminished folate absorption, since adequate absorption of this vitamin is dependent on acidity in the upper small intestine.[135] Finally, the elderly frequently take one or more drugs, some of which (e.g., phenytoin) can block folate absorption (see below).

Ascorbic acid is normally consumed by most adults at levels above the generous RDA of 60 mg daily for men and women.[65] Thus, in the Baltimore study,[67] elderly men consumed an average of more than 100 mg per day. However, some low-income groups studied in the Ten-State Survey[74] reported low intakes of the vitamin, coupled with low plasma levels in 10 per cent of the elderly surveyed. Of some interest is the finding among hospitalized elderly women in Britain[136] of low plasma and white cell levels of ascorbic acid. This could be corrected by increasing ascorbic acid intake substantially. However, similar supplementation studies failed to improve the clinical status of these elderly[137] or produced only small increases in body weight and plasma protein levels.[138]

THE NUTRITIONAL STATUS OF THE ELDERLY

Evidence from Surveys

As mentioned earlier, a combination of food intake measurement, biochemical assessment, and clinical examination allows the evaluation of a population for the frequency of malnutrition. In Great Britain, such surveys[75] have shown an incidence of malnutrition in 6 per cent of men and in 5 per cent of women aged 70 to 80 years and in 12 per cent of men and 8 per cent of women over 80 years of age. While protein-calorie malnutrition was the most frequent form, intakes of iron, thiamine, ascorbic acid, and vitamin D were considered to be frequently inadequate. Inspection of the case details in this report shows that almost all these cases of malnutrition had one or more diseases (e.g., bronchitis, emphysema) likely to diminish appetite and increase nutrient needs.

In addition to national nutrition surveys, surveys of specific groups of elderly have been conducted. Thus Baker et al.[140] evaluated the nutritional status of elderly people living at home or in nursing homes in New Jersey by comparing their blood levels of vitamins. Among the free-living elderly, the blood levels of vitamins A and E and of riboflavin, biotin, and pantothenate were adequate, whereas the levels of ascorbic acid, thiamine, folate, and vitamin B_{12} were often low. Among the institutionalized elderly, a different spectrum was observed. Levels of niacin and vitamin B_6 were low in one third of cases, and levels of the other vitamins were less frequently unacceptable. In Belfast, Northern Ireland, Vir and Love[128] compared intakes of nutrients and blood levels of vitamins and minerals for free-living elderly, nursing-home residents, and hospitalized elderly. Again, the spectrum of deficiency varied from one group to another, but the degrees of deficiency in the free-living elderly and the institutionalized subjects were not the same as in New Jersey. This undoubtedly reflects differences in nutrient intake in the two locations. The effect of nutrient intake on blood nutrient levels can be readily established in surveys such as the Boston Survey,[141] in which biochemical indicators of nutrient status were significantly better among vitamin supplement users for vitamin E, riboflavin, vitamin B_{12}, folic acid, and ascorbic acid. Furthermore, almost all the marginal to deficient blood vitamin levels in the survey were found among persons not using vitamin supplements.

Factors Affecting Nutritional Status

Factors affecting nutrient status need not all be negative. Among the positive factors is the taking of supplements of vitamins and minerals. In the Boston Survey[129] about 40 per cent of elderly men and 55 per cent of elderly women were taking supplements. In Garry's survey in New Mexico[117] 57 per cent of men and 61 per cent of women were receiving supplements, in some cases raising intakes of vitamins to several times the RDA values. Regarding factors increasing malnutrition among the elderly, Exton-Smith[139] has divided these into socioeconomic factors and physical and mental disorders. The *primary* causes of malnutrition he recognizes among the elderly include:

1. Ignorance of the need for a balanced diet, notably common among elderly widowers.
2. Restriction on the range of foods through poverty, which is reflected in the Boston Survey[129] by the lower nutrient intakes of people of lower socioeconomic status.
3. Social isolation, which reduces interest in food as evidenced by a higher frequency of anemia and of low leukocyte ascorbic acid levels in men living alone. This is reversible through congregate feeding.
4. Physical disability which can restrict the possibility of purchasing a good variety of foods, as evidenced by lower intakes of some nutrients by the house-bound elderly with osteoarthritis and other crippling disabilities.[139]
5. Mental disorder, common among the elderly, which is incompatible with selection of a good, balanced diet.

Secondary causes of malnutrition among the elderly include:

1. Malabsorption from various intestinal conditions. The major nutrients affected are fat-soluble vitamins, vitamin B_{12}, folic acid, and calcium. Absorption of the latter two nutrients is impaired by the achlorhydria common in the elderly.
2. Alcoholism, which can affect the nutritional status of the elderly by substituting alcohol for nutrient-rich calorie sources and by reducing absorption of folic acid and some other nutrients.
3. Therapeutic drugs, which can interfere with the absorption and metabolism of nutrients.

The last of these factors, therapeutic drugs, covers a wide range of chemicals used extensively by the elderly. Roe[142] has provided a well-organized classification of the types of adverse effects of drugs on absorption and metabolism of nutrients (Table 7–11). In addition to depressing appetite in some

TABLE 7–11. Drug-Nutrient Interactions

Nutrient	Drug	Cause of Reduced Nutrient Availability
Absorption from Intestine		
Folacin	Cholestyramine	Adsorption to drug
	Bicarbonate	Reduced acidity
	Sulfasalazine	Enteral enzyme inhibition
Calcium	Tetracycline	Chelation
	Neomycin, methotrexate	Mucosal damage
Phosphate	Aluminum hydroxide	Precipitation
Vitamins A, K	Cholestyramine	Adsorption to drug
Vitamin B_{12}	Cimetidine	Achlorhydria
Metabolism		
Folate	Aspirin	Inhibits red cell uptake
	Phenytoin	Increased catabolism
Vitamin D	Isoniazid	Inhibits hydroxylation
	Phenytoin, phenobarbital	Increases catabolism
Vitamin K	Cephalosporin	Inhibits prothrombin carboxylation
Vitamin B_6	Isoniazid	Inhibits pyridoxal kinase

Adapted from Roe. Drug-Nutrient Interactions 1985; *4*:117–135.

cases, specific drugs can reduce absorption of nutrients by suppressing acidity in the upper small intestine (e.g., antacids affecting folate and calcium absorption), by precipitation of a nutrient in a nonabsorbable form (e.g., phosphate by aluminum hydroxide), and by adhesion of the nutrient to a nonabsorbable resin (e.g., cholestyramine binding vitamins A, D, K, and B_{12} and folic acid). In addition, the metabolism of a number of vitamins can be affected adversely by drugs, in particular folic acid and vitamins B_6, D, and K. The mechanisms of these actions vary according to the metabolic pathway of the vitamin. In a number of cases, the precise action of the drug remains uncertain.[142]

Since the elderly are extensive chronic users of drugs, it is desirable for the clinician to be aware of these effects of nutrient utilization and to be able to recognize clinical signs of nutritional deficiency. In the case of drugs cited in Table 7–11, it may be desirable to monitor nutrient status if the patient is to continue on the therapy. Table 7–12 recommends increasing the intakes of certain vitamins for individuals receiving specific drugs known to affect their utilization. Finally, the clinician should be aware that

TABLE 7–12. Recommended Vitamin Intakes for Individuals Receiving Specific Drugs

Drug	Recommended Daily Vitamin Intake	
Phenytoin	Vitamin D	800–1200 IU
	Vitamin K	2–5 mg
	Folacin	0.8–1.2 mg
Sulfasalazine	Folacin	0.8–1.2 mg
Cholestyramine	Vitamin A	5000–10,000 IU
Colestipol	Vitamin D	800–1200 IU
	Folacin	0.8–1.2 mg

From Roe DA. Drug-Nutrient Interactions 1985; *4*:117–135. Reproduced with permission.

a few elderly people presenting in a confusional state may be suffering from acute vitamin deficiencies, especially thiamine and folate deficiencies, which are sometimes precipitated by an acute infection.[125, 143]

Nutritional Evaluation of the Elderly Patient

The preceding section emphasizes risk factors that should alert the clinician to the possibility of malnutrition in an elderly person. Attempts have been made to formalize evaluation of patients of all ages. For example, Mullen et al.[144, 145] propose a Prognostic Nutritional Index constructed from a combination of serum albumin, triceps skinfold thickness, transferrin concentration in plasma, and delayed hypersensitivity in grades of reactivity. Other clinicians have developed similar formulas that are described in the last section of this volume. However, the elderly patient has additional risk factors that contribute to the clinical evaluation of nutritional status.

Prendergast[146, 147] has devised an approach that recognizes the characteristics of target groups of elderly at special risk of malnutrition. First, from a consideration of age, marital status, living arrangements, financial resources, social relationships, patient's perception of his or her health, and living activities, the physician can establish how well the patient can maintain adequate nutrition. This is followed by an analysis of symptoms that relate to general malnutrition and to specific deficiency diseases. Symptoms of particular relevance to malnutrition include a history of vomiting, diarrhea, difficulty in eating and chewing, recent weight loss, food allergies, and the presence of decubitus ulceration. Factors suggesting malnutrition are explored, including overweight and underweight and recent weight loss. It is also claimed that deficiencies of individual vitamins and minerals may be suspected at this stage because of specific classic signs and symptoms observed during clinical examination; many of these, however, are not specific for nutrient deficiencies and could be misleading. A dietary history is now taken by a trained dietician, while exploration of past medical history can indicate disease (cirrhosis, pancreatitis, gastrectomy, etc.) that affect nutrient utilization. Next, certain basic indicators like those of Mullen[144] and others can be useful in nutritional assessment of the elderly, including weight for height, triceps skinfold thickness, midarm muscle circumference, complete blood count, albumin and transferrin levels, and delayed hypersensitivity. Finally, the drugs used by older patients, including ethanol, can be significant factors in nutrient utilization, especially since chronic therapeutic drug use is common among the elderly.

In conclusion, the evaluation of the nutritional status of the elderly involves more factors than are needed for young patients. The above description provides a screen for identifying risk factors as well as nutrient intakes, and thus alerts the physician to the multifactorial nature of nutritional deficiency in the elderly. For other aspects of evaluating the nutritional status of the elderly, the reader can consult a recent Ross Round-Table report.[148]

References

1. Rowe JW. Health care of the elderly. N Engl J Med 1985; 312:827–835.
2. Katz S, Branch LG, Branson, et al. Active life expectancy. N Engl J Med 1983; 309:1218–1224.
3. Hutchinson M, Munro HN (eds). Nutrition and Aging. Fifth Annual Bristol Myers Symposium on Nutrition Research. New York, Academic Press, 1986.
4. Forbes GB, Reina JC. Adult lean body mass declines with age: some longitudinal observations. Metabolism 1970; 19:653–663.
5. Forbes GB. The adult decline in lean body mass. Hum Biol 1976; 48:161–173.
6. Steen GB, Isaksson B, Svanberg, A. Body composition at 70 and 75 years of age: a longitudinal population study. J Clin Exp Gerontol 1979; 1:185–200.
7. Cohn SH, Vartsky D, Yasumura S, et al. Compartmental body composition based on total body nitrogen, potassium and calcium. Am J Physiol 1980; 239:E524–530.
8. Munro HN, Young VR. Urinary excretion of N^τ-methylhistidine (3-methylhistidine): a tool to study metabolic responses in relation to nutrient and hormonal status in health and disease in man. Am J Clin Nutr 1978; 31:1608–1614.
9. Uauy R, Winterer JC, Bilmazes C, et al. The changing pattern of whole body protein metabolism in aging humans. J Gerontol 1978; 33:663–671.
10. Korenchevsky, V. Physiological and Pathological Aging. New York, Hafner, 1961.
11. Borkan GA, Hults DE, Gerzof SG, et al. Age changes in body composition revealed by computed tomography. J Gerontol 1983; 38:673–677.
12. Lexell J, Henriksson-Larsson K, Sjostrom M. Distribution of different fibre types in human skeletal muscles. 2. A study of cross-sections of whole m. vastus lateralis. Acta Physiol Scand 1983; 117:115–122.
13. Stalberg E, Fawcett PR. Macro EMG in healthy subjects of different ages. J Neurol Neurosurg Psychiatry 1982; 45:870–878.
14. Larsson L, Grimby G, Karlsson J. Muscle strength and speed of movement in relation to age and muscle morphology. J Appl Physiol 1979; 46:451–456.
15. Aniansson A, Gustafsson E. Physical training in elderly men with special reference to quadriceps muscle strength and morphology. Clin Physiol 1981; 1:87–98.
16. Shock NW. Energy metabolism, caloric intake, and physical activity of the aging. In Carlson LA (ed). Nutrition in Old Age (10th Symposium of the Swedish Nutrition Foundation). Uppsala, Almqvist & Wiksell, 1972: 12–23.
17. Silverberg AB. Carbohydrate metabolism and diabetes in the aged. In Ambrecht HJ, Prendergast JM, Coe RM (eds). Nutritional Intervention in the Aging Process. New York, Springer, 1984: 191–208.
18. Keen H, Fuller JH. The epidemiology of diabetes. In Exton-Smith AN, Caird FC (eds). Metabolic and Nutritional Disorders in the Elderly. Bristol, John Wright & Sons, 1980: 146–160.
19. Rowe JW, Minaker KL, Pallotta JA, et al. Characterization of the insulin resistance of aging. J Clin Invest 1983; 71:1581–1587.
20. Kritchevsky D. Diet, lipid metabolism, and aging. Fed Proc 1979; 38:2001–2006.
21. The Lipid Research Clinics Population Studies Data Book, Vol. I. The Prevalence Study. NIH Publication no. 80–1527. U.S. Dept. of Health and Human Services, 1980: 28–81.
22. Robert J, Bier D, Scholler D, et al. Effect of intravenous glucose on whole body leucine dynamics studied with 1-^{13}C-leucine in healthy young adult and elderly subjects. J Gerontol 1984; 39:673–681.
23. Golden MHN, Waterlow JC. Total protein synthesis in elderly people: a comparison of results of ^{15}N-glycine and ^{14}C-leucine. Clin Sci 1977; 53:227–238.
24. Gersovitz M, Munro HN, Udall J, et al. Albumin synthesis in young and elderly subjects using a new stable isotope methodology: response to level of protein intake. Metabolism 1980; 29:1075–1086.
25. Shock N, Greulich RC, Andres R, et al. Normal Human Aging: The Baltimore Longitudinal Study of Aging. NIH Publication no. 84–2450. U.S. Dept. of Health and Human Services, 1984.
26. Miles WR. In Gerard RN (ed). Methods in Medical Research. Chicago, Year Book Medical Publishers, 1950: 154–156.
27. Carlson LA. Introduction. In Carlson LA (ed). Nutrition in Old Age (10th Symposium of the Swedish Nutrition Foundation). Uppsala, Almqvist & Wiksell, 1972: 9–11.
28. Minaker KL, Meneilly GS, Rowe JW. Endocrine systems. In Finch CE, Schneider EL (eds). Handbook of the Biology of Aging. 2nd ed. New York, Van Nostrand–Rheinhold, 1985: 433–456.
29. Adelman RC. Impaired hormonal regulation of enzyme activity during aging. Fed Proc 1975; 34:179–182.
30. Hausman PB, Weksler ME. Changes in the immune response with age. In Finch CE, Schneider EL (eds). Handbook of the Biology of Aging. 2nd ed. New York, Van Nostrand–Rheinhold, 1985: 414–432.
31. James SJ, Makinodan T. Nutritional intervention during immunological aging: past and present. In Armbrecht HJ, Prendergast JM, Coe RM (eds). Nutritional Intervention in the Aging Process. New York, Springer, 1984: 209–227.
32. Chandra RK, Joshi P, Au B, et al. Nutrition and immunocompetence of the elderly: effect of short-term nutritional supplementation on cell-mediated immunity and lymphocyte subsets. Nutr Res 1982; 2:223–232.
33. Finch CE, Schneider EL (eds). Handbook of the Biology of Aging. 2nd ed. New York, Van Nostrand–Rheinhold, 1985.

34. Finch CE, Landfield PW. Neuroendocrine and autonomic functions in aging mammals. *In* Finch CE, Schneider EL (eds). Handbook of the Biology of Aging. 2nd ed. New York, Van Nostrand–Rheinhold, 1985: 567–594.

35. Duara R, London ED, Rapoport SI. Changes in structure and energy metabolism of the aging brain. *In* Finch CE, Schneider EL (eds). Handbook of the Biology of Aging. 2nd ed. New York, Van Nostrand–Rheinhold, 1985: 595–616.

36. Cotman CW, Holets VR. Structural changes at synapses with age: plasticity and regeneration. *In* Finch CE, Schneider EL (eds). Handbook of the Biology of Aging. 2nd ed. New York, Van Nostrand–Rheinhold, 1985: 617–644.

37. Rogers J, Bloom FE. Neurotransmitter metabolism and function in the aging nervous system. *In* Finch CE, Schneider EL (eds). Handbook of the Biology of Aging. 2nd ed. New York, Van Nostrand–Rheinhold, 1985: 645–691.

38. Dement W, Richardson G, Prinz P, et al. Changes of sleep and wakefulness with age. *In* Finch CE, Schneider EL (eds). Handbook of the Biology of Aging. 2nd ed. New York, Van Nostrand–Rheinhold, 1985: 692–717.

39. Wurtman RJ. Nutrients that modify brain function. Sci Am 1982; *246*:50–59.

40. Cherkin A. Effects of nutritional factors on memory function. *In* Armbrecht HJ, Prendergast JM, Coe RM (eds). Nutritional Intervention in the Aging Process. New York, Springer, 1984: 229–249.

41. Guigoz Y, Munro HN. Nutrition and aging. *In* Finch CE, Schneider EL (eds). Handbook of the Biology of Aging. 2nd ed. New York, Van Nostrand–Rheinhold, 1985: 878–893.

42. McCay CM, Crowell MF, Maynard LA. The effect of retarded growth upon the length of the life-span and upon ultimate body size. J Nutr 1935; *10*:63–79.

43. Nolen GA. Effect of various restricted dietary regimens on the growth, health and longevity of albino rats. J Nutr 1972; *102*:1477–1494.

44. Weindruch R, Walford RL. Dietary restriction in mice beginning at 1 year of age: effect on life-span and spontaneous cancer incidence. Science 1982; *215*:1415–1418.

45. Goodrick CL, Ingram DK, Reynolds MA, et al. Effects of intermittent feeding upon growth, activity, and lifespan in rats allowed voluntary exercise. Exp Aging Res 1983; *9*:203–209.

46. Berg BN. Pathology and aging. *In* Everitt A, Burgess JA (eds). Hypothalamus, Pituitary and Aging. Springfield, IL, Charles C Thomas, 1976: 43–67.

47. Ross MH. Nutrition and longevity in experimental animals. *In* Winick M (ed). Nutrition and Aging. New York, John Wiley & Sons, 1976: 23–41.

48. McCarter RJM, Masoro EJ, Yu BP. Rat muscle structure and metabolism in relation to age and food intake. Am J Physiol 1981; *242*:R89–R93.

49. Bertrand HA, Lynd FT, Masoro EJ, et al. Changes in adipose mass and cellularity through the adult life of rats fed ad libitum or a life-prolonging restricted diet. J Gerontol 1980; *35*:827–835.

50. Liepa GU, Masoro EJ, Bertrand HA, et al. Food restriction as a modulation of age-related changes in serum lipids. Am J Physiol 1980; *238*:E253–E257.

51. Voss KH, Masoro EJ, Anderson W. Modulation of age-related loss of glucagon-promoted lipolysis by food restriction. Mech Ageing Dev 1982; *18*:135–149.

52. Yu BP, Bertrand HA, Masoro EJ. Nutrition-aging influence of catecholamine-promoted lipolysis. Metabolism 1980; *29*:438–444.

53. Reaven EP, Reaven GM. Structure and function changes in the endocrine pancreas of aging rats with reference to the modulating effects of exercise and calorie restriction. J Clin Invest 1981; *68*:75–84.

54. Segall PE, Ooka H, Rose K, et al. Neural and endocrine development after chronic tryptophan deficiency in rats.

55. Levin P, Janda JK, Joseph JA, et al. Dietary restriction retards the age-associated loss of rat striatal dopaminergic receptors. Science 1981; *241*:561–562.

56. Merry BJ, Holehan AM. The endocrine response to dietary restriction in the rat. *In* Woodhead AD, Blackett AD, Hollaender A (eds). Molecular Biology of Aging. New York, Plenum, 1985: 117–141.

57. Weindruch R, Gottesman SR, Walford RL. Modification of age-related immune decline in mice dietarily restricted from or after mid-adulthood. Proc Natl Acad Sci USA 1982; *79*:898–902.

58. Weindruch RH, Suffin SC. Quantitative histologic effects on mouse thymus of controlled dietary restriction. J Gerontol 1980; *35*:525–531.

59. Good RA. Nutrition and immunity. J Clin Immunol 1981; *1*:3–11.

60. Liu JJ, Segre D, Gelberg HB, et al. Effects of long-term treatment of mice with anti-J-monoclonal and life-span. Mech Ageing Dev 1984; *27*:359–372.

61. Miller DS, Payne PR. Longevity and protein intake. Exp Gerontol 1968; *3*:231–234.

62. Kayser J, Neumann J, Lavolley, J. Effets favorables exerces sur la longevite du rat Wistar par divers types de restrictions vitaminiques. CR Acad Sci (D) (Paris) 1972; *274*:3593–3596.

63. Hurd ER, Johnston JM, Okita JR, et al. Prevention of glomerulonephritis and prolonged survival in New Zealand black/New Zealand white F_1 hybrid mice fed on essential fatty acid–deficient diet. J Clin Invest 1981; *67*:476–485.

64. Beach RS, Gershwin ME, Hurley LS. Nutritional factors and autoimmunity. Prolongation of survival in zinc-deprived NZB-W mice. J Immunol 1982; *128*:308–313.

65. Energy and protein requirements. Report of a joint FAO/WHO/UNU meeting, 1981. WHO Technical Report Series. No. 724. Geneva, World Health Organization, 1985.

66. Recommended Dietary Allowances. 9th revised edition. Washington, DC, National Academy of Sciences, 1980.

67. McGandy RB, Barrows CH, Spanias A, et al. Nutrient intakes and energy expenditure in men of different ages. J Gerontol 1966; *21*:581–587.

68. Elahi VK, Elahi D, Andres R, et al. A longitudinal study of nutritional intake in men. J Gerontol 1983; *38*:162–180.

69. Stiedemann M, Jansen C, Harrill I. Nutritional status of elderly men and women. J Am Diet Assoc 1978; *73*:132–139.

70. Exton-Smith AN, Stanton BR. Report of an Investigation into the Dietary of Elderly Women Living Alone. London, King Edward's Hospital Fund, 1965.

71. Debry G, Bleyer R, Martin JM. Nutrition of the elderly. J Hum Nutr 1977; *31*:195–204.

72. Munro HN. An introduction to nutritional aspects of protein metabolism. *In* Munro HN, Allison JB (eds). Mammalian Protein Metabolism. Vol. 2. New York, Academic Press, 1964: 3–39.

73. Prentice AM, Davies HL, Black AE, et al. Unexpectedly low levels of energy expenditure in healthy women. Lancet 1985; *1*:1419–1422.

74. Ten-State Survey: Highlights. DHEW Publication no. HSM 72–8134. U.S. Dept. of Health, Education and Welfare, 1972.

75. Department of Health and Social Security: A Nutrition Survey of the Elderly. Reports on Health Soc. Subj. no. 16. London, Her Majesty's Stationery Office, 1979.

76. Munro HN. Protein nutriture and requirement in elderly people. Bibl Nutr Dieta 1983; *33*:61–74.

77. Munro HN. Historical perspective on protein requirements. *In* Blaxter K, Waterlow JC (eds). Nutritional Adaptation in Man. London, Libby, 1985: 155–167.

78. Munro HN, Young VR. New approaches to the assessment of protein status in man. *In* Howard AN, Baird IM (eds). Recent Advances in Clinical Nutrition. London, Libby, 1981: 33–41.

I. Brain monoamine and pituitary responses. Mech Ageing Dev 1978; *7*:1–7.

79. Cuthbertson DP, Munro HN. A study of the effect of overfeeding on the protein metabolism of man. III. The protein saving effect of carbohydrate and fat when superimposed on diet adequate for maintenance. Biochem J 1937; *31*:694–705.

80. Munro HN. General aspects of the regulation of protein metabolism by diet and by hormones. *In* Munro HN, Allison JB (eds). Mammalian Protein Metabolism. Vol. 1. New York, Academic Press, 1964: 381–481.

81. Kishi K, Miyatani S, Inoue G. Requirement and utilization of egg protein by Japanese young men with marginal intakes of energy. J Nutr 1978; *108*:658–669.

82. Cheng AHR, Gomez A, Gergan JC, et al. Comparative nitrogen balance study between young and aged adults using three levels of protein intake from a combination of wheat-soy-milk mixtures. Am J Clin Nutr 1978; *31*:12–22.

83. Zanni E, Calloway DH, Zezulka AY. Protein requirement of elderly men. J Nutr 1979; *109*:513–524.

84. Uauy R, Scrimshaw NS, Young VR. Human protein requirements: nitrogen balance response to graded levels of egg protein in elderly men and women. Am J Clin Nutr 1978; *31*:779–785.

85. Gersovitz M, Motil K, Munro HN, et al. Human protein requirements: assessment of the adequacy of the current recommended dietary allowance for dietary protein in elderly men and women. Am J Clin Nutr 1982; *35*:6–14.

86. Tuttle SG, Bassett SH, Griffith, WH, et al. Further observations on the amino acid requirements of older men. II. Methionine and lysine. Am J Clin Nutr 1965; *16*:229–231.

87. Watts JW, Mann AN, Bradley L, et al. Nitrogen balances of men over 65 fed the FAO and milk patterns of essential amino acids. J Gerontol 1964; *19*:370–378.

88. Tontisirin K, Young VR, Rand WM, et al. Plasma threonine response curve and threonine requirements of young men and elderly women. J Nutr 1974; *104*:495–505.

89. Tontisirin K, Young VR, Miller M, et al. Plasma tryptophan response curve and tryptophan requirements of elderly people. J Nutr 1973; *103*:1220–1228.

90. Brenner BM, Meyer TW, Hostetter TH. Dietary protein and the progressive nature of kidney disease. N Engl J Med 1982; *307*:652–659.

91. Riggs BL, Wahner HW, Seeman E, et al. Changes in bone mineral density of the proximal femur and spine with aging. Differences between the postmenopausal and senile osteoporosis syndromes. J Clin Invest 1982; *70*:716–723.

92. Gern SM. Bone loss and aging. *In* Farmer A (ed). Nutrition of the Aged. Calgary, University of Calgary, 1977: 73–90.

93. Heaney RP, Gallagher JC, Johnston CC, et al. Calcium nutrition and bone health in the elderly. Am J Clin Nutr 1982; *36*:986–1013.

94. Nordin BEC. Calcium metabolism and bone. *In* Exton-Smith AN, Caird FI (eds). Metabolic and Nutritional Disorders in the Elderly. Bristol, John Wright & Sons, 1980: 123–145.

95. Markovic V, Kostial K, Simonovic I, et al. Bone status and fracture rates in two regions of Yugoslavia. Am J Clin Nutr 1979; *32*:540–549.

96. Horsman A, Gallagher JC, Simpson M, et al. Prospective trial of oestrogen and calcium in postmenopausal women. Br J Med 1977; *2*:789–792.

97. Recker RR, Saville PD, Heaney RP. Effect of estrogens and calcium carbonate on bone loss in postmenopausal women. Ann Intern Med 1977; *87*:649–655.

98. Heaney RP, Recker RR, Saville PD. Menopausal changes in calcium balance performance. J Lab Clin Med 1978; *92*:953–963.

99. Horsman A, Jones M, Francis R, et al. The effect of estrogen dose on postmenopausal bone loss. N Engl J Med 1983; *309*:1405–1407.

100. Anand CR, Linksweiler HM. Effect of protein intake on calcium balance of young men given 500 mg calcium daily. J Nutr 1974; *104*:695–700.

101. Bengoa JM, Sitrin MD, Wood RJ, et al. Amino acid induced hypercalciuria in patients on total parenteral nutrition. Am J Clin Nutr 1983; *38*:264–269.

102. Spencer H, Kramer L, Osis D, et al. Effect of a high protein (meat) intake on calcium metabolism in man. Am J Clin Nutr 1978; *31*:2167–2180.

103. Heaney RP, Recker RR. Effects of nitrogen, phosphorus and caffeine on calcium balance in women. J Lab Clin Med 1982; *99*:46–55.

104. Parfitt AM, Gallagher JC, Heaney RP, et al. Vitamin D and bone health in the elderly. Am J Clin Nutr 1982; *36*:1014–1031.

105. Gallagher JC, Riggs BL, Eisman J, et al. Intestinal calcium absorption and serum vitamin D metabolites in normal subjects and osteoporotic patients. J Clin Invest 1979; *64*:729–736.

106. Slovik DM, Adams JS, Neer RM, et al. Deficient production of 1,25-dihydroxyvitamin D in elderly osteoporotic patients. N Engl J Med 1981; *305*:372–374.

107. Armbrecht HJ, Wongsurawat N, Zenser TV, et al. Differential effects of parathyroid hormone on the renal 1,25-dihydroxy-vitamin D_3 and 24,25-dihydroxyvitamin D_3 production of young and adult rats. Endocrinology 1982; *111*:1339–1344.

108. Aloia JF, Cohn SH, Babu T, et al. Skeletal mass and body composition in marathon runners. Metabolism 1978; *27*:1793–1796.

109. Aloia JF, Cohn SH, Ostuni, et al. Prevention of involutional bone loss by exercise. Ann Int Med 1978; *89*:356–358.

110. Krølner B, Toft B, Nielse SP, et al. Physical exercise as prophylaxis against involutional vertebral bone loss: a controlled trial. Clin Sci 1983; *64*:541–546.

111. Smith EL, Reddan W, Smith PE. Physical activity and calcium modalities for bone mineral increase in aged women. Med Sci Sports Exerc 1981; *13*:60–63.

112. Lynch SR, Finch CA, Monsen ER, et al. Iron status of elderly Americans. Am J Clin Nutr 1982; *36*:1032–1045.

113. Cook JD, Finch CA, Smith NJ. Evaluation of the iron status of a population. Blood 1976; *48*:449–455.

114. Dallman PR, Yip R, Johnson C. Prevalence and causes of anemia in the United States, 1976–1980. Am J Clin Nutr 1984; *39*:437–445.

115. Gershoff SN, Brusis OA, Nino HV, et al. Studies of the elderly in Boston. I. The effects of iron fortification on moderately anemic people. Am J Clin Nutr 1977; *30*:226–234.

116. Lipschitz DA, Mitchell CO, Thompson C. The anemia of senescence. Am J Hematol 1981; *11*:47–54.

117. Garry PJ, Goodwin JS, Hunt WC, et al. Nutritional status in a healthy elderly population: dietary and supplemental intakes. Am J Clin Nutr 1982; *36*:319–331.

118. Dibble MV, Brin M, Thiele VF, et al. Evaluation of the nutritional status of elderly subjects with a comparison between fall and spring. J Am Geriatr Soc 1967; *15*:1031–1061.

119. Sandstead HJ, Henriksen LK, Greger JL, et al. Zinc nutriture in the elderly in relation to taste acuity, immune response and wound healing. Am J Clin Nutr 1982; *36*:1046–1059.

120. Golden MHN. Trace elements. *In* Exton-Smith AN, Caird FI (eds). Metabolic and Nutritional Disorders in the Elderly. Bristol, John Wright & Sons, 1980: 45–58.

121. Henzel JH, DeWeese MS, Lichti EL. Zinc concentrations in healing wounds. Arch Surg 1970; *100*:349–357.

122. Cuthbertson DP, Fell GS, Smith CM, et al. Metabolism after injury. I. Effects of severity, nutrition and environmental temperature on protein, potassium, zinc, and creatine. Br J Surg 1972; *59*:925–931.

123. Haeger K, Lanner E, Magnusson PO. Oral zinc sulfate in the treatment of venous leg ulcer. *In* Pories WJ, Strain WH, Hsu JM (eds). Clinical Applications of Zinc Metab-

olism. Springfield, IL, Charles C Thomas, 1974: 158–167.

124. Hallbook T, Lanner E. Serum-zinc and healing of venous leg ulcers. Lancet 1972; 2:780–782.

125. Exton-Smith AN. Vitamins. In Exton-Smith AN, Caird FI (eds). Metabolic and Nutritional Disorders in the Elderly. Bristol, John Wright & Sons, 1980: 26–38.

126. Iber FL, Blass JP, Brin M, et al. Thiamin in the elderly—relation to alcoholism and to neurological degenerative disease. Am J Clin Nutr 1982; 36:1067–1082.

127. Sauberlich HE, Herman YF, Stevens CO, et al. Thiamin requirement of the adult human. Am J Clin Nutr 1979; 32:2237–2248.

128. Vir SC, Love AHG. Nutritional status of institutionalized and noninstitutionalized aged in Belfast, Northern Ireland. Am J Clin Nutr 1979; 32:1934–1947.

129. McGandy RB, Russell BM, Jacob RA, et al. Nutritional status survey of healthy non-institutionalized elderly: nutrient intakes from 3-day diet records and nutrient supplements. Nutr Res, in press.

130. Danford DE, Munro HN. The liver in relation to the B vitamins. In Arias I, Popper H, Schachter D, et al. (eds). The Liver: Biology and Pathobiology. New York, Raven Press, 1982: 367–384.

131. Rosenberg IH, Bowman BB, Cooper BA, et al. Folate nutrition in the elderly. Am J Clin Nutr 1982; 36:1060–1066.

132. Nutrition Canada: Food Consumption Patterns Report. Ottawa, Department of National Health and Welfare, 1977.

133. Jagerstad M, Westesson E-K. Folate. Scand J Gastroenterol 1979; 14(suppl 52):196–202.

134. Russell RM, Rosenberg IH, Wilson PD, et al. Increased urinary excretion and prolonged turnover time of folic acid during ethanol ingestion. Am J Clin Nutr 1983; 38:64–70.

135. Russell RM, Kraskinski SD, Samloff IM. Correction of impaired folic acid (PTE GLU) absorption by orally administered HCl in subjects with gastric atrophy. Am J Clin Nutr 1984; 39:656 (abstr).

136. Andrews J, Letcher M, Brook M. Vitamin supplementation in the elderly: 17 month trial in an old person's home. Br Med J 1969; 2:416–418.

137. Burr ML, Hurley RJ, Sweetman PM. Vitamin C supplementation of old people with low blood levels. Gerontol Clin 1975; 17:236–243.

138. Schorah CJ, Tormey WD, Brooks GH, et al. The effect of vitamin C supplements on body weight, serum proteins, and general health of an elderly population. Am J Clin Nutr 1981; 34:871–876.

139. Exton-Smith AN. Nutritional status: diagnosis and prevention of malnutrition. In Exton-Smith AN, Caird FI (eds). Metabolic and Nutritional Disorders in the Elderly. Bristol, John Wright & Sons, 1980: 66–76.

140. Baker H, Frank O, Thind IS, et al. Vitamin profiles in elderly persons living at home or in nursing homes versus profiles in healthy young subjects. J Am Geriatr Soc 1979; 27:444–450.

141. Jacob RA, Hartz SC, Russell RM, et al. The effects of vitamin supplement usage on biochemical indicators of nutritional status in the elderly. Fed Proc 1982; 42:830 (abstr).

142. Roe DA. Drug effects on nutrient absorption, transport and metabolism. Drug-Nutrient Interactions 1985; 4:117–135.

143. Carney MWP. Vitamin deficiencies and excesses: behavioral consequences in adults. In Galler JR (ed). Nutrition and Behavior: Human Nutrition, Vol. 5. New York, Plenum, 1984: 193–222.

144. Mullen JL, Busby JP, Waldman MT, et al. Prediction of operative morbidity and mortality by preoperative nutritional assessment. Surg Forum 1979; 30:80–82.

145. Busby GP, Mullen JL, Matthews DC, et al.: Prognostic Nutritional Index in gastrointestinal surgery. Am J Surg 1980; 139:160–167.

146. Prendergast JM. Nutritional evaluation of the institutionalized elderly. In Armbrecht JH, Prendergast JM, Coe RM (eds). Nutritional Intervention in the Aging Process. New York, Springer, 1984: 289–292.

147. Wolinsky FD, Prendergast JM, Miller DK, et al. A preliminary validation of a nutritional risk measure for the elderly. Am J Prevent Med 1985; 1:53–59.

148. Redfern DE (ed). Addressing the Nutrition State of the Elderly—State of the Art. Columbus, OH, Ross Laboratories, 1982.

8

OBESITY

OLIVER E. OWEN

DEFINITION OF OBESITY

Obesity is the excessive accumulation of fat in the adipose tissue. It is a normal variant among humans of different body types. In most humans it develops in the absence of disease, including endocrine disorders. However, when the mass of adipose tissue fat exceeds 30 per cent of the body weight and is largely distributed to upper parts of the body (such as the nape of the neck, shoulders and abdomen), it constitutes a health hazard. The accumulated fat increases body weight. Thus, obesity and overweight are related, but not necessarily interdependent: overweight signifies increased body weight relative to height and can be induced by enlargement of any tissue, such as occurs with muscle hypertrophy; obesity reflects an increased proportion of body weight induced by excessive fat mass.

Fat is a normal constituent of the body; it serves as a cushion for viscera, as an insulator for the body, and as an energy depot. Human survival depends on the ability to ingest food rapidly and to store nutrients in an economical form.[1] The most efficient nutrient or fuel depot should have the highest calorie:weight ratio, should be able to supply the substrate requirements for all tissues, and should be expendable without adverse effects.[1] Fat has the highest caloric potential per unit of weight and is readily expendable. During starvation, fat catabolism either directly or indirectly furnishes almost all of the various tissue energy requirements.[1] Even the energy utilized to synthesize glucose from amino acids and glycerol, and the energy from recycled lactate and pyruvate are derived from the oxidation of free fatty acids (FFA).[2]

The fat deposited as fuel is stored primarily in adipose tissue. The maximum capacity of adipose tissue to enlarge is undefined but is known to be huge.

ETIOLOGY OF OBESITY

In his 1962 presidential address to the Endocrine Society,[3] Astwood stated: "Obesity is a disorder which, like venereal disease, is blamed upon the patient. The finding that treatment doesn't work is ascribed to lack of fortitude. Corpulence in America is regarded along with narcotic addiction as something wicked." He proposed that "obesity is an inherited disease and due to a genetically determined defect." Although everyone recognizes that stature, skin color, and foot size are largely determined by genes, Astwood was sure that his concept that obesity or one's shape was primarily influenced by genes would "be accepted with reluctance." Astwood acknowledged the roles of physical inactivity and excessive eating. Nonetheless, he stressed that obesity among humans, like selective breeding among animals, was genetically determined. He further suggested that our societal conviction that gluttony was primarily responsible for obesity had discouraged genetic investigation, and meaningful information pertaining to the inheritance of obesity was scant.[3] Subsequently, genetic studies of twins suggested that human obesity is highly heritable.[4]

In 1986 Stunkard and co-workers examined the contributions of genetic factors and the family environment to human body fat content in 540 adult adoptees.[4] Using the body mass index as an indicator of leanness and fatness, they divided the adoptees into four weight classes: thin, median, overweight, and obese. Their results showed a strong relation between the weight class of the adoptees and the body mass index of their biological parents. On the other hand, no relation existed between the weight class of the adoptees and the body mass index of their adoptive parents. The genetic influences manifested in this study extended across the whole range of body composition from very thin to morbidly obese. This is extremely strong evidence that genetic influences are primary in determining fatness in adult humans, and family environment alone has limited influences. However, obesity tissue and thus fatness can be manifested only in an environment that provides nutritional abundance: Caloric intake must exceed caloric expenditure to induce gains in obesity tissue.

There are varying degrees of inherited influences from polygenic and/or major genic sources, and, therefore, differing efforts are needed to prevent the wide-ranging expression of obesity. In mild forms of obesity body fatness can be easily regulated by dietary intake and exercise, whereas in extreme forms of obesity maintenance of body fat reduction is awesomely difficult. Nonetheless, abdominal (android) obesity is accompanied by a heightened incidence of morbidity and mortality, and legitimate means should be employed to reduce body fat. Invariably, oxidizable caloric intake over a protracted time must be less than metabolic requirements. This is accomplished by decreasing food consumption and/or augmenting energy expenditure.

DISTRIBUTION AND NATURE OF ADIPOSE TISSUE

Subcutaneous adipose tissue is distributed over the entire body, with some extra deposits in the breasts, buttocks, and thighs in women and in the abdomen in men. There are also large deposits of adipose tissue located deep in the body. These depots are primarily located in the mesenteric, perirenal, and pericardial areas. There are differences among the adipose tissue depots. Adipocytes around the waist and flanks appear to be metabolically more active than those located in the buttocks and thighs.[5] These fat cells have increased catecholamine receptors, which facilitate lipolysis.[5]

Adipocytes are composed of thin, pliable rims of cell wall and cytoplasm surrounding relatively large droplets of liquid fat. The area of the cell containing the nucleus is thickened and gives the cell the appearance of a signet ring in a microscopic section. Adipocytes have the unique responsibility of storing the esters of long-chain fatty acids. This fuel depot is commonly referred to as intracellular neutral lipids or triglycerides. The deposition of triglycerides in adipocytes induces enlargement of adipose tissue, manifested by an increase in fat cell size and fat cell number. In childhood obesity there is an increased number of adipocytes (hyperplasia). Apparently, hyperplasia decreases with age until adolescence. Thereafter, the number of fat cells increases very little. Therefore, in most obese adults, gains in adipose tissue masses are accompanied by increased sizes of the adipocytes (hypertrophy). However, in persons with extreme obesity there may be both hypertrophy and hyperplasia of fat cells.[6] Adipocytes increase in weight (size) to a maximum weight of about 0.7 to 0.8 μg/cell. An increase in adipocyte number occurs after the "maximal" adipocyte weight (size) has been obtained.[6]

Women have more body fat then men at any relative body weight. With obesity, more of the feminine body fat is distributed over the gluteal and femoral regions of the body. This form of obesity is referred to as peripheral or lower body obesity. It characterizes the gynoid pattern of fat distribution. With masculine obesity, more of the body fat is located in the abdomen, shoulders, and nape of the neck. This form of obesity is referred to as upper body obesity. It characterizes the android pattern of fat distribution. Although there is a general difference in fat distribution between the sexes, there is a high percentage of overlap, especially at the two extremes of the life span.[6–8]

Another system of subgrouping the apparent heterogeneity of human obesity is based on the cellular characteristics of the adipose tissue: hypertrophic obesity, which is due to enlarged fat cells, and hyperplastic obesity, which is due to an increased number of fat cells.[9,10] However, as noted above, there is also overlap within this system.

The vast majority of the adipose tissue in humans is white fat. There is a small amount of brown fat in infants, but the presence and the role of this form of adipose tissue in adults are poorly defined.

MEASUREMENTS OF ADIPOSE TISSUE

The information related to body fat and obesity gathered during the first two thirds of this century is limited by the available techniques to measure body composition. Furthermore, the diagnosis of obesity is arbitrary, and judgment varies among different societies. Thus, the presence or absence of obesity is formulated in the mind of the examiner. Visual appraisal is the most frequent means of assessment: If a person looks fat, that person is fat, according to the examiner.[11]

Body fat can be assessed by height:weight ratio, direct chemical analysis, densitometry, skinfold thickness, total body water, total exchangeable potassium, and fat-soluble (inert) gas uptake.[12] Validation of all these techniques is questionable, and variability among the methods is wide. Thus, current methods for estimating body fat are useful but not always exact.

The diagnosis of obesity is frequently based on the comparison of a subject's weight to a standard reference table.[12] Sex, age, and frame are taken into consideration. The comparison is usually expressed as a percentage of relative body weight: The individual's weight is a percentage of the mean weight of a reference population. If an individual is grossly heavier than an average reference human, it is reasonable to assume that he or she is overweight and fat. However, except in extreme cases, relative body weight is not a reliable index of fatness.[12]

The Metropolitan Life Insurance Company has formulated height and weight tables for many years. The most recently available tables were developed in 1983, and were based on pooled data of 25 United States and Canadian insurance companies with about 4.2 million policies.[13] People with known heart disease, cancer, and diabetes were screened out to isolate the effects of weight on longevity. However, nutritional factors, tobacco consumption, and other activities in life were not eliminated. Tables 8–1 (English system) and 8–2 (metric system) present weights based on the lowest mortality for men and women between 25 and 59 years of age. Males and females are presented according to weight, height, and body frame. Elbow breadth is highly correlated with anthropometric measurements, and weight tables are shown for small, medium, and large frames. Instructions for determining frame size are given in Table 8–3.[13]

It should be noted that in 1983 values of body weights of adult men and women were greater than those published in the 1959 Metropolitan Life Insurance Table without any adverse effects on lon-

TABLE 8–1. 1983 Metropolitan Height and Weight Tables for Men and Women
According to Frame, Ages 25–59

Height (In Shoes)†		Weight in Pounds (In Indoor Clothing)*		
Feet	Inches	Small Frame	Medium Frame	Large Frame
MEN				
5	2	128–134	131–141	138–150
5	3	130–136	133–143	140–153
5	4	132–138	135–145	142–156
5	5	134–140	137–148	144–160
5	6	136–142	139–151	146–164
5	7	138–145	142–154	149–168
5	8	140–148	145–157	152–172
5	9	142–151	148–160	155–176
5	10	144–154	151–163	158–180
5	11	146–157	154–166	161–184
6	0	149–160	157–170	164–188
6	1	152–164	160–174	168–192
6	2	155–168	164–178	172–197
6	3	158–172	167–182	176–202
6	4	162–176	171–187	181–207
WOMEN				
4	10	102–111	109–121	118–131
4	11	103–113	111–123	120–134
5	0	104–115	113–126	122–137
5	1	106–118	115–129	125–140
5	2	108–121	118–132	128–143
5	3	111–124	121–135	131–147
5	4	114–127	124–138	134–151
5	5	117–130	127–141	137–155
5	6	120–133	130–144	140–159
5	7	123–136	133–147	143–163
5	8	126–139	136–150	146–167
5	9	129–142	139–153	149–170
5	10	132–145	142–156	152–173
5	11	135–148	145–159	155–176
6	0	138–151	148–162	158–179

*Indoor clothing weighing 5 pounds for men and 3 pounds for women.

†Shoes with 1-inch heels.

Source of basic data. Build Study, 1979, Society of Actuaries and Association of Life Insurance Medical Directors of America, 1980.

Courtesy of Statistical Bulletin, Metropolitan Life Insurance Company.

gevity,[13] even though these tables were designed to examine the effects of obesity on longevity.

The degree of obesity can be expressed as percentage over average weight for sex, height, and frame. Although the assessment of obesity is judgmental, individuals with body weights that exceed average body weight by 15 to 30 per cent, 30 to 50 per cent, 50 to 100 per cent, or more than 100 per cent are classified as having mild, moderate, severe, or morbid obesity, respectively.

Another method for establishing body fat or the degree of obesity is calculation of the body mass index, which is the weight in kilograms divided by the square of the height in meters. However, body composition varies widely among humans with different somatotypes: endomorphy (roundness), mesomorphy (muscularity), and ectomorphy (leanness). In the extreme example, men who compete

TABLE 8–2. 1983 Metropolitan Height and Weight Tables for Men and Women on Metric Basis
According to Frame, Ages 25–59

Height (In Shoes)† Centimeters	MEN Weight in Kilograms (In Indoor Clothing)*			Height (In Shoes)† Centimeters	WOMEN Weight in Kilograms (In Indoor Clothing)*		
	Small Frame	Medium Frame	Large Frame		Small Frame	Medium Frame	Large Frame
158	58.3–61.0	59.6–64.2	62.8–68.3	148	46.4–50.6	49.6–55.1	53.7–59.8
159	58.6–61.3	59.9–64.5	63.1–68.8	149	46.6–51.0	50.0–55.5	54.1–60.3
160	59.0–61.7	60.3–64.9	63.5–69.4	150	46.7–51.3	50.3–55.9	54.4–60.9
161	59.3–62.0	60.6–65.2	63.8–69.9	151	46.9–51.7	50.7–56.4	54.8–61.4
162	59.7–62.4	61.0–65.6	64.2–70.5	152	47.1–52.1	51.1–57.0	55.2–61.9
163	60.0–62.7	61.3–66.0	64.5–71.1	153	47.4–52.5	51.5–57.5	55.6–62.4
164	60.4–63.1	61.7–66.5	64.9–71.8	154	47.8–53.0	51.9–58.0	56.2–63.0
165	60.8–63.5	62.1–67.0	65.3–72.5	155	48.1–53.6	52.2–58.6	56.8–63.6
166	61.1–63.8	62.4–67.6	65.6–73.2	156	48.5–54.1	52.7–59.1	57.3–64.1
167	61.5–64.2	62.8–68.2	66.0–74.0	157	48.8–54.6	53.2–59.6	57.8–64.6
168	61.8–64.6	63.2–68.7	66.4–74.7	158	49.3–55.2	53.8–60.2	58.4–65.3
169	62.2–65.2	63.8–69.3	67.0–75.4	159	49.8–55.7	54.3–60.7	58.9–66.0
170	62.5–65.7	64.3–69.8	67.5–76.1	160	50.3–56.2	54.9–61.2	59.4–66.7
171	62.9–66.2	64.8–70.3	68.0–76.8	161	50.8–56.7	55.4–61.7	59.9–67.4
172	63.2–66.7	65.4–70.8	68.5–77.5	162	51.4–57.3	55.9–62.3	60.5–68.1
173	63.6–67.3	65.9–71.4	69.1–78.2	163	51.9–57.8	56.4–62.8	61.0–68.8
174	63.9–67.8	66.4–71.9	69.6–78.9	164	52.5–58.4	57.0–63.4	61.5–69.5
175	64.3–68.3	66.9–72.4	70.1–79.6	165	53.0–58.9	57.5–63.9	62.0–70.2
176	64.7–68.9	67.5–73.0	70.7–80.3	166	53.6–59.5	58.1–64.5	62.6–70.9
177	65.0–69.5	68.1–73.5	71.3–81.0	167	54.1–60.0	58.7–65.0	63.2–71.7
178	65.4–70.0	68.6–74.0	71.8–81.8	168	54.6–60.5	59.2–65.5	63.7–72.4
179	65.7–70.5	69.2–74.6	72.3–82.5	169	55.2–61.1	59.7–66.1	64.3–73.1
180	66.1–71.0	69.7–75.1	72.8–83.3	170	55.7–61.6	60.2–66.6	64.8–73.8
181	66.6–71.6	70.2–75.8	73.4–84.0	171	56.2–62.1	60.7–67.1	65.3–74.5
182	67.1–72.1	70.7–76.5	73.9–84.7	172	56.8–62.6	61.3–67.6	65.8–75.2
183	67.7–72.7	71.3–77.2	74.5–85.4	173	57.3–63.2	61.8–68.2	66.4–75.9
184	68.2–73.4	71.8–77.9	75.2–86.1	174	57.8–63.7	62.3–68.7	66.9–76.4
185	68.7–74.1	72.4–78.6	75.9–86.8	175	58.3–64.2	62.8–69.2	67.4–76.9
186	69.2–74.8	73.0–79.3	76.6–87.6	176	58.9–64.8	63.4–69.8	68.0–77.5
187	69.8–75.5	73.7–80.0	77.3–88.5	177	59.5–65.4	64.0–70.4	68.5–78.1
188	70.3–76.2	74.4–80.7	78.0–89.4	178	60.0–65.9	64.5–70.9	69.0–78.6
189	70.9–76.9	74.9–81.5	78.7–90.3	179	60.5–66.4	65.1–71.4	69.6–79.1
190	71.4–77.6	75.4–82.2	79.4–91.2	180	61.0–66.9	65.6–71.9	70.1–79.6
191	72.1–78.4	76.1–83.0	80.3–92.1	181	61.6–67.5	66.1–72.5	70.7–80.2
192	72.8–79.1	76.8–83.9	81.2–93.0	182	62.1–68.0	66.6–73.0	71.2–80.7
193	73.5–79.8	77.6–84.8	82.1–93.9	183	62.6–68.5	67.1–73.5	71.7–81.2

*Indoor clothing weighing 2.3 kilograms for men and 1.4 kilograms for women
†Shoes with 2.5 cm heels
Source of basic data Build Study, 1979. Society of Actuaries and Association of Life Insurance Medical Directors of America
Courtesy of Statistical Bulletin, Metropolitan Life Insurance Company.

in physical exhibitions to demonstrate their muscularity after prolonged power-lifting to develop huge hypertrophic muscles may be grossly overweight for their heights and frames but have below normal body fat content.[14] Furthermore, tall athletes such as professional basketball players may have body mass indices that erroneously suggest excessive body fat based on height and weight tables. This is most likely due to muscle and bone densities and masses of aerobically trained, and especially black, athletes which are greater than those of normal reference humans used to estimate body mass indices or body compositional variables. Nonetheless, on the whole, body mass indices are a useful tool for estimating obesity, and a nomogram is available[15] (Fig. 8–1). The normal values for body mass indices range from 20 to 25. A body mass index between 25 and 30 usually reflects borderline to moderate excessive body fat, and a body mass index greater than 30 reflects obesity.

Fatness can also be expressed as a percentage of the body mass. In adults, a percentage of fat greater than 20 per cent of body mass for males and greater than 25 per cent for females characterizes obesity. The percentage of body fat can be calculated for men and women from body mass indices:[11,16]

Male % body fat

$$= 1.218 \times \text{body mass index} - 10.13$$

Female % body fat

$$= 1.48 \times \text{body mass index} - 7$$

Direct estimates of body fat can be made using the Archimedes principle. The method is based on the assumption that the body can be considered as two compartments: the fat compartment, which has a density of about 0.91, and the fat-free compartment,

TABLE 8–3. How to Determine Your Body Frame by Elbow Breadth

To make a simple approximation of your frame size:

Extend your arm and bend the forearm upwards at a 90-degree angle. Keep the fingers straight and turn the inside of your wrist toward the body. Place the thumb and index finger of your other hand on the two prominent bones on either side of your elbow. Measure the space between your fingers against a ruler or a tape measure. (For the most accurate measurement, have your physician measure your elbow breadth with calipers.) Compare this measurement with the measurements shown below.

These tables list the elbow measurements for men and women of medium frame at various heights. Measurements lower than those listed indicate that you have a small frame while higher measurements indicate a large frame.

MEN

Height (In 1-inch Heels)	Elbow Breadth (Inches)	Height (In 2.5 cm. Heels)	Elbow Breadth (Centimeters)
5'2"–5'3"	2½"–2⅞"	158–161	6.4–7.2
5'4"–5'7"	2⅝"–2⅞"	162–171	6.7–7.4
5'8"–5'11"	2¾"–3"	172–181	6.9–7.6
6'0"–6'3"	2¾"–3⅛"	182–191	7.1–7.8
6'4"	2⅞"–3¼"	192–193	7.4–8.1

WOMEN

Height (In 1-inch Heels)	Elbow Breadth (Inches)	Height (In 2.5-cm. Heels)	Elbow Breadth (Centimeters)
4'10"–4'11"	2¼"–2½"	148–151	5.6–6.4
5'0" –5'3"	2¼"–2½"	152–161	5.8–6.5
5'4" –5'7"	2⅜"–2⅝"	162–171	5.9–6.6
5'8" –5'11"	2⅜"–2⅝"	172–181	6.1–6.8
6'0"	2½"–2¾"	182–183	6.2–6.9

Source of basic data: Data tape, HANES I–Anthropometry, goniometry, skeletal age, bone density, and cortical thickness ages 1–74. National Health and Nutrition Examination Survey, 1971–75. National Center for Health Statistics.

Courtesy of Statistical Bulletin, Metropolitan Life Insurance Company.

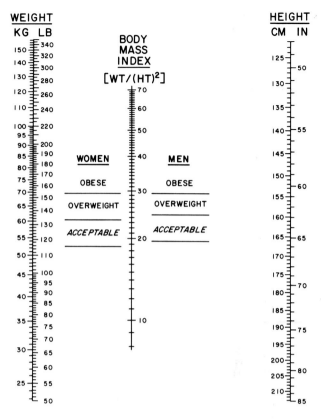

FIGURE 8–1. Nomogram for determining body mass index. A straight edge is attached from the individual's weight on the left side to the point on the right hand line, which corresponds to his or her height. The body mass index is the point at which this line connecting weight and height crosses the central vertical lines. (Reproduced with permission of G. A. Bray, 1986.)

which has a density of about 1.10. The reference densities of the fat compartment and the fat-free compartment are the average values derived from direct body analysis of three male cadavers that had substantial variability in their water and protein content. Work done on body composition is far from complete because an insufficient quantity of data was averaged to formulate the widely used "reference body." Yet the classic techniques of densitometry to determine the percentages of body that are assumed to be fat or fat-free are based on the "reference body." In addition, the lack of knowledge pertaining to the effects of varying masses or densities of bone in different races and ages, of muscle in aerobically trained athletes, and of small and large adipocytes[12] on the assessment of body fat is worrisome. Nonetheless, densitometry is used to calculate the per cent of the body that is assumed to be fat.

Body density is determined from the specific gravity of the body: Weight of the body completely submerged under water is divided by the body weight out of water; corrections for gastrointestinal and respiratory gases are made. No universal formula is used to calculate the body composition, but the for-

mulas developed by Brozek and co-workers give results similar to those of others.[11,17,18]

Underwater weighing for densitometric analysis is conducted in a large tank in which a heavy chair of known weight is suspended from a scale.[17,19] The underwater weighing procedure is repeated several times until three readings within 25 g are obtained. Residual lung volume is determined by the nitrogen washout technique,[17] and body composition is computed:[17,19]

$$\text{Fat mass (kg)} = \text{kg wt} \times \frac{4.570}{\text{density} - 4.142}$$

$$\text{Density} = \text{kg wt in air} \div$$
$$\left(\frac{\text{kg wt in air} - \text{kg under water}}{\text{water density}} \right.$$
$$\left. - \text{residual lung volume} - 0.10 \right)$$

$$\text{Fat-free mass (kg)} = \text{kg wt} - \text{fat mass (kg)}$$

Skinfold thickness is the most convenient and widely used method to diagnose obesity. Through this indirect technique estimates of body density and, therefore, body fat and fat-free masses can be made.

On average about one half of the total body fat is distributed just beneath the skin. Deep deposits of fat in the abdominal and chest cavities and in the retroperitoneal spaces make up the other half. However, the fraction of subcutaneous fat varies from 0.1 to 0.7. Age, sex, and ethnic differences influence body fat distribution. Thus, estimates of body fat based on skinfold thickness have a wide potential for error. Therefore, it is important to visually examine any individual to add perspective to the values obtained from skinfold thickness measurements. Sometimes weight may be more useful than skinfold measurements. With these qualifications in mind, skinfold measurements made by trained observers usually estimate body fat within 4 or 5 per cent of that estimated by densitometry.[20] However, the fatter the person, the greater the error in estimating body fat.

Standardization of calipers and methods used for measuring skinfold thickness is necessary for universal comparability of results. Skinfold thickness should be measured to the nearest 0.5 mm. The measurement is made on a double thickness of "pinched-up" skin and subcutaneous adipose tissue held between the thumb and index finger and gently pulled away from the body. The calipers should be placed about 1 cm away from the examiner's thumb and finger tips toward the underlying muscle. The caliper should exert a constant pressure of 10 g/mm^2 on a contact surface of 20 to 40 mm.^{2} If the skinfold is extremely thick, the reading from the measuring dial should be made 3 seconds after applying the calipers.[21]

Measurements of skinfold thickness over the biceps, triceps, subscapular, and suprailiac areas provide responsible estimates of body fat and obesity. Although the use of these four sites best correlates to body fat, an acceptable method employs only the triceps and/or the subscapular areas.[21] In general, there is little difference when a single skinfold site has been used to construct a table to estimate body fat. The triceps skinfold is located midway between the shoulder and elbow. The nondominant arm should be used to make the measurement, and the arm should hang freely during the procedure.

Table 8–4 relates the skinfold thickness over the triceps area to percentiles for whites in the United States.[22]

Tables of height:weight ratio, densitometry, and skinfold thickness are frequently used to estimate body fat percentages or masses. Other techniques are more esoteric and demand skilled personnel and equipment available only in special laboratories. Dilutional techniques are rarely used but can partition the body into water-soluble (fat-free) and fat-soluble (fat) components. The volume of water in the fat-free compartment of the body can be measured by isotopic dilutional methods employing radioactive hydrogen (^{3}H or ^{2}H). By dividing the concentration of water into the total water content of the body, an estimate of fat-free mass can be made. The fat mass of the body can be calculated as the difference between total body mass and fat-free mass. The reliability of these estimates depends upon the accuracy of measuring the volume of water in the body and the concentration of water in the fat-free tissues. Both measurements have limitations and collectively induce twofold errors in body fat estimates.[23]

Estimates of the high-energy-requiring and potassium-containing mass (fat-free mass, lean body mass, body cell mass) reflecting active protoplasmic tissues can be made either by isotope dilution of exchangeable radioactive potassium (^{42}K) or by determining potassium (^{40}K) in the body by using a whole body counter. About 97 per cent of total body potassium is intracellular. Approximately 90 per cent of the body potassium is exchangeable with its isotope, and total body potassium can be counted in a whole body counter with an error of about 5 per cent. The value widely used as the potassium content of fat-free body tissue is based on the analysis of four adult cadavers and is 68.1 mEq/kg (range 66.5 to 72.0 mEq/kg). Grande and Keys suggested values of 64.4 mEq/kg for men and 57.7 mEq for women, while others have proposed values of 63.3 mEq/kg for men and 64.0 mEq/kg for women.[23] Body potassium concentration changes with sex, age, hydration, disease states, and nutritional status.[23] In addition, the potassium concentration of lean tissue is not constant. Therefore, estimates of lean body mass based on assumed potassium concentration in fat-free tissue have serious limitations. Nevertheless, measurements of body potassium for estimating the fat-free mass are useful although not absolute values. Estimates for lean body (fat-free) mass can be calculated:

$$\text{Fat free mass} = \frac{\text{total body potassium}}{68}$$

Fat-soluble gas uptake has been used to estimate total body fat mass. Gases that are highly soluble in lipids but not in water separate the fat compartment from the aqueous, fat-free compartment. This method uses partition coefficients of substances at equilibrium on two sides of diffusing membranes. By knowing the partition coefficient of the gas between the aqueous and lipid compartments, estimates of body fat can be calculated.[23] However, the body is not composed of two compartments, one aqueous and the other lipid. The partition coefficients for brain, liver, kidney, muscle, and adipose tissue are each different for the many gases employed.[23] Some gases used (e.g., cyclopropane) induce deep anesthesia. In addition, they may require airtight systems and need extended periods of time

TABLE 8–4. Percentiles for Triceps Skinfold for Whites of the United States Health and Nutrition Examination Survey I of 1971 to 1974

Age Group	Triceps Skinfold (mm) Percentiles															
	n	5	10	25	50	75	90	95	n	5	10	25	50	75	90	95
	Males								Females							
1–1.9	228	6	7	8	10	12	14	16	204	6	7	8	10	12	14	16
2–2.9	223	6	7	8	10	12	14	15	208	6	8	9	10	12	15	16
3–3.9	220	6	7	8	10	11	14	15	208	7	8	9	11	12	14	15
4–4.9	230	6	6	8	9	11	12	14	208	7	8	8	10	12	14	16
5–5.9	214	6	6	8	9	11	14	15	219	6	7	8	10	12	15	18
6–6.9	117	5	6	7	8	10	13	16	118	6	6	8	10	12	14	16
7–7.9	122	5	6	7	9	12	15	17	126	6	7	9	11	13	16	18
8–8.9	117	5	6	7	8	10	13	16	118	6	8	9	12	15	18	24
9–9.9	121	6	6	7	10	13	17	18	125	8	8	10	13	16	20	22
10–10.9	146	6	6	8	10	14	18	21	152	7	8	10	12	17	23	27
11–11.9	122	6	6	8	11	16	20	24	117	7	8	10	13	18	24	28
12–12.9	153	6	6	8	11	14	22	28	129	8	9	11	14	18	23	27
13–13.9	134	5	5	7	10	14	22	26	151	8	8	12	15	21	26	30
14–14.9	131	4	5	7	9	14	21	24	141	9	10	13	16	21	26	28
15–15.9	128	4	5	6	8	11	18	24	117	8	10	12	17	21	25	32
16–16.9	131	4	5	6	8	12	16	22	142	10	12	15	18	22	26	31
17–17.9	133	5	5	6	8	12	16	19	114	10	12	13	19	24	30	37
18–18.9	91	4	5	6	9	13	20	24	109	10	12	15	18	22	26	30
19–24.9	531	4	5	7	10	15	20	22	1060	10	11	14	18	24	30	34
25–34.9	971	5	6	8	12	16	20	24	1987	10	12	16	21	27	34	37
35–44.9	806	5	6	8	12	16	20	23	1614	12	14	18	23	29	35	38
45–54.9	898	6	6	8	12	15	20	25	1047	12	16	20	25	30	36	40
55–64.9	734	5	6	8	11	14	19	22	809	12	16	20	25	31	36	38
65–74.9	1503	4	6	8	11	15	19	22	1670	12	14	18	24	29	34	36

From Frisancho, AR. Am J Clin Nutr *34*:2540–2545, 1981. © Am J Clin Nutr, American Society for Clinical Nutrition. Reproduced with permission.

to equilibrate in the tissues. In today's milieu it is unlikely that the Institutional Review Board for the protection of human welfare will permit all the research needed to validate fat-soluble gas uptake techniques for measuring body composition.

Many measurements of body fat (adipose tissue) rest upon multiple layers of uncertainties. For example, the use of skinfold thickness to estimate body fat depends on the uncertain accuracy of body densitometry. Furthermore, potassium concentrations in lean tissues are not constant, and fat-soluble gases are not limited to adipose tissue. Accurate means to measure body fat are needed.

Newer anthropometric measurements for characterizing obesity continue to evolve. One technique employs measurements of the circumference of the waist and hips (and thighs) and calculates the waist/hip circumference ratio. It is a simple way to depict obesity, and allows the professional health provider to determine body fat distribution. Waist circumference, in centimeters or inches, is highly dependent upon the size of the individuals examined. Using the ratio of the waist to hip circumferences overcomes the body size variable and estimates central and peripheral fat distribution. The circumferences of body parts should be measured with the person in the erect position, around the waist at a height one-third of the distance between the xiphoid process and the umbilicus, and around the hips at a point 4 cm below the superior anterior iliac spine.[6] The available information suggests that men and women with a waist/hip ratio of greater than 1.0 and 0.8, respectively, have upper body (android) obesity and should lose body fat.[24]

CALORIC VALUE OF ADIPOSE TISSUE

Isolated adipocytes of white fat from well-nourished humans are about 85 per cent pure fat. Unfortunately, this observation has led to a confusion about changes in caloric value of the body during weight gain or loss. Changes in adipose tissue mass are associated with several changes in other tissue masses not confined to adipocytes. For example, during weight gain more muscle, blood, extracellular fluid, connective tissue, and skin are needed to support and maintain the increased adipose tissue mass. The obesity tissue that develops during weight gain as a consequence of overeating consists of about 62 per cent pure fat, 24 per cent active protoplasmic tissue, and 14 per cent extracellular water.[23] In normal men and women with a pure fat mass of 15 and 25 per cent of body weight, respectively, the quantity of active protoplasmic tissue associated with it is not large. However, the quantity of the pure fat mass is among the most variable components of the body, and with morbid obesity may reach weights exceeding 100 kg. In such distorted individuals the accompanying active protoplasmic tissue can be estimated to be about 39 kg. This is in addition to the other lean tissues (muscle, heart, liver, kidney, etc.) of the body. Thus, humans with massive obesity have large quantities of active protoplasmic tissue masses associated with their huge amounts of pure fat. This is becoming generally recognized as more humans undergo body compositional measurements (Fig. 8–2).

In acknowledging the fact that lean tissue or active protoplasmic mass increases as body fat increases, it should be evident that the caloric value of obesity tissue is less than the widely held value of 7700 kcal/kg (3500 kcal/lb). Since gains in obesity tissue are about 14 per cent fluid, 62 per cent fat, and 24 per cent active protoplasmic tissue, of which only 20 per cent of the latter is protein, the caloric value of weight loss should be about equal to the caloric value of weight gain. Thus, the energy equivalent of obesity tissue is about 5772 kcal/kg (2624 kcal/lb), assuming a caloric value of 9 kcal/g for fat and 4 kcal/g for protein.

ADIPOSE TISSUE METABOLISM

The metabolic requirements of adipose tissue (but not obesity tissue) per unit of weight are low because about 85 per cent of the mass is due to the weight of the stored triglycerides. However, the rims of the active protoplasmic tissue that encase the fat droplets have energy requirements comparable to those of hepatocytes when expressed per unit of cell protein. The cytoplasmic masses of the adipocytes are actively storing triglycerides and mobilizing fatty acids and glycerol continuously.

In good or excessive nutritional states the adipose tissue is the fuel depot of the body. Its chemical reserve in gross obesity can exceed a million calories.

Adipose tissue is in a continuous state of flux, storing and mobilizing lipids. The vast majority of lipid stored in adipose tissue is from dietary sources. Dietary lipids are mostly in the form of triglycerides. These triglycerides contain saturated and unsaturated long-chain fatty acids. Ingested fat is crushed in the mouth, churned in the stomach, digested in the duodenum, and absorbed in the small intestine. Lipids are absorbed as fatty acids and monoglycerides and are bound to intracellular proteins. The immediate metabolism of intracellular lipid is influenced by the lengths of the fatty acid chains. Long-chain fatty acids and monoglycerides are reesterified to triglycerides and packaged with cholesterol and phospholipids in apoprotein envelopes to form chylomicrons. These chylomicrons are secreted into the lacteals of the lymphatic system and are destined for distribution to the capillaries of the adipose tissue. Short-chain fatty acids are released into the portal blood, bound to albumin, transported to the liver, elongated, combined with phospholipids, cholesterol, and apoproteins to form a very low density lipoprotein, and released into the blood. They are also transported to the capillaries of the adipose tissue.

The C-II apoproteins of the chylomicrons and the very low density lipoproteins serve to guide these water-soluble lipids to specific tissue receptor sites located on the surface walls of the capillary endothelium of adipose tissue. Thus, as the blood traverses the white fat of the body, the triglyceride core of chylomicrons and very low density lipoproteins are delivered to their target tissue.[25]

The capillary endothelium of adipose tissue (and muscle) possesses lipoprotein lipase, which is activated by insulin and C-II apoproteins contained in

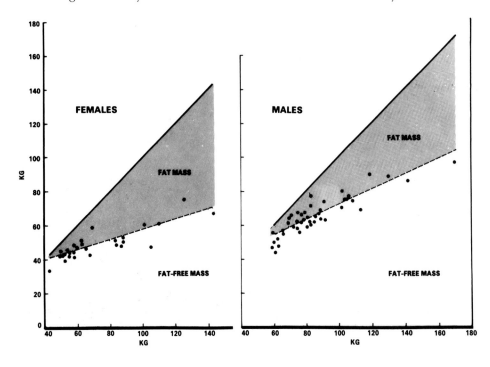

FIGURE 8–2. Total body weight, fat-free mass, and fat mass in healthy lean and obese females and males. (From Owen OE, Holup J, D'Alessio DA, et al. Am J Clin Nutr, in press, 1987. © Am J Clin Nutr, American Society for Clinical Nutrition. Reproduced with permission.)

the envelope of the chylomicrons and the very low density lipoproteins. Triglyceride-rich chylomicrons and very low density lipoproteins bind to the capillary walls, and the activated lipase liberates fatty acids and monoglycerides. The fatty acids and monoglycerides pass through the endothelium into the adipocytes and undergo reesterification to form stored triglycerides.[25]

After a meal containing carbohydrates as well as fat, postprandial hyperglycemia stimulates insulin secretion, and in addition, contributes to the formation of glycerol-3-phosphate (alpha-glycerol phosphate). The insulin augments glucose translocation from the extracellular space to the intracellular space. Glycolysis produces alpha-glycerol phosphate. This glycerol serves as the intracellular backbone for the reesterification of intracellular fatty acids.[25]

The net balance of the dynamic flux of fatty acids into and out of adipocytes in healthy humans is dependent upon the quantity and the caloric value of food consumed during a given observation time. When macronutrients exceed energy requirements during the postprandial period, lipid deposition occurs, and during caloric deprivation lipid depletion occurs.

After a meal laden with calories is eaten, the energy expenditure of the body rises (Fig. 8–3). This is known as the thermic effect of food (specific dynamic action), and was described about 100 years ago. The thermic effect of food depends upon the nature[26] and the quantity of food ingested.[27] It occurs in all healthy individuals, whether lean or obese. When a usual mixed meal is eaten, the caloric challenge is so large that most of the nutrients are disposed of by nonoxidative (storage) pathways during the first few postprandial hours. The greater the caloric challenge, the greater the storage becomes as a means of depositing nutrient excess. The storage

of food requires energy and is probably the main determinant of the thermic effects of food.

Figure 8–4 displays carbohydrate, fat, and protein storage in healthy lean males after four different breakfasts containing different caloric contents but constant proportions of carbohydrates, fat, and protein. Although the protein content of meals in most industrialized nations is only 15 per cent of the caloric load, when a large meal is eaten the protein load is large. In contrast to the potentially massive caloric stores of lipid in adipose tissue and the small yet significant storage of carbohydrates as glycogen in liver and muscle, there is no specific depot for proteins or amino acids. Nonetheless, once protein repletion occurs and there is no further gain in protein storage, the excessive amino acids can be converted into glucose and/or into lipids. Therefore, total protein storage resembles glucose storage in that they are both linearly related to intake.[28,29] Once oxidative requirements are met and storage depots are repleted, the excessive carbon skeletons of amino acids in glucose can be converted into long-chain fatty acids and stored as triglycerides in adipose tissues. The majority of the nonoxidative disposition of glucose is via glycogen synthesis and storage in liver and muscle. The postprandial nonprotein respiratory quotient only transiently rises above unity (1). Therefore, the net quantity of carbohydrate converted into fat is probably trivial. Postprandial lipid storage is also linearly related to intake. Thus, in a manner similar to the storage of protein and carbohydrate, when mixed meals are eaten that contain large caloric intakes, the vast majority of the ingested fat is stored as triglycerides.[28,29] Regardless of body weight, caloric excess predisposes the human body to gains in "obesity tissues."

The importance of the adipose tissue fuel depot in sustaining energy requirements was recognized long before it was discovered that free fatty acids (FFA) were released from stored triglycerides[30] and

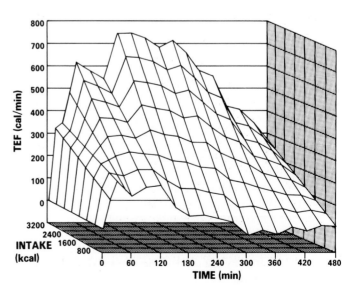

FIGURE 8–3. Three-dimensional response surface generated from resistant regression lines relating caloric intake to the thermic effects of food during an 8-hr study period.

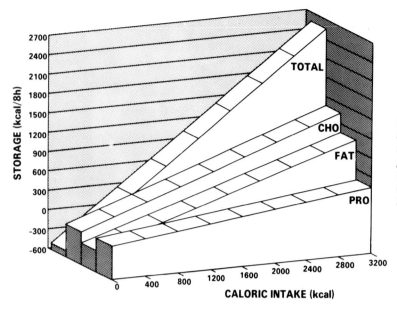

FIGURE 8–4. The relationships between carbohydrate, fat, and protein storage and caloric intake of mixed meals displayed with resistant regression lines. Quantities of carbohydrate, fat, protein, and total equivalents of macronutrients were summed over 8 hr following the ingestion of progressively increasing caloric content of the mixed meals.

served as the primary transport of lipids destined for oxidative metabolism during caloric deprivation. FFA represents the only form of lipid released from adipose tissue triglyceride stores. They travel in the blood stream tightly bound, but not covalently bound, to albumin. Physiologically, plasma FFA concentrations vary from 0.1 mmol/L after a carbohydrate meal to 2.0 mmol/L during starvation. After an overnight fast the plasma FFA concentration is about 0.5 mmol/L and composes about 10 per cent of the total plasma lipid concentration. Their turnover rates are extremely rapid in all nutritional states.

In 1956 it was discovered that FFA mobilized from stored triglycerides served as the primary transport form,[30] and subsequently it was shown[28] that there was a reciprocal relationship between carbohydrate and FFA oxidation by many tissues: When carbohydrate oxidation is high, fatty acid oxidation is low, and vice versa.[28] An increased release rate of FFA from adipose tissue is associated with an increased activity of hormone-sensitive lipase. A wide variety of hormones (catecholamines, glucagon, vasopressin, growth hormone, cortisol, and ACTH) stimulate lipolysis through a GTP-binding N protein and adenylate cyclase, which activates the cyclic AMP cascades to turn on hormone-sensitive lipase.[30] The importance of hormone-sensitive lipase regulation during starvation resides in its control of FFA mobilization, since the uptake of FFA from the plasma for energy-yielding oxidation by muscle, liver, kidney, and other tissues, is largely, but not completely, dependent upon the plasma concentration of FFA.[31]

The catecholamines play the cardinal role of hormones in mobilizing FFA. The availability of these hormones, specifically norepinephrine, is continuously modulated by the tone of the sympathetic nervous system. Beta$_1$ and alpha$_2$ adrenergic receptors are located on the plasma membranes of human adipocytes. Both of these adrenergic receptors are coupled to the adenylate cyclase system, but they have opposing influences on lipolysis by activating different plasma membrane GTP-binding N proteins that either stimulate (beta$_1$-adrenergic receptors) or inhibit (alpha$_2$-adrenergic receptors) the catalytic unit that activates the cyclic AMP cascade.[32] The anatomical distribution of the sympathetic nervous system and the preponderance of alpha$_2$- or beta$_1$-adrenergic receptors influence the deposition and mobilization of adipocyte triglycerides; thus, the differential location and size of the body fat depots are influenced by the sympathetic nervous system as reflected by the relative activities of receptors inhibiting or stimulating mobilization of FFA from adipocytes.

Progressing from the postabsorptive state into the prolonged starved state, there is a gradual decrease in the blood glucose concentration from about 70 to 80 down to 50 to 60 ml/dl during the initial 3 days of fasting. The decrease in blood glucose is paralleled by a decrease in serum insulin concentration.[2] During starvation the facilitated translocation of glucose by insulin from the extracellular to the intracellular space is diminished, intracellular availability of alpha-glycerophosphate from catabolized glucose is low, reesterification of intracellular fatty acids is diminished, and augmented FFA release occurs. In addition, fasting enhances the lipolytic effects of epinephrine and norepinephrine[33] by increasing the beta-adrenergic receptor sensitivity to catecholamines. During total starvation norepinephrine secretion may increase and reinforce lipolysis.[33,34]

Growth hormone secretion is episodic during starvation.[2] It is the primary stimulus for the production of somatomedins, and changes in plasma growth hormone and somatomedins occur in parallel.[35] Since malnutrition reduces serum somatomedin concentrations, it is unlikely that they induce lipolysis directly or indirectly. Synergistic with norepinephrine, glucagon and perhaps vasopressin act directly and in concert to augment lipolysis.[30] Iodothyronines and glucocorticoids apparently act permissively to stimulate the release of FFA from adipose tissue. T_4 and/or T_3 increase the concentrations of both alpha-adrenergic and beta-adrenergic receptors.[32] In addition, these iodothyronines augment receptor coupling to the adenylate cyclase system.[32] Thus, thyroid hormonal influences on receptor number and function explain the well known augmented adrenergic responsiveness that occurs in hyperthyroidism.

The possible roles of beta-lipotropin, beta-endorphin, and delta-melanocyte as stimulators of lipolysis are unclear.

In the presence of physiologic hypoglycemia, hypoinsulinemia, and hyperglucagonemia the heightened sensitivity to the lipolytic effect of norepinephrine becomes manifest. The plasma venous FFA concentration increases, and the oxidation rate of FFA increases two- to threefold, changing the caloric delivery from about 40 per cent to 85 to 90 per cent of total body requirements.

Total starvation has been used not only as a therapeutic but also as a research tool to induce weight loss in obese humans. Weight lost during states of caloric deprivation is complex because the caloric value of tissue lost during weight reduction is not constant. This is most evident in but not limited to patients undergoing total starvation for weight reduction. During the initial days of fasting, diuresis ensues and weight loss is large. Thus, the caloric value per unit of weight is relatively low. However, as starvation progresses beyond a week or two and fluid balance develops, the caloric value per unit of weight is high.[36] During this period of starvation, fat is supplying 85 to 90 per cent of body energy requirements, either by direct oxidation of FFA or by indirect oxidation of ketone bodies, acetoacetate, beta-hydroxybutyrate, and acetone.[36]

In addition to changes in fluid loss and changes in the nature and quantity of fuel oxidized by obese humans undergoing periods of starvation, the hormonal profile alters in a manner that diminishes caloric expenditure per unit of body mass. The sum of these influences results in a gradual decrease in percentage of body weight lost as starvation progresses. Figure 8–5 shows the curvilinear nature of weight loss among men and women undergoing various lengths of starvation.

The diminished caloric requirements of humans undergoing weight reduction is frequently stated and overemphasized. Figure 8–6 reveals data averaged from two morbidly obese women with Type II diabetes mellitus and hypertension. They drank water and took small quantities of Na, K, and Cl while undergoing 23 days of total caloric starvation. Figure 8–6 shows their averaged resting metabolic requirements (RMR), and nature and quantity of glucose, fat, and protein oxidized during their periods of total starvation. It should be noted that their RMR were large. Although their RMR diminished during starvation, the decreases per unit body weight were small. During the initial day their average overnight fasting RMR was 1.603 kcal/min/155.4 kg or 10.35 cal/min/kg. After 23 days their overnight fasting RMR was 1.28 kcal/min/141.5 kg or 9.07 cal/min/kg. Thus, the average reduction in their RMR per unit of body mass was only 13 per cent.

METABOLIC REQUIREMENTS

The regulation of energy metabolism is a matter of increasing importance in the understanding of obesity. Recent studies of energy expenditure in normal adult men and women are presented in Chapter 2. The findings differ significantly from the energy expenditure when calculated from commonly used predictive equations. Because of the importance of this material as background for discussing the development of obesity, much of the information in the following section is repeated from Chapter 2.

The total daily caloric requirements are indicated by body size and state of activity. The RMR of adult humans vary from about 800 to 3000 kcal/day.[28,37,39] Superimposed on this wide range of resting energy requirements are those associated with exercise. Physical activity usually accounts for about 20 to 30 per cent of the daily caloric expenditure.[40] However, the quantity of energy used for physical activity has a large variance. Competitive athletes can consume 10 to 20 times their RMR for minutes to hours during forceful exercise. Although smaller quantities of fuels are expended by those unable to participate in such strenuous activities, nonetheless, considerable amounts of energy stored as fat can be mobilized by exercise in anyone capable of doing augmented physical activity. The effects of exercise on energy requirements, body composition, and changes in body weight are reviewed in Chapter 11.

The RMR for normal humans are based on three large and authoritative studies done during the first half of this century. In 1919, Harris and Benedict published their classic monograph on RMR of males and females.[41] They developed regression formulas for predicting the RMR of men and women based on height, weight, age, and sex. DuBois and DuBois measured the body surface area (BSA) of humans and derived a formula for calculating BSA based on height and weight.[42] Boothby and colleagues (Mayo Foundation) studied males and females[43] and reported in 1922 that the RMR could best be predicted from BSA.[44] Between 1930 and 1950, Robertson and Reid studied males and females and derived regression formulas for predicting RMR based on sex, age, and BSA.[45]

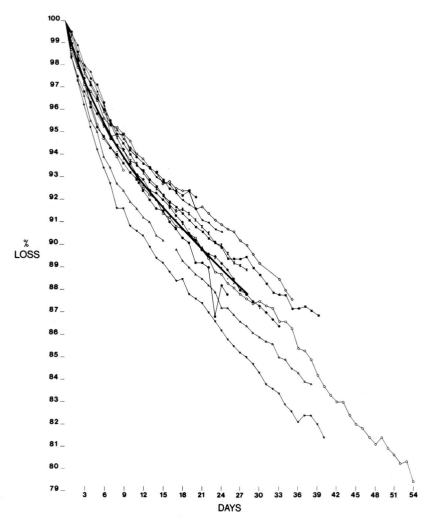

FIGURE 8–5. Weight loss, expressed as percentage of initial body weight in ten obese male and female volunteers who fasted for 9 to 54 days. (From Owen OE, Starvation. In DeGroot LJ [ed]. Endocrinology. 2nd ed. Orlando, Grune & Stratton, in press. Reproduced with permission.)

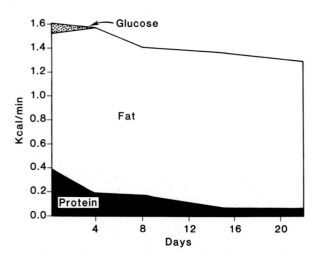

FIGURE 8–6. Caloric and fuel requirements of two morbidly obese Type II diabetic patients undergoing 22 days of total starvation.

The RMR may be the best predictor of overall requirements and usually accounts for 65 to 70 per cent of the daily energy requirements.[37] Values in tables widely used for predicting RMR are smoothed means derived from the studies done in the first half of this century[41–45] and are expressed as calories per m^2 of BSA per hour or day for men and women of given ages.[46] However, modern studies have shown that the Harris and Benedict[41,47] and Mayo[44] equations and the Roberston and Reid tables[45] overestimate the measured RMR of normal lean and obese women[28] and men,[29] of morbidly obese humans,[48] and of malnourished patients.[49] Moreover, the influence of age in mentally and physically healthy humans has little impact on the RMR of females[28] and males.[29]

Figure 8–7 displays modern-day measured RMR contrasted against the most commonly used prediction equations of Harris and Benedict for predicting RMR of men and women. The overestimations are greatest for younger adults, both men and women. As age increases, the overestimations become trivial, absent, or negative. Thus, current studies[28,29] would suggest that the use of antiquated equations and tables for predicting RMR should cease.

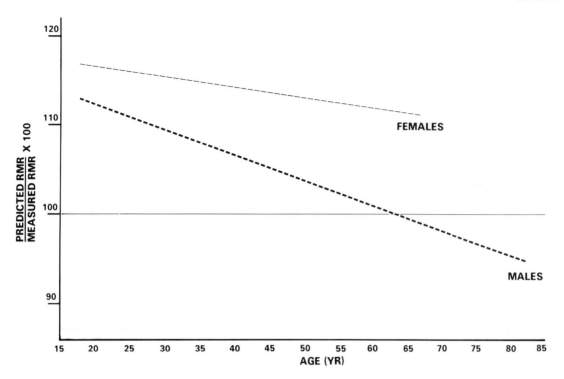

FIGURE 8–7. *The measured RMR of women and men, displayed as 100 per cent, are contrasted against the predicted RMR for women and men based upon the Harris-Benedict equations. (From Owen OE, Holup J, D'Alessio DA, et al. Am J Clin Nutr, in press, 1987. © Am J Clin Nutr, American Society for Clinical Nutrition. Reproduced with permission.)*

A reapprasial of the resting caloric requirements of healthy lean and obese women, some of whom were trained athletes, and men was reported.[28,29] The caloric expenditures were measured by indirect calorimetry. Body compositions were determined by skinfold thickness and densitometric techniques. Ages ranged from 18 to 82 years and body weights from 43 to 171 kg. Stepwise and multiple regression analyses were used to determine whether one or several variables of weight, height, age, or body composition best predicted the RMR of women and men.

It was found that body compositional variables reflecting active protoplasmic tissue such as weight, body surface area, fat free mass as measured by skinfold thickness or by densitometry, lean body mass, and body cell mass were all highly interrelated.[28,29] Therefore, it is extremely difficult to identify which of these variables truly reflects active protoplasmic tissue. Furthermore, the use of combinations of variables to predict RMR is comparable to weight alone in predicting the RMR of women and men. Since weight is the most easily and accurately measured variable and is highly correlated with RMR of humans, it should be used if estimates of RMR are needed for adults. This is not to deny the existence of minor differences among variables that reflect active protoplasmic tissues and RMR. This claim brings forth another issue because it does not support the frequently made claim that RMR correlates best with lean body mass.[50–57] In retrospect, this is not surprising, because the resting energy requirements of various aerobic tissues are vastly different per unit of mass.[58,59] In normal-weight adults the brain and liver constitute about 4 to 5 per cent of total body weight and are responsible for about 40 per cent of the RMR.[23,59] Muscle composes 35 to 40 per cent of body weight but accounts for about 20 per cent of the RMR.[23,59] Adipose tissue constitutes about 15 to 25 per cent of body weight but accounts for only 2 to 5 per cent of RMR.[23,59] These disproportionate rates of energy requirements per mass of different tissues partly explain why the bulk quantity of heterogeneously active protoplasmic tissue correlates about as well with the RMR as does total body weight. These same considerations should be extended to obese and athletic humans. Although the absolute RMR is greater the heavier the man or woman,[40,51,60] there are reduced energy expenditures per kilogram of body weight for lean and obese nonathletic men and women and for athletic women as weight increases. Large variances in body weight occur, not because of major differences in high-energy-requiring brain and liver masses, but because of large differences in the amount of moderate-energy-requiring skeletal muscle mass in athletes, or because of huge differences in the amount of low-energy-requiring adipose tissue mass in obese nonathletes. Thus, a major portion of the RMR in adults is relatively constant because of brain and liver metabolism, but the increases in RMR per kilogram of body weight depend primarily on other body components, particularly skeletal muscle and adipose tissue.

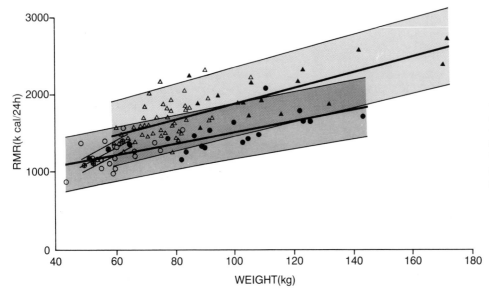

FIGURE 8–8. *The RMR (kcal/24 hr) are contrasted against the weights (kg) of the 44 lean (○) and obese (●) healthy women, 8 of whom were athletes (⊕) and 60 lean (△) and obese (▲) healthy men.*

Figure 8–8 displays the relation between measured RMR and body weight. The slopes of the regression lines for the RMR and weight for nonathletic lean and obese women or for lean and obese men are statistically indistinguishable. Therefore, single regression lines with their 95 per cent confidence limits were developed for the nonathletic healthy lean and obese women (RMR = 795 + 7.18 × weight kg) or lean and obese men (RMR = 879 + 10.2 × weight kg). Note that both nonathletic women and men have wide 95 per cent confidence limits, reflecting the heterogeneous nature of the RMR for lean and obese nonathletic women and men. The regression line for the athletic women (RMR = 50.4 + 21.1 × weight kg) is clearly different from the nonathletic women (p < 0.05), and the 95 per cent confidence limits for the regression line for the athletes are narrow. Similar data for men are not available.

When weight is used as the variable to predict RMR of men or women, the energy requirements per unit of mass are different for the sexes. However, there is no difference between the slopes of the regression lines for predicting the RMR of women and men when fat-free mass (FFM) is used as the variable for predicting RMR. Figure 8–9 shows that the apparent influence of sex on RMR is eliminated when fat-free mass by densitometry or skinfold thickness is used as the variable: male RMR = 290 + 22.3 FFM kg; female RMR = 334 + 19.7 FFM kg. The elimination of the influence of gender on RMR when fat-free mass is used to predict RMR can be explained by the fact that adult women have more stored, relatively inert triglycerides than men per unit of body weight. Correcting for this difference in body composition abolishes the dissimilarity in RMR per unit of weight. However, determining body fat in live humans is difficult. For practical reasons the authors prefer using body weight as a predictor of RMR.

FIGURE 8–9. *The RMR (kcal/24 hr) are contrasted against the fat-free masses (FFMD) by densitometry for 44 lean (○) and obese (●) healthy women, 8 of whom were athletes (⊕), and for 60 lean (△) and obese (▲) healthy men. (From Owen OE, Holup J, D'Alessio DA, et al. Am J Clin Nutr, in press, 1987. © Am J Clin Nutr, American Society for Clinical Nutrition. Reproduced with permission.)*

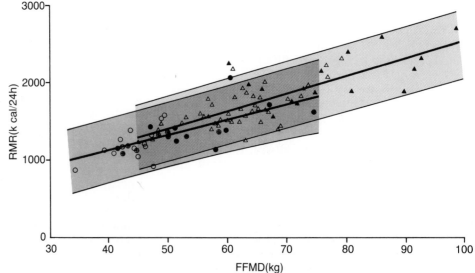

It should be emphasized that, owing to the large variations in measured RMR, the predicted RMR based on weight may over- or underestimate the measured RMR of nonathletic women by 21 to 33 per cent[28] and nonathletic men by 18 to 29 per cent.[29] Closer estimates can be made for athletes. The predicted RMR of a well-trained competitive athlete estimates RMR within 8 to 10 per cent. Athletic women have greater increases in RMR per gain in body weight than nonathletic women (Fig. 8–7). Body weight is also more highly correlated with RMR among athletes (r = 0.94) than among nonathletes (r = 0.74).

The newly developed prediction equations for the RMR of healthy women and men are better than those previously available for humans. The use of weight as the variable for both men and women, which is easily and accurately measured, and eliminating age, simplifies predicting the RMR of humans. However, the usefulness of any RMR prediction equation derived from a population with large 95 per cent confidence limits is questionable. Therefore, if possible, the metabolic requirements of humans should be measured rather than predicted. This added information is most useful in formulating weight reduction programs. Actually measuring rather than predicting should receive strong support because the RMR per kilogram of body weight varies widely among both lean and obese humans. This recently confirmed observation conclusively demonstrates that a metabolic condition such as heightened metabolic efficiency is not necessarily or exclusively related to obesity. Instead, it suggests that both lean and obese healthy humans have wide ranges of metabolic requirements, and some lean as well as some obese humans have a greater predisposition for developing and maintaining body fat.

The postprandial state is also associated with augmented energy expenditure. This heightened metabolic requirement state accompanying food ingestion is referred to as the thermic effects of food (TEF). In humans, TEF has been divided into obligatory energy expenditure associated with eating, digesting, absorbing, and storing food[61] and facultative energy expenditure associated with hormone secretion,[62,63] sodium-potassium-ATPase pump activity,[64] protein synthesis,[65] and substrate recycling.[66,67] TEF is usually considered to account for about 10 to 15 per cent of the total daily energy requirements. However, this differs tremendously, depending upon the nature and quantity of nutrients ingested.

TEF is another component of energy expenditure, and the postprandial rise in caloric expenditure and its relationship to obesity have been the subject of intensive studies during the last decade. Numerous studies have reported that the rise in metabolic rate that follows food ingestion is blunted in obese humans. The authors of these reports claimed that because less nutrients were oxidized, obese people have an increased metabolic efficiency that results in aug-

mented storage of nutrients in body fat.[40,68–70] However, other researchers have failed to show a difference in the TEF between lean and obese humans.[51,71,72] The discrepancies in these reports can largely be explained by inadequate assessment of postprandial thermogenesis in obese humans. Hill and co-workers showed that the TEF increased as the caloric content of the meal increased.[27] Many of the early studies used too small a caloric challenge and too short a postprandial study period to properly assess the differences, if any, in the TEF between lean and obese humans.[73,74] A recent study avoided these problems by investigating TEF in lean and obese males randomly fed mixed meals containing 0, 8, 16, 24, and 32 kcal/kg fat-free mass and measured oxidative and nonoxidative disposal rates of carbohydrate, fat, and protein.[75] Among these males were 3 lean and 3 obese men who coincidentally received similar amounts of foods for 4 different meals. Figure 8–10 is a three-dimensional display of their augmented postprandial resting energy requirements and the time course of the TEF. The data show that the TEF are linearly related to caloric intake, and that the magnitude and duration of augmented postprandial thermogenesis increases linearly with caloric consumption. This study clearly demonstrated that postprandial oxidative macronutrient disposal is not related to body weight or fat-free mass. In fact, postprandial energy expenditure over RMR is independent of leanness and obesity. Thus, a more efficient postprandial metabolism is not a characteristic of obesity. It is of interest to note that in lean and obese humans TEF can be equal to or greater than 30 per cent of the RMR when a huge caloric challenge is ingested.

The nature and quantity of fuels oxidized after eating mixed meals is of general interest. Sitting in the resting state following an overnight fast and eating a small to a large breakfast meal containing 43 per cent carbohydrate, 42 per cent fat, and 15 per cent protein induces rapid changes in macronutrient oxidation rates. Figure 8–11 shows three-dimensional response surfaces generated from resistant regression lines relating the nature and quantity of fuels oxidized by 10 men who ingested 8, 16, 24, and 32 kcal/kg of their fat-free masses. There was a progressive increase in quantity and a delay in maximum amounts of carbohydrate and fat oxidized. A reciprocal relationship between carbohydrate and lipid postprandial oxidation rates developed: as postprandial carbohydrate oxidation increased, lipid oxidation simultaneously decreased, and vice versa. Glucose is preferentially oxidized and fat is preferentially stored during the early postprandial period.[75]

A large proportion of ingested macronutrients are disposed of by nonoxidative (storage) pathways. When energy requirements are met and proteins are repleted, direct or indirect storage of excessive macronutrients is the most important route of fuel dis-

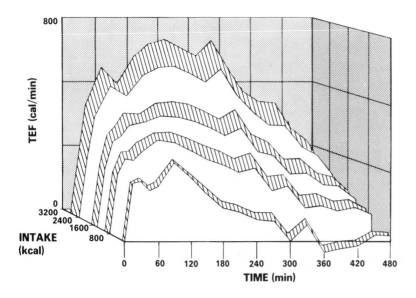

FIGURE 8–10. Mean ± SEM of TEF in three lean and three obese males who ingested four different caloric challenges (490 to 563, 981 to 1127, 1374 to 1552, and 1962 to 2255 kcal) containing 43 per cent carbohydrate, 42 per cent fat, and 15 per cent protein.

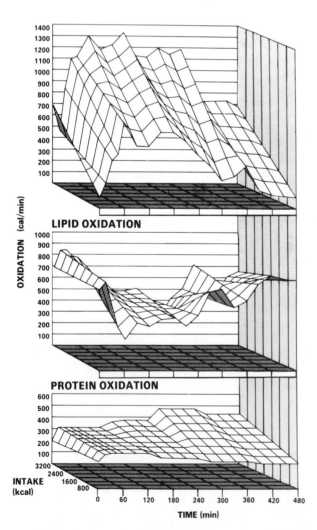

FIGURE 8–11. Three-dimensional response surfaces generated from resistant regression analysis of data from 10 men relating carbohydrate, fat, and protein oxidation with mixed-meal caloric intake.

posal. The larger the incremental increase in caloric intake over expenditure, the greater the quantities of fuels destined for adipose tissue and accompanying fat mass. (See Adipose Tissue Metabolism.) Figure 8–4 shows the relationship between mixed-meal caloric intake and storage of macronutrients. Carbohydrate, fat, and protein storage increase linearly with caloric intake, and nonoxidative disposal of these macronutrients is completed within 8 hours after huge caloric intakes (32 kcal/kg fat-free mass).

Several interrelated hormonal systems influence thermogenesis. The iodothyronines play a cardinal role in regulating the basal and resting metabolic rates but do not change the exercise-induced or diet-induced energy expenditure.[76] The central nervous system is integrated with the sympathadrenomedullary system, and both interrelate with the iodothyronines. Cortisol promotes the release and thermogenic response of the body to norepinephrine and epinephrine, and the catecholamines augment the thermogenic response of the body to L-triiodothyronine.[77] Special emphasis has been attributed to the beta-adrenergic activity of norepinephrine as being responsible for the rise in facultative energy expenditure associated with carbohydrate metabolism.[78,79] Although insulin per se does not exert a thermogenic effect,[80] insulin facilitates intracellular translocation, oxidation, and storage of glucose, reduces lipolysis and augments lipogenesis, and promotes amino translocation and protein synthesis. Furthermore, the heightened circulating postprandial insulin concentration could stimulate the ventromedial hypothalamus and enhance norepinephrine secretion.[78,80] The bioactivity of iodothyronine hormones is considered normal,[37] whereas the bioactivity of catecholamines is controversial in obesity.[51,69,80–82] However, insulin secretion does increase as weight and adiposity increase.[83] Nonetheless, the progressive increase in the RMR and TEF among healthy women with weights ranging from 43 to 143 kg discredits any hypothesis suggesting a uniformly altered or defective thermogenic mechanism related to hormonal secretion, sodium-potassium-ATPase pumping, substrate recycling, or synthetic processing as causes for less or more energy efficient states and, thus, secondary leanness or obesity.

In summary, it has been been demonstrated that (1) the expression of obesity is primarily determined by genetic inheritance and secondarily influenced by the availability of food; (2) the resting metabolic rates of healthy humans are lower than previously recognized; (3) increased metabolic efficiency should no longer be considered as an important cause of obesity in humans; (4) the nature and quantities of nutrients oxidized change dramatically after a mixed meal, with a reciprocal relationship between carbohydrate and fat oxidation; and (5) the storage of excessive macronutrients is approximately proportional to intake.

COMPLICATIONS OF OBESITY

The amount of body fat in the general population varies from inadequate to excessive quantities, and forms a continuum of the percentage of body weight. The risks of developing or having disabilities or illnesses associated with body fat contents are not clearly demarcated. Nevertheless, the stimulus to arbitrarily classify humans as having excessive body fat is based upon the clinical belief that obesity is associated with suffering and death. The primary reason to convert a measurement of body weight into the diagnosis of obesity is the need for a diagnosis to support a decision to initiate therapy.[84] Weight reduction appears to prevent some of the diseases associated with excessive body fat.

Obesity in both men and women is associated with mortality from various causes. Some reports show a U-shaped or J-shaped association, with death rates higher at the upper and the lower extremes of body weight. However, other studies report either monotonic increase or decrease in mortality as weight increases.[84] Nevertheless, the idea that obesity is a risk factor for such medical diseases as ischemic heart disease,[85–87] strokes,[85,87] hypertension,[87,88] diabetes mellitus,[89,90] peripheral atherosclerosis,[85,86,91] cancer,[92] pulmonary dysfunction,[93] digestive diseases,[93] gallstones,[93] gout,[93] degenerative joint disease,[93] cutaneous disease,[93] and other disorders is widely held. Furthermore, obesity is associated with adverse social and psychological consequences.[94] Collectively, death from all causes associated with obesity is probably curvilinearly related to overweight. At weights 60 per cent or more above standard insurance weights, morbidity and mortality are approximately double those of the general population.[87]

Cardiovascular Disease

In addition to smoking, diet, physical activity, and diabetes, regional patterns of fat distribution impose a risk factor for cardiovascular disease. Prospective epidemiological studies in men and women have shown that abdominal (android) obesity is associated with increased risk for ischemic heart disease, strokes, and death independent of the total degree of obesity.[6–8,24] Even moderate obesity is a health hazard when men and women accumulate excessive fat in the upper body region. In android or upper body segmental obesity the fat cells from the abdominal wall are hypertrophied.[6,8] These adipocytes exhibit differences in hormonal sensitivities to insulin[6] and corticosteroids[6,95] when compared with other subcutaneous fat cells. Hypertrophic abdominal obesity is associated with other metabolic aberrations such as hyperinsulinemia,[6,96] hyperlipidemia,[6,97,98] hypertension,[87,88] and diabetes mellitus.[89,90,99,100] The direct impact of obesity with its augmented cardiovascular workload and the indirect influences of atherosclerosis and hypertension are probably synergistic in causing heightened morbidity and mortality in obese humans.

Twenty years ago we made an interesting but anecdotal observation that patients with android obesity and symptoms of angina who underwent 5 to 6 weeks of therapeutic starvation had tortuous but patent coronary arteries on angiographic studies after fasting. Unfortunately, the influence of weight reduction on obese humans with coronary artery disease was not adequately evaluated.

Hypertension has been coupled to obesity for many decades,[88,101] but there is no understanding of the pathophysiology of this relationship.[88] Hypertension improves or normalizes with weight reduction in a significant number of obese patients. In parallel, as body weight increases, arterial pressure rises. Hypertension occurs frequently in industrialized nations that have populations that gain weight with age.[88,101,102] Furthermore, hypertensive patients have a predisposition to gain weight. This suggests the possibility that obesity and hypertension have a common link.[88] However, this relationship may be modified by race, sex, and environmental factors. For example, body mass index is related to hypertension among white women but not among black women.[88]

Normotensive and hypertensive obese humans have increased cardiac output rates and elevated blood volumes compared with normal-weight controls. The role of peripheral vascular resistance in the development of hypertension in obese patients is controversial, but the hemodynamic fault in obesity hypertension may be similar to that present in essential hypertension without obesity.[87]

The possible roles of salt intake, neuroendocrine abnormalities, or altered plasma renin activity have not provided a clear explanation for the elevated arterial blood pressure observed in obese humans. Nonetheless, several investigative groups have reported that the arterial blood pressure is reduced into the normal ranges in about 60 to 80 per cent of patients who achieve substantial weight losses.[8]

Diabetes Mellitus and Hyperlipidemia

The well-recognized association of diabetes mellitus and obesity was observed by physicians over 100 years ago.[89,90,103] In 1936 Joslin and co-workers suggested that obesity might precipitate the manifestation of diabetes or worsen the prognosis of diabetes.[103] These early observations have adequately been substantiated. Of adults about 35 to 55 years of age with moderate obesity, some 8 to 10 per cent will manifest diabetes mellitus.[104] As age and duration of obesity progress, there is an increase in the incidence of diabetes. About 50 per cent of grossly obese middle-aged adults have diabetes. The majority of these patients have non–insulin-dependent (Type II) diabetes mellitus.[103] Among middle-aged adults, more women than men are fat and women manifest diabetes more frequently than men. However, at a similar degree of relative overweight, men have higher blood glucose, insulin, and triglyceride concentrations.[6] Thus, men are more vulnerable to the metabolic aberration of obesity than women. This is especially noted at moderate degrees of obesity (30 to 40 kg body fat). Greater increases in body fat do not further predispose men to the adversities of obesity, whereas metabolic and cardiovascular risks are continuously increased with weight gain among women. Blacks may be slightly more likely to have diabetes than whites, especially at the older ages in the more obese individuals.[105]

Although the amount of total body fat has a major influence on the metabolic abnormalities seen among obese patients, for the degree of fatness, upper body (abdominal or android) obesity is seen to play the commanding role. Hypertrophic adipocytes develop with abdominal obesity, and these enlarged fat cells are associated with diminished biological action of insulin on glucose oxidation, presumably owing to a decrease in the number of insulin receptors or to a postreceptor defect.[106–108] Adipose tissue, however, accounts for only a small fraction of glucose disposal,[109] and therefore impaired insulin action on hypertrophic adipocytes is unlikely to be directly responsible for glucose intolerance. However, these hypertrophic cells exhibit augmented lipolysis,[8,110] and increased plasma FFA decreases glucose oxidation by other tissues, especially muscle.[111,112] Compensatory hyperinsulinemia down-regulates insulin receptors on several target organs, notably the liver and muscle.[108,113] In addition, increased FFA flux stimulates hepatic synthesis and release of triglycerides (very low density lipoproteins). Thus, hypertrophic abdominal adipocytes that develop as a consequence of relative overnutrition are a significant factor in the development of glucose intolerance, hyperinsulinemia, and hypertriglyceridemia

associated with abdominal or android obesity.[6,8] This form of obesity is readily identified by visual inspection and is confirmed by demonstrating an increased waist/hip ratio for men (> 1.0) and women (> 0.8). Treatment should be designed to reduce body (abdominal) fat and eliminate the metabolic (hyperglycemia, hypertriglyceridemia, and hypercholesterolemia) and cardiovascular (hypertension, occlusive arterial lesions, and peripheral venous stasis) abnormalities.

Caloric restriction and weight reduction have remarkably beneficial effects on reducing hyperglycemia and hypertriglyceridemia. However, long-standing therapeutic success rates in accomplishing these objectives are astonishingly low.

Gastrointestinal Disorders

Digestive diseases, primary gallbladder stones and hepatic steatosis, are highly related determinants when weight is excessive.

The association between gallstones and obesity has been documented in several studies,[93,114] and the incidence of gallstones increases with the degree of obesity, age, and parity.[93,115] Abnormalities in hepatic function are common in obese patients.[93] However, hepatic steatosis may be present in liver biopsy specimens although hepatic function studies are within normal ranges.[93]

Respiratory Disorders

Pulmonary dysfunction is common in obesity. It varies from respiratory impairment during physical exertion to the pickwickian syndrome: the syndrome characterized by marked obesity, hypoventilation, and somnolence.[93] Obese humans have a fairly uniform respiratory pattern; they breathe rapidly and shallowly. Functional residual capacity and expiratory reserve volume are low. Lung compliance appears to be normal, but the mechanics of breathing require increased energy requirements associated with the workload of moving a massive chest wall.[93,116] Ventilation primarily occurs in the upper lung segments, whereas perfusion primarily occurs in the lower lung segments, creating a ventilation-perfusion mismatch.[11,117] Some grossly obese patients have a diminished sensitivity of the respiratory center to the stimulatory effects of CO_2.

The pickwickian syndrome may be associated with two forms of sleep apnea: one develops with transient cessation of the neural impulses originating in the central nervous system to the muscles of respiration; another occurs with mechanical obstruction of the airway system due to a collapsed tongue that occludes the glottis.[93] Advanced respiratory failure associated with obesity requires, firstly, emergency treatment and, subsequently, medical intervention with aggressive weight reduction therapy and medicinal agents such as progestational or antidepressant drugs.[93,118,119] Such malignant forms of obesity frequently require surgical treatment.

Arthritis

Overweight individuals have degenerative joint disease. The knees and feet seem to be the most frequently involved joints. However, the prevalence of osteoarthritis of the hands (non-weightbearing joints) is also increased in obese men and women.[93] Weight reduction may be the single most important therapeutic measure for a chronically traumatized knee or foot joint subjected to the burden of body overweight.

The incidence of gout is a well-recognized complication of obesity. The relative risk for the prevalence of gout is two to three times greater in obese than in normal humans.[93] Starvation can induce severe hyperuricemia and precipitate gouty arthritis. A weight reduction diet with 50 to 100 g of carbohydrates daily and adequate hydration prevents the hyperuricemia associated with total caloric deprivation.

Dermatological and Endocrine Diseases

Skin diseases are frequent among obese humans. There is a heightened prevalence of stasis dermatitis on the legs and around the ankles; superficial fungal infection located in the intertriginous areas and bacterial abscesses are common. In addition, hirsutism, acne, and stria are common accompaniments of obesity. Acanthosis nigricans deserves specific attention in obese humans. Dark, hypertrophic, velvety skin areas on the lateral areas of the neck and in the axillary areas, and dark, hypertrophic skin over the knuckles are frequently associated with malignant cancers.[120] When acanthosis nigricans occurs in obesity, endocrine disorders are likely to be present. The prevalence of acanthosis nigricans is increased in obese individuals, most of whom are also mildly to moderately insulin-resistant.[121,122] In addition, acanthosis nigricans is associated with other insulin-resistant states. In Type B extreme insulin resistance, acanthosis nigricans is associated with severe insulin resistance, other biochemical or clinical signs of autoimmune disorders such as systemic lupus erythematosus, and the presence in blood of high titers of anti–insulin receptor antibodies.[121] This condition is very rare and appears to afflict predominately females over 20 years of age. In Type A extreme insulin resistance, acanthosis nigricans and insulin resistance occur together with virilization and polycystic ovaries in young females. This condition is more common than the Type B extreme insulin resistance. Several different defects at the level of

the insulin receptor have been described in these patients whose blood does not contain anti–insulin receptor antibodies.[123,124]

Primary or secondary endocrine disorders accompany obesity. One of the most extensively studied changes in body metabolism is insulin resistance in obese humans. Investigations not only have included whole-body responses to insulin but have also been focused on specific target cells.

Hyperinsulinemia is a characteristic of human obesity.[125,126] Human forearm perfusion studies[125] and steady-state glucose insulin infusion studies[127–129] showed that relative hyperinsulinemia is needed to induce the usual metabolic responses of tissues to insulin. In addition, diabetologists have long recognized that the insulin requirements of obese patients are greater than those of normal-weight diabetic patients. Collectively, the hyperinsulinemia in otherwise normal, obese humans and the excessive insulin requirements of Type II obese diabetic humans are considered ample evidence for stating that insulin resistance exists when body fat mass is enlarged. Furthermore, the insulin receptor numbers are reduced on blood monocytes[130] and on hepatocytes in obese humans with hyperinsulinemia. However, linking "down regulation" of insulin receptors on organs exposed to high blood insulin concentrations and the presence of insulin resistance in Type II diabetes mellitus with recognized postreceptor defects[130] to insulin resistance in obese humans may have generated some conclusions that should be cautiously received. Hyperinsulinemia may or may not indicate that adipocytes from non-diabetic, obese individuals are insulin resistant. No consensus has been reached regarding the status of the adipocyte insulin receptor in obesity.[130] A number of studies have not found a change in the total cellular content of the receptor,[130–134] whereas others have described an overall decrease.[128,130,135–138] All studies agree that the number of receptors per cell surface area is reduced in the obese condition, but the possibility that this reduction induces insulin resistance is speculative.[130] Insulin availability (quantity of insulin in the extracellular fluid and time required to disperse insulin to the receptor sites in adipose tissue) as related to the adipose tissue mass may not be excessive in obesity. To conclude that insulin resistance exists in the peripheral tissues (adipocytes) of obese humans without considering the delivery rate of insulin to the adipocyte may be erroneous. Nonetheless, at this stage of research, obesity is generally considered to be an insulin-resistant state.

Gonadal dysfunction is also associated with obesity. The concentration of testosterone is reduced, and estradiol and estrone are increased in a manner directly related to weight in obese men.[93] The reduction in plasma testosterone concentration is probably due to a reduction in the plasma sex hormone–binding globulin concentration. Testicular size and pituitary releasing and gonadotropin hormones are normal.[93]

The onset of menarche frequently occurs at a younger age in obese girls, and as age progresses irregular menstrual cycles with amenorrhea, functional uterine bleeding, and infertility are common. Premature menopause is common among women who experienced early menarche. Hirsutism and anovulatory cycles as well as polycystic ovaries are frequently observed. Estrogen-linked abnormalities associated with obesity may be secondary to altered hydroxylation of estradiol[93] and may be related to the development of endometrial carcinoma.[93] Unbound plasma androgens may also be elevated and may be responsible for the virilization of obese women. Some of the hormonal peculiarities are alleviated with adequate weight reduction.

Thyroidal dysfunction may induce weight gain, and iodothyronine hormones are frequently evaluated in obese humans. However, the prevalence of primary thyroid abnormalities (various hypothyroid states) associated with obesity in the general population is overstated. Obesity, hypertension, and diabetes mellitus not infrequently lead to diagnostic studies to define adrenal diseases, specifically Cushing's syndrome, but adrenal dysfunction is exceptional.

Cancer

Certain types of malignancies exist at unusual prevalence in overweight men and women.[92] Men who weigh 40 per cent or more over standard values have a mortality ratio for cancer 1.33 times greater than a normal-weight, matched male population. These overweight men have significantly higher mortality ratios for colorectal and prostate cancer. Women who are equally overweight have a 1.55 times greater risk for death from cancer than do normal-weight women. Higher rates of endometrial, cervical, and gallbladder cancer occur in overweight women; in addition there is a higher prevalence of ovarian and breast cancer in obese women.[92]

Accidents

Obesity not only increases the risk of death from cardiovascular and respiratory failures, from digestive tract diseases, and from malignancies, but contributes significantly to health hazards related to functional impairments of daily living. Obesity increases pain and contributes to physical limitations and propensities for fatal accidents.[87,139]

Social and Psychological Adversities

Adverse social and psychological consequences of obesity are readily acknowledged. Early studies viewed psychological disturbances as a cause of obesity. Overeating and diminished physical activities do occur secondarily to emotional stresses. However, social and psychological aberrations are more frequently consequences of obesity rather than vice versa.[94] "The social prejudice and discrimination directed at overweight persons and the effects of dieting lead to the disturbances."[94]

In developed countries there is strong, harsh, brutal prejudice directed toward obese humans, regardless of age, sex, race, or socioeconomic status.[94] Young children, adults, and even physicians condemn the "lazy, ugly, self-indulging, immoral" obese persons. The obese are discriminated against in educational and marriage opportunities, in the work force, and in job security.[94] Therefore, it is surprising that "there is no evidence of an increased prevalence of major psychiatric disorders in obese persons when strictly defined diagnostic criteria are used."[140] This statement should, however, not be misconstrued to imply that obese persons are free of psychological problems.

Women and adolescent girls suffer more than men and boys do from the deleterious consequences of society's contempt for obesity,[94] even though the prevalence of obesity in females and males is equal. In addition, women are frequently displeased with their "figures," although their body weights are normal. The predilection for women to suffer unduly because of body image or obesity should be worrisome.

Severely obese (75 to 100 percent overweight) individuals receive the worst degree of directed prejudice and discrimination.[94] Unlike mildly to moderately obese humans, the severly obese person rarely escapes some psychological insult.[94] Intelligent societies should be able to eliminate discriminatory attitudes that are detrimental to psychological health.

THERAPY FOR OBESITY

When caloric expenditure exceeds caloric intake, the body tissue masses decrease. The caloric value of obesity tissues is about 5772 kcal/kg (2624 kcal/1b). This is significantly less than the caloric value of adipose tissue, 7700 kcal/kg (3500 kcal/1b). Therefore, the caloric deficit required to lose a kilogram or pound of weight is less than that required to lose the same unit of fat stored in adipose tissue triglycerides. On the other hand, the caloric requirements of humans are also less than those stated.[28,50] Therefore, the overestimation of the caloric value of obesity tissue is balanced by the overestimation of energy requirements.

Most people who think they are overweight because of obesity do not seek professional advice. Instead, they generally limit their caloric intake or augment their caloric expenditure through physical activity. Decreased caloric intake and increased caloric expenditure allows these individuals with a small degree of undesired obesity tissue to accomplish their weight loss goals.

A common approach to weight reduction is limitation of certain high-calorie foods from the diet and substitution of low-calorie foods and beverages. In essence, this is a form of "counting calories" consumed. It takes self-discipline, and for the person requiring only modest restrictions it usually accomplishes the desired results. As the obesity problem enlarges, the actions taken to induce loss of obesity tissue become more taxing. Fat humans may find protracted reduction in the size of food portions and abstinence from between-meal snacks difficult to maintain. Frequently such individuals will turn to the use of monotonous dietary preparations. Other obese humans seek professional help to reduce their body masses. Once the patient seeks medical advice for losing weight, the reduction program should no longer be left to the patient's own discretion. An acknowledged physician and his delegates should prescribe the treatment course after evaluating the patient as an individual and establishing goals and criteria for success. Therapeutic guidelines should be developed and the patient's clinical course closely monitored. A combination of diet, exercise, and behavior modification seems to be the most sensible approach for weight reduction. The program should be tailored specially for each patient, recognizing the importance of genetic inheritance. One should be judicious with therapeutic objectives and not create false hopes and expectations. Obese humans should not be tortured with dietary restrictions, exercise regimens, and behavior modifications that are counter to the biology of survival.

Professional therapy for many other obese individuals is directed at the prevention or reversal of complications as frequently as it is toward reduction of obesity tissue per se.

Currently, about 10 billion dollars is spent annually on obesity and related problems. The number of obese adults in America amounts to about 34 million. There is an extraordinary high prevalence among certain groups, for example, black women[141] and Pima Indians.

Reduced caloric intake and augmented energy expenditure are the cornerstones of therapy for decreasing the obesity tissues and body mass. Although this is simple in principle, it is difficult to accomplish in those individuals who have been unsuccessful when left to their own devices.

Dietary Therapy

Owen and co-workers reported the urinary excretory rates of the major nitrogenous compounds of obese human(s) drinking water and taking only sodium, potassium, chloride, and vitamins during prolonged starvation.[2] Although humans progressively excrete less and/or conserve relatively more nitrogen (protein) during prolonged starvation, a large negative nitrogen (protein) balance develops during prolonged periods of total caloric deprivation.[2] Blackburn and co-workers recognized the importance of this negative nitrogen balance and introduced the concept and technique of modifying total starvation by adding small quantities of protein to the intake of patients undergoing caloric deprivation for weight reduction. They gave supplementary dietary protein to obese individuals who were otherwise calorie-restricted and showed that negative nitrogen balance was minimal during weight loss. They coined the phrase "protein-sparing modified fast" for this form of dietary therapy for obesity. Out of Blackburn and colleagues'[142–144] original contributions to the dietary management of obesity have sprung a series of commercial dietary amino acid preparations.

Obese individuals frequently try regimens that promise rapid weight loss. Both starvation and very-low-calorie diet induce quick weight loss. Numerous packaged forms of very-low-calorie diets containing about 300 to 500 kcal/day are available on the open market. These very-low-calorie diets, usually formulated as "liquid protein" products, are frequently consumed without professional guidance and fortunately usually without any acknowledged adverse side effects. However, such a safety record should not obscure the fact that under protracted use these drastically restricted diets are extremely hazardous and are associated with cardiac dysfunction and lethal complications in some obese but otherwise healthy individuals.[145] Although collagen and gelatin hydrolysates were the sources for these low-calorie liquid protein diets, some of those who died were consuming products with high-biological-value protein.[145] Publicity pertaining to the deaths of these unfortunate people resulted in a drastic decrease in the use of such diets. Nonetheless, very-low-calorie diets continue to appear on the market.

Van Itallie and Yang wrote a scholarly review pertaining to use of very-low-calorie diets composed primarily of protein hydrolysates for the treatment of obesity.[145] They stressed use of caution with any very-low-calorie or protein- and calorie-deficient diet because of the recognized cardiac dysfunction manifested by low QRS voltage and prolonged QT interval that occurs after 7 weeks of therapeutic starvation.[146] The protein-sparing modified fast does not prevent cardiac atrophy with weight loss, fiber attenuation, myofibril fracture, and lipofuchsin deposition. Summary evidence shows that cardiac dysfunction and death were directly related to the length of time that the very-low-calorie diets were used for weight reduction.[145,147] Van Itallie and Yang recommended that all patients who embark on a program of fasting or a very-low-calorie diet for rapid weight reduction (1) be made aware of the risks associated with protracted adherence to such drastic measures, and (2) remain under a physician's care during such treatment.[145]

The foregoing does not contradict the fact that restriction of dietary intake remains a cornerstone for weight reduction. The dietary prescription should satisfy all nutrient needs except energy and should be acceptable to the patient and readily available. A balanced hypocaloric diet containing complex carbohydrates, unsaturated fats, and high-biological-value proteins (0.5 g/kg of ideal body weight) with adequate minerals and vitamins is recommended. It is difficult to accomplish these requirements with a diet containing less than 800 to 1000 kcal/day. Novelty diets with alleged mystical properties should be avoided.

Obese individuals usually have larger resting metabolic requirements than do lean humans.[28] A diet containing less than 14 to 18 kcal/kg/day for women and 16 to 20 kcal/kg/day for men should induce desirable weight loss in obese humans who are otherwise healthy and have normal mobility. Exceptions occur but are rare. A reasonable and safe rate of weight loss for dieters is about 1 per cent of body weight per week.[148]

The production and consumption of artificial sweeteners have produced a major commercial industry in the United States. However, artificial sweeteners are not an essential element of the diet and may have serious adverse health effects. Therefore, few people need to use them.

Fructose is a nutritive sweetener with a caloric value that is approximately equal to that of glucose; therefore, it is of no value in weight-reducing programs. Sorbitol, mannitol, and xylitol are sugar alcohols which contribute sweetness but are poorly absorbed from the gut. When they are consumed in amounts of 30 or more grams per day, diarrhea develops. Saccharin, a nonnutritive sweetener, may have a possible role as a carcinogen. Until the Food and Drug Administration decides the fate of this sweetener, its use should be limited. There are too many unresolved problems about cyclamates at this time to permit its re-emergence on the open market. Aspartame, a dipeptide, appears acceptably safe for most people. Exceptions are pregnant women and young children, who are urged not to consume large amounts of aspartame-sweetened products. Another shortcoming of aspartame is that its sweetness is lost during cooking.

Physical Therapy

Chapter 11 provides information pertaining to physical exercise and weight control. Increasing energy expenditure through exercise is especially important for individuals with sedentary lifestyles. Although common sense implies that exercise might decrease body fat and increase muscle mass, apparently fat-free mass measured by densitometric techniques does not change appreciably. However, when exercise is part of the weight loss program, muscle mass as well as bone mineral content are spared.[149–151] We have long recommended to our patients undergoing weight reduction that they participate in activities that are enjoyable and not harmful to their bodies. They are more likely to continue such activities after their weight reduction goals are obtained.

Cardiovascular and musculoskeletal systems must be guarded against injury. If an exercise program is to be initiated, the American College of Sports Medicine recommends a cardiac stress test for all individuals over 35 years of age or those less than 35 years of age if they have hypertension, diabetes mellitus, hyperlipidemia, or a strong family history of atherosclerotic cardiovascular disease.[15]

Excessive trauma to joints, especially the ankles, knees, and hips, should be avoided. Walking, pedaling a stationary bicycle, or swimming may be good forms of exercise in the obese with compromised joints in the lower extremities.

Exercise should be done 3 to 5 times weekly at an intensity of 60 to 85 per cent the maximum heart rate (estimated at 220/min minus one's age)[153] for at least 30 minutes.[154]

Psychological Therapy

Behavior modification may also be helpful in weight-reducing programs. Restricting the places where food can be eaten, walking rather than riding, developing an awareness of eating patterns, and correcting undesirable habits can be most beneficial to some people.[155,156]

Drug Therapy

The role of drug therapy in the treatment of obesity is controversial. Nonetheless, central nervous system effectors are likely to produce useful therapeutic medicinal agents in the future. Drugs could be developed that alter genetic expression and predispositions to developing adiposity.

Surgical Therapy

Surgical intervention has been extensively used to treat morbidly obese patients. Individuals with either 100 per cent or 100 pounds above ideal body weight and who have tried self-help groups or sought professional help and failed to reduce their weight may be candidates for surgical procedures to control obesity.[157–160]

Surgical control of obesity is designed to enforce caloric restriction through gastric obstruction or intestinal malabsorption. The initial attempt at surgical control of obesity was the jejunoileal bypass. A segment of the proximal jejunum is anastomosed to a segment of the terminal ileum; the lengths of these segments are variable. The defunctionalized remaining small intestine is drained into the transverse colon. The initial weight loss during the first 6 months is mostly regained. Numerous different complications universally develop, making jejunoileal bypass surgery the most dangerous weight-reduction technique employed today. At least 20 per cent of the patients require takedown of the bypass.[157] Early serious complications induced perioperative mortality, thromboembolic disease, wound infection, renal failure,[160,161] and wound dehiscence. Diarrhea invariably occurs and may be associated with incapacitating electrolyte imbalance and dehydration. Late serious complications are renal stones, liver disease, pancreatitis, cholecystitis, intestinal obstruction, osteoporosis, and arthritis. Relatively minor complications are anemia, hypokalemia, and hypoproteinemia.[15,157,161]

Jejunoileal bypass has been largely abandoned and replaced by gastric bypass or plication (stapling) procedures, which create small gastric reservoirs but allow the passage of food into the distal stomach through a small channel. Gastric bypass and partitioning by plication share the same principle of limiting the size of the meal intake. Nausea and vomiting frequently occur after gastric surgery for controlling obesity. However, constant nibbling and consumption of high-calorie liquid foods sabotage the surgical procedures. Gastric stapling is associated with gastric leaks,[157] and gorging stretches the size of the small stomach pouch. Failure of treatment, defined as less than 25 per cent weight reduction, occurs in 62 per cent of patients who undergo gastric stapling (partitioning). However, successful weight reduction is the rule among patients with gastrojejunostomies. Rosato[157] believes gastric bypass is the surgical procedure of choice for the treatment of morbid obesity. Long-term follow-up studies are needed to complete the evaluation of surgical gastrojejunostomies for the control of morbid obesity.

SUMMARY

Obesity is inherited and becomes manifested when caloric intake exceeds caloric expenditure. It is associated with a variety of diseases leading to morbidity and mortality. Medical, psychological, and surgical forms of therapy are associated with complications and limited success rates. Nonetheless, imperative judgment suggests it is prudent to reduce excessive body fat when it impairs the quality of life and threatens the health of humans.

REFERENCES

1. Owen OE, Morgan AP, Kemp HG, et al. Brain metabolism during fasting. J Clin Invest 1967; 46:1589–1595.
2. Owen OE, Felig P, Morgan AP, et al. Liver and kidney metabolism during prolonged starvation. J Clin Invest 1969; 48:574–583.
3. Astwood EB. The heritage of corpulence. Endocrinology 1962; 71:337–341.
4. Stunkard AJ, Sorenson TIA, Hanis C, et al. An adoption study of human obesity. N Engl J Med 1986; 314:193–198.
5. Leibel RL, Hirsch J. Metabolic characterization of obesity. Ann Intern Med 1985; 103:1000–1002.
6. Krotkiewski M, Bjorntorp P, Sjostrom L, et al. Impact of obesity on metabolism in men and women. Importance of regional adipose tissue distribution. J Clin Invest 1983; 72:1150–1162.
7. Vague J. The degress of masculine differentiation of obesities: a factor determining predisposition to diabetes, atherosclerosis, gout, and uric calculous disease. Am J Clin Nutr 1956; 4:20–34.
8. Kissebah AH, Vydelingum N, Murray R, et al. Relation of body fat distribution to metabolic complications of obesity. J Clin Endocrinol Metab 1982; 54:254–260.
9. Hirsch J, Knittle JL. Cellularity of obese and nonobese human adipose tissue. Fed Proc 1970; 29:1516–1521.
10. Bjorntorp P, Sjostrom L. Number and size of adipose tissue fat cells in relation to metabolism in human obesity. Metab Clin Exp 1971; 20:703–713.
11. Foster DW. Eating disorders: obesity and anorexia nervosa. In Wilson JD, Forster DW (eds). Williams' Textbook of Endocrinology. 7th ed. Philadelphia, WB Saunders, 1985: 1081–1107.
12. Grande F. Assessment of body fat in man. In Bray GA (ed). Obesity in Perspective. Bethesda, MD, National Institutes of Health 1975: 189–203.
13. Metropolitan Life Foundation Statistical Bulletin. New York, Metropolitan Life Foundation, 1983; 64:2–9.
14. Segal KR, Gutin B, Nyman AM, et al. Thermic effect of food at rest, during exercise, and after exercise in lean and obese men of similar body weight. J Clin Invest 1985; 76:1107–1112.
15. Bray GA. Obesity: benefits and risks of treatment. Drug Therapy 1984; 14:60–65.
16. Black D, James WPT, Besser GM, et al. Obesity. A report of the Royal College of Physicians. J R Coll Phys Lond 1983; 17:5–65.
17. Brozek J, Grande F, Anderson R, et al. Densitometric analysis of body composition: revision of some quantitative assumptions. Ann NY Acad Sci 1963; 110:113–140.
18. Pearson AM, Purchas RW, Reineke EP. Theory and potential usefulness of body density as a predictor of body composition. In Body Composition in Animals and Man. Publication 1958. Washington, National Academy of Science, 1968: 153–169.
19. Goldman RF, Buskirk ER. Body volume measurement by underwater weighing: description of a method. In Brozek J, Henschel A (eds). Techniques for Measuring Body Composition. Washington, National Academy of Science, 1961: 78–89.
20. Garrow JS. Energy Balance and Obesity in Man. 2nd ed. New York, Elsevier/North-Holland, 1978: 125.
21. Mayer J. Obesity. In Goodhart RS, Shils ME (eds). Modern Nutrition in Health and Disease. 6th ed. Philadelphia, Lea & Febiger, 1980: 721–470.
22. Frisancho AR. New norms of upper limb fat and muscle areas for assessment of nutritional status. Am J Clin Nutr 1981; 34:2540–2545.
23. Grande F, Keys A. Body weight, body composition and calorie status. In Goodhart RS, Shils ME (eds). Modern Nutrition in Health and Disease. 6th ed. Philadelphia, Lea & Febiger, 1980: 3–34.
24. Bjorntorp P. Regional patterns of fat distribution. Ann Intern Med 1985; 103:994–995.
25. Goldstein JL, Brown MS. Familial hypercholesterolemia: a genetic receptor disease. Hosp Pract 1985; 20:35–46.
26. Horton ES, Danforth E Jr. Energy metabolism and obesity.

In Brodoff NB, Bleicher SJ (eds). Diabetes Mellitus and Obesity. Baltimore, Williams & Wilkins, 1982: 261–268.

27. Hill JO, Heymsfield SB, McMannus C III, et al. Meal size and thermic response to food in male subjects as a function of maximum aerobic capacity. Metabolism 1984; 33:743–749.

28. Owen OE, Kavle E, Owen RS, et al. A reappraisal of caloric requirements in healthy women. Am J Clin Nutr 1986; 44:1–19.

29. Owen OE, Holup J, D'Alessio DA, et al. A reappraisal of caloric requirements of men. Am J Clin Nutr, in press.

30. Khoo JC, Steinberg D. Hormone-sensitive lipase of adipose tissue. *In* Boyer PD (ed). The Enzymes. Vol. 16. New York, Academic Press, 1983: 183–204.

31. Owen OE, Reichard GA Jr., Kinney JM, et al. Metabolism during catabolic states of starvation, diabetes, and trauma in humans. *In* Brodoff BN, Bleicher SJ (eds). Diabetes Mellitus and Obesity. Baltimore, Williams & Wilkins, 1982: 172–184.

32. Lefkowitz RJ, Caron MG, Stiles GL. Mechanisms of membrane-receptor regulation: biochemical, physiological, and clinical insights derived from studies of the adrenergic receptors. N Engl J Med 1984; 310:1570–1579.

33. Arner P, Engfeldt P, Nowak J. In vivo observations on the lipolytic control of noradrenaline during therapeutic fasting. J Clin Endocrinol Metab 1981; 53:1207–1212.

34. Leiter LA, Grose M, Yale JF, et al. Catecholamine responses to hypocaloric diets and fasting in obese human subjects. Am J Physiol 1984; 247:E190–197.

35. Merimee TJ, Froesch ER. Insulin-like growth factors in the fed and fasted states. J Clin Endocrin Metab 1982; 55:999–1002.

36. Owen OE. Starvation. *In* DeGroot LJ (ed). Endocrinology. 2nd ed. Orlando, Grune & Stratton, in press.

37. Ravussin E, Burnand B, Schutz Y, et al. Twenty-four hour energy expenditure and resting metabolic rate in obese, moderately obese, and control subjects. Am J Clin Nutr 1982; 35:566–573.

38. Jequier E. Long-term measurement of energy expenditure in man: direct or indirect calorimetry. *In* Bjorntorp P, Cairella M (eds). Recent Advances in Obesity Research III. London, John Libbey, 1981: 130–135.

39. Bogardus C, Lillioja S, Ravussin E, et al. Familial dependence of the resting metabolic rate. N Engl J Med 1986; 315:96–100.

40. Jequier E, Schutz Y. Long-term measurements of energy expenditure in humans using a respiration chamber. Am J Clin Nutr 1983; 38:989–998.

41. Harris JA, Benedict FG. A Biometric Study of Basal Metabolism in Man. Washington, Carnegie Institute, 1919: 1–266.

42. DuBois BS, DuBois EF. Clinical calorimetry: a formula to estimate the approximate surface area if height and weight be known. Arch Intern Med 1916; 17:863–871.

43. Boothby WM, Berkson J, Dunn HL. Studies of the energy of metabolism of normal individuals: a standard for basal metabolism, with a nomogram for clinical application. Am J Physiol 1936; 116:468–484.

44. Boothby WM, Sandiford I. Summary of the basal metabolism data on 8,614 subjects with especial reference to the normal standards for the estimation of the basal metabolism rate. J Biochem 1922; 54:783–803.

45. Roberston JD, Reid DD. Standards for the basal metabolism of normal people in Britain. Lancet 1952; 1:940–943.

46. DuBois EF. Basal energy metabolism at various ages: man. *In* Altman PL, Dittmer DS (eds). Metabolism. Bethesda, MD, Federation of American Societies for Experimental Biology, 1968: 345.

47. Daly JM, Heymsfield SB, Head CA, et al. Human energy requirements: Overestimation by widely used prediction equation. Am J Clin Nutr 1985; 42:1170–1174.

48. Feurer ID, Crosby LO, Buzby GP, et al. Resting energy expenditure in morbid obesity. Ann Surg 1983; 197:17–21.

49. Roza AM, Shizgal HM. The Harris-Benedict equation re-evaluated: resting energy requirements and the body cell mass. Am J Clin Nutr 1984; 40:168–182.

50. Cunningham JJ. A reanalysis of the factors influencing basal metabolic rate in normal adults. Am J Clin Nutr 1980; 33:2372–2374.

51. Felig P, Cunningham FP, Levitt M, et al. Energy expenditure in obesity in fasting and postprandial state. Am J Physiol 1983; 244:E45–51.

52. Miller A, Blyth C. Lean body mass as a metabolic reference standard. J Appl Physiol 1953; 5:311–316.

53. Behnke AR. Relationship of lean body weight to metabolism and some consequent systematizations. Ann NY Acad Sci 1953; 56:1095–1142.

54. Keys A, Taylor HL, Grande F. Basal metabolism and age of adult man. Metabolism 1973; 22:579–587.

55. Tzankoff S, Norris A. Effect of muscle mass decrease on age-related BMR changes. J Appl Physiol 1977; 43:1001–1006.

56. Tzankoff S, Norris A. Longitudinal changes in basal metabolism in man. J Appl Physiol 1978; 45:536–539.

57. Bernstein RS, Thornton JC, Yang MU, et al. Prediction of resting metabolic rate in obese patients. Am J Clin Nutr 1983; 37:595–601.

58. Brozek J, Grande F. Body composition and basal metabolism in man: correlation analysis versus physiological approach. Human Biol 1955; 27:21–31.

59. Cahill GF, Owen OE. Some observations on carbohydrate metabolism in man. *In* Dickens F, Randle FJ, Whelan WJ (eds). Carbohydrate Metabolism and Its Disorders. Vol. 1. New York, Academic Press, 1968: 497–518.

60. James WPT, Davies HL, Bailes J, et al. Elevated metabolic rates in obesity. Lancet 1978; 1:1122–1125.

61. Trayburn P, James WPT. Thermogenesis: dietary and non-shivering aspects. *In* Cioffi LA, James WPT, van Itallie TB (eds). The Body Weight Regulatory System: Normal and Disturbed Mechanisms. New York, Raven Press, 1981: 97–105.

62. Himms-Hagen J. Thermogenesis in brown adipose tissue as an energy buffer: implications for obesity. N Engl J Med 1984; 311:1549–1558.

63. Bray GA, York DA. Hypothalamic and genetic obesity in experimental animals: an autonomic and endocrine hypothesis. Physiol Rev 1979; 59:719–809.

64. Guernsey DC, Stevens DD. The cell membrane sodium pump as a mechanism for increasing thermogenesis during cold acclimation in rats. Science 1977; 196:908–910.

65. Miller BG, Otto WR, Grimble RF, et al. The relationship between protein turnover and energy balance in lean and genetically obese (ob/ob) mice. Br J Nutr 1979; 41:185–199.

66. Newsholme EA, Crabtree B. Substrate cycles in metabolic regulation and in heat generation. Biochem Soc Symp 1976; 41:61–109.

67. Katz J. Energy balance and futile cycling. *In* Kinney JM, Lense E (eds). Assessment of Energy Metabolism in Health and Disease. Columbus, OH, Ross Laboratories, 1980: 63–66.

68. Kaplan ML, Leveille GA. Calorigenic response in obese and nonobese women. Am J Clin Nutr 1976; 29:1108–1113.

69. Shetty PS, Jung RT, James WPT, et al. Postprandial thermogenesis in obesity. Clin Sci 1981; 60:519–525.

70. Schwartz RS, Halter JB, Bierman E. Reduced thermic effect of feeding in obesity: role of norepinephrine. Metabolism 1983; 32:114–117.

71. Sharief NN, Macdonald I. Differences in dietary-induced thermogenesis with various carbohydrates in normal and overweight man. Am J Clin Nutr 1982; 32:267–272.

72. Welle SL, Campbell RG. Normal thermic effect of glucose in obese women. Am J Clin Nutr 1983; 37:87–92.

73. Pittet PH, Chappius PH, Acheson K, et al. Thermic effect of glucose in obese subjects studied by direct and indirect calorimetry. Br J Nutr 1976; 35:281–292.

74. Golay A, Schutz Y, Meyer HU, et al. Glucose-induced ther-

mogenesis in nondiabetic and diabetic obese subjects. Diabetes 1982; *31*:1023–1028.

75. D'Alessio DA, Kavle EC, Mozzoli MA, et al. Oxidative and nonoxidative macronutrient disposal in lean and obese men. Submitted for publication.

76. Acheson K, Jequier E, Burger A, et al. Thyroid hormones and thermogenesis: the metabolic cost of food and exercise. Metabolism 1984; *33*:262–265.

77. Owen OE, Reichard GA, Boden G, et al. Interrelationships among key tissues in the utilization of metabolic substrates. *In* Katzen HM, Mahler RJ (eds). Diabetes, Obesity, and Vascular Disease. Part II: Metabolic and Molecular Interrelationships. Washington. Hemisphere, 1978: 517–550.

78. Anand BK, Chhina GS, Sharma KN, et al. Activity of single neurons in the hypothalamic feeding centers: effects of glucose. Am J Physiol 1964; *207*:1146–1154.

79. Young JB, Landsberg L. Catecholamines and the sympathoadrenal system: the regulation of metabolism. *In* Ingbar SH (ed). Contemporary Endocrinology. Vol 1. New York, Plenum Press, 1979: 245–303.

80. Acheson KJ, Ravussin E, Wahren J, et al. Thermic effect of glucose in man: obligatory and facultative thermogenesis. J Clin Invest 1984; *74*:1572–1580.

81. Welle S, Campbell RG. Stimulation of thermogenesis by carbohydrate overfeeding: evidence against sympathetic nervous system mediation. J Clin Invest 1983; *71*:916–925.

82. Acheson K, Jequier E, Wahren J. Influence of betaadrenergic blockage on glucose-induced thermogenesis in man. J Clin Invest 1983; *72*:981–986.

83. Cahill GF. Obesity. *In* Brodoff BN, Bleicher SI (eds). Diabetes Mellitus and Obesity. Baltimore, Williams & Wilkins, 1982: 215–218.

84. Stallones RA. Epidemiologic studies of obesity. Ann Intern Med 1985; *103*:1003–1005.

85. Hubert HB, Feinleib M, McNamara PM, et al. Obesity as an independent risk factor for cardiovascular disease: A 26-year follow-up of participants in the Framingham Heart Study. Circulation 1983; *67*:968–977.

86. Barrett-Connor EL. Obesity, atherosclerosis, and coronary artery disease. Ann Intern Med 1985; *103*:1010–1019.

87. Kral JG. Morbid obesity and related health risks. Ann Intern Med 1985; *103*:1043–1047.

88. Dustan HP. Obesity and hypertension. Ann Intern Med 1985; *103*:1047–1049.

89. Cahill GF Jr. Obesity and diabetes. *In* Bray G (ed). Recent Advances in Obesity Research: II, Proceedings of the 2nd International Congress on Obesity. Westport, CT, Technomic Publishing Co, 1979: 101–110.

90. National Diabetes Data Group. Classification and diagnosis of diabetes mellitus and other categories of glucose intolerance. Diabetes 1979; *28*:1039–1057.

91. Nelius SJ, Heyden S, Hansen J, et al. Lipoprotein and blood pressure changes during weight reduction at Duke's Dietary Rehabilitation Clinic. Ann Nutr Metab 1982; *26*:384–392.

92. Garfinkel L. Overweight and cancer. Ann Intern Med 1985; *103*:1034–1036.

93. Bray GA. Complications of obesity. Ann Intern Med 1985; *103*:1052–1062.

94. Wadden TA, Stunkard AJ. Social and psychological consequences of obesity. Ann Intern Med 1985; *103*:1062–1067.

95. Krotiewski M, Blohme B, Lindholm N, et al. The effects of adrenal corticosteroids on regional adipocyte size in man. J Clin Endocrinol Metab 1976; *42*:91–97.

96. Bjorntorp P, Berchtold P, Tibblin G. Insulin secretion in relation to adipose tissue in man. Diabetes 1971; *20*:65–70.

97. Bjorntorp P, Gustafsson A, Persson B. Adipose tissue fat cell size and number in relation to metabolism in endogenous hypertriglyceridemia. Acta Med Scand 1971; *190*:363–367.

98. Stern MP, Olefsky J, Farquhar JW, et al. Relationship between fasting plasma lipid levels and adipose tissue morphology. Metab Clin Exp 1973; *22*:1311–1317.

99. Bjorntorp P, Jonsson A, Berchtold P. Adipose tissue cellularity in maturity onset diabetes mellitus. Acta Med Scand 1972; *191*:129–132.

100. Leonhardt W, Haller H, Hanefeld M. The adipocyte volume in human adipose tissue. II. Observations in diabetes mellitus, primary hyperlipoproteinemia and weight reduction. Int J Obesity 1978; *2*:429–439.

101. Symonds B. The blood pressure of healthy men and women. JAMA 1923; *80*:232.

102. Chiang BN, Perlman LV, Epstein FH. Overweight and hypertension. Circulation 1969; *39*:403–421.

103. Berger M, Muller WA, Renold AE. Relationship of obesity to diabetes: some facts, many questions. *In* Katzen HM, Mahler RJ (eds). Diabetes, Obesity and Vascular Disease, Metabolic and Molecular Interrelationships, Part I. New York, John Wiley and Sons 1978:6:211–228.

104. West K, Kalbfleisch M. Influence of nutritional factors on prevalence of diabetes. Diabetes 1971; *20*:99–108.

105. Bonham GS, Brock DB. The relationship of diabetes with race, sex, and obesity. Am J Clin Nutr 1985; *41*:776–783.

106. Salans LB, Knittle JL, Hirsch J. The role of adipose cell size and adipose tissue insulin sensitivity in the carbohydrate intolerance of human obesity. J Clin Invest 1968;*47*:153–165.

107. Harrison LC, King-Roach AP. Insulin sensitivity of adipose tissue in vitro and the response to exogenous insulin in obese human subjects. Metab Clin Exp 1976; *25*:1095–1101.

108. Olefsky JM. Insulin resistance and insulin action: an in vitro and in vivo perspective. Diabetes 1981; *30*:148–162.

109. Bjorntorp P, Sjostrom L. Carbohydrate storage in man: speculation and some quantitative considerations. Metab Clin Exp 1978; *27*:1853–1865.

110. Smith U, Hammerstein J, Bjorntorp P, et al. Regional differences and effect of weight reduction on human fat cell metabolism. Eur J Clin Invest 1979; *9*:327–334.

111. Owen OE, Reichard GA Jr. Human forearm metabolism during prolonged starvation. J Clin Invest 1971; *50*:1536–1545.

112. Owen OE, Reichard GA Jr. Fuels consumed by man: the interplay between carbohydrates and fatty acids. Biochem Pharmacol 1971; *6*:177–213.

113. Bar RS, Harrison LC, Muggeo M. Regulation of insulin receptors in normal and abnormal physiology in humans. Adv Intern Med 1979; *24*:23–52.

114. Leijd B. Cholesterol and bile acid metabolism in obesity. Clin Sci 1980; *59*:203–206.

115. Lew EA, Garfinkel L. Variations in mortality by weight among 750,000 men and women. J Chron Dis 1979; *32*:563–576.

116. Sharp JT, Barrocas M, Chokroverty S. The cardiorespiratory effects of obesity. Clin Chest Med 1980; *1*:103–118.

117. Luce JM. Respiratory complications of obesity. Chest 1980; *78*:626–631.

118. Strohl KP, Saunders NA, Feldman NT, et al. Obstructive sleep apnea in family members. N Engl J Med 1978; *299*:969–973.

119. Whitcomb ME, Altman N, Clark RW, et al. Central and obstructive sleep apnea: pulmonary disease conference at the Ohio State University, Columbus. Chest 1978; *73*:857–860.

120. Brown J, Winkelmann RK. Acanthosis nigricans: a study of 90 cases. Medicine (Baltimore) 1968; *47*:33–51.

121. Kahn CR, Flier JS, Bar RS, et al. The syndromes of insulin resistance and acanthosis nigricans. Insulin-receptor disorders in man. N Engl J Med 1976; *294*:739–745.

122. Kahn RC, Baird KL, Flier JS, et al. Insulin receptors, receptor antibodies, and the mechanism of insulin action. Recent Prog Horm Res 1981; *37*:477–538.

123. Shimoyama R, Ray TK, Savage CR Jr. et al. In vivo and in

vitro effects of anti-insulin receptor antibodies. J Clin Endocrinol 1984; *59*:916–923.

124. Boden G, Shimoyama R, Savage R, et al. Carbohydrate (CHO) oxidation in patients with type B insulin resistance. Diabetes 1985; *34*:498–502.

125. Rabinowitz D, Zierler KL. Forearm metabolism in obesity and its response to intra-arterial insulin. Characterization of insulin resistance and evidence for adaptive hyperinsulinism. J Clin Invest 1962; *41*:2173–2181.

126. Karam JH, Grodsky GM, Forsham PH. Excessive insulin response to glucose in obese subjects as measured by immunochemical assay. Diabetes 1963; *12*:197–204.

127. Bogardus C, Lillioja S, Mott DM, et al. Relationship between degree of obesity and in vivo insulin in man. Am J Physiol 1985; *248*:E286–E291.

128. Kolterman OG, Insel J, Saekow M, et al. Mechanisms of insulin resistance in human obesity: evidence for receptor and postreceptor defects. J Clin Invest 1980; *65*:1272–1284.

129. Nagulesparan M, Savage PJ, Unger R, et al. A simplified method using somatostatin to assess in vivo insulin resistance over a range of obesity. Diabetes 1979; *28*:980–983.

130. Amatruda JM, Livingston JN, Lockwood DH. Cellular mechanisms in selected states of insulin resistance: human obesity, glucocorticoid excess, and chronic renal failure. Diabetes Metab Rev 1985; *1*(3):292–317.

131. Pederson O, Hijollunk E, Schwartz N. Insulin receptor binding and insulin action in human fat cells: effect of obesity and fasting. Metabolism 1982; *31*:884–895.

132. Lonnroth P, DiGirolamo M, Krotkiewski M, et al. Insulin binding and responsiveness in fat cells from patients with reduced glucose tolerance and type II diabetes. Diabetes 1983; *32*:748–754.

133. Livingston JN, Lerea KM, Bolinder J, et al. Binding and molecular weight properties of the insulin receptor from omental and subcutaneous adipocytes in human obesity. Diabetologia 1984; *27*:447–453.

134. Kashiwagi A, Bogardus C, Lillioja S, et al. In vitro insensitivity of glucose transport and antilipolysis to insulin due to receptor and postreceptor abnormalities in obese Pima Indians with normal glucose tolerance. Metabolism 1984; *33*:772–777.

135. Harrison LC, Martin FIR, Melick RA. Correlation between insulin receptor binding in isolated fat cells and insulin sensitivity in obese human subjects. J Clin Invest 1976; *58*:1435–1441.

136. Olefsky JM. Decreased insulin binding to adipocytes and circulating monocytes from obese subjects. J Clin Invest 1976; *57*:1165–1172.

137. Kolterman OG, Reaven GM, Olefsky JM. Relationship between in vivo insulin resistance and decreased insulin receptors in obese man. J Clin Endocrinol Metab 1979; *48*:487–494.

138. Ciaraldi TP, Kolterman OG, Olefsky JM. Mechanism of the postreceptor defect in insulin action in human obesity. J Clin Invest 1981; *68*:875–880.

139. Drenick EJ, Bale GS, Seltzer F, et al. Excessive mortality and causes of death in morbidly obese men. JAMA 1980; *243*:443–445.

140. Halmi KA, Long M, Stunkard AJ. Psychiatric diagnosis of morbidly obese gastric bypass patients. Am J Psychiatry 1980; *137*:470–472.

141. Van Itallie TB. Health implications of overweight and obesity in the United States. Ann Intern Med 1985; *103*:983–988.

142. Blackburn GL, Flatt JP, Clowes GHA Jr, et al. Protein-sparing therapy during periods of starvation with sepsis or trauma. Ann Surg 1973; *177*:588–594.

143. Flatt JP, Blackburn GL. The metabolic fuel regulatory system: implications for protein-sparing therapies during caloric deprivation and disease. Am J Clin Nutr 1974; *27*:175–187.

144. Blackburn GL, Greenberg I. Multidisciplinary approach to adult onset of obesity therapy. Int J Obesity 1978; *2*:35–44.

145. Van Itallie TB, Yang MU. Cardiac dysfunction in obese dieters: a potentially lethal complication of rapid, massive weight loss. Am J Clin Nutr 1984; *39*:695–702.

146. Pringle TH, Scobie IN, Murray RG, et al. Prolongation of the QT interval during therapeutic starvation: a substrate for malignant arrhythmias. Int J Obesity 1983; *7*:253–261.

147. Talbot JM. Research Needs in Management of Obesity by Severe Caloric Restriction. Bethesda, MD, Life Sciences Research Office, Federation of American Societies for Experimental Biology, 1979.

148. Van Itallie TB. The overweight patient. Clin Implic Nutr 1985; *1*:1–7.

149. Sydney KH, Shepard RJ, Harrison J. Endurance training and body composition of the elderly. Am J Clin Nutr 1977; *30*:326–333.

150. Brewer V, Meyer BM, Keele MS, et al. Role of exercise in prevention of involutional bone loss. Med Sci Sports Exerc 1983; *15*:445–449.

151. Krolner B, Toft B, Nielsen SP, et al. Physical exercise as prophylaxic against involutional vertebral bone loss: a controlled trial. Clin Sci 1983; *64*:541–546.

152. American College of Sports Medicine. Guidelines for graded exercise testing and exercise prescription. 2nd ed. Philadelphia, Lea & Febiger, 1980.

153. Pollock ML. The recommended quantity and quality of exercise for developing and maintaining fitness in healthy adults: position statement of the American College of Sports Medicine. Med Sci Sports Exerc 1978; *10*:8–10.

154. Weinsier RL, Wadden TA, Ritenbaugh C, et al. Recommended therapeutic guidelines for professional weight control programs. Am J Clin Nutr 1984; *40*:865–872.

155. Wadden TA, Stunkard AJ, Brownell KD, et al. Treatment of obesity by behavior therapy and very low caloric diet. J Consult Clin Psychol 1984; *52*:692–694.

156. Stunkard AJ. Obesity. *In* Kaplan HI, Freedman AM, Sadock BJ (eds). Comprehensive Textbook of Psychiatry. Baltimore, William & Wilkins, 1985: 1133–1142.

157. Rosato FE. Gastric stapling as a treatment of massive obesity. *In* Day W (ed). Eating Disorders Throughtout the Life Span. New York, Praeger, in press.

158. Drenick E. Risk of obesity and surgical indications. Int J Obesity 1981; *5*:387–398.

159. Kral JG. Obesity surgery—state of the art. *In* Van Itallie TB, Hirsch J (eds). Recent Advances in Obesity Research IV. London, John Libbey, 1985.

160. Pasulka PS, Bistrian BR, Benotti PN, et al. The risks of surgery in obese patients. Ann Intern Med 1986; *104*:540–546.

161. Bray GA. Obesity. *In* Current Concepts. A Scope Publication. Kalamazoo, Upjohn Co, 1982; May:3–52.

9

STARVATION: SOME BIOLOGICAL ASPECTS

GEORGE F. CAHILL, JR.

Starvation implies total cessation of food (caloric) intake and survival on endogenously stored substrates. Humans are well adapted to both partial and total starvation for long periods of time, and it is obvious that biochemical and physiological alterations have been derived from considerable evolutionary pressure. In fact, one can surmise from modern-day metabolic data that total starvation of 1 to 2 months was not a rare event in ancient times. As an extreme, a very large man with a much-increased muscle mass coupled with a marked accumulation of triglyceride in adipose tissue can survive for over a year without any exogenous intake, and this has been irrefutably documented more than once.[4, 6-9] Thus an American professional football lineman would be the ideal candidate to outlive the remainder of the population were all food intake to cease.

Even normal-weight males without excess muscle or triglyceride can withstand prolonged periods of complete starvation, as evidenced by the 33 Irish political objectors who in 1980 and 1981 survived total deprivation for over 2 months during a hunger strike. Ten others died in the process. Nevertheless, although well adapted, humans are not as fit as many marine mammals who annually starve for as long as 9 months. Also, the North American black bear, which in its winter den fasts for up to 6 months without urination, defecation, or any caloric or fluid intake, certainly does far better than humans.[10-13] But one has to appreciate that humans are, nevertheless, fairly tough creatures in the wild, especially in regard to nutritional aberrations such as episodic starvation.

NORMAL BODY COMPOSITION

To place the function of caloric reserves in humans or any living creatures in proper perspective, a few broad words concerning the relative biological roles of fat, carbohydrate, and protein are in order. Fat stores in almost all living organisms are in the form of triglyceride, the ester of three fatty acids and glycerol. Human triglyceride is an oil, chemically and physically almost identical to olive oil and thus immiscible with water and stored mainly in specialized cells, the adipocytes.[14] In non-homotherms triglyceride may be accumulated in other cells, such as hepatocytes or skin cells, but in mammals it is almost solely in the adipocyte. With fat mobilization, as in starvation or exercise, hydrolysis of triglyceride produces three free fatty acids per triglyceride molecule. These are transported tightly bound to albumin in the circulation to fatty acid–using tissues such as heart, skeletal muscle, liver, and kidney. The other product, glycerol, is removed mainly by the liver either for glucose synthesis, as in fasting, or for energy and/or fat synthesis, as in the fed state.

From an overall caloric aspect, the greatest importance of triglyceride is not its high energy content but rather its extra-aqueous nature, meaning that as it accumulates in adipocytes there is little need for any increase in electrolytes, water, or other intracellular components. Triglyceride is, however, an excellent means of energy storage in terms of calories per unit weight. Pure triglyceride yields 9.4 kcal/g. As adipose tissue expands with its concomitant minimal increase in water, protein, and electrolytes, the accumulated tissue yields between 6 and 8 kcal/g; this again is a very efficient form of energy storage, especially where mobility is significant.

Carbohydrate storage is a different matter. The large branching chain molecules of glucose that make up glycogen are accumulated inside cells with stored water and electrolytes between the chains. In other words carbohydrate is not stored as a dry, dehydrated molecule but rather as a gel of glycogen and water, each molecule being several million daltons in molecular weight and surrounded and mixed with water and electrolytes as well as proteins and other intracellular components. It was shown almost 50 years ago that as cells build up glycogen 2 to 4 g of water are stored per gram of glycogen.[15] In fact, this phenomenon is one of the reasons why potassium levels in the circulation are decreased during

carbohydrate uptake into cells, especially after insulin administration. The potassium is removed to keep the expanded intracellular water both isotonic and isosmotic with intracellular fluid. The significant phenomenon, calorically, is that carbohydrate stored as glycogen is a poor source of energy per unit weight, yielding about 1 kcal/g or less of total accumulated tissue instead of the approximately 4 kcal/g of pure anhydrous glycogen, were it to be stored as such (Fig. 9–1).

Organisms for which mobility plays a role in survival must use fat as their dominant means of energy storage. The best example is the triglyceride depots in insects and birds prior to long migratory flights. The rubythroated hummingbird (A. colubris) is over 50 per cent triglyceride by weight before it crosses the Gulf of Mexico for its annual migration.[16] The same is true for migrating insects such as the monarch butterfly (Danaus plexippus)[17] prior to its annual flight. Conversely, a sessile animal such as a clam need store little, if any, triglyceride. The principle even applies to the plant kingdom, where triglyceride is stored for energy in seeds and nuts. The smaller size permitted by lipid instead of carbohydrate storage allows easier physical distribution away from the parental plant or tree. In contrast carbohydrate is solely used to sustain a sessile life style and a reproductive process not needing mobility.

Human evolutionary selection has involved two essentially contradictory processes, one being the expanding brain and its accompanying intellect, and the other being mobility and survival in a nutritionally, environmentally, and socially hostile milieu. A big brain is an energetic liability and therefore threatens survival in a deprived environment, yet the intellectual advantage provided by the brain is obviously the most significant component of man's biological success in dominating nature.[18]

A normal middle-aged man weighing 75 kg is composed of 15 kg of fat, the greatest majority (perhaps 12 kg) as triglyceride, 12 to 13 kg of protein, and about 42 kg of water. Minerals and glycogen add up to 4.2 kg, and a reasonable approximation is that 3.5 kg is minerals and about 0.5 to 0.8 kg is

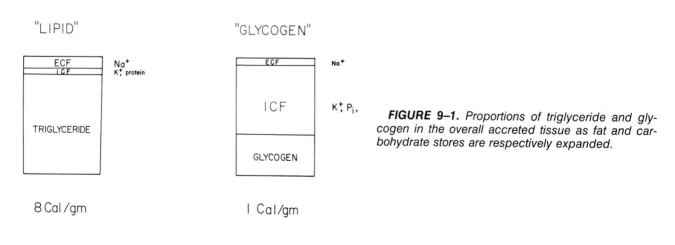

FIGURE 9–1. Proportions of triglyceride and glycogen in the overall accreted tissue as fat and carbohydrate stores are respectively expanded.

glycogen,[19, 20] the latter amount being obviously extremely variable. Rounding the numbers and giving an approximation of potential energy stores in a random normal human, one can construct a simple table of fuels (Table 9–1), dividing those tissues available for consumption, meaning relatively or easily expendable, versus those essentially unexpendable or, in biological terms, "constitutive."

With starvation, every tissue (even brain, but probably to a very small degree) contributes something for fuel. It is adipose tissue and skeletal muscle that provide the bulk of calories, particularly the former. Adipose tissue stores provide a 2-months' supply of calories for basal energy expenditure in a normal human, but the amount of muscle protein that can (and does) provide calories is significant and is critical in the transition between the fed state and starvation. The amount of muscle also plays a critical role in the duration of long-term starvation itself. One other point of interest relating to fuels in this 75-kg man, if one considers muscle to be between 20 and 25 per cent protein, is that his total muscle mass would provide about 30 kg net weight protein or 25,000 kcal, whereas his adipose tissue mass, using an approximate number of 80 per cent of adipose tissue being triglyceride, would be 12 kg or over 100,000 kcal. This again emphasizes the overriding economy of fat as fuel. It should also be pointed out that the muscle and liver glycogen,[19, 20] totaling about 600 g, would require another 1.5 to 2.5 kg of water to keep the glycogen in its intracellular gel state, as discussed above; tallying calories, glycogen in muscle and liver is only just over a day's supply of energy. In the total picture, glycogen is an evanescent source of fuel, but obviously crucial for anaerobic glycolysis during acute stress, where it may be life-saving.

ENERGY DEMANDS

In the basal state, a normal adult man consumes energy at the rate of about 1 kcal/minute, roughly equivalent to 0.1 horsepower or to a 75-watt light-bulb or motor.[6–9] If only basal energy is being expended, all of the calories are lost as heat. In spite of much opinion to the contrary, the efficiency of humans in converting stored fuel into metabolically available energy is extremely uniform. No humans are super-efficient or super-wasteful. There are a few extremely rare exceptions to the latter, such as individuals with inborn errors of mitochondrial metabolism who may lose energy even in the basal state; the Luft-Ernster syndrome[21] is one of only a few reported examples.

The organ that appears to have the most constant energy demand is the brain, which consumes one fifth of the basal calories. It is true that there are focal areas in the brain of both increased oxygen consumption and fuel utilization, such as a strip of the motor cortex involved in exercise of a muscle group. But the total mass of the brain so overrides these regional variabilities in metabolic activity that overall oxygen consumption changes little unless there is a diffuse generalized discharge of numerous brain cells as in a major convulsive seizure. Thus the brain, like a large computer with only some circuits in use at any given time, uses almost a constant supply of energy, whether the owner is sleeping, playing chess, jogging, or daydreaming.

The armor that protects the brain from the environment obviously prevents it from expanding or contracting with energy accumulation or mobilization, so that the brain cannot store calories. The brain is so critically dependent on the rest of the body for energy that interruption of perfusion for more than a minute or so is incompatible with physiological function, and interruption for more prolonged periods is incompatible even with viability of neurons. This dependency is so extreme that when total perfusion is compromised, for example, with acute amputation of a leg and subsequent hemorrhage, the compensatory response of the sympathetic nervous system and arteries throughout the body is to redirect blood flow to the head, so that essentially what remains is a heart-lung-brain circulation. It is known to military surgeons that soldiers in their third and fourth decades can survive the severance of a peripheral artery as with an amputated limb thanks to the compliance of the blood system and its capacity to respond to sympathetic stimulation and vasoconstriction, whereas older individuals, with a little early atherosclerosis and slightly stiffer vessels, not only continue to hemorrhage from the severed artery but also are less able to redirect the remaining blood flow. The younger soldier survives the injury; the older one dies.

Concerning energy requirements of the rest of the body, the heart consumes about 5 per cent, the kidneys 10 per cent, the liver and viscera about 30 per cent, and the resting muscle and other tissues the balance. In contrast, during vigorous exercise, muscle may increase its oxygen consumption 10- to 20-fold and consume up to 90 per cent of total energy expenditure. The remaining tissues continue to consume about the same energy as during the resting state.

There is another major anatomical and resulting metabolic hurdle that must be surmounted, which

TABLE 9–1. Fuels in a 75-Kilogram Man

	Kilograms	Kilocalories
Adipose tissue triglyceride	12	110,000
Protein		
Muscle	6	25,000
Others*	6	25,000
Carbohydrate		
Muscle glycogen	0.5	2,000
Liver glycogen	0.1	400
Free glucose	0.02	80

*Mainly non-utilizable

poses a particular problem to humans in addition to the size of the brain, and that is the selective control of permeation by the blood-brain barrier.[22] This physiological partition between the circulating blood and the central nervous system is present in all vertebrates and probably extends even to peripheral nerve. In other words, all neural tissues are excluded from direct contact with blood and extracellular fluid. There are of course some exceptions, such as areas of the hypothalamus and the optic nerve where it enters the optic globe, but generally speaking, nerve is bathed by its own private and unique milieu, the cerebrospinal fluid.

It is interesting to speculate why this segregation of nerve tissue from the rest of the body fluids exists. One hypothesis is that cells destined to evolve into the nervous system became exquisitely sensitive to electrical and substrate variations and segregated from other cells in early multicellular organisms. A reasonable speculation is that these first progenitor neural cells evolve as external receptors in the simple creatures living in the primeval sea. Those organisms were exposed to extremely low concentrations of various stimulating factors in the environment. If a signal was interpreted as food or friendly, the organism would respond in a positive tropic manner, whereas if a signal was interpreted as noxious or hostile, the organism would be induced to go in the opposite direction. Primitive motile organisms such as bacteria and lower animals retain this chemosensitivity and response, and the most fascinating problem is how they can recognize the gradients of these environmental cues and respond accordingly.[23, 24]

Small molecules, originally environmental and now endogenous and in very low concentrations, appear to have been retained throughout vertebrate evolution as the primary neurotransmitters; glutamate, GABA, aspartate, and dopamine are examples. The concentration of glutamate ranges between 5 and 20 mmol inside nerve cells, is about 50 μmol in blood, and ranges between 3 and 5 μmol in cerebrospinal fluid, as obtained by lumbar puncture.[25] Its concentration directly on the surfaces of brain cells in situ is not known but is probably even less, perhaps under 1 μmol. The only amino acid that approximates equal concentrations in spinal fluid and blood or other extracellular fluids is glutamine, at about 0.5 mmol, and it is safe to say that glutamine plays no modulating role in neurotransmission. Of interest, proline, the concentration of which in blood plasma is about 0.1 mmol, is undetectable in spinal fluid by standard ion exchange chromatography. One might guess that proline may also be an exquisite neurotransmitter, but there are no data in the neuroscience literature for or against this hypothesis.

The anatomical basis for sequestration of the central nervous system from the peripheral circulation is the vascular endothelial cell. Brain capillaries, like other capillaries throughout the body, are lined with endothelium. Unique to brain and one or two other areas, for example the testis, is the presence of tight junctions between the endothelial cells.[22] In fact, there are several tight junctions in series between adjacent capillary endothelial cells, and this structure essentially prevents the exchange of fluid and electrolytes between the brain and the circulation. Any material other than water that has to cross from the peripheral circulation to the brain cell must be transported through the endothelial cells, since free diffusion is essentially prohibited. Thus excluded from brain are large molecules such as lipoproteins or immunoglobulins. Water-soluble substrates present in blood and for which there are transport processes across the membranes of the endothelial cell (or else easy permeability, perhaps by nonionic diffusion) include glucose, lactate, pyruvate, acetate, glycerol, and of course the various amino acids present in the circulation. Under normal circumstances there is only one component in blood that crosses the barrier and is of sufficient concentration to provide the brain with water-soluble fuel, and that one substance is glucose. There is some evidence, even in humans, that lactate and pyruvate,[26, 27] when markedly elevated, can provide a significant amount of fuel for brain, but generally speaking, glucose is the only substrate. This was shown 40 years ago by Sokoloff[28] and Kety[29] in their classic studies on the determination of cerebral blood flow and substrate utilization in man.

The entry of glucose into brain is by the process of facilitated diffusion, meaning that it is not uphill but rather down a concentration gradient. Yet it has all the specificities of enzymatic carrier transport, namely, substrate specificity, competition between substrates, and saturation of the system. The entry of glucose into brain cells occurs by a similar process; thus there are two facilitated diffusions in series, each requiring a given "pressure" or substrate concentration to permit adequate glucose uptake. Both processes appear to be insulin-independent; however, it has been known for years that there appears to be an adaptation to ambient glucose concentration by brain, though the precise physiology of this adaptation remains to be defined.

Clinicians treating diabetes have noted since insulin became available that if a patient had an ambient glucose concentration of 200 mg/dl or so, a reduction of glucose by insulin might produce significant cerebral symptoms of glucose deprivation, even with arterial levels of glucose over 100 mg/dl. Thus a true physiological "hypoglycemia" can be induced even in the presence of some degree of hyperglycemia. On the other hand, and in support of the adaptability concept, it has been observed that patients with islet cell tumors and protracted hypoglycemia, as well as extremely well controlled or overenthusiastically controlled diabetics, can have ambient glucose concentrations of 30 or 40 mg/dl without any symptoms. This is also true occasionally of children with inborn errors of carbohydrate homeostasis such as von Gierke's disease, in whom dramatically low glucose concentrations can be observed. Recently McCall and colleagues[30] and Gjedde and Crone[31] have demonstrated in experimental animals an adaptation of glucose transport into brain as a function of ambient glucose concentrations, thus giving a more scientific basis to the inferences drawn from the above-mentioned anecdotal observations. To summarize, with prolonged hypoglycemia, brain has an apparently easier access to blood glucose, but how remains to be defined.

Since the brain has to have continuous perfusion by oxygen and glucose, as well as having to eliminate its metabolically produced carbon dioxide, there must be a strong biochemical and physiological priority for an organism to maintain brain metabolic activity. As previously mentioned, the cardiovascular system is attuned to defend brain circulation as its last-ditch effort. The sympathetic nervous system and the direct adrenal output of adrenalin and noradrenalin play extremely important roles in this process.[32] Likewise, metabolically there are a number of systems, some primary and some as backup, that are designed to maintain glucose output to keep the brain going. Again, the sympathetic nervous system and the direct adrenal output into the circulation of adrenalin (epinephrine) and noradrenalin (norepinephrine) are responsible players in this life-saving effort. The first event, of course, is to stimulate glycogen breakdown by the liver. In addition to sympathetic nerve endings directly in liver, as well as elevated levels of catecholamines, there is a significant part played by pancreatic alpha cell release of glucagon in accelerating glycogen breakdown. These all increase the activity of liver glycogen phosphorylase, and the net result is an outpouring of glucose from liver glycogen. It has also been demonstrated that glucagon and catecholamines alter the rate-controlling gluconeogenic enzymes in liver in the direction of glucose production. The glucagon and catechol effects on glycogenolysis start almost instantaneously and peak within a minute or two, whereas the gluconeogenic effects are more prolonged, taking minutes to start and lasting hours. These latter adapt the animal for a stressful situation that might continue beyond the acute emergency. The third glucogenic wave is the delivery of peripheral substrates to liver to maintain gluconeogenesis and, again, the sympathetic nervous system as well as circulating catecholamines play fundamental roles by initiating muscle glycogen breakdown with an outpouring of lactate and alanine, which are carried to the liver as excellent substrates for glucose synthesis.[33]

It should also be added that elevation of free fatty acids by the acute emergency situation inhibits glucose uptake by a number of tissues,[34, 35] particularly muscle and heart, and these in turn spare glucose for consumption by brain or by ischemic muscle, a topic covered in Chapter 11.

PROGRESSIVE STARVATION

The Postprandial Phase

As a mixed meal is ingested, complex carbohydrates in the gut are broken down into simple sugars, of which the most significant is glucose, coming primarily from starch but also from the two dominant disaccharides in the human diet, sucrose and lactose. The other two sugars from these ingested disaccharides, namely fructose from the sucrose and galactose from the lactose, are also rapidly taken up into the portal circulation, removed by specific enzyme systems in the liver, and converted into the usual intermediates of hepatic glucose metabolism.

The glucose that is absorbed is distributed by the circulation throughout the body, with a number of tissue priorities for its uptake. These appear to be a function of the relative level of insulin, which in turn is a function of the amount of glucose absorbed. The first priority, of course, is to maintain brain metabolism, requiring 100 to 125 g of glucose per day or 400 to 500 kcal/day. Should the rate of glucose entry into blood surpass this constant rate of glucose uptake by brain, the next priority is replenishment of liver glycogen. The amount of glycogen stored in the liver is widely variable and can be as low as 0.5 per cent of liver weight, or 5 g, or as high as 10 to 15 per cent, or 150 to 200 g. Liver glycogen serves a role not only in carbohydrate storage but also and equally important as a buffer or capacitor for large glucose inputs into the body. This is particularly the case when a meal containing adequate carbohydrate has not been consumed in the recent past and lipogenic enzymes have decreased in activity. Thus, the liver serves as a kind of overflow holding tank for excess calories which may eventually be destined for fat.

The proteins in the diet are broken down into amino acids by hydrolysis, and these amino acids also have priorities in their disposition. The first, of course, is to replenish the constitutive protein reserves in liver and muscle, replacing protein broken down since the previous meal. In mammals there is no protein depot purely for storage alone. Extra amino acids, mainly the nonessentials, are deaminated in liver and the carbohydrate residues used either for liver energy and fat synthesis or for gluconeogenesis. The branched-chain amino acids are primarily metabolized in the periphery and used by adipose tissue for fat synthesis in times of caloric excess, or in times of overall body catabolism (as in starvation or trauma) are deaminated and oxidized by muscle.[36]

Dietary fat enters as triglyceride, which in conjunction with a number of proteins and endogenous fat, the lipoproteins, forms a particle that passes via the lymph into the general circulation. This particle, the chylomicron, has two general alternatives for its disposition. In the fasting state it is utilized by muscle as fuel, and in the fed state it is removed primarily by adipose tissue for incorporation into fat droplets as a major component of overall energy storage.[14]

In the postprandial state, presuming that the mixed meal contained excess substrate in all three categories (carbohydrate, protein, and fat), the body continues in an anabolic phase as long as calories are entering via the gastrointestinal tract. The signal for this process is an elevated insulin concentration, and, as will be discussed in the case of liver, a slightly elevated glucose concentration probably also plays a significant role.

Muscle glycogen appears to be relatively stable in concentration postprandially unless the muscle is stimulated with vigorous activity.[20] Should a muscle have been utilized and its glycogen depleted, one of the first priorities for glucose in muscle after its uptake would be re-expansion of that specific muscle's glycogen pool. Should liver glycogen be replenished and muscle glycogen also be fully stocked, the next priority for glucose utilization is its metabolic use by muscle as substrate. Thus in the postprandial state, as glucose enters the body, the elevated insulin level signals muscle (both heart and skeletal muscle) to utilize glucose as its basal fuel. At the same time adipose tissue is signaled to decrease its rate of free fatty acid release, so free fatty acid levels fall. In other words, the entire body is using glucose. Even with mild exercise in the postprandial state, the main substrate being used by the body is glucose derived from the diet, rather than any fat, either exogenous or endogenous.

Finally, if glucose entry is more rapid than needed for replenishment of glycogen reserves as well as for its first priority, brain metabolism, and is sufficient for utilization as fuel by muscle, the excess calories are converted into fat in liver and adipose tissue. Not yet certain is the relative role of human liver versus adipose tissue in de novo fat synthesis. Human adipose tissue is capable of synthesizing long-chain fatty acids from glucose; this has been shown in vivo and in vitro. Its metabolic rate in this process, however, appears to be much less than that of experimental animals such as the rat and mouse. Of course, these small animals have much higher total metabolic rates and turnovers of various substrates and storage depots, so that one would expect any process to be more rapid in these small creatures as compared with larger humans. Nevertheless, it is felt by most investigators that the liver probably plays the central role in human fat synthesis from carbohydrate. Liver, however, not being a fat-storing organ, exports fat as triglyceride in the form of aggregates of lipid and apolipoproteins (to form the beta lipoprotein or endogenous fat particle, in contrast to the larger and exogenously derived fat particle, the chylomicron).

As the end of the meal is finally digested by the gastrointestinal tract and the various contents are delivered to the circulation, insulin levels fall, serving as the signal for glucose removal by adipose tissue and muscle to decrease. Finally, as the rate of glucose entry into the blood from the gut equals that of removal by the brain, adipose tissue and muscle and finally the liver are signaled not to take up any more glucose. The liver then becomes a glucose-producing organ. It is still not quite clear how the normal human maintains such a narrow range of glucose homeostasis in spite of the fact that daily glucose excursions are many times the amount of free glucose in the body, and three or four times the amount stored as glycogen in the liver.

One explanation for the remarkable glucose homeostasis is the unique characteristic of the glucose phosphorylating system in liver, namely, glucokinase.[37–39] It was shown 30 years ago that liver has a glucose phosphorylating enzyme with a K_m equivalent to the glucose concentration in the circulation. It was also shown that maintenance of this enzyme's activity is a function of insulin levels. In the fasted state glucokinase decreases in activity, and in the fed state it increases. Moreover, glucokinase is characterized by unique kinetics: glucose not only is a substrate but also allosterically activates the enzyme.[40] Thus there is a remarkable amplifying system whereby small increases in glucose concentration increase insulin, which increases glucokinase activity; the glucose then allosterically activates the enzyme directly, and finally, because of the unique K_m of the enzyme at the physiological level of glucose, the glucose concentration itself augments the rate of glucose phosphorylation. The net result allows a rapid change in the direction and rate of uptake or production of glucose with only a minor change in blood glucose concentration. To emphasize this, a healthy young individual after a large carbohydrate meal of 100 g, five times the amount of free glucose in the body, may have an elevation of arterial glucose concentration to only 6 to 7 mmol from the pre-meal concentration of 4 to 5 mmol. After the meal it may fall to as low as 3 to 4 mmol and then gradually return to its original starting point.

One might ask why the range of glucose concentrations should be restricted so closely. One answer is the renal glucose threshold of 9 to 10 mmol. Glycosuria is detrimental not only because of some caloric wastage but also probably because it predisposes the urinary tract to infection. Other reasons for maintaining a narrow range of glucose concentration are the sensitivity to infection of other tissues in the body in the presence of hyperglycemia, the teratogenicity of hyperglycemia in the pregnant female, and the altered half-lives and functional problems (such as antigenicity) of many proteins in the body with continued exposure to high levels of blood glucose due to nonenzymatic glycosylation. There are evolutionary selective pressures to prevent hyperglycemia, to which can be added the tendency of the body to maintain some degree of stability in its osmolality. The reason why the body should prevent hypoglycemia, as already described, is to provide the brain with adequate substrate via its two facilitated diffusion barriers in series, the blood-brain barrier and a second process transferring glucose from brain extracellular fluids into brain cells.

The Postabsorptive Phase

The postabsorptive phase is best exemplified in the human after an overnight fast. All the food from the previous meal has been absorbed and the small intestine is empty. Glucose consumption is now mainly by brain, but other tissues, particularly skeletal muscle, are still deriving about one fourth to one third of their energy from glucose, and this amount is progressively diminishing. Free fatty acids are beginning to be mobilized from adipose tissue to provide the other two thirds to three fourths of muscle substrate, and free fatty acid levels are rising in the blood.[35, 41-43] Liver glycogen, which had been perhaps 100 to 150 g following the absorption of the meal, is now falling. The source of hepatic glucose production may vary depending on the individual and on the size of and interval since the last meal, with as much as three fourths or as little as one fourth coming from liver glycogen and the balance from gluconeogenesis. As the morning progresses, gluconeogenesis becomes more and more significant in all individuals, so that after 24 hours of abstinence from caloric intake (particularly carbohydrate intake) gluconeogenesis is the prime contributor of hepatic glucose production.

The primary signal early in fasting seems to be the lower insulin level, which in the presence of normal or, in some studies, even elevated levels of glucagon, provokes not only hepatic glycogenolysis but also initiation of gluconeogenesis (Fig. 9–2). The lower insulin level also initiates proteolysis in skeletal muscle with release of amino acids, mainly glutamine and alanine,[44] the optimal nitrogenous substrates for gluconeogenesis in liver (and also in kidney).

Early Starvation

As liver glycogen falls to a nadir of approximately 0.5 g/dl, gluconeogenesis becomes the sole supporter of hepatic glucose production. Thus at 2 to 3 days of starvation ("early" starvation) brain is living primarily off glucose produced from muscle protein. This is no problem in an animal with a small brain and a large muscle mass, such as a bear or an emperor penguin, at least for a brief period of time, and even in humans it is no major problem, provided

the individual has been appropriately nourished from the start. Total urinary nitrogen excretion in the fed state is simply a function of nitrogen intake, provided that the subject is in nitrogen balance. However, with the initiation of caloric deprivation, nitrogen excretion falls off in a day or two. Then the body begins to depend on gluconeogenesis from muscle protein as its primary source of glucose for brain, and urinary nitrogen excretion may again rise until the next phase of starvation, in which glucose utilization in brain is displaced by ketone body utilization.[45] Thus in early starvation there is a stimulation of muscle protein breakdown by the low insulin level and an outpouring of amino acids, primarily alanine and glutamine. The levels of the branched-chain amino acids are increased in the circulation even though they are principally metabolized directly inside the muscle. Since the branched-chain amino acids, leucine, isoleucine, and valine, are not accumulated inside cells relative to extracellular concentrations, this rise in blood is paralleled by a rise inside cells.[46-48] Their levels in blood may double, as if protein had been ingested. In all metabolic states, the rate of nitrogen excretion in the urine appears to parallel the level of branched-chain amino acids in the circulation, suggesting that their catabolism in muscle is regulated primarily by their levels in cells and blood. Inasmuch as branched-chain amino acids are not concentrated to any significant degree inside muscle, their levels in muscle would parallel those in the circulation, and this makes easily understandable the parallelism of blood levels to urinary nitrogen excretion.

By the second or third day of starvation, about 75 g of muscle protein is catabolized daily. This is an insufficient amount to provide all of the substrate for glucose utilization by the brain, and other sources of fuel must be available. One of these is glycerol derived from adipose tissue triglyceride hydrolysis. If 180 to 200 g of triglyceride is broken down daily to maintain caloric needs, then about 18 to 20 g of glycerol is available for glucose synthesis by the liver (and to a lesser degree by the kidney) (Fig. 9–3). Another non-nitrogenous source of glucose precursor is lactate and pyruvate coming from muscle glycogen. As stated above, muscle glycogen is mainly used in brisk exercise, but there is some evidence that with prolonged starvation there is a mild progressive decrease in muscle glycogen, even if the muscle is not exercised vigorously. This lactate and pyruvate contribute carbohydrate to the precursor pool for hepatic gluconeogenesis. In any case, even the consumption of 75 g of muscle protein, meaning four to five times that amount as wet muscle (about ⅔ lb of muscle per day), would be incompatible with survival for more than a week or two if allowed to persist. The fine regulation of these processes is evidenced by the extremely stable blood glucose concentration. In the normal individual this approximates 3.5 to 4.0 mmol at 2 to 3 days of total

MUSCLE PROTEIN METABOLISM

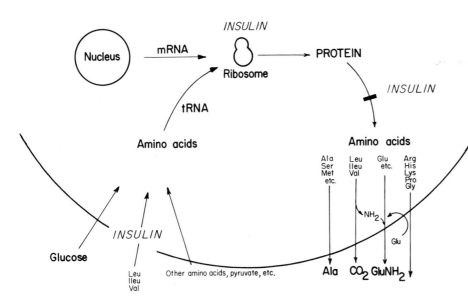

FIGURE 9–2. Effect of insulin in promoting glucose and amino acid uptake into muscle, activation of protein synthesis at the ribosome, and inhibition of proteolysis. Also shown is the predominant release of alanine (Ala) and glutamine ($GluNH_2$).

starvation.[41] It will then remain at this level throughout starvation until the terminal event, at which time it may fall precipitously, but for obvious ethical reasons this observation is from studies of experimental animals and not of humans.

The most significant event of starvation concerning substrate utilization and nitrogen conservation is the development of a mild but regulated and balanced ketoacidosis.[4, 41] As the liver enters a gluconeogenic mode of operation in the presence of low insulin levels and the permissive presence of glucagon, glucocorticoids, and thyroid hormone, it also begins to produce acetoacetate and beta-hydroxybutyrate.

A few sentences are in order here concerning ketogenesis and its energetics. As long-chain fatty acids are oxidized to acetyl CoA, about one third of their total energy becomes available from the reduced pyridine nucleotides, NADH and NADPH, that are produced in this process. Thus during ketogenesis, liver is provided with more than adequate substrate.[49] What does it then do with the excess acetate? A number of biochemical processes have been clarified by which the acetate so produced is exported to the periphery for oxidation as ketoacids or "ketone bodies." Normally, acetate would condense with oxaloacetate to be burned by the tricarboxylic acid (Krebs) cycle inside the liver. With accelerated glu-

FIGURE 9–3. Glucose production from various precursors by liver and kidney in starving humans. Not shown is the 10 to 15 g of glucose derived from ketoacids after the first week or so of starvation.

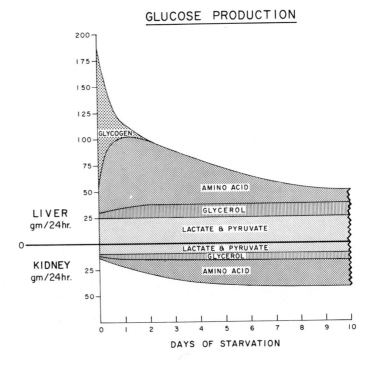

GLUCOSE PRODUCTION

coneogenesis the oxaloacetate is instead used for synthesis of phosphoenolpyruvate, the initial step in the gluconeogenic process. It should also be added that alanine coming in from the periphery generates pyruvate. In the fasting state, however, pyruvate dehydrogenase is markedly diminished in activity and the pyruvate instead is carboxylated to oxaloacetate, which, as just stated, is swept into glucose again by the accelerated gluconeogenic process. Thus, to summarize, gluconeogenic precursors coming from the periphery are pushed into gluconeogenesis with almost 100 per cent efficiency and are not used by the liver's tricarboxylic acid cycle for energy or for fat synthesis. Instead the liver derives its own energy directly from the dehydrogenation of the long-chain fatty acids to acetate, and then finally exports the acetate as ketone bodies for oxidation by peripheral tissues. The liver tricarboxylic acid cycle essentially stops, and this is reflected by the extremely low respiratory quotient shown by liver in fasting states or in diabetic ketoacidosis, which really is a "super-fasted" state.

Later Starvation

Normally, blood levels of acetoacetate and beta-hydroxybutyrate are barely detectable even with very sensitive enzymatic procedures.[41] A reasonable estimate would be between 20 and 30 μmol for each of these. The levels of these substrates in blood gradually increase over the first week of starvation up to approximately 1.5 mmol acetoacetate and 6 mmol beta-hydroxybutyrate. These levels then persist throughout the next several weeks of starvation until the fat depots are exhausted just prior to death. Garber and colleagues[42] have shown that hepatic ketone body production is maximal after 2 days of starvation and that the subsequent rise in blood level is primarily due to a diminution in utilization by tissues, except, of course, brain. There is also a slight decrease in renal excretion.[9] In other words, skeletal muscle and particularly heart are active consumers of ketoacids at days 2 to 3 of starvation, but soon afterwards their consumption of these fuels diminishes, permitting a greater proportion to be used by brain. Göttstein some 20 years ago demonstrated that the enzymatic apparatus for the oxidation of beta-hydroxybutyrate and acetoacetate by human brain is always available (constitutive), since brain can utilize both of these substrates immediately after their acute infusion into a normal human.[50] Thus what dictates the amount of ketoacid used by brain is the ambient level in the circulation and, as has been mentioned above, the level reaches a plateau at a total of about 7.5 mmol after a week of starvation, permitting two thirds to three fourths of brain oxygen consumption to be derived from ketoacid oxidation. As brain consumes more and more ketone bodies as its primary fuel, glucose oxidation is di-

minished accordingly; the decrease has been demonstrated to take place at the point of glucose phosphorylation through inhibition of brain hexokinase by products of ketoacid oxidation.[45] The most significant point, however, is that, as brain diminishes its glucose utilization, there is less and less need for hepatic gluconeogenesis and pari passu a diminished need for muscle proteolysis to produce gluconeogenic amino acid. Thus, instead of 75 g/day of muscle protein, after 2 weeks of starvation only some 20 to 30 g of muscle protein is lost daily, contributing 4 to 5 g of urinary nitrogen (Fig. 9–4). This diminished amount obviously permits maintenance of a large proportion of muscle mass, permitting starvation to continue as long as there is some amount of triglyceride to produce free fatty acids and glycerol from adipose tissue.

A dictum of biochemistry is that acetate once produced cannot be recaptured for entry into carbohydrate. The explanation is that pyruvate dehydrogenase is essentially irreversible from a thermodynamic aspect. Occasionally it is also asked why acetate cannot condense with oxaloacetate, go around the tricarboxylic acid cycle, and then be incorporated into glucose. The answer is that two carbons are lost per turn of the cycle, so it is essentially impossible for the cycle to produce net carbohydrate precursor unless products of amino acids enter into the cycle to generate new oxaloacetate or its precursors. In fact, this is the route that the gluconeogenic amino acids other than alanine and serine use to promulgate gluconeogenesis.

It was shown many years ago that ruminants can use ketoacids or short-chain lipids and their oxida-

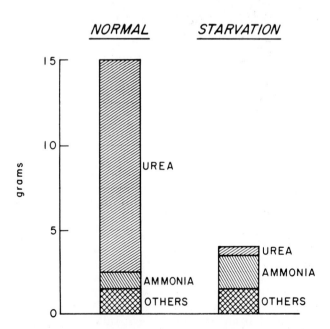

FIGURE 9–4. *Urinary nitrogen constituents in the fed state (left column) and after several weeks of starvation (right column). The extremely small amount of urea excreted with starvation is apparent.*

tive products for incorporation into glucose.[51] Reichard and Owen and colleagues have shown that this can also take place in humans, and it is now known that about 10 to 15 g of glucose per day can be produced from acetoacetate, probably by reduction of acetoacetate to propanediol and its eventual conversion into pyruvate.[52–54] Thus about 10 to 15 g of gluconeogenetically produced glucose per day is derived from fatty acids. Although this seems trivial on the surface, after a month or so of starvation, it could provide a tremendous selective advantage by sparing several pounds of muscle from catabolism during each starvation-refeeding cycle.

ENERGETICS OF STARVATION

Benedict, in his classic treatise on starvation, in which he studied a 30-day fast in a normal volunteer, Mr. Levanzin, noted a progressive decrease in oxygen consumption, indicating a corresponding decrease in energy expenditure.[55] This decrease approximated 10 to 15 per cent by the end of the first week and another 5 to 10 per cent subsequently. Of course part of this decrease is a result of a smaller metabolic body mass. Ingbar and colleagues and others demonstrated that fasting or even nonspecific illness decreases the conversion of thyroxine to triiodothyronine, resulting in a kind of mild hypometabolism, and this explains part of the decrease in overall caloric expenditure as evidenced by the decreased oxygen consumption.[56] The other component is a mild but significant decrease in basal catechol levels, and this has been shown by Landsberg and colleagues[57] to be related to the presence or absence of carbohydrate intake. There is some evidence that the increase in oxygen consumption noted with high calorie and especially high carbohydrate intake is related to increased catechol production and possibly also to increased conversion of thyroxine (T_4) to triiodothyronine (active T_3); this state is termed "luxus consumption," meaning a decreased metabolic efficiency with hypercaloric intakes.

Another component of energy conservation with starvation is physical torpor. The transient hyperactivity of hungry animals in early starvation is well documented, but this is followed by physical inactivity as the fast proceeds, and the same appears to hold true for humans. Starving populations become compliant, a fact that has been used for political as well as military advantages over the millennia. Totally fasting humans, however, like the black bear awakened from its winter sleep, still can perform physical feats; the author was acquainted with one marathon runner who fasted for a week prior to the race and yet finished in 3½ hours—not an excellent time, but still remarkable in that it could be achieved.

FINAL COMMENTS

So far in this chapter *Homo sapiens* has been dealt with as a single entity with some comparisons to bears, birds, and others. Knowing the metabolism of starvation, could there be some degree of genetic heterogeneity in the challenge of starvation? Firstly, nothing has been said of scaling in normal humans. One fifth of the oxygen consumed in the model 70- to 75-kg male is used by the brain, whereas in a child up to 50 per cent of basal energy may be used by the brain (Fig. 9–5). From this it is easy to understand how the human child is at such risk to develop hypoglycemia with even normal brief periods of deprivation. Some feel that even the mild hypoglycemia seen with gastrointestinal upsets such as car sickness in some children may represent the edge of a normal gaussian distribution rather than a disease entity. The child usually has only one or two of these hypoglycemic episodes and always grows out of the problem.

Are there racial differences? One wonders whether the tendency to obesity (and to diabetes) in the American Indian or in the Polynesian may not result from a blunting of caloric homeostasis, permitting obesity to occur more easily in order to face the challenge of intermittent starvation. There is no question but that the Polynesian floating across the Pacific for several months was better adapted if he or she fattened up prior to the excursion. As in the professional football player, an increased muscle mass would be a cofactor in providing the selective advantage. Perhaps this is why dances, athletic events, war games, and other physical activities are common among primitive peoples during harvests and other hypercaloric times. This activity certainly increased protein accretion which otherwise would have gone to triglyceride. What a contrast to modern

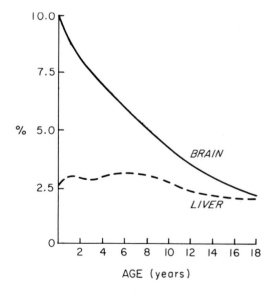

FIGURE 9–5. *Relative sizes of brain and liver in man as a function of age.*

man who sits, drinks, and watches television after festive hypercaloric events!

As a final observation, caloric homeostasis in lower animals is usually governed by external events (day/night ratios, changing seasons, temperature, etc.), as is reproduction. Subhuman primates are noted for their monthly instead of seasonally related sexual cycles, and many studies have shown emotional and environmental effects on primate sexual periodicity. For example, a monkey colony in a hostile environment does not breed, indicating that reproductive behavior comes under intellectual control. In a similar manner, humans have probably more or less lost physiological control of caloric homeostasis and eat mainly for emotional (hedonistic) needs, especially in the third and later decades of life. This supersedence of voluntary over physiological control was probably crucial to primitive man, since it allowed a preplanned fattening up prior to anticipated prolonged starvation. The penalty, however, is today's overnutrition and its morbid sequelae such as maturity-onset diabetes, atherosclerosis, and hypertension. Nevertheless, the hypothesis that humans lost an appetite–body calorie feedback loop for a selective reason is understandable from the data discussed in this chapter.

References

1. Keys A, Brozek J, Henschel A, Mickelsen O, et al. The Biology of Human Starvation. Vol. I and II. Minneapolis, University of Minnesota Press, 1950.
2. Winick M. Hunger Disease. Studies by the Jewish Physicians in the Warsaw Ghetto. New York, John Wiley & Sons, 1979.
3. Helweg-Larsen P, Hoffmeyer H, Keiler J, et al. Famine disease in German concentration camps: complications and sequels. Acta Med Scand 1952; 144(Suppl 274):3–460.
4. Cahill GF Jr. Starvation in man. N Engl J Med 1970; 282:668–675.
5. Felig P. Starvation. In DeGroot LJ, Cahill GF Jr, Odell WD, et al. (eds). Endocrinology. Vol. 3. New York, Grune & Stratton, 1979: 1927–1940.
6. Grande F, Keys A. Body weight, body composition and caloric status. In Goodhart RS, Shils ME (eds). Modern Nutrition in Health and Disease. Philadelphia, Lea & Febiger, 1980: 3–34.
7. Ravussin E, Burnand B, Schutz Y, et al. Twenty-four hour energy expenditure and resting metabolic rate in obese, moderately obese, and control subjects. Am J Clin Nutr 1982; 35:566–573.
8. Felig P, Cunningham J, Levitt M, et al. Energy expenditure in obesity in fasting and postprandial state. Am J Physiol 1983; 244:E45–51.
9. Sapir DG, Owen OE. Renal conservation of ketone bodies during starvation. Metabolism 1975; 24:23–33.
10. Nelson RA. Polar bears—active yet hibernating? In Stone GB (ed). Spirit of Enterprise. The 1981 Rolex Awards. San Francisco, WH Freeman, 1981: 245–247.
11. Nelson RA, Wahner HW, Jones JD, et al. Metabolism of bears before, during and after winter sleep. Am J Physiol 1973; 224:491–496.
12. Nelson RA, Jones JD, Wahner HW, et al. Nitrogen metabolism in bears: urea metabolism in summer and in winter sleep and role of urinary bladder in water and nitrogen conservation. Mayo Clin Proc 1975; 50:141–146.
13. Nelson RA. Protein and fat metabolism in hibernating bears. Fed Proc 1980; 39:2955–2958.
14. Renold AE, Cahill GF Jr. Metabolism of isolated adipose tissue: a summary. In Renold AE, Cahill GF Jr (eds). Handbook of Physiology. Sec. 5. Baltimore, Williams & Wilkins, 1965: 483–490.
15. Fenn WO, Haege LF. The deposition of glycogen with water in the livers of cats. J Biol Chem 1940; 136:87–101.
16. Odum EP. Adipose tissue in migratory birds. In Renold AE, Cahill GF Jr (eds). Handbook of Physiology. Sec. 5. Baltimore, Williams & Wilkins, 1965: 37–43.
17. Tietz A. Metabolic pathways in the insect fat body. In Renold AE, Cahill GF Jr (eds). Handbook of Physiology. Sec. 5. Baltimore, Williams & Wilkins, 1965: 45–54.
18. Lewin R. How did humans evolve big brains? Science 1982; 216:840–841.
19. Nilsson L. Liver glycogen content in man in the postabsorptive state. Scand J Clin Lab Invest 1973; 32:317–323.
20. Hultman E. Muscle glycogen in man determined in needle biopsy specimens. Scand J Clin Lab Invest 1967; 19:209–217.
21. Luft R, Ikkos D, Palmieri G, et al. A case of severe hypermetabolism of non-thyroid origin with a defect in the maintenance of mitochondrial respiratory control: a correlated clinical, biochemical, and morphological study. J Clin Invest 1962; 41:1776–1804.
22. Rapoport SI. Blood-brain barrier in physiology and medicine. New York, Raven Press, 1976.
23. Morse DE, Hooker N, Duncan H, et al. γ-Aminobutyric acid, a neurotransmitter, induces planktonic abalone larvae to settle and begin metamorphosis. Science 1979; 204:407–410.
24. Manahan DT, Wright SH, Stephens GC. Simultaneous determination of net uptake of 16 amino acids by a marine bivalve. Am J Physiol 1983; 244:R832–838.
25. Cahill GF Jr, Aoki TT, Smith RJ. Glucagon and amino acid metabolism. In Lefebvre PJ (ed). Handbook of Experimental Pharmacology. Vol. 66/I. Heidelberg, Springer Verlag, 1983: 339–417.
26. Fernandes J, Berger R, Smit GPA. Lactate as energy source for brain in glucose-6-phosphatase deficient child. Lancet 1982; 1:113.
27. Nemoto EM, Hoff JT, Severinghaus JW. Lactate uptake and metabolism by brain during hyperlactatemia and hypoglycemia. Stroke 1974; 5:48–53.
28. Sokolov L. Metabolism of the central nervous system in vivo. In Handbook of Physiology. Sec. I. Neurophysiology. Baltimore, Waverly Press, 1960: 1843.
29. Kety SS. The general metabolism of the brain in vivo. In Richter D (ed). The Metabolism of the Nervous System. 2nd International Neurochemical Symposium, The Metabolism of the Nervous System. London, Pergamon Press, 1957: 221.
30. McCall AL, Millington W, Wurtman R. Metabolic fuel and amino acid transport into the brain in experimental diabetes mellitus. Proc Natl Acad Sci USA 1982; 79:5406–5410.
31. Gjedde A, Crone C. Blood-brain glucose transfer: repression in chronic hyperglycemia. Science 1981; 214:456–457.
32. Cryer P. Does central nervous system adaptation to antecedent glycaemia occur in patients with insulin dependent diabetes mellitus? Ann Intern Med 1985; 103:284–286.
33. Felig P. The glucose-alanine cycle. Metabolism 1973; 22:178–207.
34. Randle AJ, Hales PB, Garland D, et al. The glucose fatty acid cycle, its role in insulin sensitivity and the metabolic disturbances of diabetes mellitus. Lancet 1963; 1:785–789.
35. Owen OE, Reichard GG Jr. Fuels consumed by man: the interplay between carbohydrates and fatty acids. Progr Biochem Pharmacol 1971; 6:199.
36. Matthews DE, Bier DM, Rennie MJ, et al. Regulation of leucine metabolism in man: a stable isotope study. Science 1981; 214:1129–1131.
37. Vinuela E, Salas M, Sols A. Glucokinase and hexokinase in liver in relation to glycogen synthesis. J Biol Chem 1963; 238:1175–1177.

38. Sharma C, Manjeshwar R, Weinhouse S. Effects of diet and insulin on glucose-adenosine triphosphate phosphotransferases of rat liver. J Biol Chem 1963: 238:3840–3845.

39. Salas M, Vinuela E, Sols A. Insulin-dependent synthesis of liver glucokinase in the rat. J Biol Chem 1963; 238:3535–3538.

40. Storer AC, Cornish-Bowden A. Kinetics of rat liver glucokinase. Biochem J 1976; 159:7–14.

41. Cahill GF Jr, Herrera MG, Morgan AP, et al. Hormone-fuel interrelationships during fasting. J Clin Invest 1966; 45:1751–1769.

42. Garber AJ, Menzel PH, Boden G, et al. Hepatic ketogenesis and gluconeogenesis in humans. J Clin Invest 1974; 54:981–989.

43. Owen OE, Felig P, Morgan AP, et al. Liver and kidney metabolism during prolonged starvation. J Clin Invest 1969; 48:574–583.

44. Marliss EB, Aoki TT, Pozefsky AS, et al. Muscle and splanchnic glutamine and glutamate metabolism in postabsorptive and starved man. J Clin Invest 1971; 50:814–817.

45. Ruderman NB, Ross PS, Berger M, et al. Regulation of glucose and ketone-body metabolism in brain of anaesthetized rats. Biochem J 1974; 138:1–10.

46. Askanazi J, Carpentier YA, Michelsen CB, et al. Muscle and plasma amino acids following injury. Influence of intercurrent infection. Ann Surg 1980; 192:78–85.

47. Askanzi J, Elwyn DH, Kinney JM, et al. Muscle and plasma amino acids after injury. The role of inactivity. Ann Surg 1978; 188:797–803.

48. Askanazi J, Fürst P, Michelson CB, et al. Muscle and plasma amino acids after injury. Hypocaloric glucose vs. amino acid infusion. Ann Surg 1980; 191:465–472.

49. Flatt JP. On the maximal possible rate of ketogenesis. Diabetes 1972; 21:50–53.

50. Göttstein U, Held K, Müller W, et al. Utilization of ketone bodies by the human brain. In Meyer JS, Reivich M, Lechner H, et al. (eds). Research on the Cerebral Circulation. 5th International Salzburg Conference. Springfield, IL, Charles C Thomas, 1972: 137–145.

51. Argiles JM. Has acetone a role in the conversion of fat to carbohydrate in mammals? TIBS 1986; 11:61–63.

52. Reichard GA Jr, Owen OE, Haff AC, et al. Ketone-body production and oxidation in fasting obese humans. J Clin Invest 1974; 53:508–515.

53. Reichard GA Jr, Haff AC, Skutches CL, et al. Plasma acetone metabolism in fasting humans. J Clin Invest 1979; 63:619–626.

54. Owen OE, Trapp VE, Skutches CL, et al. Acetone metabolism during diabetic ketoacidosis. Diabetes 1982; 31:242–248.

55. Benedict FG. A study of prolonged fasting. Washington, DC, Carnegie Institute of Washington, Publication 203, 1915.

56. Vagenakis AG, Burger A, Portnay GI, et al. Diversion of peripheral thyroxine metabolism from activating to inactivating pathways during complete fasting. J Clin Endocrinol Metab 1975; 41:181–194.

57. Landsberg L, Young JB. Dietary intake and sympathoadrenal activity. In Frankle DG, Dwyer J, Moragne L, et al. (eds). Dietary Treatment and Prevention of Obesity. London, John Libbey, 1985: 87–95.

10

EATING DISORDERS

PAUL E. GARFINKEL / DAVID M. GARNER
GARY RODIN

This chapter will provide an overview of the recent understanding of anorexia nervosa and bulimia, and will consider briefly disordered eating behavior that may occur in other metabolic disorders.

ANOREXIA NERVOSA AND BULIMIA

Anorexia nervosa is a condition found predominantly in adolescent females and is characterized by severe weight loss due to self-imposed dietary restriction and fears of fatness or even normal body size. This illness has become common and may present to physicians in various forms and pose serious psychological and social problems. Bulimia is a closely related disorder in which dieting and the desire for thinness may alternate with periods of overeating. The ingestion of large quantities of food is frequently followed by further efforts to reduce weight (vomiting, laxative misuse, or dieting) and feelings of self-deprecation. Bulimia may occur as an isolated disorder without significant weight loss, in association with anorexia nervosa, or as a symptom of other physical or emotional illnesses.

Clinical Features

The anorexic's pursuit of thinness begins with dieting, generally by curtailing the ingestion of sweets, desserts, and high-calorie snacks. Many patients avoid carbohydrate-containing foods and become inflexible in their eating habits, dividing foods into "good" and "bad" categories. When the initial weight goal has been attained feelings of being overweight persist and a new lower weight goal is established that requires further restriction of intake. Indeed, a weight goal shifting steadily downward is one of the early signs of the syndrome.

Although Gull[79] originally emphasized the loss of appetite in the disorder and chose the name "anorexia" on this basis, most patients maintain a normal awareness of hunger, but are terrified of giving in to the impulse to eat.[53] By contrast, the perception of satiety may be distorted. Many patients report severe bloating, nausea, and distention after consuming even small amounts of food. In addition, instead of feeling satisfied after eating, they often feel guilty for having given in to the impulse to eat and fear being unable to stop. Recent studies have demonstrated delayed gastric emptying, which may contribute to these altered satiety feelings.[42,138]

In spite of the progressive and severe weight loss, many anorexic women deny that they are emaciated. This denial reflects a disturbance of body image which typically takes one of two forms: a lack of awareness of the extent of the weight loss or a distorted belief that a particular body part is still too large. Associated with these misconceptions of the body are attitudes of self-loathing and mistrust of bodily functions.

Rather than feeling exhausted while starving, these people often experience excess energy. Many anorexics will rigorously exercise, engaging in extensive self-prescribed calisthenics daily. However, this apparent energy is often limited to exercise and school work, while other activities are neglected. Social relationships are avoided and the individual may become secretive and irritable. Life within the family becomes strained with increasing but futile pressure directed toward the girl to eat.

There are significant differences between anorexic patients who lose weight only by restricting their intake (restrictors) and those whose rigorous dieting alternates with episodes of bulimia. The bulimic group are predisposed to obesity through their family history and a past history of being overweight themselves. On presentation, they may not be emaciated. During bulimic episodes they eat large amounts of foods "forbidden" by their diets. Patients may interrupt this gorging several times a day to induce vomiting. Others will misuse large quantities of laxatives with the intent of preventing absorption of the ingested food. The amount of money needed to buy food can become considerable; some patients may begin to steal money or food. This group of bulimic patients commonly display other impulsive behavior including misuse of alcohol and street drugs, suicide attempts and self-mutilation.[60] They also tend to be more socially outgoing and have more variability in their moods. Depression may occur more commonly in this group and they are prone to a variety of metabolic complications due to hypokalemia.

Recently, attention has been drawn to a group of women who have recurrent bulimia and purge themselves with vomiting or laxatives but never become emaciated. Studies in a nonclinical population have found this behavior in about 4 per cent of young women.[46,116] A recent study by our group[64] has shown that although these women never lose much weight, they share many features with the bulimic group of anorexics; these include the tendency to premorbid obesity, a family history of obesity, and compulsivity in their personal lives. This form of bulimia, like that associated with anorexia nervosa, tends to be chronic with a propensity to metabolic and gastrointestinal complications.

Presentation

Patients with anorexia nervosa generally present to physicians with weight loss and fear of gaining any weight. Bloating, early satiety, amenorrhea, and family disputes concerning the patient's weight loss are also common reasons for seeking medical attention. When weight loss is minimal, the presenting symptoms such as diarrhea alternating with severe constipation, hypokalemia, tetany and convulsions may be due to the affects of repeated vomiting and laxative misuse. Some request diuretics to relieve "bloated" feelings while others wish to obtain diet pills to reduce their appetite. Anorexic women may consult physicians because of amenorrhea or infertility, and some present to sexual dysfunction clinics with vaginismus and frigidity. Others present with low mood and social withdrawal. Dentists may first recognize bulimics because of the erosion of dental enamel that occurs with chronic vomiting. With increasing public awareness of the syndrome, more patients are presenting to doctors following self-diagnosis. However, a careful assessment is always required to rule out other physical and psychiatric disorders.

Differential Diagnosis

A number of other illnesses must be differentiated from anorexia nervosa and bulimia. These are chronic wasting diseases such as tumors or tuberculosis, hypothalamic diseases, regional enteritis, and several primary endocrine disturbances, such as anterior pituitary insufficiency, Addison's disease, hyperthyroidism, and diabetes mellitus. Several psychiatric disorders may also be confused with anorexia nervosa. These include depression, schizophrenia, and conversion disorders.

MEDICAL DISORDERS

The somatic causes of weight loss can usually be distinguished from anorexia nervosa or bulimia with a thorough history and physical examination. Of diagnostic importance in anorexia nervosa are the patient's desire for the weight loss, her conviction that her emaciated body is not too thin, and her deliberate dieting. Often there will also be evidence of disposing of food, self-induced vomiting, laxative misuse, and the marked drive for activity with excess energy. If such a clear history is available, one can be reasonably certain of the diagnosis.

While weight loss and amenorrhea are common in hypothalamic tumors, it is rare for a tumor to present with the other symptoms of anorexia nervosa. An EEG, a skull x-ray, and, at times, a CAT scan will be required to clarify the diagnosis. The latter is indicated if the clinical picture does not resemble "typical" anorexia nervosa, if urological signs are present, or if the illness begins to take an unexpected course. In anterior pituitary insufficiency a reduced BMR and amenorrhea are usually the only major resemblance to anorexia nervosa. There is rarely serious weight loss in Simmond's disease, which is distinguished from anorexia nervosa by the loss of secondary sexual characteristics. Laboratory testing will also be useful since end organ hypofunction such as hypothyroidism or deficiency of growth hormone (growth hormone is often elevated in starving anorexics) will be evident in pituitary insufficiency.

In hyperthyroidism, significant weight loss may occur but the hypermetabolic state (elevated pulse, respiration, and blood pressure, sweaty warm extremities, etc.) is generally quite different from most presentations of anorexia nervosa. Bulimic patients may display some of these features—a hot flushed appearance, tachycardia, and restlessness after periods of prolonged overeating[31]—but their thyroid function tests will definitely not be in the hyperthyroid range. Occasionally a physician who measures serum thyroxine and finds it low in anorexic patients will consider the individual hypothyroid and treat her with thyroxine. While it is true that anorexic patients may display a thyroid conservation response to starvation, this is not a true hypothyroid state. Thyroxine has no place in the management of anorexia nervosa.

Diabetes mellitus may be suspected when there is weight loss, polydipsia, and polyuria. However, in anorexia nervosa, large volumes of fluid may be ingested not because of thirst but to control hunger with low calorie intake.

Of all the endocrine disorders, Addison's disease may resemble anorexia nervosa most closely in that weight loss, vomiting, reduced food intake, hypotension, and occasionally hypoglycemia may occure. Skin pigmentation, which may occur in addisonian patients, has on occasion been observed in anorexics as well.[37] However, the weight loss of adrenal insufficiency is due to anorexia, not to an aversion to weight gain as in anorexia nervosa. Addisonian patients are inactive and have markedly reduced energy, at times being bedridden. On laboratory testing, the elevated potassium and reduced sodium are different from the potassium depletion that is common in anorexia nervosa. If uncertainty exists, provocative and suppressive tests of adrenocortical function will confirm the diagnosis.

PSYCHIATRIC DISORDERS

In addition to these medical disorders there are three functional illnesses that may resemble anorexia nervosa but should be distinguished because of differing treatments. Table 10–1 compares clinical features of anorexia, conversion disorder, schizophrenia, and depression.

Conversion Disorder. There are a group of patients whose presenting features resemble those of anorexia nervosa but who on close clinical examination are found to lack the core features.[57] Although such patients were described in the older literature as having "atypical" anorexia nervosa,[21] the symptoms of some of these patients are now thought to represent conversion disorders. Such patients may vomit and lose weight, not primarily to achieve a thin body size, but because of the symbolic association between food or vomiting and specific conflictual psychological issues. For example, vomiting may signify revulsion or disgust related to sexual or other concerns. These symptoms may serve to control others or to avoid unconscious conflicts but seem less related to the problems with self-control and identity that are seen in the anorexic.[21]

The conversion disorder group likely represents a small proportion of the young women who have chronic vomiting and weight loss. Garfinkel et al.[59] have described 20 such patients out of 360 referred over 10 years with a provisional diagnosis of anorexia nervosa. The frequency of this disorder both in the general population and in a psychiatric or medical population is not known. Unlike anorexics, these patients do not engage in deliberate means to lose weight such as extreme exercise and laxative and diuretic abuse. They also do not report the active pursuit of thinness that is typical for patients with anorexia nervosa. With the conversion patients there is often a specific identifiable traumatic event or series of events that precipitates the symptoms and causes food and digestion to assume symbolic significance. The psychological disturbances are more circumscribed in these patients who seem to function normally except for their presenting symptoms. In comparison with the anorexic patients they report being more involved and satisfied in relationships with the opposite sex. The anorexia nervosa patients seem to have a more pervasive psychological disturbance, with restricted functioning in many areas unrelated to eating. On objective psychometric testing, we have found less evidence of disturbances in body image in the conversion disorder group compared with the anorexia nervosa sample. In contrast to the anorexics, the conversion disorder group have a stronger sense of self-control, less obsessive-compulsive behavior, and more consistent social relationships, all of which indicate less pervasive psychosocial deficits.[59]

Schizophrenia. Occasionally schizophrenic patients lose large amounts of weight because of a refusal to eat. This may be due to delusions about food (e.g., the food has been poisoned), the effects of food on the body (e.g., causing the stomach or intestines to rot), or, rarely, from the negativistic behavior as-

TABLE 10–1. *Functional Disorders Associated with Weight Loss and Vomiting: Clinical Features*

	Anorexia Nervosa	Conversion Disorder	Schizophrenia	Depression
Intense drive for thinness	+ +	—	—	—
Self-imposed starvation	+ +(Due to fear of body size)	—	+ +(Due to delusions about food)	—
Disturbance in body image	+(Lack of awareness of change in body size and lack of satisfaction or pleasure in the body)	—	—	—
Appetite	Maintained (but fear of giving in to impulse)	Variable	Maintained	True "anorexia"
Satiety	Usually bloating, nausea, early satiety	Variable	Variable	Variable
Avoidance of specific foods	Carbohydrates or foods presumed high in calories	—	Foods that may be thought to be poisoned	Loss of interest in all food
Bulimia	Present in 30 to 50%	May occur	Rare	Rare
Vomiting	+(To prevent weight gain)	+(Expresses some symbolic meaning)	Rare (to prevent food having presumed undesirable effects on the body)	—
Laxative misuse	+(To prevent weight gain)	Infrequent (expresses some symbolic meaning)	—	—
Activity level	Increased	Reduced	—	Reduced
Amenorrhea	+	+	+	+

sociated with catatonia. Historically, some writers have postulated a more fundamental association between schizophrenia and anorexia nervosa,[121] and some features of schizophrenia may be observed in anorexia nervosa. Specifically, the social withdrawal, negativism, and indecisiveness seen in anorexia nervosa may superficially resemble the defect of volition characteristic of schizophrenia. Also, the distorted bodily self-perceptions of the anorexic may resemble the psychotic perceptions of schizophrenics. However, in the anorexic these distorted perceptions are limited to the patient's own body. A few anorexic patients describe a sense of helplessness and a lack of personal control, which are considered to be "first rank" symptoms of schizophrenia. However, a careful mental status examination will indicate that such frank delusions are absent in the anorexic and that they do not have the other characteristic disturbances in thought process or affect that are seen in schizophrenia. Furthermore, there is no increased risk for schizophrenia in the families of anorexics.[149]

The differential diagnosis of anorexia nervosa and schizophrenia may be complicated by the fact that a few anorexics develop frank psychoses. Grounds[78] reported that 5 per cent of inpatient anorexics developed transient psychoses. These are generally secondary to metabolic imbalance in severe starvation[37] or to an underlying personality disorder, such as the borderline personality, in which "micropsychotic episodes" have been described. Whether the coexistence of these two disorders is greater than would occur by chance is not known. Theander[149] and Dally[37] found that only 1 per cent of anorexics eventually developed schizophrenia (a figure very similar to the estimated lifetime prevalence of schizophrenia in the general population).

Depression. Anorexia nervosa and depression may be difficult to distinguish from each other clinically because there are common signs and symptoms, familial tendencies and neuroendocrine abnormalities. These similarities have caused some to suggest that anorexia nervosa is actually a variant of affective illness.[25] Kay[99] noted "depressive mood" in 50 per cent of his anorexic patients, and Rollins and Piazza[136] reported depressive symptoms in 74 per cent of their sample. Shared vegetative and other features are listed in Table 10–2. It is easy to see why blurring between these two syndromes may occur.

Anorexia, weight loss and insomnia occur in the typical "endogenous depression." The mirror triad of bulimia, weight gain, and hypersomnia may be found with depressive illness in adolescence or young adulthood. Why some depressed patients overeat while most lose their appetite is not clear. Herman and Polivy[86] postulate that the nature of the eating behavior before the onset of depression may be a determining factor in the eating disturbance with depression. This is supported by the observation that unrestrained eaters (non-dieters) develop anorexia when depressed, while restrained eaters lose their control over eating and gain weight. In contrast to the depressed group, patients with anorexia nervosa do not truly lose their appetite until late in the starvation process.

A further difference between the anorexic and the depressed patient is the relationship between self-esteem and eating behavior. For the anorexic patient, control over eating is used to enhance self-

TABLE 10–2. Similar Characteristics of Anorexia Nervosa and Depression

	Depression	Anorexia Nervosa
Cognitive features		
Poor concentration	+	+ *
Indecisiveness	+	+ *
Lack of interests	+	+ *
Lack of pleasure	+	+
Social withdrawal	+	+ *
Affective changes		
Sad, despairing mood	+	± (or indifference)
Guilt	+	+
Self-esteem	reduced	tied to low body weight
Vegetative features		
Insomnia, fragmented sleep	+ (or hypersomnia)	+ *
Loss of libido	+	+ *
Amenorrhea	+	+ *
Weight loss	+ (or weight gain)	+
Constipation	+	+ *
Motor features		
Activity level	↑ or ↓	↑
Family history		
Affective disorder	↑	↑
Alcoholism	↑	↑
Neurohormonal changes		
Blunting of TRH stimulation	+	+ *
DST nonsuppression	+	+ *
MHPG excretion	↓	↓ *

*Features that are likely to be related to starvation.

esteem. With primary depression, disinterest in eating may be secondary to a generalized sense of worthlessness. Many of the vegetative symptoms, cognitive disturbances, and neurohumoral abnormalities described in depressed patients also occur in patients with anorexia nervosa (Table 10–2). It seems likely that these effects in anorexic patients are mediated by starvation since many of the cognitive and vegetative changes disappear with weight restoration. For example, reported abnormalities in urinary 3,methoxy-4,hydroxyphenylglycol (MHPG) excretion in anorexia nervosa have been shown to be related to body fat[94] and to body weight increases.[38] While similar low levels of secretion of MHPG may occur in depression, they have not been related to low body fat in this condition.

Additional support for a link between the two syndromes comes from follow up and family studies. Cantwell et al.[25] reported an increased incidence of depression on long-term follow-up of anorexic patients. First-degree relatives of anorexic patients also have an overrepresentation of depressive illness and alcoholism.[56,90,128,165]

Effects of Starvation on Attitudes, Emotions, and Behavior

Recently, investigators have recognized that many of the symptoms of anorexia nervosa are not specific to the disorder but are actually secondary to starvation.[56] Anorexic patients' food-related attitudes and behavior may appear to be puzzling or even paradoxical. They restrict their intake despite an intense interest in food and eating. Many have collected and assiduously read books on nutrition and cooking; some are avid gourmet cooks and enjoy feeding others while denying themselves food. It is not uncommon for anorexic patients to enter food-related professions (e.g., dietician, cook, or waitress). Peculiar eating rituals are typical at mealtime. Some patients refuse to eat in the presence of anyone. Often they cut up food into tiny pieces and linger over each meal for hours. Spices and condiments are used liberally on unusual combinations of food. There is a remarkable parallel between many of these behaviors observed in patients with anorexia nervosa and those of individuals exposed to semistarvation conditions. Differentiation of starvation symptoms from the primary psychopathology of anorexia nervosa has important implications for understanding of both the physical and psychological aspects of these eating disorders.

Probably the most systematic study of the effects of starvation in man was conducted during World War II at the University of Minnesota.[103] The experiment involved restricting the caloric intake of 36 young, healthy, and psychologically normal volunteers for 6 months. The men lost, on the average, 25 per cent of their original body weight; changes in attitudes, emotions, and behavior as well as metabolic and anthropometric parameters were assessed. The volunteers displayed many of the attitudes and behaviors that have been identified in anorexia nervosa. Most of the men became intensely preoccupied with food and eating. Eating habits underwent remarkable changes that served to prolong the ingestion and appeal of food. The men made unusual concoctions by mixing foods together, and they demanded that the food be served hot. Consumption of coffee and tea increased so dramatically that they had to be limited during the experiment. Food became the principle topic of conversation, and the men would spend hours planning how they would consume their daily meal allotment. Toward the end of the starvation regimen the men would spend 2 hours over a meal which previously they would have consumed in minutes. Many of the men began collecting recipes, cookbooks, menus, and cooking utensils as a result of their growing obsession with food. Despite little interest in culinary matters prior to the experiment, almost 90 per cent of the men mentioned cooking as part of their post-experiment plans. For some, the fascination was so great that they actually changed occupations after the experiment; three became chefs and one went into agriculture.

Bulimia, which is common in anorexia nervosa, may be linked to semi-starvation. During the Minnesota experiment several of the volunteers failed to adhere to their diets and reported episodes of bulimia followed by remorse.[141] Even after 12 weeks of rehabilitation, a number of the men complained that they experienced an increase in hunger immediately following a large meal. They found it difficult to stop eating, and some reported consuming between 8000 and 10,000 calories per day without feeling satisfied. After about 5 months of rehabilitation, the majority of men reported some normalization of their eating patterns; however, for some the extreme overconsumption persisted. Factors that distinguished between men whose eating normalized rapidly from those who continued to eat prodigious amounts were not identified. The important point is that there were a wide range of responses to the semi-starvation experience, with a subset of men developing bulimia that persisted many months after they were permitted free access to food.

Anorexic patients often find refeeding distressful because of increased hunger following a large meal. They assume that they will be unable to stop overconsuming and will ultimately attain their worst fear—obesity. They must be reassured that although normal satiety does not return immediately, with months of consistent eating and weight restoration, the intense urges to overeat recede.

Cognitive and perceptual changes were observed among the subjects in the Minnesota experiment. The volunteers reported decreased concentration, alertness, comprehension, and judgment; however, on formal intelligence testing there were no signs of diminished intellectual abilities. Hyperacuity to noise and light was observed in some subjects. Others reported visual disturbances including an inability to focus, eye aches, and "spots" in the visual fields. Auditory disturbances were also evident in some

subjects (e.g., ringing in the ears). Most subjects experienced a reduced tolerance for cold temperatures. These symptoms are not uncommon in anorexia nervosa patients and must be considered to be secondary to starvation.[56] Compulsive behavior and obsessional thinking may be initiated or enhanced by the starvation process. The observation of personality changes as a result of starvation has obvious implications for anorexia nervosa. Although psychological disturbance undoubtedly antedates the development of the disorder, the starvation process may dramatically alter the manifest symptoms. This underscores the need for renourishment as essential to the psychological treatment of anorexia nervosa since the patients' genuine personality traits may be obscured by starvation.

Emotional changes occurred in the majority of the Minnesota volunteers. Although the subjects were psychologically healthy prior to the experiment, most experienced significant changes in mood during semi-starvation. Some reported transitory and others protracted periods of depression, with an overall lowering of the threshold for depression. Significant lability in mood was evident in a small minority of subjects. Anxiety was common; as the experiment progressed many of the formerly even-tempered men began smoking and nail-biting. Standardized personality testing revealed significant increases in depression and psychopathology. These emotional aberrations did not vanish immediately during rehabilitation but persisted for several weeks, with some men deteriorating even further.

Social and sexual changes were also evident during semi-starvation. The Minnesota volunteers became more socially withdrawn and reported a marked decline in social contact with women. Masturbation, sexual fantasies, and sexual impulses either decreased or were much less intense. Thus the lack of sexual interest often observed in anorexia nervosa may be partially attributed to the starvation process and its effect on the hormonal substrate of normal sexual functioning. Hoarding of food-related items is common in anorexia nervosa and may be part of the starvation state. The volunteers in the Minnesota study not only collected cookbooks and cooking utensils but also accumulated other non–food-related items such as second-hand clothing and old books. This behavior was not typical prior to the experiment.

Sleep changes occurred in some of the semi-starvation subjects. This parallels findings of sleep disturbances in anorexia nervosa, especially early morning awakening and insomnia, which are independent of mood changes.[35] It should also be noted that food-related dreams observed in anorexia nervosa[107] are similar to those found in starvation subjects.[141]

SIGNIFICANCE OF STARVATION IN TREATMENT

As is evident from the foregoing discussion, many of the symptoms assumed to be specific to anorexia nervosa are actually complications of starvation. These are not limited to food but extend to virtually all areas of psychological and social functioning. Therefore, it is absolutely essential for weight restoration to occur to accurately assess and ameliorate the emotional disturbances in anorexia nervosa. This often becomes a contentious point in treatment. Even when the patient expresses a sincere desire to recover from the disorder, she routinely persists in her belief that she must be thin.[61] This belief must be gently challenged with the evidence that body weight tends to be homeostatically regulated around a predetermined "set point."[100,101] Diet-induced deviations from the organism's "natural weight" are met by metabolic adaptations designed to restore former weight levels. The precise mechanism by which this defense of body weight operates is a matter of speculation and controversy; however, the concept of "set point" has received growing empirical support.[101]

The treatment of anorexia nervosa must take into consideration the profound effects of starvation on attitudes, emotions, and behavior while at the time being sensitive to the fear that the patient feels at the prospects of weight gain. Weight gain alone, without attendance to psychological issues, may be counterproductive. Psychotherapy aimed at the establishment of trust and autonomy through the correction of faulty assumptions in various areas of functioning is the cornerstone of treatment.[56,61]

Pathogenesis

Anorexia nervosa can be viewed as a disorder with risk factors in the individual, the family, and the culture. These factors interact to produce dieting to enhance one's sense of self-control and self-worth. However, with progressive weight loss, starvation and other factors may result in a self-perpetuating cycle. Various risk factors will be briefly described here; they have been more completely discussed elsewhere.[56]

Cultural Factors. A cultural component to the pathogenesis of anorexia nervosa is suggested by epidemiological data. This disorder was once considered to be rare, but recent studies have documented a prevalence of one serious case in 100 to 150 adolescent girls.[35] Bulimia without weight loss is even more common. Anorexia nervosa has increased in frequency in the past 15 years, and this increase has been in females only. About 95 per cent of cases occur in females. While anorexia nervosa was once limited to upper and middle class individuals of a particular age (12 to 25), there is evidence that as it has become more common it has become more equally distributed through all the social classes and now occurs with increasing frequency in women over 25.[56]

There is some evidence to link two cultural factors to the pathogenesis. These are (1) the idealization of the thin female form and (2) pressures on women to achieve, often for others rather than for oneself. Garner and Garfinkel[62] hypothesized that if pressures to be slim were a risk factor to the illness, anorexia nervosa would be more common in women who had to be slim because of career choice. They found an increased prevalence of the disorder in dance and modeling students. Moreover, the frequency of anorexia nervosa developing within dance settings varied greatly; anorexia nervosa was almost twice as common in those dance settings that were intensely achievement- and performance-oriented.

Family Factors. Family risk factors may be genetic or psychological or due to family interactions.

1. With regard to genetic factors, it is known that some illnesses are overrepresented in families with an anorexic member, i.e., depression, alcoholism, and anorexia nervosa.[56] It is not known whether the clustering of these illnesses in families of patients with anorexia nervosa occurs because of shared genetic features, biological vulnerabilities, or psychological factors. The reported monozygous twin concordance rate of 50 per cent as compared with the 10 per cent rate in dizygous twins suggests a genetic component.[56]

2. There have been few empirical studies of the psychological characteristics of anorexics' parents. Two recent studies have documented an increase in obsessionality or conscientiousness in fathers of anorexics.[34,58] This finding might be important, in view of the postulated etiological significance of heightened expectations for achievement and in view of the anorexics' strong need to please others.

3. Specific familial interaction patterns have been noted, but their significance has not been substantiated by empirical studies. Garfinkel et al.[58] recently compared families with an anorexic member in Canada and Ireland with controls matched for social class in each country. They found that, in both countries, the families with an anorexic individual perceived more problems in areas of performance expectations, role adaptability, style of communication, and expression of feelings. At present, we do not know if this finding is part of the pathogenesis or is entirely due to the effects of a chronically ill family member.

Individual Factors. Since not everyone exposed to familial and cultural risk factors develops the disorder, factors within the individual must be important:

1. Difficulties separating from the family and functioning autonomously have been commented on by many.[56] There are many psychological factors that may impede the development of a sense of identity or the capacity to live independently. Individuals who fail to develop a sense of mastery or control over their lives may feel a sense of personal helplessness and use dieting as an isolated area in which personal control may be experienced.

2. Difficulties in self-perception are common and are closely linked to this sense of helplessness. Experimentally this has been assessed using measures of visual self-perception and recognition of inner feelings.[63] If there is little awareness of inner states or changes in one's body, than the body is experienced as something foreign that must be artificially controlled rather than as a source of feedback and comfort.

3. Obesity may be a predisposing factor, particularly for the bulimic subgroup of anorexia nervosa patients. An individual who has been obese may be very sensitive to past humiliations that she attributes to her obesity. This may serve as a potent stimulus to relentless dieting, especially if her self-worth is largely determined by appearance.

4. Personality characteristics are important as they relate to the regulation of self-worth. Anorexics are generally individuals whose self-esteem is closely bound to external standards for performance and appearance. Expectations are less internally derived but are tied to pleasing others.

5. Conceptual development may be a further risk factor, although it has received less study to date. Bruch[22] has suggested that anorexics remain fixed at early levels of cognitive functioning. A clinical manifestation of this cognitive arrest may be the anorexic's "all or nothing" style of thinking.[61] There are likely other important individual risk factors to the illness, but they have not been clarified.

Many of the precipitating factors for the clinical appearance of anorexia nervosa may be nonspecific. These include such psychological stressors in adolescence as separations and losses, or other situations which represent a threat to self-esteem. Factors that sustain the illness may be very different from those that are predisposing or initiating. Common sustaining factors include the presence of the starvation syndrome, vomiting as a means of controlling weight, the familial relationships that have changed because of the illness, social and vocational skills, and others.[56] Starvation itself perpetuates the illness because the associated cognitive, affective, and behavioral changes are experienced by the anorexic as a direct threat to her sense of self-control and self-esteem; as a result she increases her dieting to feel more in control. Vomiting and other purging behavior also perpetuate the illness: they are reinforcing in that they allow the person to eat and yet to prevent any weight gain. Furthermore, vomiting is a means of expressing emotion for those unable to tolerate more direct emotional expression.

Hypothalamic-Pituitary Function. Disturbances in hormonal patterns have long been recognized in anorexia nervosa and at times have contributed to the view that anorexia nervosa is a primary hypothalamic disturbance. In the past 15 years considerable research has led to the identification of factors related to the observable hypothalamic abnormalities. At this time, the evidence suggests that these disturbances are related either to the emotional turmoil that precedes the onset of the disorder or to the weight loss or the reduced dietary intake.

Prolactin. Since hyperprolactinemia is a common cause of secondary amenorrhea,[12] many studies have been conducted to examine whether abnormal prolactin (PL) secretion plays a role in the amenorrhea of anorexia nervosa. Resting PL levels are normal.[56] There is no relationship between basal PL and body weight, estradiol, or gonadotropins.[157] Chlorpromazine and other dopamine (DA) receptor blockers stimulate normal PL secretion in anorexia nervosa.[82] PL responses to thyrotropin releasing hormone (TRH) are quite variable, being reported as totally normal,[157] reduced,[91] or normal in magnitude but delayed in time.[157]

In normal adults, plasma PL levels rise shortly after the onset of nocturnal sleep. This is generally followed by a series of even larger secretory episodes, resulting in progressively higher plasma concentrations during the night, with peak values occurring during the end of the sleep period.[163] There is often a suppression of the sleep-induced rise in PL in anorexia nervosa.[95] However, this may be related to dietary differences in anorexics since nocturnal PL can be reduced by a vegetarian diet.[87]

Growth Hormone. Starving patients with anorexia nervosa often have elevated basal GH levels, but once caloric intake is increased GH levels return to normal.[54] Interestingly, this return of GH levels precedes weight gain. Changes in the hypothalamic-pituitary-gonadal axis and in plasma GH of patients with anorexia nervosa are probably related to different factors. Reproductive changes are related to loss of body weight and are reversed by an increase in body weight, while changes in GH are apparently related only to caloric intake. These changes may be more general since elevated basal GH also occurs in other conditions in which there is decreased food intake, including kwashiorkor and marasmus.[127]

Glucose usually produces a drop in the elevated GH levels, although a paradoxical rise following oral glucose has also been observed.[27] The latter becomes normal with improved nutritional intake. Elevation of GH following oral glucose is blunted by the DA agonist bromocriptine in anorexia nervosa and also in acromegaly.[82] A reduced response to another DA agonist, apomorphine, has been found in anorexia nervosa; this reverts to normal following weight restoration.[27] However, the flattened response to L-dopa may not become normal following weight restoration.[143] The GH response to insulin-induced hypoglycemia has also been reported as attenuated in anorexia nervosa.[39] Normally, GH secretion is not altered by TRH, while in anorexia nervosa GH release may occur;[110] however, this phenomenon may occur in a variety of other diseases.[18] In addition, normal responses to arginine have been reported in anorexia nervosa as well as normal rises in GH during sleep.[154]

Hypothalamic-Pituitary-Thyroid Axis. Thyroxine (T_4) levels in anorexia nervosa are within the low normal range, and they do not rise after weight gain.[157] Thyroxine binding protein as assessed by serum triiodothyronine (T_3) resin uptake is also normal.[20] T_3 levels are reduced in anorexia nervosa, while there is an increase in the inactive reverse form of T_3.[24] Levels of T_3 correlate linearly with body weight; both reduced T_3 and elevated reverse T_3 return to normal after weight gain. The alteration in T_3 and reverse T_3 is likely related to fasting since it is seen in other forms of acute starvation and carbohydrate deprivation prior to weight loss.[152] Furthermore, glucose feeding rapidly reverses the fall in T_3 that occurs after fasting.[23] Low T_3 and increased reverse T_3 in these situations serve an adaptive function; the target cells for thyroid hormones have regulatory mechanisms based on metabolic needs.[119] Conversion of T_4 to T_3 at the cellular level may be regulated by need, so that deprivation of calories would alter cellular mechanisms involved in regulation of deiodination of T_4. This would reduce production of T_3 and increase reverse T_3. Since the latter is a much less calorigenic hormone, this would result in lowering of metabolic rate and conservation of energy. Since a relative hypothyroidism serves an adaptive function, treatment of anorexia nervosa patients with thyroid hormone replacement is not recommended. One review of a consultation practice revealed that 5 per cent of anorexics were being treated incorrectly with L-thyroxine at the time of the psychiatric assessment.[56]

Resting levels of thyroid stimulating hormone (TSH) are within normal limits.[155] TSH responses to TRH are of normal magnitude in anorexia nervosa, and the response correlates with the resting TSH level as it does in normal subjects.[20] Maximal TSH response also correlates with body weight. A delay in the TSH response to TRH has been noted, but this reverts to normal after weight gain.[155]

Pituitary-Adrenal Regulation. Morning levels of plasma cortisol have been frequently reported to be elevated in anorexia nervosa, but normal levels have also been reported.[20] Cortisol levels in the CSF have also been reported to be elevated.[68] The circadian rhythm of cortisol in such patients is preserved at higher levels, but may also appear flattened.[16] Cortisol production rate is increased relative to body size.[158] There is incomplete suppression of cortisol by dexamethasone in some but not all patients; this is related to low body weight.[56] In fact, obese subjects and normal volunteers have been found to become nonsuppressors when they lose weight.[6,43] Adrenal responses to ACTH are normal or increased in anorexia nervosa.[159] The most likely explanation for these abnormalities appears to be a reduction in the sensitivity to negative feedback from adrenal steroids.[158]

Metabolism of cortisol is also altered in anorexia nervosa; specifically, the metabolic clearance rate is decreased, urinary free cortisol levels are increased, and levels of urinary 17-ketosteroids are low.[15,158] Studies of cortisol metabolism have shown an increase in the tetrahydrocortisol-tetrahydrocortisone ratio.[14] These alterations in cortisol metabolism seem to be related to low levels of T_3, since administration of T_3 to these patients causes an improvement of these metabolic abnormalities.[16] However, as the relative hypothyroid state may serve an adaptive function, treatment with T_3 is not recommended.

Hypothalamic-Pituitary Axis. Many studies have evaluated gonadotropins in anorexia nervosa because of the amenorrhea attending this disorder. Amenorrhea in anorexia nervosa occurs within the context of low and noncyclic levels of ovarian sex steroids.[152] The low estrogen levels are the cause of the vaginal atrophy seen in these patients and the dyspareunia reported by some who are sexually active.

Amenorrhea in anorexia nervosa appears to be due to hypogonadotropic hypogonadism. Markedly underweight patients with anorexia nervosa have low levels of plasma gonadotropins.[20] Resting luteinizing hormone (LH) correlates positively with body weight, and LH levels normalize as weight is regained.[20] Furthermore, baseline follicle-stimulating hormone (FSH) values return to normal as weight increases.[143]

The 24-hour secretory patterns of gonadotropins in those emaciated patients resemble patterns in normal prepubertal girls. These 24-hour patterns are characterized either by low LH levels throughout the 24-hour period or by a circadian rhythm in LH in which mean levels during sleep are lower than daytime mean values.[17] Following clinical remission, the LH secretory pattern may reveal a pattern more characteristic of mature adult females, namely high mean LH levels and no circadian rhythm. However, immature patterns may also persist.[16] Interestingly, the adult pattern is not present in those who have regained weight but who remain symptomatic.[98]

The LH response to luteinizing hormone releasing hormone (LHRH) may be greatly reduced or absent in patients with anorexia nervosa. This response is also correlated with body weight.[56] Normal release of LH after LHRH occurs in patients when body weight is normalized even though circadian patterns may remain immature.[98] The FSH response to LHRH has a prepubertal pattern that is higher than the LH response.

The response to LHRH in an anorexia nervosa patient with minimal LH responses and normal FSH responses is comparable to that of a normal prepubertal child.[123] Repeated treatment with LHRH in patients with anorexia nervosa restores normal ovarian steroid secretion and a normal ovarian cycle with follicular growth and maturation, ovulation, and corpus luteum formation. During repeated therapy there is a progressive increase in the LH response to LHRH, with a progressive decrease in the FSH response so that the prepubertal-like pattern reverts to normal. Moreover, FSH responses to LHRH return to normal prior to the return of LH responses.

A delay in the time course of response of plasma LH and FSH to a bolus of LHRH has been noted.[155] Delay appears to be related to weight loss, since it is also found in patients with weight loss and secondary amenorrhea who do not have anorexia nervosa.[156] The peak LH response to clomiphene also is related to body weight in patients with anorexia nervosa. Clomiphene is effective in releasing LH only in those patients who have regained weight.[10] Similarly, feedback effects of estrogen given to anorexia nervosa patients become apparent only following some weight gain. With weight restoration there is an increase in LH resting levels and negative feedback effects of estrogen are then apparent. The positive feedback effects of estrogen, however, remain impaired in the majority of patients. Abnormal responses to clomiphene citrate and to estrogen provide further evidence supporting hypothalamic dysfunction.

Anorexia nervosa in males is also accompanied by hypogonadotropic hypogonadism, although males represent less than 5 per cent of patients with this disorder. Males may show complete impotence and loss of all sexual interest. Low urinary testosterone, plasma gonadotropin, and testosterone levels have been reported, as well as a pubertal LH secretory pattern.[54,129]

In patients with anorexia nervosa, the metabolism of testosterone is altered: the ratio of 5-α-reductase activity to 5-β-reductase activity is reduced, so that the urinary metabolites of testosterone show a reduction in androsterone and an increase in etiocholanolone. This alteration is identical to that seen in hypothyroidism and presumably is due to the same cause, that is, a reduction in plasma T_3.[14] Although administration of T_3 reverses the alteration, it is not clinically warranted.

Monoamines (MA). The neurotransmitter monoamines are of interest in anorexia nervosa and bulimia for several reasons:

1. They exert significant control over the release or inhibition of release of various neurohumors.

2. They exert significant regulatory control over eating behavior.[55]

3. Recently, several investigators have implicated abnormalities in MA function in the pathophysiology of anorexia nervosa.[3,114,134]

Plasma norepinephrine (NE) concentration and urinary excretion of the catecholamine metabolites methoxyhydroxyphenylglycol (MHPG) and homovanillic acid (HVA) are low in untreated patients with anorexia nervosa,[77] suggesting reduced activity in both central and peripheral sympathetic nervous system. Reduced MHPG excretion in anorexic patients has been linked to depressive symptoms,[83] and reduced MHPG is not uncommon in depression.[144] However, the various contributors to the low MHPG

in anorexics have not been definitely determined. Gerner and Gwirstman[67] reported the very low levels to be independent of the anorexic's depressed mood. Plasma NE and the urinary metabolites return to normal when refeeding has resulted in weight gain to normal levels.[77,83]

There is some evidence to suggest that this increase in catecholamine metabolite excretion is due to weight gain rather than food intake. Johnston, et al.[94] found that the excretion of MHPG, dehydroxyphenylglycol (DHPG), and vanillylmandelic acid (VMA) were all reduced to about 60 per cent of control values, while HVA was reduced only marginally in emaciated anorexics. They found that there was a strong association between the excretion of these MA metabolites and body mass; body size and fatness were much more closely related to these MA metabolites than was daily energy intake. By contrast, there is evidence that sucrose refeeding of a sympathetically innervated organ, the heart, increases sympathetic activity.[106]

Johnston et al.[94] found a normal fasting plasma tyrosine to neutral amino acid ratio in anorexics. This suggests that the availability of the MA precursor is not a limiting factor in the reduced MA synthesis. However, they confirmed the earlier finding of Coppan et al.[29] of reduced plasma tryptophan in anorexics as well as elevated plasma valine. Together these findings suggest a possible reduction in brain tryptophan availability and hence serotonin synthesis which may play a role in some of the described neuroendocrine changes.

Menstrual Function and Fertility

For many patients loss of menses occurs shortly after the onset of the weight loss.[52] However, in a significant proportion (estimates vary between 7 and 24 per cent), amenorrhea appears to precede the weight loss.[52] It is not clear whether this is due to the emotional upheaval preceding the dieting or to an independent hypothalamic abnormality. However, it is premature to conclude that there is a primary hypothalamic dysfunction because of the retrospective bias in reporting the temporal relationship between dieting behavior and amenorrhea and because of the known effects of emotional disturbance on menstrual function. Earlier studies of women in concentration camps demonstrated that for most with amenorrhea the cessation of menses occurred immediately after internment, before the nutritional status had been seriously impaired.

For most anorexic patients, amenorrhea is related to the degree of weight loss. This is also true for the female population as a whole. Weight is not the only critical factor determining menstruation, however. Studies of female athletes have suggested that amenorrhea may relate more to the percentage of body fat, the extent of exercise, or the degree of emotional stress than to the actual weight. Therefore, weight is only one of the several important variables in the development of amenorrhea.

Patients with anorexia nervosa usually, but not always, resume menstruation after their weights are restored. Between 50 and 75 per cent of patients menstruate regularly at the time of follow-up studies.[56] Return of menses is quite common, but not invariable, when patients regain weight to more than 90 per cent of average for their age and height. Most of the evidence suggests that anorexics are normally fertile after weight restoration and resumption of menses. When Garfinkel and Garner[56] reviewed outcome studies of anorexia nervosa there were many studies that documented normal fertility in recovered individuals.

Patients with anorexia nervosa who wish to have children should be counseled to wait until they have recovered. Active symptomatology may be exacerbated by pregnancy. For this reason clomiphene or other fertility-inducing agents should not be used unless (1) the patient has gained weight to a level greater than 90 per cent of average; (2) her eating behavior and attitudes to her body have stabilized; and (3) she has maintained this state for 1 year. Most patients will not require clomiphene if these criteria are met. Sexually active patients may choose to use oral contraceptives; there is no evidence that anorexic patients have untoward responses to oral contraceptives. However, the use of such compounds to produce withdrawal bleeding and therefore a semblance of normal hormonal function in sexually inactive amenorrheic patients should be strongly discouraged, as this may foster the denial of illness and may prevent recognition of the natural return of menses.

Treatment

Gull[80] recognized that the illness could be fatal and felt that this clinical point had to guide all treatment. He observed that the family had no control over the situation and that the patient had to be separated from family and friends; someone else had to assume control. He also recognized that food must be given according to the physician's instructions: "The inclination of the patient must be in no way consulted." He noticed that many other medical attendants would say, "Let her do as she likes, don't force foods." Gull himself had earlier thought that this was reasonable advice, but he learned from experience the danger in doing so.

Weight restoration must be considered the first phase of treatment in anorexia nervosa. There are two reasons for this: 1. The starvation symptoms must be reversed before the patient can benefit from psychotherapy. 2. The patient must face her phobia—her increased body size—to overcome the panic this induces and to deal with emotional problems

that have predisposed the individual to develop the syndrome.

People with anorexia nervosa lack a sense of trust of themselves and others; they fear being misunderstood by physicians who will be interested only in having them gain weight. The management of the anorexic patient must begin with an emphasis on developing a treatment alliance based on mutual trust. This occurs through an approach that is patient, noncritical, and firm, through consistency and a sensitivity to the patient's needs, and through a demonstration that the problem and its treatment involve factors other than her weight.

An initial weight range should be set as a goal, usually about 90 per cent of average for age and height. The patient should be reassured that, as far as possible, she will not be allowed to lose control and gain too much or too rapidly. Most patients can tolerate gains of 1 to 2 kg per week. Although some patients can gain weight outside the hospital with regular weighing and support, about one half will need hospitalization. The indications for hospital admission include severe weight loss, marked bulimia and vomiting that requires a controlled environment, the need for diagnostic evaluation, the development of medical complications (e.g., hypokalemia), transient crises, and serious denial of illness.

Several different methods of restoring weight appear to be effective. Some patients will gain weight when removed from their families and when reassured by the controlled hospital environment and consultation with a dietician. For many, however, bed rest may be required as well since it tends to erode the patient's denial by emphasizing that she is ill. Moreover, the restriction of activity may be used as part of a reward system to encourage weight gain.

We generally allow the patient out of bed for increasing periods of time as weight is being restored, although other clinicians recommend keeping the patient in bed until she has attained her target weight. Sometimes anxiety interferes with eating. This may be treated with relaxation exercises, drugs such as a relatively short-acting benzodiazepine (lorazepam or oxazepam) before meals for a few weeks, or a sedating neuroleptic in small doses (e.g., chlorpromazine 25 mg t.i.d.). If larger doses are required a neuroleptic that produces less hypotension (e.g., haloperidol) may be preferable. Using these approaches means that tube or intravenous feeding, with associated complications, is seldom necessary. The goals and method of weight restoration must be clearly understood by all hospital staff, so that the kinds of conflicts and pathological interactions that the patient may have experienced in her family do not occur in hospital.

Dietary management to reverse the starvation syndrome is important. Dietary re-education must be provided to dispel myths or strange beliefs about food and to begin a well-balanced diet. To prevent gastric dilatation the patient should initially be placed on about 1500 kcal/day. This should be increased to 2500 to 3500 kcal over 2 weeks. With this calorie intake and bed rest most patients slowly achieve their agreed weight goal. Some patients may fear that if they become accustomed to consuming a greater volume of food, they will be unable to reduce their intake to a maintenance level later. A more normal-sized meal with a 600-kcal liquid supplement may allay these fears. It should be explained that the upper limit on daily calories will be closely monitored so that the patient will not be allowed to overeat or gain excess weight.

Hospitalization or a day care program should continue for about 2 weeks after weight has been restored to about 90 per cent of average for the patient's age and height, to demonstrate to the patient that control over food intake can be maintained. During this phase she should be allowed more control over the choice of diet in consultation with the dietician.

By the time of discharge, a minimum acceptable weight should be agreed upon and weighing should be carried out weekly. The patient must understand that if this level of weight is not maintained she will be readmitted to hospital. During and after hospitalization, the patient must begin to deal with the underlying psychological problems including the sense of helplessness, confusion about inner feelings, and conflicts related to control and autonomy. For most patients, this requires the development of a trusting and supportive relationship with a skilled psychotherapist. Psychotherapy for anorexics should focus more on the establishment of a sense of control and trust in feelings and abilities than on the traditional psychodynamic concepts of insight. The parents and siblings of the anorexic patient often need to be included in psychotherapy for progress to occur. There are few conditions that generate such panic, anger, and guilt in parents as seeing their starving child refuse to eat. Psychotherapy sessions should provide emotional support, education about the disorder, and a forum for the clarification and correction of the distorted family relationships that frequently develop. It is important to allow the anorexic patient to experience herself as separate and distinct from her family. The development of this sense of autonomy is essential for the patient to begin to pursue her own interests.

Role of Medication

The value of medications in the treatment of anorexia nervosa is unclear. Chlorpromazine, once the mainstay of treatment because of its antipsychotic, antiemetic, and appetite-stimulating properties, now has only a very limited role. The resistance of patients to such sedating medications and side effects as hypotension and a reduced convulsive threshold restrict the value of neuroleptics. Such medications, of course, do not alter distorted beliefs about the body. A recent controlled trial of another neuroleptic, pimozide, suggested that the rate of weight gain induced by a behavioral program and the change in attitude of anorexics was modestly enhanced by this drug.[153] However, these results must be interpreted cautiously until further studies have been reported. A small dose of chlorpromazine (25 to 50 mg) or a short-acting benzodiazepine such as lorazepam 0.5 mg may be used when marked anxiety before meals persists in spite of continued emotional support and interferes with the patient's willingness to increase food intake. We have been reluctant to use minor tranquilizers in the bulimic subgroup because of the propensity of such patients to develop addictions. Other drugs have aroused the interest of workers in this field. Cyproheptadine, lithium, bromocriptine, naloxone, and cannabis have all been studied, but clear evidence of benefit has not been found. The role of anticonvulsants in treating bulimia is also quite unclear. Following initial favorable reports[75] of treatment with diphenylhydantoin, larger controlled series[76,164] have found that there is a subgroup not clearly related to EEG abnormalities but who are responsive to anticonvulsants. This work must be pursued as should a preliminary report that carbamazepine may useful for bulimics who also have displayed disordered mood.[96]

Of all drug treatments, the role of antidepressants remains the most controversial. The existence of depressive symptoms in patients with anorexia nervosa has been recognized for many years.[99] Recently, by using a semi-structural interview, the Schedule for Affective Disorders and Schizophrenia, Piran found that 85 per cent of anorexics and bulimics at some time in their past met rigorous criteria for an affective disorder.[128] This type of information has led some authors to view anorexia nervosa as a variant of affective disorder,[25] and more recently similar claims have been advanced about bulimia.[90] This work has been supported by evidence that affective disorder and alcoholism are more common in these families than one would expect to occur by chance alone. For example, Piran et al.[128] found a prevalence of affective disorder of 50 per cent in parents of anorexics (which is as high as that of the parents of bipolar probands), and of alcoholism of 27 per cent. The evaluation of depressive symptoms is complicated by direct effects of starvation on subjective mood state, energy level, interest, and concentration. Antidepressant medications have been considered in our unit when symptoms of major depression persist after refeeding, especially when there is also a positive family history of affective disorder. Patients who respond to antidepressants often have had a previous history of depressive episodes not related to weight and starvation and a strong family history of affective disorder.

Antidepressants may not improve the rate of weight gain, and with amitriptyline, in fact, the reported increased carbohydrate craving[126] may make the patient more at risk for developing bulimia. The tricyclic antidepressants may pose other problems in this group; for example, hypotension may be potentiated. Glassman[70] has presented some evidence to suggest nortriptyline may produce less hypotension than other tricyclics. Sedating tricyclics are often unacceptable to anorexics and bulimics because this side effect stimulates fears of losing control. Patients may be more likely to continue taking medications that are less sedating, such as those with the least antihistaminic and anticholinergic properties. Preliminary results with the MAO inhibitor isocarboxozide in bulimics demonstrated significant improvements in depression and anxiety ratings, as well as improved eating behavior.[102] This relationship between responses to tricyclics and MAO inhibitors in terms of both mood and eating behavior, requires clarification.

Complications

The complications of anorexia nervosa and bulimia may be due to the starvation process itself, to artificial attempts to control weight (by vomiting or misuse of laxatives or diuretics), to the complications of weight-restoring treatments, and to the psychological sequelae. These complications have been described in more detail elsewhere.[56]

Changes in serum electrolytes are among the most common and potentially serious complications. Hyponatremia is not frequent; when it does occur it is generally due to salt restriction and water intoxication as well as excess loss of sodium. A number of case reports of convulsions secondary to hyponatremia have been described. Hypokalemia is much more frequent and potentially serious. It has been found in some reports in up to one third of patients. It may result in tetany, renal tubular vacuolation, cardiac arrhythmias, and even death, but at times extreme potassium deficiency develops gradually in the absence of striking symptoms or signs.[166] It has been suggested that cardiac arrhythmias secondary to hypokalemia are currently the most common cause of death in anorexia nervosa. Hypokalemia chiefly occurs in women with multiple routes of electrolyte depletion, such as vomiting, laxative misuse, and diuretic misuse. To avoid dangerous hypokalemia, regular monitoring of electrolytes is warranted and potassium supplements may be required. If such supplements are being vomited up, hospitalization becomes necessary.

Russell, et al.[137] have described depletion of total body potassium and nitrogen in emaciated patients with anorexia nervosa. In untreated patients, there is a disproportionate loss of total body nitrogen. With refeeding total body potassium increases faster than total body nitrogen. Before refeeding, the mean potassium to nitrogen ratio was 1.30 mmol K per gram N which was 76 per cent of normal. Re-

feeding rapidly restored this ratio so that by 8 weeks it was 95 per cent of the normal. Russell et al.[137] related these abnormalities in total body potassium to functional abnormalities in skeletal muscle cellular function. Abnormalities in muscle function in anorexics related to their inability to generate normal power, easy fatiguability, and slow relaxation. These all reverted to normal with 8 weeks of refeeding.

Edema is frequent, especially when severely emaciated patients are rapidly refed. The mechanisms responsible for the edema are not well defined. In the past, reduced plasma proteins were considered responsible. However, these are generally normal in anorexia nervosa.[56,137] At times the edema may be related to the deliberate ingestion by the anorexic of large quantities of salt in order to provide rapid weight gain to avoid hospitalization. A few patients drink large quantities of fluid to reduce their sense of hunger, and this may also play a role. Some patients may stand all the time (even when reading or eating) in the belief that this will expend more calories than sitting, and postural factors may contribute to their edema.[41] Also, alterations in membrane permeability to sodium that occur in kwashiorkor[125] may be a factor.

Bradycardia and hypotension occur commonly. Bradycardia is widely reported and may be due to (1) lowered circulating norepinephrine from the starvation itself,[106] (2) a decreased triiodothyronine level, and (3) the effects of vigorous exercise as seen in trained athletes. Fohlin[48] observed that the oxygen uptake at rest was about 20 per cent lower for anorexics than would be predicted for other individuals of comparable age, sex and body surface area. Fohlin et al.[49] reported a close correlation between body weight and cardiac volume, although it was infrequent that the heart volume was significantly below the range for healthy children. However, cardiac chamber dimensions and left ventricular mass may be reduced in patients with anorexia nervosa when there has been a correction for body surface area. Gottdiener et al.[74] described smaller end-diastolic and end-systolic left ventricular dimensions, reduced left ventricular wall thickness, and smaller left atrial and aortic root dimensions than in normals. These improve markedly with weight gain.

Electrocardiographic changes are common and have been reported in about 60 per cent of an anorexic sample.[56] Common ECG changes include sinus bradycardia, extremely low voltage, T wave inversion, AV block, and several other arrythmias. These have been previously observed in experimental semi-starvation.[103] The presence of arrythmias during exercise is of even greater significance. These include, infrequently, weight-related supraventricular premature beats and, occasionally, runs of ventricular tachycardia or occasional ventricular premature beats during exercise. Thurston and Marks[150] reported a prolonged QT interval in several of their patients, a finding also described in experimental starvation. Many of the abnormalities described above occur in the presence of normal serum electrolytes, although hypokalemia from repeated vomiting or from laxative and diuretic misuse, and severe weight loss increase the risk of these arrhythmias.[41] Undoubtedly, many deaths due to starvation in anorexia nervosa are related to these cardiac changes.

Less frequently, heart functioning may be altered by the ingestion of emetine-containing emetics (e.g., ipecac). These are widely available without prescription. Recently, several patients have been described with chronic ingestion of these emetics following bulimic periods.[19] Emetine is a general poison for muscle, and such patients may present with a progressive skeletal and cardiac myopathy. Death as a result of ventricular tachycardia following repeated emetine use has been reported.[1]

Significant reductions in glomerular filtration rate (GFR) may occur in anorexia nervosa, and this has also been described in obese subjects who are fasting.[44] This reduced GFR is likely related to a reduced plasma flow, although it has also been suggested that there might be a defect in the water permeability of the capillary wall.[48] Several groups have observed reduced concentrating capacity of the kidneys in anorexia nervosa.[48,139] It has been suggested that this reversible defect is of renal rather than central origin, since administration of vasopressin does not improve the ability to concentrate urine. Reversible changes in concentrating capacity have been reported in protein-calorie malnutrition but these have been suggested to be vasopressin-responsive. Other infrequent renal disorders include urinary calculi,[8] possibly related to fluid restriction. Furthermore, severe protracted potassium deficiency has been known to produce renal tubular vacuolation in patients with anorexia nervosa.

Gastric emptying has been shown to be delayed in anorexia improved after some weight gain, but was still significantly different from normal and may account for the early bloating and other satiety-related symptoms that many anorexic patients experience. Metoclopramide has been shown to improve significantly the gastric emptying in anorexic subjects.[140] However, it may also produce depression in these individuals. Domperidone, a DA blocking agent that facilitates gastric emptying and does not cross the blood-brain barrier, may be beneficial in this regard.[138]

Acute gastric dilatation has been shown to occur in starving people who are fed rather rapidly under a variety of circumstances. Similar dilatation may occur in patients with anorexia nervosa early in their treatment. Numerous case reports gave documented gastric dilatation, which at times leads to perforation with a significant mortality.[56] Other gastrointestinal complications include constipation and the habitual reliance on laxatives. Some patients have been known to develop an ileus. This may be facilitated by use of phenothiazines, with their anticholinergic properties. Some patients with bulimia who induce vomiting develop parotid gland enlargement.

Neurological complications include convulsions, cerebral atrophy, and peripheral neuropathy. Convulsions have been reported in about 10 per cent of anorexics in large series.[31,37] These are generally due to metabolic changes such as electrolyte disturbances, low blood sugar, or use of medications such as phenothiazines and insulin. Occasionally they may relate to alcohol withdrawal states. Air encephalograms have generally been normal, but a few instances of cerebral atrophy have been noted. More recently, cerebral atrophy has been documented by CT scans. While this cerebral atrophy has usually been reversible with weight gain, in a few instances it persisted.[56] Occasionally a peripheral neuropathy or a lateral popliteal palsy may occur.

While a variety of hematologic changes occur, these are generally of a mild degree. Normochromic anemia of a mild nature is common, but hypochromic anemia has also been described. Bone marrow hypoplasia is frequent. Here the marrow is characterized by an absence of fat spaces in the presence of an apparently gelatinous material in which marrow cells are embedded. There is often a relative increase in histiocytes and reticulum cells in the marrow. This hypoplasia is readily reversed after several weeks of refeeding. A mild thrombocytopenia may occur which, on several occasions, has been reported in association with generalized petechiae and ecchymoses. Total iron binding capacity may be lowered in starving anorexics. Cholesterol levels and carotene levels are generally increased and there have been reports of lowered levels of zinc in plasma.

Total peripheral leukocyte counts and absolute neutrophil counts are significantly lower in patients with anorexia nervosa. Assessment of marrow granulocyte reserve was found to be normal in spite of neutropenia, and this may help explain why anorexic patients do not more often suffer from infections. The susceptibility to infection in these patients has not been clearly established. Traditionally, anorexics have been thought to be at high risk for serious infections. However, it has been suggested that viral infections may be rare in this group but that the susceptibility to bacterial illnesses may be increased.[8,13,37] Abnormalities in the antimicrobial defense system have been noted by some. These include reduced levels of plasma complement and reduced polymorphonuclear bactericidal capacity in some patients. Responses to cellular immune tests such as tuberculin and macrophage inhibitions have produced variable results. In general, however, when patients are severely depleted nutritionally, anergy is common.[134]

Prognosis

The outcome of anorexia nervosa is extremely varied. For many it occurs as a single, relatively mild illness in adolescence, while for others it is a lifelong disorder with recurrences or persistent symptoms; the latter type has a high mortality.[30] Studies evaluating patients 4 to 10 years after initial treatment show that over 40 per cent of patients have totally recovered while a further 30 per cent are considerably improved at follow-up. However, about 20 per cent are unimproved or seriously impaired and about 9 per cent have died as a result of the illness. In those who have chronic forms of the illness, depressive symptoms, social phobias and the symptoms of anorexia nervosa can be incapacitating. One interesting trend is of a reduced mortality to 3 per cent in several large studies[89,117] utilizing a combined treatment approach of weight gain and psychotherapy. This may reflect a true reduction due to the consistent safe approach to weight restoration and ongoing care employed in these studies.

A number of factors have been demonstrated to be related to a good outcome. Most clearly related is the development of the syndrome at an early age of onset. Good results have been reported in up to 85 per cent of patients whose illness begins before age 16. Features associated with poor outcomes include chronicity; the presence of bulimia, vomiting, and laxative abuse; a premorbid history of obesity; and poor educational and vocational adjustment. More pronounced familial difficulties also suggest a poor prognosis, as does a poor response to treatment after 1 year.

DISORDERED EATING IN THE MEDICALLY ILL

Disturbed eating behavior is an important and often overlooked cause of malnutrition and metabolic imbalance in the medically ill. Food intake may be inappropriate in relation either to normal dietary requirements or to the special dietary requirements of conditions such as diabetes mellitus or end-stage renal disease. Disturbed eating behavior in the medically ill may result from psychological or organic factors that produce alterations in appetite, a fear of eating, an inability to ingest or absorb sufficient oral intake, or an inability or unwillingness to comply with particular dietary restrictions.

This section will focus on the psychological aspects of disturbed eating in the medically ill, although it is recognized that organic factors frequently affect appetite and food intake. Medical illness may precipitate functional eating disorders such as anorexia nervosa or other psychiatric disorders such as depression in which anorexia is prominent. Also, noncompliance with dietary instructions is common and often hazardous in certain medical conditions.

Organic Aspects of Disturbed Eating Behavior

The organic factors in medical illness that contribute to alterations in appetite and food intake are poorly understood and will be alluded to only briefly here. Anorexia is a common and nonspecific symptom in a wide variety of medical disorders,[92] although in certain hypothalamic disorders food intake may increase.[50] In other conditions, such as regional enteritis with partial obstruction, food intake may be curtailed because of a fear of eating in spite of a normal appetite.[92] In conditions such as cancer, anorexia has been attributed to a variety of psychological and metabolic factors.[93,118]

Patients who are unable to eat or to absorb sufficient nutrients to maintain homeostasis or who deteriorate on oral feeding may require long-term parenteral nutrition. This method of feeding is discussed at length in Chapter 43. The availability of nutritional support by this means is a major medical advance, and this treatment appears to be well tolerated by many patients. However, there have been few systematic psychological studies of patients who have been maintained on long-term total parenteral nutrition. Psychological sequelae that have been described in patients on long-term TPN include grief reactions, depression, organic brain syndromes, drug dependency, and body image changes.[80,109,112,133] Now that this procedure has become relatively safe and widely accepted, further investigations may help to elucidate the psychological ramifications and the factors that contribute to a satisfactory adjustment.

Medical Illness As a Precipitant of Anorexia Nervosa and/or Bulimia

At present, it is not known whether anorexia nervosa and bulimia occur with increased frequency in the medically ill. There have been some case reports of physical illness precipitating anorexia nervosa,[10,37] but systematic studies have not yet been carried out. Physical illness may represent a nonspecific stress that precipitates anorexia nervosa or bulimia in a susceptible individual. On the other hand, physical illness may be a more specific stressor for individuals who are susceptible to anorexia nervosa because it so often represents an assault on areas of particular vulnerability in such patients. For example, physical illness often results in a disturbed body image,[4] a lowering of self-esteem,[145,151] increased dependency upon and conflict with family members,[104,115] and disturbances in mood.[40,130,142] All of these psychological disturbances have been described in individuals with anorexia nervosa. Alterations in eating behavior due to functional psychiatric disorders may be even more common in the medically ill than has been appreciated, because anorexia in such patients is usually attributed to physical factors.

Insulin-dependent diabetes mellitus (IDDM) is a condition that is common in the population at risk for anorexia nervosa and bulimia, namely adolescent females. It has been estimated that by age 18, one in 300 to 400 white children in the United States will develop IDDM.[73,105] IDDM also has many features that are shared with the functional eating disorders, including the reduction in carbohydrate consumption, disturbances in body image,[146] low self-esteem and depression,[145] and family conflict.[115] Case reports have increasingly appeared in the literature regarding the association of anorexia nervosa and bulimia with IDDM.[45,66,72,88,124,132,135,147] Some suggest that the coexistence of these two disorders is no more frequent than would be expected based on the prevalence of each in the population.[30] Others postulate that eating disorders frequently remain undiagnosed in diabetics and may be much more common than has been suspected.[66,72]

Suggestions that have appeared in the literature regarding the possible association between diabetes mellitus and anorexia nervosa include the following:

1. The preoccupation with food and the need to limit carbohydrate consumption in diabetes mellitus may contribute to the development of a carbohydrate phobia.[132] This phenomenon, which may occur in diabetes, has been considered by some to be an important aspect of anorexia nervosa.[33]

2. Individuals who are prone to develop anorexia nervosa are more likely to do so when alterations in diabetic control provide a means of adjusting weight.[124] Whereas nondiabetic anorexics must starve themselves strenuously to reduce weight, diabetics have a ready albeit dangerous means of losing weight through noncompliance with their insulin administration or their diabetic diet.

3. Diabetes may represent a nonspecific emotional stress that could precipitate anorexia nervosa in an individual at risk.[135]

4. Pathological family interactions may result in the exacerbation of the symptoms of both anorexia nervosa and diabetes mellitus. Dietary noncompliance in the diabetic child has been considered by some to be the outcome of disturbances in family interaction patterns, as has been postulated with the disordered eating behavior of anorexia nervosa.[115]

All theories described that attempt to explain the relationship between IDDM and functional eating disorders must be considered speculative. Further research is needed to elucidate more definitively the nature and significance of this relationship.

Disturbed Eating Associated with Psychiatric Complications of Medical Illness. Systematic studies have demonstrated that psychiatric disorders are common in the medically ill. Approximately 25 per cent of general practice patients[71] or medical inpatients[111] have been found to suffer from a psychiatric disorder, most often depression. Depressive symptoms, not necessarily associated with an overt psychiatric disorder, may be found in up to one half of some medical patient populations.[28]

It has recently been emphasized that a variety of psychiatric disorders may be associated with anorexia and weight loss.[57] Depression associated with these symptoms may be more common in the medically ill than is often appreciated. A review of medical charts revealed that the primary physicians failed to diagnose depression and other significant psychological disturbances in about 50 per cent of cases.[122] The failure to recognize depression in medical patients may be common because symptoms such as anorexia, weight loss, lethargy, and insomnia can be secondary either to the physical effects of an illness or to a lowering of mood. Too strong a reliance on physical explanations for anorexia and weight loss may cause the physician to neglect psychological causes for these symptoms.

Disturbed eating behavior in medical patients may also occur because of confusion. It has been estimated that about 25 per cent of elderly medical patients who are considered intact in their cognitive functions on admission to the hospital may develop delirium during the first month of hospitalization.[108] Patients who are confused may neglect dietary intake or may develop specific delusions that cause them to avoid food.

Dietary Noncompliance

Compliance in the health care setting has been defined as "the extent to which a person's behavior (in terms of taking medications, following diets or executing lifestyle changes) coincides with medical or health advice."[85] Compliance with a prescribed diet may be essential to maintain metabolic and nutritional homeostasis in medical disorders such as end-stage renal failure and IDDM. Unfortunately, compliance is often poor with regard to prescribed diets or other aspects of recommended medical treatment. It is estimated that approximately half of all patients on any long-term regimen become noncompliant.[85] The degree of dietary compliance reported in patients with various medical conditions varies, in part, depending upon which measures of compliance are used. Estimates of dietary compliance in hemodialysis patients have ranged from 28 to 70 per cent of that population.[85]

Psychological, environmental, and social factors and characteristics of the therapeutic regimen and of the physician-patient relationship may all be important determinants of compliance.[69] Attempts to identify specific personality types that can be correlated with compliance or noncompliance with diet or other aspects of medical treatment have not been successful.[11,131] Neither age, sex, socioeconomic status, education, religion, marital status, nor race have been shown to predict compliance.[113] Also, knowledge of the disease has not correlated well with compliance with treatment.[7,160,162] It may be that the patient's attitude toward the disease and its treatment are more important than factual knowledge with regard to the degree of compliance. It has been suggested that noncompliers tend to perceive themselves as less susceptible to or less threatened by actual or potential illness.[5]

A variety of psychological factors may contribute to dietary noncompliance. In diabetic children, dietary abuse and "cheating" on reports of urine tests have been attributed to the expression of anger, depression, the fear of "large" doses of insulin, magical thinking, and attempts to relieve anxiety.[161] Other factors may also contribute to noncompliance with the diet. Mothers in a pediatric clinic who were dissatisfied with their doctor's friendliness or ability to carry out an exchange or to understand their concerns were less likely to comply with the doctor's instructions.[51] Family attitudes and coping mechanisms within the family may also affect compliance. Pathological coping mechanisms in the family have been associated with poor diabetic control.[104] With diabetic adolescents, diet may become the focus of family conflict.[148] The adolescent's need to assert himself at this stage of development may be heightened by parental overprotectiveness and may cause rebellion in the form of dietary noncompliance. The psychological aspects of dietary compliance have also been studied in end-stage renal disease. Although there have been few consistent findings, patients who comply poorly with the dietary regimen have been found to demonstrate low tolerance for frustration and evidence of gain from the sick role.[97] Overall, socioeconomic factors have not helped to predict noncompliance, except that patients who live alone tend to be less compliant with regard to medication and diet.[2,131]

Acknowledgments

The authors wish to acknowledge grant support from the Ontario Mental Health Foundation (Grant No. 810). and the Medical Research Council (Grant No. MA 7914). Dr. David Garner is a scholar of the Medical Research Council of Canada. Miss Barbara Bridle provided valuable technical assistance.

References

1. Adler AG, Walinsky P, Krall RA, et al. Death resulting from ipecac syrup poisoning. JAMA 1980; 243:1927–1928.
2. Archer M, Rinzler S, Christakis C. Social factors affecting participation in a study of diet and coronary heart disease. J Health Soc Behav 1967; 8:22–31.
3. Barry VC, Klawans HL. On the role of dopamine in the pathophysiology of anorexia nervosa. J Neural Transm 1976; 38:107–122.
4. Baumann S. Physical aspects of the self. A review of some aspects of body image development in childhood. Psychiatr Clin North Am 1981; 4:445–469.
5. Becker MH, Maiman LA. Sociobehavioral determinants of compliance with health and medical care recommendations. Med Care 1975; 13:10–24.
6. Berger M, Pirke KM, Doerr P, et al. Influence of weight loss on the dexamethasone suppression test. Arch Gen Psychiatr 1983; 40:584–585.
7. Bergman AB, Warner RJ. Failure of children to receive penicillin by mouth. N Engl J Med 1963; 268:1334–1338.
8. Berkman JM: Anorexia nervosa, anterior-pituitary insufficiency, Simmonds' cachexia, and Sheehan's disease: including some observations on disturbances in water metabolism associated with starvation. Postgrad Med 1948; 3:237–246.
9. Beumont PJV, Abraham SF, Argall WJ, et al. The onset of anorexia nervosa. Aust NZ J Psychiatr 1978; 12:145–149.
10. Beumont PJV, Carr PJ, Gelder MG. Plasma levels of luteinizing hormone and of immunoactive oestrogens (oestradiol) in anorexia nervosa: response to clomiphene citrate. Psychol Med 1973; 3:495–501.
11. Blackwell B. The drug defaulter. Clin Pharmacol Ther 1972; 13:841–848.
12. Bohnet HG, Dahlen HC, Wuttke W, et al. Hyperprolactinemic anovulatory syndrome. J Clin Endocrinol Metab 1976; 42:132–143.
13. Bowers TK, Eckert E. Leukopenia in anorexia nervosa. Lack of increased risk of infection. Arch Intern Med 1978; 138:1520–1523.
14. Boyar RM, Bradlow HL. Studies of testosterone metabolism in anorexia nervosa. In Vigersky R (ed). Anorexia Nervosa. New York, Raven Press, 1977: 271–276.
15. Boyar RM, Hellman LD, Roffwarg H, et al. Cortisol secretion and metabolism in anorexia nervosa. N Engl J Med 1977; 296:190–193.
16. Boyar RM, Katz, J. Twenty-four hour gonadotrophin secretory patterns in anorexia nervosa. In Vigersky R (ed). Anorexia Nervosa. New York, Raven Press, 1977: 177–187.
17. Boyar RM, Katz J, Finkelstein JW, et al. Anorexia nervosa: immaturity of the 24-hour luteinizing hormone secretory pattern. N Engl J Med 1974; 291:861–865.
18. Brambilla F, Smeraldi E, Sacchetti E, et al. Abnormal anterior pituitary responsiveness to hypothalamic hormones in depression. In Muller EE, Aanolyi A (eds). Neuroendocrine Correlates in Neurology and Psychiatry. Amsterdam, Elsevier, 1979: 239–254.
19. Brotman MC, Forbath N, Garfinkel PE, et al. Ipecac syrup poisoning in anorexia nervosa. Can Med Assoc J 1981; 125:453–454.
20. Brown GM, Garfinkel PE, Jeuniewic N, et al. Endocrine profiles in anorexia nervosa. In Vigersky R (ed). Anorexia Nervosa. New York, Raven Press, 1977: 123–135.
21. Bruch H. Eating Disorders: Obesity, Anorexia Nervosa and the Person Within. New York, Basic Books, 1973.
22. Bruch H: Anorexia nervosa. In Wurtman RJ, Wurtman JJ (eds). Nutrition and the Brain. Vol. 3. New York, Raven Press, 1979: 101–115.
23. Burman KD, Diamond RC, Harvey GS, et al. Glucose modulation of alterations in serum iodothyronine concentrations induced by fasting. Metabolism 1979; 28:291–299.
24. Burman KD, Vigersky RA, Loriaux DL. Investigations concerning thyroxine deiodinative pathways in patients with anorexia nervosa. In Vigersky R (ed). Anorexia Nervosa. New York, Raven Press, 1977: 255–269.
25. Cantwell DP, Sturzenburger S, Burroughs J, et al. Anorexia Nervosa: An affective disorder? Arch Gen Psychiatr 1977; 34:1087–1093.
26. Caron HS, Roth HP. Patients' cooperation with a medical regimen. Difficulties in identifying the noncooperator. JAMA 1968; 203:922–926.
27. Casper RC, Davis JM, Pandey CN: The effect of nutritional status and weight changes on hypothalamic function tests in anorexia nervosa. In Vigersky R (ed). Anorexia Nervosa. New York, Raven Press, 1977: 134–147.
28. Cavanaugh SA. The prevalence of emotional and cognitive dysfunction in a general hospital population using the MMSE, GHQ and BDI. Gen Hosp Psychiatr 1983; 5:15–24.
29. Coppen AM, Gupta RK, Eccleston EG, et al. Letter: Plasmatryoptophan in anorexia nervosa. Lancet 1976; 1:961.
30. Crisp AH. Clinical and therapeutic aspects of anorexia ner-

vosa: A study of thirty cases. J Psychosom Research 1965; 9:67–78.

31. Crisp AH. The possible significance of some behavioral correlates of weight and carbohydrate intake. J Psychosom Res 1967; 11:117–131.

32. Crisp AH. Premorbid factors in adult disorders of weight, with particular reference to primary anorexia nervosa (weight phobia). J Psychosom Res 1970; 14:1–22.

33. Crisp AH. Anorexia Nervosa: Let Me Be. New York, Grune & Stratton, 1980.

34. Crisp AH, Harding B, McGuinness B. Anorexia nervosa: psychoneurotic characteristics of patients. J Psychosom Res 1974; 18:167–173.

35. Crisp AH, Palmer RL, Kalucy RS. How common is anorexia nervosa? A prevalence study. Br J Psychiatr 1976; 218:549–554.

36. Crisp AH, Stonehill E. Aspects of the relationship between psychiatric status, sleep, nocturnal motility and nutrition. J Psychosom Res 1971; 15:501–509.

37. Dally P. Anorexia Nervosa. New York, Grune & Stratton, 1969.

38. Darby PL, VanLoon G, Garfinkel PE, et al. LH, growth hormone, prolactin and catecholamine responses to LHRF and bromocriptine in anorexia nervosa. (Abstract) Psychosom Med 1980; 41:585.

39. Devlin JG. Obesity and anorexia nervosa, a study of growth hormone release. Ir Med J 1975; 68:227–231.

40. Dovenmuehle RH, Verwoerdt A. Physical illness and depressive symptomatology. I. Incidence of depressive symptoms in hospitalized cardiac patients. J Am Geriatr Soc 1962; 10:932–946.

41. Drossman DN, Ontjes DA, Heizer WD. Anorexia Nervosa. Gastroenterology 1979; 77:1115–1131.

42. Dubois A, Gross HA, Ebert MH, et al. Altered gastric emptying and secretion in primary anorexia nervosa. Gastroenterology 1979, 77:319–323.

43. Edelstein CK, Roy-Byrne P, Fawzy FI, et al. Effects of weight loss on the dexamethasone suppression test. Am J Psychiatr 1983; 140:338–341.

44. Edgren B, Wester PO. Impairment of glomerular filtration in fasting for obesity. Acta Med Scand 1971; 190:389–393.

45. Fairburn CG. Self-induced vomiting. J Psychosom Res 1980; 24:193–197.

46. Fairburn CG, Cooper PJ. Self-induced vomiting and bulimia nervosa: an undetected problem. Br Med J 1982, 284:1153–1155.

47. Fairburn CG, Steel JM. Anorexia nervosa in diabetes mellitus. Br Med J 1980; 28:1167–1168.

48. Fohlin L. Body composition, cardiovascular and renal function in adolescent patients with anorexia nervosa. Acta Pediatr Scand (Suppl) 1977; 268:1–20.

49. Fohlin L, Freyschuss U, Bjorke B, et al. Function and dimensions of the circulatory system in anorexia nervosa. Acta Paediatr Scand 1978; 67:11–16.

50. Foster DW. Gain and loss of weight. In Petersdorff RG, Adams RD, Braunwald E, et al. (eds). Harrison's Principles of Internal Medicine. 10th ed. New York, McGraw-Hill, 1983.

51. Francis J, Korsch VM, Morris MJ. Gaps in doctor-patient communication. N Engl J Med 1969; 280:535–540.

52. Fries H. Studies on secondary amenorrhea, anorectic behavior and body-image perception: importance for the early recognition of anorexia nervosa. In Vigersky RA (ed). Anorexia Nervosa. New York, Raven Press, 1977: 163–176.

53. Garfinkel PE. Perception of hunger and satiety in anorexia nervosa. Psychol Med 1974; 4:309–315.

54. Garfinkel PE, Brown GM, Stancer HC, et al. Hypothalamic-pituitary function in anorexia nervosa. Arch Gen Psychiatr 1975; 32:739–744.

55. Garfinkel PE, Coscina DV. The biology and psychology of hunger and satiety. In Zales MR (ed). Eating, Sleeping

and Sexuality: Treatment of Disorders in Basic Life Functions. New York, Brunner/Mazel, 1982.

56. Garfinkel PE, Garner DM. Anorexia Nervosa: A Multidimensional Perspective. New York, Brunner/Mazel, 1982.

57. Garfinkel PE, Garner DM, Kaplan AS, et al. Differential diagnosis of emotional disorders that cause weight loss. Can Med Assoc J 1983; 129:939–945.

58. Garfinkel PE, Garner DM, Rose J, et al. A comparison of characteristics in the families of patients with anorexia nervosa and controls. Psychol Med 1983; 13:821–828.

59. Garfinkel PE, Kaplan AS, Garner DM, et al. The differentiation of vomiting/weight loss as a conversion disorder from anorexia nervosa. Am J Psychiatr 1983; 140:1019–1022.

60. Garfinkel PE, Moldofsky H, Garner DM. The heterogeneity of anorexia nervosa: bulimia as a distinct subgroup. Arch Gen Psychiatr 1980; 37:1036–1040.

61. Garner DM, Bemis KM: A cognitive-behavioral approach to anorexia nervosa. Cog Ther Res 1982; 6:1–27, 1982.

62. Garner DM, Garfinkel PE. Socio-cultural factors in the development of anorexia nervosa. Psychol Med 1980; 10:647–656.

63. Garner DM, Garfinkel PE. Body image in anorexia nervosa: Measurement, theory and clinical implications. Int J Psychiatr Med 1981; 11:263–284.

64. Garner DM, Garfinkel PE, O'Shaughnessy M. The validity of the distinction between bulimia with and without anorexia nervosa. Am J Psychiatr 1985; 142:581–587.

65. Garner DM, Garfinkel PE, Schwartz D, et al. Cultural expectations of thinness and women. Psych Rep 1980; 47:483–491.

66. Garner S. Anorexia nervosa in diabetes mellitus. Br Med J 1980; 281:1144.

67. Gerner RH, Gwirtsman HE. Abnormalities of dexamethasone suppression test and urinary MHPG in anorexia nervosa. Am J Psychiatr 1981; 138:650–653.

68. Gerner RH, Wilkins JN. CSF cortisol in patients with depression, mania or anorexia nervosa and in normal subjects. Am J Psychiatr 1983; 140:92–94.

69. Gillum RF, Barsky AJ. Diagnosis and management of patient noncompliance. JAMA 1974; 228:1563–1567.

70. Glassman A. Tricyclic antidepressants. In Stancer, HC, Garfinkel PE, Rakoff VM (eds). Guidelines for the Use of Psychotropic Drugs. New York, SP Publications, 1983.

71. Goldberg DP, Blackwell B. Psychiatric illness in general practice. A detailed study using a new method of case identification. Br Med J 1970; 2:439–443.

72. Gomez J, Dally P, Isaacs AJ. Anorexia nervosa in diabetes mellitus. Br Med J 1980; 281:62–63.

73. Gorwitz K, Howen GG, Thompson T. Prevalence of diabetes in Michigan school-age children. Diabetes 1976; 25:122–127.

74. Gottdiener JS, Gross HA, Henry WL, et al. Effects of self-induced starvation on cardiac size and function in anorexia nervosa. Circulation 1978; 58:425–433.

75. Green RS, Rau JS. Treatment of compulsive eating disturbances with anticonvulsant medication. Am J Psychiatr 1974; 131:428–432.

76. Green RS, Rau JH: The use of diphenylhydantoin in compulsive eating disorders: further studies. In Vigersky RA (ed). Anorexia Nervosa. New York, Raven Press, 1977: 377–382.

77. Gross HA, Lake CR, Ebert MH, et al. Catecholamine metabolism in primary anorexia nervosa. J Clin Endocrinol Metab 1979; 49:805–809.

78. Grounds A. Transient psychoses in anorexia nervosa: a report of 7 cases. Psychol Med 1982; 12:107–113.

79. Gull WW. The address in medicine delivered before the annual meeting of BMA at Oxford. Lancet 1868; 2:171.

80. Gull WW. Anorexia nervosa. Transactions of the Clinical Society of London, 1974; 7:22–28. Reprinted in Kaufman RM, Heiman M (eds). Evolution of Psychosomatic Concepts. Anorexia Nervosa: A Paradigm. New York, International Universities Press, 1964.

81. Gulledge AD, Gipson WT, Steiger E, et al. Home parenteral nutrition for the short bowel syndrome. Psychological issues. Gen Hosp Psychiatry 1980; 2:271–281.

82. Hafner RJ, Crisp AH, McNeilly AS. Prolactin and gonadotrophin activity in females treated for anorexia nervosa. Postgrad Med 1976; 52:76–79.

83. Halmi KA, Dekirmenjian H, Davis JM, et al. Catecholamine metabolism in anorexia nervosa. Arch Gen Psychiatr 1978; 35:458–460.

84. Harrower ADB, Yap PL, Nairn IM, et al. Growth hormone, insulin, and prolactin secretion in anorexia nervosa and obesity during bromocriptine treatment. Br Med J 1977; 2:156–159.

85. Haynes RB, Taylor DW, Sackett DL (ed). Compliance in Health Care. Baltimore, Johns Hopkins University Press, 1979.

86. Herman CP, Polivy J. Anxiety, retraint and eating behavior. J Personality 1975; 84:666–672.

87. Hill P, Wynder F. Diet and prolactin release. Lancet 1976; 2:806–807.

88. Hillard J. Bulimia and diabetes: a potentially life-threatening combination. Psychosomatics 1983; 24:294–295.

89. Hsu LKG, Crisp AH, Harding B. Outcome of anorexia nervosa. Lancet 1979; 1:61–65.

90. Hudson JI, Pope HG JR, Jonas JM, et al. Family history study of anorexia nervosa and bulimia. Br J Psychiatr 1983; 142:133–138.

91. Isaacs AJ, Leslie RDG, Gomez J, et al. The effect of weight gain on gonadotrophins and prolactin in anorexia nervosa. Acta Endocrinol 1980; 94:145–150.

92. Isselbacher JK. Anorexia, nausea and vomiting. In Petersdorff RG, Adams RD, Braunwald E, et al. (eds). Harrison's Principles of Internal Medicine. 10th ed. New York, McGraw-Hill, 1983.

93. Johnson J. Anorexia in the cancer patient. In Wolland J (ed). Nutritional Management of the Cancer Patient. New York, Raven Press, 1979.

94. Johnston JL, Lieter LA, Burrow GN, et al. Excretion of urinary catecholamines in anorexia nervosa: effects of body composition and energy intake. Am J Clin Nutr 1984; 40:1001–1006.

95. Kalucy RC, Crisp AH, Chard T, et al. Nocturnal hormonal profiles in massive obesity, anorexia nervosa and normal females. J Psychosom Res 1976; 20:595–604.

96. Kaplan AS, Garfinkel PE, Darby PL, et al. Carbamazepine in the treatment of bulimia. Am J Psychiatr 1983; 140:1225–1226.

97. Kaplan de Nour A, Czaczkes JW. Personality factors in chronic hemodialysis patients causing noncompliance with medical regimen. Psychosom Med 1972; 34:333–344.

98. Katz JL, Boyar RM, Roffwarg H, et al. Weight and circadian luteinizing hormone secretory pattern in anorexia nervosa. Psychosom Med 1978; 40:549–567.

99. Kay DWK. Anorexia nervosa: A study in prognosis. Proc Roy Soc Med 1953; 46:669–674.

100. Keesey RE. A set point analysis of the regulation of body weight. In Stunkard AJ (ed). Obesity. Philadelphia, WB Saunders, 1980.

101. Keesey RE. A hypothalamic syndrome of body-weight regulation at reduced levels. In Understanding Anorexia Nervosa and Bulimia. Report of the Fourth Ross Conference on Medical Research. Columbus, OH, Ross Laboratories, 1983: 60–66.

102. Kennedy S, Piran N, Owens M, et al. Anorexia nervosa and bulimia—response to MAOI therapy. J Clin Psychopharmacol 1985; 5:279–285.

103. Keys A, Brozek J, Henschel A, et al. The Biology of Human Starvation. Vol I. Minneapolis, University of Minnesota Press, 1950.

104. Koski ML. Coping processes in childhood diabetes. Acta Pediatr Scand Suppl 1969; 19:6–56.

105. Kyllo CJ, Nuttall RQ. Prevalence of diabetes mellitus in school age children in Minnesota. Diabetes, 1978; 27:57–60.

106. Landsberg L, Young JB. Fasting, feeding and regulation of the sympathetic nervous system. N Engl J Med 1978; 298:1295–2301.

107. Levitan H. Implications of certain dreams reported by patients with anorexia nervosa syndrome. Post-graduate board, Royal Victoria Hospital and McGill University, Montreal, April, 1979.

108. Lipowski ZJ. Transient cognitive disorders (delirium, acute confusional states) in the elderly. Am J Psychiatr 1983; 140:1426–1436.

109. MacRitchie KJ. Parenteral nutrition outside hospital. Psychosocial styles of adaptation. Can J Psychiatry 1980; 25:303–313.

110. Maeda K, Kato Y, Yamaguchi N, et al. Growth hormone release following thyrotropin-releasing hormone injection into patients with anorexia nervosa. Acta Endocrinol (Copenh) 1976; 81:8.

111. Maguire GP, Julier DL, Hawton KE, et al. Psychiatric morbidity and referral on two general wards. Br Med J 1974; 1:268–270.

112. Malcolm R, Robson JRK, Vandereen TW, et al. Psychosocial aspects of total parenteral nutrition. Psychosomatics 1983; 21:115–125.

113. Marston M. Compliance with medical regimens: a review of the literature. Nurs Res 1970; 19:312–323.

114. Mawson AR. Anorexia nervosa and the regulation of intake: A review. Psychol Med 1974; 4:289–308.

115. Minuchin S, Baker L, Rosman B, et al. A conceptual model of psychosomatic illness in children: Family organization and family therapy. Arch Gen Psychiatr 1975; 32:1031–1038.

116. Mitchell JE, Pyle RL. The bulimic syndrome in normal weight individuals: a review. Int J Eating Disord 1982; 2:61–73.

117. Morgan HG, Russell GFM. Value of family background and clinical features as predictors of long-term outcome in anorexia nervosa: four-year follow-up study of 41 patients. Psychol Med 1975; 5:355–371.

118. Morrison SD. Anorexia and the cancer patient. In Eys JV, Seelig MS, Nichols BL Jr (eds). Nutrition and Cancer. New York, Spectrum Publications, 1979.

119. Moshang T Jr, Parks JS, Bader L, et al. Low serum triiodothyronine euthyroidism in anorexia nervosa. J Clin Endocrinol 1975; 40:470–473.

120. Moshang T Jr, Utiger RD. Low triiodothyronine euthyroidism in anorexia nervosa. In Vigersky R (ed). Anorexia Nervosa. New York, Raven Press, 1977: 263–270.

121. Nicolle G. Prepsychotic anorexia. Proc Roy Soc Med 1939, 32:153–162.

122. Nielson AC, Williams TA. Depression in ambulatory medical patients. Arch Gen Psychiatr 1980; 37:999–1004.

123. Nillius SJ, Wide L. The pituitary responsiveness to acute and chronic administration of gonadotrophin-releasing hormone in acute and recovery stages of anorexia. In Vigerksy R (ed). Anorexia Nervosa. New York, Raven Press, 1977.

124. O'Gorman EC, Eyre DG. A case of anorexia nervosa and diabetes mellitus. Br J Psychiatr 1980; 137:103.

125. Patrick J. Oedema in protein energy malnutrition: the role of the sodium pump. Proc Nutr Soc 1979; 38:61–68.

126. Paykel ES, Mueller PS, De LaVergne P: Amitriptyline, weight gain and carbohydrate craving: a side effect. Br J Psychiatr 1973; 123:501–507.

127. Pimstone EL, Becker DJ, Hansen JDL. Human growth hormone in protein calorie malnutrition. In Pecile A, Muller EE (eds). Growth and Growth Hormone. Amsterdam, Excerpta Medica, 1973: 389–401.

128. Piran N, Kennedy S, Owen M, et al. The presence of affective disorder in patients with anorexia nervosa and bulimia. J Nerv Ment Dis 1985; 173:395–400.

129. Pirke MK, Fichter M, Lund P, et al. Twenty-four hour sleep-awake pattern of plasma LH in patients with anorexia nervosa. Acta Endocrinol (Copenh) 1979; 92:193–204.

130. Plumb M, Holland J. Comparative studies of psychological

function in patients with advanced cancer. II. Inteviewer-rated current and past psychological symptoms. Psychosom Med 1981; 43:243–254.

131. Porter AMW. Drug defaulting in a general practice. Br Med J 1969; 1:218–222.

132. Powers FS. Anorexia nervosa and diabetes mellitus. J Clin Psychiatr 1983; 28:219–223.

133. Price BS, Levine EL. Permanent total parenteral nutrition: psychological and social responses of the early stages. JPEN 1979; 3:48–52.

134. Redmond DE Jr, Swann A, Heninger GR. Letter: Phenoxybenzamine in anorexia nervosa. Lancet 1976; 2:307.

135. Roland JM, Bhanj S. Anorexia nervosa occurring in patients with diabetes mellitus. Postgrad Med J 1982; 58:354–356.

136. Rollins N, Piazza E. Diagnosis of anorexia nervosa. A critical reappraisal. J Am Acad Child Psychiatr 1978; 17:126–137.

137. Russell DM, Prendergast PJ, Darby PL, et al. A comparison between muscle function and body composition in anorexia nervosa: the effect of refeeding. Am J Clin Nutr 1983; 38:229–237.

138. Russell DM, Freedman ML, Feiglin DHI, et al. Delayed gastric emptying and improvement with domperidone in a period with anorexia nervosa. Am J Psychiatr 1983; 140:1235–1236.

139. Russell GFM, Bruce JT. Impaired water diuresis in patients with anorexia nervosa. Am J Med 1966; 40:38–48.

140. Saleh JW, Lebwohl P. Metoclopramide-induced gastric emptying in patients with anorexia nervosa. Am J Gastroenterol 1980; 74:127–132.

141. Schiele BC, Brozek J. "Experimental neurosis" resulting from semistarvation in man. Psychosom Med 1948; 10:31–50.

142. Schiffer RB, Caine Ed, Bamford MS, et al. Depressive episodes in patients with multiple sclerosis. Am J Psychiatr 1983; 140:1498–1500.

143. Sherman BM, Halmi KA. Effect of nutritional rehabilitation of hypothalamic-pituitary function in anorexia nervosa. In Vigersky R (ed). Anorexia Nervosa. New York, Raven Press, 1977: 211–223.

144. Stancer HC, Warsh JJ, Tang SW, et al. In Youdim MHB, Usdin E, Sourkes TL (eds). Enzymes and Neurotransmitters and Mental Disease. Chichester, England, Wiley, 1980: 221.

145. Sullivan BJ. Self-esteem and depression in adolescent diabetic girls. Diabetes Care 1978; 1(1):18–22.

146. Sullivan BJ. Adjustment in diabetic adolescent girls: I. Development of the Diabetic Adjustment Scale. Psychosom Med 1979; 41:119–126.

147. Szmukler GI, Russel GFM. Diabetes mellitus, anorexia nervosa and bulimia. Br J Psychiatr 1983, 142:305–308.

148. Tattersall RB, Lowe J. Diabetes in adolescence. Diabetologia 1981; 20:517–523.

149. Theander S. Anorexia nervosa: a psychiatric investigation of 94 female cases. Acta Psychiatr Scand (Suppl) 1970; 214:1–194.

150. Thurston J, Marks P. Electrocardiographic abnormalities in patients with anorexia nervosa. Br Heart J 1974; 36:719–723.

151. Tietz W, Vidmar T. The impact of coping style on the control of juvenile diabetes. Int J Psychiatr Med 1972; 3:67–74.

152. Vagenakis AG. Thyroid hormone in prolonged experimental starvation in man. In Vigersky R (ed). Anorexia Nervosa. New York, Raven Press, 1977: 243–252.

153. Vandereycken W, Pierloot R. Combining drugs and behavior therapy in anorexia nervosa: a double-blind placebo/pimozide study. In Darby PL, Garfinkel PE, Garner DM, et al (eds). Anorexia Nervosa: Recent Developments in Research. New York, Alan R. Liss, 1983: 365–376.

154. Vigersky RA, Andersen AE, Thompson RH, et al. Hypothalamic dysfunction in secondary amenorrhea associated with simple weight loss. N Engl J Med 1977; 297:1141–1145.

155. Vigersky RA, Loriaux DL. Anorexia nervosa as a model of hypothalamic dysfunction. In Vigersky R (ed). Anorexia Nervosa. New York, Raven Press, 1977: 109–122.

156. Vigersky RA, Loriaux DL, Andersen AE, et al. Delayed pituitary hormone response to LRF and TRF in patients with anorexia and with secondary amenorrhea associated with simple weight loss. J Clin Endocrinol Metab 1976; 43:893–900.

157. Wakeling A, DeSouza VA, Gore MBR, et al. Amenorrhea, body weight and serum hormone concentrations, with particular reference to prolactin and thyroid hormones in anorexia nervosa. Psychol Med 1979; 9:265–272.

158. Walsh BT, Katz JL, Levin J, et al. Adrenal activity in anorexia nervosa. Psychosom Med 1978; 40:499–506.

159. Warren MP, Van de Wiele RL. Clinical and metabolic features of anorexia nervosa. Am J Obstet Gynecol 1973; 117:435–449.

160. Watkins JD, Williams TF, Martin DA, et al. A study of diabetic patients at home. Am J Public Health 1967; 57:452–459.

161. Wats FN. Behavioral aspects of the management of diabetes mellitus: education, self-care and metabolic control. Behav Res Ther 1980; 18:171–180.

162. Weintraub M, Au WYW, Lasagna L. Compliance as a determinant of serum digitoxin concentration. JAMA 1973; 224:481–485.

163. Weitzman ED. Circadian rhythms and episodic hormone secretion. Annu Rev Med 1976; 27:225–243.

164. Wermuth BM, Davis KL, Hollister LE, et al. Phenytoin treatment of the binge-eating syndrome. Am J Psychiatr 1977; 134:1249–1253.

165. Winokur A, March V, Mendels J. Primary affective disorder in relatives of patients with anorexia nervosa. Am J Psychiatr 1980; 137:695–698.

166. Wolff WP, Vecsei P, Kruck F, et al. Psychiatric disturbances leading to potassium depletion, sodium depletion, raised plasma-renin concentration and secondary hyperaldosteronism. Lancet 1968; 1:257–261.

11

EXERCISE

JOHN T. DEVLIN / EDWARD S. HORTON

ENERGY EXPENDITURE AND CALORIC REQUIREMENTS

Components of Energy Expenditure

Energy expenditure can be subdivided into several components. These include resting metabolic rate (RMR), the thermic effect of food, the thermic effect of exercise, and adaptive thermogenesis. Adaptive thermogenesis refers to changes in metabolic rate that are the result of environmental influences such as changes in the quantity or composition of the diet, cold acclimation, and responses to drugs or hormones.[1]

There are a number of methods to determine energy expenditure accurately, including direct and indirect calorimetry and the use of the doubly labeled water ($^2H_2^{18}O$) technique. Of these, indirect calorimetry is the most widely available. Measurements of energy expenditure may be useful for many individuals engaging in a physical exercise program. Obese subjects who wish to exercise as an adjunct to dietary therapy can quantitate the impact of the exercise program on energy balance and better estimate the rate of weight loss to be anticipated. Subjects who are below ideal or desired body weight can determine the additional caloric intake required to produce optimal amounts of lean body weight accretion while minimizing increases in body fat.

In clinical practice, reliable methods for measuring metabolic rates, such as indirect calorimetry, are seldom available for widespread use. Caloric expenditure can be estimated by adding the calculated expenditure of exercise to the sedentary levels. Estimates of resting metabolic rate (RMR) in kilocalories per 24 hours can be made with reasonable accuracy using the Harris-Benedict formulas, derived from measurements made in adult men and women by indirect calorimetry:

Men: $66.5 + 13.8 \times$ Wt (kg) $+ 5 \times$ Ht (cm) $- 6.8$
$\times$ Age (yr)

Women: $655 + 9.6 \times$ Wt $+ 1.8 \times$ Ht $- 4.6 \times$ Age

225

Multiplying the RMR by 1.3 gives an estimate of the caloric needs for weight maintenance in a sedentary individual. The additional energy expenditure involved in various physical activities can be estimated by referring to standard tables. There are many tables that give caloric expenditures for various activities in kcal/min, but these do not take into account differences in body mass. For this reason, using multiples of the resting oxygen consumption (MET's) to plan an exercise program may be advantageous. One MET is defined as the equivalent of the resting oxygen consumption. This either can be measured directly or can be estimated at 3.5 ml/kg/min. Representative energy costs of various activities in MET's are shown in Table 11–1.

Any increased caloric requirements during physical training should be met with a balanced increase in all elements of the diet rather than in a single category of food (e.g., meats). Exercise training appears to result in relatively small losses in total body weight, moderate-to-large losses in body fat, and small-to-moderate increases in lean body weight. If significant weight loss is the goal, an intake of energy that is less than the total energy expenditure should be planned. During the early stages of a weight reduction diet (less than 10 days), the caloric equivalent of weight loss is approximately 3200 to 3400 kcal/kg. Later, however, the caloric value of the weight change rises to approximately 7000 kcal/kg.[2] Thus, a daily caloric deficit of 1000 kcal/day will result in approximately 1 kg of weight loss per week.

Effects of Diet on Metabolic Rates

Numerous studies have demonstrated a change in basal metabolic rate induced by alterations in caloric intake. Overfeeding in normal volunteers has been associated with increases in basal energy expenditure. This phenomenon, called dietary-induced thermogenesis, may result in a 10 to 15 per cent increase in RMR. In contrast, underfeeding results in a decrease in resting metabolic rate.[1] This helps explain some of the difficulty encountered with the dietary treatment of obesity. Since underfeeding has been shown to increase levels of metabolically inactive 3,3′,5′-triiodothyronine (reverse T_3), and to decrease free 3,5,3′-triiodothyronine (T_3) levels, with opposite changes during overfeeding,[3] thyroid hormones appear to play an important role in dietary-induced thermogenesis. Sympathetic nervous system activity has also been shown to be altered by changes in caloric intake[4] and may have an important effect on metabolic rates. Other factors that may affect energy expenditure during altered dietary intake include insulin, futile substrate cycles, and Na-K ATPase activity.

Effects of Exercise on Oxygen Consumption

One of the rationales for adding an exercise program to the dietary treatment of obesity is to prevent the decrease in metabolic rate seen with underfeeding. In one study, obese females on a weight-reduction diet were found to have a decrease in oxygen consumption ($\dot{V}O_2$) both at rest and during low-intensity cycle exercise. However, at higher intensities of cycle exercise, there was no difference in $\dot{V}O_2$ between the baseline and underfeeding periods, suggesting the ability of higher-intensity exercise to offset the reduced metabolic rate seen during underfeeding.[5] Another recent study has shown that the addition of a physical exercise regimen is able to prevent the decrease in RMR that normally occurs during low-calorie diets.[6] When exercise was added to a 500-kcal diet, there was a rapid increase in metabolic rate back to the control levels, which preceded any possible increase in lean body mass.

Not only is $\dot{V}O_2$ increased during acute exercise, but there is also a sustained increase in $\dot{V}O_2$ following exercise. This has been reported to be as high as 23 per cent above pre-exercise levels 13 hours after the completion of exercise,[7] and elevations of 8 to 10 per cent have been measured as long as 48 to 72 hours following very intense exercise, although these early studies were not well controlled for dietary intake. The increase in $\dot{V}O_2$ following exercise was initially explained by Hill and Lupton in 1923 by the "oxygen debt" hypothesis, and was thought to represent the oxidation of lactate and other metabolites that accumulated during exercise. It is probable that the increase in metabolic rate following exercise is regulated by several factors such as concentrations of catecholamines, thyroid hormones, free fatty acids, and calcium, as well as by increased body temperature, with the latter perhaps being the most important.[8] Hormones may increase membrane permeability to sodium and potassium and thereby increase Na-K pump activity, which along with persistent increases in "futile" substrate cycling may account for the prolonged increases in $\dot{V}O_2$ seen after intense exercise. Recent data suggest that RMR may

TABLE 11–1. Energy Costs of Exercise in MET's

	Mean	Range
Cycling		
10 mph	7.0	—
Dancing (aerobic)	—	6–9
Handball	—	8–12+
Skiing		
Downhill	—	5–8
Cross-country	—	6–12+
Running		
12 min/mile	8.7	—
10 min/mile	10.2	—
8 min/mile	12.5	—
7 min/mile	14.1	—
Swimming	—	4–8+
Tennis	6.5	4–9+

be elevated for at least 12 hours in normal control subjects, but there may be a defect in this thermic response to exercise in obese subjects.[9]

Several authors have examined the interactions of physical exercise and food intake on total energy expenditure. Miller[10] has shown that energy expenditure during exercise and following a meal was greater than the sum of the independent effects of the meal and exercise. This led him to speculate that exercise may potentiate the thermic effect of food (TEF) and help to dissipate extra calories. These results could not be confirmed by Bray,[11] who found no additive effect of work on the thermic response following either a 1000 or a 4000 kcal meal. Recently, Segal[12] has shown that bicycle exercise could potentiate the thermic effect of food in lean women (2.54× elevation in TEF), but not in obese subjects (1.01× increase). This raises the possibility that there is a defect in the potentiating effect of exercise on the thermic effect of food in obesity.

Finally, the literature is very divided on the effect of physical training on resting metabolic rate. Early studies by Schneider[13] found that physical training raised RMR in two subjects and lowered it in a third subject. More recent work by Terjung[14] has failed to show any effect of physical training on RMR.

SUBSTRATE UTILIZATION AND HORMONAL RESPONSES TO EXERCISE

Patterns of carbohydrate and lipid oxidation can be accurately determined using the technique of indirect calorimetry. The respiratory exchange ratio (RER) is the ratio of moles of CO_2 produced for each mole of O_2 consumed. Estimating the respiratory quotient (RQ) from measurements of the RER during steady-state conditions, and correcting for the contribution made from protein oxidation, allows for determination of fuel oxidation rates. An RQ of 0.7 indicates lipid oxidation, whereas carbohydrate oxidation yields an RQ of 1.0, with intermediate levels found when a mixture of these two fuels is being oxidized.[15]

In the postabsorptive state, the RQ of muscle is close to 0.7, suggesting that resting muscle utilizes primarily lipid as an energy source. The pattern of fuel consumption during exercise depends on the duration, type, and intensity of exercise as well as on the subject's level of physical training.

During the earliest phases of exercise, muscle glycogen is the major fuel consumed. Within 10 to 40 minutes, circulating glucose becomes of greater importance, with a capacity for muscle glucose uptake during exercise of 7 to 20 times the basal extraction rate. The relative contribution to energy expenditure from glucose peaks between 90 and 180 minutes of exercise and then declines slightly, while free fatty acid (FFA) utilization continues to increase during prolonged exercise. Thus, the relative contribution of FFA to total oxygen consumption is approximately 37 per cent after 40 minutes of cycle exercise at 30 per cent of maximal oxygen consumption ($\dot{V}O_2$ max), but increases to 50 per cent and 62 per cent of total energy expenditure after 3 and 4 hours of exercise, respectively.[16] The importance of FFA oxidation to total energy expenditure is thus seen to increase with the duration of exercise at least at relatively low workloads (30 per cent $\dot{V}O_2$ max).

In addition to duration of exercise, the intensity of exercise is also an important determinant of fuel utilization. RQ measurements of 0.87, 0.90, and 0.93 have been obtained with exercise at workloads of 25, 50, and 80 per cent of $\dot{V}O_2$ max. This indicates a greater reliance on carbohydrate as an energy source at increasing relative workloads. Finally, the ability of an individual to utilize FFA during heavy work depends on the subject's level of physical fitness. In trained subjects any given workload is performed at a lower percentage of $\dot{V}O_2$ max than in untrained subjects. RQ is lower, indicating a greater utilization of lipids for oxidation. When trained and untrained subjects are compared at the same relative workload, the trained subject can exercise at a lower RQ than the untrained subject. Potential explanations for this include increases in lipoprotein lipase activity, increased mitochondrial oxidative capacity, and FFA-mediated increase in citrate concentration with inhibition of phosphofructokinase,[17] all favoring increased lipid oxidation and a relative decrease in carbohydrate oxidation.

In normal subjects, blood glucose levels vary little during exercise, despite up to a 20-fold increase in glucose uptake in exercising muscle. During moderate exercise, the precise regulation of hepatic glucose production to meet the needs of exercising muscle is responsible for the maintenance of euglycemia. With more severe exercise, blood glucose may increase 20 to 30 mg/dl. In contrast, exercise that continues 90 minutes or longer causes a decrease of 10 to 40 mg/dl. Genuine hypoglycemia (blood glucose <40 mg/dl) is rare, but has been observed in marathon runners, in patients on low-carbohydrate diets, and in insulin-treated diabetic patients.[16]

The hormonal milieu responsible for this enhanced hepatic delivery of glucose consists of adrenergic inhibition of insulin release, increased plasma glucagon levels, and, possibly, the local release of norepinephrine from sympathetic nerves. Epinephrine levels increase only in response to high-intensity exercise or declining blood glucose levels. Although plasma cortisol and growth hormone levels increase late in exercise, the significance of these alterations is uncertain.

The hormonal changes during exercise also promote lipolysis and free fatty acid delivery to exercising muscle. The advantage of using lipid as an energy source is apparent when one considers the body energy stores available. In a 70-kg subject, fat stores may average 14 kg, with a potential energy yield of 120,000 kcal. The energy available from carbohydrate is less than 2000 kcal, with less than 1600 kcal supplied by muscle and 400 kcal by liver glycogen. Since the central nervous system requires a constant delivery of blood glucose, sparing of carbohydrate stores would be advantageous in long-term exercise. Total body protein has a caloric value of 30,000 to 40,000 kcal, although this is of limited usefulness as an energy source because it subserves either a structural or a functional role in muscle and visceral tissues, and protein losses of 20 per cent or greater are associated with marked debility or death.

EFFECTS OF PHYSICAL TRAINING ON BODY COMPOSITION, AEROBIC CAPACITY, AND PROTEIN TURNOVER

Because of wide variations in lean body mass in subjects of the same height, the use of standard tables for estimating "ideal body weight" may be misleading, and should preferably be replaced with some measurement of body composition. Although several methods are quite accurate, including measurements of body density by underwater weighing, of total body potassium with ^{40}K, and of total body electrical conductivity, these are usually available only in a research setting. The use of skinfold calipers for estimating body fat has become a practical method for widespread use. In order to optimize the accuracy of skinfold measurements, they should be peformed by someone skilled in the technique using an instrument such as the Lange calipers. Accuracy of body fat estimations can be increased by taking measurements from multiple sites, such as the triceps, subscapular, biceps, pectoral, and suprailiac regions.[18] Ranges of percentage of body fat considered normal are 10 to 20 per cent for men, and 12 to 25 per cent for women. Fat as a percentage of body weight in highly trained subjects ranges from 5 to 10 per cent in men and 7 to 10 per cent in women.

Several studies have examined the effects of differing types of physical training on body composition and on $\dot{V}O_2$ max. Gettman[19] compared the effects of circuit weight training (CWT) with the effects of a running program over a 20-week period. Weight training was designed as a "circuit" in which moderate amounts of weight were lifted with several repetitions and minimum rest periods between stations, in the expectation of stimulating cardiorespiratory fitness. CWT resulted in a greater increase in muscle strength and in lean body mass, whereas the cardiorespiratory response to such training ($\dot{V}O_2$ max) increased only in proportion to the increase in lean body mass. In contrast, the running program produced smaller increases in lean body mass but significantly increased $\dot{V}O_2$ max. This and other studies suggest that weight training programs are most effective if the goal is to increase lean body mass and muscle strength. However, if the aim of the exercise training program is to increase aerobic capacity and cardiovascular fitness, then endurance training with activities such as running, swimming, and cycling is preferable.

Physical training increases the ability of skeletal muscle to oxidize glucose, long-chain fatty acids, and ketone bodies. Increases in mitochondrial protein are due to increases in both the size and number of mitochondria. Training has resulted in significant increases in tricarboxylic acid enzymes such as citrate synthase, NAD-specific isocitrate dehydrogenase, and succinate dehydrogenase. In addition, muscles of trained individuals produce less lactate during exercise, which may help to delay fatigue during brief, strenuous exercise. Decreased lactate production in trained subjects is due both to a greater reliance on FFA as an oxidative fuel and to an increased capacity for pyruvate removal through conversion to alanine via the alanine transaminase reaction.[17]

Several studies have examined the adaptations to physical training in different types of muscle fiber. White fibers (with lower respiratory capacity and hexokinase activity, and the highest glycogenolytic capacity) undergo the smallest increases in respiratory capacity and hexokinase activity with little or no changes in glycolytic activity. Fast-twitch red fibers, which have the highest respiratory capacity and hexokinase activity, undergo the largest absolute increase in oxidative capacity and hexokinase activity after endurance training. Although training may increase respiratory enzymes sufficiently in certain white fibers to give them a red appearance on staining, normal endurance exercise does not appear to result in interconversion of fiber types.[20]

Endurance exercise training produces an adaptive increase in maximum cardiac output. However, maximum blood flow to the working muscles, expressed as milliliters per gram of muscle per minute, is not increased in the trained state. Physical training results in an enhanced ability to extract oxygen, which is reflected in a greater arteriovenous O_2 difference. Skeletal muscles' increased content of mitochondria and myoglobin, rather than improved O_2 delivery, is responsible for the trained individual's lower lactate levels and lower RQ during submaximal exercise. In contrast to skeletal muscle, heart muscle does not undergo an adaptive increase in respiratory capacity in response to endurance exercise. However, physical training does result in cardiac muscle hypertrophy, enhanced myocardial contractility, and increased resistance to hypoxia. On the average, an increase in maximum cardiac output appears to account for approximately 50 per cent of the rise in $\dot{V}O_2$ max that occurs in response to training. The other 50 per cent of the increase is accounted for by increased extraction of O_2 by the working muscles, as reflected in an increased arteriovenous O_2 difference.

One of the more prevalent beliefs in the field of

physical training, especially among bodybuilders, is that excess quantities of dietary protein are needed to meet the additional requirements of exercise and for increases in lean body mass. The average American diet supplies 80 to 110 g of protein per day, which is more than adequate to meet the RDA of 0.8 g protein/kg body weight for adults (1.5 g/kg in adolescents). Although many authors feel this requirement is not increased in subjects undergoing physical training, this opinion is not uniform[21] and the area is in need of further research.

Traditionally, it has been stated that muscle mass could be increased by isometric exercise but not by increases in dietary protein. However, one study[22] reported that increasing dietary protein from 1.4 to 2.8 g/kg/day in young adults undergoing intensive training did result in greater increments in lean body weight over a 40-day period. Notably, the additional dietary protein did not enhance endurance work performance, and the authors concluded that 100 g of protein was an adequate daily intake for men performing heavy work.

Potential sources of increased protein losses during exercise include urinary and fecal elimination and sweat. There is no evidence for any increase in urinary or fecal nitrogen losses due to exercise, but sweat losses may increase from nonexercising levels of 2 g protein/day to an additional 7 to 8 g during 4 hours of strenuous exercise.[23] The additional protein needs necessitated by even this heavy degree of physical activity should be met by the typical American diet.

New insights into the effects of exercise on protein metabolism have been provided by the use of tracer infusions of [14]C- and ^{15}N-labeled amino acids to determine rates of whole-body protein turnover. Under steady-state conditions, nitrogen balance is the result of equal rates of protein synthesis and breakdown. When excess dietary protein is administered, protein oxidation, but not protein synthesis, is increased.[24] However, a different result is obtained when dietary protein is inadequate. Subjects given a low-energy diet containing protein were able to maintain their protein synthetic rate at control levels, whereas on a protein-free diet the synthetic rate fell by 40 per cent within 48 hours, with a smaller decrease in protein breakdown rate. Thus, it appears that adequate protein is needed to maintain a normal protein synthesis rate. However, giving increased amounts of protein will not increase the rate of protein synthesis but will merely result in increased protein oxidation.

Physical activity has been shown to produce favorable effects on protein metabolism. Children have a more rapid recovery from malnutrition when they are given a program of physical exercise to accompany the refeeding.[25] Conversely, immobilizing subjects up to the neck in plaster of Paris caused a fall in the rate of whole-body protein synthesis.[26] This provides a rationale for the use of physio-

therapy in the prevention of muscle wastage in the chronically ill, hospitalized patient.

Because of the ability of continuous muscular work to increase the rate of whole-body protein synthesis, attempts have been made to minimize the losses of lean body mass through an exercise program in obese subjects maintained on a hypocaloric diet. Warwick[27] found that adding a regimen of cycle exercise to an 800 kcal/day weight-reducing diet had no effect on either the rate of weight loss or cumulative nitrogen balance during the 3- to 4-week study period. Recently, Bogardus[28] reported similar findings in obese subjects on a mixed hypocaloric diet, in whom exercise training was able to improve VO_2 max but had no additive effect on the body compositional changes induced by the diet.

The effect of repeated, long-term exercise to favor protein anabolism, at least in subjects on unrestricted diets, is in contrast to the acute effects of exercise on protein and amino acid metabolism. Rennie[29] has shown that exercise acutely causes a substantial rise in amino acid catabolism, which is associated with a decrease in whole-body protein synthesis and a rise in protein breakdown. The large increases in protein catabolism are probably confined to the period of exercise. During exercise, there is an increased muscle uptake of branched-chain amino acids (BCAA's) associated with an increased output from the splanchnic bed, implying an increased rate of oxidation of BCAA's in the active muscle. In addition, there is an increase in muscle alanine output with enhanced hepatic uptake of this amino acid. Alanine can be considered a vehicle for nitrogen transport to the liver from muscle, where it can donate its nitrogen to urea. Alanine also serves as a gluconeogenic precursor, which takes on increased significance with prolonged exercise, since gluconeogenesis plays a progressively greater role in hepatic glucose production as glycogen stores become depleted. Thus, there is an increased rate of protein oxidation and urea formation and excretion induced by acute exercise; this effect, along with reduced plasma amino acid concentrations, is similar to the changes observed during prolonged starvation. It is noteworthy that the protein catabolism induced by acute exercise may be increased by prior feeding of a low-carbohydrate diet. Under these conditions of reduced carbohydrate availability, hepatic and muscle glycogen stores are reduced and amino acids, as well as FFA, are substituted as oxidative fuels in the presence of reduced carbohydrate availability.

Following acute exercise, a positive whole-body nitrogen balance is re-established by an increase in protein synthesis that exceeds degradation.[29] It appears that, despite the protein catabolic effects of acute exercise, sustained physical exercise over the long term has an anabolic effect on muscle protein. This does not appear to require additional dietary protein, except possibly in the early stages of a training program, when muscle bulk is increasing.

EFFECTS OF NUTRITION OF PHYSICAL PERFORMANCE

Antecedent Diet

Christensen and Hansen[30] were the first to show that antecedent diet has a major effect on work performance. They found that men maintained on a high-carbohydrate diet for 3 days could perform heavy work for more than twice as long as men on a high-fat diet for the same time period. Since the work of Bergstrom, Hultman, and others[31,32] in the 1960's, it has been known that muscle glycogen depletion correlates with exhaustion in prolonged, high-intensity exercise (greater than 70 per cent $\dot{V}O_2$ max). During this intensity of exercise, carbohydrate oxidation provides the major source of energy, and endurance has been shown to correlate with the initial muscle glycogen content. Although lipid can substitute for carbohydrate as an oxidative fuel during prolonged excercise at low intensities (less than 50 per cent $\dot{V}O_2$ max), carbohydrate continues to play an important role at higher work intensities. Since the rate of glycogen consumption is related to the carbohydrate oxidation rate, the importance of muscle glycogen content at the beginning of an endurance event is of obvious importance.

In general, muscle glycogen synthesis is proportional to the amount of carbohydrate in the diet. The muscle glycogen varied from 0.6 to 4.7 g/100 g muscle in subjects refed a carbohydrate-restricted or carbohydrate-rich diet following exercise.[32] The observation that refeeding a high-carbohydrate diet following exhaustive exercise could result in very high concentrations of muscle glycogen led to the regimen of "carbohydrate loading," as originally described by Ahlborg. To "supercompensate" muscle glycogen prior to an endurance event requires the depletion of glycogen with an exhaustive bout of exercise, resulting in maximal stimulation of glycogen synthase activity. Some athletes prefer to maintain low muscle glycogen concentrations, and maximal glycogen synthase activation, by consuming a low-carbohydrate (100 g) diet for a 3-day period beginning 6 days prior to an endurance event. Then, for the 3 days immediately preceding the event, a high-protein, low-fat, and high-carbohydrate (250 to 525 g) diet is consumed to produce supernormal muscle glycogen concentrations. More recent studies suggest that the 3-day low-carbohydrate phase of this regimen is not necessary. Restricting exercise during the final 3 days before the event also helps to prevent further glycogen depletion. Muscle glycogen levels of approximately two times normal can be achieved using this technique. Several studies, including one examining endurance performance during a 30-km running race[33] and another during high-intensity cycle exercise,[32] have demonstrated the ability of the "carbohydrate loading" technique to improve performance.

Although carbohydrate loading may enhance performance in prolonged, high-intensity exercise, it is of no benefit and may actually be deleterious for certain types of physical performance. Since muscle glycogen content is a limiting factor only in prolonged exercise, short-term (less than 30 to 60 minutes) exercise performance will not be improved by this technique. Additionally, carbohydrate oxidation assumes greater importance with increasing workloads, especially over 70 per cent $\dot{V}O_2$ max. Physical exercise at below 50 per cent $\dot{V}O_2$ max can utilize lipid as the primary substrate, and will rarely be limited by muscle glycogen depletion. Those events most likely to be dependent on the size of the muscle glycogen stores include distance running, cross-country skiing, cycle racing, and possibly some team sports such as ice hockey and soccer.

Some adverse side effects of carbohydrate loading include feelings of heaviness and stiffness in the exercised muscle, probably due to binding of water to glycogen when the latter is stored in skeletal musculature.[34] Less common but potentially more serious has been the report of temporary chest pain, EKG changes, and arrhythmias associated with the technique. Carbohydrate loading should therefore probably be avoided in subjects with cardiovascular disease, diabetes mellitus, or hypertriglyceridemia.

Feeding before and during Exercise

Usually, subjects undergoing physical exercise programs are advised to eat a light meal approximately 3 to 4 hours prior to vigorous exercise, in order to prevent a decrease in liver glycogen such as might occur with more prolonged fasting. Muscle lacks the enzyme glucose-6-phosphatase, and cannot serve as a source of plasma glucose. Hepatic glucose production, largely from glycogenolysis, therefore plays a key role in the euglycemia during prolonged exercise.

Several studies have examined the ability of glucose feeding, either in the immediate pre-exercise period or during exercise, to enhance exercise performance. It might be expected that increasing the availability of glucose by ingestion during exercise would slow the depletion of muscle glycogen, and thereby delay exhaustion. Although early studies[35] did show that a glucose infusion slowed muscle glycogen depletion during cycle exercise, these studies were done at exercise intensities below 50 per cent $\dot{V}O_2$ max, where glucose oxidation does not play a critical role in overall fuel utilization.

More recently, glucose ingestion during high-intensity (74 per cent $\dot{V}O_2$ max) cycle exercise has been found to prevent any decrease in plasma glucose concentration during exercise, and to improve endurance times in 7 out of 10 subjects.[36] This is in contrast to a study by Felig,[37] who reported that, although glucose ingestion during exercise could prevent the fall in plasma glucose that occurred with placebo ingestion, there was no significant improvement in endurance times. Part of the difference between these two studies may be the lower exercise intensity (60 to 65 per cent $\dot{V}O_2$ max) of the latter study.

In contrast to the potentially beneficial effects of glucose ingestion during exercise, recent studies have demonstrated a worsening of endurance performance[38] and more rapid glycogen consumption[39] if a glucose polymer is ingested 30 minutes before high-intensity cycle exercise. It has been postulated that pre-exercise glucose ingestion may result in initial elevations of plasma glucose and insulin concentrations at the onset of exercise, with resultant inhibition of lipolysis. The decreased availability of FFA's was then postulated to result in increased consumption of muscle glycogen during exercise. More recently, we[39a] and others[38] have found that pre-exercise snack feedings, containing both carbohydrate and fat, result in no impairment in endurance performance.

Part of the increased endurance capacity found in physically trained subjects is due to an enhanced capacity for fatty acid oxidation. Techniques that elevate plasma FFA levels, such as the administration of a fatty meal combined with heparin to induce lipolysis, have resulted in decreased muscle glycogen consumption and improved endurance performance.[39] Caffeine ingestion (330 mg, or approximately 2.5 cups of coffee) has resulted in 50 to 100 per cent increases in plasma FFA levels, along with significant improvements in endurance during cycle exercise.[40] Since the latter subjects also reported decreased subjective feelings of exertion after caffeine ingestion, it is possible that CNS stimulation due to caffeine was partly responsible for the enhanced endurance capacity.

Fluids

Because the mechanical efficiency of cycle exercise and running is only about 25 to 30 per cent, 70 to 75 per cent of the energy expenditure is converted into heat. This is of major importance during prolonged exercise, where as much as 1.5 to 2 L of fluid may be lost through sweat. Although water and electrolytes come primarily from the extracellular space, the losses are made up from intracellular water to maintain the plasma volume. The result may be intracellular dehydration, which can impair work ability, and increase body temperature and pulse rate. Since thirst may not be a reliable indicator of fluid losses during intense exercise, a weigh-in before and after heavy exercise may be very helpful for determining fluid losses. Sweat becomes progressively more hypotonic as exercise is prolonged, so that the major loss (over two thirds) in sweat is free water. In addition to being well-hydrated prior to exercise, the individual can take small portions of an isotonic or hypotonic solution at frequent intervals during prolonged exercise. An additional source of fluid during exercise is the water released as glycogen is hydrolyzed, since 2 to 3 L of water may be bound when glycogen stores are filled to a maximum.[42]

The use of rapid weight programs for "making weight" in sports such as wrestling and boxing should be strongly discouraged. Rapid weight loss is usually in the form of body fluids and lean tissue, and may also result in decreased muscle glycogen concentrations. Several studies have shown that a reduction in body water equaling 1 per cent of body weight may adversely effect work ability. If fluid losses equal 4 to 5 per cent of body weight, the capacity for very hard muscular work decreases by 20 to 30 per cent.[34] In addition, sports such as wrestling that involve isometric contractions are dependent on muscle glycogen stores.

Vitamins and Minerals

Food fads incorporating increased vitamins and minerals are especially common among subjects engaged in physical training programs. Although there may be some psychological benefits to augmented intakes, there are no proven physiological benefits. Whereas the use of "megavitamin" therapy is of no benefit to the training program, clearly a vitamin-deficiency syndrome can have deleterious consequences on excercise performance. This is unlikely to occur on a balanced diet that is adequate in total calories.

Iron deficiency has been shown to impair performance owing to a decrease in the oxygen-carrying capacity of the blood.[43] There is no specific increased need for dietary iron with exercise. However, in menstruating women and adolescent boys, dietary iron may be insufficient, and periodic blood hemoglobin levels should be monitored. Recent reports of occult intestinal blood loss in marathon runners[44] suggest one possible mechanism for the anemia sometimes seen during physical training programs, in addition to the dilutional effect of increased plasma volume which is known to occur.

Thiamine requirements are proportional to the total energy intake and expenditure, increasing by 0.5 mg for each additional 1000 kcal. Similarly, the RDA for riboflavin and niacin are based on total caloric intake. One recent study[45] reported an increased requirement for riboflavin in normal-weight women after they begin participating in an exercise program. Individual riboflavin requirements ranged from 0.62 to 1.21 mg/1000 kcal before exercise training, and 0.63 to 1.4 mg/1000 kcal during the exercise periods. There is no evidence that increased intake of vitamin C or vitamin E can enhance stamina or improve muscle peformance, and excessive intakes may produce undesired side effects. Nicotinic acid taken in excess can inhibit uptake of fatty acids by cardiac muscle during exercise.

Prolonged exercise during Olympic marathon trials has been shown to raise plasma zinc and copper levels, possibly owing to tissue redistribution of these minerals.

TREATMENT OF SPECIFIC MEDICAL CONDITIONS WITH EXERCISE

Obesity

The ability of an exercise program to minimize the decrease in metabolic rate that usually accompanies a hypocaloric diet has already been discussed. In a frequently quoted study by Mayer,[46] caloric intake in exercised rats was proportional to energy expenditure over a wide range of exercise levels, although reduction of exercise to less than 1 hour per day resulted in a paradoxical increase of feeding and body weight gain. Epidemiological studies show a strong correlation between the percentage of men in sedentary occupations and the occurrence of obesity. Whether inactivity in general precedes or follows obesity, however, is not clear.

Woo[47] has shown that obese women engaging in moderate physical exercise do not compensate by an increase in caloric intake, which produces a sustained negative energy balance and weight loss.

Because exercise training is often promoted as an adjunct to diet in the treatment of obesity, several authors have examined the capacity for cycle exercise in persons on hypocaloric diets. Phinney[48] found no impairment in endurance treadmill performance at 60 per cent $\dot{V}O_2$ max after a period of adaptation to a protein-supplemented modified fast. In contrast, Bogardus[49] described a 50 per cent reduction in cycle endurance at 75 per cent $\dot{V}O_2$ max in subjects on a similar carbohydrate-restricted, ketogenic diet, with no impairment in endurance in subjects on a carbohydrate-containing, hypocaloric diet. In both studies, the low-carbohydrate, ketogenic diets resulted in reduced pre-exercise muscle glycogen concentrations. It is probable that subjects on low-carbohydrate diets will have reduced endurance capacities if they exercise at higher intensities (over 60 to 70 per cent $\dot{V}O_2$ max), at which muscle glycogen content plays an important role. In addition, endurance capacity may be more limited for types of exercise that place a greater demand on specific muscle groups (e.g., cycling) than for other forms of exercise (e.g., running or walking).

Diabetes Mellitus

Individuals with Type II, non–insulin dependent diabetes mellitus (NIDDM) are frequently obese and exhibit insulin resistance. In addition, insulin resistance is now known to be a feature of Type I, insulin-dependent diabetes (IDDM). Efforts to overcome insulin resistance have focused primarily on hypocaloric dieting in overweight subjects and on increased physical exercise. Physical training programs in NIDDM have resulted in improved insulin sensitivity and lowered plasma glucose levels and hemoglobin A_{1C} concentrations. The addition of a physical training program to a hypocaloric diet has resulted in greater improvements in insulin sensitivity than treatment with diet alone. Weight-reduction diets in obese, NIDDM subjects should be based on the energetic principles outlined above, while following the American Diabetes Association's recommendations for a diet low in saturated fat, high in carbohydrate (55 to 60 per cent of total calories), and high in dietary fiber.

In contrast, physical training has not resulted in improved diabetic control, assessed by mean plasma glucose or hemoglobin A_{1C} concentrations, in IDDM subjects. Optimal insulin replacement is of primary importance in insulin-deficient diabetics, although regular exercise may provide numerous other benefits to these individuals also. Potential benefits of physical exercise programs include lowered systolic blood pressure; lower LDL and VLDL, and increased HDL, cholesterol levels; improved cardiovascular fitness; and increased sense of well-being. However, IDDM subjects are at risk of exercise-associated hypoglycemia, and poorly controlled subjects may develop increased ketosis and hyperglycemia if they exercise. Because of these special risks of exercise in insulin-deficient diabetics, and the finding by several authors that diabetic control is not improved after training, most diabetologists would not consider exercise to be a necessary part of the therapeutic regimen in IDDM subjects, particularly in those individuals who have diabetic complications such as proliferatve retinopathy, nephropathy, or neuropathy that may be worsened by strenuous exercise. Rather, exercise and meal plans should be devised to allow insulin-deficient diabetics who wish to exercise to do so safely.

Cardiovascular Conditions

Several other medical conditions may be improved by a regular physical exercise program. As mentioned above, hypertension and hyperlipoproteinemias may be significantly improved by exercise. Reduction of cardiovascular risk factors by frequent exercise is expected to have a major influence on the prevalence of cardiovascular disease in the general population. Exercise is also finding a major role in cardiac rehabilitation programs, although these subjects are beyond the scope of this chapter.

References

1. Horton ES. Introduction: an overview of the assessment and regulation of energy balance in humans. Am J Clin Nutr 1983; 38:972–977.
2. Brozek J, Grande F, Taylor HL, et al. Changes in body weight and body dimensions in men performing work on a low calorie carbohydrate diet. J Appl Physiol 1957; 10:412–420.
3. Danforth E. The role of thyroid hormones and insulin in the regulation of energy metabolism. Am J Clin Nutr 1983; 38:1006–1017.
4. Landsberg L, Young JB. The role of the sympathetic nervous system and catecholamines in the regulation of energy metabolism. Am J Clin Nutr 1983; 38:1018–1024.
5. Apfelbaum M, Brigant L, Joliff M. Effects of severe diet restriction on the oxygen consumption of obese women during exercise. Internat J Obesity 1977; 1:387–393.
6. Stern JS, Schultz C, Mole P, et al. Effect of caloric restriction and exercise on basal metabolism and thyroid hormone. Nutr Metab 1980; 1:361.
7. Edwards HT, Thorndike A, Dill DB. The energy requirement in strenuous muscular exercise. N Engl J Med 1935; 213:532–535.
8. Gaesser GA, Brooks GA. Metabolic bases of excess post-exercise oxygen consumption: a review. Med Sci Sports Exerc 1984; 16:29–43.
9. Devlin JT, Horton ES. Potentiation of the thermic effect of insulin by exercise: differences between lean, obese, and non–insulin-dependent diabetic men. Am J Clin Nutr 1986; 43:884–890.
10. Miller S, Mumford P, Stock MJ. Gluttony. 2. Thermogenesis in overeating man. Am J Clin Nutr 1967; 20:1223–1229.
11. Bray GA, Whipp BJ, Koyal SN. The acute effects of food intake on energy expenditure during cycle ergometry. Am J Clin Nutr 1974; 27:254–259.
12. Segal KR, Gutin B. Thermic effects of food and exercise in lean and obese women. Metabolism 1983; 32:581–589.
13. Schneider EC, Foster AO. The influence of physical training on the basal metabolic rate of man. Am J Physiol 1931; 98:595–601.
14. Terjung RL, Tipton CM. Exercise training and resting oxygen consumption. Int Z angew Physiol 1970; 28:262–272.
15. Lusk G. Animal calorimetry: analysis of the oxidation of mixtures of carbohydrate and fat. J Biol Chem 1924; 59:41–42.
16. Felig P, Wahren J. Fuel homeostasis in exercise. N Engl J Med 1975; 293:1078–1084.
17. Holloszy JO, Booth FW. Biochemical adaptations to endurance exercise in muscle. Ann Rev Physiol 1976; 38:273–291.
18. Durnin JVGA, Womersley J. Body fat assessed from total body density and its estimation for skinfold thickness: measurements on 481 men and women aged from 16 to 72 years. Br J Nutr 1974; 32:77.
19. Gettman LR, Ayres JJ, Pollock ML, et al. The effect of circuit weight training on strength, cardiorespiratory function, and body composition of adult men. Med Sci Sports 1978; 10:171–176.
20. Gollnick PD, Armstrong RB, Saltin B, et al. Effect of training on enzyme activity and fiber composition of human skeletal muscle. J Appl Physiol 1973; 34:107–111.
21. Young VR, Torun B. Physical activity: impact on protein and amino acid metabolism and implications for nutritional requirements. In XIIth International Congress of Nutrition. New York, Alan R. Liss, 1981.
22. Consolazio CF, Johnson HJ, Nelson RA, et al. Protein metabolism during intensive physical training in the young adult. Am J Clin Nutr 1975; 28:29–35.
23. Lemon PWR, Mullin JP. Effect of initial muscle glycogen levels on protein catabolism during exercise. J Appl Physiol 1980; 48:624–629.
24. Waterlow JC, Jackson AA. Nutrition and protein turnover in man. Br Med Bull 1981; 37:5–10.
25. Torun B, Schutz Y, Viteri F, et al. Growth, body composition and heart rate/$\dot{V}o_2$ relationship changes during the nutritional recovery of children with two different physical activity levels. Bibl Nutr Dieta 1979; 27:55–56.
26. Schonheyder F, Heilskov NSC, Olesen K. Isotopic studies on the mechanism of the negative nitrogen balance produced by immobilization. Scand J Clin Lab Invest 1954; 6:178–188.
27. Warwick M, Garrow JS. The effect of addition of exercise to a regime of dietary restriction on weight loss, nitrogen balance, resting metabolic rate and spontaneous physical activity in three obese women in a metabolic ward. Int J Obesity 1981; 5:25–32.
28. Bogardus C, Ravussin E, Robbins DC, et al. Effects of physical training and diet therapy on carbohydrate metabolism in patients with glucose intolerance and non–insulin-dependent diabetes mellitus. Diabetes 1984; 33:311–318.
29. Rennie MJ, Edwards RHT, Krywawych S, et al. Effect of exercise on protein turnover in man. Clin Sci 1981; 61:627–639.
30. Christensen E, Hansen O. Arbeitsfähigkeit und Ernährung. Scand Arch Physiol 1939; 81:160–171.
31. Ahlborg B, Bergstrom J, Ekelund L-G, et al. Muscle glycogen and muscle electrolytes during prolonged physical exercise. Acta Physiol Scand 1967; 70:129–142.
32. Bergstrom J, Hermansen L, Hultman E, et al. Diet, muscle glycogen and physical performance. Acta Physiol Scand 1967; 71:140–150.
33. Karlsson J, Saltin B. Diet, muscle glycogen, and endurance performance. J Appl Physiol 1971; 31:203–206.
34. Olsson K-E, Saltin B. Variations in total body water with muscle glycogen changes in man. Acta Physiol Scand 1970; 80:11–18.
35. Bergstrom J, Hultman E. A study of the glycogen metabolism during exercise in man. Scand J Clin Lab Invest 1967; 19:218–228.
36. Coyle EF, Hagberg JM, Hurley BF, et al. Carbohydrate feeding during prolonged strenuous exercise can delay fatigue. J Appl Physiol 1983; 55:230–235.
37. Felig P, Cherif A, Minagawa A, et al. Hypoglycemia during prolonged exercise in normal men. N Engl J Med 1982; 306:895–900.
38. Foster C, Costill DL, Fink WJ. Effects of preexercise feedings on endurance performance. Med Sci Sports 1979; 11:1–5.
39. Costill DL, Coyle E, Dalsky G, et al. Effects of elevated plasma FFA and insulin on muscle glycogen usage during exercise. J Appl Physiol 1977; 43:695–699.
39a. Devlin JT, Calles-Escandon J, Horton ES. Effects of preexercise snack feeding on endurance cycle exercise. J Appl Physiol 1986; 60:980–985.
40. Ivy JL, Costill DL, Fink WJ, et al. Influence of caffeine and carbohydrate feedings on endurance performance. Med Sci Sports 1979; 11:6–11.
41. Whipp BJ, Wasserman K. Efficiency of muscular work. Am J Physiol 1969; 26:644–648.
42. Saltin B. Aerobic work capacity and circulation of exercise in man. Acta Physiol Scand 1964; 62(Suppl 230):1–52.
43. Gardner GW, Edgerton VR, Senewiratne B, et al. Physical work capacity and metabolic stress in subjects with iron deficiency anemia. Am J Clin Nutr 1977; 30:910–917.
44. Stewart JG, Ahlquist DA, McGill DB, et al. Gastrointestinal blood loss and anemia in runners. Ann Intern Med 1984; 100:843–845.
45. Belko AZ, Obarzanek E, Kalkwarf HJ, et al. Effects of exercise on riboflavin requirements of young women. Am J Clin Nutr 1983; 37:509–517.
46. Mayer J, Marshall NB, Vitale JJ, et al. Exercise, food intake and body weight in normal rats and genetically obese adult mice. Am J Physiol 1954; 177:544–548.
47. Woo R, Garrow JS, Pi-Sunyer FX. Voluntary food intake during prolonged exercise in obese women. Am J Clin Nutr 1982; 36:478–484.
48. Phinney SD, Horton ES, Sims EAH, et al. Capacity for moderate exercise in obese subjects after adaptation to a hypocaloric, ketogenic diet. J Clin Invest 1980; 66:1152–1161.
49. Bogardus C, LaGrange BM, Horton ES, et al. Comparison of carbohydrate-containing and carbohydrate-restricted hypocaloric diets in the treatment of obesity. J Clin Invest 1981; 68:399–404.

ROLE OF NUTRITION IN SPECIFIC DISORDERS

12

PEPTIC ULCER

M.B. DESAI / K.N. JEEJEEBHOY

A circumscribed loss of mucosa adjacent to an acid-secreting area of the stomach is called a peptic ulcer. It usually occurs in non–acid secreting areas of gastric mucosa, in the esophagus and duodenum, and in the small intestine when anastomosed to stomach. The two opposing factors involved in the process of ulcerogenesis are acid peptic secretion, which is injurious to the mucosa, and protective factors such as mucus and glycoprotein secretion, collectively called the gastric mucosal barrier. Though the precise role of each factor is not defined, an imbalance between the two causes an ulcer. Higher acid output than normal,[1] increased secretory drive in the nonstimulated state,[2] rapid gastric emptying uninhibited by acid,[3] and reduced duodenal pH may be associated with the formation of a duodenal ulcer. In contrast, patients with gastric ulcer have normal or low acid output[4] plus factors decreasing mucosal defense, such as bile salt–induced mucosal injury,[5] aspirin ingestion,[6] and altered mucosal blood flow.[7]

Whatever the cause, it is now known that reducing acid secretion with the new H_2-blockers heals the ulcer in most patients.

DIET AND EATING HABITS IN ULCEROGENESIS

There is little scientific evidence to support the belief that diet contributes to peptic ulcer disease. However, there are some interesting observations. Duodenal ulcer is less common in North India, where wheat is the main staple of the diet, contrasted with rice-eating South India.[8] In a randomized trial the recurrence rate of ulcer was significantly lower in subjects given wheat than in those given their usual rice diets.[9] The difference is attributed to the need for secreting more saliva in order to chew wheat; the same author found increased ulcer formation with a liquid diet.[10] Furthermore, Gregory[11] has shown that saliva has an epidermal growth factor, urogastrone,[12] which inhibits acid secretion and enhances healing of experimental ulcers.[13] Finally, fiber in wheat may play a role, since a high-fiber diet may also protect against gastric ulceration.[14]

Beverage intake may influence ulcerogenesis. Coffee is a strong stimulant of acid secretion[15] quite apart from its caffeine content. It also aggravates or induces nonspecific symptoms of abdominal discomfort.[16] Furthermore, a higher incidence of peptic ulcer is noted with increased consumption of coffee.[17] Though no evidence is available to show that other caffeine-containing beverages (colas, Tab, etc.) induce peptic ulcer, they certainly increase acid secretion.[18]

The role of alcohol in ulcerogenesis is uncertain, and although patients in whom ulcers healed using placebos were less likely to take alcohol,[19] alcohol ingestion per se has not been shown to increase the incidence of peptic ulceration.[20] In contrast, there is a strong relationship between cigarette smoking and ulcerogenesis. Cigarette smoking is associated with increased risk of duodenal and gastric ulceration, reduced ulcer healing and increased relapse after treatment.[21,22]

DIET THERAPY OF PEPTIC ULCER DISEASE

Despite the evidence that strict diet has probably very little effect on the healing of peptic ulcers, Isenberg[22] found that about 77 per cent of hospitals

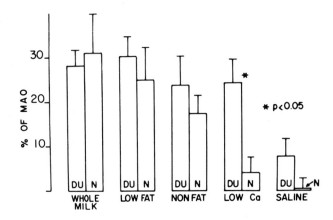

FIGURE 12–2. *Increase in acid output in response to ingestion of whole, low-fat, nonfat, and low-calcium milk and 0.15 molar NaCl in patients with duodenal ulcer (DU) and normal subjects (N). Increase above basal level of acid output expressed as percentage of maximal acid output (MAO) produced in response to administration of betazole or pentagastrin. Vertical bars represent 1 standard error of the mean. (From Ippoliti AF, Maxwell V, Isenberg JI. Ann Intern Med 1976; 84:286–289. Reproduced with permission.)*

surveyed in the United States still prescribe "peptic ulcer diets."

Historically, diets have been used for years for the treatment of peptic ulcer. Celsus in the first century prescribed smooth diets, and later practitioners wrote about the special healing properties of milk.[23] Sippy in 1915 advocated a rigidly outlined program of milk, cream, and soft foods.[24] Even today soft bland diets are advocated[25] without scientific proof of efficacy.

To understand why a diet cannot aid the healing of peptic ulcer, it is useful to observe the effects of a mixed meal on gastric secretion and duodenal pH. With each meal, the buffer effect of the meal raises the pH for about an hour.[26] A meal alone has only a little or a very brief effect in raising the pH above 3.[27] However, mixing antacids with a meal is of value. Intragastric pH is raised more when antacids are taken 1 to 3 hours after a meal than when taken hourly on an empty stomach[28] (Fig. 12–1). Milk, after a transient buffering action for 20 minutes,[29] increases the secretion of acid to a greater extent than it can buffer because of milk's calcium content[30] (Fig. 12–2). Thus clinical trials of peptic ulcer diets have failed to show an effect on peptic ulcer healing,[31–33] but use of antacids 1 and 3 hours after meals has promoted ulcer healing. However, the use of antacids in such quantity is difficult for the patient and may cause diarrhea.

In short, there is no rationale for a specific diet in uncomplicated peptic ulcer disease. Raising the intragastric pH with H_2-blockers and avoidance of ag-

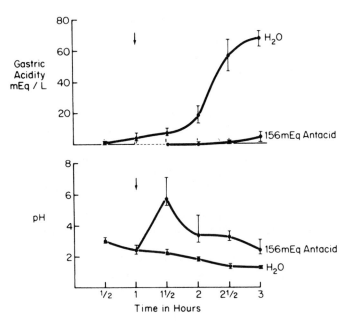

FIGURE 12–1. *Effect of ingestion of 156 mEq of antacid or 60 ml of water on changes in gastric acidity, as measured in mEq/L and pH, in response to a meal. Arrows indicate time of ingestion of antacid or water. Results are means ± 1 standard error in 7 patients with duodenal ulcer. (From Fordtran JS, Morawski SG, Richardson CT. N Engl J Med 1973; 288:923–928. Reproduced with permission.)*

gravating factors such as smoking result in rapid healing of the ulcer, and such a regimen is convenient and of proven efficacy. Additionally, avoidance of smoking, coffee, and other caffeine-containing beverages may prevent abdominal discomfort because of acid reflux.

NUTRITION IN PATIENTS WITH COMPLICATIONS DUE TO PEPTIC ULCER

Since two of the complications, hemorrhage and perforation, are emergencies, and penetration and obstruction affect the ability to eat, all four complications of peptic ulcer create problems in maintaining the nutrition of the patient.

Hemorrhage. During acute hemorrhage, the patient is monitored through nasogastric suction, so feeding is impossible. However, patients who have had mild bleeding that has ceased need not be starved. Feeding should be started immediately. Meulengracht[34] showed that early feeding was beneficial to patients with hemorrhage. Once the bleeding has stopped, the patient should be refed as quickly as possible, to replace the protein and iron that have been lost. In addition, iron supplementation may be necessary, especially if there was a prior deficiency. Patients who are operated upon for hemorrhage do not automatically need parenteral nutrition. In the event of postoperative complications preventing oral feeding for more than a week, parenteral nutrition should be begun. In this situation, it is better to give nutritional support early because of the evidence that functional changes occur within 2 weeks of nutrient deprivation and precede significant weight loss.[35]

Perforation. Since this is a surgical emergency, the question of nutritional support arises only in the postoperative period. The guidelines given above are appropriate. Peritonitis may result in prolonged ileus, necessitating parenteral nutrition in the postoperative period.

Gastric Outlet Obstruction. Early satiety and vomiting, both caused by the obstruction, reduce the intake of food and prevent its entering the small bowel. The only way to treat this problem is to correct the obstruction surgically. However, in a malnourished patient not suitable for surgery, preoperative nutritional support may have to be considered. Again, there are no controlled trials to prove or disprove the benefits of preoperative preparation. Nevertheless, the following are practical guidelines.

Patients with less than 10 per cent body weight loss who are not hypoproteinemic should be prepared for surgery by correcting dehydration and potassium deficits due to vomiting and by correction of any anemia.

In patients with more than 10 per cent weight loss, preoperative nutritional support is advisable. Initially it is necessary to evacuate retained gastric contents by stomach lavage through an Ewald tube. After that, a liquid diet should be started orally or by continuous intragastric infusion. The latter permits greater intake of calories, since the uniform rate of infusion into the stomach makes inflow equal outflow and avoids gastric distention.

In those with complete pyloric obstruction, or those with severe vomiting, a period of TPN is advisable to improve the nutritional status of the patient while giving time for edema in the obstructed stomach to subside.

NUTRITION AND SURGERY FOR PEPTIC ULCER

An operation for peptic ulcer may alter the anatomical configuration and physiological functions of the stomach, thus affecting the ability to eat.

The stomach serves the following functions:

1. *Reservoir.* The stomach can hold up to 1 liter of contents, and it relaxes receptively to receive a meal.[36]

2. *Trituration of food.* The antrum grinds food into small particles, and only those smaller than 2 mm are released into the duodenum.[37] It has been shown in animals that digestion proceeds much more rapidly when ingested liver is reduced to particles below 1 mm.[37]

3. *Controlled release of ingested food.* Gastric contents are made iso-osmotic before they enter the duodenum. Complex interactions between pressures and resistance control gastric emptying.[38]

4. *Digestion of protein.* Protein is degraded to polypeptides by gastric acid and pepsin.

5. *Intrinsic factor and R protein.* Fundic parietal cells secrete intrinsic factor, which combines farther on with exogenous vitamin B_{12} to facilitate its absorption in the terminal ileum. Another substance called R protein also binds cobalamin—but at an acid pH, so that in the stomach R protein has more affinity for vitamin B_{12} than has intrinsic factor. Pancreatic proteases release vitamin B_{12} from R protein in the proximal small intestine. Here, at the higher intestinal pH, vitamin B_{12} binds to intrinsic factor. The ileal mucosa is then better able to absorb vitamin B_{12} from this complex. Pancreatic insufficiency can thus cause malabsorption of vitamin B_{12} because the B_{12} is not released from its complex with R protein. The major portion of vitamin B_{12} is absorbed in the terminal ileum, so that resection of this portion causes serious B_{12} malabsorption.

Clinical Effects of Gastric Surgery

Dumping. This is the commonest effect of all gastric surgical procedures that injure or bypass the pyloric mechanisms. Within 20 to 90 minutes of eating, the patient develops upper abdominal pain, distention, and possibly nausea and vomiting. Distention of the proximal jejunum probably causes these symptoms.[39] Vasomotor symptoms, which follow the abdominal symptoms, are flushing, palpitations, sweating, dizziness, and hypotension. Following the ingestion of a meal, copious diarrhea may relieve symptoms. The causes of these symptoms are multiple. Extravascular fluid depletion, as a result of the rapid influx of fluid into the jejunum, contributes to hypotension and dizziness. It is caused by the entry of hypertonic gastric contents requiring dilution. However, these symptoms are not entirely abolished by simultaneous expansion of the vascular and extracellular fluid volume by intravenous infusions.[40,41] Release of intestinal hormones is also believed to contribute to the production of these symptoms.[42]

Postoperative diarrhea may be an important symptom. It is worse after ingestion of liquids. Hypertonic liquids like soup, "pop," and syrups are likely to cause the most marked symptoms. Patients with severe symptoms may develop a functional lactase deficiency because rapid intestinal transit prevents hydrolysis of lactose.[43] The diarrhea is especially observed after ingestion of milk and milk products.

These patients also have a high output of bile acids.[44] Bile acids reaching the colon may be a factor in the pathogenesis of postvagotomy diarrhea, since bile acids stimulate peristalsis and also prevent the colon from absorbing salt and water. Diarrhea after gastric surgery may also be due to unmasking of subclinical celiac sprue[43] or to inadvertent gastroileostomy, short-circuiting the bowel.

Malabsorption. Malabsorption may be of macronutrients such as proteins, fats, and carbohydrates, or may be selective for micronutrients such as calcium, vitamin D, or vitamin B_{12}.

Macronutrients. Acid reduction has to be marked in order to influence digestion, and by itself is not the cause of malabsorption. Even when gastric secretions are impaired, pancreatic secretions can complete hydrolysis of food. On the other hand, reduced acid plus stasis in the afferent loop can cause bacterial overgrowth and a stagnant loop syndrome.[45] A gastrocolic fistula following a recurrent ulcer may also cause bacterial contamination of the upper bowel. In some cases, there may be an asynchrony between the release of food from the stomach and pancreatic secretion, resulting in functional pancreatic insufficiency.

Despite all the above possibilities, steatorrhea rarely exceeds 15 g/day unless there is pre-existing celiac sprue, short bowel, or inadvertent gastroileostomy. The fecal nitrogen output rarely exceeds 20 per cent of nitrogen intake in the postgastrectomy state without another cause.

Micronutrients. Iron deficiency is very common after gastric surgery,[46] especially in menstruating women.[47] A major cause is the lack of gastric acid, which reduces the release of iron bound to protein.[48]

Imbalance of calcium metabolism is also common after gastric surgery, and 30 per cent of such patients have osteoporosis. Although this abnormality is usually subclinical,[49,50] there is an increased tendency for bones to fracture with only moderate trauma, in patients with long-standing gastrectomy.[51] While serum vitamin B_{12} levels are low, pernicious anemia is rare[51] unless the patient has had a total gastrectomy.

Nutritional Consequences of the Postgastrectomy State

Weight Loss. After gastric resection, significant weight loss is common.[52] It is not as great following vagotomy and pyloroplasty unless dumping is severe. Total gastrectomy causes very major weight loss, often in the range of 25 to 30 per cent. This loss of weight is unlikely to be due to malabsorption alone, because that can be overcome by increasing the food intake. Nevertheless, substantial weight can be lost over a year if daily small deficits are not made up.

Nutritional Therapy of Postsurgical Patients

The dietetic treatment of early satiety and dumping is based on the fact that these symptoms are largely caused by the entry of hypertonic fluids into the upper jejunum. Thus the output of liquid gastric contents will decrease if a dry solid meal, low in simple sugars but high in complex carbohydrates and pectin,[53] is administered. Avoidance of simple sugars will reduce the tonicity of the contents leaving the stomach, since most of it will be composed of large molecular starch, peptides, dextrins, and triglycerides. Milk and milk products should be avoided because of the likelihood of a functional lactase deficiency.

A drink of a hypotonic fluid (like water or tea without sugar) about 2 hours after a dry meal is recommended. An increase in the intake of red meat should be encouraged to provide more heme iron, which is readily absorbed.

While small frequent meals are popularly recommended to patients with dumping syndrome, it should be recognized that, in the absence of major gastric resection, the main problem is jejunal distention with hypertonic fluid. Instead of advising frequent meals, therefore, separation of solids and fluids should be advised. Otherwise it becomes difficult to obtain sufficient time for one meal to leave the stomach before the next is taken. Also, the intake of fiber and complex carbohydrate should be increased. Since the output of bile salts increases after gastric surgery, causing choleretic diarrhea, administration of a bile salt–binding agent such as cholestyramine resin has been shown to be useful in such patients.

In patients who do not respond to these simple measures, associated celiac disease, pancreatic insufficiency, or abnormal small bowel anatomy should be ruled out.

Oral supplements of iron and folic acid should be given.

In the presence of significant malabsorption, treatment should be directed toward correcting celiac disease with a gluten-free diet, correcting bacterial overgrowth with antibiotics, and correcting anatomical abnormalities with reoperation.

Patients with a small gastric remnant, severe dumping malabsorption, or total gastrectomy are the most difficult to treat. Such patients, especially if they have marked weight loss (more than 25 per cent) and are unable to gain weight, need artificial nutritional support; this may take two forms, home enteral feeding or home parenteral feeding.

Home Enteral Nutrition. Although these patients have difficulty handling a liquid osmotic load, so that nasogastric feeding of a formula diet is not well tolerated, some patients tolerate a defined formula diet without diarrhea if the nutrients are given through a nasogastric tube by continuous regulated infusion using a pump. The regulation of the infusion avoids peak loading of the jejunum with hypertonic fluids and contributes to successful feeding.

Home Parenteral Nutrition. Patients with gastric resection associated with small bowel resection or pancreatic insufficiency may need home parenteral nutrition, since the combined disability causes intractable diarrhea and/or severe malabsorption.

In a few severely affected patients who survive total gastrectomy, home parenteral nutrition may be required to maintain normal body weight and to provide sufficient nutrition.

Nutritional Supplementation

Deficiencies. Iron deficiency, the commonest problem, needs the greatest attention. It can be prevented by eating red meat and by iron supplements, especially in those at risk because of additional blood loss, such as menstruating women and those previously anemic. Treatment with chelated iron is better tolerated when given at night after the patient has been lying down.[47]

Calcium intake should be especially encouraged, since these patients often have difficulty taking dairy products. Low-lactose dairy products such as hard cheese should be taken. Medium-chain triglycerides increase the absorption of calcium after gastrectomy[54] and are preferable to long-chain triglycerides.

Vitamin B_{12} should be given parenterally to all patients who have had a total gastrectomy.

Weight Loss. While this is mainly due to early satiety, it is also because dumping and diarrhea cause an aversion to eating. The treatment is to control dumping and diarrhea.

Gastric Retention. Patients who complain of early satiety, constant upper abdominal pain, and pain immediately postprandially may have a bezoar. Treatment of the bezoar consists of washing it out through a large-bore tube. Afterwards fruits and vegetables may have to be blended prior to consumption in order for some patients to avoid forming a bezoar.

When the occasional patient experiences retention despite blending of food, all fruits and vegetables should be avoided. Vitamins B and C, and especially folic acid, should be given to avoid a deficiency of these nutrients. Since hematological features of vitamin B_{12} deficiency are masked by an intake of folate, serum vitamin B_{12} levels should be checked in patients taking folic acid and the vitamin should be administered if required.

References

1. Kirkpatrick JR, Lowrie JH, Forrest APM, et al. The short pentagastrin test in the investigation of gastric disease. Gut 1969; *10*:760–762.
2. Hunt JM, Kay AW. The nature of gastric hypersecretion of acid in patients with duodenal ulcer. Br Med J 1954; *2*:1444–1446.
3. Lam SK, Isenberg JI, Grossman MI, et al: Rapid gastric emptying in duodenal ulcer patients. Dig Dis Sci 1982; *27*:598–604.
4. Grossman MI, Kirsner JB, Gillespie IE. Basal and Histalog-stimulated gastric secretion in control subjects and in patients with peptic ulcer or gastric cancer. Gastroenterology 1963; *45*:14–26.
5. Rhodes J, Barvardo DE, Phillips SF, et al. Increased reflux of bile into the stomach in patients with gastric ulcer. Gastroenterology 1969; *57*:241–252.
6. MacDonald WC. Correlation of mucosal histology and aspirin intake in chronic gastric ulcer. Gastroenterology 1973; *65*:381–389.
7. Ritchie WP Jr. Ischemia and the gastric mucosal barrier. A note of caution. Surgery 1974; *76*:363–366.
8. Pulvertaft CN. Peptic ulcer in town and country. Br J Prev Soc Med 1959; *13*:131–138.
9. Malhotra SL. A comparison of unrefined wheat and rice diets in the management of duodenal ulcer. Postgrad Med J 1978; *54*:6–9.
10. Malhotra SL. Peptic ulcer in India and its aetiology. Gut 1964; *5*:412–416.
11. Gregory H. Isolation and structure of urogastrone and its relationship to epidermal growth factor. Nature 1975; *257*:325–327.
12. Elder JB, Ganguli PC, Gillespie IE, et al. Effect of urogastrone on gastric secretion and plasma gastrin levels in normal subjects. Gut 1975; *16*:887–893.
13. Koffman CG, Berry J, Elder JB. A comparison of cimetidine and epidermal growth factor in the healing of experimental gastric ulcers. Br J Surg 1977; *64*:830–836.
14. Cleave TL. Peptic Ulcer. Bristol, John Wright, 1962.
15. Cohen S, Barth GH. Gastric acid secretion and lower esophageal sphincter pressure in response to coffee and caffeine. N Engl J Med 1975; *293*:897–899.
16. Cohen S. Pathogenesis of caffeine-induced gastrointestinal symptoms. N Engl J Med 1980; *303*:122–124.
17. Paffenbarger RS Jr, Wing AL, Hyde RT. Chronic disease in

former college students. Am J Epidemiol 1974; *100*:307–315.

18. McArthur K, Hogan D, Isenberg JI. Relative stimulatory effects of commonly ingested beverages on gastric acid secretion in humans. Gastroenterology 1982; *83*:199–203.

19. Koo J, Lam S-K. Individual prediction of ulcer recurrence after vagotomy for chronic duodenal ulcer by discriminant analysis. Gastroenterology 1983; *85*:413–419.

20. Friedman GD, Siegelaub AB, Seltzor CC. Cigarettes, alcohol, coffee and peptic ulcer. N Engl J Med 1974; *290*:469–473.

21. Sonnenberg A, Muller-Lissner SA, Vogel E, et al. Predictors of duodenal ulcer healing and relapse. Gastroenterology 1981; *81*:1061–1067.

22. Isenberg JI. Peptic ulcer: epidemiology, nutritional aspects, drugs, smoking, alcohol and diet. *In* Winick M (ed). Nutrition and Gastroenterology. New York, John Wiley & Sons, 1980: 141–151.

23. Williams SR. Nutrition and diet therapy. *In* Gastrointestinal Diseases. St. Louis, CV Mosby, 1981: 512–592.

24. Sippy BW. Gastric and duodenal ulcer: medical cure by an efficient removal of gastric juice corrosion. JAMA 1915; *64*:1625–1630.

25. Spiro HM. Is milk all that bad for the ulcer patient? (Editorial.) J Clin Gastroenterol 1981; *3*:219–220.

26. Lennard-Jones JE, Barbouris M. Effect of different foods on the acidity of the gastric contents in patients with duodenal ulcer. Gut 1965; *6*:113–117.

27. Peterson WL, Barnett C, Feldman M, et al. Reduction of twenty-four-hour gastric acidity with combination drug therapy in patients with duodenal ulcer. Gastroenterology 1979; *77*:1015–1020.

28. Fein HD. Nutrition in disease of the stomach, including related areas of the esophagus and duodenum. *In* Goodhart RS, Shils ME (eds). Modern Nutrition in Health and Disease. 6th ed. Philadelphia, Lea & Febiger, 1980: 892–911.

29. Bingle JP, Lennard-Jones JE. Some factors in the assessment of gastric antisecretory drugs by a sampling technique. Gut 1960; *1*:337–349.

30. Ippoliti AF, Maxwell V, Isenberg JI. The effect of various forms of milk on gastric acid secretion: studies in patients with duodenal ulcer and normal subjects. Ann Intern Med 1976; *84*:286–289.

31. Baron JH, Wastell C. Medical treatment. *In* Wastell C (ed). Chronic Duodenal Ulcer. London, Butterworth, 1972; 117–133.

32. Evans PRC. Value of strict dieting, drugs and "Robaden" in peptic ulceration. Br Med J 1954; *1*:612–616.

33. Doll R, Pygott F. Factors influencing the rate of healing of gastric ulcer: admission to hospital, phenobarbitone and ascorbic acid. Lancet 1952; *1*:171–175.

34. Meulengracht E. Treatment of haematemesis and melaena with food; mortality. Lancet 1935; *2*:1220–1222.

35. Russell DM, Leiter LA, Whitwell J, et al. Skeletal muscle function during hypocaloric diets and fasting: a comparison with standard nutritional assessment parameters. Am J Clin Nutr 1983; *37*:133–138.

36. Guyton AC. Movement of food through the alimentary tract. *In* Textbook of Medical Physiology. 6th ed. Philadelphia, WB Saunders, 1981: 792.

37. Meyer JH, Thomson JB, Cohen MB, et al. Sieving of solid food by the canine stomach and sieving after gastric surgery. Gastroenterology 1979; *76*:804–813.

38. Miller J, Kauffman G, Elashoff J, et al. Search for resistances controlling canine gastric emptying of liquid meals. Am J Physiol 1981; *241*:G403–G415.

39. Machella TE. Mechanism of the post-gastrectomy dumping syndrome. Gastroenterology 1950; *14*:237–252.

40. Butz R. Dumping syndrome studied during maintenance of blood volume. Ann Surg 1961; *154*:225–234.

41. LeQuesne LP, Hobsley M, Hand BM. The dumping syndrome. I. Factors responsible for the symptoms. Br Med J 1960; *1*:141–147.

42. Editorial: Dumping syndrome and gut peptides. Lancet 1980; *2*:1173–1174.

43. McKelvey STD. Gastric incontinence and post-vagotomy diarrhoea. Br J Surg 1970; *57*:741–747.

44. Allan JG, Gerskowitch VP, Russel RI. The role of bile acids in the pathogenesis of postvagotomy diarrhoea. Br J Surg 1974; *61*:516–518.

45. Booth CC, Brain MC, Jeejeebhoy KN. Late post-gastrectomy syndromes. Hypoproteinemia after partial gastrectomy. Proc Roy Soc Med 1964; *57*:582–585.

46. Clark CG. Medical complications of gastric surgery for peptic ulcer. Compr Ther 1981; *7*:26–32.

47. Hobbs JR. Iron deficiency after partial gastrectomy. Gut 1961; *2*:141–149.

48. Wheldon EJ, Venables CW, Johnston IDA. The relationship of anaemia to gastric secretion more than 15 years after vagotomy and gastroenterostomy. Br J Surg 1975; *62*:356–359.

49. Eddy RL. Metabolic bone disease after gastrectomy. Am J Med 1971; *50*:442–449.

50. Deller DJ, Witts LJ. Changes in the blood after partial gastrectomy with special reference to vitamin B_{12}. Q J Med 1962; *3*:71–88.

51. Nilsson BE, Westlin NE. The fracture incidence after gastrectomy. Acta Chir Scand 1971; *137*:533–534.

52. Goligher JC, De Dombal FT, Pulvertaft CM, et al. Five to eight year results of Leeds/York controlled trial of elective surgery for duodenal ulcer. Br Med J 1968; *2*:781–787.

53. Ralphs DNL, Mertz G, Dilaware JB. Pectin in dumping syndrome: reduction of symptoms and plasma volume changes. Lancet 1981; *1*:1075–1078.

54. Agnew JE, Holdsworth LD. The effect of fat on calcium absorption from a mixed meal in normal subjects, patients with malabsorptive disease, and patients with a partial gastrectomy. Gut 1971; *12*:973–977.

13

ENTEROCUTANEOUS FISTULAS

RIYAD TARAZI / EZRA STEIGER

An enterocutaneous fistula is defined as an abnormal passage or communication leading from an internal organ to the surface of the body.[1] This word is derived from the Latin *fistula* meaning "pipe" or "flute" and presumably referred to a long, narrow suppurating canal connecting normally unrelated structures.[2] Fistulas of the gastrointestinal tract have been described since the ancient days. William Beaumont's experiments on the famous gastric fistula of St. Alexis Martin marked the beginning of the scientific approach to the study of gastrointestinal fistulas in humans.[3]

Enterocutaneous fistulas most commonly appear secondary to abdominal surgery, which various studies have shown to be the etiology in 51 to 100 per cent of cases.[4-16] Other causes include inflammatory bowel disease in 1.8 to 44 per cent,[4,8,10,11,13-16] cancer in 1.8 to 11 per cent,[4,6,8] radiation in 2 to 17 per cent,[10,13,15] and trauma in 1.8 to 6.5 per cent.[4-7,10] Rare cases are due to foreign bodies, hernias, and unusual infections.[17-22] Other etiological considerations include hypoalbuminemia and malnutrition, which can lead to impaired wound healing and anastomotic disruption.

The mortality rate for gastrointestinal fistulas in most recent series ranges between 6 to 20 per cent.

Since the work by Chapman et al.,[6] it has been recognized that adequate nutritional support is an integral part in the management of gastrointestinal fistulas. In their series the mortality of patients suboptimally nourished was 58 per cent, compared with 17 per cent when adequate calories were supplied. Roback et al.[16] noted a 74 per cent mortality in malnourished patients with gastrointestinal fistulas compared with 17 per cent if the patient's nutritional status was good. Coutsoftides et al.,[23] studying patients with enterocutaneous fistulas, noted a mortality of 31.8 per cent in malnourished patients as compared with 3.63 per cent in patients who were well nourished. Sheldon et al.[11] similarly noted a mortality of 45 per cent in inadequately nourished patients versus 14 per cent in those who were adequately nourished.

The anatomical location of the fistula and the volume of drainage also contribute to increased mortality. In 1975 Edelmann et al.[24] reported a collective series of 384 patients with gastrointestinal fistulas in which mortality was 20 per cent if fistula output was less than 500 ml. The mortality was doubled when the fistula output increased to more than 500 ml. Fazio et al.[25] studied 174 patients with enterocutaneous fistulas and reported the following mortalities: High-output jejunal and ileal fistulas carried a mortality of 48.3 and 23.7 per cent, respectively, with a total mortality of 30.3 per cent. With low-output fistulas, jejunal fistula mortality was zero and ileal fistula mortality was 5.9 per cent, with a total mortality of 4.8 per cent. Edmunds et al.[4] noted a 62 per cent mortality for gastroduodenal fistulas (46 per cent for end-duodenal fistulas and 67 per cent for lateral duodenal fistulas). They also noted a 54 per cent mortality in small bowel fistulas with profuse drainage and 16 per cent mortality in distal ileal and colonic fistulas. Tables 13–1 and 13–2 summarize reported mortalities of gastrointestinal fistulas from selected series in the literature from 1960 to 1983.

Sheldon et al.[11] noted a 16 per cent mortality with high-output small bowel fistulas compared with no mortality with low-output fistulas. Reber et al.[37] reported a 67 per cent mortality with high-output fistulas compared with 33 per cent mortality for low-output fistulas. Soeters et al.[39] noted a mortality of 25 per cent if fistula output was more than 500 ml and a mortality of 12 per cent if fistula output was less than 500 ml. Edmunds et al.[4] in 1960 published their classic paper on external fistulas rising from the gastrointestinal tract. They noted that the treatment was associated with a high mortality and morbidity ranging from 40 to 65 per cent. Of the 68 deaths in 157 patients with external fistulas, 78 per cent were related to electrolyte and fluid imbalance, 61 per cent to malnutrition, and 67 per cent to sepsis. Today with improvements in monitoring and management of fluid and electrolyte abnormalities, and the recognition, prevention, and treatment of malnutrition, sepsis plays the major role in mortality.

EARLY STAGES OF FISTULA MANAGEMENT

Diagnosis and Early Treatment

When there is clinical suspicion of a fistula, the fluid from the midline incision or drain site and the patient's blood is sent for BUN, bilirubin, amylase, and electrolyte determination. These tests will help to differentiate serum, pancreatic, biliary, small bowel, or urinary tract origins of the drainage. A plain film of the abdomen is obtained to look for

TABLE 13–1. Mortality Due to Gastrointestinal Fistulas (Selected Series 1960–1983)

Author, Year, Reference	Small Bowel Only		All Fistulas	
	No.	%	No.	%
Edmunds et al., 1960[4]	25/46	54.3	68/157	43.3
West et al., 1961[26]	4/23	17.4	17/67	25.4
Bowlin et al., 1962[5]	5/15	33.3	26/79	32.9
Chapman et al., 1964[6]	15/23	65.2	25/65	44.6
Halversen et al., 1969[27]	11/31	35.5	22/55	40.0
Nassos et al., 1971[9]	4/15	26.7	5/23	21.7
Roback et al., 1972.[16]	17/55	30.9	17/55	30.9
Voitk et al., 1973[14]	5/13	38.5	8/29	27.6
Himal et al., 1974[28]	2/25*	8.0	24/91	26.4
	22/66	33.3		
Rocchio et al., 1974[29]	4/16	25.0	6/37	16.2
Aguirre et al., 1974[15]	5/26	19.2	8/37	21.6
Athanassiades et al., 1975[30]	4/26	15.4	25/81	30.9
Blackett and Hill, 1978[31]	4/19	21.1	5/25	20.0
N-Fekete et al., 1978[32]	2/25†	8.0	2/25	8.0
Allardyce, 1983[33]	20/52	38.5	20/52	38.5
Sheldon et al., 1971[11]	—‡		6/51	11.8
MacFadyen et al., 1973[13]	—‡		4/61	6.5
Deitel, 1976[34]	—‡		12/30*	40.0
			8/86	9.3
Graham, 1977[35]	—‡		3/39	7.7
Sitges-Serra et al., 1982[36]	—‡		16/75	21.3

*Himal reported 8.0% mortality with nutritional support and 33.3% with no nutritional support. Similarly Deitel reported a 40% mortality pre-TPN and 9.3% with TPN use.
†All 25 patients reported were children.
‡Mortality due to small bowel fistulas not determined.

TABLE 13-2. Mortality Due to Duodenal Fistulas (Selected Series 1960-1983)

Author, Year, Reference		No.	%
Edmunds et al., 1960[4]	Side	6/9	67.0
	End	14/28	50.0
	Total	20/37	54.1
Bowlin et al., 1962[5]	Side	7/11	63.6
	End	1/8	12.5
	Total	8/19	42.1
Chapman et al., 1964[6]		4/7	57.0
Nassos et al., 1971[9]	Side	0/5	0
	End	1/3	33.3
	Total	1/8	12.5
Reber et al., 1978[37]	Side		0
	End		25.0
Tarazi et al., 1983[38]	Side		25.0
	End		42.0

signs of an abscess or bowel obstruction. A water-soluble dye is injected into the fistulous tract to radiographically localize its origin and any associated abscesses or bowel abnormalities. This must be done in the presence of a physician familiar with the patient and with previous operations performed. Other simple diagnostic modalities to help localize the site of origin of the fistula include diluted methylene blue per nasogastric tube, grape juice enemas, or indigo carmine intravenously. Occasionally a barium study is performed if no intraperitoneal leak is found. After the fistulogram is reviewed, additional studies may include an upper gastrointestinal series, a barium enema, or both. Enterocutaneous fistulas are usually associated with either localized or generalized sepsis and peritonitis secondary to fistula leak in the abdominal cavity. If generalized peritonitis is found, external drainage has to be instituted surgically. No attempts at primary repair of the fistula should be done, as the rate of operative failure is high when definitive therapy is undertaken in the face of uncontrolled sepsis.[37] Usually the abscess can be drained at the bedside with the patient under local anesthesia by probing through the fistulous tract and inserting a sump catheter. Cultures of the retrieved fluid are sent. With improvement in the techniques of computerized axial tomography and guided percutaneous drainage of intra-abdominal abscesses, a very small percentage of patients will require surgery in the initial phase of management;[40] however, undrained sepsis, peritonitis, intestinal hemorrhage, or bowel ischemia will dictate urgent operation irrespective of the state of nutrition or the timing of the first operation.[25]

Also involved in making the decision for early operation are associated findings (Table 13-3) that will dictate a less likely chance of spontaneous closure. Once this is determined, early operation is performed if the fluid, electrolyte, and nutritional status is adequate. However, if the patient is deemed nutritionally unfit for a major operation, intensive nutritional support is started until positive nitrogen balance is achieved. Generally at least 7 days of nutritional support giving 35 kcal/kg/day and 1.5 g of amino acid/kg/day is necessary to achieve significant reduction in postoperative morbidity and mortality in the severely malnourished patient.[41]

Conservative Therapy

FLUIDS AND ELECTROLYTES

Fluids and electrolyte resuscitation is an integral part of the conservative therapy of patients with gastrointestinal fistulas and is initiated in the early stages of fistula management. Blood and plasma are used to replenish the patient's blood volume if they are required to assure hemodynamic stability. Hypoalbuminemia (arbitrarily defined as an albumin of less than 2.7 g/dl) is treated with 12.5 to 25 g of salt-poor albumin twice daily to decrease tissue edema and improve healing. Parenteral fluid replacement is calculated by adding fistula output per day, plus 1500 ml for urine output, plus 500 ml for insensible fluid loss, plus the equivalent of other losses such as from the nasogastric tube. This determines the total fluid volume required per day, assuming the patient has normal renal function. Requirements for electrolytes are estimated by sending aliquots of urine, nasogastric output, and fistula output for electrolyte and mineral determinations.[42] With knowledge of the daily volume and electrolyte requirements, fluid and electrolyte replacement is started. A knowledge of gastrointestinal tract secretion provides useful information to diagnose and treat gastrointestinal fistulas.

The main function of the gastrointestinal tract is secretion and absorption. While the upper gastrointestinal tract is mainly secretory, the small intestine is primarily absorptive. Ingested fluid (2000 ml/day),

TABLE 13-3. Factors That Decrease Chance of Spontaneous Closure of Fistula

Loss of bowel continuity, such as complete disruption of a gastrojejunal anastomosis

Unremitting small bowel obstruction secondary to adhesions, tumor, or the local inflammatory process associated with the fistula causing stricturing of the bowel

Adjacent abscess cavity through which the fistula drains to the skin

Underlying inflammatory bowel disease, radiation, or malignancy. To confirm the diagnosis of cancer, it is sometimes possible to obtain a biopsy specimen of the mucosa through the fistula tract using a pediatric bronchoscope or cystoscope[10]

Epithelization of the fistulous tract down to the opening into the bowel with a fistulous tract less than 2 cm

Presence of a foreign body such as suture or prosthetic material

An opening in the bowel greater than 1.0 cm²

High-output fistulas and multiple complicated fistulas

TABLE 13–4. Salivary Secretion

Characteristics	Electrolytes	Stimulation				Inhibition		
500–2000 ml/day	Na 2–10 mEq/L (5–100)*	Parasympathetic (acetylcholine)				Atropine		Scopolamine
		Sympathetic (norepinephrine)						
Osmolarity 50–300 mOsm/L†	K 20 mEq/L (40–20)‡	β-Amylase α- ↑K + ↑H_2O					ACTH	
		Food					Aldosterone	
Specific gravity 1.002–1.012	Cl 8–18 mEq/L (5–70)	Taste	Touch	Smell	Ideas			
							ADH§	
		Nausea		Cigarette smoking				
	HCO_3–30 mEq/L (30–60)							
		Neostigmine				Sleep Dehydration	Fatigue	Fear

*(a–b): a, concentration at low flow rates; b, concentration at high flow rates.
†At low flow rates Osm = 50 mOsm/L, and at high flow rates Osm 300 = Osm/L.
‡Saliva has the highest K^+ concentration of any digestive juice.
§Salivary Na levels are depressed by the administration of ACTH and to a lesser degree desoxycorticosterone, aldosterone, and ADH.

salivary (1500 ml/day), gastric (2500 ml/day), biliary (500 ml/day), pancreatic (1500 ml/day), and intestinal secretion (1000 ml/day) present approximately 5–9 L to the absorptive surface of the small intestine per day. Ninety-eight per cent of this volume is absorbed, and 200 ml is excreted in stools. The duodenum, mainly jejunum, constitutes the major site of water absorption, about 5.5 L/day. Of the remaining 3.5 L, 2 L is absorbed by the ileum, and 1.3 L of the amount delivered to the colon is absorbed. Tables 13–4 through 13–10 summarize the basic

mechanism of stimulation and inhibition of gastrointestinal tract secretions.

DRAINAGE AND SKIN PROTECTION

Adequate fistula drainage must be provided. If the fistula is draining intraperitoneally, surgical drainage is performed; however, if the fistula is draining into an abscess cavity, adequate drainage can be performed by inserting a sump catheter through the fistulous tract into the abscess cavity.

TABLE 13–5. Stimulation of Gastric Acid Secretion

Characteristics	Electrolyte		Acetylcholine-Mediated (ACh)	Gastrin-Mediated	Histamine-Mediated	Direct Effect	Unknown Mechanism
1000–2500 ml/day	Na 75 mEq/L (10–40)	ACh		Gastrin		Caffeine	
			Parasympathomimetic				
Osmolarity isotonic	K 10 mEq/L (0–30)		Taste	Pentagastrin			
			Smell		Histamine		
		Cephalic phase	Chewing			Amino acids and peptides	Morphine and enkephalins
	Cl 125 mEq/L (10–150)		Swallowing				
			Thought of food	Amino acids and peptides			
		Gastric distention					
	HCO_3^- (—) mEq/L (0–25)	Hypoglycemia				NH_3	
		3-Methylglucose		Duodenal gastrin			
		2-Deoxyglucose					

TABLE 13–6. Inhibition of Gastric Acid Secretion

Characteristics	Electrolyte	Acetylcholine-Mediated (ACh)	Gastrin-Mediated	Histamine-Mediated	Direct Effect	Unknown Mechanism
1000–2500 ml/day	Na 75 mEq/L (10–140)	Atropine	Cholecystokinin (CCK)*	Atropine	Prostaglandins	Enteroxyntin
			Atropine	H2 receptor blockers		
Osmolarity isotonic	K 10 mEq/L (0–30)	H2 receptor blockers	H2 receptor blockers	Serotonin	H2 receptor blockers	Enterogastrone (acid, fat, and hyperosomolar solution in duodenum)
	Cl 125 mEq/L (10–150)		Secretin† Bulbogastrone	Somatostatin (weak)		Urogastrone
				GIP‡ (weak)		
	HCO3⁻ (—) mEq/L (0–25)	Somatostatin	Glucagon Somatostatin	Somatostatin	Somatostatin	Serotonin Naloxone
			VIP			GIP
			Neurotoxin			

*Cholecystokinin and secretin inhibit gastrin-mediated acid release by inhibition phenomenon.
†Secretin, although it inhibits gastrin-mediated acid secretion, it increases pepsinogen secretion.
‡Release of gastrin by antral distention is resistant to antral acid and is enhanced by atropine; however, this is a weak stimulus.

TABLE 13–7. Gastrin Secretion

Acetylcholine-Mediated		Direct Effect	
Stimulation	Inhibition	Stimulation	Inhibition
Atropine		Amino acids and peptides	pH <3.0
	Acetylcholine		
Antral distention		Ca⁺⁺	Secretin
		Foods Pr>CHO>Fat	
Vagus stimulation in cephalic and gastric phase		Bombesin	Somatostatin
	Somatostatin	Food buffers	
			VIP

TABLE 13–8. Bile Secretion

Characteristics	Electrolytes	Stimulation	Inhibition
250–1110 ml/day	Na 151 mEq/L (131–164)	Secretin*	Decreased rate of return of bile acids to the liver†
		CCK	
Osmolarity— isotonic	K 4.6 mEq/L (3.6–5.2)	Cerulein*	H2 receptor antagonists
		Gastrin*	
		Vagus (ACH)‡	
Specific gravity 1.008–1.016	Cl 102 mEq/L (83–112)		Anticholinergic drugs
		Histamine	
		Increased rate of return of bile acids to the liver	VIP§
	HCO3 26 mEq/L (19–29)		

*Stimulation by secretin, cerulein, and gastrin increases bile volume, raises HCO3 concentration and decreases Cl concentration.
†ACH stimulates gallbladder contraction. Cholecystokinin (CCK) plays a similar role.
‡This is seen in patients with biliary fistulas or ileal resection.
§VIP inhibits CCK-induced gallbladder contraction.

ROLE OF NUTRITION IN SPECIFIC DISORDERS

TABLE 13–9. Pancreatic Secretions

Characteristics	Electrolytes (mEq/L)	Stimulation Volume		Stimulation Enzymes		Inhibition Volume		Inhibition Enzymes	
		+++	*+*	*+++*	*+*	*+++*	*+*	*+++*	*+*
500–1000 ml/day	Na 140 mEq/L (113–185)	Secretin	VIP	CCK	Gastrin	Glucagon	Somatostatin	Glucagon	Bile acids
Osmolarity— 300 mOsm	K 5 mEq/L (2–8)	Intestinal phase of gastric secretion (acid in duodenum)		Cephalic and gastric phase of gastric secretion (vagus)	Bombesin	Isoproterenol	Prostaglandins	Somatostatin	Trypsin
	Cl 75 mEq/L (54–95)				Chymodenin		Vasopressin		
					Prostaglandins		Pancreatic polypeptide		
	HCO₃ 115 mEq/L (60–150)			Cerulein	Trypsin inhibitors				

TABLE 13–10. Intestinal Secretion

Characteristics	Electrolytes	Stimulation	Inhibition
	Duodenum	Acetylcholine	Alpha-adrenergics
Duodenum 100–2000 ml/day	Na 145 mEq/L (136–150)	Gastrin	Epinephrine and norepinephrine
		Glucagon	
Small bowel 100–9000 ml/day	K 6.3 mEq/L (4.5–8.0)	VIP	Somatostatin
			Atropine
Average 1000–3000 ml/day	Cl 136 mEq/L (130–140)	GIP	Glucocorticoids
		Secretin	
Osmolarity—isotonic	HCO₃ (14–22)	Cholecystokinin	Opiate receptor agonists
		Serotonin	
	Small Bowel		
	Na 140 mEq/L (80–150)	Calcitonin Prostaglandins	
	K 5.0 mEq/L (2–8)	5-HT	
	Cl 105 mEq/L (43–137)	Substance P	
	HCO₃ 30 mEq/L (20–40)	Metylxanthines	
		Bombesin	
		Vasopressin	
		Neurotensin	
		Bile salts and acids in lumen	

Antibiotics are not used unless the sepsis is present, but oral mycostatin swallow is used to prevent *Candida* overgrowth. Fistula drainage from the small bowel has activated pancreatic enzymes that are corrosive to the skin. Protection against skin maceration is done using sump suction, stoma bags, and skin barriers such as Stomahesive or karaya paste (Figs. 13–1 to 13–3). Multiple techniques of fistula containment have been described.[43–48]

METHODS OF DECREASING FISTULA OUTPUT

The use of continuous nasogastric suction to decrease fistula output is still controversial. While a nasogastric tube is inevitable in patients with ileus or distal small bowel obstruction, some authors believe that its routine use is not warranted all the time as no definite decrease in fistula output has been shown with its use.[4,49] Moreover, Fischer[49] advocates the use of a gastrostomy tube placed with the use of local anesthesia if prolonged intubation is anticipated to avoid pharyngitis, otitis, and occasionally esophageal stricture secondary to esophagitis. Cimetidine, in doses of 300 to 600 mg given four times a day, has been shown to decrease fistula output.[10,37] The role of somatostatin is still debatable, although DiCostanzo et al. showed decreased fistula output with its use.[50]

NUTRITIONAL SUPPORT

Virtually all patients with gastrointestinal fistulas either are malnourished or will become malnour-

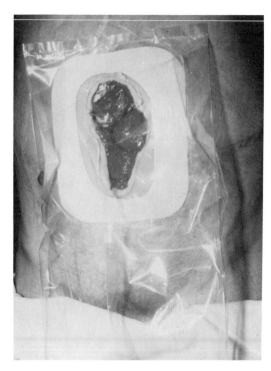

FIGURE 13–2. *Stoma bag applied.*

ished secondary to sepsis, increased catabolism, fluid and protein losses, or inability to use the intestinal tract effectively. With the diagnosis of a fistula a detailed nutritional assessment is obtained and data are entered into a computerized form for easier serial assessments (Fig. 13–4).

For patients with gastric, duodenal, jejunal, or ileal

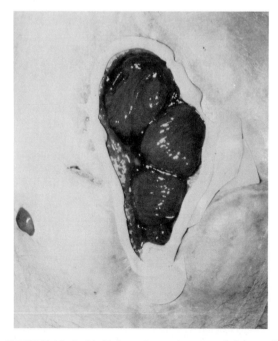

FIGURE 13–1. *Multiple enterocutaneous fistulas with a proximal jejunostomy, karaya paste.*

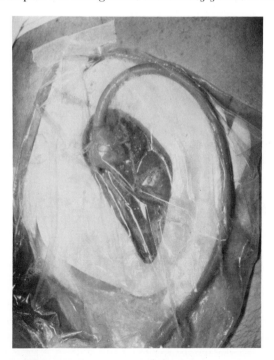

FIGURE 13–3. *Foley catheter attached to a collecting system to prevent overflow from the bag; mainly used in high-output gastrointestinal fistulas.*

```
Cleveland Clinic Foundation                          1-478-848-4
Department of General Surgery                          JANE DOE
Nutritional Support Service                          2-May-1984
                                                        STEIGER
                                                         9S06


                   Nutritional Assessment Report

Referring Physician:    STEIGER
Diagnosis:              ENTEROCUTANEOUS FISTULA
Operation:              RESECTION, ENTEROCUTANEOUS FISTUAL 12/25
Age(years):             71
Sex:                    F
Height(cm):             158
Frame type:             M
Usual weight(Kg):        63.6
Ideal weight(Kg):        50
BEE(Kcal):              1179
ECR(Kcal):              2064 to 2358
Protein Req(gms):        89 to 118



          Act
           Wt   % Wt  TSF  MUAMC      Pre                   Skin
  Date    (Kg) Change (mm) (cm) Alb Inf Alb  TLC  BUN Creat Gluc Test  PNI

11/28/83  53.0  -17%   07  20.8 2.6 156 3.1  600  17  1.3   95  0/4   78%
12/12/83  56.0  -12%   10  21.9 3.0 190 5.0  900  42  1.3   85  0/0
 1/03/84  59.0   -7%   12  23.2 3.5 247 10.1 1100 33  1.3  112  1/4   30%


Adipose Stores:        TSF:   6%ile Moderate Deficit

Somatic Protein:       MUAMC:  60%ile Adequate

Visceral Protein:      Albumin:  Adequate
                       Transferrin:  Adequate
                       Pre-Albumin:  Adequate

Immune Function:       TLC:  Moderate Deficit
                       Skin Tests:  Relatively Anergic

PNI:                          30% Low Risk


Suggest:
  50% Dextrose + 8.5% FreAmine (1 kcal/ml) --> 86 to 98 cc/hr
```

FIGURE 13–4. A 71-year-old female developed an enterocutaneous fistula after lysis of adhesions for small bowel obstruction. Serial nutritional assessments are depicted. On December 25 the patient underwent successful treatment of the fistula with resection and end-to-end anastomosis.

fistulas, nutritional support is started by intravenous hyperalimentation. Distal ileal or colonic fistula patients can often be supported with enteral feedings. Caloric requirements are calculated by multiplying basal energy expenditure by 1.5 to 2.0.

Frequent nitrogen balance determinations are performed and caloric requirements adjusted accordingly. With the institution of total parenteral nutrition (TPN), a decrease in the fistula output is usually noted. Hamilton et al.[15] noted that parenteral hyperalimentation decreased fluid losses from the fistula by 85 per cent within 48 hours providing the patient was taking nothing by mouth.

Hamilton et al.[51] noted a similar decrease of 80 to 85 per cent in fistula output within 2 to 3 days and claimed that this was very helpful in spontaneous closure. Wolfe et al.[53] in an experimental study with enterocutaneous fistulas in dogs noted an 81 per cent decrease of fistula output with elemental diet and a 93 per cent decrease with total parenteral nutrition. This is contrary to Fischer's findings of a 31.5 per cent decrease in fistula output with TPN.[49] There is slight controversy concerning the preferred method of nutritional support; however, most authors agree

that initially, when the patient is hypercatabolic and usually septic and caloric requirements are up to two times normal, parenteral nutrition is the ideal route, since full caloric and nitrogen replenishment can be achieved in a shorter period of time. This may be supplemented by enteral feeding later.

Respectable fistula closure rates have been achieved with enteral feeding. Rocchio et al.[29] reported a 50 per cent spontaneous closure rate in 16 patients with enterocutaneous fistulas using enteral feeding. Bury et al.[54] noted a 54 per cent spontaneous closure rate with a 15 per cent mortality. Voitk et al.[14] noted a 59 per cent spontaneous closure rate with 28 per cent mortality using elemental diets. The above data compare favorably with series using total parenteral nutrition alone. Fat emulsions and peripheral TPN have been used also with good results. Graham[35] noted a spontaneous closure rate of 89 per cent in 39 patients with external gastrointestinal fistulas with a mortality of 7.7 per cent. All infusions in his series were initially done via a peripheral vein; however, central venous catheters were placed in 9 patients as peripheral access decreased. Silberman et al.[55] reported a 73.3 per cent spontaneous closure rate of various gastrointestinal fistulas using the peripheral lipid system. They concluded that in the subset of patients with external gastrointestinal fistulas, the lipid system appeared equally effective as TPN.

We have been disenchanted with the use of elemental diets in nutritional support of enterocutaneous fistulas. The theoretical benefits are that enteral feeding is easier to manage, safe, and cheaper and avoids the complications associated with catheter sepsis or pneumothorax, which in our institution occur in roughly 1.5 to 2 per cent of patients. However, adequate nitrogen and caloric intake may be difficult to achieve because of gastrointestinal intolerance manifested by diarrhea or increased fistula output. Elemental diets are often markedly hyperosmolar and may even accentuate gastrointestinal intolerance. In addition, enteral diets are unpalatable, and when given through nasogastric tubes they can be associated with serious complications such as aspiration pneumonia. Moreover, in upper gastrointestinal fistulas a tube should be passed 40 cm beyond the fistula to avoid reflux of feeding out through the fistula. TPN decreases fistula output by decreasing enteral stimulation of intestinal secretion and at the same time restores the patients nutritional status to normal. Improved wound healing and increased resistance to infection will be secondary gains of improvement in nutritional status, both of which should impact favorably on the patient's clinical course. TPN adds the dimension of time to the patient's advantage by allowing for resolution of the associated inflammatory resection and the possibility of spontaneous closure during which time the patient's nutritional status is improved.

WHEN TO RESUME ORAL INTAKE

When to resume oral intake is determined clinically by observing decrease or absence of fistula drainage and radiologically by documentation of fistula closure either by a Gastrografin swallow, enema, or injection of the old fistula site. After the fistula has been demonstrated to have closed radiologically, an additional period of 7 days is allowed to pass before testing the patient with oral intake.

ENTEROCUTANEOUS FISTULAS ASSOCIATED WITH RADIATION AND CANCER

Radiation induced fistulas are notorious for the poor results of treatment with respect to both successful spontaneous closure rate and mortality. Fazio et al.[25] noted a 45.4 per cent mortality with radiation-induced fistulas. On the contrary, Reber et al.[37] noted a mortality of 19 per cent and a spontaneous closure rate of 14 per cent in such cases. Copeland et al.[56] reported on six small bowel fistulas secondary

to radiation (five enterocutaneous and one duodenocutaneous). The spontaneous closure rate was 50 per cent with a mortality of 50 per cent. Excluding the one duodenocutaneous fistula, spontaneous closure rate was 40 per cent with a mortality of 60 per cent. All patients were dead within 9 months of fistula closure. Copeland et al. concluded that intravenous hyperalimentation should be used only to prepare patients nutritionally for surgery.

The results of cancer induced fistulas are usually less dismal. Fazio et al.[25] noted a 12.5 percent mortality of small bowel fistulas associated with cancer. Reber et al.[37] noted a 9 per cent fistula-related mortality with a 26 per cent spontaneous closure rate for enterocutaneous fistulas associated with cancer. Rocchio et al.[23] noted a spontaneous closure rate of 50 per cent with a mortality of 33.3 per cent in small bowel fistulas associated with malignancy. Roback et al.[16] noted a 33.3 per cent fistula-related mortality in enterocutaneous fistula associated with malignancy, with a total mortality of 50 per cent. Of the total number of patient deaths, 66.6 per cent were due to causes unrelated to the fistula. Copeland et al.[57] in 1974 in a series of seven patients with postoperative gastrointestinal fistulas in patients with metastatic adenocarcinoma noted a spontaneous closure rate of 71.4 per cent with a mortality of 14.3 per cent. Copeland[58] later in 1977 noted a 44 per cent spontaneous closure rate in enteric fistulas associated with cancer. In two patients spontaneous closure occurred even though cancer was confirmed in the biopsy of the fistulous tract. Thomas[59] noted that if the fistulous tract was involved with cancer, the results with intravenous hyperalimentation to heal the fistula was poor. Of six patients with cancer not involving the fistulous tract, 50 percent had spontaneous closure. One had a recurrence of the fistula once oral food was resumed.

The role of nutritional support in patients with fistulas secondary to radiation or cancer is mainly to improve the patient's nutritional status in preparation for surgery and to attempt spontaneous closure if possible.

ENTEROCUTANEOUS FISTULAS ASSOCIATED WITH CROHN'S DISEASE

Enterocutaneous fistulas are characteristic of Crohn's disease and occur in 15 to 20 per cent of patients, usually through the anterior abdominal wall. According to Irving,[60] two types of fistulas occur. Type I fistulas arise from a segment of bowel, often the terminal ileum, that is involved by active Crohn's disease. Type II fistulas follow breakdown of an anastomosis following surgical resection of an involved segment of bowel. The success of TPN has been mainly in patients with Type II fistulas. Type I fistulas are notorious for their resistance to medical therapy. Shike and Jeejeebhoy[61] and Driscoll and Rosenberg[62] reviewed the literature up to 1980 and collected a report of 67 patients with 77 Crohn's fistulas treated by hyperalimentation. The combined success rate of spontaneous closure was 43 per cent. Mullen et al.[63] reported a retrospective analysis of 74 patients with inflammatory bowel disease of various types who were treated with intravenous hyperalimentation. Surgical treatment was carried out in 62 per cent of the 74 patients during intravenous hyperalimentation. In 15 per cent of the patients, the indication for surgery was an enterocutaneous fistula. Permanent fistula closure with intravenous hyperalimentation alone occurred in 33 per cent of 43 patients who had fistulas. The overall permanent fistula closure with intravenous hyperalimentation and surgery was 86 per cent.

Controversy still exists on the role of TPN in treatment of fistulas in Crohn's disease. MacFadyen et al.[13] evaluated their experience with total parenteral nutrition in the treatment of Crohn's fistulas. Their series included 31 fistulas in 23 patients. The spontaneous closure rate of small bowel fistulas with TPN was 75 per cent. Grant et al.[64] noted a 100 per cent closure rate in 2 patients treated with nutritional support. Greenberg et al.[65] reported spontaneous closure of Crohn's fistulas in 6 of 7 patients (85.7 per cent) receiving TPN and prednisone but only one (14.3 per cent) closure in patients receiving nutritional support alone. On the contrary, Elson et al.[66] noted that 1 of 4 patients (25 per cent) among their 20 patients with Crohn's disease had any long-lasting benefits from nutritional support.

Eisenberg et al.[67] found that 2 of 18 patients with Crohn's fistulas avoided surgery. Fischer et al.[68] noted that while fistulas may close, they reopen later and need surgical correction. The current knowledge concerning the treatment of Crohn's fistulas with TPN indicates that a trial of this therapy is worthwhile before surgery is contemplated, keeping in mind that the success rate of such a treatment is poor.

SPONTANEOUS CLOSURE RATE OF ENTEROCUTANEOUS FISTULAS WITH TPN

While most authors agree that increased spontaneous closure rate of fistulas has been achieved by TPN, there is still debate about the effect on mortality (see Tables 13–11 and 13–12 on the various spontaneous closure rates from selected series published from 1960 to 1983). Kaminsky et al.[69] noted a decrease in mortality from 40 to 12.5 per cent and increased spontaneous closure rate from 34.4 to 80 per cent in two groups of patients with external fistulas of the gastrointestinal tract treated with and without hyperalimentation. Himal et al.[28] reported an improvement in mortality from 33 to 8 per cent in patients receiving adequate nutrition. He also noted an improvement in spontaneous closure rate from 27 to 50 per cent. Reber et al.,[37] although noting an increase in spontaneous closure rate of enterocutaneous fistulas from 26 to 35 per cent, noted no change in mortality, which remained at 29 per

TABLE 13–11. Spontaneous Closure Rate of Enterocutaneous Fistulas (Selected Series 1960–1983)

Author, Year, Reference	Small Bowel Only		All Fistulas	
	No.	%	No.	%
Edmunds et al., 1960[4]	2/46	4.3	51/157	32.5
Bowlin et al., 1962[5]	5/15	33.0	37/71	52.0
Chapman et al., 1964[6]	NA		18/33	55.0
Halversen et al., 1969[27]	4/31	12.9	16/55	29.1
Nassos et al., 1971[9]	6/15	40.0	9/23	39.7
Sheldon et al., 1971[11]	0/29	0	14/51	27.5
Roback et al., 1972.[16]	22/55	40.0	22/55	40.0
Voitk et al., 1973[14]	10/17	58.8	18/26	69.2
MacFadyen et al., 1973[13]	18/26	69.2	45/61	73.7
Himal et al., 1974[28]	14/25	56.0	14/25	56.0
Rocchio et al., 1974[29]	8/16	50.0	24/37	64.9
Aguirre et al., 1974[15]	7/26	27.0	11/38	28.9
Graham, 1977[35]	NA		35/39	89.7
Blackett and Hill, 1978[31]	10/19	52.6	15/25	60.0
N-Fekete et al., 1978[32]	13/24	54.2	13/24	54.2
Sitges-Serra et al., 1982[36]	NA		62/87*	71.3
Allardyce, et al., 1983[33]	19/44	43.2	19/44	43.2

*The series was 87 fistulas in 75 patients; 62 fistulas healed spontaneously.
NA, not applicable.

TABLE 13–12. Spontaneous Closure Rate of Duodenal Fistulas (Selected Series 1962–1982)

Author, Year, Reference		Spontaneous Closure No.	%
Bowlin et al., 1962[5]	Side	5/11	45.5
	End	7/8	87.5
	Total	12/19	63.2
Chapman et al., 1964[6]	Total	3/7	42.9
Nassos et al., 1971[9]	Side	1/5	20.0
	End	2/3	66.6
	Total	3/8	37.5
Reber et al., 1978[37]	Side	3/11	27.3
	End	4/8	50.0
Tarzi et al., 1982[38]	Total	11/29	37.9

cent. They analyzed the course of 186 patients with external gastrointestinal fistulas treated from 1968 to 1977. A group of 82 patients treated between 1968 and 1971 was compared with a group of 104 patients treated between 1972 and 1977. In the first group 35 per cent of the patients received intravenous hyperalimentation, compared with 71 per cent in the second group. Reber et al. found that the spontaneous closure rate was 26 per cent in the period 1968 to 1971 and 35 per cent in 1972 to 1977 with a total mortality of 22 per cent and a fistula-related mortality of 10 to 13 per cent; this was unchanged over 10 years. They also noted that although there was a difference in the spontaneous closure rate it was not statistically significant. They concluded that intravenous hyperalimentation has simplified the nutritional management rather than altered the outcome of gastrointestinal fistulas.

Soeters et al.[39] in 1979 reviewed the Massachusetts General Hospital experience with 404 patients who had gastrointestinal fistulas of various kinds. They divided these patients into three therapeutic periods. During the first period, 1945 to 1960, the introduction of antibiotics occurred. The second period, 1960 to 1970, included improvement in the parasurgical critical care management. The third period, 1970 to 1975, saw the introduction of total parenteral nutrition. The mortality for the small bowel fistulas decreased from 54 per cent (1946 to 1959) to 15.1 per cent (1960 to 1970). There was no further decrease in mortality in the hyperalimented group from 1970 to 1975. Soeters et al. reported a mortality of 25.6 per cent. In their series spontaneous closure rate of gastrointestinal fistulas increased from 10 to 23.3 per cent. They concluded that the major determinant of mortality was uncontrolled sepsis. Deitel et al.[34] noted in a group of patients with external fistulas of the gastrointestinal tract divided in two periods, that the mortality decreased from 40 to 9.3 per cent with the use of nutritional support and an improvement in the spontaneous closure rate from 34.4 to 81 per cent. Although some reports have shown decreased mortality with total parenteral nutrition, mortality figures in several large series without nutritional support range from 15 to 28 per cent and with total parenteral nutrition range from 6.5 to 22 per cent.

Controlled prospective studies or the use of nutritional support in patients with gastrointestinal fistulas having varying degrees of malnutrition are difficult to devise. The effect of associated septic conditions must also be considered in assessing differences in groups studied. The results of treatment in nonseptic patients could be expected to be much better than in septic patients, and the results of treatment in relatively well-nourished patients could also be expected to be much better than in severely malnourished patients. No series has analyzed their results subclassifying their patients according to the degree of malnutrition or the presence of sepsis. Control of sepsis and maintenance of adequate nutrition are both important in maximizing the potential for recovery in patients with gastrointestinal fistulas.

SURGICAL THERAPY OF ENTEROCUTANEOUS FISTULAS

Elective surgical therapy is contemplated when infection is controlled, the patient's nutritional status is improved, and conservative measures have failed. The period of conservative management usually takes 4 to 6 weeks. Reber et al.[37] noted that in their patients 91 per cent of gastrointestinal fistulas that closed spontaneously did so in 1 month. The remaining 9 per cent of spontaneous closures occurred within an additional 2-month period. Reber advocated surgery for all fistulas that have not healed by the end of 1 month. Dunphy and Sheldon[3] noted that when intravenous hyperalimentation is continued beyond 1 month only an additional 3 to 5 per cent will close spontaneously. Fischer[49] noted that if a fistula has not closed by the end of 2 months, it is unlikely that it will ever close.

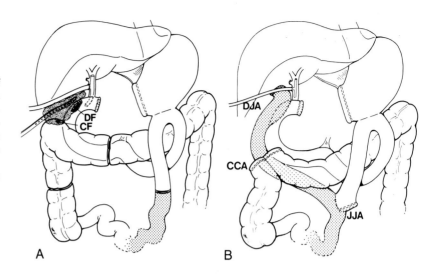

FIGURE 13–5. A, *Preoperative sketch of a duodenocolocutaneous fistula. DF, duodenal fistula; CF, colonic fistula. B, Postoperative sketch of a Roux-en-Y duodenojejunostomy with hepatic flexure resection. DJA, duodenojejunal anastomosis; CCA, colocolic anastomosis; JJA, jejunojejunal anastomosis. (Adapted from Tarazi R, Coutsoftides T, Steiger E, et al. World J Surg 1983; 7:463–473.)*

Duodenal Fistulas

The procedure of choice for fistulas of the gastrointestinal tract is resection and primary neoanastomosis. However, in the region of the duodenum anatomical restrictions prevent this option and other surgical techniques must be utilized. Fistulas arising secondary to disruption of a gastroduodenal or a gastrojejunal anastomosis may require dismantling of the anastomosis and reconstruction by different means, for example, converting a Billroth I to a Billroth II anastomosis or takedown of a Billroth II and reconstruction of a neoanastomosis. A stump duodenal fistula may be treated by debridement of the end and an attempt at a new closure.[38] Alternatively, it may be converted to a controlled stump fistula by inserting a catheter through the stump or closed and reinforced by a serosal patch[70,71] or a Roux-en-Y duodenojejunostomy.[72] Side duodenal fistulas present a challenging problem because simple suture closure may break down or compromise the lumen. This can be avoided by using a serosal patch[70,71] after repair or a defunctionalized Roux-en-Y limb of jejunum for single fistulas as advocated by Ujiki[72] (Fig. 13–5). This procedure is very helpful when it is difficult to mobilize the stomach or duodenum secondary to dense adhesions and marked inflammation. In very rare instances, the Whipple pancreaticoduodenostomy may be the only possible procedure.[73]

Small Bowel Fistulas

Operations for the treatment of small bowel fistulas include (1) simple closure, (2) incomplete or complete intestinal bypass, and (3) primary resection with an end-to-end anastomosis. Simple closure either by pursestring suture or by seromuscular ap-

proximation of apparently normal adjacent bowel over the fistulous opening is usually unsuccessful.[4,11,16,27,37,74] In Reber's series[37] direct suture closure failed in 41 per cent of 32 patients so treated. If exclusion bypass is performed, complete bypass is the procedure of choice,[6,11] especially in certain fistulas deep in the pelvis or fistulas associated with cancer or radiation or if the patient's condition is unsuitable for a prolonged operation (Fig. 13–6).

The procedure of choice for enterocutaneous fistulas is bowel resection with an end-to-end anastomosis.[4,6,11,15,16,25,27,37,74] Table 13–13 summarizes operative success rates as reported by certain selected published series from the literature, 1960 to 1983. However, in certain conditions such as multiple fistulas or fistulas associated with an abscess cavity, this procedure may be preceded by any of the following: (1) proximal stoma (Fig. 13–7), (2) exteriorization with a proximal stoma, or (3) bowel resection with a proximal stoma.

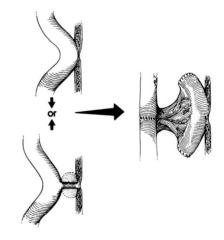

FIGURE 13–6. *Complete exclusion bypass.*

TABLE 13–13. Success of Various Methods of Surgical Treatment of External Gastrointestinal Fistulas (Selected Series 1960–1983)

Author, Year, Reference	External Fistula Location	Local Closure		Complete Bypass		Resection with EEA	
		No.	%	No.	%	No.	%
Edmunds et al., 1960[4]	Small bowel	1/4	25	1/1	100	10/11	91
Chapman et al., 1964[6]	Gastroduodenal, small bowel, colon	1/7	14	1/4	25	7/16	44
Halversen et al., 1964[27]	Gastric and small bowel	0/1	0	5/6	83	6/7	83
Sheldon et al., 1971[11]	Small bowel	—	—	—	—	22/25	88
Roback et al., 1972[16]	Small bowel	0.7	0	1/1	100	10/11	91
Reber et al., 1978[37]	Esophagus, gastroduodenal, small bowel, colon	19/32	59.4	10.10	100	57/66	86
Zera et al., 1983[75]	Small bowel	0/6	0	—	—	10/12	83

Multiple Fistulas Resistant to Conventional Medical or Surgical Therapy

Home parenteral nutrition with or without a proximal diverting jejunostomy has been a good adjunct in a small group of patients with catastrophic intraabdominal conditions that resulted in multiple external and internal fistulas not responding to conventional medical or surgical therapy.

These patients are supported with prolonged inhospital nutrition or home parenteral nutrition for a period of 4 to 6 months until the abdominal condition abates, inflammation subsides, adhesions become more pliable, and the status of the patient becomes more favorable for a major elective operation. At that time the fistula and the small bowel are excised and continuity is re-established. This is done under the coverage of a proximal jejunostomy, which is closed at a later date[76] (Fig. 13–8). Byrne et al.[77] reported, in a similar group of patients, a 50 per cent spontaneous continuous closure rate with zero mortality in small bowel fistulas treated with home parenteral nutrition alone with no diverting jejunostomy. Using this technique, the patient can return to the home setting. Otherwise he or she would have required prolonged hospitalization.

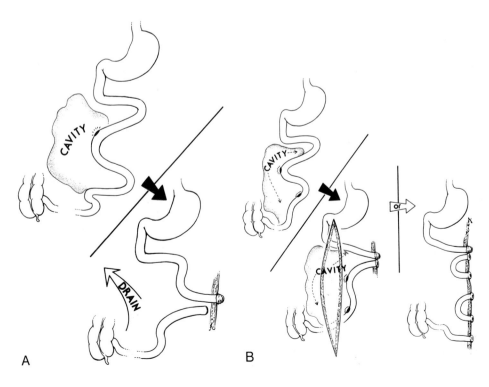

A   B

FIGURE 13–7. A, Proximal fistulas with an abscess cavity treated by proximal diversion and drainage of the abscess cavity. B, Multiple enterocutaneous fistulas managed by proximal diverting jejunostomy and drainage. Delayed restoration is possible by prolonged TPN either in hospital or at home. (Adapted from Fazio VW, Coutsoftides T, Steiger E. World J Surg 1983; 7:481–488.)

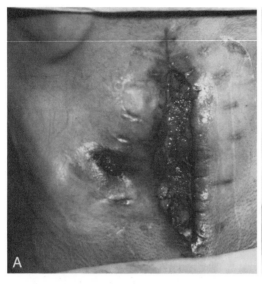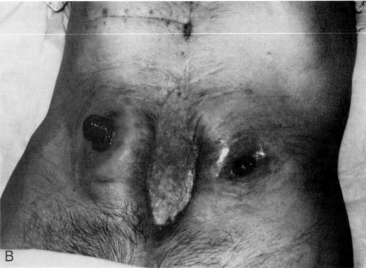

FIGURE 13–8. *Five years after total cystectomy with an ileal conduit and radiation treatment to the pelvis, a 53-year-old white male presented with a small bowel obstruction. He underwent a laparotomy with lysis of adhesions and repair of two small bowel enterotomies. On the seventh postoperative day he developed multiple enterocutaneous fistulas through the midline incision (A). A proximal diverting jejunostomy was placed and the patient was discharged on home TPN for 3 months, after which a skin graft was applied to granulation tissue in midline incision (B). Four weeks later, with documentation of fistula closure, he was readmitted and the jejunostomy was closed.*

REFERENCES

1. Dorland's Illustrated Medical Dictionary. 26th ed. Philadelphia, WB Saunders, 1981: 506.
2. Webster WM, Carey CL. Fistulae of the intestinal tract. Curr Prob Surg 1976; *13*(6):5–78.
3. Dunphy JE, Sheldon GF. Early operation versus prolonged parenteral hyperalimentation in the treatment of enterocutaneous fistulas. *In* Delaney JP, Varco RL (eds). Controversies in Surgery II. Philadelphia, WB Saunders, 1983: 374–387.
4. Edmunds LH Jr, Williams GM, Welch CE. External fistulas arising from the gastro-intestinal tract. Ann Surg 1960; *152*:445.
5. Bowlin JW, Hardy JD, Conn JH. External alimentary fistulas: analysis of seventy-nine cases, with note on management. Am J Surg 1962; *103*:6.
6. Chapman R, Foran R, Dunphy JE. Management of intestinal fistulas. Am J Surg 1964; *108*:157.
7. Welch CE, Edmunds LH. Gastrointestinal fistulas. Surg Clin North Am 1962; *42*:1311.
8. Lorenzo GA, Beal JM. Management of external bowel fistulas. Arch Surg 1969; *99*:394.
9. Nassos TP, Braasch JW. External small bowel fistulas: current treatment and results. Surg Clin North Am 1971; *51*:687.
10. Halasz NA. Changing patterns in the management of small bowel fistulas. Am J Surg 1978; *136*:61.
11. Sheldon GF, Gardiner BN, Way LW, et al. Management of gastrointestinal fistulas. Surg Gynecol Obstet 1971; *133*:385.
12. Ali SD, Leffall LD Jr. Management of external fistulas of the gastrointestinal tract. Am J Surg 1972; *123*:535.
13. MacFadyen BV Jr, Dudrick SJ, Ruberg RL. Management of gastrointestinal fistulas with parenteral hyperalimentation. Surgery 1973; *74*:100.
14. Voitk AJ, Echave V, Brown RA, et al. Elemental diet in the treatment of fistulas of the alimentary tract. Surg Gynecol Obstet 1973; *137*:68.
15. Aguirre A, Fischer JE, Welch CE. The role of surgery and hyperalimentation in the therapy of gastrointestinal-cutaneous fistulae. Am Surg 1974; *180*:393.
16. Roback SA, Nicoloff DM: High output enterocutaneous fistulas of the small bowel: an analysis of fifty-five cases. Am J Surg 1972; *123*:317.
17. Mezey E, Nicholos AW, Holt PR. Tuberculous ileoduodenal fistula. Gastroenterology 1967; *52*:83.
18. Leslie MD, Slater ND, Smallwood CI. Small bowel fistula from a Littre's hernia. Br J Surg 1983; *70*:244.
19. Sejdinaj I, Powers RC. Enterocolonic fistula from swallowed denture. JAMA 1973; *225*:994.
20. Bothra R. Late onset of small bowel fistula due to tantalum mesh. Am J Surg 1973; *125*:649.
21. Robinson KB, Levin EJ. Erosion of retained surgical sponge into the intestine. Am J Roentgenol Radium Ther Nucl Med 1966; *96*:339–343.
22. Cotler HB, Meadowcroft IA, Smink RD. Enteric fistula as a complication of a pelvic fracture. J Bone Joint Surg 1983; *65A*:854–856.
23. Coutsoftides T, Fazio VW. Small intestine cutaneous fistulas. Surg Gynecol Obstet 1979; *149*:333–336.
24. Edelman G, Maillet P, Tremolieres J. Les Fistules Externes de l'Intestin Grele. Paris, Masson, 1975.
25. Fazio VW, Coutsoftides T, Steiger E. Factors influencing the outcome of treatment of small bowel cutaneous fistula. World J Surg 1983; *7*:481–488.
26. West JP, Ring EM, Miller RE, et al. A study of the causes and treatment of external postoperative intestinal fistulas. Surg Gynecol Obstet 1961; *113*:490.
27. Halverson RC, Hogle HH, Richards RC. Gastric and small bowel fistulas. Am J Surg 1969; *118*:968.
28. Himal HS, Allard JR, Nadeau JE, et al. The importance of adequate nutrition in closure of small intestinal fistulas. Br J Surg 1974; *61*:724–726.
29. Rocchio MA, Cha C, Haas KF, et al. Use of chemically defined diets in the management of patients with high output gastrointestinal cutaneous fistulas. Am J Surg 1974; *127*:148.
30. Athanassiades S, Notis P, Tountas C. Fistulas of the gastrointestinal tract: experience with eighty-one cases. Am J Surg 1975; *130*:26.
31. Blackett RL, Hill GL. Postoperative external small bowel fis-

tulas: a study of consecutive series of patients treated with intravenous hyperalimentation. Br J Surg 1978; 65:775–778.

32. N-Fekete C, Ricour C, Duhamel JF, et al. Enterocutaneous fistulas of the small bowel in children (25 cases). J Pediatr Surg 1978; 13:1–4.

33. Allardyce DB. Management of small bowel fistulas. Am J Surg 1983; 145:593–595.

34. Deitel M. Nutritional management of external gastrointestinal fistulas. Can J Surg 1976; 19:505.

35. Graham JA. Conservative treatment of gastrointestinal fistulas. Surg Gynecol Obstet 1977; 144:512.

36. Sitges-Serra A, Jaurrieta E, Sitges-Creus A. Management of postoperative enterocutaneous fistulas: the roles of parenteral nutrition and surgery. Br J Surg 1982; 69:147.

37. Reber HA, Roberts C, Way LW, et al. Management of external gastrointestinal fistulas. Ann Surg 1978; 188:460.

38. Tarazi R, Coutsoftides T, Steiger E, et al. Gastric and duodenal cutaneous fistulas. World J Surg 1983; 7:463–473.

39. Soeters PB, Ebeid AM, Fischer JE. Review of 404 patients with gastrointestinal fistulas: impact of parenteral nutrition. Ann Surg 1979; 190:189.

40. Hau T. Percutaneous surgical drainage of abdominal abscesses. In Manual of Gastrointestinal Disease. 68th Annual Clinic Congress, American College of Surgeons, 1982: 5–7.

41. Mullen JL, Buzby GP, Mathews DC, et al: Reduction of operative morbidity and mortality by combined preoperative and postoperative nutritional support. Ann Surg 1980; 192:604.

42. Grischkan D, Steiger E, Fazio V. Maintenance of home hyperalimentation in patients with high output jejunostomies. Arch Surg 1979; 114:838–841.

43. Sonneland J. The capture of fistulous fluids. Surgery 1866; 3:598–599.

44. MacFarlane M, Frawley JE. A technique for drainage of enterocutaneous fistulas. Surg Gynecol Obstet 1975; 1141:263–264.

45. Suriyapa C, Anderson MC. A simple device to control drainage from enterocutaneous fistulas. Surgery 1971; 70:455–458.

46. Herrera-Fernandez F, Cifuentes-Leon E, Leon-Paz J. Technique to temporarily re-establish continuity in a jejunal fistula. Am J Surg March 1982; 143:386.

47. Sterza GA, Laing BJ, Gilsdorf RB. Management of enterocutaneous fistulas and problem stomas with silicone casting of the abdominal wall defect. Am J Surg 1977; 134:772–776.

48. Todd IP, Saunders B. Care of fistulous stomata. Br Med J 1971; 4:747–748.

49. Fischer JF. The management of high-output intestinal fistulas. Adv Surg 1975; 9:139.

50. DiCostanzo J, Cano N, Martin J. Somatostatin in persistent gastrointestinal fistula treated by TPN. (Letter.) Lancet 1982; 2:338–339.

51. Hamilton RF, Davis WC, Stephenson DV, et al. Effects of parenteral hyperlimentation on upper gastrointestinal tract secretions. Arch Surg 1971; 102:340–352.

52. No entry.

53. Wolfe BM, Keltner RM, Willman VL. Intestinal fistula output in regular, elemental and intravenous alimentation. Am J Surg 1972; 124:803.

54. Bury KD, Stephens RV, Randall HT. Use of a chemically defined, liquid, elemental tract. Am J Surg 1971; 121:174–183.

55. Silberman H, Granson M, Fong G, et al. Management of external gastrointestinal fistulas with glucose and lipids. Surg Gynecol Obstet 1980; 150:856–858.

56. Copeland EM, Dudrick SJ. Nutritional aspects of cancer. Curr Prob Cancer 1976; 1(3):3–51.

57. Copeland EM, MacFadyen BV, Dudrick SJ. Intravenous hyperalimentation in cancer patients. J Surg Research 1974; 16:241–247.

58. Copeland EM, Souchon EA, MacFadyen BV, et al. Intravenous hyperalimentation as an adjunct to radiation therapy. Cancer 1977; 39:609–616.

59. Thomas RJS. The response of patients with fistulas of the gastrointestinal tract to parenteral nutrition. Surg Gynecol Obstet 1981; 153:77–80.

60. Irving M. Assessment and management of external fistulas in Crohn's disease. Br J Surg 1983; 70:233–236.

61. Shike M, Jeejeebhoy KN. Low output cardiac failure in a woman with Crohn's disease receiving long-term total parenteral nutrition. Clinical Pathological Conference. Gastroenterology 1980; 78:605–619.

62. Driscoll RH, Rosenberg IH. Total parenteral nutrition in inflammatory bowel disease. Med Clin North Am 1978; 62:185–201.

63. Mullen JL, Hargrove WC, Dudrick SJ, et al. Ten years experience with intravenous hyperalimentation and inflammatory bowel disease. Ann Surg 1978; 187:523–529.

64. Grant JP. Handbook of Total Parenteral Nutrition. Philadelphia, WB Saunders, 1980: 36.

65. Greenberg GR, Haber GB, Jeejeebhoy KN. Total parenteral nutrition (TPN) and bowel rest in the management of Crohn's disease. Gut 1976; 12:828.

66. Elson CO, Layden TJ, Nemchausky BA, et al. An evaluation of total parenteral nutrition in the management of inflammatory bowel disease. Dig Dis Sci 1980; 25:42–48.

67. Eisenberg HW, Turnbull RB, Weakly FL. Hyperalimentation as preparation for surgery in transmural colitis. Dis Colon Rectum 1974; 71:469–475.

68. Fischer JE, Foster GS, Abel RM, et al. Hyperalimentation as primary therapy for inflammatory bowel disease. Am J Surg 1973; 125:165–175.

69. Kaminsky VM, Deitel M: Nutritional support in the management of external fistulas of the alimentary tract. Br J Surg 1975; 62:100.

70. Bender HW, Sebor J, Zuidema GD. Serosal patch grafting for closure of posterior duodenal defects. Am J Surg 1968; 115:103.

71. Keller TB. The serosal patch: A surgical parachute. Am J Surg 1973; 126:186.

72. Ujiki GT, Shields TW. Roux-en-Y operation in the management of postoperative fistulae. Arch Surg 1981; 116:614.

73. Musicant ME, Thompson JC. The emergency management of lateral duodenal fistula by pancreaticoduodenectomy. Surg Gynecol Obstet 1969; 128:108.

74. Sternquist JC, Bubrick MP, Hitchcock CR. Enterocutaneous fistula. Dis Colon Rectum 1979; 21:578–581.

75. Zera RT, Bubrick MP, Sternquist JC, et al. Enterocutaneous fistulas: effects of total parenteral nutrition and surgery. Dis Colon Rectum 1983; 26:109–112.

76. Oakley JR, Steiger E, Lavery IC, et al. Catastrophic enterocutaneous fistulae. The role of home hyperalimentation. Clev Clin Q 1979; 46(4):133–136.

77. Byrne WJ, Burke M, Fonkalsrud EW, et al. Home parenteral nutrition: an alternative approach to the management of complicated gastrointestinal fistulas not responding to conventional medical or surgical therapy. JPEN 1979; 3:355–359.

14

SHORT BOWEL SYNDROME

K.N. JEEJEEBHOY

Resection of small intestine becomes necessary in a variety of situations including those resulting from congenital abnormalities, trauma, inflammation, vascular insufficiency, and tumors. Frequent causes of bowel resection include Crohn's disease in young individuals and intestinal infarction in the elderly.

When short lengths of the small bowel are resected, there is little disturbance of bowel function, especially if the ileocecal junction is left intact. This ability to resect small intestine without disturbance of function is mainly due to the great degree of intestinal reserve in normal humans. In addition, even if intestine is resected in lengths that compromise absorption, adaptation of the remaining bowel increases function and restores the ability to absorb normally. However, when over 50 per cent of the bowel has been resected, impairment of absorption tends to be prolonged or permanent. The degree of malnutrition that results from bowel resection is, however, a function of a number of factors, so that simply knowing how much bowel has been resected is not sufficient to predict functional disability.

In any individual patient with bowel resection, the physician may be called upon to provide a range of nutritional support regimens depending upon the site and length of resection, the degree of adaptation, and existing disease. Thus support will change, as over time adaptation of the bowel proceeds.

NORMAL ABSORPTION AND MOTILITY OF THE SMALL INTESTINE

In order to understand the effects of resection it is necessary to review certain aspects of small bowel function that are relevant to the subsequent clinical effects of resection.

Motility. After a meal is eaten its transit through the bowel depends upon a complex relationship between the different areas of the gastrointestinal tract modulating gastric, small bowel, and colonic motility.

Gastric Emptying. The nature of the chyme entering the small intestine affects gastric emptying. In general, ingestion of nutrients, especially fat but also proteins and to a lesser extent carbohydrates, inhibits gastric emptying. Inhibition of gastric emptying depends upon stimulation not only of duodenal receptors but also of receptors that extend along the intestine, so that experimental reinfusion of chyme collected from the duodenum into the jejunoileum inhibits gastric motility. Furthermore, with a larger meal, inhibition is prolonged.[1]

Small Intestinal Motility. Small bowel transit has been studied by the use of nonabsorbable isotopes.[2] These studies have shown the striking effect of the ileum in slowing transit. The marker traverses the first 50 per cent of the bowel in one third of the time it takes to pass through the next 30 per cent. In humans, Connell[3] has also shown that passage of chyme through the jejunum is strikingly faster than through the distal intestine.

Ileocecal Valve. The nature of this valve and its control of intestinal motility is controversial; however, it appears that when the ileum is resected, removal of the valve markedly accelerates small bowel transit, and its reconstruction decreases diarrhea and fluid losses.[4,5]

Colonic Motility. Motility of the gastrointestinal tract is slowest at the level of the colon. Mean transit time through the colon varies widely (between 24 and 150 hours), depending on the fat and fiber content of the diet eaten. Thus the colon is very important in slowing intestinal transit.

Interdigestive Motility and Secretion. The stomach and small bowel become active periodically in the NPO (nil per os) state, and are swept by waves of electrical activity called interdigestive migratory myoelectrical complexes. During these episodes there is significant secretion of bile and pancreatic juice,[6] which may reach 30 per cent of the maximum.

Secretion and Absorption of Fluid and Electrolytes. The small bowel receives a total of 5 to 6 L of endogenous secretions per day, including about 1 L each of saliva and bile and 1.5 to 3 L of gastric and pancreatic juices. All of this, except for about 1 L, is absorbed in the small intestine, the site of this function depending upon the nature of the meal eaten. With a meat and salad meal, most of it is absorbed high in the jejunum, whereas with a milk and doughnut meal there is greater water secretion into the bowel and more is absorbed distally.[7]

The absorption of fluid and electrolytes is significantly different in the three major areas of the intestine, namely jejunum, ileum, and colon. These differences depend partly on the nature of the electrolyte transport processes and partly on the permeability of the intercellular spaces. An understanding of these differences is crucial to recognizing the differences in the effect of resecting proximal versus distal bowel and the role of the colon in patients with intestinal resection.

In general, water absorption is a passive process resulting from the active transport of nutrients and electrolytes. Among electrolytes, the transport of sodium is the main process that aids the creation of an electrochemical gradient across the mucosa and also drives the uptake of sugars and amino acids.

There are two main processes that result in the absorption of sodium and chloride. The first is coupled to the absorption of carbohydrates and amino acids, and the second is isotonic sodium chloride absorption. The first process dominates in the jejunum,[8] whereas the second is of importance in the ileum[9] and colon.

These mechanisms aid in transporting electrolytes across the intestinal epithelium and, because sodium transport is closely coupled to sugar and amino acid transport, they also aid in the absorption of nutrients. However, the net effect on intraluminal contents depends not only on absorption, but also upon back-diffusion through the intercellular junctions. In the jejunum these junctions are "leaky," and thus back-diffusion readily occurs, resulting in the maintenance of isotonicity of jejunal contents. In contrast, the ileal and colonic junctions progressively increase in "tightness," so that back-diffusion occurs less readily in these areas, allowing the intraluminal contents to become concentrated with respect to plasma and so conserving fluid gained from the lumen.

Nutrient Digestion and Absorption. Partly digested gastric contents are mixed with pancreatic secretions and bile in the duodenum. These secretions aid in the digestion of all major nutrients—carbohydrate, protein, and fat. The products of hydrolysis of triglycerides, beta-monoglycerides, and free fatty acids, together with fat-soluble vitamins, are finely dispersed in particles called micelles, which are made up of bile salts. These products of digestion are absorbed by the jejunum, and what remains unabsorbed is taken up by the ileum. Under normal circumstances in humans, absorption of nutrients is completed within the first 150 cm of the bowel.[10] Thus in the normal individual very little nutrient reaches the ileum.

Unique Functions of the Ileum. The ileum is concerned with the absorption of vitamin B_{12} and of bile salts. These functions are unique to this segment of the small intestine and have special implications in patients with ileal resection. Inadequate absorption of bile salts in the ileum results in altered digestion and absorption of fat in the jejunum. Normally the synthesis of bile salts does not equal the demand that fat digestion imposes on it. This need is met instead by ileal reabsorption of bile salts, which are then recycled into the jejunum. With ileal resection, bile salts are no longer recycled and synthesis increases. However, if the loss is total, synthesis never increases sufficiently to meet the needs of the whole day.

Under these circumstances bile salt synthesis adds to the bile salt pool during the night, when the bowel is quiescent, and the first meal of the day results in the bile that has been stored overnight becoming available for digestion of fat. However, since reabsorption is minimal, the bile salt pool is depleted, and fat in the subsequent meals is poorly absorbed. In addition, the malabsorption of bile acids in patients with ileal resection results in an increased load of bile salts entering the colon, so that absorption of water and sodium in the colon is reduced. The deoxy bile acids also cause fluid secretion, thus enhancing fluid and electrolyte losses from the colon.

EFFECTS OF INTESTINAL RESECTION ON MOTILITY

Gastric Motility. It was indicated earlier that the presence of nutrients in the small intestine inhibits gastric motility, and thus it is not surprising that small bowel resection increases the rate of gastric emptying.[11]

Small Bowel Motility. Since the motility of the jejunum is rapid and that of the distal ileum slow, proximal bowel resection alone does not result in an increased rate of intestinal transit.[11] In contrast, after ileal resection, the remaining bowel has a very rapid transit rate.[11,12] When the remaining bowel is the jejunum, ^{51}Cr fed as a marker is almost completely excreted within a few hours.[13]

Colonic Motility. The colon is the area of the intestinal tract with the slowest motility. Thus the presence of an intact colon is important in maintaining a transit rate that is close to normal. Consequently distal resections that include the colon tend to increase the rate of intestinal transit.

EFFECTS OF INTESTINAL RESECTION ON ABSORPTION OF FLUID AND ELECTROLYTES

The effect of intestinal resection on fluid and electrolyte absorption will depend upon both the extent and the site of resection. As long as the colon is intact, diarrhea is minimal. Fluid and electrolyte losses will not be excessive, unless (1) the fluid load delivered to the colon following small bowel resection exceeds its reserve capacity, or (2) the contents of the small intestinal dejecta entering the colon inhibit colonic absorption. Normally the reserve capacity of the colon is about 5 L per day,[14] but both bile salts[15] and free fatty acids[16] alter the ability of the colon to absorb water and sodium. Furthermore, certain forms of vegetable residue and carbohydrate can be degraded by colonic bacteria into titratable acids, which also increase osmotic load and water output.[17,18]

Thus proximal resection results in little diarrhea because the ileum can reabsorb the increased fluid and electrolyte load, and any remaining excess is taken up by the colon. The reabsorption of bile salts by intact ileum causes the colon to receive very few substances capable of impeding water and electrolyte absorption. In contrast, when the ileum is resected, the colon receives a larger fluid load because the

contents not only are isotonic but also contain substances (bile salts, fatty acids, unabsorbed carbohydrate) that reduce the reabsorption of water and electrolytes, resulting in diarrhea.

If the colon is partially or completely resected, the area of bowel capable of taking over the fluid and electrolyte absorption of the resected small bowel is lost. The importance of the colon in modulating the severity of diarrhea following resection has been emphasized in several publications.[19,20] If both ileum and colon are resected, patients are left with bowel that cannot concentrate luminal contents. In such patients isotonic water and salt loss is a major problem, resulting in dehydration, hypokalemia, and hypomagnesemia.

EFFECTS OF RESECTION ON NUTRIENT ABSORPTION

Absorption of nutrient occurs throughout the small bowel, so that removal of the jejunum alone results in a takeover by the ileum of the absorptive function and little malabsorption.[21] In contrast, resections which exceed 100 cm of ileum cause steatorrhea.[22] The degree of malabsorption increases with increasing length of resection,[23] and a variety of nutrients are malabsorbed.[13,24] Thus the effect of malabsorption on the nutritional status of the patient increases with increasing resection. Balance studies of energy absorption by bomb calorimetry and fecal fat estimation have shown that the absorptions of fat and carbohydrate are equally reduced to between 50 and 75 per cent of the intake.[13] By contrast, in another group of patients studied,[23] nitrogen absorption was also reduced, but to a lesser extent, not only averaging 81 per cent of the intake but in addition being significantly higher than the corresponding energy absorption in any given patient.

In a study by Ladefoged et al.,[24] the degree of calcium, magnesium, and zinc absorption was depressed but did not correlate with the remaining length of bowel, which varied from 30 to 200 cm. The median calcium, phosphorus, magnesium, and zinc absorptions were 8, 32, −2, and −7 per cent of their respective intakes. Thus in these patients it was recommended that parenteral replacement be mandatory. Of the eight patients studied by Woolf et al.,[13] four required parenteral supplementation. The data taken as a whole suggest that energy and nitrogen needs are easier to meet by increasing oral intake than are needs for divalent ions and electrolytes. A review of the literature indicates that while there is considerable variability, resections of up to 33 per cent result in no malnutrition and those of up to 50 per cent can be tolerated without special aids. However, when the extent of resection exceeds 75 per cent of the bowel, nutritional status cannot be maintained without special help.[25–29] When resection results in only some centimeters of jejunum remaining, survival is limited and survivors are often depleted nutritionally.[30–35]

Adaptation of the Small Intestine. Following resection, the remaining small intestine hypertrophies and also increases its absorptive function. Flint was the first to demonstrate that following small bowel resection in humans, a significant increase in villus height occurred, and he computed that the area of the absorptive surface had increased fourfold.[36] Since then, there have been studies in humans[37] and in animal models[38,39] demonstrating this phenomenon.

Associated with anatomical changes, there is an improvement in absorption in animals[40] and humans.[41] The morphological effects following resection seem to be mediated by an increase in cell proliferation[42,43] and by cell migration up the villus. The increased rate of proliferation appears to result from an increase in the size of the crypt zone, where cell replication occurs.[43,44] Morphological changes may then be responsible for the functional compensation, but in addition, each cell may also show changes in the form of increased Na-K ATPase activity.[45]

There are several possible causes of these functional and morphological changes. They can be grouped into four major categories: increased work load of the remaining bowel, local nutrition, the effect of endogenous secretion such as bile and pancreatic juice, and hormonal effects.

When ileum, which is normally not exposed to a large nutrient load, is transposed to the area of the jejunum, then hypertrophy occurs.[46] Such an effect could be due to increased local nutrition or to increased work load. Studies instilling NaCl, lactose, and alpha-methyl glucoside into intestinal sacs have shown that these non-nutrient agents, which are transported by the mucosa, are effective in promoting cell proliferation.[47] This supports the concept that increased functional demand rather than local nutrition is important for adaptation. Furthermore, since enterally fed amino acids are not taken up by the crypt cell, where stimulation would be expected to occur,[48] it is unlikely that orally fed amino acids would stimulate mucosal protein synthesis at the site of cell proliferation. In fact, parenterally administered amino acids are take up by crypt cells. The role of endogenous secretions in promoting villus hypertrophy has been demonstrated in experiments in which transportation of the duodenal papilla into the ileum resulted in ileal hyperplasia.[49] Finally, humoral factors have been suggested by observations in parabiotic animals, in which intestinal resection in one of the pair resulted in hyperplasia of the intestine of the other.[50] An interesting candidate hormone suggested by observations in the human is enteroglucagon.[51]

NUTRITIONAL TREATMENT OF INTESTINAL RESECTION

Based on the considerations already discussed, the approach to a patient with intestinal resection depends on the extent of resection, the presence of continuing intestinal disease that reduces the functional length of the intestine, the site of resected bowel, and time for adaptation. The progress of the patient with time will lead to modifications of therapy. However, there are a variety of therapeutic avenues applicable to all patients. First these general approaches are considered, and then the specific applications are discussed.

General Therapeutic Approaches

Initial Treatment after Resection: Control of Diarrhea. Diarrhea is due to a combination of increased secretions, increased mobility, and osmotic stimulation of water secretion due to malabsorption of luminal contents. Initially diarrhea is controlled by keeping the patient NPO to reduce any osmotic component. With massive secretion even when the patient is NPO, there may be substantial fluid losses due to gastric hypersecretion and malabsorbed endogenous secretions stimulated by interdigestive migratory myoelectric complexes. Reduction of secretion, especially gastric secretion, can be effected by infusing H_2 blockers. The author prefers to give the H_2 blocker initially as a continuous IV infusion (cimetidine, 300 mg over 6 hours) rather than as a bolus because of its short half-life. In addition, the use of opiates aids in slowing intestinal propulsion and in increasing ion transport.[52] Loperamide, which acts locally, should be tried in increasing doses. If loperamide is ineffective, codeine or diphenoxylate may be used instead.

Oral Feeding. The next consideration is to determine the nature and amount of oral feeds. The degree of concern and the rigor of these measures depend upon the extent of bowel resected. In patients who have more than 60 to 80 cm (>15 to 20 per cent of normal length[53,54]) of bowel remaining, refeeding should be progressive with a view ultimately to feeding a normal or modified oral diet. By contrast, in patients who have no small bowel except the duodenum, the initial target should be small liquid feeds. With those having intermediate lengths of bowel, progressive feeding should be attempted with the following plan. Initially isotonic flavored carbohydrate-electrolyte feeds should be given. These feeds contain a mixture of glucose polymer (Caloreen) 3.4 per cent, Na^+ 85 mEq/L, K^+ 12 mEq/L, HCO_3^- 9 mEq/L, and Cl^- 109 mEq/L. A similar mixture has been shown to be well absorbed by patients with massive resection who were previously dependent on intravenous fluids.[55]

The next stage is to decide whether attempts are to be made to feed a normal diet or to use artificial (defined-formula) diets. Here again, where resection leaves the patient with more than 60 to 80 cm of small intestine, a normal oral diet should be tried. When trying such feeds, the patient is given dry solids, with isotonic fluids given 1 hour after the meal. The separation of solids from liquids is important in view of the marked increase in speed of gastric emptying noted with resection. Using this approach, we have found that the fat content of the diet fed made no difference to the diarrhea or to the total malabsorption in patients with massive resection.[13]

Data from Woolf et al.[13] and from Ladefoged et al.[24] suggest that electrolyte and divalent ion replacement may be required parenterally in order to meet requirements even when the oral intake of calories and nitrogen is sufficient to meet needs. It is recommended that this caloric intake be estimated roughly as 32 kcal/kg/day of ideal body weight and that an oral intake of about 1.5 to 2 times this amount be the goal for patients who have lost 50 per cent or more of their bowel. Intake obviously has to be increased so as to reach the target gradually, depending on tolerance and degree of diarrhea. Parenteral supplementation is given to provide what is estimated to be lacking in intake. For example, if the oral intake is 40 kcal/kg/day, it can be assumed that about 20 kcal/kg/day is absorbed, and 12 kcal/kg/day needs to be given intravenously. It is recommended that electrolyte supplementation by the parenteral route be 9 to 11 mmol Ca^{++}, 7 to 15 mmol Mg^{++}, and 70 to 100 μmol Zn^{++}, together with 150 to 200 mmol Na^+ and 60 to 100 mmol K^+, depending on losses. As the intestine adapts, it is possible to supplement by mouth and reduce parenteral intake. This ability to reduce or stop parenteral feeding differs among individuals. Also, it should be recognized that minor illnesses can precipitate electrolyte and divalent ion deficiency by increasing diarrhea and causing anorexia. Hence a safety factor should be taken into account for each patient when parenteral support is withdrawn.

In contrast, patients who fail to tolerate a normal diet as indicated above and those with a very short bowel should be given a constant infusion of defined-formula diet. The important consideration here is the use of controlled, well-modulated rates of infusion, starting with a diluted diet infused at 25 ml/hour and gradually increasing to one that is full strength at 100 to 125 ml/hour. This procedure ensures that the intestine receives an osmotic load at a constant rate. Furthermore, the rate is modulated depending upon the tolerance of the bowel. Using this approach, we have found that patients who would otherwise need intravenous feeding can be managed entirely by the oral route.

Parenteral Electrolytes and Nutrients

Initially all patients need intravenous fluid and electrolyte replacement, especially sodium chloride, potassium, and magnesium. These are infused to meet needs as judged on the basis of urine flow (with a target of exceeding 1 L/day), normal serum electrolyte levels, central venous pressure, and blood pressure. In particular, there should be no postural drop in blood pressure when hydration is adequate.

The intravenous infusion is gradually decreased as the oral intake is enhanced to meet all needs orally, but this may require many weeks of adaptation.

Parenteral Nutrition. In patients in whom remaining small bowel is less than 60 to 80 cm, parenteral nutrition should be started at once to avoid the development of malnutrition while oral refeeding is being attempted. Again parenteral nutrient intake can be gradually reduced as oral intake increases. Often progress is toward the use of only electrolytes parenterally, while other nutrient requirements are met orally. During the administration of parenteral nutrition, an area that is often neglected is the provision of trace elements. We have noted that with small bowel resection and severe diarrhea the need for zinc increases to between 12 and 15 mg/day because of endogenous losses.[56] These are computed by measuring the volume of intestinal fluid lost per day in the NPO state and adding 12 to 13 mg of Zn^{++} for every liter of such loss.

Long-Term Nutritional Support

This is a dynamic process which should be re-evaluated as the patient adapts. There are four stages in this process: (1) discharge on normal or modified oral diet, separating solids from liquids; (2) use of defined-formula diets on an ambulatory basis; (3) oral diet as above with parenterally administered electrolytes and fluids; and (4) total or partial parenteral nutrition with variable oral intake.

The aim should be to progress up the options toward the first in the above list. However, it is important to use a system that, although allowing the patient to maintain normal nutritional status, is free of serious diarrhea so as to allow the patient to work and to become socially rehabilitated. For example, it is possible for patients to eat 10 to 12 meals a day, have a similar number of bowel movements, including nocturnal movements, and remain free from parenteral support. However, life for such a person is an oral-anal existence that leaves little time for rehabilitation. The option chosen must avoid such an outcome and permit social and work rehabilitation. The availability of the options of home enteral[57] and parenteral nutrition[58-60] have revolutionized the outlook for such patients.

Special Considerations Depending on Length and Site of Resection

Jejunal Resection, Leaving Intact Ileum and Colon. Patients with this type of resection can be fed immediately and rarely have any problems.

Ileal Resection <100 cm, Colon Largely Intact. Patients with this type of resection have so-called choleraic diarrhea and are best managed with the use of cholestyramine to bind the bile salts, 4 g three times a day. A vitamin B_{12} absorption study should be done, and if the results are abnormal, parenteral vitamin B_{12} should be given, 200 μg per month. Such patients may also have hyperoxaluria[61] because of enhanced colonic absorption of oxalate. They need both a low-oxalate diet and cholestyramine. Since bile salts enhance colonic oxalate absorption, the use of cholestyramine is useful in reducing it.

Ileal Resection 100 to 200 cm, Colon Largely Intact. After this type of resection patients have little difficulty in maintaining nutrition with an oral diet, but have problems because of bile salts entering the colon and causing steatorrhea with fatty acid diarrhea. In such patients, cholestyramine and a fat-restricted diet are useful. As well, they should receive dietary advice about eating dry meals and separating solids from liquids to reduce diarrhea. Hyperoxaluria and vitamin B_{12} malabsorption should be treated as indicated earlier.

Resection >200 cm of Small Bowel and Lesser Resection Associated with Colectomy. Patients with either of these resections need the graduated adaptation program indicated under general considerations earlier, and they will need different regimens depending upon the amount of bowel left and rate of adaptation.

Resection Leaving <60 cm of Small Bowel and Those with Only a Duodenum. Following these extensive resections, patients need parenteral nutrition at home on an indefinite basis. The infusion rate and caloric intake are gradually reduced as the patient becomes able to maintain his weight, as on an oral diet. The judgment as to when to reduce intravenous feeding is made from the observation that weight gain is occurring beyond desired limits and that reduced infusion does not result in electrolyte and fluid imbalance.

Remaining Problems

The question of oral micronutrients and vitamin absorption after intestinal resection is an area that needs further study. While macronutrient requirements can easily be judged by body composition, micronutrient needs and the requirement for oral supplementation have yet to be precisely defined.

References

1. Malagelada J-R. Gastric, pancreatic and biliary response to a meal. *In* Johnson LR (ed). Physiology of the Gastrointestinal Tract. New York, Raven Press, 1981: 893–924.
2. Summers RW, Kent TH, Osborne JW. Effects of drugs, ileal obstruction and irradiation on rat gastrointestinal propulsion. Gastroenterology 1970; 59:731–739.
3. Connell AM. Propulsion in the small intestine. Rend Gastroenterol 1970; 2:38–46.
4. Singelton AO, Redmond DC, McMurray JE. Ileocecal resection and small bowel transit and absorption. Ann Surg 1964; 159:690–694.
5. Ricotta J, Zuidema GD, Gadacz TR, et al. Construction of an ileocecal valve and its role in massive resection of the small intestine. Surg Gynecol Obstet 1981; 152:310–314.
6. Vantrappen GR, Peeters TL, Janssens J. The secretory component of the interdigestive migrating motor complexes in man. Scand J Gastroenterol 1979; 14:663–667.
7. Fordtran JS, Locklear TW. Ionic constituents and osmolality of gastric and small-intestinal fluids after eating. Am J Dig Dis 1966; 11:503–521.
8. Fordtran JS, Dietschy JM. Water and electrolyte movement in the intestine. Gastroenterology 1966; 50:263–285.
9. Turnberg DA, Bieberdorf RA, Morawski SG, et al. Interrelationships of chloride, bicarbonate, sodium and hydrogen transport in human ileum. J Clin Invest 1970; 49:557–567.
10. Borgstrom B, Dahlquist A, Lundh G, et al. Studies of intestinal digestion and absorption in the human. J Clin Invest 1957; 36:1521–1536.
11. Nylander G. Gastric evacuation and propulsive intestinal motility following resection of the small intestine in the rat. Acta Chir Scand 1967; 133:131–138.
12. Reynell PC, Spray GH. Small intestinal function in rat after massive resection. Gastroenterology 1956; 31:361–368.
13. Woolf GM, Jeejeebhoy KN. Diet for the patient with short bowel syndrome: high fat or high carbohydrate? Gastroenterology 1983; 84:823–828.
14. Debongnie JC, Phillips SF. Capacity of the colon to absorb fluid. Gastroenterology 1978; 74:698–703.
15. Hofmann AF, Poley JR. Cholestyramine treatment of diarrhea associated with ileal resection. N Engl J Med 1969; 281:397–402.
16. Binder HJ. Fecal fatty acids—mediators of diarrhea? Gastroenterology 1973; 65:847–850.
17. Williams RD, Olmsted WH. The effect of cellulose, hemicellulose and lignin on the weight of the stool: a contribution to the study of laxation in man. J Nutr 1936; 11:433–449.
18. Bond JH, Levitt MD. Fate of soluble carbohydrate in the colon of rats and man. J Nutr 1976; 57:1158–1164.
19. Cummings JH, James WPT, Wiggins HS. Role of the colon in ileal-resection diarrhea. Lancet 1973; 1:344–347.
20. Mitchell J, Zukerman L, Breuer RI. The colon influences ileal-resection diarrhea. (Abstract.) Gastroenterology 1977; 72:1103.
21. Booth CC, Aldis D, Read AE. Studies on the site of fat absorption. 2. Fat balances after resection of varying amounts of the small intestine in man. Gut 1961; 2:168–174.
22. Hofmann AF, Poley JR. Role of bile acid malabsorption in the pathogenesis of diarrhea and steatorrhea in patients with ileal resection. I. Response to cholestyramine or replacement of dietary long chain triglyceride by medium chain triglyceride. Gastroenterology 1972; 62:918–934.
23. Hylander E, Ladefoged K, Jarnum S. Nitrogen absorption following small intestinal resection. Scand J Gastoenterol 1980; 15:853–858.
24. Ladefoged K, Nicolaidou P, Jarnum S. Calcium, phosphorus, magnesium, zinc and nitrogen balance in patients with severe short bowel syndrome. Am J Clin Nutr 1980; 33:2137–2144.
25. Haymond HE. Massive resection of the small intestine: analysis of 257 collected cases. Surg Gynecol Obstet 1935; 61:693–705.
26. McClenahan JE, Fisher B. Physiologic effects of massive small intestinal resection and colectomy. Am J Surg 1950; 79:684–688.
27. Trafford HS. Outlook after massive resection of small intestine, with report of 2 cases. Br J Surg 1956; 44:10–13.
28. West ES, Montague JR, Judy FR. Digestion and absorption in man with 3 feet of small intestine. Am J Dig Dis 1938; 5:690–692.
29. Pilling GP, Cresson SL. Massive resection of the small intes-

tine in the neonatal period: report of 2 successful cases and review of the literature. Pediatrics 1957; *19*:940–948.

30. Martin JR, Pattee CJ, Gardner C, et al. Massive resection of small intestine. Can Med Assoc J 1953; *69*:429–433.

31. Kinney JM, Goldwyn RM, Barr JS Jr, et al. Loss of the entire jejunum and ileum and the ascending colon. Management of a patient. JAMA 1962; *179*:529–532.

32. Walker-Smith J. Total loss of mid-gut. Med J Aust 1967; *1*:857–860.

33. Clayton BE, Cotton DA. A study of malabsorption after resection of the entire jejunum and the proximal half of the ileum. Gut 1961; *2*:18–22.

34. Anderson CM. Long-term survival with six inches of small intestine. Br Med J 1965; *5432*:419–422.

35. Meyer HW. Sixteen-year survival following extensive resection of small and large intestine for thrombosis of the superior mesenteric artery. Surgery 1962; *51*:755–759.

36. Flint JM. The effect of extensive resection of the small intestine. Johns Hopkins Med J 1912; *23*:127–144.

37. Porus RL. Epithelial hyperplasia following massive small bowel resection in man. Gastroenterology 1965; *48*:753–757.

38. Booth CC, Evans KT, Menzies T, et al. Intestinal hypertrophy following partial resection of the small bowel in the rat. Br J Surg 1959; *46*:403–410.

39. Nygaard K. Resection of the small intestine in rats. III. Morphological changes in the intestinal tract. Acta Chir Scand 1967; *133*:233–248.

40. Stassoff B. Experimentelle Untersuchungen uber die kompensatorischen Vorange der Darmresektionen. Beits Klin Chir 1914; *89*:527–533.

41. Althausen TL, Doig RK, Uyeyama K, et al. Digestion and absorption after massive resection of small intestine; recovery of absorptive function as shown by intestinal absorption tests in 2 patients and consideration of compensatory mechanisms. Gastroenterology 1950; *16*:126–139.

42. Loran MR, Althausen TL. Cellular proliferation of intestinal epithelia in the rat two months after partial resection of the ileum. J Biophys Biochem Cytol 1960; *7*:667–672.

43. Obertop H, Nundy S, Malamud D, et al. Onset of cell proliferation in the shortened gut. Rapid hyperplasia after jejunal resection. Gastroenterology 1977; *72*:267–270.

44. Cairnie AB, Lamerton LF, Steel GG. Cell proliferation studies in the intestinal epithelium of the rat. I. Determination of the kinetic parameters. II. Theoretical aspect. Exper Cell Res 1965; *39*:528–553.

45. Tilson MD, Wright HK. Augmented ileal sodium and potassium stimulated adenosine triphosphatase after jejunal transposition. Surg Forum 1970; *21*:326–327.

46. Altmann GG, Leblond CP. Factors influencing villus size in the small intestine of adult rats as revealed by transposition of intestinal segments. Am J Anat 1970; *127*:15–36.

47. Clark RM. "Luminal nutrition" versus "functional work-load" as controllers of mucosal morphology and epithelial replacement in the rat small intestine. Digestion 1977; *15*:411–424.

48. Alpers DH. Protein synthesis in intestinal mucosa: the effect of the route of administration of precursor amino acids. J Clin Invest 1972; *51*:167–173.

49. Weser E, Heller R, Tawil T. Stimulation of mucosal growth in the rat ileum by bile and pancreatic secretions after jejunal resection. Gastroenterology 1977; *73*:524–529.

50. Williamson RCN, Buckholtz TW, Malt RA. Humoral stimulation of cell proliferation in the small bowel after transection and resection in rats. Gastroenterology 1978; *75*:249–254.

51. Gleeson MH, Bloom SR, Polak JM, et al. Endocrine tumour in kidney affecting small bowel structure, motility and absorptive function. Gut 1971; *12*:773–782.

52. McKay JS, Linaker BD, Turnberg MA. The influence of opiates on ion transport across rabbit ileal mucosa. Gastroenterology 1981; *80*:279–284.

53. Cook GC, Carruthers RH. Reaction of human small intestine to an intraluminal tube and its importance in jejunal perfusion studies. Gut 1974; *15*:545–548.

54. Gackman L, Hallberg D. Small-intestinal length. An intraoperative study in obesity. Acta Chir Scand 1974; *140*:57–63.

55. Griffin GE, Fagan EF, Hodgson AJ, et al. Enteral therapy in the management of massive gut resection complicated by chronic fluid or electrolyte depletion. Dig Dis Sci 1982; *27*:902–908.

56. Wolman SL, Anderson GH, Marliss EB, et al. Zinc in total parenteral nutrition: requirements and metabolic effects. Gastroenterology 1979; *76*:458–467.

57. Main ANH, Morgan RJ, Hall MJ, et al. Home enteral tube feeding with a liquid diet in the long term management of inflammatory bowel disease and intestinal failure. Scott Med J 1980; *25*:312–314.

58. Jeejeebhoy KN, Zohrab WJ, Langer B, et al. Total parenteral nutrition at home for 23 months, without complication and with good rehabilitation. A study of technical and metabolic features. Gastroenterology 1973; *65*:811–820.

59. Broviac JW, Scribner BH. Prolonged parenteral nutrition in the home. Surg Gynecol Obstet 1974; *139*:24–28.

60. Shils ME. A program for total parenteral nutrition at home. Am J Clin Nutr 1975; *28*:1429–1435.

61. Andersson H, Jagenburg R. Fat-reduced diet in the treatment of hyperoxaluria in patients with ileopathy. Gut 1974; *15*:360–366.

15

INFLAMMATORY BOWEL DISEASE

GORDON R. GREENBERG

Medical treatment of acute inflammatory bowel disease has traditionally relied upon bed rest, repletion of fluids and electrolytes, and high doses of corticosteroids. When this approach fails to achieve remission or when complications of the primary disease process arise, intestinal resection is generally considered to be the treatment of choice. However, in Crohn's disease significant recurrence rates are well recognized after surgery; indeed, with each successive operation the chance of reoperation rises and recurrences may develop faster.[1] In ulcerative colitis, surgery usually involves total colectomy and a permanent ileostomy or continent ileal reservoir.[2] Thus, any alternative form of therapy that might induce a clinical remission and avoid operation would clearly be an important advance in the therapeutic armamentarium for inflammatory bowel disease. Over the last 15 years, the use of parenteral and enteral nutritional support systems coupled with bowel rest has been the focus of much attention as a therapeutic option in the management of patients with inflammatory bowel disease. The broad rationale for utilizing this approach is twofold. Bowel rest through exclusion of standard oral diets should minimize secretory, transport, and motor activities of the diseased bowel, eliminate unwanted antigenic stimuli, and allow acute inflammation to resolve. Simultaneously, since all nutritional requirements are met, protein-calorie depletion that may be present and would rapidly progress on standard hypotonic intravenous solutions is avoided. Achieving protein anabolism and weight gain contributes to patient recovery, while the provision of essential nutrients facilitates repair of the diseased bowel. Notwithstanding initial encouraging reports, the value of nutritional support and bowel rest in the management of inflammatory bowel disease remains controversial.

NUTRITIONAL CONSEQUENCES OF INFLAMMATORY BOWEL DISEASE

Nutritional debilitation of considerable magnitude may occur in patients with inflammatory bowel disease. The major potential mechanisms include reduced dietary intake, enteric loss of nutrients, malabsorption, and the presence of active inflammation. These factors often act in concert, notably during phases of active inflammation, and can significantly influence morbidity and perhaps mortality.

Prolonged inadequate intake of calories orally as a consequence of anorexia or abdominal pain is one of the foremost mechanisms contributing to a compromised nutritional state, especially in children. Active mucosal inflammation and the accompanying diarrhea lead to substantial enteric losses of protein, blood, and minerals, particularly when there is colonic involvement, and also constitute a major mechanism for nutritional depletion. Malabsorption, however, occurs only in Crohn's disease and becomes significant when there is extensive small bowel involvement, after multiple resections, or when bacterial overgrowth is present. Increased energy expenditure associated with active inflammation has often been proposed as a further mechanism contributing to malnutrition, but recently this concept has been challenged. Chan et al.[3] reported that patients with active Crohn's disease have a resting energy expenditure, as determined by indirect calorimetry, that is not significantly different from the predicted energy expenditure for healthy subjects as estimated from the Harris-Benedict formula. No correlation was found between resting energy expenditure and disease activity. Although none of their patients had fever or sepsis, the magnitude of hypercatabolism even in this latter group appears to be substantially less than originally proposed. Baker et al.[4] noted that the actual resting energy expenditure, also determined by indirect calorimetry, in a group of critically ill patients with sepsis exceeded by only 15 per cent the estimated requirements derived from the Harris-Benedict formula. Taken together, these data suggest that increased energy expenditure as a direct consequence of the inflammatory process is at best a minor component contributing to nutritional depletion.

A broad spectrum of nutritional deficits may develop in patients with inflammatory bowel disease.[5] Weight loss is reported to occur in 20 to 75 per cent of patients, the incidence being dependent upon the severity of illness.[6,7] In active Crohn's disease, unlike starvation or anorexia nervosa, resting energy expenditure increases in relationship to the degree of weight loss. Barot et al.[8] found that Crohn's patients with weights less than 90 per cent of their ideal body weight had a higher energy expenditure per kilogram body weight than patients who were within 10 per cent of their ideal body weight. The mechanism accounting for this observation is not entirely clear, but one suggestion has been that underweight patients with Crohn's disease have a proportionally greater decrease in body fat with relative sparing of body cell mass (the total mass of metabolically active cells).[3] Reduced protein stores and low levels of serum albumin occur in 20 to 80 per cent of patients,[5] primarily as a consequence of increased enteric loss[9] and in part due to insufficient oral intake. Several additional nutritional derangements may develop in inflammatory bowel disease including: anemia due to iron, folate, and B_{12} loss and the effects of chronic active disease; electrolyte, mineral, and trace element depletion due largely to losses from diarrhea; and osteomalacia resulting from vitamin D deficiency, negative calcium balance, and the administration of corticosteroids. This global picture of macronutrient and micronutrient deficiency can lead to alterations in cellular immunity with increased risk of infection,[10,11] delayed wound healing and repair of inflamed tissues,[12] and growth retardation in children.[13]

Thus, in compromised patients with inflammatory bowel disease provision of nutritional support systems to meet the objective of restoring and maintaining lean body mass and energy stores appears well-founded. In this regard, it is pertinent to note that delivery of inordinate amounts of calories is not required to achieve this goal. Provision of 1 to 1.5 g/kg IBW/day of protein as a balanced amino acid mixture and a caloric input of 35 to 40 Kcal/kg IBW/day, equally divided as dextrose and lipid, will satisfy the energy requirements of most patients.[4,14]

THE CONCEPT OF BOWEL REST

In addition to providing nutritional support for the malnourished patient with inflammatory bowel disease, one of the proposed beneficial effects of either total parenteral nutrition or defined formula diets is the promotion of bowel rest by eliminating standard oral diets. It is therefore relevant to consider whether administration of these nutritional support systems meets the objective of minimizing stimulation of gastric, pancreatic exocrine, and motor functions.

Although total parenteral nutrition involves the delivery of a balanced input of protein as amino acids, calories as glucose and fat, electrolytes, trace elements, and vitamins, only the effects of macronutrients on gastrointestinal function have been studied in any detail. Administration of intravenous hypertonic dextrose sufficient to achieve hyperglycemia decreases pancreatic volume and enzyme secretion, as shown in patients with gastrointestinal fistulas arising from the pancreas.[15] Intravenous infusion of amino acids in humans has no effect on pancreatic bicarbonate or trypsin,[16,17] although a modest increase in gastric acid secretion by a gastrin-independent mechanism has been reported.[18] Similarly, in healthy subjects concentrations of Intralipid ranging from 5 to 20 per cent given intravenously do not significantly stimulate pancreatic bicarbonate or enzyme secretion, either alone or against a background of intravenous secretion.[19] The effects of intravenous nutrients on gastrointestinal motor activity have not been studied in humans, but in dogs the normal fasting pattern of cyclic migrating motor complexes is not altered by the administration of total parenteral nutrition.[20] In accord with these findings, a profile of several of the gastrointestinal hormones that are known to modulate gastric acid and pancreatic exocrine secretions as well as motor activity have been shown to remain at fasting basal plasma concentrations throughout a 24-hour period of total parenteral nutrition.[21] Therefore, the available evidence would indicate that intravenous nutrients as provided in TPN do not significantly stimulate gastrointestinal functions and supports the efficacy of these solutions as a therapeutic modality to achieve complete bowel rest.

Administration of defined-formula diets also facilitates bowel rest but not to the degree that is accomplished with total parenteral nutrition. Intrajejunal perfusion of these diets at doses sufficient to meet nutrient requirements evokes significant increments in pancreatic bicarbonate and enzyme secretion, which are paralleled by a rise in circulating plasma concentrations of cholecystokinin.[22] Indeed, sustained elevations have been observed of most circulating gut hormones to concentrations that can approach 70 per cent of the plasma levels observed following a normal diet.[23] Moreover, the normal cyclic motor activity occurring in the fasting state is disrupted and replaced by a pattern that is equivalent to that with oral feeding.[24] However, gastric acid secretion is lower than is observed after ingestion of standard oral diets, due in part to the elimination of the cephalic phase of acid secretion.[25,26]

Defined-formula diets are almost totally absorbed in the duodenum and proximal jejunum, with virtually no residue reaching the distal gut.[27] In this regard, it has been postulated that the etiology of Crohn's disease has two components, namely an underlying predisposition to ulceration of the gut and a secondary immunological reaction to the passage of foreign protein through the damaged gut wall.[28] It is the latter component that defined-formula diets and TPN are thought to treat by reducing or eliminating this protein, although the nature of the offending protein or proteins remains unidentified. Alterations in fecal flora, notably a reduction in enterococci, were initially described by Bounous and Devroede,[29] but subsequent studies[28,30] have been unable to confirm this finding. However, Harper et al.[31] recently demonstrated that exacerbations in disease activity can be initiated by the reintroduction of small bowel effluent into the defunctioned colon of Crohn's colitis patients treated by split ileostomy. The responsible agent appears to be larger than 0.22 microns, since ultrafiltrates of the fecal stream were without effect; the source is less clear, although dietary protein found in standard oral diets has been offered as one suggestion.[28] Whatever the exact factor, it is the medical bypass of fecal contents from

inflamed bowel achieved with either defined-formula diets or TPN that forms the basis for present concepts of the value of bowel rest in the management of inflammatory bowel disease.

Prolonged administration of TPN in animals is associated with subtotal villous atrophy of intestine[32] and reduced pancreatic exocrine function.[33] It is conceivable that similar morphological or functional alterations in humans also might occur within the gastrointestinal tract following a period of bowel rest, particularly with TPN. Kotler and Levine[34] did report on one patient who was found to have a decreased bicarbonate output in response to stimulation with intravenous secretin when studied after 2 years of home TPN. However, within 1 month of resumption of oral feedings, output had returned to normal levels. Notwithstanding the observation that TPN maintains all of the gastrointestinal hormones at fasting plasma concentrations, the subsequent gut and pancreatic endocrine hormonal responses to a standard meal in patients with Crohn's disease after 3 weeks of TPN are equivalent to plasma concentrations observed in healthy subjects.[21] Moreover, morphological recovery of atrophic jejunum in infants with protracted diarrhea has been demonstrated after 3 weeks of TPN.[35] Thus, in contrast to observations in animals, these data accord with the suggestion that in humans no long-term morphological or functional sequelae occur as a direct consequence of the administration of TPN or defined-formula diets.

NUTRITIONAL SUPPORT IN CROHN'S DISEASE

The clinical course of acute Crohn's disease may be quite different from that of ulcerative colitis. Spontaneous remissions and relapses tend to be observed more often in Crohn's disease, while, unlike ulcerative colitis, emergency surgery is an infrequent occurrence. Strictures and fistulas are more common complications of Crohn's disease, and multiple intestinal resections can result in a short bowel syndrome. Each of these settings contributes to progressive nutritional debilitation and may adversely affect clinical outcome. It is therefore preferable to consider the role of nutritional support and bowel rest in Crohn's disease independently of that of ulcerative colitis, although published series have frequently failed to make this distinction clear. Since total parenteral nutrition and defined-formula diets have each found their advocates in the management of acute inflammatory bowel disease, the clinical efficacy of these two modalities will be considered separately.

Total Parenteral Nutrition

Following the first preliminary report by Steiger et al.[36] on the successful outcome of patients with

Crohn's disease treated by TPN, several publications appeared reporting equally positive results. However, many of these studies are retrospective, nonrandomized reviews, often with small numbers of patients and inadequate follow-up. Moreover, documentation of the major end point, clinical remission with nutritional repletion, has frequently been imprecise. Although the heterogeneous nature of Crohn's disease complicates this task, the validity of clinical observations could be enhanced by the combined use of several different types of indices, as has been reported in certain more recent studies. These have included: a clinical index, such as the Crohn's Disease Activity Index,[37] which is derived primarily from subjective factors and perhaps more accurately should be designated an index of the quality of life rather than of disease activity; multiple laboratory indices of inflammation,[38] which include serum orosomucoid, one of the better indicators in the circulation of disease activity;[39] and the measurement of fecal granulocyte excretion by [111]indium granulocyte scanning, which is a specific measure of mucosal inflammation.[40] There is also the necessity for inclusion of more objective determinations of nutritional repletion. Frequently used parameters such as an increase in body weight or changes in anthropometric measures may not accurately reflect a gain in lean body mass, since both factors can record changes in tissue water. Precise methods of measuring body composition including analysis of total body nitrogen and potassium by neutron activation have been developed[41] but undertaken in only a small number of studies. Notwithstanding these limitations a composite analysis of results from retrospective and more recent prospective controlled trials, as summarized in Table 15–1, does allow for some insight into the indications and likely outcome of patients with Crohn's disease managed by TPN and bowel rest.

INDICATIONS

One of two reasons is usually given for undertaking nutritional support and bowel rest in patients with Crohn's disease. The first indication is for adjunctive therapy in the patient in whom surgery is already planned or in whom a complication has developed in the postoperative period. Here the emphasis is on the nutritional repletion provided with the aim of reducing postoperative morbidity. The second indication is for use of TPN as primary therapy in an attempt to achieve clinical remission and so avoid surgery, usually in the patient who has failed with conventional medical management including high-dose corticosteroids.

Evidence in support of TPN as adjunctive therapy to surgical management is only partially clarified. Protein-calorie malnutrition impairs wound healing and diminishes immunocompetence, thus increasing the risk of infection,[10–12] and each of these factors leads to increased morbidity and mortality in the postoperative period. Provision of TPN to meet patient requirements achieves weight gain and promotes nitrogen retention, but in functional terms the data are rather limited on whether these factors reduce the incidence of postoperative complications. Collins et al.[42] in a prospective study on patients undergoing proctocolectomy observed that provision of calories with amino acids resulted in a lower complication rate postoperatively than either the provision of amino acids alone or standard intravenous isotonic solutions. Further prospective, controlled data with specific reference to postoperative complication rates in patients with inflammatory bowel disease following TPN are lacking.

In a retrospective series initially reported by Eisenberg et al.[43] and subsequently updated by Fazio et al.[44] of 58 seriously ill malnourished patients with inflammatory bowel disease undergoing surgery, 51 were considered to have had their clinical course improved by the administration of TPN, but the incidence of postoperative complications was not stated. Rombeau et al.[45] came to similar conclusions in a retrospective, nonrandomized study of 33 matched patients with inflammatory bowel disease requiring surgery. Whereas postoperative complications developed in 5 of 11 patients receiving support for a mean of 1 day prior to surgery, only 1 of 22 patients provided with a mean of 12 days of TPN had a complicated postoperative course. It was concluded that a minimum of 5 days of preoperative TPN would reduce the incidence of both total and septic complications. However, as recently underscored by Heimann et al.,[46] nutritional depletion is only one of several factors that correlate with surgical outcome in patients with Crohn's disease. The extent of the operative procedure, the number of previous operations, and the necessity for ileostomy also play major roles in determining postoperative complication rates, particularly those that include sepsis. The relative importance of these additional factors when compared with nutritional depletion requires clarification.

Thus, there are some initial indications that TPN is an effective modality for preparing nutritionally depleted patients prior to surgery, and for maintaining postoperative nutritional status, and perhaps contributes to a reduction in postoperative complications. Further randomized, prospective trials that encompass both improved techniques of nutritional assessment and identification of patient subgroups prone to major surgical complications are required to confirm this impression.

The role of TPN as primary therapy in the management of patients with active Crohn's disease continues to be the subject of some debate. Several considerations arise initially in attempting to achieve a balanced perspective from the published literature. First is the concern frequently raised regarding what constitutes an appropriate control group. Most

TABLE 15–1. Total Parenteral Nutrition in Crohn's Disease

Series	No. of Patients	Clinical Remission in Hospital			Long-Term Remission			Length of Follow-up (Months)
Retrospective								
Anderson (1973)[56]	8	7 (88%)			1 (13%)			3
Fischer (1973)[47]	7	3 (43%)			nr			nr
Vogel (1974)[49]	8	8 (100%)			4 (50%)			4–48
Eisenberg (1974)[43]	46	nr			nr			nr
Reilly (1976)[48]	23	14 (61%)			nr			nr
Dean (1976)[54]	11	4 (36%)			nr			nr
Harford (1978)[50]	30*	23 (77%)			4/21 (19%)			27
Mullen (1978)[55]	50	19 (38%)			nr			nr
Milewski (1980)[52]	7	2 (29%)			nr			nr
Bos (1980)[51]	86	24 (28%)			7 (8%)			10–48
Houcke (1980)[58]	36	27 (75%)			22 (61%)			4–24
Holm (1981)[59]	8	7 (88%)			7 (88%)			4–48
Shiloni (1983)[53]	9	9 (100%)			6 (67%)			6–36
Ostro (1985)[62]	100	77 (77%)			50/93 (54%)			12
Prospective								
Elson (1980)[60]	20	13 (65%)			8 (40%)			12
Greenberg (1981)[61]	43	33 (77%)			29 (67%)			24
Muller (1983)[63]	30	25 (83%)			17 (57%)			3–48
Prospective, Controlled		*Controls*		*TPN*	*Controls*		*TPN*	
Dickinson (1980)[41]	9	3/3 (100%)		4/6 (67%)	0/3 (0%)		1/6 (17%)	12
Lochs (1983)[70]	20	6/10 (60%)		6/10 (60%)	6/10 (60%)		5/10 (50%)	12
Greenberg (1985)[71]	32†	9/15 (60%)		12/17 (71%)	6/15 (40%)		8/17 (47%)	12
McIntyre (1986)[69]	16	5/7 (71%)		9/9 (100%)	2/7 (29%)		3/9 (33%)	27–64
TOTALS	564‡	326 (58%)						

*Data combined with report of Fazio et al.[44]

†Control group comprised of 15 patients on partial parenteral nutrition and oral diet; does not include 19 patients randomized to elemental diet.

‡Total does not include controls.

nr, not reported.

often, the major objective of TPN when used as primary therapy is a sustained clinical remission in patients resistant to other medical therapy, notably corticosteroids. In this clinical setting, TPN is initiated in conjunction with ongoing administration of corticosteroids, since abrupt cessation of the drug is usually not possible. Although patients are considered to be their own controls, this experimental design has the limitation of not strictly providing an independent assessment of the value of TPN. An alternative approach has been the prospective comparison of the efficacy of TPN versus corticosteroids, but this also does not entirely solve the problem of a suitable control population. Corticosteroids have proven efficacy in the management of acute Crohn's disease[37] and are much simpler and cheaper to deliver than complicated nutritional support systems. Most importantly, the medical therapy of drug-resistant patients is not addressed. To date, no study of TPN has been undertaken that entirely solves the dilemma of an adequate control group for Crohn's patients in whom medical treatment has failed.

A second consideration is the outcome of patients receiving TPN as primary therapy. Not only must there be adequate documentation of short-term in-hospital remission rates, but equally important is the long-term outcome or quality of life for such patients, particularly in comparison with the usual therapeutic alternative, surgical resection. The influence on remission rates of disease location and the presence of specific complications, notably fistulas, are further considerations that requires specific emphasis. Finally, the question arises as to whether bowel rest, often regarded as a critical component of primary TPN therapy, is indeed a prerequisite for attaining clinical remission. Each of these aspects will be considered in turn.

Outcome

In 1973, Fischer et al.[47] were the first to report on a small group of 7 patients with Crohn's disease managed with total parenteral nutrition as primary therapy; they observed a 43 per cent in-hospital remission rate. This series was expanded in an update by Reilly et al.,[48] where 14 of 23 Crohn's patients (61 per cent) had remissions while on TPN in hospital. No detailed follow-up was provided in either report. However, initial indications that in-hospital remission rates achieved with TPN might not be sustained in all patients were provided in a retrospective review by Vogel et al.[49] Although all of 8 patients with Crohn's disease receiving TPN as primary therapy were discharged from hospital in clinical remission, only 3 patients remained well after 4 to 24 months of follow-up.

One of the larger retrospective series lending some support to this conclusion was undertaken by Fazio and colleagues and compiled in two separate publications.[44,50] The in-hospital remission rate and outcome in 19 patients with Crohn's disease treated by TPN as primary therapy and a further 48 Crohn's patients provided TPN as adjunctive therapy prior to planned surgery were described. In the first group receiving TPN as primary therapy 12 of 19 patients achieved clinical remission; in the second group, 11 of 48 patients also had remission and avoided surgery. In total, 23 patients with Crohn's disease were therefore considered to have received TPN as primary therapy, and 21 were available for follow-up. The relapse rate was substantial, as 14 patients (67 per cent) ultimately required surgical intervention with a mean interval of 10 months between their course of TPN and operation. Several subsequent retrospective series, in which TPN was administered for periods ranging from 3 to 6 weeks, also emphasize good nutritional repletion and frequently a rapid reduction in symptoms; however, there is considerable variation in the in-hospital remission rates and particularly in the long-term outcome.[51–59] A possible bias in patient selection is one of the factors that might contribute to these discrepant results.

Three prospective, uncontrolled trials that have evaluated the role of TPN as primary therapy in Crohn's disease have, however, reported rather similar results as regards the initial response and long-term outcome. Elson et al.[60] studied 20 patients with Crohn's disease on corticosteroids who had been considered refractory to medical management, and 13 patients (65 per cent) had a successful clinical response. After a follow-up period of 20 to 48 months, 62 per cent remained in remission: 3 patients were symptom-free and off all drugs, and 5 remained improved on medication. The remaining 5 patients required surgery.

Greenberg and Jeejeebhoy[61] also studied prospectively 43 patients with active Crohn's disease and observed a 77 per cent in-hospital remission rate; with a 2-year follow-up 29 patients (67 per cent) remained in medical remission, although the majority of patients required maintenance prednisone. Subsequently, Ostro et al.[62] extended these results in a retrospective analysis of 100 Crohn's patients in whom the presenting features included an acute inflammatory mass in 28 patients, subacute obstruction in 29, extensive small bowel disease in 19, and fistulous disease in 24. Overall, 77 patients were discharged in remission. Administration of corticosteroids did not appear to influence these results. Where TPN was the sole form of therapy 42 of 51 patients (82 per cent) achieved remission, and 35 of 49 patients (71 per cent) had remissions while receiving corticosteroids. After 1 year continued remission was observed in 50 of the 93 patients (54 per cent) who were available for follow-up.

Of particular interest is a prospective study undertaken by Muller et al.[63] in which 30 consecutive patients with complicated Crohn's disease received as the only form of therapy TPN for 3 weeks in hospital and then subsequently for 9 weeks as outpatients. No medications or food were provided during this period. A clinical remission was obtained in 25 patients (83 per cent) as defined by a symptom-free status in the absence of medication and the ability to work. A cumulative relapse rate of 35 per cent occurred at 1 year, 60 per cent at 2 years, 81 per cent at 3 years, and 85 per cent at 4 years. These results were compared with retrospective data from matched patients who had previously undergone surgical resection at the same institution. Using the same criteria for relapse, the cumulative recurrence rate with TPN was about four times higher than was noted for surgical resection. The authors concluded that TPN as primary therapy is not an alternative to surgical resection for patients with drug-resistant Crohn's disease.

Notwithstanding substantial differences reported by various centers on the early clinical response to TPN, the composite data suggest that an in-hospital remission can be achieved in 40 to 80 per cent of patients, with a mean figure of 58 per cent. Sustained long-term remission is less frequent, ranging from 17 to 67 per cent, but mean figures here are much more difficult to derive given either the absence of data or the wide variation in length of follow-up. Whether the results achieved with primary TPN therapy as regards long-term quality of life are comparable to treatment with surgical resection requires prospective evaluation.

FISTULOUS DISEASE

Following the introduction of TPN, impressive clinical results were reported with the healing of postoperative fistulas.[64] By contrast, fistulas that complicate Crohn's disease are much less amenable to any form of medical therapy, including TPN.[65] The different mechanism for fistula formation in Crohn's disease likely accounts for this finding. Unlike the postoperative setting, it has been proposed that fistulas in acute Crohn's disease occur as a consequence of the extension of a deep transmural fissure in the presence of a partially obstructed segment of bowel.[66] Permanent closure generally would not be anticipated unless the obstructive element, which usually has both acute inflammatory and chronic fibrotic components, is relieved. Although individual published series on the management of Crohn's fistulas by TPN usually involve small numbers of patients, the composite data provided in Table 15–2 suggest that a successful outcome is least often observed in this group of patients. In the absence of recent surgical intervention, for 156 pa-

TABLE 15–2. Total Parenteral Nutrition As Primary Therapy for Crohn's Disease Fistulas

Series	No. of Patients	In-Hospital Closure	Long-Term Closure
Anderson (1973)[56]	2	1	0
Vogel (1974)[49]	2	1	1
Eisenberg (1974)[43]	18	5	2
MacFayden (1974)[105]	23	13	nr
Reilly (1976)[48]	2	0	0
Harford (1978)[50]	4	0	0
Mullen (1978)[55]	37	12	10
Elson (1980)[60]	5	1	1
Milewski (1980)[52]	3	0	0
Bos (1981)[106]	33	5	nr
Muller (1983)[63]	3	2	2
Ostro (1985)[62]	24	15	11
TOTALS	156	55 (35%)	27 (17%)

nr, not reported.

tients with Crohn's disease complicated by fistulas, a successful closure rate in hospital following TPN was found in only 55 patients (35 per cent) and less than half of these responders had a sustained remission for longer than 3 months. Any attempt to stratify these data according to fistula type provides numbers that are generally too small for statistical interpretation. However, there are trends to indicate that enterovesicular and enterovaginal fistulas are most resistant to medical closure, while marginally better results may occur with enterocutaneous and most often with enteroenteric fistulas.[67,68] At the present time, the available data suggest that TPN may improve the nutritional status of patients with Crohn's fistulas, facilitate a reduction in the acute inflammatory component, and diminish drainage. Long-term permanent closure on TPN alone can, however, be expected in only a minority of cases.

CROHN'S COLITIS

An early retrospective series of Reilly et al.[48] suggested that patients with granulomatous colitis may respond less well to TPN than do patients with Crohn's disease involving the small bowel. Similar findings were subsequently reported by Bos and Weterman[51] in a larger retrospective analysis of 44 patients with Crohn's colitis, in which only 12 patients were considered to achieve remission with TPN. Two recent prospective randomized control trials lend support to the above conclusions concerning the efficacy of TPN in Crohn's colitis.

Dickinson et al.[41] undertook a prospective controlled trial of TPN and bowel rest in 36 patients with acute colitis, 9 of whom had granulomatous colitis. Patients were randomized to a group receiving only TPN and a control group that was allowed a full oral diet. All patients received prednisone 40 mg daily, which was reduced every 3 days or more depending upon the response to treatment. The trial was completed either when the prednisone was reduced to 10 mg/day or when the patients came to colectomy. Neither the control group nor the group

receiving TPN demonstrated any significant increase in body weight, although the control group lost 7.3 per cent of body protein mass while the group receiving TPN retained body protein. In the control group 1 of 3 patients came to surgery, while in the group receiving TPN 3 of 6 patients with Crohn's disease came to surgery. The numbers in this subgroup of Crohn's colitis patients are clearly too few to support any statistical conclusions, but they do allow for the inference that TPN with bowel rest has no primary therapeutic effect in Crohn's colitis.

Similar conclusions were drawn in a larger prospective randomized trial of McIntyre et al.[69] in which 16 patients with Crohn's colitis were randomly assigned to either bowel rest with total parenteral nutrition or an oral diet. Both groups of patients reveived 60 mg of prednisone daily. All 9 patients in the bowel rest group improved, but notably 5 of 7 patients in the oral diet group also achieved clinical remission. The two patients who failed on the oral diet improved with a subsequent period of TPN, and none of the 16 patients required surgery. With a median follow-up of 43 months, 11 of the 16 patients suffered relapses. Six of these patients had previously received TPN, while 5 had received the oral diet. The number of patients in this study is also small, but the data accord with the suggestion that total parenteral nutrition and bowel rest does not play a positive role in achieving remission with Crohn's colitis patients and rather should be considered an adjunctive therapeutic modality for nutritional repletion.

BOWEL REST: A PREREQUISITE FOR IMPROVEMENT?

Although it has been suggested that bowel rest is one of the major mechanisms whereby TPN or elemental diets contribute to improvement in patients with Crohn's disease, two recent prospective studies have recently cast doubt on this concept.

Lochs et al.[70] undertook a prospective trial in 20

patients with Crohn's disease treated with parenteral nutrition and no other medications. The patients were randomly divided into two groups: the first group was maintained on complete bowel rest with nothing by mouth, while the second group was allowed a low-residue oral diet ad libitum. At the end of 4 weeks of therapy not only was an equivalent improvement in nutritional status observed in both groups, but also a similar decrease in disease activity. Eight of 10 patients responded in the bowel rest group, while 7 of 10 patients in the oral diet group had remissions. Although parenteral nutrition provides nutritional repletion and reduces disease activity, these data suggest that bowel rest is not a prerequisite for improvement.

Recently, Greenberg et al.[71] also assessed the role of bowel rest in a prospective trial of 51 patients with active Crohn's disease who were resistant to other medical management including corticosteroids. Patients were randomly assigned to three groups receiving different levels of nutritional support for 21 days. Seventeen patients received total parenteral nutrition and nil per os, 19 a defined-formula diet, and 15 partial parenteral nutrition and oral food ad libitum. Clinical remission occurred in 71 per cent of patients on TPN, 58 per cent on the defined-formula diet, and 60 per cent on partial parenteral nutrition, differences that were not statistically significant. Also of note was the observation of a short mean interval to relapse requiring either drug adjustment or surgery in each of these groups after successful therapy: 9 months on TPN (4 of 12 patients), 7 months on the defined-formula diet (9 of 11 patients), and 8 months on partial parenteral nutrition (5 of 9 patients). This study indicated not only that TPN has no distinct advantage over defined-formula diets in the management of patients with active Crohn's disease but, in agreement with the findings of Lochs et al.,[70] also suggested that bowel rest is not the major determinant of clinical remission.

If bowel rest does not play a prominent role in achieving a remission, what then is the reason for clinical improvement? It is noteworthy that neither of the above-mentioned studies specifically defined the possible beneficial role of nutritional repletion. This issue was addressed by Harries et al.,[72] who undertook a controlled prospective study in 28 malnourished patients with Crohn's disease to examine the effect of a low-residue nonelemental liquid supplement on nutritional status and disease activity. Patients were randomly allocated in a crossover design to 2 months on an ordinary diet alone (control period) and 2 months when the nutritional supplement was provided in addition (treatment period). Significant improvements in clinical and biochemical parameters including serum orosomucoid occurred with the enteral supplement but not in the control period, suggesting that clinical remission was directly related to nutritional repletion. An increase in T lymphocyte counts was also observed, reflecting an improvement in cellular immunity. Since it is well recognized that both T lymphocyte numbers and cell-mediated immunity are improved by nutritional repletion in patients with protein-calorie malnutrition,[73] this factor may have indirectly contributed to a reduction in disease activity. The provision of essential nutrients that influence the metabolism and differentiation of epithelial tissue might also enhance repair of diseased mucosa. One suggested possibility was vitamin A, which initially was reported to normalize stool frequency after ileocecal resection for Crohn's disease,[74] although subsequent studies have been unable to confirm this observation.[75,76] Alternatively, one of the amino acids—for example, glutamine, which directly facilitates epithelial growth[77]—might contribute to improvement. However, clinical responses with TPN or elemental diets are often observed prior to significant changes in nutritional status, and remission has been reported in patients receiving intravenous protein-sparing therapy,[61] in which no exogenous nonprotein calories are provided.[78] Thus factors in addition to nutritional repletion seem likely. Although at present the precise mechanisms remain speculative, certain lines of evidence do favor the concept that nutritional support rather than bowel rest is one of the predominant factors.

OVERVIEW

The following conclusions may be drawn from the published literature on the value of total parenteral nutrition in the management of Crohn's disease. This therapeutic modality allows for repletion of total body protein, energy stores, and mineral, vitamin, and trace element deficiencies in patients with acute Crohn's disease. In consequence, it is a useful modality for any patient in whom disease activity precludes the maintenance of a normal nutritional state, whether or not operation is planned. Although TPN provides important adjunctive nutritional support in the preoperative patient and in patients suffering postoperative complications, a positive role in reducing postoperative complication rates remains to be established. When TPN is used as primary therapy in patients with acute Crohn's disease, in-hospital remission rates of 40 to 80 per cent can be expected after 14 to 21 days of treatment. Improved clinical responses are most likely to occur in patients with small bowel disease alone or in combination with large bowel disease; TPN has no primary role in the management of patients with Crohn's colitis. Of the various complications of Crohn's disease, patients with fistulas or major obstructive symptoms are the most resistant to medical management and most often will require surgery. The long-term outcome with at least 1 year of follow-up is less favorable, with relapse rates ranging from 25 to 85 per cent. Given this observation, prospective studies are required to determine whether provision of TPN in medically resistant patients achieves a quality of life equivalent to surgical resection, particularly when the length of in-hospital stay and associated cost of TPN are considered; one retrospective study points to a negative answer. The mechanism by which TPN achieves remission remains speculative, although initial data suggest that one of the predominant factors is nutritional repletion and not bowel rest.

Elemental Diets

Administration of elemental diets represents an alternative approach to providing nutritional support and bowel rest in patients with inflammatory bowel disease. Indeed, there may be certain possible advantages to this modality when compared with TPN. Enteral feeding is generally more widely available, is simpler to use at a lesser cost, and is associated with fewer complications. The requirement for intraluminal digestive mechanisms is diminished, and complete absorption occurs in the upper small intestine. Moreover, nutrient delivery through the portal system may be associated with enhanced protein synthesis and may permit less complex regulation of the metabolic demands placed on the patient.

In contrast to TPN, the published experience on the use of elemental diets in inflammatory bowel disease is more limited (Table 15–3). Most of these studies are nonrandomized retrospective reviews and often comprise small numbers of patients.[30,79–81] Rocchio et al.[82] provided an elemental diet to 25 patients with Crohn's disease, achieved weight gain and a positive nitrogen balance in all and a clinical remission in 10 patients (40 per cent); 10 patients ultimately required surgery, but postoperative complications were reported to be minimal. No long-

term follow-up was provided. Axelsson and Jarnum[30] treated 11 Crohn's patients considered refractory to corticosteroids with an elemental diet over an average period of 26 days. Eight patients (73 per cent) went into clinical remission. Although a significant reduction in fecal volume and sedimentation rate occurred, there was no change in hemoglobin and in particular no improvement in serum orosomucoid, suggesting incomplete resolution of the inflammatory process. However, of the 8 patients achieving remission, 4 remained symptom-free for 22 to 35 months.

O'Morain et al.[28] in reporting their initial prospective experience on 27 patients with Crohn's disease receiving an elemental diet for 4 weeks, illustrated two of the problems that may arise with enteral feeding. Two patients were withdrawn immediately because of nonpalatability of the diet and one patient was withdrawn because of obstructive symptoms. Although the remaining 24 patients achieved clinical remission, 16 patients also received drug therapy either as corticosteroids or levamisole. At 6 month's follow-up, 18 of the 24 patients remained well. These results prompted O'Morain et al.[83] to undertake a prospective controlled trial in which 21 patients with acute Crohn's disease were randomly selected to receive either prednisolone 0.75 mg/kg/day or an elemental diet for 4 weeks. Two patients in each treatment group were withdrawn; nonpalatability was the reason for both cases in the elemental diet group. In the steroid-treated group, 8 of 10 patients were considered to be in clinical remission at 4 weeks, while 9 of 11 patients receiving the elemental diet achieved remission. After 3 months' follow-up, only one patient in each group had relapsed. This study was one of the first to suggest that elemental diets are as effective as

TABLE 15–3. Elemental Diets in Crohn's Disease

Series	No. of Patients	Clinical Remission in Hospital		Long-Term Remission		Length of Follow-up (Months)
Retrospective						
Voitk (1973)[79]	7	3 (43%)		nr		nr
Rocchio (1974)[82]	25	10 (40%)		nr		nr
Axelsson (1977)[30]	11	8 (73%)		4 (36%)		22–35
Prospective						
O'Morain (1980)[83]	27	24 (89%)		18 (67%)		6
Lochs (1978)[87]	25	15 (60%)		12 (48%)		6–24
Prospective, Controlled		*Controls*	*Elemental Diet*	*Controls*	*Elemental Diet*	
O'Morain (1984)[28]	21	8/10 (80%)	9/11 (82%)	7/10 (70%)	8/11 (73%)	
Saverymutti (1985)[84]	37	16/16 (100%)	15/21 (71%)	nr		
Greenberg (1985)[71]	34*	9/15 (60%)	11/19 (58%)	6/15 (40%)	2/19 (11%)	12
TOTALS	146†	95 (65%)				

*Control group composed of 15 patients on partial parenteral nutrition and oral diet; does not include 17 patients randomly assigned to TPN.
†Total does not include controls.
nr, not reported.

corticosteroids in the initial management of patients with active Crohn's disease.

Similar conclusions were recently drawn by Saverymuttu et al.[84] In a randomized prospective trial, 16 patients with moderately active Crohn's disease received prednisolone 0.5 mg/kg/day plus a normal diet and were compared with 16 patients treated with an elemental diet plus three oral nonabsorbable antibiotics. After 10 days' treatment 15 of 16 patients on the elemental diet and all 16 patients on prednisolone achieved clinical remission and showed statistically indistinguishable falls in a disease activity index and fecal granulocyte excretion. Nausea and vomiting occurred in nearly a quarter of the patients receiving antibiotics, and it is questionable whether their use provides any additional benefit over the administration of elemental diets alone, since with the possible exception of metronidazole[85] no other antibiotics have a proven role in the management of Crohn's disease. Furthermore, the absence of long-term follow-up precludes any assessment of the possible advantages of an elemental diet over corticosteroids in prolonging remission rates. In this trial the reintroduction of solid food was accompanied by elective coverage with low doses of corticosteroids.

Although numbers of patients are small, both of these prospective studies do indicate that an elemental diet may be as effective as corticosteroids for the initial treatment of moderately acute Crohn's disease. Any advantage to this approach over drug therapy alone remains to be established, but the potential for minimizing drug (corticosteroids or azathioprine) side effects, particularly in children, has obvious clinical relevance. Perhaps equally important, neither trial addresses prospectively the question of what role elemental diets play in patients with acute Crohn's disease who have become resistant to conventional medical management, including high-dose corticosteroids.

There are few studies that address the role of elemental diets in patients with Crohn's disease specifically complicated by fistulous disease. Calam et al.[86] treated 6 patients with Crohn's disease and perianal fistulas. Although 4 patients demonstrated diminished drainage on the diet, the majority of fistulas reopened with the introduction of solid food. Axelsson and Jarnum[30] noted that 3 of 5 patients with fistulas required surgical intervention, notwithstanding elemental diet treatment, while Lochs et al.[87] found that only 1 of 11 patients obtained fistula closure. Numbers of fistula patients in all remaining studies on elemental diets and Crohn's disease are small, but clinical results, as with TPN, are generally disappointing. Permanent closure rates, however, appear to be no worse than those reported with the use of TPN.

As already noted for TPN, primary therapy with elemental diets has little role in promoting remission for patients with Crohn's colitis. Lochs et al.[87] found

by discriminant analysis that patients with colonic disease alone and fever had a 90 per cent chance of failing treatment.

The limited data available on the use of elemental diets in Crohn's disease with small bowel or combined involvement suggest that it is an effective alternative to total parenteral nutrition in achieving an early clinical remission and in the long-term outcome. Two drawbacks of this treatment modality include unpalatability of the diets, which can be circumvented by continuous nasogastric feeding, and diarrhea that occurs as a consequence of the hyperosmolality of some diets and the relatively low concentrations of sodium found in most diets. The latter problem can be partly alleviated by the addition of 70 to 110 mmol of sodium chloride to the diets, an approach that takes advantage of glucose-sodium cotransport systems to facilitate absorption of water from the jejunum.[88]

HOME PARENTERAL NUTRITION

Total parenteral nutrition or defined formula diets are usually employed for short-term nutritional support. However, in a small number of patients with Crohn's disease, gastrointestinal reserve may be insufficient for the maintenance of an adequate nutritional state on oral or enteral diets alone. Most often the clinical setting involves ongoing active inflammation following multiple small bowel resections. The remaining bowel may be incapable of absorbing sufficient nutrients to maintain nutritional homeostasis (short-bowel syndrome). Alternatively, resection of the colon and ileum, regions of the gut that are primarily responsible for concentration of intestinal contents, may result in substantial losses of isotonic fluid, electrolytes, minerals, and trace elements, but relatively normal macronutrient absorption (end-jejunostomy syndrome). Under either of these circumstances, a program of permanent home parenteral nutrition may be successfully instituted, either to provide complete nutritional support or alternatively to facilitate fluid and electrolyte balance.

Jeejeebhoy et al.[89] provided some of the initial experience on home parenteral nutrition in a report that included 3 patients with Crohn's disease and massive small bowel resection treated for an average of 28 months. Full nutritional repletion and social rehabilitation into the community was achieved with each patient.

Fleming et al.[90] also reported on their findings with 19 patients on home parenteral nutrition, 14 of whom had inflammatory bowel disease. The major indications included short bowel syndrome with an average of 80 cm of remaining bowel and extensive active Crohn's disease contributing to gastric outlet obstruction. With a duration of treatment ranging from 12 to 90 months, nutritional repletion was possible in all patients and was accompanied by a 50 per cent reduction in hospitalization after home parenteral nutrition was initiated. Of note was the observation that 6 patients required additional surgery, including 2 patients who developed fistulous disease while on home parenteral nutrition. A similar finding of the appearance of fistulas in patients with Crohn's disease on home parenteral nutrition has subsequently been reported by others.[91,92] Thus, while home parenteral nutrition has become the treatment of choice of patients who cannot restore and maintain nutrition orally, it does not appear to prevent the development of further complications related to Crohn's disease.

NUTRITIONAL SUPPORT IN ULCERATIVE COLITIS

Acute ulcerative colitis sufficiently severe to require hospital admission is relatively uncommon, but when it occurs patients are often febrile, hypercatabolic, and critically ill. Although high-dose intravenous corticosteroids are the mainstay of medical therapy, about 25 to 50 per cent of patients with severe acute ulcerative colitis come to urgent surgery that may carry mortality rates ranging from 20 to 25 per cent.[93,99] Thus, any additional medical measure that would avert the necessity for surgery is obviously desirable. Total parenteral nutrition has been advocated in this clinical setting on the premise that an improved nutritional status coupled with bowel rest would achieve clinical remission and avoid the necessity for colectomy. Unfortunately, published experience as summarized in Table 15–4 does not support this concept.

Two prospective controlled trials have examined the value of total parenteral nutrition and bowel rest in the management of ulcerative colitis. Dickinson et al.[41] randomly assigned 27 patients with acute ulcerative colitis to receive either TPN or only fluid, electrolyte, and blood replacement. In addition, all patients received prednisone. The clinical remission rate and requirements for surgery were equivalent in the two groups: 7 of 13 patients receiving TPN and 6 of 14 control patients came to colectomy.

Similar findings were more recently reported by McIntyre et al.[69] In a prospective study 27 patients with acute ulcerative colitis treated with 60 mg of intravenous prednisolone daily were randomly selected to receive either TPN and bowel rest or an oral diet. No benefit was derived from TPN and bowel rest, as 9 of 15 patients receiving TPN and 5 of 12 patients fed orally came to urgent colectomy. There was one postoperative death in each group. Moreover, within 6 months surgery was required in an additional 3 patients who had been treated with TPN and in 2 patients who had received an oral diet.

A prospective, nonrandomized study undertaken by Elson et al.[60] that included 10 patients with ulcerative colitis treated by TPN and bowel rest is of interest. Although 3 patients avoided surgery, in the remaining 7 patients undergoing colectomy an increased incidence of postoperative complications was reported. Clearly the decision to perform colectomy in the deteriorating patient should not be delayed for modest gains in nutritional status.

There are only two studies that have retrospectively assessed the role of elemental diets in the management of ulcerative colitis. Rocchio et al.[82] reported clinical remission in 3 of 9 patients, while Axelsson and Jarnum[30] observed improvement in 8 of 23 patients in whom other medical therapy was considered a failure. Thus, the mean response rate of 34 per cent in these two studies appears to be no better than would be anticipated in a prospective study undertaken with an appropriate control population.

TABLE 15–4. Total Parenteral Nutrition in Ulcerative Colitis

Series	No. of Patients	Clinical Remission in Hospital		Long-Term Remission		Length of Follow-up (Months)
Retrospective						
Fischer (1973)[47]	4	1 (25%)		1 (25%)		6
Vogel (1974)[49]	1	1 (100%)		0 (0%)		
Fazio (1976)[44]	14	5 (36%)		3 (21%)		20–41
Reilly (1976)[48]	11	1 (9%)		nr		nr
Dean (1976)[54]	5	4 (80%)		nr		nr
Mullen (1978)[55]	24	9 (38%)		4 (17%)		6–120
Prospective						
Elson (1980)[60]	10	4 (40%)		1 (10%)		44
Prospective, Controlled		*Controls*	*TPN*	*Controls*	*TPN*	
Dickinson (1980)[41]	27	8/14 (57%)	6/13 (46%)	5/14 (36%)	4/13 (31%)	12
McIntyre (1986)[69]	27	7/12 (58%)	6/15 (40%)	3/12 (25%)	2/15 (13%)	27–64
TOTALS	97*	37 (38%)				

*Does not include controls.
nr, not reported.

Although numbers of patients are small, the published data indicate that nutritional support and bowel rest are of little value in the primary management of patients with acute ulcerative colitis. This finding is perhaps not surprising, since early surgical attempts to defunction the colon in ulcerative colitis proved of little benefit,[95] and disease activity may persist in the retained rectum in patients who have undergone subtotal colectomy. In the failing patient with ulcerative colitis, surgery continues to be the treatment of choice. Indeed, protracting the need for colectomy to achieve nutritional repletion may actually lead to increased morbidity.

NUTRITIONAL SUPPORT IN INFLAMMATORY BOWEL DISEASE IN CHILDHOOD

Approximately 30 to 40 per cent of patients with inflammatory bowel disease will present under the age of 21 years. Delays of significant magnitude in linear growth and sexual maturation have now been well documented in 20 to 50 per cent of such children, with the vast majority, 75 to 85 per cent, having Crohn's disease.[96] Although growth failure has been attributed to several potential mechanisms including nutritional, hormonal, and disease-related factors, present evidence now favors the hypothesis that protein-calorie malnutrition is the major causative mechanism. Inadequate dietary intake relative to the metabolic requirements for growth, coupled with excessive intestinal losses and malabsorption, are all factors that lead to nutritional compromise. However, as a consequence of nutritional depletion, hormonal factors also play an important role. Recently Kirschner and Sutton[97] reported that growth-impaired children with active inflammatory bowel disease have low circulating levels of somatomedin C, a substance thought to mediate the anabolic effects of growth hormone on peripheral tissues including cartilage, muscle, and fat. With nutritional therapeutic intervention, somatomedin levels improved, suggesting not only a possible causal relationship but also that serial determinations of somatomedin may prove to be a useful marker for adequacy of nutritional repletion in children with inflammatory bowel disease.

Total parenteral nutrition or elemental diets have been utilized successfully in children with inflammatory bowel disease to reduce symptoms, achieve nutritional repletion, and re-establish linear growth. Kelts et al.[98] administered TPN to 7 children with Crohn's disease and growth failure for a period of 6 to 8 weeks and was able to demonstrate significant weight gain and improved growth velocity in all children. In 4 children with clinically active Crohn's disease receiving TPN for 4 to 6 weeks, Layden et al.[99] was also able to demonstrate reversal of growth arrest and sexual maturation in two patients.

Provision of TPN prior to intestinal resection may also influence postoperative growth. Lake et al.[100] reported in a nonrandomized prospective study that 4 adolescents receiving 1 month of preoperative TPN demonstrated greater postoperative growth velocity when compared with 4 matched adolescents who underwent the same type of resection without prior nutritional support. There was no difference in postoperative weight gain, sexual development, or 3-year disease control. The mechanism by which 1 month of nutritional support facilitates 2 years of growth is speculative, but one possible factor is the repletion of trace elements, notably zinc, that are essential for normal growth. Since patient selection bias may also have influenced outcome, further prospective randomized trials are required to confirm these interesting preliminary observations.

An alternative approach to the management of growth retardation in inflammatory bowel disease described by Motil et al.[101] included the administration of a commercially prepared liquid formula providing 1500 ml nightly by Silastic nasogastric feeding tube or feeding gastrostomy in adolescents with nutritional dwarfism. Significant weight gain, improved nitrogen balance, and total body potassium were demonstrated after 3 weeks. Following 7 months of nutritional supplementation, the average height and weight velocities were found to be at least five times greater than those observed during the 10 months prior to supplementation and equaled or exceeded the growth velocities of normal adolescents.

Similar successful results with defined-formula diets were observed by Morin et al.,[102] who reported complete remission of symptoms in 4 Crohn's patients as well as significant increments in height and weight during the 6 weeks of feeding. Moreover, nutritional status continued to improve for 3 months following the diet, although relapse occurred in all patients within 9 months. Recently, this same group[103] has undertaken a prospective randomized trial comparing the effect of an elemental diet with prednisone in the treatment of 18 newly diagnosed pediatric patients with active Crohn's disease. Clinical remission was observed in 6 of 9 patients on prednisone and 7 of 9 patients receiving the elemental diet alone. However, all patients receiving prednisone but only 5 of 9 patients receiving the elemental diet maintained clinical remission 6 weeks after cessation of therapy.

A program of home parenteral nutrition has been successfully employed by Strobel et al.[104] in 17 patients with severe Crohn's disease not controlled by other therapeutic modalities. Six of these 17 children had growth failure. With a mean duration of 140 days, 12 of 17 patients (70 per cent) achieved a clinical remission. Of this group, 4 children have remained in remission on no therapy with a mean follow-up of 332 days; 4 other children required surgical management upon resumption of oral feeding, while an additional 7 patients required a second course of home parenteral nutrition.

Thus, nutritional support in pediatric patients with inflammatory bowel disease will reverse growth retardation notwithstanding the presence of active disease. Elemental diets or other oral formula preparations are the preferable route of administration, but when these modalities fail, total parenteral nutrition is then indicated. As previously noted for adults with Crohn's disease, the efficacy of these nutritional support modalities in achieving an initial positive clinical response can be anticipated in the majority of cases, but considerably fewer patients will have a sustained remission. Whether nutritional support may be of some benefit in reversing growth arrest for pediatric patients with ulcerative colitis is as yet unknown. However, based on experience in the adult population it seems unlikely that this therapeutic modality would have any positive influence on the primary disease process.

References

1. Greenstein AJ, Sachar DB, Pasternack BS, et al. Reoperation and recurrence in Crohn's colitis and ileocolitis: crude and cumulative rates. N Engl J Med 1975; 293:685–690.
2. Cohen Z, McLeod RS, Stern H, et al. The pelvic pouch and ileoanal anastomosis procedure: surgical technique and initial results. Am J Surg 1985; 150:601–607.
3. Chan ATH, Fleming CR, O'Fallon WM, et al. Estimated versus measured basal energy requirements in patients with Crohn's disease. Gastroenterology 1986; 91:75–78.
4. Baker JP, Detsky AS, Stewart S, et al. Randomized trial of total parenteral nutrition in critically ill patients: metabolic effects of varying glucose-lipid ratios as the energy source. Gastroenterology 1984; 87:53–59.
5. Heatley RV. Nutritional implications of inflammatory bowel disease. Scand J Gastroenterol 1984; 19:995–998.
6. Farmer RG, Hawk WA, Turnbull RG. Clinical patterns in Crohn's disease: a statistical study of 615 cases. Gastroenterology 1975; 68:627–635.
7. Mekhjian HS, Switz DM, Melnyk CS, et al. Clinical features and natural history of Crohn's disease. Gastroenterology 1979; 77:898–906.
8. Barot LR, Rombeau JL, Steinberg JJ, et al. Energy expenditure in patients with inflammatory bowel disease. Arch Surg 1981; 116:460–462.
9. Logan RFA, Gillon J, Ferrington C, et al. Reduction of gastrointestinal protein loss by elemental diet in Crohn's disease of the small bowel. Gut 1981; 22:383–387.
10. Law DK, Dudrick SJ, Abdou NI. Immunocompetence of patients with protein-calorie malnutrition. The effect of nutritional repletion. Ann Intern Med 1973; 79:545.
11. Bistrian BR, Blackburn GL, Scrimshaw NS, et al. Cellular immunity in semi-starved states in hospitalized adults. Am J Clin Nutr 1975; 23:1148.
12. Irwin TT. Effects of malnutrition and hyperalimentation on wound healing. Surg Gynecol Obstet 1978; 146:33–37.
13. McCaffery TD, Nasr K, Lawrence AM, et al. Severe growth retardation in children with inflammatory bowel disease. Pediatrics 1970; 45:386–393.
14. Jeejeebhoy KN, Anderson GH, Nakhooda AF, et al. Metabolic studies in total parenteral nutrition with lipid in man: comparison with glucose. J Clin Invest 1976; 57:125–136.
15. Zajtchuk R, Amato JC, Shoemaker WC, et al. The relation-

ship between blood glucose levels and external pancreatic secretion in man. J Trauma 1969; 9:629–637.
16. Bivins BA, Bell RM, Rapp RP, et al. Pancreatic exocrine response to parenteral nutrition. JPEN 1984; 8:34–36.
17. Stastna R, Skala I, Hruba F, et al. The effect of some solutions for parenteral nutrition on gastric and pancreatic secretion. Nutr Metab 1979; 23:349–356.
18. Varner AA, Isenberg JE, Elashoff JD, et al. Effect of intravenous lipid on gastric acid secretion stimulated by intravenous amino acids. Gastroenterology 1980; 79:873–876.
19. Edelman K, Valenzuela JE. Effect of intravenous lipid on human pancreatic secretion. Gastroenterology 1983; 85:1063–1066.
20. Weisbrodt NW, Copeland EM, Thor PH, et al. The myoelectric activity of the small intestine of the dog during total parenteral nutrition. Proc Soc Exp Biol Med 1976; 153:121–124.
21. Greenberg GR, Wolman SL, Cristofides ND, et al. Effect of total parenteral nutrition on gut hormone release in humans. Gastroenterology 1981; 80:988–993.
22. Watanabe K, Shiratori K, Takeuchi T, et al. Release of cholecystokinin and exocrine pancreatic secretion in response to an elemental diet in human subjects. Dig Dis Sci 1986; 31:919–924.
23. Greenberg GR, Blair J. Effect of enteral and parenteral nutrition on gut hormone release in man. (Abstract.) Dig Dis Sci 1984; 29:325.
24. Schang JC, Angel F, Lambert A, et al. Inhibition of canine duodenal interdigestive myoelectric complex by nutrient perfusion of jejunal and ileal Thiry-Vella loops. Gut 1981; 22:738–743.
25. Rivilis J, McArdle AH, Wiodek GH, et al. Effect of an elemental diet on gastric secretion. Ann Surg 1974; 179:226–229.
26. Bury KD, Jambunatham G. Effects of elemental diets on gastric emptying and gastric secretion in man. Am J Surg 1974; 127:59.
27. Russell RI. Progress report: elemental diets. Gut 1975; 16:68–79.
28. O'Morain C, Segal AW, Levi AJ. Elemental diets as primary treatment of acute Crohn's disease: a controlled trial. Br Med J 1984; 288:1859–1862.
29. Bounous G, Devroede GH. Effects of an elemental diet on human fecal flora. Gastroenterology 1974; 66:210–214.
30. Axelsson C, Jarnum S. Assessment of the therapeutic value of an elemental diet in chronic inflammatory bowel disease. Scand J Gastroenterol 1977; 12:89–95.
31. Harper PH, Bennett MK, Jewell DP. Role of the faecal stream in the maintenance of Crohn's colitis. Gut 1985; 26:279–284.
32. Feldman FJ, Dowling RH, McNaughton J, et al. Effects of oral versus intravenous nutrition after small bowel resection in the dog. Gastroenterology 1976; 5:712–719.
33. Johnson LR, Schanbacher LM, Dudrick SJ, et al. Effect of long-term parenteral feeding on pancreatic secretion and serum secretin. Am J Physiol 1977; 233:E524–E529.
34. Kotler DP, Levine GM. Reversible gastric and pancreatic hyposecretion after long-term total parenteral nutrition. N Engl J Med 1979; 300:241–242.
35. Greene HL, McCabe DR, Merenstein GB. Protracted diarrhea and malnutrition in infancy: changes in intestinal morphology and disaccharidase activities during treatment with total intravenous nutrition or oral elemental diets. Pediatrics 1975; 87:695–704.
36. Steiger E, Wilmore DW, Dudrick SJ, et al. Total intravenous nutrition in the management of inflammatory disease of the intestinal tract. (Abstract.) Fed Proc 1969; 28:808.
37. Summers RW, Switz DM, Sessions JT, et al. National cooperative Crohn's disease study. Results of drug treatment. Gastroenterology 1979; 77:827–828.
38. Pettit SH, Holbrook IB, Irving MH. Comparison of clinical scores and acute phase protein in the assessment of acute Crohn's disease. Br J Surg 1985; 72:1013–1016.

39. Andre C, Descos L, Landais P, et al. Assessment of appropriate laboratory measurements to supplement the Crohn's Disease Activity Index. Gut 1981; 22:571–574.
40. Saverymuttu SH, Camilleri M, Rees H, et al. Indium 111–granulocyte scanning in the assessment of disease extent and disease activity in inflammatory bowel disease. A comparison with colonoscopy, histology, and fecal Indium 111–granulocyte excretion. Gastroenterology 1986; 90:1121–1128.
41. Dickinson RJ, Ashton MR, Axon ATR, et al. Controlled trial of intravenous hyperalimentation and total bowel rest as an adjunct to the routine therapy of acute colitis. Gastroenterology 1980; 79:1199–1204.
42. Collins JP, Oxby CB, Hill GL. Intravenous amino acids and intravenous hyperalimentation as protein-sparing therapy after major surgery: a controlled clinical trial. Lancet 1978; 1:788–791.
43. Eisenberg HW, Turnbull RB Jr, Weakley FL. Hyperalimentation as preparation for surgery in transmural colitis (Crohn's disease). Dis Colon Rectum 1974; 17:469–475.
44. Fazio VW, Kodner I, Jagelman DG, et al. Inflammatory bowel disease of the bowel: parenteral nutrition as primary or adjunctive treatment. Dis Colon Rectum 1976; 19:574–578.
45. Rombeau JL, Barot LR, Williamson LE, et al. Preoperative total parenteral nutrition and surgical outcome in patients with inflammatory bowel disease. Am J Surg 1982; 143:139–143.
46. Heimann, TM, Greenstein AJ, Mechanic L, et al. Early complications following surgical treatment for Crohn's disease. Ann Surg 1985; 201:494–498.
47. Fischer JE, Foster GS, Abel RM, et al. Hyperalimentation as primary therapy for inflammatory bowel disease. Am J Surg 1973; 125:165–175.
48. Reilly J, Ryan JA, Strole W, et al. Hyperalimentation in inflammatory bowel disease. Am J Surg 1976; 131:192–200.
49. Vogel CM, Corwin TR, Baue AE. Intravenous hyperalimentation in the treatment of inflammatory diseases of the bowel. Arch Surg 1974; 108:460–467.
50. Harfod FJ, Fazio VW. Total parenteral nutrition as primary therapy for inflammatory disease of the bowel. Dis Colon Rectum 1978; 21:555–557.
51. Bos LP, Weterman IT. Total parenteral nutrition in Crohn's disease. World J Surg 1980; 4:163–166.
52. Milewski PJ, Irving MH. Parenteral nutrition in Crohn's disease. Dis Colon Rectum 1980; 23:395–400.
53. Shiloni E, Freund HR. Total parenteral nutrition in Crohn's disease. Is it a primary or supportive mode of therapy? Dis Colon Rectum 1983; 26:275–278.
54. Dean RE, Campos MM, Barrett B. Hyperalimentation in the management of chronic inflammatory intestinal disease. Dis Colon Rectum 1976; 19:601–604.
55. Mullen JL, Hargrove WC, Dudrick SJ, et al. Ten years experience with intravenous hyperalimentation and inflammatory bowel disease. Ann Surg 1978; 187:523–529.
56. Anderson DL, Boyce HW, Jr. Use of parenteral nutrition in treatment of advanced regional enteritis. Am J Dig Dis 1973; 18:633–640.
57. Descos L, Vignal J. Total parenteral nutritional in the management of Crohn's disease. World J Surg 1980; 4:161–162.
58. Houcke P, Roger J, Blais J, et al. Exclusive parenteral nutrition. Results in 45 acute exacerbations of Crohn's disease. Nouv Presse Med 1980 9:1361.
59. Holm I. Benefits of total parenteral nutrition (TPN) in the treatment of Crohn's disease and ulcerative colitis. Acta Chir Scand 1981; 147:271–276.
60. Elson CO, Layden TJ, Nemchausky BA, et al. An evaluation of total parenteral nutrition in the management of inflammatory bowel disease. Dig Dis Sci 1980; 25:42–48.
61. Greenberg GR, Jeejeebhoy KN. Total parenteral nutrition (TPN) in the primary management of Crohn's disease. In Pena AS, Weterman IT, Booth CC, et al. (eds). Developments in Gastroenterology: Recent Advances in Crohn's Disease. The Hague, Martinus Nijhoff, 1981; 492–498.
62. Ostro MJ, Greenberg GR, Jeejeebhoy KN. Total parenteral nutrition and complete bowel rest in the management of Crohn's disease. JPEN 1985; 9:280–287.
63. Muller JM, Keller HW, Erasmi et al. Total parenteral nutrition as the sole therapy in Crohn's disease—a prospective study. Br J Surg 1983; 70:40–43.
64. Aguirre A, Fischer JF, Welch CE. The role of surgery and hyperalimentation in therapy of gastrointestinal-cutaneous fistulae. Ann Surg 1974; 180:393.
65. Driscoll RH, Jr, Rosenberg IH. Total parenteral nutrition in inflammatory bowel disease. Med Clin North Am 1978; 62:185–201.
66. Greenstein AJ, Kark AE, Dreiling DA. Crohn's disease of the colon. I. Fistula in Crohn's disease of the colon: classification, presenting features and management in 63 patients. Am J Gastroenterol 1974; 62:419.
67. Broe PJ, Bayless TM, Cameron JL. Crohn's disease: Are enteroenteral fistulas an indication for surgery? Surgery 1982; 91:249–253.
68. Givel JC, Hawker P, Allen R, et al. Entero-enteric fistula complicating Crohns' disease. J Clin Gastroenterol 1983; 5: 321–323.
69. McIntyre PB, Powell-Tuck J, Wood SR, et al. Controlled trial of bowel rest in the treatment of severe acute colitis. Gut 1986; 27:481–484.
70. Lochs H, Meryn S, Marosi L, et al. Has total bowel rest a beneficial effect in the treatment of Crohn's disease? Clin Nutr 1983; 2:61–64.
71. Greenberg GR, Fleming CR, Jeejeebhoy KN, et al. Controlled trial of bowel rest and nutritional support in the management of Crohn's disease. (Abstract). Gastroenterology 1985; 88:140.
72. Harries AD, Danis V, Heatley RV, et al. Controlled trial of supplemental oral nutrition in Crohn's disease. Lancet 1983; 1:887–890.
73. Chandra R. Rosette-forming T lymphocytes and cell-mediated immunity in malnutrition. Br Med J 1974; 3:608–609.
74. Skogh M, Sundquist T, Tagesson C. Vitamin A in Crohn's disease. Lancet 1980; 1:766.
75. Wright JP, Mee AS, Parfitt A, et al. Vitamin A therapy in patients with Crohn's disease. Gastroenterology 1985; 88:512–514.
76. Norrby S, Sjodahl R, Tagesson C. Ineffectiveness of vitamin A therapy in severe Crohn's disease. Acta Chir Scand 1985; 151:465–468.
77. Spector MH, Traylor J, Young EA, et al. Stimulator of mucosal growth by gastric and ileal infusion of single amino acids in parenterally nourished rats. Digestion 1981; 21:33–40.
78. Greenberg GR, Jeejeebhoy KN. Intravenous protein-sparing therapy in patients with gastrointestinal disease. JPEN 1979; 3:427–432.
79. Voitk AJ, Echave V, Feller JH, et al. Experience with elemental diet in the treatment of inflammatory bowel disease. Arch Surg 1973; 107:329–333.
80. Goode A, Hawkins T, Feggetter JGW, et al. Use of an elemental diet for long-term nutritional support in Crohn's disease. Lancet 1976; 1:122–124.
81. Russell RI, Hall MJ. Elemental diet therapy in the management of complicated Crohn's disease. Scott Med J 1979; 24:291–295.
82. Rocchio MA, Cha CM, Haas KF, et al. Use of chemically defined diets in the management of patients with acute inflammatory bowel disease. Am J Surg 1974; 127:469–475.
83. O'Morain C, Segal AW, Levi AJ. Elemental diets in treatment of acute Crohn's disease. Br Med J 1980; 281:1173–1175.
84. Saverymuttu S, Hodgson HJF, Chadwick VS. Controlled trial comparing prednisone with an elemental diet plus

non-absorbable antibiotics in active Crohn's disease. Gut 1985; 26:994–998.

85. Ursing B, Alm T, Barany F, et al. A comparative study of metronidazole and sulfasalazine for active Crohn's disease study in Sweden. II. Result. Gastroenterology 1982; 83:550–562.

86. Calam J, Crooks PE, Walker RJ. Elemental diets in the management of Crohn's perianal fistula. JPEN 1980; 4:4–8.

87. Lochs H, Egger-Schodle M, Schuh R, et al. Is tube feeding with elemental diets a primary therapy of Crohn's disease? Klin Wochenschr 1984; 62:821–825.

88. Halperin ML, Wolman SL, Greenberg GR. Paracellular recirculation of sodium is essential to support nutrient absorption in the gastrointestinal tract: an hypothesis. Clin Invest Med 1986; 9:209–211.

89. Jeejeebhoy KN, Langer B, Tsalles G, et al. Total parenteral nutrition at home: studies in patients surviving 4 months to 4 years. Gastroenterology 1976; 71:943–953.

90. Fleming RC, McGill DB, Berkner S, et al. Home parenteral nutrition for management of the severely malnourished adult patient. Gastroenterology 1980; 79:11–18.

91. Shike M, Jeejeebhoy KN. Low output cardiac failure in a woman with Crohn's disease receiving long-term total parenteral nutrition. Gastroenterology 1980; 78:605–619.

92. Quayle AR, Griffith CDM, Mangnall D, et al. Long term parenteral nutrition in the management of severe Crohn's disease. Clin Nutr 1985; 4:195–199.

93. Ritchie JK, Ritchie SM, McIntyre PB, et al. Management of severe acute colitis in district hospitals. J Roy Soc Med 1984; 77:465–471.

94. Jarnerot G, Rolny P, Sandberg-Gertzen H. Intensive intravenous treatment of ulcerative colitis. Gastroenterology 1985; 89:1005–1013.

95. Truelove, SC, Ellis H, Webster CU. Place of a double-barrelled ileostomy in ulcerative colitis and Crohn's disease of the colon: a preliminary report. Br Med J 1965; 1:150–153.

96. McCaffery TD, Mars K, Lawrence AM, et al. Severe growth retardation in children with inflammatory bowel disease. Pediatrics 1970; 45:386–393.

97. Kirschner BS, Sutton MM. Somatomedin-C levels in growth-impaired children and adolescents with chronic inflammatory bowel disease. Gastroenterology 1986; 91:830–836.

98. Kelts DG, Grand RJ, Shen G, et al. Nutritional basis of growth failure in children and adolescents with Crohn's disease. Gastroenterology 1979; 76:720–727.

99. Layden T, Rosenberg J, Menchausky B, et al. Reversal of growth arrest in adolescents with Crohn's disease after parenteral alimentation. Gastroenterology 1976; 70:1017–1021.

100. Lake AM, Kim S, Mathis RK, et al. Influence of preoperative parenteral alimentation on postoperative growth in adolescent Crohn's disease. J Pediatr Gastroenterol Nutr 1985; 4:182–186.

101. Motil KJ, Grand RJ, Matthews DE, et al. Whole body leucine metabolism in adolescents with Crohn's disease and growth failure during nutritional supplements. Gastroenterology 1982; 82:1359–1368.

102. Morin CL, Roulet M, Roy CC, et al. Continuous elemental enteral alimentation in children with Crohn's disease and growth failure. Gastroenterology, 1980; 79:1205–1210.

103. Seldman EG, Bouthillier L, Weber AM, et al. Elemental diet versus prednisone as primary treatment of Crohn's disease. (Abstract). Gastroenterology 1986; 90:1625.

104. Strobel CT, Byrne WJ, Ament ME. Home parenteral nutrition in children with Crohn's disease: an effective management alternative. Gastroenterology 1979; 77:272–279.

105. MacFayden BV, Dudrick SJ. The management of fistulas in inflammatory bowel disease with parenteral hyperalimentation. *In* Romieu C, Sollasal C, Joyeux H, et al. (eds). International Congress on Parenteral Nutrition. University of Montpelier, Montpelier, France, 1974: 559–562.

106. Bos LP, Nube M, Weterman IT. Total parenteral nutrition (TPN) in Crohn's disease; a clinical evaluation. *In* Pena AS, Weterman IT, Booth CC, et al. (eds). Developments in Gastroenterology: Recent Advances in Crohn's Disease. The Hague, Martinus Nijhoff, 1981: 499–506.

16

MALABSORPTION

ROBIN C. SPILLER / *DAVID B. A. SILK*

Although there are separate specific absorptive pathways for many dietary nutrients, in clinical practice isolated defects of absorption (e.g., vitamin B_{12} in pernicious anemia) are in the minority. This is either because the disease process affects many aspects of absorption (e.g., tropical sprue[1]) or because malabsorption of one dietary component (e.g., lactose in lactase deficiency) produces a secondary effect, such as intestinal hurry, that in turn induces malabsorption of fat.[2] Thus it is more convenient to classify malabsorption according to where in the digestive tract the main abnormality lies (Table 16–1) rather than by the type of nutrient that is malabsorbed. This chapter deals only with diseases affecting primarily the small bowel, excluding those marked with an asterisk in Table 16–1, since they are covered in separate chapters.

INCIDENCE

Malabsorptive diseases vary enormously in their incidence. While tropical sprue and giardiasis are endemic in some parts of the world, perhaps affecting 50 per cent of the population, and celiac disease, the commonest cause of generalized intestinal malabsorption in the United Kingdom, occurs in 0.02 to 0.03 per cent of the population, the incidence of abetalipoproteinemia must be several orders of magnitude smaller, since only a few cases have ever been described. Our coverage in this chapter to some extent reflects the incidence of disease, but space will also be given to some extremely rare malabsorption syndromes because understanding of these diseases often throws considerable light on normal absorptive processes.

NORMAL PHYSIOLOGY OF NUTRIENT ABSORPTION

Carbohydrate

Starch, sucrose, and lactose are the most important dietary carbohydrates, together accounting for

281

TABLE 16–1. Causes of Malabsorption

Site	Mechanism	Example
Gastric	Precipitate emptying Lack of intrinsic factor Excess acid secretion	Postgastrectomy dumping Pernicious anemia Zollinger-Ellison syndrome
Pancreatic	Inadequate enzyme and bi- carbonate secretion	Cystic fibrosis Chronic pancreatitis Carcinoma of pancreas
Biliary	Defective micelle formation	Chronic biliary obstruction Primary biliary cirrhosis Massive ileal resection Cholestyramine
Small bowel	Loss of absorptive surface/ damaged enterocyte	Celiac disease Tropical sprue Giardiasis Small bowel resection* Crohn's disease* Radiation enteritis Contaminated small bowel syndrome* Lymphoma
	Isolated brush border en- zyme defects	Lactase insufficiency Congenital alactasia Sucrase-isomaltase deficiency Glucose-galactose malabsorption Hartnup disease
	Impaired postabsorptive fat transport	Lymphangiectasia Abetalipoproteinemia
	Drugs	Alcohol* Neomycin*

*Discussed in other chapters.

60 per cent of the energy intake in a normal Western diet. Starch is a macromolecule (molecular weight 1×10^6) composed of glucose molecules linked mainly by alpha-1,4 bonds with occasional branching in the linear polymer formed by alpha-1,6 bonding. Pancreatic alpha-amylase is a specific enzyme capable of hydrolyzing alpha-1,4 bonds except those at the end of a polymer. It cannot hydrolyze the branching alpha-1,6 bonds, and hence the end products of amylase digestion of starch are maltose, maltotriose, and alpha-limit dextrins.[3] Brush border enzymes cleave di- and trisaccharides as well as longer chain oligosaccharides,[4] including alpha-limit dextrins, yielding glucose, which is then absorbed by a sodium-linked, carrier-mediated, energy-dependent transport system. Glucose and galactose share this transport system, exhibiting competitive inhibition, while fructose is absorbed by a noncompeting pathway.[5] Lactose is a unique disaccharide in that brush border enzyme levels are relatively low, and thus hydrolysis is the rate-limiting step in absorption.[6] Sucrose by contrast is rapidly hydrolyzed, with monosaccharide accumulating in the intestinal lumen during its absorption, though the extent of this is limited by end-product inhibition of hydrolysis.[7] Since lactase concentrations are low already, lactose malabsorption is one of the earliest signs of diffuse damage to the brush border, and it is a feature of many of the mucosal diseases that are discussed below. Polysaccharides in which the links between the glucose monomers are not alpha-1,4 bonds escape breakdown by pancreatic amylase and brush border hydrolases and enter the colon, where they are metabolized by colonic bacteria as described later in this chapter.

Fat

Approximately 40 per cent of non-nitrogen calories taken in a Western diet are in the form of fat, the average 70-kg man taking about 120 g/day, mainly as saturated and monounsaturated long-chain triglycerides (C16 and C18). Only about 5 g of dietary fat escapes absorption in the small intestine to be excreted in the stool.

After mastication and trituration in the stomach, fat is presented to the small intestine in the form of lipid droplets. The transfer of water-insoluble triglyceride from this lipid phase, via the aqueous phase of intestinal contents, to the lipid membrane of the enterocyte involves a complex series of reactions. Hydrolysis of the triglyceride begins in the stomach with the action of lingual lipase,[8] which, unlike pancreatic lipase, is not inactivated by gastric acid. Although usually quantitatively insignificant, this may account for a substantial proportion of hydrolysis in severe exocrine pancreatic insufficiency. Lipase acts at the lipid-aqueous interface to hydrolyze triglyceride to free fatty acids, mono- and diglycerides, and glycerol, a process that is catalyzed by a pancreatic protein, colipase, deficiency of which leads to steatorrhea.[9] Free fatty acid is capable of stimulating the release of cholecystokinin from the upper small intestinal mucosa, which acts together with other neural and hormonal factors, including secretin, to stimulate alkaline pancreatic and biliary secretion. This neutralizes gastric acid and creates an alkaline pH, which, in the presence of bile salts, allows the emulsification of triglycerides and the solubilization of otherwise highly insoluble long-chain fatty acids. These dissolve in micellar aggregates composed of bile salts, monoglycerides, fatty acids, and cholesterol, and in this water-soluble form lipid can diffuse across the unstirred water layer to gain access to the lipid membrane of the enterocyte. Once there, triglyceride can diffuse down its concentration gradient, intracellular accumulation of free fatty acid being prevented by esterification. Free fatty acids are transported through the cell bound to fatty acid binding protein (FABP),[10] which is located in the enterocyte cytoplasm. Once across the cell membrane, free fatty acids, bound to FABP, are transported to the smooth endoplasmic reticulum in the apical portion of the enterocyte just beneath the microvillous membrane. There triglyceride is resynthesized and then transported to the rough endoplasmic reticulum, where lipoproteins are synthesized. After combination with these apoproteins, triglyceride is stored in the Golgi apparatus in the supranuclear portion of the enterocyte prior to secretion into the extracellular space by reverse pinocytosis as chylomicrons,[11] which are transported via the lymphatic channels. This process requires synthesis of apoproteins, and in states of severe protein-calorie malnutrition with depression of protein synthesis, fat absorption may be significantly impaired.[12] Apoprotein B is essential for chylomicron synthesis, as is seen from the absence of chylomicrons in abetalipoproteinemia.[13] Medium-chain triglycerides (MCT), whose mean fatty acid chain length is 8, differ from long-chain triglycerides in that the free fatty acids are relatively water-soluble, and hence their absorption is less dependent on the presence of bile salts. Furthermore, once free fatty acids have entered the cell, some can enter the portal blood without prior esterification.[14] Thus, if enterocyte protein synthesis is impaired, there is less impairment of MCT absorption than of the normal long-chain dietary triglycerides.[14]

Nitrogen

A normal diet provides about 10 to 14 g of nitrogen as protein daily, to which must be added about 10 g of nitrogen secreted into the gastrointestinal tract as endogenous protein, about equal amounts from gastrointestinal secretions and desquamated cells. Protein macromolecules must be digested to oligopeptides and amino acids prior to uptake by the enterocyte. Competitive inhibition demonstrated between amino acids indicates that in humans there are at least three separate amino acid transport systems:[15] (1) monoamino, monocarboxylic (neutral) amino acids; (2) dibasic amino acids and cystine; and (3) dicarboxylic (acidic) amino acids. Dipeptides appear to share a common transport system,[16] with a higher maximum transport capacity than any one amino acid system. At high concentrations many amino acids are more rapidly absorbed from oligopeptide solutions than from equivalent solutions containing free amino acids.[17, 18] Further studies at Central Middlesex Hospital have shown that the optimum peptide chain length for maximizing the rate of absorption is 2 to 3 amino acid residues.[19] However, at lower, more physiologic concentrations these differences are less obvious.[20] Long-term feeding studies comparing nitrogen balance during feeding with a lactalbumin hydrolysate with that during feeding with an equivalent amino acid mixture have failed to show any nutritional benefit in patients with a normal intestine,[21] perhaps because of the enormous reserve capacity for absorption of the normal intestine. Currently we are undertaking further studies to assess whether benefit would be seen in the short bowel syndrome, in which this reserve is largely lost.

PHYSIOLOGICAL EFFECTS OF MALABSORBED NUTRIENTS

Patients who suffer from malabsorption experience symptoms due to the primary pathology as well as symptoms that can be regarded as secondary phenomena due to the presence of malabsorbed nutrients in the gastrointestinal tract. These symptoms, which could be alleviated by dietary restriction, can be more clearly identified in normal subjects and have recently been the subject of vigorous research efforts. It is known that after a homogenized liquid meal very little fat or carbohydrate escapes absorption in the upper small intestine.[22, 23] When more complex, solid meals are taken, the amount of carbohydrate escaping absorption in the small intestine rises, but is still normally less than 10 per cent of intake.[24] Patients with malabsorption differ therefore from normals in the extent to which the small bowel and colon are exposed to fat and carbohydrate. This difference may be less marked for protein, which, unlike fat and carbohydrate, is normally present in substantial amounts in the form of desquamated enterocytes and glycoproteins from intestinal secretions.

TABLE 16–2. Effect of Malabsorbed Fat

Impaired intestinal water and electrolyte absorption

Delayed absorption of calcium, magnesium, bile salts, and vitamin D

Gut peptide release and inhibition of eating, gastric emptying, and small bowel transit

Accelerated colonic transit and decreased colonic reservoir function

Fat (Table 16–2)

IMPAIRED INTESTINAL WATER AND ELECTROLYTE ABSORPTION

Unlike malabsorbed sugars, unabsorbed triglyceride exerts no appreciable osmotic effect, but it does have other important effects on intestinal water and electrolyte handling. Low concentrations of long-chain free fatty acids, when perfused into the normal intestine, cause intestinal secretion in the jejunum[25] and inhibit sodium and water absorption from the ileum[26] and colon.[27] This is especially relevant to celiac disease and tropical sprue, in which enterocyte damage, in the presence of otherwise normal digestion, allows the intraluminal accumulation of free fatty acids. Recent studies in India have confirmed an excess of long-chain fatty acids in the stools of patients with tropical sprue[28] and associated defects in colonic electrolyte absorption.[29] The authors have gone one step further and demonstrated an inhibition of colonic enterocyte ATPase by long-chain fatty acids,[28] which may provide a mechanism for this association.

The chemical similarity between the known cathartic ricinoleic acid[25] and 12-hydroxystearic acid, a bacterial metabolite of stearic acid,[30] led some authors[31] to believe that this specific metabolite was responsible for the catharsis associated with steatorrhea. Subsequently it was shown that excluding oleic acid from the diet could eliminate 12-hydroxystearic acid from the stool without altering symptoms,[32] and it is now clear that many long-chain fatty acids cause intestinal secretion. Ricinoleic acid is an especially potent cathartic by virtue of its poor absorption, which allows it to be active when taken by mouth even in normal subjects.

DELAYED ABSORPTION OF CALCIUM, MAGNESIUM, BILE SALTS, AND VITAMIN D

Although fat loading acutely increases fecal excretion of magnesium[33] in patients with steatorrhea, the long-term significance of this is uncertain owing to the compensatory increase in magnesium absorption as body Mg^{++} stores fall.[34] Fecal calcium is also increased in steatorrhea due to celiac disease,[35] some of which probably reflects increased endogenous secretion of calcium associated with increased enterocyte turnover. Impaired absorption is most likely due to failure to absorb vitamin D,[36] but the presence of unabsorbed, free, long-chain fatty acids may lead to the formation of insoluble calcium soaps, thus rendering dietary calcium unavailable for absorption.[37, 38] Unabsorbed fat may also impair vitamin D absorption, since this occurs much faster from a monomeric micellar solution than from one in which the micelles are expanded by the presence of fatty acids.[39]

Micellar bile acids cannot be absorbed before the micellar lipid,[40] so that delayed lipid absorption is also associated with delayed bile acid absorption. However, owing to compensatory slowing of intestinal transit, bile acid absorption in celiac disease appears to be delayed but intact,[41] fecal bile acids not being elevated, except in the most severe cases.[42] Experimental slowing of bile acid recycling leads to a compensatory expansion of the bile salt pool,[43, 44] a mechanism that perhaps is the reason why celiacs have a bile salt pool that is three times normal.[45]

In addition to these direct effects on absorption, unabsorbed fat stimulates the release of many regulatory peptides from mucosal endocrine cells and thus indirectly influences many aspects of gut function.

GUT PEPTIDE RELEASE AND POSSIBLE MOTOR EFFECTS

Direct intubation studies in our own laboratory, in which we simulated fat malabsorption in healthy volunteers by infusing 10 g of partially digested fat into the ileum, demonstrated a marked release of the peptide hormones neurotensin, enteroglucagon,[46] and peptide YY.[47] Postprandial release of these hormones is known to be elevated in celiac disease,[48, 49] and our fat infusions produced levels closely simulating these changes. These peptide rises produced no obvious subjective sensation but were associated with profound inhibition of jejunal motility and a corresponding prolongation of transit time of a dye bolus through the jejunum.[46] Others have reported inhibition of both gastric emptying and small bowel transit by similar infusions,[50] which the same group had also shown to inhibit eating by generating a sense of satiety.[51] All these effects may be regarded as compensatory, since by prolonging mucosal contact time they may enhance absorption, particularly if there is some defect reducing the absorptive reserve of the small intestine.

It appears unlikely that neurotensin mediates the observed inhibitory effect, since although it does delay gastric emptying,[52] its effect on the small bowel is not inhibitory.[53] Enteroglucagon also appeared an unlikely mediator, since inhibitory effects were seen without rises in this hormone.[50] Peptide YY, a recently described mucosal peptide,[54] is found in the terminal ileum and colon of humans.[55] Abnormally high levels are detectable postprandially in patients with fat malabsorption,[49] and infusion of hormone in normal subjects at rates designed to simulate these pathological levels delays gastric emptying[56] and also mouth-to-cecum transit.[57] Peptide YY release in celiac patients correlates inversely with the rate of gastric emptying[47] and may contribute to a number of features of celiac disease including anorexia, abdominal distention, and slow transit.[58]

DECREASED COLONIC RESERVOIR FUNCTION

The reservoir function of the colon appears to be diminished in steatorrhea because, although mouth-to-cecum transit is usually delayed in all but the most severe cases,[59, 60] clinical observation suggests that overall mouth-to-anus transit is usually shortened, implying accelerated colonic transit. Malabsorbed dietary fat is substantially hydrolyzed by bacterial lipases,[61] producing long-chain fatty acids in the colon. Although short-chain fatty acids are actively absorbed by the colon,[62, 63] stimulating water and electrolyte absorption in the process,[64] long-chain fatty acids are not well absorbed and actually inhibit water and electrolyte absorption.[27] In addition, as we have recently reported,[65] oleic acid emulsions infused into the cecum accelerate colonic transit, inducing mass movements, which can be seen to be associated with giant propulsive pressure waves originating near the cecal pole (Figs. 16–1 and 16–2). The oleic acid in these studies appeared to reduce the cecal volume, and this causes a loss of cecal reservoir function. The implications of this are that the normal postprandial rises in ileocolonic inflow could no longer be accommodated in the right colon and would result in urgent postcibal defecation, which is a common symptom in patients with steatorrhea.

IMPLICATIONS FOR DIETARY MANAGEMENT OF STEATORRHEA

Since most fecal fat is dietary in origin, it is apparent that a low-fat diet, or one containing fat in a more easily absorbed form, such as medium-chain triglycerides, would reduce some of the effects described above and hence provide symptomatic relief. Controlled studies have confirmed that such a diet reduces abdominal cramps and diarrhea in fat malabsorption,[66] but the benefit lies mainly in reduction of colonic symptoms, since no benefit is seen in those without colons.[67] Caution should be used in advocating such diets, since there are also distinct disadvantages including loss of palatability and calories. The need to substitute very high doses of carbohy-drates for the "lost calories" appears, in some cases, to actually prolong the diarrheal episode.[68] Furthermore, if the inhibitory effect of fat, the "ileal brake,"[46] is lost, then the compensatory changes such as the delay in gastric emptying will also be lost, and this may further exacerbate the diarrhea.

Carbohydrate

Although absorption of starch presented as rice or gluten-free wheat flour is virtually complete, normal subjects fail to absorb about 10 per cent of starch presented as oats or whole wheat flour; gluten apparently interferes with the hydrolysis of the starch.[69–71] This minor degree of malabsorption should not be regarded as undesirable, since this starch is probably essential for normal colonic function, providing as it does a substrate for colonic bacteria. These generate a range of short-chain fatty acids, some of which, such as butyrate, are a preferred energy source for colonic enterocytes.[72] Starch, having a very large molecular weight, exerts little osmotic effect in the small intestine, but is fermented to hydrogen, carbon dioxide, methane, and short-chain fatty acids by bacteria in the colon; excessive malabsorption thus produces flatus and, if severe, abdominal cramps and diarrhea. Malabsorption of low-molecular-weight carbohydrates, such as lactose, also produces flatus, colic, and diarrhea, but in this case small bowel effects are more important.[73] Isotonic solutions of nonabsorbable sugars that contain no sodium cause marked secretion of sodium and water across the highly permeable jejunal membrane.[74, 75] This markedly accelerates small bowel transit and, by reducing mucosal contact time, reduces absorption.[76] In malnourished lactase-deficient Africans, lactose loading can cause severe steatorrhea, which is abolished by a lactose-free diet.[2] This acceleration of transit appears to be an impor-

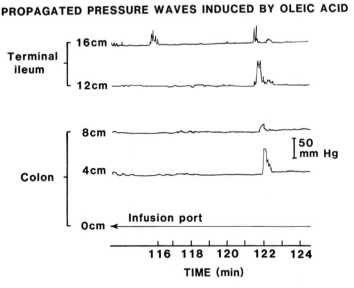

FIGURE 16–1. Graphic recording of a rapidly propagated, high-amplitude, prolonged pressure wave originating in the terminal ileum, progressing caudally down the ascending colon. Numbers in cm refer to distance of the pressure recording port from the tip of the orocecal tube, via whose end port oleic acid emulsion was infused into the right colon.

PROPAGATED PRESSURE WAVES INDUCED BY OLEIC ACID

Terminal ileum
16cm
12cm

Colon
8cm
4cm
0cm
Infusion port

50 mm Hg

TIME (min)
116 118 120 122 124

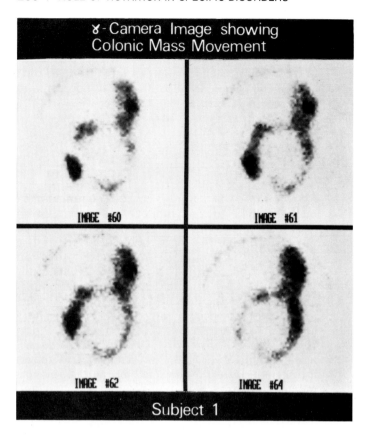

FIGURE 16-2. Gamma scans obtained by labeling the fatty acid emulsion with [111]indium DTPA. Image numbers refer to the number of minutes since the start of the infusion into the mid ascending colon. Between image 62 and 63 there has been a mass caudal movement of colonic contents which was, in each case, associated with the propagation of one of the prolonged pressure waves illustrated in Figure 16-1.

tant determinant of symptoms,[77] especially diarrhea, since the colonic tolerance for fluid loading is markedly dependent on the rate of ileocolonic inflow. Sudden boluses of as little as 500 ml cause diarrhea, whereas up to 4 L of saline can be infused over 24 hours without altering stool frequency.[78]

Malabsorbed carbohydrate in the ileum releases neurotensin and also appears to inhibit jejunal motility,[47] though to a lesser degree than fat. Gastric emptying has also been reported to be delayed in experimental carbohydrate malabsorption generated by feeding an amylase inhibitor.[79] In these recent studies the onset of the delay was compatible with an inhibitory reflex generated as malabsorbed starch reached the ileum. Ileal starch released neurotensin, which the authors suggest could mediate the inhibitory effect observed.

The laxative effect of malabsorbed carbohydrate depends upon the interaction between bacterial metabolism and colonic function, both of which show adaptation so that, with continued exposure, symptoms decrease over time.[80] Although lactase levels in jejunal biopsies of lactase-deficient subjects cannot be elevated by a high-milk diet, clinical tolerance for milk does improve if the diet is continued.[81] This is probably due, at least in part, to more efficient bacterial metabolism of unabsorbed lactose yielding short-chain fatty acids which are readily absorbed. Changes in bacterial flora may also explain why tolerance develops to the laxative effect of dietary fiber in patients with severe constipation.

Nitrogen

Generalized malabsorption of amino acids is seen only as part of a more general malabsorption syndrome in which the effects of malabsorbed fat and carbohydrate predominate. In the rare cases in which there is a specific defect in amino acid absorption large doses of the malabsorbed amino acid will induce diarrhea,[82] which is probably osmotic in origin, though secretion due to excess of malabsorbed dibasic amino acids may also play a part.[83] Diarrhea is not usually a feature of amino acid transport defects such as cystinuria or Hartnup disease, since in the normal diet the malabsorbed amino acids are probably absorbed mainly in the dipeptide form. The only obvious exception to this is lysinuric protein intolerance, in which there is a complete block to the absorption of dibasic amino acids at the basolateral membrane level[84] and the malabsorbed amino acids are known to cause intestinal secretion.[83] Malabsorbed amino acids that enter the colon are extensively metabolized to short-chain fatty acids and ammonia as well as a number of characteristic bacterial products, one of the better known of which is indigotin, a bacterial breakdown product of tryptophan that is responsible for the blue staining of the stool in the blue diaper syndrome.[85]

SPECIFIC MALABSORPTIVE DISORDERS

Having considered the basic physiology of malabsorption, we will now attempt to apply these principles to understanding the symptoms and logically managing the nutritional support of patients with malabsorption.

Celiac Disease (Gluten-Sensitive Enteropathy)

While Samuel Gee's classic description of celiac disease was made in 1888,[86] it was not until the end of the Second World War in Europe, with its attendant severe food shortages, that it was clearly shown by some Dutch physicians that wheat-free diets benefited children with this wasting disease.[87] Subsequent studies[88-90] have shown that the gluten fraction of flour contains the toxic agent, which is probably a peptide fragment of gliadin.[91] This exerts a toxic effect within a few hours of contact with the small bowel, inducing total villous atrophy within a few weeks of continuous exposure. Gluten is not toxic to normal subjects even in very large doses,[92] thus celiac disease appears to be a specific, probably inherited, sensitivity.

CLINICAL FEATURES

The clinical effects of celiac disease are a direct result of the loss of villous absorptive area, which affects mainly the duodenum and jejunum, inducing malabsorption of a range of substances. Gluten sensitivity is probably much commoner than is generally recognized; patients exhibit a wide range of sensitivity, so that the clinical presentation depends considerably on the availability and indications for jejunal biopsy. In early series jejunal biopsy was carried out only in children with steatorrhea, and thus by definition all cases involved steatorrhea.[93] More recently indications for jejunal biopsies are more liberal, and in centers with an interest in the condition there is a much higher incidence of detection and a correspondingly milder average clinical picture.[94] Current practice in the United Kingdom suggests that up to 30 per cent of patients will present without gastrointestinal complaints; in these patients the disease generally is detected by virtue of mild hematological abnormalities, such as macrocytosis or iron deficiency,[95] usually reflecting either folate or iron malabsorption, respectively. The other 70 per cent of patients exhibit steatorrhea, diarrhea, and/or weight loss. As Table 16–3 shows, celiac children with steatorrhea present primarily with growth failure, which is a highly sensitive index of malabsorption. Both diarrhea and vomiting are common. Anorexia often continues in spite of weight loss, in contrast to other diseases causing malabsorption (e.g., pancreatic exocrine insufficiency), in which weight loss is usually associated with hyperphagia. The anorexia associated with celiac disease is actually more important in determining weight loss than is steatorrhea per se, as the "lost calories" could easily

TABLE 16–3. Features of 42 Children with Celiac Disease

Feature	Number
Growth failure	36*†
Diarrhea	30
Vomiting	24
Anorexia	21
Physical findings‡	
Muscle wasting	40
Abdominal distention	33
Glossitis	26
Mouth ulcers	8
Edema	4

*Median age at diagnosis 2 years (range 1 to 9).
†26 out of 42 were below third percentile.
‡None had cutaneous manifestations of vitamin deficiencies such as bruising, hyperkeratosis or skin rash. Neither did any have rickets or evidence of peripheral neuropathy.
Data from Hamilton et al.[93]

be replaced if intake was increased.[96] One possible explanation for this impaired appetite is that malabsorbed fatty acids in the terminal ileum activate the "ileal brake," delaying gastric emptying and small bowel transit,[46] and thus induce early postprandial satiety, as has been demonstrated experimentally.[51] The laboratory features in celiacs with steatorrhea (Table 16–4) reflect the fact that the brunt of the disease is borne by the upper small intestine, gluten having been digested to nontoxic fragments by the time the meal residue reaches the ileum. Thus the commonest laboratory features reflect malabsorption of iron and folic acid, which are both absorbed optimally from the duodenum and upper jejunum, while malabsorption of substances such as vitamin B_{12} and bile salts, which are absorbed from the distal ileum, is correspondingly rare. Colonic absorption has not been directly measured but is probably unimpaired, so that malabsorption of water and electrolytes is rare.

THE MUCOSAL LESION

Villous atrophy with crypt hyperplasia, the characteristic jejunal lesion originally described by Paulley,[99] is due to accelerated cell exfoliation,[100] which results in relatively immature cells lining the tips of the stunted villi. Normally aminopeptidases, disaccharidases, and sodium/potassium ATPase levels rise

TABLE 16–4. Laboratory Features in Celiac Patients with Steatorrhea

	Hamilton et al.[93]	Cooke et al.[97]
Anemia	85%	40%
Folate deficiency	63%	61%
Iron deficiency	32%	52%
Hypocalcemia	36%	64%
Hypomagnesemia	14%	—
Hypoalbuminemia	32%	57%
Increased fecal nitrogen	—	43%[98]
Vitamin B_{12} deficiency	0%	11%

as the enterocyte matures and migrates from crypt to villous tip,[101] so it is not surprising that in celiac disease the mean enzyme levels in jejunal homogenates are depressed, as immature cells predominate.[102, 103] As yet there is no evidence of an underlying enzyme deficiency in celiac disease, since the specific activity of all these enzymes returns to normal after treatment with a gluten-free diet. Lactose intolerance due to lactase insufficiency may, however, be very slow to improve,[104] probably because, as already indicated, lactase activity, even in normal subjects, is the lowest of all the brush border enzymes.

CORRELATION BETWEEN MUCOSAL LESION AND SYMPTOMS

The severity of malabsorption depends on how far down the small bowel the villous atrophy extends.[105] Severely affected celiacs have villous atrophy extending to the ileum,[106] while in milder cases only the proximal jejunum is affected.[105] This proximal-distal gradient of villous damage is not due to a differential sensitivity to gluten, since direct ileal instillation of gluten will induce the same mucosal lesion as it does in the jejunum;[105] it probably merely reflects the fact that the proximal small bowel is exposed to the largest load of gluten. Those in whom the ileal mucosa has been damaged have lost the reserve of absorptive function normally provided by the distal small bowel[107] and hence suffer severe steatorrhea, while those in whom the ileum is spared have markedly fewer symptoms.[105] The jejunal villous atrophy seen in most untreated patients produces marked derangement of jejunal function with defective absorption of glucose,[108] amino acids,[109] water, and electrolytes; half the patients demonstrate net secretion of the last two substances.[110, 111] This malabsorption causes excessive nutrients to enter the ileum, which in other settings is associated with ileal hyperplasia.[112] Although ileal hyperplasia has not been reported in celiac disease, there are reports of ileal hyperfunction.[113, 114] The mechanism for this adaptive increase in ileal absorption is uncertain but may include activation of the "ileal brake," causing slowing of intestinal transit and prolongation of mucosal contact time.

MALABSORPTION OF SPECIFIC SUBSTANCES

Folic Acid. Since folic acid is mainly absorbed in the jejunum (ileal absorption being rather ineffective),[115] malabsorption of folic acid is a particularly sensitive index of jejunal damage in celiac disease.[116] Intestinal perfusion studies in celiac patients have shown a depressed jejunal absorption of both crystalline folic acid[115] and pteroylpolyglutamate,[117] the normal dietary form of folic acid. Since jejunal morphology correlates well with serum folate levels,[118] these are very helpful in monitoring the response to

a gluten-free diet, providing the patient is no longer taking crystalline folic acid supplements.[116]

Iron. Iron deficiency, which is common in celiac disease, usually causes an adaptive increase in iron absorption, and in some[119] but not all[120] patients this appears to compensate for the jejunal defect. In those with normal iron absorption, iron deficiency is probably due to increased losses in the form of desquamated cells, which can be substantial.[121, 122]

Xylose. Xylose is a poorly absorbed nonnutrient sugar that, like iron and folic acid, is mainly absorbed in the jejunum[123] and then excreted unchanged in the urine. Although absorption is reduced in celiac patients,[92] and urinary excretion of xylose is correspondingly low, the range in normals is so wide that appreciable overlap occurs with values seen in celiac patients, rendering the test unhelpful diagnostically.[124]

Calcium, Magnesium, and Zinc. After an oral dose of radiolabeled ^{47}Ca, ^{24}Mg, or ^{65}Zn, isotope promptly appears in the blood, and peak levels occur within 1 hour,[125–127] implying rapid absorption from the upper small intestine. More direct perfusion studies in normals and celiacs confirm that calcium absorption is much more rapid from the jejunum than from the ileum and that jejunal absorption is markedly impaired in celiac disease.[128] As for iron, intestinal losses of cations in desquamated cells are also increased[35, 37] leading to negative balance of both calcium and magnesium.[129] The binding of cations as insoluble salts can be clearly demonstrated by increased fecal excretion after fat loading;[33, 130, 131] however, because this leads to a compensatory increase in absorption, the overall significance of this effect is probably limited.

Fat. Although in normal subjects most fat is absorbed from the upper small intestine,[22, 23] after large fat loads[107] or following jejunal resection,[131] the ileum is capable of absorbing substantial quantities of fat. Thus it is not surprising that the severity of steatorrhea in celiac patients correlates better with ileal rather than jejunal morphology,[105, 106] since it is only after loss of ileal function that fat will escape absorption in the small intestine. In addition to the mucosal lesion reducing absorption, there is also maldigestion due to delayed and reduced pancreatic and biliary secretions,[132] which probably reflects impaired cholecystokinin release.[133] Fecal fat is further elevated by increased endogenous fat losses, presumably from desquamated cells.[98]

Nitrogen. Normal subjects excrete about 2 g of nitrogen daily, largely in the form of bacterial protein. Fecal nitrogen losses in celiac disease are elevated up to five fold in proportion to the severity of the steatorrhea.[98] Although there is evidence that jejunal absorption of free amino acids is impaired, dipeptide absorption is less affected,[109] so that nitrogen absorption after a normal protein meal would be predicted to be relatively normal. This is supported by studies by Crane and Neuberger,[134] who showed that although absorption of orally administered ^{15}N-labeled protein was delayed, total absorption was normal. This suggests that increased intestinal losses rather than malabsorption may be the most important factor causing a negative nitrogen balance in celiac disease.

Carbohydrate. Malabsorbed carbohydrate is rapidly metabolized by bacteria, so fecal carbohydrate is an unreliable guide to malabsorption. Certainly absorption of model, nonmetabolizable sugars, such as xylose, are impaired and jejunal perfusion studies have shown that glucose and fructose malabsorption is also present.[108] As recovery occurs, monomer absorption returns to normal, but intolerance to lactose commonly remains owing to hypolactasia.[102]

Vitamin B[12]. Blood vitamin B[12] levels are often low in severely affected celiac patients, though rarely low enough to cause anemia or neuropathy.[135] Total body absorption is in most cases normal, however, unless steatorrhea is severe.[97, 106]

Bile Salts. Increased fecal bile salts are rarely seen except in the most severe cases, implying that in the majority ileal reabsorption is normal.[42] As already described, the postprandial rise in serum bile acids occurs more slowly in celiacs, in keeping with the known sluggish enterohepatic circulation of bile salts in this condition.[136]

WATER AND ELECTROLYTES

Malabsorption of sugars and amino acids together with jejunal secretion results in an increased flow of sodium and water entering the ileum and colon. Colonic function has not been assessed, but colonic morphology is normal and function appears relatively intact, so celiacs rarely become saline- or water-depleted.

NUTRITIONAL THERAPY

Although steroid suppression of the inflammatory response to gluten can achieve a partial remission,[137, 138] in most patients a gluten-free diet is the only treatment necessary. Starch can be obtained from maize, oats, and rice,[139] which are gluten-free, but flour made from wheat, rye, and barley should be excluded.[140] Success in maintaining a gluten-free diet in the United Kingdom is aided considerably by the existence of a self-help group, the Coeliac Society (P.O. Box 181, London, NW2 2YQ, United Kingdom) which publishes a handbook, updated each year, to provide detailed information on which products contain gluten. Food manufacturers in Europe are now obliged to indicate when a product is gluten-free, using a symbol consisting of an ear of corn with a diagonal line through it.

The stricter the diet the more completely jejunal morphology recovers[41] and steatorrhea disappears.[142] Response can generally be detected clinically within 1 to 2 weeks and is often dramatic, with cessation of diarrhea and steatorrhea.[143] Deficiency states often correct more slowly, so it is usual to aid recovery by supplementing the diet with crystalline folic acid 5 mg three times daily, vitamin B[12] 1 mg intramuscularly weekly, and oral iron if indicated. Some patients, particularly adults, respond much more slowly. Pink and Creamer[144] described 54 adult patients, 38 of whom responded promptly, but 8 took more than 1 year to improve and 3 deteriorated in spite of a gluten-free diet, responding only when steroids were added. Two patients deteriorated and died in spite of all these measures. Some of the nonresponders were subsequently shown to have developed diffuse intestinal lymphoma, a well-recognized complication of celiac disease.[145, 146] Rarely patients respond initially and then relapse with evidence of intestinal perforation and at laparotomy are found to have developed ulcerative jejunoileitis,[147] which may in some cases be a manifestation of diffuse intestinal lymphoma.[148] In some patients the order of presentation may be reversed so that gluten sensitivity is demonstrable only after the lymphoma has been excised.[149]

In the majority of patients who have responded normally to gluten withdrawal, reintroducing gluten produces histological and biochemical evidence of mucosal damage within a few days,[150, 151] a fall in brush border lactase being one of the earliest markers of damage.[103, 152] There is, however, considerable variability in sensitivity to gluten, so that in some patients clinical relapse may be very delayed, some taking many months to develop histological damage on a gluten-containing diet.[153]

Tropical Sprue (Tropical Malabsorption Syndrome)

While celiac disease is the commonest cause of total villous atrophy in the temperate zones, on a worldwide basis tropical sprue is by far the most important cause. This is endemic in some tropical areas, and also occurs in epidemic form (100,000 cases being reported in a 2-year period in Southern India[154]). Visitors from temperate zones are also affected,[155] insidiously developing diarrhea some months after arrival in the tropics. Stools are bulky, frothy, and fatty, the malabsorption being associated with anorexia, weakness, and progressive weight loss. In a survey of 50 patients with the tropical malabsorption syndrome (Table 16–5), glossitis and anemia were seen in two thirds of cases, hypoproteinemic edema and muscle wasting being a feature of severe disease.[156] The diagnosis is established clinically from the appearance of the jejunal biopsy, which shows subtotal villous atrophy associated with an infiltrate of chronic inflammatory cells.[156, 157] Normal healthy subjects from the tropics show a range of jejunal abnormalities, the villi losing their normal fingerlike appearance under the dissecting micro-

TABLE 16–5. Features of Tropical Sprue

	Per Cent of Patients Affected
Clinical Features	
Diarrhea	100
Abdominal pain	50
Weakness	96
Weight loss	60
Anorexia	50
Wasting	60
Edema	30
Glossitis	60
Laboratory Features	
Anemia	68
Folate deficiency	70
Vitamin B_{12} <100 ng/L	40
Steatorrhea (6–20 g/24 hr)	50
Xylose malabsorption	75
Vitamin B_{12} malabsorption	75
Folic acid malabsorption	76

scope and developing a convoluted form associated with villous blunting. These abnormalities increase with age and are most obvious in the proximal small intestine.[157, 158] In tropical sprue these features are exaggerated, with villous edema and thickening progressing to partial and even subtotal villous atrophy.[156, 157]

SMALL INTESTINAL FUNCTION

As with gluten-sensitive enteropathy, the histological abnormalities in tropical sprue are maximal in the proximal small intestine; in a few cases in which ileal biopsies have been performed they have shown lesser degrees of villous damage than the jejunal biopsy.[155] This may explain why abnormalities of proximal small bowel function such as folic acid and xylose malabsorption are commonly seen in the absence of steatorrhea, which is found only in those with severe mucosal damage.[156] Direct assessment of jejunal function by intestinal perfusion has demonstrated defective jejunal absorption of free amino acids[159] and water and electrolytes,[160] some patients showing net jejunal secretion. Absorption of amino acids from 50 mmol/L dipeptide solutions, for example, glycyl-leucine or glycyl-glycine, is much less affected than absorption from the equivalent free amino acid solution,[161] especially when lower, more physiological concentrations are perfused.[162]

Ileal electrolyte absorption is also defective,[163] and more recently colonic perfusion studies have shown colonic absorption to be similarly impaired.[29] This is an important difference from celiac disease, and may account for the greater incidence of diarrhea in tropical sprue (100 per cent)[156] compared with celiac disease (75 per cent).[97]

Malabsorption of vitamin B_{12} is commoner than in celiac disease but does not in this case imply ileal disease. Rather, it appears to be due to bacterial consumption of dietary vitamin B_{12}, since antibiotics can normalize vitamin B_{12} absorption within 48 hours, long before the mucosal lesion has started to heal.[164]

As already mentioned, hypoalbuminemia is also common. This is mainly due to malnutrition, with depressed synthesis as the major contributory factor. Increased protein loss via the gut is a relatively insignificant factor.[165]

As already described in regard to celiac disease, lactase specific activity in the jejunal biopsy is a very sensitive indicator of disease, lactase being undetectable in 64 per cent of 50 Indian patients with tropical sprue described by Desai.[166] Gray found evidence of depressed jejunal hydrolysis and absorption of lactose with low levels of lactase, sucrase, and maltase in 100, 68, and 65 per cent, respectively, of 85 patients with tropical sprue.[167] Although after treatment sucrase and maltase activities returned to normal, lactase levels remained abnormally low in 63 per cent. These biochemical findings agree with the clinical observation that while lactose loading frequently induces abdominal cramps and diarrhea, a similar load of sucrose rarely does.[168]

ETIOLOGICAL ROLE OF SMALL BOWEL CONTAMINATION

Drinking water is often grossly contaminated with coliforms in areas where tropical sprue is endemic. This gross contamination is generally well tolerated, perhaps owing to the bactericidal action of gastric acid, and only a minority of the exposed population develop sprue, which is associated with excess numbers of coliforms in the upper jejunum.[163] More recently aerobic organisms, mainly *Enterobacter* species, have also been demonstrated in jejunal biopsy material,[169] though they do not appear to have breached the mucosa. In a detailed study of three cases, Klipstein was able to demonstrate the presence of *Klebsiella pneumoniae*, which in culture produced an enterotoxin capable of inducing secretion in a rabbit ileum.[170] Unfortunately, no other studies have implicated this organism, so it is likely that this *Klebsiella* species is just one of many possible infectious agents that may initiate the process that results in tropical malabsorption. Epidemiological evidence supports the idea that viruses can also initiate this process,[154] but as yet none have been isolated. In man, antibiotic therapy is able to reverse intestinal secretion within a few days,[163] suggesting that bacteria cause the abnormalities of intestinal function, rather than being merely secondary to the delay in small bowel transit seen in this condition.[171, 172] Just how bacteria cause malabsorption is unclear; there are probably several mechanisms, including toxin secretion, bile salt deconjugation, and interference with folate metabolism. Folate malabsorption[173] and folate depletion are universal in tropical sprue, and the villous lesion often responds well to large doses of folic acid[174] or vitamin B_{12}. Coliforms sometimes produce large amounts of ethanol, and this can directly impair folate absorption.[170] Supraphysiological doses of crystalline folic acid appear to overcome this block, and symptoms of diarrhea, anorexia, and abdominal distention often respond well[175–177] to folic acid treatment. However, unless antibiotics are also given, the long-term response to folic acid alone is disappointing, with about 50 per cent of patients progressing to a chronic malabsorption syndrome.[178] Antibiotic treatment alone, usually tetracycline 250 mg q.i.d. for 4 weeks, results in gradual folate repletion and remission of symptoms. Jejunal morphology improves first, with loss of megaloblastic changes in the crypt cells before serum folate and bone marrow morphology improves.[179] In otherwise normal individuals who have folate depletion due to inadequate intake, the bone marrow bears the brunt of the disease, containing as it does the most rapidly proliferating cell compartment in the body, while jejunal morphology is relatively normal.[180] However, in sprue this situation may be reversed, with markedly increased crypt cell turnover rendering the jejunum more vulnerable to folate depletion than the bone marrow. Conventional treatment is to give folic acid 5 mg three times daily, together with at least 1 month of tetracycline therapy, and on this regimen, if the jejunal flora can be normalized, most patients improve rapidly.[164] Vitamin B_{12}, 1 mg weekly, is also advisable to speed recovery and to avoid the risk of precipitating subacute combined degeneration of the spinal cord due to unrecognized vitamin B_{12} deficiency. Recovery in those who return to temperate zones is likely to be complete,[181] though those who remain in the tropics are likely to relapse, presumably because they continue to be exposed to the adverse environmental conditions that induced the initial attack.[178]

Giardiasis

Although usually associated with the tropics, the ubiquitous protozoan parasite *Giardia lamblia* accounts for a substantial proportion of diarrheal illnesses throughout the world. The organism has two life forms, the motile trophozoite and the encysted form. The trophozoite is a pear-shaped, bilaterally symmetrical, 10-μm organism, propelled by four pairs of flagellae. This thrives in the upper small intestine, which provides not only ample nutrients but also bile salts, which the trophozoite appears to need to enable it to take up preformed phospholipid to be incorporated into its own membranes.[182] The organism is to be found in jejunal biopsies concentrated midway between the crypts and villous tips, where it adheres to the brush border surface by means of its ventral sucking disc. A substantial proportion of the absorptive surface may be covered by the organism, which may occasionally be found within the enterocyte.[183] Passage into the lower small intestine induces encystment, 8-μm oval cysts being

shed in the feces in large numbers. Transmission of the disease is via ingestion of fecally contaminated water or food containing cysts, which release two binucleate trophozoites on coming into contact with gastric acid.[184]

Although commoner in the tropics, accounting for 23 per cent of cases of nondysenteric diarrhea in Bombay,[185] and 36 per cent of cases of chronic diarrhea in American servicemen in Vietnam,[186] it also occurs in the United Kingdom and in the continental United States, both as isolated cases[187] and as water-borne[188] and food-borne epidemics.[189] Travel to an endemic zone may be followed by acute diarrhea that develops 12 to 19 days after exposure.[190] Symptoms are usually diarrhea, fatigue, abdominal cramps, and flatulence. Spontaneous resolution occurs in about half of the cases, the rest remaining symptomatic until diagnosis and appropriate treatment.[189] While this description applies to most cases, a substantial number present with an obscure chronic diarrhea,[191] which is often diagnosed only after lengthy investigations.[187] Although immunodeficiency is often associated with malabsorption due to giardiasis,[192] and homosexuals are known to have an increased risk,[193] most isolated cases in the United States and the United Kingdom have no such predisposing factor.[187, 191]

Chronic infestation is associated with a variable degree of villous inflammation and stunting, malabsorption being proportional to the severity of histological damage.[194] In a series of 40 cases of giardiasis in Caucasian travellers visiting India and Africa, 14 had steatorrhea (8 to 30 g/24 hr), 18 had xylose malabsorption, and 18 had malabsorption of vitamin B_{12}; in 12 there was malabsorption of all three substances.[194] Steatorrhea and weight loss in this series was modest and hypoalbuminemia, low serum folate, and cutaneous signs of vitamin deficiencies were not seen. Occasionally the malabsorption may be more severe, and giardiasis in small children has been mistaken for celiac disease.[195] Some of the features of this condition resemble tropical sprue, and in the more severely affected cases small bowel contamination, with *Enterobacter* species has been reported,[196] suggesting that bacterial overgrowth exacerbates the damage caused by *Giardia lamblia*. Recent reports from India also describe mild steatorrhea in a similar proportion (17 of 63), with 8 of the 17 having significant bacterial overgrowth in their duodenal aspirates. No cases in this series were severely malnourished, and surprisingly none had malabsorption of vitamin B_{12}.[196]

The precise mechanism by which infection with *Giardia lamblia* causes malabsorption is unclear but electron micrographs show a thick layer of mucus and extruded cytoplasm, appearing to originate from the crypts, covering much of the villous surface, thus providing a mechanical barrier to absorption.[197, 198] The fact that the villous damage and inflammatory changes respond to treatment with mepacrine[199] suggest that the *Giardia* organisms rather than the associated bacterial overgrowth cause the lesion, but as yet no toxin has been identified. As with other mucosal disease, brush border enzyme levels, especially of lactase and sucrase, are depressed,[199] suggesting a functional defect in the enterocyte in spite of its relatively normal anatomical appearance. These deficiencies all appear to be secondary to the infestation, since with treatment enzyme levels return to normal.[200]

Diagnosis is best made by demonstrating the motile trophozoite in an imprint of the jejunal biopsy or in the thick mucus often noted adherent to the biopsy capsule. This technique gives a positive result in 92 per cent of cases, compared with only 64 per cent positivity for duodenal aspirates and 54 per cent for stool examination for cysts (3 to 4 stools examined per patient).[201] Recently it has become possible to reliably detect specific IgM antibody to giardial antigens using an enzyme-linked immunosorbent technique; this assay is positive only during active infection, and titers fall rapidly after eradication of the parasite.[202] This noninvasive test is unlikely to supplant jejunal biopsy in clinical practice but may well be useful in epidemiological studies and for following the success of public health programs.

Treatment with 2 g of metronidazole daily for 3 days gives a 91 per cent cure rate, a second course raising this to 95 per cent overall.[194] Newer, better-tolerated compounds are now being tested, tinidazole being highly effective, 150 mg twice daily for 7 days curing all of 35 patients.[203] Subsequent single-dose studies have shown a 90 per cent cure rate after a single 1.5 g dose.[204] Single-dose therapy achieves considerable financial savings, a highly relevant consideration given that worldwide most cases of giardiasis occur in countries where finance is the major factor limiting effective health care.

Disaccharide Intolerance

LACTOSE

As already described, hypolactasia—that is, low levels of the brush border disaccharidase, lactase—is a feature of a number of mucosal diseases. Most commonly however, it occurs as an isolated finding in an otherwise normal small intestine. Mammals generally show a steady decline in brush border lactase after weaning, and man is no exception to this rule. This decline, which is characteristic of adult-acquired hypolactasia and is also known as lactase insufficiency, is genetically determined and is inherited as an autosomal recessive trait.[205]

Different ethnic groups have widely differing incidence of lactase insufficiency. Generally Northern European races have an incidence of less than 20 per cent, while many African and Asian racial groups have an incidence of greater than 65 per cent. Within the same geographical area, for example, West Africa, ethnic groups with a tradition of dairy farming have a lower incidence of lactase insufficiency than those who traditionally have not had access to milk. This suggests that over many generations the nutritional disadvantage provided by lactase insufficiency in a milk-drinking culture has been sufficient to produce a decreased incidence of the relevant gene.[206] In groups with a high incidence of adult-acquired lactase insufficiency, lactose intolerance becomes apparent early in life (1 to 2 years in Nigeria),[207] whereas in groups with a low incidence intolerance becomes apparent only in adolescence.[208]

Lactase levels as measured on jejunal biopsy decline some years before clinical lactose intolerance (abdominal pain and diarrhea after a 50-g lactose load) becomes obvious.[209] Detailed biochemical characterization of the lactase in infants, normal adults, and those with lactase insufficiency shows no qualitative difference between the enzyme in each group; the groups differ only in the amount per gram of protein of the jejunal homogenate.[210] As already described, the specific activity of lactase in a normal jejunal biopsy is considerably lower than that of maltase and sucrase, which probably explains why lactase intolerance is a such a common feature of a range of mucosal diseases[7, 102, 168, 211] while sucrose intolerance is rare, presumably because of the much larger functional reserve for sucrose hydrolysis and absorption.

Effect of Lactose Intolerance. Ingestion of 50 g lactose in 200 ml of water results in a hypertonic sodium-free solution entering the jejunum. This causes marked influx of sodium and water down the electrochemical and osmotic gradients into the jejunum, which is highly permeable to sodium and water. If the normal lactose hydrolysis is depressed, then the normal stimulation of sodium and water absorption by glucose and galactose absorption is also depressed. This results in net water and electrolyte secretion,[73] which accelerates transit through the small bowel.[77] Fast transit per se further reduces absorption, exacerbating symptoms which consist of abdominal cramps, borborygmi, flatus, and diarrhea. These symptoms are mainly due to colonic fermentation of malabsorbed lactose, producing hydrogen, carbon dioxide, methane, and short-chain fatty acids, some of which can be absorbed from the colon and hence salvaged for use by the body (in the rat this actually accounts for about 25 per cent of lactose absorption).[212] This component of lactose metabolism is probably capable of adaptation as bacterial populations alter in response to changes in diet. Bacterial and colonic adaptation accounts for the decrease in colonic symptoms that is seen with continued lactose loading (1 L milk daily) in subjects with lactase insufficiency.[81] Similar increased tolerance has been documented with another nonabsorbable disaccharide, lactulose[80] which can be hydrolyzed only by bacteria. In man increased tolerance to lactose is not due to any alteration in brush border lactase levels,[81] though an adaptive increase has been observed in rats fed high-lactose diets.[213]

Diagnosis of Lactose Malabsorption. Diagnosis is best performed by assessing the amount of lactose entering the colon after a test dose of lactose (50 g in 200 ml of water), as indicated by the subsequent rise in breath hydrogen. This rise correlates closely with direct measures of lactose flow in the terminal ileum[214] and with the occurrence of symptoms.[215] Earlier studies assessed lactose absorption from the rise in venous blood glucose after the same load.[216] Such indirect measures are unfortunately greatly influenced by factors other than lactose absorption, including gastric emptying and glucose metabolism, and correlates less well with jejunal lactase levels than the simpler, noninvasive measurement of the breath hydrogen response.[217] Interestingly the same dose of lactose given as milk produces less symptoms[81] and a lower breath hydrogen response,[215] perhaps because the fat and protein in the milk delay gastric emptying and reduce the load per hour entering the small intestine.

Nutritional Implications of Lactase Insufficiency. Although a few subjects appear to develop symptoms with very small (3 g) doses of lactose,[218] in most cases of lactase insufficiency substantial doses must be given as a bolus to induce symptoms. Lisker reported that 750 ml of milk, taken as a single bolus, was necessary to induce symptoms in 77 of 123 subjects with lactase insufficiency, 250 ml causing symptoms in only 7 subjects.[219] Furthermore in the same study, 91 per cent of subjects who were intolerant of a particular dose of lactose were symptom-free if the same dose was given in two portions separated by 8 hours. Thus, owing to the substantial absorptive reserve of the small intestine, even lactase-insufficient subjects can tolerate lactose if the load per hour is kept low. Bolus feeding of the poorly absorbed disaccharide lactulose accelerates small bowel transit in a dose-dependent fashion.[220] This results in boluses of fluid and malabsorbed carbohydrate entering the cecum, overwhelming its capacity to metabolize the sugar and absorb fluid. Lower doses induce smaller pulses in ileocolonic inflow and allow cecal fermentation to salvage most of the malabsorbed carbohydrate, thus preventing diarrhea. It follows therefore that if enteral feeding is being given to lactase-insufficient subjects as intermittent large boluses, a high lactose content may be undesirable. This restriction is even more relevant in the presence of small bowel disease, when as we have seen, lactase insufficiency is often secondary to mucosal damage which will further impair absorption of water and electrolytes. Thus in malnourished children with infective gastroenteritis, lactose intolerance is an important factor influencing the choice of diet, being detected in 77 per cent of a group of Mexican children hospitalized because of diarrhea.[221] Clinically this presents with the passage of frothy, acidic (pH less than 6.0) loose stools containing detectable reducing sugars. These symptoms, in most cases, remit on a lactose-free diet provided by substituting glucose for lactose.[221] The more prolonged the diarrhea and the more malnourished the child, the greater the severity of carbohydrate intolerance becomes, so that in proportion there is sucrose, maltose, and even glucose intolerance.[222] These signs of carbohydrate intolerance presumably reflect severe mucosal damage, since as the diarrhea settles, evidence of sugar malabsorption disappears.[221] Young children, because of their small size and relatively poorly developed colon, appear particularly vulnerable to the effects of lactose malabsorption. Severely malnourished adults from racial groups with a high incidence of lactase insufficiency also appear to be intolerant of very high lactose diets. Daily intake of 150 g of lactose given in 5×400 ml liquid feeds induced marked increases in stool volume and fecal fats,[2] presumably because the acceleration of transit reduced mucosal contact time. Such patients often have a high incidence of mucosal abnormalities and hence a reduced absorptive reserve, whereas in healthy Americans with lactose insufficiency but otherwise normal intestines, lactose loading does not induce steatorrhea.[223]

Studies that have reported diarrhea in persons consuming diets with a very high lactose content have generally used bolus feeding of liquid diets, a technique that maximizes symptoms. As Lisker clearly showed,[219] dividing up the lactose dose allows better tolerance. In the United Kingdom it is our experience that when diets containing 21 g of lactose per 24 hours are infused continuously via a nasogastric tube, diarrhea is not a problem, even in those with biochemical evidence of lactase insufficiency.[224] In Third World countries where malnutrition is a common problem, milk is a cheap, valuable nutritional resource and the extra expense of removing lactose from the feed is rarely justified except during acute diarrheal episodes. Although diets containing 1.2 g of lactose per kg body weight given as 5 daily boluses do cause increased stool volumes, controlled clinical trials have shown that there is no nutritional advantage to replacing the lactose by glucose and galactose.[225] Malnourished children gain weight equally well on lactose-containing or lactose-free diets because the amount of energy lost owing to lactose malabsorption is nutritionally insignificant. Thus when economy is an important consideration a milk-based diet should be tried first, and only if this results in severe diarrhea should a lactose-reduced diet be used. If continuous (24-hr) nasogastric enteral feeding is used, only very rarely will lactose intolerance be clinically evident even in subjects with lactase insufficiency.

Congenital Lactase Deficiency. This is an extremely rare condition in which mucosal lactase levels are low at birth and remain low throughout life.

Presentation is within the first few days of life with diarrhea, abdominal distention, and failure to thrive.[226, 227] Acidic, frothy stools that are positive to ward testing for reducing sugars are characteristic, as is the rapid resolution of symptoms on a lactose-free diet. This rare syndrome must be distinguished from the transient lactase deficiency of premature babies[228] and from the even rarer glucose-galactose malabsorption, which presents similarly. Transient lactase deficiency of prematurity resolves within a few weeks, while glucose-galactose malabsorption can be identified by performing a glucose tolerance test. Lactase-deficient subjects have a normal blood sugar rise after 50 g of glucose, while glucose-galactose malabsorbers show no rise.[229] The symptoms in congenital lactase deficiency are due to an isolated defect in absorption and are readily treated by a lactose-free diet, there being no other systemic features. This should be distinguished from a subgroup of patients with congenital lactose intolerance, who have numerous metabolic disorders including lactosuria, vomiting, diarrhea, aminoaciduria, and renal acidosis.[227] Most such children reported in the literature have died within the first year of life, with only about 50 per cent responding symptomatically to a low-lactose diet. Only a few of the patients in the literature have had formal lactose tolerance tests, but when done these have suggested a normal absorption of lactose.

SUCRASE-ISOMALTASE DEFICIENCY

Sucrose, which accounts for nearly 30 per cent of carbohydrate intake in a Western diet, can be absorbed only after hydrolysis by the enzyme sucrase-isomaltase. This enzyme is absent in sucrase-isomaltase deficiency,[230] a genetic defect inherited as an autosomal recessive trait. Although rare in North America (0.2 per cent),[231] in some parts of the world with inbred populations it is quite common; for example, the incidence is 10.5 per cent in Eskimos in Western Greenland.[232] Watery diarrhea develops as the child is weaned onto sucrose-containing foods, particularly sucrose-sweetened fruit juices.[233] Sucrose exclusion cures the diarrhea, while a sucrose tolerance test (loading dose 2 g/kg) results in a flat blood glucose curve and acidic watery stools. A glucose tolerance test shows a normal blood sugar response. Malabsorbed sucrose can be detected in the stool by heating to accelerate its breakdown to glucose, which can then be detected with a Clinitest tablet.[233] Less invasively, malabsorption of sucrose can be detected by a rise in breath hydrogen of greater than 20 parts per million after 50 g of sucrose, normal subjects showing no significant rise even after 100 g.[234] While some authors suggest symptoms improve with age,[235] others have found no improvement. Indeed sucrose intolerance may be first diagnosed in adult life[236] and should be considered in cases of obscure watery diarrhea whatever the patient's age.

TREHALASE DEFICIENCY

This is an interesting, but nutritionally trivial disorder of absorption of the disaccharide trehalose, which comprises 1.4 per cent of fresh young mushrooms. Case reports have indicated that low levels of brush border trehalase produce intolerance of large doses of mushrooms. A father and son have been described in whom 50 g of trehalose (representing nearly 4 kg of mushrooms) produced abdominal pain, vomiting, and diarrhea, whereas the same dose in most individuals produces no untoward effects. Jejunal biopsy showed absent trehalase activity but normal sucrase and maltase levels.[237]

Monosaccharide Intolerance

GLUCOSE-GALACTOSE MALABSORPTION

This is a rare genetic defect, inherited as an autosomal recessive trait in which both glucose and galactose are malabsorbed.[229, 238] Initiation of oral feeds results in severe diarrhea, dehydration, acidosis, and malnutrition beginning in the first few days of life. Substitution of fructose for glucose and lactose results in prompt remission of symptoms and allows normal development.[229] Untreated, dehydration, acidosis, and nephrocalcinosis leads to an early demise. Jejunal biopsy reveals normal morphology and disaccharidase levels but failure of glucose uptake.[239] This defect has been confirmed by in vivo perfusion studies showing that in spite of normal disaccharide hydrolysis, glucose absorption is very low.[240] Oral loading with either glucose or galactose fails to induce a rise in blood sugar and induces diarrhea, about two thirds of the galactose and one third of the glucose load appearing in the stool within 6 hours of dosing.[229] While the infant remains on a liquid diet all glucose and galactose must be excluded, but once a solid diet is achieved, diarrhea becomes less marked and the diet can be liberalized. In later life patients with this condition still remain intolerant of large doses of glucose and galactose solutions and some forms of starch, but tolerance is surprisingly variable and depends on the form of starch; for example, a patient may tolerate normal amounts of potatoes but develop violent diarrhea after a few slices of white bread. Although most cases are diagnosed in infancy, some, like sucrase-isomaltase deficiency, are first diagnosed in adults with obscure diarrhea.[240] Defective monosaccharide absorption cannot be compensated for by uptake of disaccharides as is the case for isolated amino acid transport defects;[241] this may explain why such severe symptoms result from defects in monosaccharide transport when equivalent defects in free amino acid absorption produce virtually no gastrointestinal symptoms (see below).

FRUCTOSE MALABSORPTION

Fructose is a common dietary sugar whose energy-dependent, carrier-mediated uptake is inhibited by sorbose and to a lesser extent by glucose.[242] Absorption rates are slower than those seen during intestinal perfusion of equal concentrations of glucose,[243] and even in healthy subjects there is incomplete absorption after a large oral load (50 g as 20 per cent solution).[244] Indeed, excessive fructose intake in the form of fruit juices can be the cause of chronic diarrhea in children who are otherwise healthy.[245] This limited capacity for absorption in normal subjects is to be clearly distinguished from the metabolic disorder of fructose intolerance. This rare autosomal recessive defect is due to an absence of the hepatic enzyme fructose-1-phosphate aldolase.[246, 247] Oral or intravenous fructose loading produces marked hypoglycemia[247] with associated faintness. There is no defect of fructose absorption in this condition, which presents in neonates with hepatomegaly, jaundice, and postprandial hypoglycemia after fructose-containing foods.

GENERALIZED MONOSACCHARIDE INTOLERANCE

These rare specific monosaccharide intolerances described above must always be distinguished from the generalized monosaccharide intolerance, which appears as a transient defect in children from impoverished tropical regions presenting with severe diarrhea. In a study of 403 Mexican children hospitalized because of acute diarrhea, 23 were transiently intolerant of glucose, fructose, and galactose.[221, 222] Small bowel contamination with coliforms was found in 18 of these 23, and antibiotic treatment produced a prompt clinical response suggesting that the bacteria were responsible for the diarrhea. All of these children had normal monosaccharide tolerance tests 2 months later.[222]

Less Common Malabsorptive Disorders

COW'S MILK ALLERGY

This syndrome of malabsorption, diarrhea, and vomiting associated with variable villous atrophy attributable to an allergy to cow's milk protein is a disease of neonates.[248] Exclusion of cow's milk results in clinical and histological remission, while challenge produces villous atrophy and inflammatory changes within 24 hours.[249, 250] Additional symptoms include urticaria, asthma, and anaphylaxis after milk challenge. Some patients also exhibit a low-grade colitis responding to milk elimination.[251] Challenge with lactose produces no symptoms, but the same amount of lactose given as milk produces diarrhea with acid stools positive for reducing sugars.[252] This syndrome is essentially a feature of the neonatal period[249] and is perhaps related to increased intestinal permeability, since after the age of 2 most children previously intolerant of cow's milk become tolerant.[253]

ISOLATED DEFECTS IN AMINO ACID ABSORPTION

These are extremely rare genetic defects, usually inherited as autosomal recessive traits and generally presenting in infancy. Since enterocytes and renal tubular cells exhibit common amino acid transport mechanisms, defects in intestinal absorption are often first suspected because of the presence of aminoaciduria, which may, as in cystinuria[254] and the "blue diaper syndrome,"[85] be a major clinical feature. Malabsorption of amino acids is generally not a feature of these diseases, since the transport defect does not involve dipeptide-bound amino acids, which are absorbed normally,[255] the only exception to this general rule is lysine in lysinuric protein intolerance.[256]

CYSTINURIA

This autosomal recessive inherited disorder is characterized by a defect in the transport of cystine, lysine, ornithine, and arginine in both the intestinal and the renal tubule. Symptoms are solely due to the insolubility of cystine, resulting in the formation of cystine stones in acid urine. Oral dosing with 5 g of cystine fails to elevate plasma cystine levels,[254] while 10 g of lysine or ornithine by mouth produces a rise in fecal amino acids.[82] Direct measurement of absorption by jejunal perfusion shows that, at low concentrations simulating those likely to be seen postprandially, lysine, arginine,[255] and cystine[257] absorption is impaired. At higher concentrations, using large unphysiological oral loads, the absorptive defect is less obvious, perhaps because, at high concentrations, passive diffusion may be more important than active transport.[258] The lack of nutritional deficit and normal amino acid absorption from protein hydrolysates but not of free amino acids[259] is explained by the finding that absorption of dipeptide-bound arginine[255] or lysine[260] is normal. Thus the specific transport defect spares the separate dipeptide transport and absorption of the basic amino acids from dietary proteins is preserved. Most patients present with renal calculi as the sole manifestation,[261] and analysis of the stones shows them to contain substantial amounts of cystine. Twenty-four-hour urinary cystine, lysine, ornithine, and arginine are all increased. Heterozygotes do not develop calculi but may have modest rises in urinary cystine excretion. Treatment is by oral bicarbonate together with a high fluid intake (3 L/day) to ensure a good flow of dilute alkaline urine, thus minimizing the chances of cystine precipitating out of solution. Existing stones may need surgical extraction, while penicillamine, which binds cystine, rendering it more soluble, may be required for long-term prophylaxis. Recently a number of less toxic mercaptan and thiol compounds have been tested and show some promise.[16]

HARTNUP DISEASE

Routine screening of neonates for aminoaciduria reveals that 1 in 33,000 children have defective tubular reabsorption of the neutral amino acids glycine, valine, alanine, cystine, leucine, isoleucine, taurine, phenylalanine, and tryptophan.[262] This tubular defect has been shown to be associated with defective intestinal absorption of tryptophan,[263] phenylalanine, and histidine when presented as free amino acids, but near-normal absorption when they are presented as dipeptides.[264, 265] Thus it appears that intact dipeptide absorption prevents clinical deficiency of these essential amino acids. Indeed, the classic, nicotinamide-responsive, pellagra-like syndrome due to tryptophan deficiency is in practice rare, occurring in only 1 of 15 cases of Hartnup disease detected by antenatal screening.[262] Case reports have tended to emphasize the more dramatic pellagra-like clinical presentation, which appears to be precipitated by periods of borderline dietary tryptophan deficiency.[266] Minor growth retardation has been noted, and on average patients are 5 cm shorter than predicted for age and sex.[266] Review of available case reports suggests that of those who are symptomatic, about half have a light-sensitive rash, half have ataxia, and about one fifth are mentally retarded;[267] however, this may reflect case selection, since mental development appeared normal in the one available prospective study.[262] The only treatment needed is nicotinamide supplementation, which reduces photosensitivity. Malabsorption would be apparent only if nitrogen was provided as free amino acids; oligopeptide-based diets would be absorbed normally.

LYSINURIC PROTEIN INTOLERANCE

Marked renal wasting of dibasic amino acids, especially lysine, is associated with inadequate urea formation and hyperammonemia after a protein load in this rare transport defect.[84] The basic defect is failure to absorb lysine, arginine, and ornithine, which is shown by below-normal increases in the plasma levels of these amino acids after oral loading.[268] This is associated with vomiting and diarrhea that begins after weaning from the breast, as protein-rich foods are introduced. Low-protein diets diminish the symptoms but lead to failure to grow normally.[84] This transport defect appears also to affect the hepatocyte, resulting in steatosis, hepatomegaly, and a defective production of urea after protein load. Lack of ornithine within the hepatocyte interrupts the urea cycle, so that deamination of amino acids after a protein load leads to hyperammonemia rather than the normal production of urea. The hyperammonemia is probably responsible for the vomiting, while the diarrhea appears to be due to malabsorption of amino acids. Oral arginine or ornithine, if tolerated, will prevent hyperammonemia and will, by allowing a more normal protein intake, result in marked growth spurt.[84] Since absorption and transport of another component of the urea cycle, citrulline, is normal, oral citrulline may well prove the most rational treatment.[268] The absorption of both dipeptide-bound and free amino acids appears equally affected, so the defect must lie beyond the brush border at the basolateral membrane.[256] Routine histology in this condition is normal, and there is no evidence of malabsorption of fat or carbohydrate.[84]

OTHER RARE DISORDERS

Other rare disorders of amino acid absorption include iminoglycinuria,[269] isolated tryptophan malabsorption (blue diaper syndrome),[85] methionine malabsorption (oasthouse syndrome)[270] and arginine and lysine malabsorption seen in Lowe's syndrome.[271] An isolated defect in proline, hydroxyproline, and glycine transport appears to cause no symptoms,[272] but oral loading with one of these amino acids does appear to impair absorption of the other two, providing evidence for competition for a common transport system. These syndromes are complex and, owing to their rarity, the true nature of the transport defect is unclear, as is its relationship to the other symptoms, such as mental deficiency, seen in many affected children.

The nutritional implications of such defects are limited owing to their excessive rarity, but obviously in such patients free amino acid solutions should not be used, as whole protein–based or oligopeptide-based diets will be better tolerated. The only exception to this rule is that in patients with lysinuric protein intolerance, citrulline should be added to the diet regardless of its degree of polymerization.

WHIPPLE'S DISEASE

The true incidence of Whipple's disease is impossible to assess accurately but has been estimated at less than 1 per 100,000.[273] Disproportionate interest has been generated by this rare disease because of the demonstration by Paulley[274] that it could be cured by antibiotic therapy, implying that the intracellular bacteria observed by Whipple in intestinal macrophages[275] were the causative agent of the malabsorption observed. The bacterium has subsequently been shown on electron micrographs to have, in addition to the usual bacterial inner plasma membrane and cell wall, a unique outer trilaminar membrane[273] that may be important in enabling this infective organism to remain as an intracellular parasite in the body for decades. Presentation is insidious, with anorexia, abdominal fullness, cough, polyarthralgia, and fever leading to weight loss, diarrhea, and abdominal pain.[276] This is predominantly a disease of males, and patients usually present in their fourth or fifth decade. The advanced stage is characterized by weight loss (in 95 per cent of patients), fat malabsorption (75 per cent), hyperpigmentation of sun-exposed skin (40 per cent), peripheral lymphadenopathy (50 per cent), splenomegaly, and various neurological features, including seizures, meningitis, and uveitis.[276] The pathognomonic lesion, however, is found in the jejunum, which, in the original case described by Whipple, was found at autopsy to be "oedematous, flecked with little yellowish grains." These have been shown to be patches of blunted edematous villi, infiltrated with macrophages, with appearances ranging from mild to severe villous atrophy. Radiological study shows nonspecific changes with dilated jejunal loops and coarse mucosal folds.[277] The diagnosis is made from the pathognomonic changes in the jejunal biopsy, which may need to be repeated since the changes are patchy.[278] Routine light microscopy shows characteristic foamy macrophages which stain positively with periodic acid–Schiff's reagent. The brunt of the disease is borne by the small intestine,[279] though rarely the disease may extend to the colon.[280] Other organs, including bone marrow, liver, meninges, and muscle, may also exhibit these PAS-positive macrophages, stuffed with small rod-shaped bacilli which may also be seen free in the tissue.[273]

Routine blood tests show a normocytic hypochromic anemia, high erythrocyte sedimentation rate, and hypoalbuminemia, while a 3-day fecal fat collection confirms fat malabsorption in 90 per cent of cases. Although Whipple believed that this was due to partial lymphatic obstruction, it now appears that the defect resides in the enterocyte.[281] After a corn oil meal, lipid droplets fail to accumulate in the endoplasmic reticulum as would be predicted with lymphatic obstruction.[281] Furthermore, the same study also showed defective uptake of amino acids and reduced esterification of long-chain fatty acids, suggesting that there is a generalized impairment of jejunal enterocyte metabolism. This disorder manifests itself in routine laboratory tests as xylose malabsorption, low serum cholesterol, prolonged prothrombin time, and low serum iron and folate, usually associated with normal serum vitamin B_{12}.[277] Hypoalbuminemia reflects both increased gastrointestinal loss and decreased synthesis, itself probably secondary to diminished protein intake.[282] Antibiotic treatment promptly alleviates steatorrhea even though histological recovery is much slower, suggesting that direct bacterial toxicity to enterocytes is a major cause of malabsorption.[283] Parenteral penicillin and an aminoglycoside should be given for 2 weeks followed by oral co-trimoxazole or tetracycline for 1 year to minimize the chances of relapse.[283, 284] Remission of fever, diarrhea, and steatorrhea is usually prompt, but relapses may occur when antibiotics are stopped, even after 1 year of treatment.

INTESTINAL LYMPHANGIECTASIA

Dilated lymphatics are a feature of only minor importance in Whipple's disease, whereas in intestinal lymphangiectasia this is the major pathophysiological feature. Such patients often have a generalized defect in the development of their lymphatic system,[285] usually presenting with generalized or localized peripheral edema, chylous pleural or ascitic effusions, and hypoalbuminemia. Albumin turnover studies show a markedly reduced half-life (4 to 5 days, compared with a normal of 17 days) and an abnormal loss of albumin in the stool.[286] Lymphangiograms show generalized abnormalities with atresia in some areas and blocked dilated lymphatics in other sites, and in some reports contrast material has been seen spilling into the gut lumen via abnormally dilated mucosal lymphatics.[287] Absorbed fat is presumably also lost via this mechanism, and a modest degree of steatorrhea is found in 3 out of 4 patients.[288] The diagnosis may be strongly suspected on clinical grounds or may be a surprise finding on jejunal biopsy. It is worth noting, however, that a negative biopsy should be repeated if clinical suspicion is high, as the abnormality is often patchy. Treatment by excision of the affected bowel may occasionally be successful, but such an approach is rarely justified. A low-fat diet, or one based on medium-chain rather than long-chain fatty acids, may help some patients,[289, 290] the logic being to reduce the postprandial rise in lymphatic flow, which is especially large after meals containing long-chain fatty acids.[291]

ABETALIPOPROTEINEMIA

This very rare condition is mentioned only because elucidation of its pathophysiology has markedly increased our understanding of lipoprotein metabolism. Patients who lack apoprotein B are unable to secrete chylomicrons or to export hepatic triglyceride. Their postprandial blood lacks chylomicrons and has very low levels of low-density and very-low-density lipoproteins, associated with low levels of plasma cholesterol, triglycerides, and free fatty acids, especially linoleic and arachidonic acid.[292] There is complete absence of apoprotein B in the enterocyte,[13] which accumulates triglyceride. Jejunal morphology is otherwise quite normal, although lactase levels are low with associated lactose malabsorption. The first clue to the diagnosis is usually the finding of acanthosis of the red cells in a patient with profound neurologic defects including ataxia and retinitis pigmentosa.[293] Less severe deficiencies of apoprotein B secretion are occasionally detected in asymptomatic subjects who exhibit acanthosis with very low serum cholesterol and triglycerides.[294] Intermediate forms have also been reported,[295] the severity being proportional to the apoprotein deficit. Malabsorption of fat appears to be secondary to lipid accumulation in the enterocyte, since fat, xylose, and lactose malabsorption are seen only in those in whom the jejunal biopsy shows lipid accumulation.[294]

RADIATION ENTERITIS

The critical dose for causing radiation injury to the small intestine, 4500 rads, lies close to the dose required to treat ovarian, uterine, and rectal cancer (4500 to 8000 rads). It follows that clinically apparent enteritis can be expected in 5 to 50 per cent of patients undergoing such treatment, depending on whether the higher or lower dose is used.[296] About one third of patients experience mild diarrhea with evidence of malabsorption of lactose, fat, and bile salts during therapy,[297] but this usually rapidly subsides.[298] Over the next few months radiation scarring develops with marked submucosal edema, hyalinization, and deposits of dense collagen in the lamina propria, and there is subsequent slower development of vascular abnormalities, including telangiectasia and obliterative endarteritis.[299] This may result in the development of stricturing, intestinal obstruction, and marked steatorrhea.[300] Further complications such as intestinal infarction and perforation are often fatal. Surgical correction is often unsuccessful owing to difficulty in operating in a pelvis full of adhesions and the extremely poor healing seen after resection of radiation-damaged bowel. The use of elemental diets may allow conservative treatment of episodes of obstruction.[301] Although this does not alter the underlying anatomical problem, it may improve nutrition, rendering subsequent surgical procedures better tolerated.

PROTEIN-CALORIE MALNUTRITION

The small intestine and pancreas are metabolically very active, requiring large amounts of protein for all cell division and enzyme secretion. It is not surprising therefore that protein deprivation produces malfunction in these organs. Widespread malnutrition is a common occurrence in some tropical countries in which diarrheal illnesses commonly precipitate the hospitalization of severely malnourished children. Even in the absence of overt diarrhea, such children commonly demonstrate mild to moderate defects in absorption of fat, protein,[302] and carbohydrate.[303] Jejunal morphology is often abnormal, ranging from mild to severe villous atrophy and inflammatory infiltration similar to that seen in tropical sprue.[304] Giardiasis[305] and contamination of the upper small bowel with enterobacteria and gram-positive cocci is common,[306] and this is often associated with evidence of bile salt deconjugation,[302] all of which damage enterocytes and contribute to defective absorption. The villous abnormalities are, as expected, associated with depressed disaccharidase levels, lactase being more affected than sucrase and maltase.[307] This is associated with clinical lactose intolerance in some but not all patients. Pancreatic

dysfunction may also impair absorption in such patients.[309] Refeeding with milk-based diets may provoke exacerbation of diarrhea, and in these children, or those with such severe malnutrition that refeeding is a medical emergency, a low-lactose diet should be used and if necessary even parenteral feeding for the first week or so. Treatment of respiratory or gastrointestinal infection with antibiotics is also important to hasten the return to normal gastrointestinal function, subsequent refeeding being done using a less expensive polymeric diet.

References

1. Jeejeebhoy KN, Desai HG, Noronha JM, et al. Idiopathic tropical diarrhoea with or without steatorrhoea (tropical malabsorption syndrome). Gastroenterology 1966; 51:333–344.
2. O'Keefe SJD, Adam JK, Cakata E, et al. Nutritional support of malnourished lactose intolerant African patients. Gut 1984; 25:942–947.
3. Gray GM. Carbohydrate digestion and absorption. Gastroenterology 1970; 58:96–107.
4. Kelly JJ, Alpers DH. Properties of human intestinal glucoamylase. Biochim Biophys Acta 1973; 315:113–122.
5. Holdsworth CD, Dawson AM. The absorption of monosaccharides in man. Clin Sci 1964; 27:371–379.
6. McMichael HB, Webb J, Dawson AM. The absorption of maltose and lactose in man. Clin Sci 1967; 33:135–145.
7. Gray GM, Santiago NA. Disaccharide absorption in normal and diseased small bowel. Gastroenterology 1966; 51:489–498.
8. Hamosh M, Klaeveman HL, Wolf RO, et al. Pharyngeal lipase and digestion of dietary triglyceride in man. J Clin Invest 1975; 55:908–913.
9. Hildebrand H, Borgstrom B, Bekassay A, et al. Isolated colipase deficiency in two brothers. Gut 1982; 23:243–246.
10. Ockner RK, Manning JA. Fatty acid binding protein: role in esterification of absorbed long chain fat in rat intestine. J Clin Invest 1976; 58:632–641.
11. Glickman RM. Fat absorption and malabsorption. Clin Gastroenterol 1983; 12:323–334.
12. Theron JJ, Wittmann W, Prinston JG. The fine structure of the jejunum in kwashiorkor. Exp Mol Path 1971; 14:184–196.
13. Glickman RM, Green PHR, Lees RS, et al. Immunofluorescent studies of apolipoprotein B in intestinal mucosa. Absence of abetalipoproteinaemia. Gastroenterology 1979; 76:288–292.
14. Greenberger NJ, Rodger JB, Isselbacher KJ. Absorption of medium and long chain triglycerides: Factors influencing their hydrolysis and transport. J Clin Invest 1966; 45:217–227.
15. Matthews DM. Protein absorption. J Clin Pathol 1971; 5(Suppl 24):29–40.
16. Silk DBA. Disorders of nitrogen absorption. Clin Gastroenterol 1982; 11:47–72.
17. Adibi SA, Morse EL. Intestinal transport of dipeptides in man: relative importance of hydrolysis and intact absorption. J Clin Invest 1971; 50:2266–2275.
18. Silk DBA, Mass TC, Addison JM, et al. Absorption of amino acids from an amino acid mixture simulating casein and a tryptic hydrolysate of casein in man. Clin Sci Mol Med 1973; 45:715–719.
19. Grimble GK, Rees RG, Keohane PP, et al. Effect of peptide chain length on absorption of egg protein hydrolysates in the normal human jejunum. Gastroenterology 1987; 92:136–142.
20. Hegarty JE, Fairclough PD, Moriarty KJ, et al. Effects of

concentration on in vivo absorption of a peptide-containing protein hydrolysate. Gut 1982; *23*:304–309.

21. Moriarty KJ, Hegarty JE, Fairclough PD, et al. Relative nutritional value of whole protein, hydrolysed protein and free amino acids in man. Gut 1985; *26*:694–699.

22. Borgstrom B, Dahlqvist A, Lundh G, et al. Studies of intestinal digestion and absorption in the human. J Clin Invest 1957; *36*:1521–1536.

23. Johansson C. Studies of gastrointestinal interactions. VII. Characteristics of the absorption patterns of sugar, fat and protein from composite meals in man. A quantitative study. Scand J Gastroenterol 1975; *10*:33–42.

24. Stephen AM, Haddad AC, Phillips SF. Passage of carbohydrate into the colon. Direct measurements in humans. Gastroenterology 1983; *85*:589–592.

25. Ammon HV, Thomas PJ, Phillips SF. Effects of oleic acid and ricinoleic acid on net jejunal water and electrolyte movement. J Clin Invest 1974; *53*:374–379.

26. Ammon HV, Phillips SF. Inhibition of ileal water absorption by intraluminal fatty acids. J Clin Invest 1974; *53*:205–210.

27. Ammon HV, Phillips SF. Inhibition of colonic water and electrolyte absorption by fatty acids in man. Gastroenterology 1973; *65*:744–749.

28. Tiruppathi C, Balasubramanian KA, Hill PG, et al. Faecal free fatty acids in tropical sprue and their possible role in the production of diarrhoea by inhibition of ATPases. Gut 1983; *24*:300–305.

29. Ramakrishna BS, Mathan VI. Water and electrolyte absorption by the colon in tropical sprue. Gut 1982; *23*:843–846.

30. Thomas PJ. Identification of some enteric bacteria which convert oleic acid to hydroxystearic acid in vitro. Gastroenterology 1972; *62*:430–435.

31. Soony CS, Thompson JB, Poley JR, et al. Hydroxy fatty acids in human diarrhoea. Gastroenterology 1972; *63*:748–756.

32. Wiggins HS, Cummings JH, Pearson JR. Hydroxystearic acid and diarrhoea following ileal resection. Gut 1974; *15*:392–395.

33. Booth CC, Hanna S, Babouris N, et al. Incidence of hypomagnesaemia in intestinal malabsorption. Br Med J 1963; *3*:141–144.

34. Graham LA, Caesar JJ, Burgen ASV. Gastrointestinal absorption and excretion of ^{28}Mg in man. Metabolism 1960; *9*:641–659.

35. Melvin KEW, Hapner GW, Bordier P, et al. Calcium metabolism and bone pathology in adult coeliac disease. Q J Med 1970; *39*:83–113.

36. Schoen MS, Lindenbaum J, Roginsky MS, et al. Significance of serum levels of 25-hydroxycholecalciferol in gastrointestinal disease. Am J Dig Dis 1978; *23*:137–142.

37. Harrison JE, Hitchman AJW, Finlay JM, et al. Calcium kinetic studies in patients with malabsorption syndrome. Gastroenterology 1969; *56*:751–757.

38. Bliss CM, Small DM, Donaldson RM. The excretion of calcium and magnesium fatty acid soaps in steatorrhoea. Gastroenterology 1972; *62*:724.

39. Hollander D, Muralidharak S, Zimmerman A. Vitamin D-3 intestinal absorption in vivo: influence of fatty acids, bile salts and perfusate pH on absorption. Gut 1978; *19*:267–273.

40. Schiff ER, Small NC, Dietschy JM. Characterisation of the kinetics of the passive and active transport mechanisms for bile acid absorption in the small intestine and colon of the rat. J Clin Invest 1972; *51*:1351–1362.

41. Spiller RC, Frost PE, Stewart JS, et al. Delayed postprandial plasma bile acid response in coeliac patients with slow-caecum transit. Clin Sci 1987; *72*:217–223.

42. Vuoristo M, Tarpila S, Miettinen TA. Serum lipids and faecal steroids in patients with celiac disease: effects of gluten-free diet and cholestyramine. Gastroenterology 1980; *78*:1518–1525.

43. Duane WC, Bond JH. Prolongation of intestinal transit and

44. Motson RW, Hammerman KJ, Admirand WH, et al. Effect of chronic changes in rate of enterohepatic cycling on bile acid kinetics and biliary lipid composition in the rhesus monkey. Gastroenterology 1981; *80*:655–660.

45. Low-Beer TS, Heaton KW, Pomare EW, et al. The effect of coeliac disease upon bile salts. Gut 1973; *14*:204–208.

46. Spiller RC, Trotman IF, Higgins BE, et al. The ileal brake—inhibition of jejunal motility after ileal fat perfusion in man. Gut 1984; *25*:365–374.

47. Spiller RC. The influence of fat on human small bowel motility. MD Thesis, Cambridge University, 1985.

48. Besterman HS, Sarson DL, Johnson DI, et al. Gut hormone profile in coeliac disease. Lancet 1978; *1*:785–788.

49. Adrian TE, Savage AP, Bacarase-Hamilton AJ, et al. Peptide YY abnormalities in gastrointestinal disease. Gastroenterology 1986; *90*:378–384.

50. Read NW, McFarlane A, Kinsman RI, et al. The effect of infusion of nutrient solutions into the ileum on gastrointestinal transit and plasma levels of neurotensin and enteroglucagon. Gastroenterology 1984; *86*:274–280.

51. Welch I, Saunders K, Read NW. Effect of ileal and intravenous infusions of fat emulsions on feeding and satiety in human volunteers. Gastroenterology 1985; *89*:1293–1297.

52. Blackburn AM, Bloom SR, Long RG, et al. Effect of neurotensin on gastric function in man. Lancet 1980; *1*:987–989.

53. Thor K, Rosell S, Rokaeus A, et al. Gln^4-neurotensin changes the motility pattern of the duodenum and proximal jejunum from a fasting-type to a fed-type. Gastroenterology 1982; *83*:569–574.

54. Tatemoto K, Mutt V. Isolation of two novel candidate hormones using a chemical method for finding naturally occurring polypeptides. Nature 1980; *285*:417–418.

55. Adrian TE, Ferri G-L, Bacarase-Hamilton AJ, et al. Human distribution and release of a putative new gut hormone, peptide YY. Gastroenterology 1985; *89*:1070–1077.

56. Allen TE, Fitzpatrick ML, Yeats JC, et al. Effect of peptide YY and neuropeptide Y in gastric emptying in man. Digestion 1984; *30*:255–262.

57. Savage AP, Adrian TE, Carolan G, et al. Effects of peptide PYY on mouth to caecum transit time and on the rate of gastric emptying in healthy volunteers. Gut, in press.

58. Spiller RC, Lee YC, Edge C, et al. Functional significance of the ileal brake in coeliac disease. Gut 1984; *25*:A545.

59. Snell AM, Camp JD. Chronic idiopathic steatorrhoea—roentgenologic observations. Ann Intern Med 1934; *53*:615–629.

60. Perman G, Mattson O. Small intestinal transit time in steatorrhea. Acta Med Scand 1962; *171*:273–281.

61. Bliss CM, Small DM. A comparison of ileal and faecal lipid in pancreatic steatorrhoea. Gastroenterology 1970; *58*:928.

62. Rupin H, Bar-Meir S, Soergel KH, et al. Absorption of short-chain fatty acids. Gastroenterology 1980; *78*:1500–1507.

63. Hoverstad T, Vohmer T, Fausa O. Absorption of short-chain fatty acids from the human colon measured by the $^{14}CO_2$ breath test. Scand J Gastroenterol 1982; *17*:373–378.

64. Roediger WEW, Moore A. Effect of short-chain fatty acids on sodium absorption in isolated human; perfused through the vascular bed. Dig Dis Sci 1981; *26*:100–106.

65. Spiller RC, Brown ML, Phillips SF. Decreased fluid tolerance, accelerated transit, and abnormal motility of the human colon induced by oleic acid. Gastroenterology 1986; *91*:100–107.

66. Andersson H, Isaksson B, Sjogren B. Fat-reduced diet in the symptomatic treatment of small bowel disease. Gut 1974; *15*:351–359.

67. Woolfe GM, Miller C, Kurian R, et al. Diet for patients with

a short bowel colon. High fat or high carbohydrate? Gastroenterology 1983; *84*:823–828.

68. Cohen SA, Hendricks KM, Mattis RA, et al. Chronic non-specific diarrhoea; dietary relationships. Pediatrics 1979; *64*:402–407.

69. Levine AS, Levitt MD. Malabsorption of starch moiety of oats, corn and potatoes. Gastroenterology 1981; *80*:1209.

70. Levitt MD, Ellis CJ, Fetzer CA, et al. Causes of malabsorption of flour. Gastroenterology 1984; *86*:1162.

71. Anderson IH, Levine AJ, Levitt MD. Incomplete absorption of the carbohydrate in all-purpose wheat flour. N Engl J Med 1981; *304*:891–892.

72. Roediger WEW. Role of anaerobic bacteria in the metabolic welfare of the colonic mucosa in man. Gut 1980; *21*:793–798.

73. Christopher NL, Bayless TM. Role of the small bowel and colon in lactose-induced diarrhoea. Gastroenterology 1971; *60*:845–852.

74. Fordtran JS, Rector FC, Ewton MG, et al. Permeability characteristics of the human small intestine. J Clin Invest 1965; *44*:1935–1944.

75. Fordtran JS, Rector FC, Carter NW. The mechanism of sodium absorption in the human small intestine. J Clin Invest 1968; *47*:884–900.

76. Launiala K. The effect of unabsorbed sucrose and mannitol on the small intestinal flow rate and mean transit time. Scand J Gastroenterol 1968; *3*:665–671.

77. Ladas S, Papanikos J, Arapakis G. Lactose malabsorption in Greek adults; correlation of small bowel transit time with the severity of lactose intolerance. Gut 1982; *23*:968–973.

78. Debongnie JC, Phillips SF. Capacity of the human colon to absorb fluid. Gastroenterology 1978; *74*:698–703.

79. Layer P, Zinsmeister AR, DiMagno EP. Effects of decreasing intraluminal amylase activity on starch digestion and postprandial gastrointestinal function in humans. Gastroenterology 1986; *91*:41–48.

80. Florent C, Flourie B, Le Blond A, et al. Influence of chronic lactulose ingestion on the colonic metabolism of lactulose in man (an in vivo study). J Clin Invest 1985; *75*:608–613.

81. Gilt E, Rousso S, Gelman-Malaichi D, et al. Lactase in man; a non-adaptable enzyme. Gastroenterology 1972; *62*:1125–1127.

82. Milne MD, Asatoor AM, Edwards KPJ, et al. The intestinal absorption defect in cystinuria. Gut 1961; *2*:323–337.

83. Hegarty JE, Fairclough PD, Cark ML, et al. Jejunal water and electrolyte secretion induced by L-arginine in man. Gut 1981; *22*:108–113.

84. Simell O, Perheentupa J, Rapola J, et al. Lysinuric protein intolerance. Am J Med 1975; *59*:229–240.

85. Drummond KN, Michael AF, Ulstrom RA, et al. The blue diaper syndrome; familial hypercalcaemia with nephrocalcinosis and indicanuria. Am J Med 1964; *37*:928–948.

86. Gee S. On the coeliac affection. St. Bartholomews Hospital Report 1888; *24*:17–20.

87. Dicke WK, Weijers HA, Van der Camer JH. Coeliac disease. 2. The presence in wheat of a factor having a deleterious effect in cases of coeliac disease. Acta Paediatrica 1953; *42*:34–42.

88. Anderson CM, Frazer AC, French JM, et al. Coeliac disease—gastrointestinal studies and the effect of dietary wheat flour. Lancet 1952; *1*:836–842.

89. Fraser AC, Fletcher RF, Roth CAC, et al. A gluten-induced enteropathy. The effect of partially digested gluten. Lancet 1959; *2*:252–255.

90. Rubin CE, Brandborg LL, Flick AL, et al. Studies of celiac sprue. III. The effect of repeated wheat instillation into the proximal ileum of patients on a gluten free diet. Gastroenterology 1962; *43*:621–632.

91. Dissanayake AJ, Jerrome DW, Offord RE, et al. Identifying toxic fractions of wheat gluten and their effect on the jejunal mucosa in coeliac disease. Gut 1974; *15*:931–946.

92. Levine RA, Briggs GW, Harding RS, et al. Prolonged gluten administration in normal subjects. N Engl J Med 1966; *274*:1109–1114.

93. Hamilton JR, Lynch MJ, Reilly BJ. Active coeliac disease in childhood. Q J Med 1969; *38*:135–157.

94. Swinson CM, Levi AJ. Is coeliac disease underdiagnosed? Br Med J 1980; *281*:1258–1260.

95. Logan RFA, Tucker G, Rifkind EA, et al. Changes in clinical features of coeliac disease in adults in Edinburgh and the Lothians 1960–1979. Br Med J 1983; *286*:95–97.

96. Gent AE, Creamer B. Faecal fats, appetite and weight loss in the coeliac syndrome. Lancet 1968; *1*:1063–1064.

97. Cooke WT, Fone DJ, Cox EV, et al. Adult coeliac disease. Gut 1963; *4*:279–291.

98. Cooke WT, Thomas G, Mangall D, et al. Observations on faecal excretion of total solids, nitrogen, sodium, potassium, water and fat in the steatorrhoea syndrome. Clin Sci 1953; *12*:223–234.

99. Paulley JW. Observations on the aetiology of idiopathic steatorrhoea. Br Med J 1954; *2*:1318–1321.

100. Watson AJ, Wright NA. Morphology and cell kynetics of the jejunal mucosa in untreated coeliac patients. Clin Gastroenterol 1974; *3*:11–31.

101. Gell DG, Chapman G, Kelly M, et al. Na+ transport in jejunal crypt cells. Gastroenterology 1977; *72*:452–456.

102. Arthur AB. Intestinal disaccharidase deficiency in children with coeliac disease. Arch Dis Child 1966; *41*:519–524.

103. Berg NO, Dahlqvist A, Lindberg T, et al. Intestinal dipeptidases and disaccharidases in celiac disease in adults. Gastroenterology 1970; *59*:575–582.

104. Pena AS, Truelove SC, Whitehead R. Disaccharidase activity and jejunal morphology in coeliac disease. Q J Med 1972; *41*:457–476.

105. MacDonald WC, Brandborg LL, Flick AL, et al. Studies of celiac sprue. IV. The response of the whole length of the small bowel to a gluten-free diet. Gastroenterology 1964; *47*:573–589.

106. Stewart JS, Pollock DJ, Hoffbrand AV, et al. A study of proximal and distal intestinal structure and absorptive function in idiopathic steatorrhoea. Q J Med 1967; *36*:425–444.

107. Booth CC, Read AE, Jones E. Studies on the site of fat absorption. 1. The site of absorption of increasing doses of ^{131}I-labelled triolein in the rat. Gut 1961; *2*:23–31.

108. Holdsworth CD, Dawson AM. Glucose and fructose absorption in idiopathic steatorrhea. Gut 1965; *6*:387–391.

109. Silk DBA, Kumar PJ, Perrett D, et al. Amino acid and peptide absorption in patients with coeliac disease and dermatitis herpetiformis. Gut 1974; *15*:1–8.

110. Fordtran JS, Rector FC, Locklear TW, et al. Water and solute movement in the small intestine in patients with sprue. J Clin Invest 1967; *46*:287–298.

111. Russell RI, Allen JG, Gerskowitch VP, et al. A study by perfusion techniques of the absorption abnormalities in the jejunum in adult coeliac disease. Clin Sci 1972; *42*:735–741.

112. Dowling RH. Small bowel adaptation and its regulation. Scand J Gastroenterol (Suppl) 1983; *74*:53–74.

113. Silk DBA, Kumar PJ, Webb JPW, et al. Ileal function in patients with untreated adult coeliac disease. Gut 1975; *16*:261–267.

114. MacKinnon AM, Short MD, Elias E, et al. Adaptive changes in vitamin B_{12} absorption in coeliac disease and after proximal small bowel resection in man. Dig Dis 1975; *20*:835–840.

115. Hepner GW, Booth CC, Kowan J, et al. Absorption of crystalline folic acid in man. Lancet 1968; *2*:302–306.

116. Weir DJ, Hourihane D. Coeliac disease during the teenage period: The value of serial serum folate estimations. Gut 1974; *15*:450–457.

117. Hoffbrand AV, Douglas AP, Fry L, et al. Malabsorption of dietary folate (pteroylopolyglutamates) in adult coeliac disease and dermatitis herpetiformis. Br Med J 1970; *4*:85–89.

118. Fry L, Keir P, McMion RMH, et al. Small intestinal structure

and function and haematological manifestations of dermatitis herpetiformis. Lancet 1968; 1:557–561.

119. Webb MGT, Taylor MRH, Gatenby PBB. Iron absorption in coeliac disease of childhood and adolescence. Br Med J 1967; 2:151–152.

120. Badenoch T, Callender ST. Effect of corticosteroids and gluten-free diets on absorption of iron in idiopathic steatorrhoea and coeliac disease. Lancet 1960; 1:192–194.

121. Croft DW, Loehry CA, Creamer B. Small bowel cell loss and weight loss in coeliac syndrome. Lancet 1968; 2:68–70.

122. Sutton DR, Baird IM, Stewart JS, et al. Free iron loss in atrophic gastritis, post gastrectomy states and adult coeliac disease. Lancet 1970; 2:387–391.

123. Fordtran JS, Soergel KH, Ingelfinger FJ. Intestinal absorption of D-xylose in man. New Engl J Med 1962; 267:274–279.

124. Sladen GE, Kumar PJ. Is the xylose test still a worth-while investigation? Br Med J 1973; 2:223–226.

125. Agnew JE, Kehayoglou AK, Holdsworth CD. Comparison of three isotopic methods for the study of calcium absorption. Gut 1969; 10:590–597.

126. Graham LA, Caesar JJ, Burgen ASU. Gastrointestinal absorption and excretion of Mg^{++} in man. Metabolism 1960; 9:646–649.

127. Andersson KE, Braith L, Dencker H, et al. Some aspects of the intestinal absorption of zinc in man. Eur J Clin Pharm 1976; 9:423–428.

128. Wensel RH, Rich C, Brown AC, et al. Absorption of calcium measured by intubation and infusion of the intact human small intestine. J Clin Invest 1969; 48:1768–1775.

129. Goldman AS, Van Fossan DD, Baird EE. Magnesium deficiency in celiac disease. Pediatrics 1962; 29:948–952.

130. Agnew JE, Holdsworth CD. The effect of fat on calcium absorption from a mixed meal in normal subjects, patients with malabsorption disease and patients with a partial gastrectomy. Gut 1971; 12:973–977.

131. Booth CC, Aldis D, Read AE. Studies on the site of fat absorption. II. Fat balances after resection of varying amounts of the small intestine in man. Gut 1961; 2:168–174.

132. DiMagno EP, Go VLW, Summerskill WHJ. Impaired cholecystokinin-pancreozymin secretion; intraluminal dilution and maldigestion of fat in sprue. Gastroenterology 1972; 63:25–32.

133. Maton PN, Selden AC, Fitzpatrick ML, et al. Defective gall bladder emptying and cholecystokinin release in coeliac disease. Reversal by a gluten-free diet. Gastroenterology 1985; 88:391–396.

134. Crane CW, Neuberger A. Absorption and elimination of ^{15}N after administration of isotopically labelled yeast protein and yeast protein hydrolysate to adult patients with coeliac disease. Br Med J 1960; 2:816–822.

135. Hoffbrand AV. Anaemia in adult coeliac disease. Clin Gastroenterol 1974; 3:71–89.

136. Low-Beer TS, Heaton KW, Heaton ST, et al. Gall bladder inertia and sluggish enterohepatic circulation of bile salts in coeliac disease. Lancet 1971; 1:991–994.

137. Taylor AB, Wollaeger EE, Comfort MW. The effect of cortisone on non-tropical sprue (idiopathic steatorrhoea). Gastroenterology 1952; 20:203–228.

138. Wall AJ, Douglas AP, Booth CC, et al. Response of the jejunal mucosa in adult coeliac disease to oral prednisolone. Gut 1970; 11:7–14.

139. Dissanayake AS, Truelove SC, Whitehead R. Lack of harmful effect of oats on small intestinal mucosa in celiac disease. Br Med J 1974; 4:189–191.

140. Anand BS, Piris J, Truelove, SC. The role of various cereals in coeliac disease. Q J Med 1978; 185:101–110.

141. Dissanayake AS, Truelove SC, Whitehead R. Jejunal mucosal recovery in coeliac disease in relation to the degree of adherence to a gluten-free diet. Q J Med 1974; 170:161–185.

142. Benson GD, Kowlessar OD, Sleisenger MH. Adult coeliac disease with emphasis upon response to the gluten-free diet. Medicine 1964; 43:1–40.

143. Shiner M. Effect of a gluten-free diet in seventeen patients with idiopathic steatorrhoea. A follow up study. Am J Dig Dis 1963; 8:969–983.

144. Pink IJ, Creamer B. Response to a gluten-free diet of patients with the coeliac syndrome. Lancet 1967; 1:300–304.

145. Cooper BT, Holmes GKT, Ferguson R, et al. Celiac disease and malignancy. Medicine 1980; 59:249–261.

146. Swinson CM, Slavin G, Coles EC, et al. Coeliac disease and malignancy. Lancet 1983; 1:111–115.

147. Jeffries GH, Steinberg H, Sleisenger MH. Chronic idiopathic ulcerative (non-granulomatous) jejunitis. Am J Med 1968; 44:47–59.

148. Issacson P, Wright DH. Malignant histiocytosis of the intestine: its relationship to malabsorption and ulcerative jejunitis. Hum Pathol 1978; 9:661–677.

149. Freeman HJ, Chiu K. Multifocal small bowel lymphoma and latent celiac sprue. Gastroenterology 1986; 90:1992–1997.

150. Pollock DJ, Nagle RE, Jeejeebhoy KN, et al. The effect on jejunal mucosa of withdrawing and adding dietary gluten in cases of idiopathic steatorrhoea. Gut 1970; 11:567–585.

151. Schenk EA, Samloft IM. Clinical and morphological changes following gluten administration to patients with treated coeliac disease. Am J Pathol 1968; 52:579–585.

152. McNicholl B, Egan-Mitchell B, Fottrel PF. Variability of gluten intolerance in treated childhood coeliac disease. Gut 1970; 20:126–132.

153. Kumar PJ, O-Donoghue DP, Steven D, et al. Re-introduction of gluten in adults and children with treated coeliac disease. Gut 1979; 20:743–749.

154. Baker SJ, Mathan VI. An epidemic of tropical sprue in southern India. II. Epidemiology. Ann Trop Med Parasitol 1970; 64:453–467.

155. O'Brien W, England NWJ. Military tropical sprue from South East Asia. Br Med J 1966; 2:1157–1162.

156. Jeejeebhoy KN, Desai HG, Noronha JM, et al. Idiopathic tropical diarrhoea with or without steatorrhoea (tropical malabsorption syndrome). Gastroenterology 1966; 51:333–344.

157. England NWJ, O'Brien W. Appearances of the jejunal mucosa in acute tropical sprue in Singapore. Gut 1966; 7:128–139.

158. Chacko CJG, Paulson KA, Mathan VI, et al. The villous architecture of the small intestine in the tropics; a necropsy study. J Pathol 1969; 98:146–151.

159. Philipstein FA, Corseino JJ. Malabsorption of central amino acids in tropical sprue. Gastroenterology 1975; 68:239–244.

160. Corcino JJ, Maldonado M, Klipstein FA. Intestinal perfusion studies in tropical sprue. Transport of water, electrolytes and D-xylose. Gastroenterology 1973; 65:192–198.

161. Adibi SA, Fogel MR, Agrawal RM. Comparison of free amino acids and dipeptide absorption in the jejunum of sprue patients. Gastroenterology 1974; 67:586–591.

162. Hellier MD, Radhakrishnan AN, Ganapathy V, et al. Intestinal perfusion studies in tropical sprue. Gut 1976; 17:511–516.

163. Gorbach SL, Banwell JG, Mitra R, et al. Bacterial contamination of the upper small bowel in tropical sprue. Lancet 1969; 1:74–77.

164. Tomkins AM, Smith T, Wright SG. Assessment of early and delayed responses in vitamin B_{12} absorption during antibiotic therapy in tropical malabsorption. Clin Sci Mol Med 1978; 55:533–539.

165. Jeejeebhoy KW, Sarwal AM, Singh B, et al. Metabolism of albumin and fibrinogen in patients with tropical sprue. Gastroenterology 1969; 56:252–267.

166. Desai HG, Chitre AV, Parek HDV, et al. Intestinal disaccharidase in tropical sprue. Gastroenterology 1967; 53:375–380.

167. Gray GM, Walter WM, Colver EH. Persistent deficiency of intestinal lactase in apparently cured tropical sprue. Gastroenterology 1968; 54:552–558.

168. Sheehy TW, Anderson R, Baggs BE. Carbohydrate intolerance in tropical sprue. Am J Dig Dis 1966; 11:461–473.

169. Tomkins AM, Drasar BS, James WPT. Bacterial colonisation of jejunal mucosa in acute tropical sprue. Lancet 1975; 1:59–68.

170. Klipstein FA, Engert RF. Enterotoxogenic intestinal bacteria in tropical sprue. III. Preliminary characterisation of Klebsiella pneumoniae enterotoxin. J Infect Dis 1975; 132:200–203.

171. Cook GC. Delayed small intestinal transit in tropical malabsorption. Br Med J 1978; 2:238–240.

172. Cook GC. Aetiology and pathogenesis of postinfective tropical malabsorption (tropical sprue). Lancet 1984; 1:721–723.

173. Hoffbrand AV, Necheles TF, Maldonado N, et al. Malabsorption of folate polyglutamates in tropical sprue. Br Med J 1969; 2:543–547.

174. Swanson VL, Wheby MS, Bayless TM. Morphologic effects of folic acid and vitamin B$_{12}$ on the jejunal lesion of tropical sprue. Am J Pathol 1966; 49:167–171.

175. Manson-Bahr P, Clarke O. Folic acid in tropical sprue. Lancet 1946; 2:903–904.

176. Webb JF, Simpson B. Tropical sprue in Hong Kong. Br Med J 1966; 2:1162–1166.

177. Davidson LSP, Girdwood RH, Innes EM. Folic acid in the treatment of the sprue syndrome. Lancet 1947; 1:511–515.

178. Sheehy TW, Baggs B, Perez-Sandiago E, et al. Prognosis of tropical sprue. A study of the effect of folic acid on the intestinal aspects of acute and chronic sprue. Ann Intern Med 1962; 57:892–908.

179. Klipstein FA, Schenk EA, Samloff IM. Folate repletion associated with oral tetracycline in tropical sprue. Gastroenterology 1966; 51:317–332.

180. Winawer SJ, Sullivan LW, Herbert V, et al. The jejunal mucosa in patients with nutritional deficiency and megaloblastic anaemia. N Engl J Med 1965; 272:892–896.

181. Lindenbaum J, Gerson CD, Kent TH. Recovery of small intestinal structure and function after residence in the tropics. Ann Int Med 1971; 74:218–222.

182. Farthing MJG, Varon S, Keusch GT, et al. Bile salts stimulate growth and multiplication of Giardia lamblia by facilitating uptake of preformed membrane phospholipid. Gastroenterology 1983; 84:1148.

183. Morecki R, Parker JG. Ultrastructural studies of the human Giardia lamblia and subjacent jejunal mucosa in a subject with steatorrhoea. Gastroenterology 1967; 52:151–164.

184. Bingham AK, Jarrol JE, Meyer EA. Giardia species. Physical factors of excystation in vivo and excystation vs eosin exclusion as determinants of viability. Exp Parasitol 1979; 47:284–291.

185. Antia FP, Desai HG, Jeejeebhoy KN, et al. Giardiasis in adults—incidence, symptomatology and absorption studies. Indian J Med Sci 1966; 20:471–477.

186. Butler T, Middleton FG, Earnest DL, et al. Chronic and recurrent diarrhoea in American servicemen in Vietnam. Arch Int Med 1973; 132:373–377.

187. Eastham EJ, Douglas AP, Watson AJ. Diagnosis of Giardia lamblia infection as a cause of diarrhoea. Lancet 1976; 2:950–951.

188. Jephcott AE, Begg NT, Baker IA. Outbreak of giardiasis associated with mains water in the United Kingdom. Lancet 1986; 1:730–732.

189. Osterholm MT, Forfang JC, Ristinen TL, et al. An outbreak of foodborne giardiasis. N Engl J Med 1981; 304:24–28.

190. Jokipii AM, Hemila M, Jokipii L. Prospective study of acquisition of Cryptosporidium, Giardia lamblia and gastrointestinal illness. Lancet 1985; 2:857–859.

191. Chester AC, MacMurray FG, Restifo MD, et al. Giardiasis as a chronic disease. Dig Dis Sci 1985; 30:215–218.

192. Ament ME, Rubin CE. Relation of giardiasis to abnormal intestinal structure and function in gastrointestinal immunodeficiency syndromes. Gastroenterology 1972; 62:216–226.

193. Schmein MJ, Jones TC, Klein H. Giardiasis: association with homosexuality. Ann Intern Med 1978; 88:801–803.

194. Wright SG, Tomkins AK, Ridley DS. Giardiasis. Clinical and therapeutic aspects. Gut 1977; 80:343–350.

195. Cortner JA. Giardiasis, A cause of celiac syndrome. Am J Dis Child 1959; 98:311–316.

196. Tandon BN, Tandon RK, Satpathy BK, et al. Mechanism of malabsorption in giardiasis: a study of bacterial flora and bile salt deconjugation in upper jejunum. Gut 1977; 18:176–181.

197. Takano J, Yardley JH. Jejunal lesions in patients with giardiasis and malabsorption. An electron microscopic study. Bull Johns Hopkins Hosp 1965; 116:413–429.

198. Poley JR, Rosenfield S. Giardiasis and malabsorption: presence of an organic mucosal barrier. A scanning (SEM) and transmission (TEM) electron microscopic study of small bowel mucosa. Gastroenterology 1981; 80:1254.

199. Alp MH, Hislop IG. The effects of Giardia lamblia infestation on the gastrointestinal tract. Aust Ann Med 1969; 18:232–237.

200. Hartong WA, Gourley WK, Arvanitakis C. Giardiasis: clinical spectrum and functional-structural abnormalities of the small intestinal mucosa. Gastroenterology 1979; 77:61–69.

201. Desai HG, Kelro RH, Zaveri MP, et al. Giardiasis: an evaluation of diagnostic methods. Indian J Gastroenterol 1983; 3:135–137.

202. Goka AKJ, Rolston DDK, Mathan VI, et al. Diagnosis of giardiasis by specific IgM antibody enzyme-linked immunosorbent assay. Lancet 1986; 2:184–186.

203. Andersson T, Forsell J, Sterner G. Outbreak of giardiasis: effect of a new anti-flagellate drug, tinidazole. Br Med J 1972; 2:449–451.

204. Jokipii L, Jokipii AM. Treatment of giardiasis: comparative evaluation of ornidazole and tinidazole as a single oral dose. Gastroenterology 1982; 83:399–404.

205. Sahi T, Iskoski M, Jussila J, et al. Recessive inheritance of adult type lactose malabsorption. Lancet 1973; 2:823–826.

206. Kretchmer N, Ranson-Kuti OJ, Hurwitz R. Intestinal absorption of lactose in Nigerian ethnic groups. Lancet 1971; 2:392–395.

207. Simoons FJ. Geographical hypothesis and lactose malabsorption: a weighing of the evidence. Am J Dig Dis 1978; 23:963–980.

208. Kaskey DA, Payne-Bose D, Welsh JD, et al. Effects of age on lactose malabsorption in Oklahoma Native Americans as determined by breath H$_2$ analysis. Am J Dig Dis 1977; 22:113–116.

209. Newcomer AD, Thomas PT, McGill D, et al. Lactose deficiency: a common genetic trait of the American Indian. Gastroenterology 1977; 72:234–237.

210. Lebenthal E, Tsuboi K, Kretchmer N. Characterisation of human intestinal and hetero-beta-galactosidases of infants and adults. Gastroenterology 1974; 67:1107–1113.

211. Sutton RE, Hamilton JR. Tolerance of young children with severe gastroenteritis to dietary lactose: a controlled study. Can Med Assoc J 1968; 99:980–982.

212. Dahlqvist A, Thomson DL. The digestion and absorption of lactose by the intact rat. Acta Physiol Scand 1964; 61:20–33.

213. Bolin TD, Tirola RC, Davis AE. Adaptation of intestinal lactase in the rat. Gastroenterology 1969; 57:406–409.

214. Bond JH, Levitt MD. Quantitative measurement of lactose absorption. Gastroenterology 1976; 70:1058–1062.

215. Solomns NW, Garcia-Ibenes R, Viteri FE. Hydrogen breath test of lactose absorption in adults—the application of physiological doses and cow's milk sources. Am J Clin Nutr 1980; 33:545–554.

216. Newcomer AD, McGill DB. Lactose intolerance tests in

adults with normal lactase activity. Gastroenterology 1966; *50*:340–346.

217. Newcomer AD, McGill DB, Thomas PT, et al. Prospective comparison of indirect methods of detecting lactase deficiency. N Engl J Med 1975; *293*:1232–1235.

218. Bedine MS, Bayless TM. Intolerance of small amounts of lactose by individuals with low lactase levels. Gastroenterology 1973; *65*:735–743.

219. Lisker R, Aguiler AR, Zavala C. Intestinal lactase deficiency and milk drinking capacity in the adult. Am J Clin Nutr 1978; *31*:1499–1503.

220. Read NW, Miles CA, Fisher D, et al. Transit of a meal through the stomach, small intestine and colon in normal subjects and its role in the pathogenesis of diarrhoea. Gastroenterology 1980; *79*:1276–1282.

221. Lifshitz F, Coello-Ramirez P, Gutierrez-Topet G, et al. Carbohydrate intolerance in infants with diarrhoea. J Pediatr 1971; *79*:760–767.

222. Lifshitz F, Coello-Ramirez P, Contreras-Gutierrez ML. The response of infants to carbohydrate oral foods after recovery from diarrhoea. J Pediatr 1971; *79*:612–617.

223. Callway DH, Chenoweth WL. Utilisation of nutrients in milk-and-wheat–based diets by men with adequate and reduced abilities to absorb lactose. I. Energy and nitrogen. Am J Clin Nutr 1973; *26*:939–951.

224. Keohane PP, Attrill H, Jones BMJ, et al. The role of lactose and *Clostridium difficile* in the pathogenesis of enteral feeding associated diarrhoea. Clin Nutr 1973; *1*:259–264.

225. Torun B, Solomons MW, Caballero B, et al. The effect of dietary lactose on the early recovery from protein-energy malnutrition. II. Indices of nutrient absorption. Am J Clin Nutr 1984; *40*:601–610.

226. Hozel A, Schwarz FV, Sutcliffe KW. Defective lactose absorption causing malnutrition in infancy. Lancet 1959; *1*:1126–1128.

227. Lifshitz F. Congenital lactase deficiency. J Pediatr 1966; *69*:229–237.

228. MacLean WC, Fink BB. Lactose malabsorption by premature infants: magnitude and clinical significance. J Pediatr 1980; *97*:383–388.

229. Meeuwisse GW, Melin K. Studies in glucose-galactose malabsorption. A clinical study of six cases. Acta Paediatr Scand (Suppl) 1969; *18*:1–18.

230. Gray GM, Conklin KA, Townley RRW. Sucrase-isomaltase deficiency. Absence of an inactive enzyme variant. N Engl J Med 1976; *294*:750–753.

231. Peterson ML, Herber R. Intestinal sucrase deficiency. Trans Assoc Am Phys 1967; *82*:273–283.

232. McNiar A, Gudmand-Hoyer E, Jarnum S, et al. Sucrose malabsorption in Greenland. Br Med J 1972; *2*:19–21.

233. Arment ME, Perera DR, Estager LJ. Sucrase-isomaltase deficiency—a frequently misdiagnosed disease. J Paediatr 1973; *83*:721–727.

234. Metz G, Jenkins DGA, Newman A, et al. Breath hydrogen in hyposucrasia. Lancet 1976; *1*:119–120.

235. Burgess EA, Levin B, Mahalanabis D, et al. Hereditary sucrose intolerance: levels of sucrase activity in jejunal mucosa. Arch Dis Child 1964; *39*:431–443.

236. Neale G, Clark M, Levin B. Intestinal sucrose intolerance in adult life. Br Med J 1985; *2*:1223–1225.

237. Madzarovova-Nohejelora J. Trehalase deficiency in a family. Gastroenterology 1973; *65*:130–133.

238. Melin K, Meeuwisse GW. Glucose-galactose malabsorption. Acta Paediatr Scand (Suppl) 1969; *188*:19–24.

239. Meeuwisse GW, Cahlquist A. Glucose-galactose malabsorption. A study with biopsy of the small intestinal mucosa. Acta Paediatr Scand 1968; *57*:273–280.

240. Hughes WS, Senior JR. The glucose-galactose malabsorption syndrome in a 23 year old woman. Gastroenterology 1975; *68*:142–145.

241. Fairclough RD, Clark ML, Dawson AM, et al. Absorption of glucose and maltose in congenital glucose-galactose malabsorption. Pediatr Res 1978; *12*:1112–1114.

242. Gracey M, Burke V, Oshin A. Active intestinal transport of D-fructose. Biochim Biophys Acta 1972; *66*:397–406.

243. Holdsworth CD, Dawson AM. The absorption of monosaccharides in man. Clin Sci 1964; *27*:371–379.

244. Ravich WJ, Bayless TM, Thomas M. Fructose: incomplete intestinal absorption in humans. Gastroenterology 1983; *84*:26–29.

245. Hyams JS, Leichtner AM. Apple juice. An unappreciated cause of chronic diarrhea. Am J Dis Child 1985; *139*:503–505.

246. Cox TM, Camilleri M, O'Donnell MW, et al. Pseudodominant transmission of fructose intolerance in an adult and three offspring—heterozygote detection by intestinal biopsy. N Engl J Med 1982; *307*:537–540.

247. Black JA, Simpson K. Fructose intolerance. Br Med J 1967; *4*:138–141.

248. Visakorpi JK, Immonen P. Intolerance to cow's milk and wheat gluten in the primary malabsorption syndrome in infancy. Acta Paediatr Scand 1967; *56*:49–56.

249. Iyngkaran N, Robinson MJ, Prathap K, et al. Cow's milk protein–sensitive enteropathy, combined clinical and histological criteria for diagnosis. Arch Dis Child 1978; *53*:20–26.

250. Goldman AJ, Anderson DW, Fellows W, et al. Milk allergy. Pediatrics 1963; *32*:425–437.

251. Gryboski JD. Gastrointestinal milk allergy in infants. Pediatrics 1967; *40*:254–261.

252. Liu HY, Tsao MU, Moore B. Bovine milk protein–induced malabsorption of lactose and fat in infants. Gastroenterology 1967; *54*:27–34.

253. Walker-Smith J. Diseases of the small intestine in childhood. Tunbridge Wells, England, Pitman Medical, 1975, Chapter 5.

254. Dent CE, Heathcote JG, Joran GE. The pathogenesis of cystinuria 1. Chromatographic and microbiological studies of the metabolism of sulphur-containing amino acids. J Clin Invest 1954; *33*:1210–1215.

255. Silk DBA, Perrett D, Clark ML. Jejunal and ileal absorption of dibasic amino acids and an arginine-containing dipeptide in cystinuria. Gastroenterology 1975; *78*:1426–1432.

256. Rajantie J, Simell O, Perheentupa J. Basolateral-membrane transport defect for lysine in lysinuric protein intolerance. Lancet 1980; *1*:1219–1221.

257. Silk DBA, Perrett D, Stevens AD, et al. Intestinal absorption of cystine and cysteine in normal human subjects and patients with cystinuria. Clin Sci Mol Med 1974; *47*:393–397.

258. Hellier MD, Holdsworth CD, Perrett D. Dibasic amino acid absorption in man. Gastroenterology 1973; *65*:613–618.

259. Asatoor AM, Crouchman MR, Harrison AR, et al. Intestinal absorption of oligopeptides in cystinuria. Clin Sci 1971; *41*:23–33.

260. Hellier MD, Holdsworth CD, Perrett D, et al. Intestinal dipeptide transport in normal and cystinuric subjects. Clin Sci 1972; *43*:659–668.

261. Dahlberg PJ, Van den Berg P, Kurtz SB, et al. Clinical features and management of cystinuria. Mayo Clin Proc 1977; *52*:533–542.

262. Wilcken B, Yu JS, Brown DA. Natural history of Hartnup disease. Arch Dis Child 1977; *52*:38–40.

263. Milne MD, Crawford MA, Girao CB, et al. The metabolic disorder in Hartnup disease. Q J Med 1960; *24*:407–421.

264. Asatoor AM, Cherry BD, Edwards KDG, et al. Intestinal absorption of two dipeptides in Hartnup disease. Gut 1970; *11*:380–387.

265. Asatoor AM, Bandoh JK, Lant AF, et al. Intestinal absorption of carnosine and its constituent amino acids in man. Gut 1970; *11*:250–254.

266. Navab F, Asatoor AM. Studies on intestinal absorption of amino acids in a case of Hartnup disease. Gut 1970; *11*:373–379.

267. Jepson JB. Hartnup disease. *In* Stanbury JB, Wyngaarden A, Frederickson DS (eds). The Metabolic Basis of Inherited Disease. New York, McGraw-Hill, 1972.

268. Rajantie J, Simmell O, Perheentupa J. Intestinal absorption in lysinuric protein intolerance: impaired for diamino acids, normal for citrulline. Gut 1980; *21*:519–524.

269. Whelan DT, Scriver CR. Cystathioninuria and renal iminoglycinuria in a pedigree. N Engl J Med 1968; *278*:924–927.

270. Hooft CJ, Timmermans J, Snoeck J, et al. Methionine malabsorption in a mentally defective child. Lancet 1964; *2*:20–21.

271. Bartsocas CS, Levy HL, Crawford JD, et al. A deficiency in intestinal amino acid transport in Lowe's syndrome. Am J Dis Child 1969; *117*:93–95.

272. Morikawa T, Tada K, Ando T, et al. Prolinuria: deficient intestinal absorption of amino acids and proline. J Exp Med 1966; *90*:105–116.

273. Dobbins WO. Whipple's disease: an historical perspective. Q J Med 1985; *221*:523–531.

274. Paulley JW. A case of Whipple's disease (intestinal lipodystrophy). Gastroenterology 1952; *22*:128–133.

275. Whipple GH. A hitherto undescribed disease characterised anatomically by deposits of fat and fatty acid in the intestinal and mesenteric lymphatic tissue. Bull Johns Hopkins Hosp 1907; *18*:382–391.

276. Comer TM, Brandt LJ, Abissi CJ. Whipple's disease: a review. Am J Gastroenterol 1983; *78*:107–114.

277. Maizel H, Ruffin JM, Jobbins WO. Whipple's disease. A review of nineteen patients from one hospital and a review of the literature since 1950. Medicine 1970; *49*:175–205.

278. Crane S, Schlippert W. Duodenoscopic findings in Whipple's disease. Gastrointest Endosc 1978; *24*:248–249.

279. Riemann JF, Rosch W. Synopsis of endoscopic and related morphological findings in Whipple's disease. Endoscopy 1978; *10*:98–103.

280. Enzinger FM, Helwig BB. Whipple's disease: a review of the literature and report of fifteen patients. Virchows Archiv (Pathol) 1963; *336*:238–269.

281. Brice RS, Owen EE, Tyor NP. Amino acid uptake and fatty acid esterification by intestinal mucosa from patients with Whipple's disease and non-tropical sprue. Gastroenterology 1965; *48*:584–592.

282. Laster L, Waldmann TA, Fenster F, et al. Albumin metabolism in patients with Whipple's disease. J Clin Invest 1966; *45*:637–644.

283. Bayless TM. Whipple's disease: newer concepts of therapy. Adv Intern Med 1970; *16*:171–189.

284. Keinath RD, Merrell DE, Vlietstra R, et al. Antibiotic treatment and relapse in Whipple's disease. Gastroenterology 1985; *88*:1867–1873.

285. Pomerantz M, Waldmann TA. Systemic lymphatic abnormalities associated with gastrointestinal protein loss secondary to intestinal lymphangiectasia. Gastroenterology 1963; *45*:703–711.

286. Waldmann, TA, Steinfield JL, Dutcher TF, et al. The role of the gastrointestinal system in idiopathic hypoproteinemia. Gastroenterology 1961; *41*:197–207.

287. Mistilis SP, Skyring AP, Stephen DD. Intestinal lymphangiectasia. Mechanisms of enteric loss of plasma protein and fat. Lancet 1965; *1*:77–89.

288. Waldmann TA. Protein-losing enteropathy. Gastroenterology 1966; *50*:422–443.

289. Jeffries GH, Chapman A, Sleisenger MH. Low fat diet in intestinal lymphangiectasia. Its effect on albumin metabolism. N Engl J Med 1964; *270*:761–766.

290. Holt P. Dietary treatment of protein loss in intestinal lymphangiectasia. Pediatrics 1964; *34*:629–635.

291. Simmonds WJ. The effect of fluid, electrolyte and food intake on thoracic duct lymph flow in unanaesthetised rats. Aust J Exp Biol Med Sci 1954; *32*:285–291.

292. Isselbacher KJ, Scheig R, Plotkin GR, et al. Congenital beta lipoprotein deficiency, hereditary disorder involving a defect in the absorption and transport of lipids. Medicine 1964; *43*:347–363.

293. Bassen FA, Kornzweig AL. Malformation of the erythrocytes in a case of atypical retinitis pigmentosa. Blood 1950; *5*:381–387.

294. Van Buchen FSP, Pol G, Degier J, et al. Congenital beta-lipoprotein deficiency. Am J Med 1966; *40*:794–804.

295. Scott BB, Miller JP, Losowsky MS. Hypolipoproteinemia: A variant of the Bassen-Kornzweig syndrome. Gut 1979; *20*:163–168.

296. Morgenstern L. Radiation enteropathy. *In* Bouchier IAD, Allan RN, Hodgson HJF, et al. (eds). Textbook of Gastroenterology. London, Balliere Tindall, 1984.

297. Kinsella TJ, Bloomer WD. Tolerance of the intestine to radiation therapy. Surg Gynecol Obstet 1980; *151*:273–284.

298. Reeves RJ, Sanders AP, Isley JK, et al. Fat absorption from the gastrointestinal tract in patients undergoing radiation therapy. Radiology 1959; *73*:398–401.

299. Tankle HI, Clark DH, Lee FD. Radiation enteritis with malabsorption. Gut 1965; *6*:560–569.

300. Smith AN, Douglas N, McLean N, et al. Intestinal complications of pelvic irradiation for gynecologic cancer. Surg Gynecol Obstet 1968; *127*:721–728.

301. Haddad H, Bounous G, Tahan WT, et al. Long-term nutrition with an elemental diet following intensive abdominal irradiation. Dis Colon Rectum 1974; *17*:373–379.

302. Mehta HC, Saini AS, Singh H, et al. Biochemical aspects of malabsorption in marasmus. Br J Nutr 1984; *51*:1–6.

303. James WPT. Comparison of three methods used in assessment of carbohydrate absorption in malnourished children. Arch Dis Child 1972; *47*:531–536.

304. Stanfield JP, Hutt MSR, Tunnicliffe K. Intestinal biopsy in kwashiorkor. Lancet 1965; *2*:519–523.

305. Barbezat GO, Bouie MD, Kaschula ROC, et al. Studies on the small intestinal mucosa of children with protein-calorie malnutrition. S Afr Med J 1967; *41*:1031–1036.

306. Gracey M, Suharjono MD, Sunoto MD, et al. Microbial contamination of the gut: another feature of malnutrition. Am J Clin Ntur 1973; *26*:1170–1174.

307. James WPT. Jejunal disaccharidase activities in children with marasmus and kwashiorkor: response to treatment. Arch Dis Child 1971; *46*:218–220.

308. Prinslow JG, Wittman WW, Pretorius PJ, et al. Effects of different sugars on diarrhoea of acute kwashiorkor. Arch Dis Child 1969; *44*:593–599.

309. Tandon BN, Banks DA, George PK, et al. Recovery of exocrine pancreatic function in adult protein-calorie malnutrition. Gastroenterology 1970; *58*:358–362.

17

DISEASES OF THE COLON

DAVID J.A. JENKINS

The major colonic disorders include constipation, irritable bowel syndrome, diverticular disease, inflammatory bowel disease (ulcerative colitis and Crohn's disease), and colonic cancer. Apart from trials of total parenteral nutrition (TPN)[1] to allow bowel rest during acute attacks of Crohn's disease (see Chapter 15), little specific nutritional research has been undertaken to define a role for nutritional treatment in the acute phase of any of the colonic disorders. However, in regard to long-term management the situation is very different. During the last two decades there has been considerable interest in the relationship of nutrition to the etiology of colonic disease and the role of nutritional modification in prophylaxis and treatment. Much of this attention has focused on dietary fiber, and with it has come a great deal of activity devoted to investigating hitherto largely neglected areas of colonic function of possible relevance to disease.

This chapter discusses long-term dietary management strategies for colonic disease in the context of the dietary fiber hypothesis, with special reference to the physiological data that have been adduced by studies of fiber and related issues.

NUTRITIONAL FUNCTIONS OF THE COLON

Nutrients entering the colon include fat, protein, carbohydrate (starch and sugars), water, and minerals. Mean figures derived from ileostomate studies are shown in Table 17–1. Also, depending on the

TABLE 17–1. 24-Hour Ileostomy Outputs (Grams)*

Wet weight	363–507
Dry weight	32–41
Fat	1.0–2.2
Protein	5.6–12.5
Carbohydrate (starch and sugars)	11.8–(25)*
Ash	5.3–6.6

From studies in the literature of patients whose colectomy followed ulcerative colitis rather than Crohn's disease.[85,86]
*Estimated.

diet, quantities of additional carbohydrate in the form of dietary fiber will pass through the ileocecal valve. The amounts may vary from 20 g on a typical Western diet to 40 to 50 g among vegetarian subgroups of the population and to over 100 g/day among more primitive tropical societies.

However, the surprising aspect of this is the magnitude of the starch and sugar losses to the colon. The figures shown in Table 17–1 refer to ileostomates. Nevertheless studies in healthy volunteers, in which carbohydrate losses have been assessed by breath H_2 measurement, have indicated that perhaps between 10 and 20 per cent of the starch in bread was not absorbed, possibly owing to a protein-starch interaction,[22] since such incomplete starch absorption was not seen with gluten-free bread. Subsequent studies have confirmed these findings. Stephen and associates,[23] using normal subjects intubated to the cecum with a triple lumen tube, demonstrated that between 2 and 20 per cent of the meal carbohydrate (approximately three fourths as starch) entered the cecum. At the same time further studies in ileostomates indicated 7 per cent available carbohydrate losses after wholemeal bread and as much as 18 per cent losses after cooked split red lentils.[24] These results agreed with indirect assessments made in normal volunteers using breath H_2 measurement.[24] Since the fiber content of red lentils is only 11 per cent, the starch losses may have constituted a substantial proportion of the total carbohydrate entering the colon.

The picture that is emerging is one in which potentially large amounts of fermentable carbohydrate substrates may be presented to the colon. Carbohydrate foods may therefore be major determinants of colonic function and metabolism and result in colonic retrieval of calories not absorbed in the small intestine.

Thus the major variables in terms of dietary residue arriving in the colon are the carbohydrate components (fiber, starch, and sugars), the amounts of protein and fat entering the colon being relatively small over a wide range of dietary intakes. Carbohydrate components form the major substrates for colonic bacterial fermentation. If unfermented they may continue to trap water and also result in the elimination of bound minerals. This is of great importance, since entering the colon are substantial quantities of water, electrolytes, minerals (e.g., Ca^{++} and Mg^{++}), and bile acids.

It has been suggested that daily the colon absorbs as much as 1350 to 1700 ml water, 175 to 215 mEq Na^+, and 115 to 155 mEq Cl^- and secretes 4 to 8 mEq K^+ and 60 mEq HCO_3^-. Dietary constituents such as fiber acting directly, or through bile acid sequestration, may influence these functions of the colon. In addition the colon has the ability to absorb metal ions such as Ca^{++} and Mg^{++}. In the pig, whose digestive tract is said to resemble man's physiologically, the colon plays a major role in mineral ab-

sorption. Again the fermentability of the carbohydrate substrate will determine how available these nutrients are.

Fiber and the carbohydrate modality of the diet thus play a major role in determining the physiological and metabolic state of the colon. It is because of this that manipulation of fiber intakes has become a theme that provides the basis for many of the newer therapeutic measures proposed for the treatment of colonic disease.

DIETARY FIBER

Dietary fiber has been defined as the plant polysaccharides and lignin that are resistant to the digestive enzymes of man, although they may be degraded to varying extents by colonic bacterial enzymes. Regrettably only crude fiber (cellulose and lignin) content is available in most commonly used food tables.

Historical Overview

Interest in dietary fiber in terms of research and clinical application is largely attributable to the observations and the hypothesis evolved by Denis Burkitt and Hugh Trowell.[2] Both practiced for many years following World War II as surgeon and physician, respectively, at Makareree University in Kampala, Uganda, before returning to Britain. They noted differences that existed in the pattern and nature of diseases affecting the affluent West as opposed to more primitive communities. They were especially impressed with differences in diet and bowel habit. In Uganda much bulky vegetable material was consumed, and constipation was unknown. Their attention therefore focused on the unabsorbable material in the diet, which they recognized as dietary fiber. They concluded that this not only was responsible for the increase in fecal bulk but was directly or indirectly related to the different pattern of diseases seen.[2]

Dietary Fiber Hypothesis

As a result Burkitt and Trowell formulated their "fiber hypothesis." They suggested that the consumption of unrefined, high-fiber carbohydrate foods protected against many Western ailments including colonic cancer, diverticular disease, appendicitis, constipation, hemorrhoids, hiatus hernia, varicose veins, diabetes, heart disease, gallstones, and obesity.[2] As they stood, these claims appeared too extensive to be realistic. Detractors suggested that the incidence of these diseases was related as well to availability of food, patterns of exercise, the motor car, television, and those variables that divide the more from the less developed communities throughout the world. Fecal bulk, on the other hand, might be related also to infections of the gastrointestinal tract, which are seen in more primitive societies where the availability of clean water is a problem. However, with the passage of time, basic laboratory data and clinical evidence have been gathered to support much of the original hypothesis. The hypothesis has had its greatest impact upon management of constipation,[3,4] diverticular disease,[5,6] diabetes,[7–13] hyperlipidemia,[14–15] and, to some extent, obesity.[18] In addition, evidence has been adduced to suggest a use for high-fiber diets in the treatment of Crohn's disease,[19] gallstones,[20] and peptic ulcers.[21]

Nevertheless in view of the many nutritional differences that exist between Western and less developed communities, the exact importance of dietary fiber per se will be debated for some time to come. It may be that in the long term the greatest value of this hypothesis will be in increasing awareness of the possible differences among foods, their degree of processing, the form in which they are eaten, and the contents of their other non- or antinutrient components. All these factors may influence digestibility and gastrointestinal function.

Physiological Effects of Fiber

Many effects of fiber have been described that have relevance to colonic function, but the action of the fiber will depend on the nature of the fiber (Table 17–2) and the food source. Fibers can be divided broadly into the categories of "soluble" and "insoluble." Thus pectin and the gums would be considered soluble, while the fiber in wheat bran is largely insoluble because it is composed to a considerable extent of cellulose and pentosan polysaccharides rendered insoluble by their combination with lignin.

In practice different foods contain characteristically different proportions of soluble and insoluble fiber sources.

The insoluble fibers such as wheat bran are relatively resistant to degradation along the length of the gastrointestinal tract. However, bran contributes to fecal bulk and in the presence of phytates, which are also found in association with fiber, may enhance losses of metal ions. At the other extreme water-soluble fibers such as the gums are largely fermented in the colon to short-chain fatty acids, contribute little to fecal bulk, and have much less impact on mineral balance. Furthermore, the presence of fiber in a food (as opposed to addition of fiber to a meal) may alter the absorption of the other major nutrient components (fat, protein, and starch).

NUTRITIONAL THERAPY OF SPECIFIC DISEASES

Constipation

The laxative effect of whole-meal bread was noted in the writings of Hippocrates. The pioneer studies were carried out in the 1930's[25] and 1940's.[26] However, the use of fiber preparations as laxatives remained a relatively underexplored area until further interest was stimulated by the formulation of the fiber hypothesis. It is now well recognized that certain types of fiber have a marked laxative effect, increase stool weight, enhance the output of fecal water and electrolytes, and reduce transit time. In general, much simple constipation can be helped by increasing the fiber content of the diet, especially by the use of whole-meal or whole-wheat products (bread, biscuits, breakfast cereals) that are high in cereal fiber.

TABLE 17–2. *Physicochemical, Physiological, and Clinical Aspects of Fiber*

Physicochemical Property	Type of Fiber	Physiological Effect	Clinical Implication
Viscosity			
Particle formation and water-holding capacity	Insoluble complexes, e.g., wheat bran, high pentosan polysaccharide + lignin mixtures	↑ Gastric emptying ↓ Mouth to cecum transit ↓ Total GI transit time ↓ Colonic intraluminal pressure ↑ Fecal bulk	↓ Constipation ↓ Diverticular disease Dilute potential carcinogens
Cation exchange	Acid polysaccharides (e.g., pectins)	↑ Small intestinal losses of minerals (±), trace elements (±), heavy metals	Negative mineral balance, probably compensated for by colonic salvage, after fermentation of fiber Antitoxic effect
Antioxidant	Lignin (reducing phenolic groups)	↓ Free radicals in digestive tract	Anticarcinogenesis(?)
Degradability (colonic bacteria)	Polysaccharides (especially pectin, gums, and mucilages)	↑ Gas and SCFA production ↓ Cecal pH	Flatus, energy production

Modified from Eastwood and Kay[83] and Kay and Strasberg.[84]

Of the commonly available fiber sources, wheat bran remains the fiber of choice for the treatment of constipation through its ability to increase fecal bulk and reduce transit time[2,3] more than other commonly available food products. In addition pharmaceutical preparations of psyllium husk (Metamucil) and ispaghula (Isogel) are in common use. Owing to differences in physiochemical properties, studies using purified fiber have demonstrated large differences in the fecal bulking ability of different fibers.[2,3,27–30] Their lignin-pentosan content may be an important determinant,[27] and the importance of particle size has been emphasized.[29,30] Bran of coarse particle size was shown to be more effective than fine bran. Fibers that are largely metabolized in the colon, such as the pectins, contribute little to fecal output.[26,27] In this respect fine bran is more metabolized than coarse bran.[32] A further reason for the deficient fecal bulking effect of finely divided bran may relate to its reduced ability to trap water.[33] Other fiber sources, such as cabbage fiber, although metabolized by the colonic bacteria, contribute to fecal bulk by increasing bacterial mass in the stool. Thus fiber may be metabolized and therefore have little effect on fecal bulk, or be relatively unmetabolized and increase fecal bulk through trapping water and electrolytes, or may increase fecal bulk though increasing bacterial mass.

In most instances current treatment of constipation therefore includes advice to increase fiber consumption from a range of foods, possibly with the additional use of bulk laxatives.

Devroede has recommended a dietary trial in which a crude fiber intake of 14.4 g daily is the goal.[34] This would be considerably higher in terms of dietary fiber content, but with the exception of McCance and Widdowson's tables,[35] dietary fiber values (which include the noncellulosic polysaccharides) are not generally available.[7] The advice of Bockus[36] complements this, emphasizing that individualization is required in a dietary prescription the principles of which are "ample fluid, sufficient fiber and enough laxative foods."

Concern has been expressed that the most obstinate types of nonspastic constipation may be associated with colonic irritability induced by laxative abuse and enemas.[36] In this situation a bland diet with a hydrophilic colloid such as Metamucil (psyllium husk) has been advised.[36]

The emphasis, therefore, has been on the use of fiber both in the diet (food fiber) and supplements (vegetable mucilloids) in the management of simple constipation. A wide range of vegetable mucilloids or vegetable gums have been used including agar, gum arabic, acacia, tragacanth, and sterculia. In addition modified dietary fibers or cellulose products have been developed for the treatment of constipation (and induction of satiety) including methylcellulose, carboxymethyl cellulose, and ethylhydroxyethyl cellulose.

In practical terms, if food is to be used to relieve constipation, a change from white to whole-meal products may prove useful, and additional bran may be taken in high-fiber breakfast cereals. If further bran is required, this may be sprinkled over breakfast cereals or mixed with yogurt or mashed banana. The dose should be increased gradually, one dessert spoonful at a time, since abdominal distention and flatulence may make the treatment unacceptable. A large intake of bran may also give rise to pruritus ani. This is likely to be due to the abrasive nature of the coarse bran particles. The problem may be relieved by dilution of the bran through consumption of additional fiber sources such as cabbage, which leads to an increase in fecal bulk that is largely bacterial in origin,[27,37] or by the addition of legumes to the diet as a source of nonparticulate fiber. In the case of patients with celiac disease rice bran is an acceptable source of fiber, although its fecal bulking effect is less pronounced.

Irritable Bowel

Fiber has been advocated for the treatment of the irritable bowel syndrome. Both success[38] and failure[39] have been reported. Other factors independent of fiber intake are obviously involved, and it is perhaps not surprising that total fiber intakes in women diagnosed as suffering from irritable bowel have been reported as similar to those in controls.[40] Despite this, vegetable fiber intake (as opposed to fruit and cereal) was reported as significantly lower,[40] and an early study by Fantus[41] demonstrated that addition of bran to the diet reduced mucus production. It therefore seems reasonable to continue to place patients with irritable bowel syndrome on a trial of high cereal fiber intake.

In the irritable bowel, especially when dominated by constipation, use of fiber in the form of hydrophilic mucilloids has been recommended.[34] As with pain in diverticular disease, there is a suggestion that the increased bulk induced by fiber may reduce intraluminal pressures within the colon.[38] Although not all studies have yielded convincing results, a controlled study of 26 patients supplemented with 20 g of wheat bran daily (either as bran or as 170 g [four slices] of whole-meal bread, or as a combination to make 20 g of bran) demonstrated some improvement in symptoms and reduced colonic motor activity.[38]

On the other hand, where diarrhea proves a problem it has been shown that as well as accelerating slow transit bran may also decelerate rapid transit.[42,43] In addition in this situation kaolin and pectin have been recommended in mild cases, and diphenoxylate (Lomotil) in the more severe.[44] The use of the purified fiber pectin here is of interest in emphasizing the differences among different sources. With pectin, a fiber metabolized in the colon, fecal bulk is not increased and its addition to the diet may be constipatory.

Diverticular Disease

Until relatively recently diverticular disease was treated in the long term by low-residue diets in order to "rest" the bowel.[45] The use of high-fiber diets of the type used in the treatment of constipation and the irritable bowel in the outpatient management of diverticular disease therefore represents a dramatic reversal of the established clinical practice.

In 1971 Painter and Burkitt[46] published their hypothesis linking reduced fiber consumption in the West with the increased incidence of diverticular disease. It was suggested that fiber, by maintaining intraluminal bulk, reduced the development of high intracolonic pressures. Hence it prevented the production of diverticula produced by mucosal evagination along the track of blood vessels piercing the bowel's muscular coat.[47] As Almy noted[48] the law of Laplace may apply to the bowel: tension in the wall (t) must be greater to exert a given pressure (p) when the radius of the bowel (r) is large: $p = t/r$.

In the absence of infection and diverticulitis, it was suggested, much of the pain experienced in diverticulosis originates from the raised intraluminal pressures.

The association of dietary fiber deficiency in the etiology of diverticular disease has been criticized. Epidemiological studies in Africa suggesting a protective role for dietary fiber were followed by studies in Greece that appeared to refute the relationship between fiber intake and the incidence of diverticular disease.[49] However, only cellulosic intake was assessed in the Greek studies, and this is unlikely to give a meaningful picture of fiber consumption.[50] In addition, the population with a low incidence of diverticular disease (rural) had higher fecal weights and faster transit times than the population with a higher incidence (urban, Western diet), suggesting that true dietary fiber intakes may well have been different.[50] Subsequently Brodribb and Humphreys[51] demonstrated that the fiber intake of 40 British patients with symptomatic disease was half that of matched controls, and similar results have been obtained using vegetarian groups.[52] Most recently further reports from Japan suggest that a reduction in fiber intake in the population relates well to the increasing incidence of diverticular disease.[53] Such changes may possibly also be explained by other dietary changes such as the increase in fat and protein in the diet.[54]

Nevertheless over the last decade there has been a general change from the low-fiber diets once advocated in the management of diverticular disease[55] to therapeutic trials of high-fiber diets. This has been the result of the importance placed on colonic volume in the hypothesized mechanisms for the generation of diverticula, the implication of fiber in the epidemiology, and to a lesser extent the findings of clinical trials.

One of the first trials was that of Painter and colleagues,[6] in which a high-fiber, low-sugar diet with enough bran to ensure defecation at least once daily showed 88 per cent improvement of symptoms over 22 months of follow-up. Others have shown similar results.[51,56-61]

The first double-blind controlled trial also indicated a reduction in pain score, although other symptoms (nausea, vomiting, heartburn, eructation, and abdominal distention) or bowel function scores (excessive flatulence and defecation-related problems) were not significantly different.[62]

More recently the use of fiber has been questioned as a result of a trial involving bran, ispaghula, and placebo in which just over 4.5 or 6.5 g of dietary fiber was added to the diets of patients with symptomatically mild diverticular disease. No significant improvement in symptoms was observed over a 4-month period despite a 15 to 30 per cent increase in fecal weight.[63]

In both of these controlled studies the increase in fecal weight was relatively small, and for consistency larger fiber intakes may be required. In addition it is possible that in the second study the relatively milder symptoms and absence of pain as a dominant feature may be reasons why a significant change was not seen. Flatulence and abdominal distention from the fiber itself may also have produced some of the milder symptoms in the treatment group. However, such studies caution that future advice may focus on other types of fiber, in addition to wheat bran, and possibly other dietary modifications (e.g., in terms of fat or protein).

Nevertheless Smith and colleagues[64] in a prospective trial demonstrated that 5 years after sigmoid myotomy only patients who had been placed on bran maintained their reduced mean motility indices. Many other studies have also indicated reduction in segmenting pressures upon fiber supplementation.[51,59-61] In view of our understanding of pain and the proposed etiology of the diverticula in diverticular disease, there appears good reason to recommend high-fiber diets in the management of diverticulosis of the sort advocated in the treatment of constipation and the irritable bowel.

Crohn's Disease

In exacerbations of both ulcerative colitis and Crohn's disease, bland low-residue diets are advised. In ulcerative colitis, in which depressed lactose levels may exist, an attempt is often made to reduce further the fermentable carbohydrate substrates entering the colon by use of milk elimination or low-lactose diets. In Crohn's disease the presence of strictures would appear to be a logical contraindication to the use of high-fiber diets for fear of causing obstruction, and in the acute phase complete bowel rest has been advocated.

There is evidence that in the acute phase both TPN and elemental diets have a significant beneficial impact on the disease process. However, elemental diets are not palatable and their tonicity may limit their tolerance in some patients owing to gastrointestinal hurry, bloating, and diarrhea. For this reason there is now interest in low-residue enteral supplements to treat the chronic malnutrition common in inflammatory bowel disease. A number of studies have indicated success.[65,66] In one, Ensure Plus (Abbott Laboratories; protein 15.2 per cent, fat 33 per cent, carbohydrate 51.8 per cent) was used with a low-residue diet to increase calories to approximately 3000/day. This resulted in increases in serum proteins and circulating T cells and a reduction in serum orosomucoid levels.[65] Although not so impressive, use of a lower-protein supplement (Precision, Wander; protein 10 per cent, lipid 0.8 per cent and carbohydrate 81 per cent) was better tolerated.[66] The initial beneficial effects in terms of the disease process were not maintained with time.

The long-term dietary management of Crohn's disease is therefore still open to debate. Nevertheless it has been reported that, as with diverticular disease, patients with Crohn's disease also consumed less fiber and more sugar prior to diagnosis than did controls.[67,68] Such retrospective evidence prompted a prospective trial of dietary modification including a reduction in sugar intake and an increase in fiber consumption in Crohn's disease patients. No fiber supplements were advocated, but fiber intake was increased by the use of whole-grain foods and increased fruit and vegetable consumption. White flour products were eliminated and sugar intake reduced. Over a 5-year period the test group required one fifth the time in hospital of the control group and was subjected to fewer operations.[19] The trial was undertaken irrespective of the presence of strictures, although, as stated earlier, these would seem an obvious contraindication. The apparent success of this trial suggested that the role of fiber in the outpatient management of Crohn's disease warranted further attention. Unfortunately more recent studies have failed to show clear-cut evidence of benefit.[68a]

Colonic Cancer

There are many associations linking colonic cancer with diet, and many theories have been advanced to explain these. Diets high in fat and protein and low in fiber are found in those populations in which the incidence of colonic cancer is highest.[69,70] Dietary fat, it has been suggested, acts either directly by the toxic effect of unabsorbed long-chain fatty acids or by enhancing colonic bile acid losses. Fecal bile acid concentrations are highest in populations with the greatest risk of colonic cancer[72] and may act directly on the colonic mucosa or after bacterial degradation to promote neoplastic change.

The reason for the association with protein may also be secondary to the bacterial metabolism of protein within the lumen of the colon with the production of volatile derivatives of amino acids, nitrosamines, or ammonia. Ammonia has been proposed as a promoter of tumor growth. It has been suggested that with increased protein intake colonic bacterial production of volatile phenols and ammonia will increase to fulfill this role.[74,75]

Despite the fact that epidemiological associations are not as strong for fiber as for fat and protein, many more hypotheses have been put forward to suggest a rationale for a protective role of fiber in relation to colonic cancer. In fact most of the properties of fiber have been ascribed a function in this respect. These include the ability of fiber to increase fecal bulk, reduce gastrointestinal transit time, trap or bind materials within the bowel lumen, lower colonic pH, and provide substrates for colonic mucosa and for bacterial cell growth.

The ability of fiber to increase fecal bulk has resulted in the suggestion that fiber may dilute potential carcinogens in the colon. Where careful measurements have been made between increased fecal bulk and freedom from colonic cancer,[76] this relationship holds true. More recently comparisons made in four Scandinavian populations with a threefold to fourfold difference in risk of colonic cancer showed a significant negative relationship between fecal weight and incidence of colonic cancer.[76] The dietary data on fiber intake supported the physiological measurements.[76] In this same study it was of interest that no relationship was seen with gastrointestinal transit time despite the hypothesis that the more rapid the transit time the less time was available for the bacterial production of potential carcinogens. A similar lack of differences was seen between the Japanese in Hawaii and the inhabitants of Japan,[77] although the Japanese in Hawaii are more prone to colonic cancer. Part of the reason for this lack of differences may lie in the fact that at fecal outputs of more than 140 g/day the significant relationship between fecal weight and transit time no longer exists.

Fiber and other nonabsorbed carbohydrate sources, on being metabolized by bacteria to short chain fatty acids reduce colonic pH.[78,79] This in turn may limit uptake of ammonia by epithelial cells.[80,81] Low pH may also reduce alpha-dehydroxylation of bile acids to potential carcinogens.[82]

In addition the provision of energy in the form of fermentable carbohydrate may promote bacterial growth and so result in the lowering of possible toxic compounds in the colon either through their metabolism to nontoxic forms or through their uptake for bacterial synthetic purposes (e.g., incorporation of ammonia into bacterial protein).

All these considerations remain as speculation in relation to carcinogenesis in the human colon. They may be relevant to long-term dietary counseling of the patients from whom adenomatous polyps have been removed. Currently the advice would include an increase in fiber and unrefined carbohydrates in the diet and a reduction in fat and perhaps protein. For the present we must await the results of the prospective trials of such diets currently being undertaken in postpolypectomy patients.

References

1. Muller JM, Keller HW, Erosini A, et al. TPN as the sole therapy for Crohn's disease—a prospective study. Br J Surg 1983; 70:40–43.
2. Trowell HC, Burkitt DP. Concluding considerations. *In* Burkitt DP, Trowell HC (eds). Refined Carbohydrate Foods and Disease. Some Implications of Dietary Fibre. London, Academic Press, 1975: 333–345.
3. Eastwood MA, Kirkpatrick JR, Mitchell WD, et al. Effects of dietary supplements of wheat bran and cellulose on faeces and bowel function. Br Med J 1973; 4:392–394.
4. Cummings JH, Hill MJ, Jenkins DJA, et al. Changes in fecal composition and colonic function due to cereal fiber. Am J Clin Nutr 1976; 29:1468–1473.
5. Brodribb AJM, Humphreys DM. Diverticular disease: Three studies. Part III. Metabolic effect of bran in patients with diverticular disease. Br Med J 1976; 1:428–430.
6. Painter NS, Almeida AZ, Colebourne KW. Unprocessed bran in treatment of diverticular disease of the colon. Br Med J 1972; 1:137–140.
7. Anderson JW, Ward K. High-carbohydrate, high-fiber diets for insulin-treated men with diabetes mellitus. Am J Clin Nutr 1979; 32:2312–2321.
9. Dori K, Matsuura M, Kawara A, et al. Treatment of diabetes with glucomanan (Konjac mannan). Lancet 1979; 1:978–988.
10. Jenkins DJA, Leeds AR, Gassull MA, et al. Unabsorbable carbohydrates and diabetes: decreased post-prandial hyperglycaemia. Lancet 1976; 2:172–174.
11. Jenkins DJA, Wolever TMS, Nineham R, et al. Guar crispbread in the diabetic diet. Br Med J 1978; 2:1744–1746.
12. Jenkins DJA, Wolever TMS, Taylor RH, et al. Diabetic glucose control, lipids, and trace elements on long term guar. Brit Med J 1980; 1:1353–1354.
13. Kiehm TG, Anderson JW, Ward K. Beneficial effects of a high carbohydrate, high fiber diet in hyperglycemic diabetic men. Am J Clin Nutr 1976; 29:895–899.
14. Kritchevsky D. Fiber, lipids, and atherosclerosis. Am J Clin Nutr 1978; 31:S65–S74.
15. Miettinen TA, Tarpila S. Effect of pectin on serum cholesterol, fecal bile acids and biliary lipids in normolipidemic and hyperlipidemic individuals. Clin Chim Acta 1977; 79:471–477
16. Jenkins DJA, Reynolds D, Slavin B, et al. Dietary fiber and blood lipids: treatment of hypercholesterolemia with guar crispbread. Am J Clin Nutr 1980; 33:575–581.
17. Thiffault C, Bélanger M, Pouliot M. Traitement de l'hyperlipoprotéinémie essentielle de type II par un nouvel agent thérapeutique, la celluline. Can Med Assoc J 1970; 103:165–166.
18. Van Itallie TB. Dietary fiber and obesity. Am J Clin Nutr 1978; 31:S43–S52.
19. Heaton KW, Thornton JR, Emmett PM. Treatment of Crohn's disease with an unrefined carbohydrate, fibre-rich diet. Br Med J 1979; 2:764–766.
20. Pomare EW, Heaton KW, Low-Beer TS, et al.: The effect of wheat bran upon bile salt metabolism and upon the lipid composition of bile in gallstone patients. Am J Dig Dis 1976; 21:521–525.
21. Malhotra SL. A comparison of unrefined wheat and rice diets in the management of duodenal ulcer. Postgrad Med J 1978; 54:6–9.
22. Anderson IH, Levine AS, Levitt MD. Incomplete absorption of the carbohydrate in all-purpose wheat flour. N Engl J Med 1981; 304:891–892.
23. Stephen AM, Haddad AC, Phillips SF. Passage of carbohydrate into the colon: direct measurements in humans. Gastroenterology 1983; 85:589–595.
24. Wolever TMS, Thorne MJ, Thompson LU, et al. Digestibility of carbohydrate from bread and lentils using a breath hydrogen technique and a human ileostomy model. Proc Nutr Soc 1984; 43:15A.
25. Williams RD, Olmsted WH. Effect of cellulose, hemicellulose and lignin on weight of stool: contribution to study of laxation in man. J Nutr 1936; 11:433–449.
26. Werch SG, Ivy AC. Study of metabolism of ingested pectin. Am J Dis Child 1941; 62:499–511.
27. Cummings JH, Branch W, Jenkins DJA, et al. Colonic response to dietary fibre from carrot, cabbage, apple bran, and guar gum. Lancet 1978; 1:5–9.
28. Cummings JH, Southgate DAT, Branch WJ, et al. The digestion of pectin in the human gut and its effect on calcium absorption and large bowel function. Br J Nutr 1979; 41:477–485.
29. Brodribb AJM, Groves C. Effect of bran particle size on stool weight. Gut 1978; 19:60–63.
30. Kirwan WO, Smith AN, McConnell AA, et al. Action of different bran preparations on colonic function. Br Med J 1974; 4:187–189.
31. Kay RM, Truswell AS. Effect of citrus pectin on blood lipids and fecal steroid excretion in man. Am J Clin Nutr 1977; 30:171–175.
32. Heller SN, Hackler LR, Rivers JM, et al. Dietary fiber: the effect of particle size of wheat bran on colonic function in young adult men. Am J Clin Nutr 1980; 33:1734–1744.
33. Cummings JH. Consequences of the metabolism of fiber in the human large intestine. *In* Vahouny GV, Kritchevsky D (eds). Dietary Fiber in Health and Diesase. New York, Plenum Press, 1982: 9–21.
34. Devroede G. Constipation: mechanism and managment. *In* Sleisenger MH, Fordtran JS (eds). Gastrointestinal Disease. Philadelphia, WB Saunders, 1978: 368–386.
35. Paul AA, Southgate DAT. McCance and Widdowson's The Composition of Foods. 4th ed. Medical Research Council Special Report Series No. 297. London, HMSO, 1978.
36. Bockus HL. Diarrhea and constipation. Part III. Simple constipation. *In* Bockus HL (ed). Gastroenterology. 3rd ed. Vol II. Philadelphia, WB Saunders, 1976: 936–953.
37. Stephen AM, Cummings JH. Mechanism of action of dietary fibre in the human colon. Nature 1980; 284:283–284.
38. Manning AP, Heaton KW, Harvey RF, et al. Wheat fibre and irritable bowel syndrome. A controlled trial. Lancet 1977; 2:417–418.
39. Soltoft JE, Kray B, Gudman-Hoyer E, et al. A double-blind trial of the effect of wheat bran on symptoms of irritable bowel syndrome. Lancet 1976; 1:270–272.
40. Hillman LC, Stace NH, Fisher A, et al. Dietary intakes and stool characteristics of patients with the irritable bowel syndrome. Am J Clin Nutr 1982; 36:626–629.
41. Fantus B, Wozasek O, Steigman KW. Studies on colon irritation; examination of feces. Am J Dig Dis 1941; 8:296–298.
42. Harvey RF, Pomare EW, Heaton KW. Effects of increased dietary fibre on intestinal transit. Lancet 1973; 1:1278–1280.
43. Payler PK, Pomare EW, Heaton KW, et al. The effect of wheat bran on intestinal transit. Gut 1975; 16:209–213.
44. Haubrich WS. Functional bowel disorders. *In* Bockus HL

(ed). Gastroenterology. 3rd ed. Vol. II. Philadelphia, WB Saunders, 1976: 895–917.

45. Littlewood ER, Ornstein MH, Baird IM, et al. Doubts about diverticular disease. Br. Med J 1981; 283:1524–1526.

46. Painter NS, Burkitt DP. Diverticular disease of the colon: a deficiency disease of Western civilization. Br Med J 1971; 2:450–454.

47. Painter NS. The aetiology of diverticulosis of the colon with special reference to the action of certain drugs on the behaviour of the colon. Ann Roy Coll Surg 1964; 34:98–119.

48. Almy TP. Diverticular disease of the colon—the new look. Gastroenterology 1965; 49:109–112.

49. Manonsos ON, Vrachliotis G, Papaevangelow G, et al. Relations of diverticulosis of the colon to environmental factors in Greece. Am J Dig Dis 1973; 18:174–176.

50. Brodribb AJM. Dietary fiber in diverticular diseases of the colon. In Spiller GA, Kay RM (eds). Medical Aspects of Dietary Fiber. New York, Plenum Medical, 1980: 43–66.

51. Brodribb AJM, Humphreys DM. Diverticular disease: three studies. Part I. Relation to other disorders and fibre intake. Br Med J 1976; 1:424–425.

52. Gera JSS, Ware A, Fursdon P, et al. Symptomless diverticular disease and intake of dietary fibre. Lancet 1979; 1:511–514.

53. Olin G, Minowa K, Oyama T, et al. Changes in dietary fiber intake amongst Japanese in the 20th century: a relationship to the prevalence of diverticular disease. Am J Clin Nutr 1983; 38:115–121.

54. Mendeloff AI. A critique of "fiber deficiency." Am J Dig Dis 1976; 21:109–112.

55. de la Vega JM. Diverticular disease of the colon. In Bockus HC (ed). Gastroenterology. 3rd ed. Vol II. Philadelphia, WB Saunders, 1976: 973–1000.

56. Plumley PE, Francis B. Dietary management of diverticular disease. J Am Diet Assoc 1973; 63:527–530.

57. Hodgson J. Effect of methylcellulose on rectal and colonic pressures in treatment of diverticular disease. Br Med J 1972; 3:729–731.

58. Parks TG. Diet and diverticular disease. Proc R Soc Med 1974; 67:1037–1040.

59. Srivastava GS, Smith AN, Painter NS. Sterculia bulk-forming agent with smooth muscle relaxant versus bran in diverticular disease. Br Med J 1976; 1:315–318.

60. Taylor I, Duthie HL. Bran tablets and diverticular disease. Br Med J 1976, 1:988–990.

61. Tarpila S, Miettinen TA. High fibre diet in patients with diverticulosis (abstract). Scand J Gastroenterol 1975; 10(Suppl 34):27.

62. Brodribb AJM. Treatment of symptomatic diverticular disease with a high-fibre diet. Lancet 1977; 664–666.

63. Ornstein MH, Littlewood ER, Baird IM, et al. Are fibre supplements really necessary in diverticular disease of the colon? A controlled clinical trial. Br Med J 1981; 282:1353–1356.

64. Smith AN, Kirwan WO, Shariff S. Motility effects of operations performed for diverticular disease. Proc Roy Soc Med 1974; 67:1041–1043.

65. Hames AD, Davis V, Heatley RV, et al. Controlled trial of supplemented oral nutrition in Crohn's disease. Lancet 1983; 1:887–90.

66. Brignola C, Lanfranchi GA, Pasquali R, et al. Calorie supplementation and Crohn's disease [letter]. Lancet 1983; 2:47.

67. Kasper H, Somner H. Dietary fiber and nutrient intake in Crohn's disease. Am J Clin Nutr 1979; 32:1898–1901.

68. Thornton JR, Emmett PM, Heaton KW. Diet and Crohn's disease: characteristics of the pre-illness diet. Br Med J 1979; 2:762–764.

68a. Ritchie JK, Wadsworth J, Lennard-Jones JR, et al. Controlled multicentre therapeutic trial of an unrefined carbohydrate, fibre rich diet in Crohn's disease. Br Med J 1987; 295:517–520.

69. Armstrong B, Doll R. Environmental factors and cancer incidence and mortality in different countries, with special reference to dietary practices. Int J Cancer 1975; 15:617–631.

70. Doll R, Peto R. The causes of cancer: quantitative estimates of available risks of cancer in the United States today. J Natl Cancer Inst 1981; 6:1191–1308.

71. Newmark HL, Wargovich MJ, Bruce WR. Colon cancer and dietary fat, phosphate, and calcium: a hypothesis. J Natl Cancer Inst 1984; 72:1323–1325.

72. Hill MJ, Draser BS, Hawksworth G, et al. Bacteria and aetiology of cancer of large bowel. Lancet 1971; 1:95–100.

73. Visek WJ, Clinton SK, Truex CR. Nutrition and experimental carcinogenesis. Cornell Vet 1978; 68:3–39.

74. Bone E, Tamm A, Hill MJ. The production of urinary phenols by gut bacteria and their possible role in the causation of large bowel cancer. Am J Clin Nutr 1976; 29:1448–1454.

75. Cummings JH, Branch WJ, Bjerrum L, et al. Colon cancer and large bowel function and metabolism. II. Bacterial metabolites in feces and urine. Am J Clin Nutr 1979; 32:2094–2101.

76. Cummings JH, Branch WJ, Bjerrum L, et al. Colon cancer and large bowel function in Denmark and Finland. Nutr Cancer 1982; 4:61–66.

77. Glober GA, Klein KL, Moore JO, et al. Bowel transit-times in two populations experiencing similar colon-cancer risks. Lancet 1974; 2:80–81.

78. Walker ARP, Walker BF, Segal I. Faecal pH value and its modification by dietary means in South African black and white schoolchildren. S Afr Med J 1979; 55:495–498.

79. Brown RL, Gibson JA, Sladen EE, et al. Effects of lactulose and other laxatives and ileal and colonic pH as measured by a radiotelemetric device. Gut 1974; 15:999–1004.

80. Down PF, Agnostini L, Murison J, et al. The interrelationships of faecal ammonia, pH and bicarbonate: evidence of colonic absorption of ammonia by non-ionic diffusion. Clin Sci 1972; 43:101–114.

81. Brown RL, Gibson JA, Fenton JC, et al. Ammonia and urea transport by the excluded human colon. Clin Sci Mol Med 1975; 48:279–287.

82. Narisawa T, Magadia NE, Weisburger JH, et al. Promoting effects of bile acids on colon carcinogenesis, after intrarectal instillation of N-methyl-N'-nitro-N-nitrosoguanidine in rats. J Natl Cancer Inst 1974; 53:1093–1097.

83. Eastwood MA, Kay RM. An hypothesis for the action of dietary fiber along the gastrointestinal tract. Am J Clin Nutr 1979; 32:364–367.

84. Kay RM, Strasberg SM. Origin, chemistry, physiological effects and clinical importance of dietary fiber. Clin Invest Med 1978; 1:9–24.

85. Kramer P, Kearney MM, Ingelfinger FJ. The effect of specific foods and water loading on the ileal excreta of ileostomized human subjects. Gastroenterology 1962; 42:535–546.

86. Sandberg AS, Anderson H, Hallgren B, et al. Experimental model for in vivo determination of dietary fibre and its effect on the absorption of nutrients in the small intestine. Br J Nutr 1981; 45:283–294.

18

DISEASES OF THE LIVER AND BILIARY TRACT

SUM P. LEE

The liver is the powerhouse of the body. It contains large numbers and quantities of enzymes involved in the metabolism of carbohydrates, lipids, and proteins. Anatomically, the liver is made up of lobules, the center of each lobule being occupied by a small branch of the hepatic vein. These central veins are fed by blood draining from the periphery of the lobules fed by portal venous blood (approximately 70 per cent of total hepatic blood flow) and blood from the hepatic arteries (approximately 30 per cent of total hepatic blood flow). The tributaries of the portal vein, together with branches of the hepatic artery and the bile ducts, are situated in the peripheral junctions of these lobules and are sometimes referred to as the "portal tract." The liver is the single largest organ in the body and is responsible for some 20 per cent of the body's basal metabolism. It is the first organ to process nutrients absorbed from the digestive tract; for example, it removes approximately 80 per cent of the amino acids from the portal circulation, and more than 90 per cent of ethanol is metabolized here. The liver detoxifies both endogenous and exogenous toxic substances, and conversely it may convert some nontoxic substances into toxic metabolites. In addition, the liver synthesizes a number of important plasma proteins and also secretes bile through the bile ducts into the duodenum, where bile salts play a major role in the digestion and absorption of fat and soluble vitamins.

The liver therefore has continuous interactions with not only exogenous and endogenous protein, carbohydrate, and fat but also with various hormones, vitamins, and trace minerals, and imbalance in the nutritional input will affect the integrity of the organ. Conversely, the disordered organ will also have major impact on the nutritional profile of the host.

NUTRITIONAL FACTORS IN THE PATHOGENESIS OF LIVER DISEASES

Alcoholic Liver Disease

Alcohol is the most commonly abused substance in Western communities. The evidence incriminating ethanol as a cause of liver disease is overwhelming, and the enormity of the cost associated with alcoholic cirrhosis of the liver is well recognized.[1] Ethanol may affect the nutritional profile of the host in diverse ways, and these depend in part on the many levels at which alcohol and nutrition interact. It can directly alter the level of intake of nutrients through a displacement of other food nutrients and a decrease in appetite (empty calories) or by causing injury to every aspect of the gastrointestinal tract. Within the digestive system, the most important target organ is the liver. It has been said that "alcohol licks the gut, but bites the liver." Cirrhosis of the liver is the third most common cause of death due to disease during the most productive years of American males.

The normal human liver can metabolize 80 to 100 g of ethanol per day in man, and considerably less (30 to 60 g) in women. It takes a great deal of alcohol, such as daily consumption of more than 150 g for more than 8 years, to result in cirrhosis of the liver. There is a gradation of abnormalities with their associated morbidity and mortality. The earliest form of alcoholic liver disease is a "fatty liver" or asymptomatic alcoholic hepatitis. Fatty infiltration of the liver is histologically reversible, if abstinence from alcohol can be achieved, and therefore the prognosis at this stage of the disease is good. As the severity of the disease progresses, it produces a spectrum of alcoholic hepatitis, characterized histologically by liver cell necrosis, increase in fibrous tissue formation, appearance of Mallory bodies, and pericellular and subsinusoidal fibrosis, with leukocytic inflammatory reaction in the perivenular zone. The disease at this stage is still reversible, requiring varying periods for recovery. With continuing damage, the end result is a scarred liver with disruption in architecture and nodular formation. Even with cirrhosis of the liver, prognosis may be greatly improved by abstinence, and hence every effort should be made to stop drinking of alcohol. The liver with advanced alcoholic cirrhosis does not revert to normal, and the patient may die of complications of cirrhosis. The clinical aspects of alcoholic liver disease have been reviewed by Fallon.[2]

While previous studies have suggested that malnutrition may be a common and predominant factor in the production of alcoholic liver diseases, more recent studies have shown that ethanol itself has a direct toxic effect on hepatocytes and can induce cell necrosis with fibrosis even in the presence of adequate nutritional intakes.[3] For example, in baboons, isocaloric replacement with ethanol in the presence of a normal diet induced a spectrum of hepatic changes indistinguishable from human alcoholic diseases.[4] There are also other epidemiological studies that have failed to demonstrate a relationship between malnutrition and the development and progression of liver diseases.[5,6]

Apart from producing abnormalities in the liver, ethanol also interferes with metabolism of other nutrients through its effect on hepatic function. This aspect is summarized in Chapter 23.

Nonalcoholic Fatty Liver Disease

Fatty liver may result from other causes than an excessive consumption of alcohol. For example, it can be induced with an excessive caloric intake, and is often associated with obesity. It is sometimes seen in pregnancy and in patients receiving corticosteroids, tetracyclines, or total parenteral nutrition (TPN). The fatty liver in obesity and pregnancy is rarely accompanied by any clinical or functional impairment of the liver and improves rapidly with weight reduction or after parturition. In obesity, there are often other variables such as diabetes and alcoholism complicating the picture.[7]

A hepatic lesion resembling alcoholic hepatitis can also occur in nondrinkers, and these individuals are often moderately obese women with mild diabetes.[8,9]

Malnutrition

As mentioned above, although malnutrition has previously been considered important in the production of alcoholic liver cirrhosis, it is now accepted that ethanol itself can exert a toxic action on hepatocytes and can cause all the features of cirrhosis. Nevertheless, nutritional factors do play a contributory role in the induction of liver disease. In animals, experimental diets deficient in choline, various proteins, and vitamins can induce liver cirrhosis. Mice fed a cholesterol-supplemented diet developed fatty liver with increased collagen production.[10] Patients undergoing intestinal bypass surgery for obesity can develop hepatic lesions clinically and histologically indistinguishable from alcoholic liver disease, even without alcohol consumption.[11] This form of liver injury occurs most commonly in those who have lost the greater amount of weight following surgery, suggesting a nutritional element in its pathogenesis. In kwashiorkor, a disease affecting both children and adults (see Chapter 9) in which gross protein malnutrition predominates, there is hepatomegaly with steatosis. However, progression to cirrhosis in the above conditions is rare unless there are other factors involved.

Total Parenteral Nutrition (TPN)

TPN has been a life-saving treatment for a variety of disease conditions in which malnutrition complicates the primary pathological process and is responsible for much of the morbidity and mortality. A spectrum of hepatobiliary disorders has been encountered in patients receiving TPN.

Elevation of serum transaminase and alkaline phosphatase is common,[12] and clinically the liver may be enlarged and mildly tender owing to steatosis. For some as yet unexplained reason, infants seem to be much more susceptible to developing hepatic abnormalities. The spectrum of abnormalities can range from steatosis to cholestasis,[13] to occasional fibrosis[14] and even cirrhosis.[15] In addition, complications of TPN, such as septicemia, often aggravate cholestasis, and opportunistic infections by unusual organisms, including fungi, can cause hepatitis of microbial origin.

Fatty liver, or triglyceride accumulation in the liver, may be observable as early as a few days after commencement of TPN. The cause of this is still unclear. It has been suggested to be caused by the constituents of the infusate, including an excess of glucose[16] or lipid,[17] inadequate lipid,[18] imbalance of amino acid,[9] and presence of toxic amino acids. Deficiencies in essential fatty acids, protein, and choline have also been incriminated. Hall et al., studying a rat model, suggested triglyceride accumulation was due to an increased hepatic synthesis of fatty acid and reduced triglyceride secretion.[20]

In adults, steatosis and cholestasis are the commonest abnormalities associated with TPN. In contrast to infants, in whom progression to fibrosis has been observed, the adult on TPN rarely has progression of the liver abnormalities beyond the stage of steatosis and cholestasis. Cholestasis occurs chiefly at the level of the bile canalicular microvilli, where blunting and vacuolation strongly suggest a failure of bile secretion in the mechanism of the cholestasis. Cholestasis, acalculous cholecystitis, biliary sludge, and gallstone formation during TPN are discussed later in this chapter.

Inborn Errors of Metabolism

HEMOCHROMATOSIS

Genetically determined hemochromatosis is the result of a specific metabolic abnormality. However, iron overload may also be caused by a number of other conditions, such as the ingestion of excessive quantities of iron, repeated blood transfusion, porphyria cutanea tarda, or portacaval shunting.

The normal total body iron is in the order of 3 to 4 g. Approximately 65 per cent of the iron is in the form of hemoglobin, myoglobin, and tissue enzymes. The rest is distributed in various tissues as stores. Storage iron can be either in a diffuse soluble fraction as ferritin, or in an insoluble aggregate as hemosiderin.

The liver is considered the most important storage organ for iron, containing about 30 per cent of the total body iron content. The amount of dietary iron that is absorbed is partially regulated by the amounts that are lost from the body. During childhood and adolescence, there is a positive iron balance. However, in adulthood, the iron store is relatively constant.[21] The obligatory daily iron loss is approximately 1 mg per day in adult males.[22] In females, through menstruation, the daily iron loss is on the order of 1.5 to 2.5 mg. Absorption of iron depends on the quantity of iron in the diet and its bioavailability. Heme iron in food is easily absorbed. In contrast, nonheme food iron is not absorbed efficiently. Nonheme iron in the intraluminal milieu is exposed to competitive binding with tannins and phytates to form absorbable complexes. On the other hand, ascorbic acid enhances its absorption. In communities consuming little meat or fish, ascorbic acid in the diet becomes the limiting factor of iron absorption.

From a practical standpoint, it is impossible to have pathological iron overloading from taking a balanced diet. The exception is the injudicious and excessive supplementation of iron, either by self-medication or by contamination with iron cooking utensils, as has been reported in African blacks.[23] Idiopathic hemochromatosis is an inherited autosomal recessive disease. In this condition, there is an abnormally large proportion of iron taken up by the mucosal cells of the gut and transferred into the body.[24] It has also been suggested that the intestinal mucosal cells and the reticuloendothelial cells are unable to store iron, leading to an abnormal amount of iron delivered to the hepatocytes and other parenchymal cells.

In addition to this genetic predisposition, the development of hemochromatosis is influenced by the amount of iron in the diet and by alcohol consumption.[23] By the time the diagnosis is established, patients have an iron store 20 to 50 times normal. Cirrhosis of the liver is almost always present, often with diabetes mellitus, skin pigmentation, and cardiomyopathy. The diagnosis and clinical features have been summarized elsewhere.[25] It is important to consider the diagnosis of hemochromatosis in patients with liver disease, since this is a treatable and preventable disease.

WILSON'S DISEASE

Like hemochromatosis, Wilson's disease is a genetically linked disorder via a recessive gene on one of the autosomes and is manifested as a multisystem disorder with heavy metal toxicity. Involvement of the liver and neurological symptoms are the two most important features (hepatolenticular degeneration). The disease may also present as the ocular signs of Kayser-Fleischer rings in the periphery of the iris and sunflower cataracts, or as renal abnormalities such as proteinuria and aminoaciduria. Involvement of the blood and endocrine system are also seen.

A normal Western diet contains 2 to 5 mg of copper per day. Approximately 50 per cent of this is absorbed from the proximal small bowel. A portion of this is transported in plasma bound to albumin and probably also to amino acids or peptides.[26] This circulating fraction, constituting about 5 to 10 per cent of the total plasma copper, is promptly removed by the liver. However, it is mobilization of the copper from hepatocytes that appears to be the most important step determining copper distribution and elimination. Approximately 0.5 mg of newly absorbed copper is incorporated into ceruloplasmin, and this is released into the bloodstream.[27] More importantly, the excretion of copper into bile, which accounts for approximately 1.5 mg of copper per day, determines the level of hepatic copper concentration.[28] There is no evidence for an enterohepatic circulation of this metal. The pathogenesis of copper accumulation in patients with Wilson's disease is still unsettled. However, based on the sequence of events described above, the following hypotheses have been proposed:

1. An increased net absorption of copper from the diet resulting in copper overloading. However, there has been no convincing evidence to support this.

2. Abnormal synthesis of ceruloplasmin, resulting in a diminished ability to mobilize hepatic copper. However, there is a lack of correlation between the amount of copper and the quantity of ceruloplasmin. Although plasma concentration of ceruloplasmin is lowered in most patients with Wilson's disease as an isolated finding, this is not diagnostic.

3. The presence of an abnormal binding protein (metallothionein) resulting in an increased affinity and segregation for the metal in the liver. This has not been substantiated by study of hepatic copper uptake, which has suggested that in fact patients with Wilson's disease have less uptake compared with normal subjects.

4. A decreased excretion of biliary copper. This appears to be a feasible explanation, and the hypothesis has been supported by a number of experimental results.[29] The spectrum of hepatic involvement in Wilson's disease is wide and variable and has been reviewed elsewhere.[30]

OTHER METABOLIC DEFECTS AFFECTING THE LIVER

Several of these conditions, such as tyrosinosis, galactosemia, and hereditary fructose intolerance, are manifested early in life. Their management depends on early recognition of the condition and exclusion of the offending substance from the diet.

Self-medication with megadoses of vitamin A can result in hypervitaminosis.[21] Exfoliative dermatitis, headache, hepatomegaly, and hypercalcemia are the most important findings in this disorder.[32] Histologically, the liver shows steatosis and lipid inclusion bodies in lipocytes (Ito cells). Hepatotoxicity can progress to fibrosis and portal hypertension with or without cirrhosis.

A number of foods contain hepatotoxins. For example, the mushroom *Amanita phalloides* causes a toxic hepatitis; plants of the genera *Crotalaria* and *Senecio* can cause an obliterative obstruction of the centrilobular hepatic veins; peanuts contaminated with *Aspergillus flavus*, which produces aflatoxins, can cause hepatitis and in certain cases can even be a cause of cirrhosis and hepatocellular carcinoma.

EFFECTS OF LIVER DISEASE ON NUTRITION

Digestion and Absorption

The amount of food intake by patients with liver disease is usually subnormal. This is often due to accompanying anorexia and lethargy. In particular, alcoholics often neglect other nutrients, having most of the caloric intake represented by ethanol. Gastrointestinal malabsorption of nutrients in advanced liver disease is common. This often is associated with the cause of liver disease itself (i.e., alcoholism and malnutrition) or due to hepatocellular dysfunction.

Alcoholics with only hepatomegaly and hepatic steatosis frequently have abnormalities in intestinal absorption. The administration of ethanol can result in hemorrhagic erosions of the gastric mucosa and tips of the jejunal villi, as well as in decreases in the villous lactase, sucrase, and alkaline phosphatase activities.[33] Similar changes have also been observed in the jejunal mucosa of patients given ethanol in the presence of an adequate diet.[34] Exocrine pancreatic function in alcoholic cirrhosis is often abnormal.[35] Some of the abnormalities in absorption and pancreatic function are due to malnutrition itself. With nutritional replacement, the absorption of xylose and folic acid can return to normal together with the disappearance of steatorrhea.[36] Likewise, exocrine pancreatic function can also return to normal after nutritional replacement.[37] In normal clinical situations, it is almost impossible to dissect out the effect of alcohol and the effect of malnutrition. These two factors almost always work in combination.

Cirrhosis of the liver itself can produce malabsorption, and this can be independent of the effect of alcohol. Steatorrhea is the commonest manifestation of malabsorption in cirrhosis of the liver. It can occur in about 50 per cent of patients with cirrhosis of all causes. The steatorrhea usually is mild and does not exceed 10 g/day. However, in 10 per cent of cases it exceeds 30 g/day. The absorptive capacity of the small intestine is impaired in cirrhosis. Although there is little or no change in jejunal histology, functional measurements of absorption of long-chain fatty chains can be abnormal.[38] It has been suggested that portal hypertension, leading to congestion of the mucosal circulation as well as lymphatic drainage, may contribute to this abnormality.

Other possible causes for steatorrhea in liver disease include pancreatic insufficiency and the decrease in intraluminal bile salt concentration. Most assessment of exocrine pancreatic function in cirrhosis of the liver was done in alcoholic cirrhosis, in which chronic pancreatitis itself may complicate the picture. In nonalcoholic cirrhosis of the liver, exocrine pancreatic secretion was found to be increased, using Lundh's test meal or secretin infusion.[39] In all studies, there was a poor correlation between the degree of steatorrhea and exocrine pancreatic insufficiency. It is therefore unlikely that exocrine pancreatic insufficiency occurs in any significant extent in nonalcoholic hepatic cirrhosis.

In cirrhosis of the liver, synthesis and excretion of bile salts can be diminished, resulting in a decrease in bile salt concentration. In patients with cirrhosis, the bile salt pool is diminished as well.[40] These findings suggested that steatorrhea is due to a decrease in the concentration of bile salts and poor micellar formation. In patients with chronic intrahepatic cholestasis complicating the cirrhosis, such as in primary biliary cirrhosis, there is a marked reduction in biliary excretion of bile salts. In such a case, steatorrhea is common and severe and there is associated malabsorption of fat-soluble vitamins. Clinical symptoms of the deficiency of these fat-soluble vitamins can include night blindness due to vitamin A deficiency, osteoporosis and osteomalacia in association with vitamin D deficiency, and bleeding tendency due to vitamin K deficiency. Severe vitamin E deficiency can be associated with hemolysis and deposition of peroxidized lipid pigments in the intestines. This gives a brownish discoloration to the gut, referred to as the "brown bowel syndrome." There is some evidence that this pigment accumulation leads to malfunction of the mitochondria of the enterocytes and in itself may aggravate the steatorrhea.[41,42] However, clinical signs of vitamin E deficiency are often unrecognizable.

Substrate Utilization

As a consequence of cirrhosis of the liver, the patient may have alterations in handling of fuel homeostasis. In a group of alcoholic cirrhotics, the difference in substrate concentration across the liver, gut, and kidney was obtained by catheterization studies to calculate the net flux of free fatty acids, ketone bodies, triglycerides, and glucose. It was found that in cirrhotics, the pattern of hepatic metabolism mimics that seen in normal subjects with prolonged starvation. In the cirrhotic patients, hepatic glycogen store was diminished, probably as a consequence of extensive hepatic fibrosis. After an overnight fast, hepatic glucose production in these patients was diminished as a result of low rates of glycogenolysis. Hepatic ketogenesis was increased.[43] Using the combined techniques of direct calorimetry and radioisotope tracer analysis, these findings have been reproduced and extended.[44] The available data suggested that after an overnight fast, the caloric requirements of patients with alcoholic cirrhosis are normal, but the nature of fuels oxidized are similar to those in normal human subjects undergoing much longer periods of total starvation. Thus, patients with alcoholic cirrhosis develop the catabolic state of starvation much more readily and rapidly. This disturbed but compensated pattern for maintaining fuel homeostasis may be partly responsible for the cachexia observed in some patients with cirrhosis.

In patients with cirrhosis, the fuel profile derived from ketone and glucose by the liver is altered, especially after fasting.[43] This may be due to a decreased total body energy requirement. Alternatively, if the total energy requirement is normal, the needs can be supplied by fuels other than glucose and ketone bodies. For example, elevation of plasma free fatty acids in patients with cirrhosis may represent an increase in mobilization and utilization of these substrates.[44] An increase in amino acid breakdown to meet such caloric demands may also result in muscle wasting, a condition commonly observed in patients with cirrhosis. More research is required to define the equation of energy source and expenditure in hepatocellular dysfunction.

Alteration in Metabolism

PROTEIN SYNTHESIS

The liver is the most important site of plasma protein synthesis. In an average 70-kg adult, total body protein is approximately 12 kg. Protein turnover is the net balance of the synthesis and degradation and is approximately 200 to 300 g/day. When dietary protein is adequate, liver and muscle can utilize amino acids released by local protein degradation for up to 50 per cent of the synthesis. However, when dietary supply is restricted, this may increase to 90 per cent. Therefore, during starvation, approximately 250 g of body protein plus dietary proteins are being broken down daily in order to make available the amino acids for protein synthesis. The liver synthesizes proteins and enzymes to maintain its structural and functional integrity. In addition, it manufactures and delivers into the plasma a variety of proteins and coagulation factors. Approximately half of the hepatic protein synthesis is designed for extrahepatic delivery.

Albumin is synthesized exclusively in the liver. Approximately 12 g of albumin, representing 25 per cent of total hepatic protein synthesis, is made by the liver daily. As in other metabolic alterations, there has to be a substantial loss of hepatic parenchymal tissues before these disturbances are noticed. Apart from hepatocellular function, other factors that regulate albumin synthesis are nutrition, hormonal balance, and osmotic pressure.[46] With advanced cirrhosis of the liver and with excessive alcohol consumption, hepatic albumin synthesis is depressed. This is aggravated by a deficiency of dietary protein and an increased gastrointestinal loss of albumin, probably related to portal hypertension.[47]

Abnormalities in coagulation in patients with cirrhosis is common. In one study, 85 per cent of patients with liver disease had at least one abnormal clotting test, and 15 per cent had abnormal bleeding.[48] The clotting factors most likely to be depressed are factors II, VII, IX, and X. When parenchymal disease is severe, factor V and fibrinogen may also be reduced. Decreased hepatic synthesis is the main cause of low clotting factor levels. However, the decrease in availability of vitamin K also contributes to the low synthesis of prothrombin. Bile salts are essential for the absorption of vitamin K. There is only a very small hepatic reserve for vitamin K, which can be depleted in 10 days without replenishment. Therefore, in the presence of severe cholestasis or complete extrahepatic biliary obstruction, vitamin K deficiency should be corrected with vitamin K supplements. Coagulation factors may also be depleted because of excessive consumption in the presence of disseminated intravascular coagulation.[49]

UREA SYNTHESIS

The nitrogen in amino acids is metabolized by the liver by transamination, with glutaminic acid as the product. Ammonia produced in other tissues can also be utilized by amination of glutamic acid with the formation of glutamine. The nitrogen is then released in the liver as ammonia and enters the urea cycle with the eventual formation of urea. In patients with cirrhosis of the liver, maximal rates of urea synthesis have been shown to be decreased and there is accumulation of ammonia.[50] The hepatic activity of enzymes of the Krebs-Henseleit urea cycle are also depressed. This may be complicated by changes in hepatic blood flow, hepatic mass and alternative pathways for removal of ammonia.[51]

CARBOHYDRATE METABOLISM

Absorbed carbohydrates reach the liver before they are delivered to other organs. An average of 55 to 60 per cent of an oral glucose load is taken up by the liver and used for glycogen synthesis, triglyceride formation, and glycolysis. In the fasted state, the liver produces and releases glucose by glycogenolysis and gluconeogenesis. The normal glycogen store is approximately 70 g, and this would be depleted after 20 hours of fasting, following which the liver continues to produce glucose by gluconeogenesis. In cirrhosis of the liver, the glycogen store is depleted and the cirrhotic assumes a pattern of metabolism similar to normal subjects after prolonged starvation.[44] Glucose homeostasis in the liver is controlled by the opposing effects of insulin and glucagon. In general, hypoglycemia is observed in severe acute liver disease. while glucose intolerance occurs more commonly in established cirrhosis.

Hypoglycemia is an uncommon finding in cirrhosis. However, in acute fulminant hepatitis, hypoglycemia is common and often persistent and requires large quantities of parenteral glucose to maintain an adequate blood glucose level. The mechanism in this condition is the decreased hepatic glucose production due to diminished glycogen store, a failure of glycogen repletion, and diminished gluconeogenesis. Inappropriate increases in the insulin level may also contribute to the hypoglycemia. In patients with liver disease, hypoglycemia is sometimes aggravated by alcohol ingestion, especially after a period of fasting. Apart from the rapid depletion of glycogen store during fasting, alcohol inhibits hepatic gluconeogenesis by increasing the NADH/NAD+ ratio. Fasting hypoglycemia is also common in children presenting with encephalopathy and fatty degeneration of the liver (Reye's syndrome) and is also occasionally found in primary hepatocellular carcinoma.

Glucose intolerance is common in cirrhosis. It is probably due to insulin resistance in the presence of high plasma insulin levels. The high insulin level is probably due to insulin hypersecretion rather than decreased degradation, and this may result in down regulation of insulin receptors in the liver, producing resistance.[52] Elevated levels of free fatty acids, fasting growth hormone, and glucagon, as well as hepatic damage, may also be contributing causes of the insulin resistance. Occasionally hypokalemia aggravates the glucose intolerance, although the mechanism is not well understood.

LIPID METABOLISM

The liver is also an important organ in the synthesis and transport of lipids. It is the principal source of cholesterol, very-low-density lipoproteins (VLDL), and high-density lipoproteins (HDL), and it also synthesizes the apoproteins of other lipoprotein classes. The liver also provides the enzyme lecithin-cholesterol acyltransferase (LCAT). Low-density lipoproteins (LDL) are not synthesized by the liver but are derived from VLDL in the presence of lipoprotein lipase. LCAT is activated by HDL and esterified cholesterol by the transfer of fatty acids from lecithin to cholesterol. In patients with acute hepatocellular dysfunction such as in viral hepatitis, the plasma HDL decreases and plasma triglyceride and cholesterol levels increase, but there is a decrease in the level of cholesterol esters.[53] These changes have been shown to occur in association with a decrease in the lipolytic activity and a decreased removal of fatty acids. In addition, the proportion of esterified cholesterol in the serum is often diminished, and this is probably due to a low LCAT activity.[53]

Alcohol ingestion is commonly associated with an accumulation of triglycerides in the liver and the development of a histologically demonstrable fatty liver. This is probably secondary to an increased availability of fatty acids in the liver. The source of the fatty acid depends on the dose of alcohol and also the fat content of the diet. In acute drinking, the fatty acids are derived from the host adipose tissue. In chronic drinking, the synthesis of fatty acids is increased by an increased amount of NADPH, while the oxidation of fatty acids is reduced because of an increase in NADPH/NAD+, which depresses the Krebs cycle. Plasma triglycerides are also increased in alcohol ingestion because of stimulation of hepatic production and release of lipoproteins; the latter is due to an inhibition of lipoprotein lipase by alcohol. Increased intestinal lipid output by the lymph, produced by acute drinking, contributes to the hyperlipidemia and fatty infiltration of the liver.[54,55]

In prolonged cholestasis, there is an elevation in plasma unesterified cholesterol and phospholipids. This is due to the presence of the lecithin and cholesterol complex, which has the properties of a low-density lipoprotein and unusual physical-chemical characteristics and morphologically has been shown to appear as a rouleau of discs. This abnormal lipoprotein has been termed "lipoprotein X." Recent experiments have suggested that this is a result of the regurgitation of biliary lipoprotein complexes into the plasma compartment in the presence of chronic bile secretory obstruction. When such biliary lipoprotein is incubated with plasma albumin, the characteristic rouleau of discs could be reproduced in vitro.[56]

HORMONE METABOLISM

The liver is involved in hormone biotransformation, inactivation, and secretion. Therefore, in the presence of hepatocellular failure, many hormones and regulatory peptides may not be degraded, resulting in an increased expression of their biological function. This effect on glucagon leads to hyperglucagonemia, which, by stimulating hyperinsulinemia with down regulation of insulin receptors, may aggravate glucose intolerance.[57] Steroid hormones are taken up from the circulation by the liver and then metabolized by hepatic enzymes, leading to their hydroxylation and oxidation. Estrogen and estrogenic

metabolites are poorly degraded by the liver in cirrhosis, and this may lead to clinical signs of gynecomastia and testicular atrophy. Aldosterone metabolism may also be impaired, leading to secondary hyperaldosteronism with hypokalemia and fluid retention. Secondary hyperaldosteronism may be responsible for resistance to diuretic therapy in cirrhosis of the liver. Antagonists to aldosterone often produce synergistic effects in combination with diuretics.

VITAMIN METABOLISM

Liver disease may also have an effect on vitamin balance. A survey of a group of nonalcoholic liver disease patients showed that although the incidence of disturbance in vitamin profile was lower than in alcoholics, there were nevertheless significant abnormalities.[58] Approximately 40 per cent had evidence of fat-soluble vitamin deficiency (vitamins A and E and carotene); about 8 to 10 per cent had deficiency of vitamin B_{12}, nicotinic acid, thiamine, or riboflavin; and 17 per cent had folate deficiency. These abnormalities were attributed to the disordered liver function, since they were shown not to be due to dietary inadequacy, age, or interference with fat absorption. The above abnormalities are amplified in alcoholics, and in a number of patients will be manifested as florid nutritional deficiency with accompanying beriberi, scurvy, folate deficiency, and peripheral neuropathy. Besides poor dietary intake, malabsorption, decreased storage, defects in metabolism, and increased requirement in the presence of liver injury all contribute to the deficiency state.

Storage and Increased Requirements. These two factors often coexist and are synergistic in bringing out a vitamin deficiency state. In patients with cirrhosis, hepatic reserve of a number of vitamins is diminished.[59] These include folate, riboflavin, nicotinamide, pantothenic acid, and vitamins B_6, B_{12}, and A. In cirrhosis, there is often a decrease in the total hepatic nitrogen content. This suggests a displacement of functional storage space due to deposition of fibrous tissue and fat. Together with cellular degeneration in cirrhosis, these two factors are the major cause of the low vitamin concentrations. Other causes include a decrease in the hepatic avidity for the vitamin and a decreased hepatic uptake of absorbed vitamins.

The liver also has a great potential of cell regeneration after tissue damage. During the regenerative phase, requirements for folic acid and vitamins B_6 and B_{12} are increased, as these vitamins are essential for cell replication. In one study of alcoholic hepatitis in the presence of a normal diet, serum folate as well as hepatic DNA synthesis was depressed. This could be reversed by folate supplement even if alcohol intake is continued. It appears that small extra amounts of vitamins may be required to meet the increased demand of tissue repair in chronic active liver disease.

Altered Metabolism of Specific Vitamins. In many cases changes in vitamin metabolism result from decreases in the availability of the active form of the vitamin. The following abnormalities in vitamin metabolism have been described.

Pyridoxine. Subnormal levels of pyridoxine phosphate, the major active form of pyridoxine, are found in patients with alcoholic cirrhosis. This is also occasionally associated with a mild anemia, and sideroblastic changes in the bone marrow. When these patients have actively ingested alcohol for 2 weeks, the low pyridoxine phosphate level is not correctable by parenteral pyridoxine. The administration of pyridoxine phosphate, however, promptly restores the serum pyridoxine phosphate level to normal and reverses the bone marrow sideroblastic changes.[60] These observations suggest that the conversion of pyridoxine to pyridoxine phosphate is inhibited by alcohol. There is also the suggestion that acetaldehyde, a metabolite of ethanol, may enhance the degradation of phosphorylated pyridoxine.[61]

Thiamine. A heavy intake of alcohol may increase the thiamine requirement, and deficiency of thiamine may lead to Wernicke's disease (mental confusion, ocular disturbances, ataxia, and sometimes polyneuropathy) and Korsakov's psychosis (impaired memory and cognition, often accompanied by fabrication of information). These coexistent diseases due to vitamin deficiency are treatable if they are recognized. Often the response to treatment with thiamine is rapid and gratifying, but severe neurological damage may be irreversible. The presence of liver disease may also interfere with the response to vitamin therapy. This is because the absorption of vitamins and their conversion into the active compounds may be impaired when the liver is damaged.[62] Patients with advanced cirrhosis may have a decreased absorption of water-soluble thiamine derivatives, but can absorb allithiamines, probably by simple diffusion. The phosphorylation of thiamine in the presence of severe liver diseases may be impaired. The absorption of pyridoxine may also be diminished. Pyridoxal-5-phosphate is an important pyridoxine derivative, which is essential for many enzymatic reactions. Plasma levels of pyridoxine are low in patients with cirrhosis, and the clearance of pyridoxal-5-phosphate from the plasma is increased. This may explain that with an intravenous infusion of pyridoxine, the rise in plasma level is lower in cirrhotics than in control subjects.

Thiamine deficiency is usually measured by blood thiamine level as well as transketolase activity in the red cells. The former reflects hepatic storage and the latter is dependent on hepatic phosphorylation of thiamine. In thiamine-deficient alcoholics the addition of thiamine increases blood thiamine levels but causes no change in red cell transketolase level. In thiamine-deficient patients without any liver disease, the in vitro addition of thiamine pyrophosphatase increased the red cell transketolase activity, but no changes were observed in thiamine-deficient cirrhotics. These results also support the view that the symptoms of thiamine deficiency in liver disease are in part due to a decrease in the hepatic conversion of thiamine to its active form or poor utilization of the active form.

Folic Acid and Vitamin B$_{12}$. Both folic acid and vitamin B$_{12}$ are stored in the liver, and in chronic liver disease the storage capacity is diminished. However, the storage time for vitamin B$_{12}$ is much longer than that of folate, and consequently folic acid deficiency is more common in patients with liver disease. Folic acid deficiency is also the most common vitamin deficiency in patients with alcoholic liver disease. In normal individuals, tissue folate stores can last 3 months without any dietary folate intake. Without any dietary intake, there is a fall in the serum folate ($<$ 3 mg/ml) within 3 weeks, followed by a decrease in the red cell folate level and the appearance of hypersegmented neutrophils. Megaloblastic anemia usually does not occur until 4 or 5 months after an absence of folate intake. In sharp contrast to this, in alcoholic subjects there is a much faster fall in serum folate levels, and megaloblastic anemia can develop in as little as 5 to 10 weeks in the presence of a diet deficient in folate.[63]

All the mechanisms of vitamin deficiency can be operative in folic acid deficiency. This process involves decreased absorption, decreased hepatic uptake, decreased storage of folate, and a decreased metabolic conversion of folate to its active form. 5-methyltetrahydrofolic acid is the major storage and circulating form. It also serves as the donor of methyl groups during the conversion of deoxyuridylate to methyldeoxyuridylate (thymidylate), which is necessary for the synthesis of deoxyribonucleic acid. The liver takes dietary folic acid (pteroylglutamic acid) to 5-methyltetrahydrofolic acid. In the patient with folate deficiency and anemia, ethanol suppresses the hematological recovery in the presence of folate supplement. In addition, the acute administration of alcohol results in a fall in serum folate levels in both normal subjects and patients with alcoholic liver disease. This suggests that ethanol interferes with the formation or release of 5-methyltetrahydrofolic acid.[64]

Vitamin B$_{12}$ levels can also be low in chronic liver disease, and this, either singly or in combination with folate deficiency, causes anemia and neurological abnormalities such as peripheral neuropathy and subacute combined degeneration of the spinal cord. In the treatment of neurological complications of these vitamin deficiencies, it is important to recognize that multiple vitamin deficiencies can occur, and replacement should include all the deficient vitamins. In conditions in which there is active hepatocellular inflammation, serum vitamin B$_{12}$ levels can actually be higher than normal. The conditions include viral hepatitis, chronic hepatitis, fatty infiltration of the liver, and carcinoma of the liver. The elevation in these conditions is most probably due to the release of vitamin B_{12} from damaged hepatocytes, but other mechanisms may also be involved. In fibromedullary carcinoma of the liver, the vitamin B_{12} level is markedly elevated. This is due to the production of an abnormal protein by the tumor cell. This protein co-migrates with the vitamin B_{12} binding protein and gives a falsely elevated result of vitamin B_{12} level in routine biochemical assays.

Vitamin A. Dark adaptation abnormality is common in patients with cirrhosis. This condition is underrecognized, and not all cases improve with the administration of vitamin A. Vitamin A is absorbed and transported to the liver by a retinol-binding prealbumin complex. In patients with acute and chronic hepatocellular dysfunction, levels of the complex are decreased. Plasma vitamin A level also decreases, and this is more commonly observed than the decrease in liver content of vitamin A. These results suggest that patients with liver disease may have an inability to release vitamin A from the liver, partly due to a diminished synthesis of the retinol-binding protein and free albumin.[65]

Vitamin D. Vitamin D_3 is transported to the liver and converted into the more active form, 25-hydroxy vitamin D_3. This in turn is converted in the kidney into 1,25-dihydroxy vitamin D, the most active form of vitamin D. In patients with chronic liver disease, there is an increased incidence of osteoporosis associated with a low serum 25-hydroxy vitamin D level.[66] In cholestatic liver disease, in which the intraluminal bile salt concentration in the gut is decreased, there is malabsorption of calcium. In such cases, metabolic bone disease is common, especially in primary biliary cirrhosis. Calcium malabsorption correlates with the serum 25-hydroxy vitamin D_3 level, and treatment with oral 25-hydroxy vitamin D_3 has been shown to improve calcium absorption.[67] Osteomalacia can also occur in some cases and can be reversed by the use of oral 25-hydroxy vitamin D.[69,70] Treatment of these patients with either oral or parenteral vitamin D was found to be unsuccessful in increasing the serum levels of 25-hydroxy vitamin D or in improving bone mineralization. Failure to increase the level of 25-hydroxy vitamin D following parenteral administration of vitamin D has also been observed in patients with alcoholic cirrhosis.[66] These data suggest that in cirrhosis there is either impaired hepatic hydroxylation or impaired hepatic release of 25-hydroxy vitamin D. Ethanol itself may contribute to 25-hydroxy vitamin D deficiency by its induction of microsomal enzymes that convert 25-hydroxy vitamin D to biologically inactive metabolites.

MINERAL METABOLISM

Hepatocellular dysfunction is associated with alteration in body concentrations of a number of minerals. The best-studied changes are of sodium and potassium. Other minerals affected include calcium, phosphorus, iron, and magnesium.

Sodium. Hyponatremia is common in patients with cirrhosis. This occurs in the presence of an increase in the total body sodium. Water retention occurs in cirrhosis in conjunction with sodium retention, and there is a net retention of water due to a diminished free water clearance secondary to an increase in circulating antidiuretic hormone. The increase in total body sodium is due mainly to increased tubular reabsorption of sodium. In cirrhosis of the liver there is secondary hyperaldosteronism, although other factors may also be involved. The increase in aldosterone level is aggravated by an excessive stimulation of the adrenal cortex by angiotensin. In cirrhosis, increased amounts of renin are released by the juxtaglomerular apparatus of the kidney in response to renal redistribution of blood flow and diminished perfusion of the renal cortex. Renin then acts on angiotensinogen to form angiotensin, leading to increased levels of aldosterone. Hepatic degradation of aldosterone is impaired in cirrhosis.

Potassium. Hypokalemia is common in cirrhosis. It is also commonly associated with alkalosis. Hypokalemic alkalosis, sometimes with hyponatremia, precipitates and aggravates hepatic encephalopathy. Serum potassium levels are usually poor indicators of the presence of potassium deficiency or the degree of deficiency. However, when this falls below 3.5 mEq/L, the total body potassium deficit is approximately 300 to 500 mEq.

Calcium. Deficiencies in calcium and metabolic bone disorders are due to abnormalities in vitamin D metabolism and reduced absorption of calcium. These have been discussed in previous sections.

Phosphorus. In patients with alcoholism and cirrhosis the serum phosphorus level has been shown to be low. Hypophosphatemia was found in 50 per cent of alcoholic patients admitted to hospital.[71] In children with encephalopathy and fatty degeneration of the viscera (Reye's syndrome), serum phosphorus has also been found to be low. Poor dietary intake (malabsorption) and increased urinary excretion of phosphorus have been suggested as causes of hypophosphatemia.

Iron. Serum iron levels are usually elevated in patients with hepatitis. The maximum values are not usually attained until both the serum bilirubin and transaminase levels have reached their peak. Serum ferritin is also increased and this may be due to the release from damaged liver cells. However, this would account for only a small part of the rise in serum iron. Transferrin levels are also raised, but the reason is not clear. For this phenomenon, decreased utilization of iron for heme synthesis, excessive hemolysis, impaired reticuloendothelial uptake, and impaired hepatic storage of iron may all play a part. The increase in serum iron may cause some diagnostic difficulties in differentiating cirrhosis with increased iron deposition from hemochromatosis. In hemochromatosis, the total iron-binding capacity is reduced and fully saturated. A liver biopsy may be helpful in differentiating hemochromatosis from simple iron overload. In hemochromatosis, iron deposition precedes fibrosis and the iron is found mainly in the hepatocytes. In cirrhosis, iron deposition is chiefly in the Kupffer cells.

In a proportion of patients with cirrhosis of the liver, there is a decreased storage of iron. In a group of patients with nonalcoholic liver disease, there was evidence of iron deficiency in approximately 25 per cent. This is largely related to an increase in gastrointestinal blood loss, and insufficient dietary intake may also contribute.[58]

Magnesium. The main symptoms of magnesium deficiency are weakness, neuromuscular hyperexcitability, and anorexia. Magnesium deficiency is common in alcoholism as well as in patients with cirrhosis of the liver. Serum magnesium levels are poor indicators of total body magnesium. A number of factors including poor diet, secondary hyperaldosteronism, and diuretic therapy aggravate magnesium deficiency.

Other Trace Minerals. Zinc, copper, manganese, nickel, cadmium, selenium, chromium, and cobalt are required as an integral part of the molecular structure of many enzymes and coenzymes. In cirrhosis of the liver, these minerals may be deficient owing to a poor hepatic storage and increased excretion.[72] A deficiency in these trace minerals may account for some of the neuropsychiatric symptoms in chronic liver disease. They may also contribute to poor tissue repair and wound healing, since some of these trace minerals, such as copper, play a major role in the biosynthesis and cross-linking of glycoaminoglycans.

NUTRITIONAL FACTORS IN THE TREATMENT OF LIVER DISEASES

The liver may be damaged acutely, as in viral hepatitis or drug- or alcohol-induced hepatitis, or chronically, as in cirrhosis of the liver. The consideration of nutritional factors in these two different presentations is different. One often overlooked factor in the dietary management of liver diseases is that, in the zest for producing a nutritionally sound diet, the food is often presented in an unattractive manner. Patients with liver diseases often have nausea, vomiting, and/or abdominal pain. A rigid regimen of an unattractive diet sometimes may induce more symptoms. The same amount of calories and nutrients can often be presented in frequent small and attractive helpings.

Uncomplicated Acute Hepatitis

Anorexia is a major symptom of acute hepatitis in the early stages, irrespective of whether this is due to viral infection or drug or alcohol reaction. With uncomplicated hepatitis, this phase is usually short and it is unusual to require intravenous supplements. As soon as appetite has begun to return, simple foods may be consumed as desired. Many patients have received advice of doubtful value. At this convalescent phase, it is important not to impose any dietary restrictions, and the patient should be encouraged to eat normally. In uncommon cases, patients may have severe anorexia and food may induce nausea and vomiting; in these cases food may be given by tube feeding.

Fat restriction, a condition often religiously practiced, is unnecessary. Low-fat diets often are more bulky for the same caloric value and are generally unappetizing and in fact may aggravate anorexia. When convalescent patients were allowed a high-fat, high-protein diet, they consumed more calories than those allowed only a low-fat diet.[73] Patients gained more weight and the convalescent phase was also shortened. Other studies also suggest that a high food (including fat) intake may be advantageous in the convalescent phase of hepatitis. Servicemen with acute viral hepatitis were force-fed to achieve a daily diet containing at least 3000 kcal with 150 g of both protein and fat. A control group was allowed to eat ad lib, with subsequently a lower caloric intake. The convalescent phase was shortened by an average of 6 days.[74] The benefit gained is relatively small and does not justify force-feeding of all patients with acute hepatitis. However, it would be reasonable to encourage patients to take as high a caloric intake as they can tolerate. The presence of fat in the diet in the amount of 30 to 40 per cent of calories per day also allows an adequate ingestion of fat-soluble vitamins. In general, it is wiser to provide fat through dairy products and eggs rather than fried foods and fatty meats.

An adequate protein diet of 1 g/kg body weight or above is usually easily achievable with a well-planned mixed diet. The protein should contain both animal and vegetable proteins. Amino acid supplements are unnecessary, as digestion and absorption of protein is normal in hepatitis and should be sufficient in a mixed diet. Supplements of vitamins, choline, inositol, and methionine, which have been advised previously at random, are also unnecessary. In a few patients with acute fulminant hepatitis, usually those associated with massive necrosis, normal or high protein intake may aggravate the syndrome of hepatic coma. When hepatic precoma develops, the protein in the diet should be restricted (see below).

With a diet high in calories, insulin secretion is increased. Increased insulin administration, especially together with glucagon, has been reported to protect liver cell damage and assist regeneration in mice with fulminant viral hepatitis.[75] Good control studies in the human are lacking. Usually, sodium and water retention is not a problem in uncomplicated acute hepatitis. Some patients with severe acute hepatitis cannot excrete a normal water load.[76] Even so, they can take fluid orally and so control their own intake, and again this is usually not a serious problem. However, if these patients are given excessive water intravenously, this may aggravate water retention and hyponatremia. Recovery from acute hepatitis is often accompanied by a diuresis. In severely ill patients in whom sodium retention is a problem, dietary regulation of salt and sodium containing food is then required (see below).

There is continuing controversy concerning advice to patients to abstain from alcohol during an attack of hepatitis and subsequently. It is sensible and responsible to highlight to the patient the potential hepatotoxicity of alcohol at a time when the patient is both interested and concerned about his own liver. However, alcohol abstinence is often overstressed without a firm basis to such advice. There have been no good control studies that have demonstrated that alcohol in moderation has a deleterious effect during the recovery phase of viral hepatitis. In general, however, on the theoretical grounds that an inflamed liver may be more vulnerable to the toxic effect of other exogenous chemicals, alcohol should be avoided during the acute stage of the inflammatory process. Therefore it is reasonable to advise abstinence during the acute phase of hepatitis until the biochemical indices (transaminase, alkaline phosphatase, and bilirubin levels) have returned to normal. During this time, other hepatotoxic substances, including general anesthetics for elective operations, should be avoided. When the patient is both clinically and "biochemically" normal, it is unreasonable to persist with the demand for abstinence. Moderation in alcohol intake is always sound and good advice, and it would be a good opportunity to introduce such advice to the patient after a period of abstinence. For patients with viral hepatitis who have recovered but in whom the biochemical profile and/or the serological markers (such as hepatitis B surface antigen) are still abnormal, there is evidence that their liver would be more susceptible to the toxic effects of ethanol.[77] In such cases, restriction to a daily intake of 20 g of ethanol or total abstinence would be advisable. The above discussion applies to acute viral hepatitis. Alcohol itself can induce hepatitis. Alcohol abuse and liver disease is a major cause of morbidity and mortality in the Western world. Patients who have suffered from repeated attacks of alcoholic hepatitis must be advised to stop alcohol. Any advice to consume alcohol in moderation almost always results in a loss of control. In these patients, the message should be clear and firm, and given with accompanying counseling and support.

Cirrhosis of the Liver

In contrast to acute uncomplicated hepatitis, in which dietary restriction is seldom necessary, dietary control may be of critical importance in cirrhosis of the liver. This will be discussed in relation to the major complications occurring with chronic hepatocellular dysfunction.

HEPATIC ENCEPHALOPATHY

With cirrhosis of the liver, there is shunting of blood from the portal circulation to the systemic circulation, and this phenomenon is associated with either intermittent or chronic signs of cerebral dysfunction. The clinical manifestations of "hepatic encephalopathy" are protean. Its most severe form terminates in coma. There is a sickly sweet, putrid odor to the breath of these patients (fetor hepaticus). However, the whole spectrum of hepatic encephalopathy includes loss of concentration and memory, confusion, apathy, personality changes, and other psychiatric symptoms. The neurological features include spasticity, muscle spasms, choreiform movements, athetoid postures, and lead-pipe and cogwheel rigidity of the limbs with flexion withdrawal of the lower limbs. Ankle clonus with plantar flexor responses is common. Often, hepatic encephalopathy is complicated by the neurological disturbances associated with chronic alcoholism, such as delirium tremens and Korsakov's psychosis.

Since the liver plays an important role in metabolism, a severely compromised hepatocellular function with shunting of blood away from the liver is accompanied by a number of nutritional and metabolic abnormalities. These have been causally linked to the pathogenesis of hepatic encephalopathy. Excessive ammonia and nitrogenous waste, accumulation of false neurotransmitters, and a deficiency in branched-chain amino acids have all been implicated. Of these, the most important and central abnormality is related to protein metabolism. In many patients with cirrhosis with portosystemic shunting, the administration of large loads of dietary protein can cause a reversible stupor or coma with neurological manifestations of hepatic precoma. There is some evidence to suggest that some protein or catabolic product of proteins is acted upon by intestinal bacteria to produce toxic substances to the brain. By the same principle, intestinal flora may produce excessive ammonia and other nitrogenous wastes, short-chain fatty acids, and mercaptans that would be bypassed from the liver and exert their damaging effects on the brain. Some of these products, such as short-chain fatty acids and mercaptans, account for the smell in fetor hepaticus when excreted by the lungs. The presence of toxic substances acting on the brain in the presence of hepatic failure is the basis of the "neurotoxin hypothesis."[78] The other hypothesis focuses on the presence of "false" neurotransmitters or the malfunctioning or inappropriate receptor reaction with "true" neurotransmitters. These include abnormalities of the inhibitory neurotransmitters (serotonin) and deficiency of excitatory neurotransmitters (dopamine and nor-epinephrine). Gamma-aminobutyric acid with associated abnormal energy metabolism in the brain has also been implicated.[79] A deficiency in the branched-chain amino acids (leucine, isoleucine, and valine) and increased levels of aromatic aminoacids (phenylalanine, tyrosine, free tryptophan, and methionine) has been implicated to contribute to hepatic encephalopathy.[80,81] The mechanism of production of hepatic coma is a complex and as yet incomplete story. However, there is a large body of evidence to indicate that dietary protein restriction is of undoubted value in these patients.

With the onset of encephalopathy, protein intake should be completely stopped. It is also advisable to facilitate the elimination of existent protein in the intestinal contents by the use of purgatives. This is particularly so if there has been recent gastrointestinal hemorrhage, which constitutes a large protein load to the gut and in itself may precipitate hepatic coma. Complete protein restriction should be imposed only on a short-term basis. After 3 to 5 days of no protein intake, this should be reintroduced gradually in the diet. Careful and slow increments of 10 to 20 g, depending upon the patient's progress, can be given. The objective is to give just enough protein to prevent negative nitrogen balance. Patients with encephalopathy can usually tolerate 30 to 40 g of protein per day. This should be given in small doses throughout the day, as a sudden single load may aggravate the encephalopathy. Some patients can be stabilized on 50 g of protein per day. This intake can be increased by the concomitant use of a nonabsorbable neomycin or a synthetic disaccharide lactulose. These two agents act in the gut, altering the metabolic activities of the intestinal flora and hence the production and absorption of "toxic" metabolites. Either neomycin or lactulose has been found to be associated with improved cerebral function in patients with chronic hepatic encephalopathy.[82] Using these agents, some patients may even be able to tolerate 70 to 100 g of protein daily.

Because of the abnormal amino acid profile in patients with chronic encephalopathy, it has been suggested that an intravenous infusion of branched-chain amino acids would confer beneficial effects in these patients. Rossi-Fanelli et al.[83] found that branched-chain amino acid administration intravenously is as effective as lactulose in hepatic encephalopathy. However, the groups of patients receiving these infusions were not nutritionally equivalent. Wahren et al.[84] found that administration of a solution of amino acids and glucose did not significantly increase rates of clinical improvement in patients with hepatic encephalopathy; furthermore, the survival rate was higher in the control group of patients who received a glucose placebo than in those who received the amino acid and glucose solution. Another study[84a] found that amino acid infusion produced a better response in hepatic encephalop-athy when compared with glucose infusion plus neomycin. The results of these three studies are not exactly comparable, and although there is a tendency to suggest that branched-chain amino acid solutions are of value, further convincing data are required.

Equally, there is conflict in the results of oral adminstration of branched-chain amino acid supplements. Oral supplements with branched-chain amino acids have been found to be effective in treating chronic hepatic encephalopathy in some studies,[85,86] while others found negative results.[87,88] To promote the anabolic effects of administered protein, a carbohydrate intake amounting to 1500 to 2000 kcal is feasible, and whenever possible, given orally.

FLUID RETENTION

Subclinical fluid retention, ranging to frank edema and ascites, is a common complication of cirrhosis, and is usually associated with nutritional, endocrinological, and secondary metabolic disturbances. The manifestations of malnutrition are commonly seen as loss of muscle mass and glossitis as well as other signs of vitamin deficiency. Endocrinological abnormalities include testicular atrophy, gynecomastia, amenorrhea or menorrhagia, and a loss of libido. These are attributed to the inability of a deranged liver to metabolize normally circulating androgenic or estrogenic hormones. Aldosterone is also poorly metabolized, leading to secondary aldosteronism. Metabolic defects have been reviewed in previous sections and include abnormalities in protein synthesis, depressed levels of blood coagulation factors, and electrolyte imbalance. Fluid retention in cirrhosis is multifactorial and is a manifestation of a complex interplay between increased portal pressure, increased antidiuretic hormone, secondary aldosteronism, hypoalbuminemia, abnormalities in tissue permeability, and poor renal function with impaired ability to excrete salt and to clear free water. Just as in hepatic encephalopathy, in which there is a lack of clear understanding of the etiology, but protein restriction can help the patient, so in fluid retention, dietary salt and water restriction are imposed on an empirical basis. For example, restriction of dietary sodium to a level about equal to that lost by the body from the skin, urine, and feces (approximately 200 mg/day) would prevent most ascitic accumulation.

Restriction of sodium has been a useful component of the management of fluid retention. The amount of sodium restriction can be assessed arbitrarily by the ability of the kidneys to excrete sodium and free water. Although it is possible to reduce dietary sodium to 200 mg or less per day, this degree of low sodium intake also reduces protein intake. A low-sodium diet can be planned to include high-protein foods, some of which have to be processed commercially to remove sodium. The resultant diet is rather unpalatable as well as uneconomical. Hidden sources of sodium in intravenous fluids, plasma, and blood transfusions, or in the diet, such as in bread or drinking water that has been artificially softened, can complicate the sodium balance and often are unnoticed. Even simple medications such as antacids may have a high sodium content and may cause an unexpected reaccumulation of fluid in patients who are otherwise stable. To control the sodium intake in the diet, it is necessary to monitor the intake and output balance. One of the simplest and most accurate ways is to record the patient's weight every day. Rapid weight gain usually indicates sodium and water retention.

With the use of diuretics, particularly the combination of a chlorothiazide and spironolactone, severe restriction of sodium may not be necessary at all times. However, the injudicious use of diuretics may actually be harmful. It can produce postural hypotension and aggravate hyponatremia and other fluid and electrolyte abnormalities and in so doing may precipitate hepatic encephalopathy. Since salt restriction itself may be unpleasant for the patient and treatment with potent diuretics can be potentially hazardous, only selected patients should be treated.

Fluid retention is common in patients with cirrhosis. It is often asymptomatic and does not carry any risk or threat to life. Therefore if fluid retention in the form of tissue edema or ascites is not causing troublesome symptoms that distress the patient, vigorous treatment is unwise. It is also important to test and monitor renal function before restricting sodium. Quantifying urinary sodium excretion may also be helpful. Sometimes it is wise to reduce sodium intake carefully and slowly. If a patient is "water tolerant" (able to generate free water) and urinary sodium excretion is normal, the patient will usually respond to dietary sodium restriction alone by diuresis and disappearance of the fluid retention. Some patients are "water tolerant" but have low urinary sodium excretion. In these patients sodium restriction in combination with diuretics is often used, and most respond to such a therapy. Some patients are "water intolerant" and have low urinary sodium excretion. Management is usually difficult. Despite the combination of sodium restriction and the use of diuretics, fluid retention is usually a problem. In these patients, sometimes restriction of fluid intake to less than 1000 ml/24 hr can reduce the severity of fluid retention. However, the overall prognosis is poor.

NUTRITIONAL FACTORS IN THE PATHOGENESIS OF BILIARY TRACT DISEASES

Of all the congenital, metabolic, infective, and neoplastic diseases affecting the biliary tract, the single most important disorder in relation to human nutrition is gallstones. Stones have galled mankind for more than 30 centuries and continue to be a major health problem.[89] In a survey, gallstone-related symptoms accounted for nearly half a million hospital admissions per year, the highest among all gastroenterological disorders.[90] Most of the gallstones in Western communities are rich in cholesterol, and there is general agreement that, together with atheromatous cardiovascular disease, they are causally related to an abnormal nutritional balance. Conversely, disorders of the biliary tract may have important consequences on host nutrition. For example, the abnormal or decreased secretion of bile, which plays an important role in fat digestion and absorption, often leads to malabsorption and its sequelae.

Gallstones

In the study of medicine, there are few areas more confusing and frustrating than the topic of diet in the causation and the treatment of gallstones. The idea is not at all new. In his sixteenth century doctrine of "tartarus," Paracelsus proposed that digestive disturbances produced an "acidulation of the blood," leading to gallstone formation.[91] Sylvius (1614–1672) is quoted to have held that abuse of beer and spirits was the cause of gallstones.[92] Frerichs deduced that the observed increased prevalence of gallstones in women was due to a "diet containing a larger proportion of vegetables."[93] Hypotheses and suggestions proliferated and were debated such that "All kinds of particular aliments have, at one time or another, been accused of causing these concretions, but have in turn been again completely exonerated."[93] Budd remarked that "gallstones of cholesterine are seldom found in conjunction with the granular disease of the liver produced by spirit drinking" and that gallstones are "most frequent in fat persons, and in those who live richly and lead indolent lives."[94] Thus by the beginning of the twentieth century, it was well recognized that lifestyle factors were involved in the etiology of gallstones.

However, numerous conflicting claims still exist today and have not been vigorously reviewed and defined. The following is an analysis of the role of nutrition in the formation of gallstones. Although these research activities have not followed a temporal sequence, the review has been grouped under three categories which follow logically from each other: (1) descriptive epidemiological studies, which have drawn attention to the importance of lifestyle factors such as diet in the etiology of gallstones; (2) metabolic studies of the effects of dietary nutrients on bile cholesterol saturation, which have attempted to elucidate the dietary mechanisms involved in the pathogenesis of gallstones; and (3) case-control studies, which have compared the dietary intakes of persons with and without gallstones, and thus provide an empirical test of the results and conclusions of the previous two categories.

DESCRIPTIVE EPIDEMIOLOGY

The importance of the descriptive epidemiology of gallstones has been to emphasize that factors related to lifestyle, of which diet is one of the major components, are involved in the causation of gallstones. The great international variations in the prevalence of gallstones, changes in prevalence over time, and changes in prevalence associated with migration all support a role for lifestyle in the etiology of gallstones.

There are many difficulties in accurately measuring the prevalence of gallstones. Because the disease is nonfatal and often asymptomatic ("silent stones"), diagnosis of the presence of gallstones in an individual is not always made prior to death. Indeed, those autopsy series which contain information on the number of gallbladders absent (symptomatic stones) as well as the number of stones present (asymptomatic stones) suggest that approximately two thirds of persons with gallstone population are asymptomatic.[96] The two most commonly used methods to measure prevalence of gallstones are autopsy series and cholecystectomy rates.

International Variations in Prevalence of Gallstones. The international variations in gallstone prevalence provide some of the strongest evidence that lifestyle (or dietary) factors are involved in the etiology of gallstones. To control for temporal variations, Table 18–1 shows the age-standardized percentage of gallstones reported in autopsy series published since 1950 that contained information on age and sex sufficient for age-standardization. Of the populations reported in these studies, those with the highest rates of gallstone formation are the Pima Indians of North America, Chileans, and whites in the United States. Next are the populations of a group of northern and central European countries—Sweden, Czechoslovakia, Germany, and Austria—followed by New Zealand, Australia, England, Scotland, Norway, Ireland, and Greece. At the bottom of this list are the Asian populations in Singapore and Thailand.

In addition to the variations in gallstone prevalence that exist between populations, it is significant that the type of gallstone varies between cultures. In developed countries, cholesterol gallstones are most common and usually occur in the gallbladder. In Africa and Asia, where the gallstone prevalence is low, pigment stones, which usually occur in the bile ducts, are most common.[111]

Comparisons between national per capita food consumption and gallstone prevalence have been carried out, but with little success. Because all the dietary nutrients that theoretically may cause gallstones (e.g., excess intakes of calories, fat, refined carbohydrate, and cholesterol, and lack of fiber) are highly correlated, it is difficult to separate out their individual effects. For example, in a multicenter study involving seven countries,[112] total caloric intake, animal protein, and animal fats were all positively correlated with prevalence of gallstones. Deciding which of these three dietary factors is (are) causing gallstones is impossible because of their collinearity (especially between animal fats and animal protein). Descriptive studies such as these may provide information on the mean consumption of food by the total population of a country; however, there is no information on the dietary consumption of the individuals who have gallstones. It is always possible that the diet of people with gallstones is different from that of the remainder of the population.

Temporal Variations in Prevalence of Gallstones. Progressive increases in the prevalence of gallstone rate during this century are thought to support a role for lifestyle and dietary factors in the etiology of gallstones. Because cholecystectomy rates partially reflect the provision of medical services, and because autopsy gallstone prevalence rates may vary between populations within the same country during the same period of time, this summary of temporal changes in prevalence of gallstones will concentrate on single autopsy series, or separate, time-interval studies of the same reference population (Table 18–2).

The first study to describe a temporal increase in the prevalence of gallstones is that of Ehrstrom,[113] who reported for males and females combined that the crude rate of prevalence of gallstones in Helsinki, Finland, increased from 0.3 per cent during the decade 1859–1869 to 4.0 per cent during the 1930's. Over this period, food consumption changed from a subsistence diet based on bark and bread to a typical modern Western diet, with increased intakes of meat, dairy products, and sugar. At Innsbruck, Austria, during the period 1930–1964, the age-standardized prevalence of gallstones increased by 50 per cent in women and 25 per cent in men.[107] The authors offered no dietary explanation for this finding. In Athens, Kalos et al.[103] described an increase in the crude prevalence rate of gallstones in both sexes from 3.0 per cent during 1925–1939 to 8.9 per cent during 1950–1974, which they attributed to an increased consumption of sugar and white flour.

In Japan, the postwar Westernization has provided a unique example of the interplay between lifestyle and disease. Since the late 1940's, the prevalence of gallstones in Tokyo has more than doubled.[114] As well, the type of gallstone has changed from the once common pigment stone situated in the bile duct to the now common cholesterol stone in the gallbladder. These changes are most likely due to the major changes that have occurred in the Japanese diet. During the postwar period, per capita consumption of fat, animal protein, cholesterol, and

TABLE 18–1. *International Variations in Prevalence of Gallstones at Autopsy (since 1950)*

Rank*	Nationality	Reference	Study Period	Age-Standardized Percentage		
				Male	*Female*	*Ratio F/M*
Presence of Stones and Absence of Gallbladder						
1	Pima Indians	96	1966	25.9	62.2	2.4
2	Chile	97	1960–1969	20.5	47.1	2.3
4	Sweden	95	1969	17.5	35.4	2.0
5	Czechoslovakia	98	1963–1966	17.5	29.7	1.7
8	New Zealand	99	1965–1969	11.1	18.4	1.7
9	Australia†		1958–1974	11.1	18.2	1.6
11	Scotland	100	1953–1973	6.8	15.3	2.3
12	Norway	101	1952–1957	7.3	14.4	1.9
13	Ireland	102	1969–1975	4.9	13.7	3.0
15	Greece (Athens)	103	1925–1974	4.4	9.0	2.1
17	Thailand	104	1954–1958	2.9	5.3	1.8
Presence of Stones Only						
3	United States whites	105	1959	13.1	27.7	2.1
4	Sweden	95	1969	12.8	27.0	2.1
6	Germany	106	1957	9.5	24.1	2.5
7	Austria	107	1955–1964	6.2	17.2	2.8
9	Australia†		1958–1974	9.7	12.5	1.3
10	England	108	1950–1954	4.9	10.8	2.2
14	Chinese (Singapore)	109	1962–1966	6.1	8.4	1.4
15	Greece (Athens)	110	1973	3.1	4.3	1.4
16	Indians and Pakistanis (Singapore)	109	1962–1966	4.7	3.7	0.8

*Descending order of prevalence in females.
†Scragg R. Personal communication.

sugar have all greatly increased. At the same time, vegetable intake has decreased while per capita consumption of total calories has changed little since the 1910's.[115]

Summary of Descriptive Studies. The descriptive epidemiological studies described above have shown conclusively that the prevalence of gallstones varies between cultures and over time. Their findings strongly support a role for lifestyle factors in the etiology of gallstones. Of these lifestyle factors, diet is likely to be one of the most important because it varies between cultures, over time, and with migration. However, the descriptive studies are not able to identify which dietary components are causative, since they provide information about the total population and not specifically the diseased persons in that population.

METABOLIC STUDIES

Metabolic studies are defined here as studies of humans that measure in a clinical setting the effect

TABLE 18–2. *Temporal Changes Showing an Increase in Prevalence of Gallstones in Autopsy Series from the Same City*

Country	City	Reference	Study Period	Gallstone Prevalence (%)	
				Crude Rate, Combined Sexes	
Finland	Helsinki	113	1859–1869	0.3	
			1930–1939	4.0	
Greece	Athens	103	1925–1939	3.0	
			1940–1949	4.4	
			1950–1974	8.9	
Japan	Tokyo	114	1949–1953	2.7*	
			1955–1959	4.8*	
			1960–1964	5.5*	
				Age-Standardized Rate	
				Male	*Females*
Austria	Innsbruck	107	1930–1939	4.9	12.3
			1945–1954	5.5	14.8
			1955–1964	6.2	17.2
Scotland	Dundee	100	1953–1964	5.5	13.3
			1965–1973	8.0	18.2

*Calculated from graphed data.

produced on the biliary lipids by varying the intake of dietary nutrients. They are important because of their contribution in elucidating the biological mechanisms associated with those dietary nutrients which the descriptive epidemiological studies have suggested may be important in causing gallstones.

The nutrients that have been investigated in metabolic studies are fat (saturated and unsaturated), cholesterol, fiber, refined carbohydrate, alcohol, and total caloric intake. Theoretically, total caloric intake is not a specific nutrient but represents the energy taken in from all nutrients combined. Although these nutrients will be discussed separately, there exists a strong interrelationship between some of them such that variation in the intake of a particular nutrient is often accompanied by a changed intake of another. For instance, diets containing high quantities of refined carbohydrates usually contain less fiber, and vice versa. Because refined carbohydrates, particularly sucrose, are an efficient source of energy, increasing their intake usually results in an increased caloric intake. In addition, saturated fats and cholesterol occur in the same types of foods, especially red meats, so that variations in their intake are often in the same direction.

In reviewing the effects of the various dietary intakes on bile lipid metabolism, evidence will be presented primarily from studies of bile, in which measurements have been made of secretion rates and concentrations of the three major biliary lipids, cholesterol, bile acids, and phospholipids, in addition to the cholesterol saturation index.[116]

Total Caloric Intake. The well-recognized observation that obesity increases the risk of gallstones has led some researchers, perhaps on the assumption that there is a positive correlation between caloric intake and obesity, to postulate an increased risk of gallstones among whose who eat high-calorie diets.[117]

Sarles et al. studied cholecystectomized patients with T-tubes in the common bile duct.[118,119] Postoperative bile was collected over a period of 3 to 37 days, during which dietary intakes of protein, carbohydrate, fat, and total calories were varied every 3 to 6 days. For the total period of the study, there was a significant positive correlation between mean caloric intake and mean biliary cholesterol concentration for subjects with gallstones (r = 0.81, p<0.001), but not for controls. There was also a significant positive correlation between mean daily cholesterol concentration and caloric intake of the preceding day for 6 out of the 13 cases and 2 out of 5 controls. A second study on 4 patients with gallstones found that a change from a low-calorie diet (range 900 to 1300 kcal/day) to a high-calorie diet (range 2200 to 2800 kcal/day) caused an elevation in the biliary cholesterol saturation in all 4 subjects. No details are given of how caloric intake was increased in these studies, so it is possible that the changes observed above were due to changes in the absolute (or proportional) intake of the major

nutrients (e.g., fat, carbohydrate). Also, no mention is made as to whether during the study period weight changes occurred. This in itself may alter cholesterol saturation.

The effects of caloric restriction are opposite to the findings described above. Bennion and Grundy[120] found that when obese subjects were put on a low-calorie diet, in which the proportions of the major nutrients were unchanged, both the secretion of cholesterol into bile and the saturation index were reduced. These changes, which were simultaneous with a lowering of body weight, were probably due to a reduced liver synthesis of cholesterol. However, when slim persons ate the same high-calorie diet as the obese subjects, they were unable to increase their body weight, biliary cholesterol secretion, and saturation to the same level as the obese. Bennion and Grundy concluded that obesity per se, in addition to a raised caloric intake, increases the cholesterol saturation of bile.

Dietary Fats. The studies that have investigated the effect of dietary fat on biliary metabolism are of two types: those comparing the effect of polyunsaturated fats with saturated fats (a major stimulus for these studies has been the attempt to elucidate the mechanism of the blood cholesterol–lowering effect of polyunsaturated fats) and those comparing high and low intakes of fat.

Studies that have compared the effects of saturated versus polyunsaturated fats on biliary lipids show that there is variability in response to the type of fat, which may be associated with the presence of hypertriglyceridemia in study subjects. For instance, Dam et al.[121] found in healthy normolipemic volunteers that substituting margarine for butter in their diets did not significantly alter the ratio of cholesterol to bile acids in bile.

However, patients with hypertriglyceridemia who changed from a saturated fat diet after 1 month to a polyunsaturated fat diet for another month were found to have an increased biliary cholesterol saturation.[122] This increase in cholesterol saturation was due to an increased hepatic secretion of cholesterol and not from a diminished bile acid pool (the bile acid was actually also increased). Van der Linden and Nakayama[123] found that when a single intravenous infusion of polyunsaturated soy bean oil emulsion (Intralipid) was given preoperatively to patients with gallstones, who typically have an increased prevalence of hypertriglyceridemia, cholesterol saturation increased and crystals appeared more frequently in their bile than in bile from gallstone patients given an infusion of saline.

On the other hand, earlier studies that compared the effects on bile of saturated and unsaturated fats suggested that unsaturated fats lowered the cholesterol saturation of bile. Lewis[124] found that the oral administration of sunflower-seed oil over 4 days to patients with gallstones or pancreatitis lowered cholesterol secretion and increased cholic acid secretion, when compared with a diet of hydrogenated coconut fat. In another study, gallstone patients who were put on various dietary fats were found after a period of 3 weeks to have bile with an increased cholesterol holding capacity while on unsaturated fat diets than while on a saturated fat diet.[125]

If the level of fat intake, rather than the type of fat, is considered, nearly all studies that have investigated the effect of the level of fat intake on biliary metabolism have substituted fat for carbohydrate and vice versa; these studies have produced results that are inconsistent. In patients with hyperlipidemia who changed their fat intake from 5 to 40 per cent of calories, the liver secretion of all three major bile lipids (cholesterol, bile acids and phospholipids) was increased, so it is unlikely that their biliary cholesterol saturation had undergone any major changes.[126]

However, a low-fat, high-carbohydrate diet was found to lower the molar cholesterol concentration and increase the molar bile acid concentration of bile in patients with hyperlipidemia.[127,128] In another study, a low-fat, low-protein diet, supplemented with sugar, increased the bile acid pool in patients with gallstones and healthy subjects because of a decreased turnover of both primary bile acids and not because of a change in their synthesis.[129]

These latter two studies suggest that a low-fat, high-carbohydrate diet protects against gallstone formation. However, one cannot conclude which of the two nutrients is responsible for the alterations to biliary metabolism, since the proportions of fat and carbohydrate intake have been changed simultaneously. Also, a major criticism of some of these studies is that the proportion of fat and carbohydrate ingested by subjects was much higher than the usual 40 per cent for either fat or carbohydrate that is consumed in a typical Western diet (e.g., 60 per cent fat or carbohydrate).[128]

Dietary Cholesterol. Dietary cholesterol has often been thought to have a role in the etiology of gallstones ever since Aschoff[130] first proposed that cholelithiasis was a metabolic disorder due to excess cholesterol in bile.

Cholesterol homeostasis, in response to an increased dietary intake of cholesterol, involves three mechanisms: (1) suppression of liver cholesterol synthesis, (2) increased secretion of cholesterol or its major metabolite, bile acid, via the feces, and (3) decreased absorption of dietary cholesterol from the gut. Their combined effect is to limit the body pool of cholesterol.

The studies that have investigated these mechanisms have often found conflicting results for each homeostatic mechanism, possibly owing to variation between individuals in their response to dietary cholesterol. With regard to liver cholesterol synthesis, patients with liver disease[131] and patients with hypercholesterolemia as well as healthy volunteers[132-134] responded to increased dietary choles-

terol with decreased synthesis. Contrary to this, Wilson and Lindsey[135] found that two healthy men did not exhibit suppression of liver synthesis.

Regarding the changes in the fecal excretion of cholesterol and bile acids that occur after increasing dietary cholesterol, Quintao et al.[132] found an increase for both cholesterol and bile acids, Nestel and Poyser[133] found an increase for both cholesterol and bile acids, and Lin and Conner[134] found an increase for bile acids, while Wilson and Lindsey[135] found no change in excretion for bile acids. With regard to absorption of dietary cholesterol from the gut, Wilson and Lindsey[135] found that this was limited to 10 to 15 per cent of total ingested cholesterol in two healthy subjects. Quintao et al.[132] found that absolute cholesterol absorption increased up to a maximum of 1 g/day as dietary cholesterol increased, while the percentage absorbed decreased from 50 per cent at low cholesterol intakes (500 mg/day) down to 30 per cent for high intakes (3000 mg/day). Conner and Lin[136] and Lin and Conner[134] found no relationship between percentage absorption, which averaged 40 to 45 per cent, and level of cholesterol intake.

Through the mechanism of decreased absorption, cholesterol homeostasis limits the effect of dietary cholesterol on biliary cholesterol saturation. In addition, only about 300 mg/day of cholesterol is absorbed on a typical Western diet, yet liver synthesis is approximately 1 g/day. Thus, as a source for cholesterol entering the bile, the liver is likely to be of much greater importance than diet. Since diet contributes only 25 per cent of the cholesterol entering the body pools each day, and because dietary cholesterol can influence the liver, which is the major source of the body's cholesterol, it is likely that any effect dietary cholesterol has on biliary cholesterol occurs indirectly via the liver.

The other important implication of cholesterol homeostasis is that the three mechanisms described above allow for individual variation in the response to dietary cholesterol, either by means of one mechanism alone or by combinations of the three mechanisms to a varying degree. This individual variation in response to dietary cholesterol may explain the inconsistent results reported by studies which have investigated the relationship of dietary cholesterol and biliary cholesterol saturation.

Three studies have reported that increases in dietary cholesterol do not alter the cholesterol saturation of bile. Dam et al.[137] studied young healthy volunteers and, on increasing their dietary cholesterol from 1 to 2 g/day, found that the ratios of the concentrations of total bile acids/cholesterol and phospholipid/cholesterol slightly increased after 3 weeks on each intake, which suggests that biliary cholesterol saturation decreased. Further, the response to increased dietary cholesterol varied between individuals, with both increases and decreases occurring in bile cholesterol concentration. Sarles et al.[138] found that a dietary intake of 1.5 g of cholesterol per day for 6 days did not increase the cholesterol saturation of a 60-year-old female gallstone patient. The third study to report no increase in the cholesterol saturation of bile after an increase in dietary cholesterol is that of Andersen and Hellstrom.[127] They studied postmenopausal normolipidemic and hyperlipidemic women and found that a diet of five eggs per day for 2 weeks did not alter the mean cholesterol saturation index of their group, although there was variation between individuals in their response to cholesterol.

In contrast with the three studies above, three further studies have found that increasing dietary cholesterol increases biliary cholesterol saturation. DenBesten et al.[139] found that the daily addition of 750 mg of cholesterol over a period of 3 weeks to the diets of young healthy men without gallstones caused a statistically significant (p<0.01) lowering in the ratio of phospholipids and bile acids to cholesterol (12.2 to 9.1). They also found in patients with gallstones on a diet of 750 mg of cholesterol per day that liver secretion of cholesterol phospholipids and bile acids all increased, but that the percentage increase in cholesterol (34.3 per cent) was greater than for bile acids (20.6 per cent). In another experiment reported in the same study, a woman with hypercholesterolemia who was maintained on a diet containing 1000 mg of cholesterol per day for 3 months, developed cholesterol crystals in her bile. Maudgal et al.[140] confirmed the above findings in a study of patients with gallstones taking chenodeoxycholic acid, who were given a normal diet containing 600 mg of cholesterol per day for 1 month followed by a low-cholesterol diet of 100 mg per day for a further month. This resulted in a significant (p<0.01), but small, lowering of the saturation index. The final study is that of Cohen et al.,[141] who found in subjects with gallstones that diets containing 500 mg, 750 mg, and 1000 mg of cholesterol per day for three consecutive periods of 3 weeks, caused successive increases in the mean bile saturation index for the group.

It is difficult to reconcile the opposite findings from those studies which have examined the effect of dietary cholesterol on cholesterol saturation. However, one can say that studies involving a comparison between patients with gallstones and matched controls, as well as studies of the possible cholesterol homeostatic mechanisms used by subjects with gallstones, have not yet been carried out. Given that individuals respond differently to increased intakes of dietary cholesterol, it is quite possible that patients with gallstones as a group respond by a different homeostatic mechanism to increased dietary cholesterol compared to persons without gallstones.

There is some indirect evidence that particular homeostatic mechanisms may be associated with gallstone disease. The Masai of East Africa, who have a higher intake of dietary cholesterol than North Americans, also have a more efficient negative feedback control of exogenous cholesterol synthesis. This may explain their low prevalence of gallstones and low bile cholesterol saturation.[142] Studies of cholesterol turnover have found no difference between patients with gallstones and controls in the rate of cholesterol input into the rapidly exchangeable pool.[143,144] Since this rate of input comprises both endogenous cholesterol synthesis and absorbed exogenous cholesterol, and since cholesterol synthesis is increased in patients with gallstones, this suggests that cholesterol absorption from the gut is diminished in patients with gallstones.[144]

Dietary Fiber. Dietary fiber has been defined as "plant polysaccharides and lignin which are resistant to hydrolysis by alimentary enzymes of man."[145] It comprises pectins, hemicelluloses, all of which are carbohydrate polymers, and lignin, which is an aromatic polymer. In addition, there are fiber-associated substances, which include phytic acid, silica, cell wall protein, and vitamins. The combination of dietary fiber and fiber-associated substances is known as the dietary fiber complex.[145] The term crude fiber is also used. This is made up mainly of cellulose and lignin, and thus is not synonymous with dietary fiber.

A role for dietary fiber in the etiology of gallstone disease was first put forward by Heaton,[146] and subsequently by Burkitt.[147] Burkitt's epidemiological observations on the rarity of gallstones among black Africans led him to hypothesize that many of the Western diseases, including gallstones, were the result of overconsumption of refined carbohydrates. Burkitt's contribution was to shift the emphasis away from an excess of refined carbohydrates to a deficiency of dietary fiber.[145]

Since the publication of the hypothesis associating gallstones with a deficiency in fiber intake, a number of studies have been carried out to examine the effect of fiber on biliary metabolism. Most of these studies have used wheat bran.

Bran, which is composed mainly of hemicelluloses, appears to lower the cholesterol saturation of bile in those with supersaturated bile but not in those whose bile is marginally saturated or who have colonic disease. The mean saturation index in subjects with gallstones decreased from 1.49 to 1.29 after they ate an average of 57 g of bran per day for 4 to 6 weeks.[148] Another group of subjects with gallstones also lowered their mean saturation index from 1.43 to 0.76 after 4 weeks on a diet that was supplemented by 50 g of wheat bran per day.[149] People without gallstones who consumed 30 g of wheat bran per day for 2 months were also able to lower their saturation index only if it was initially above 1.0.[150]

Other studies have found that the addition of bran to the diet has no effect on biliary cholesterol saturation. The mean saturation index in a group of young healthy men remained at about 0.6 after the addition of 30 g wheat bran per day to the diet for 6 weeks.[151] Another group of young healthy males were also unable to change their saturation index away from an average initial level of about 1.0 after adding approximately 30 g/day of wheat bran to the diet for 4 to 8 weeks.[152] People with diverticular disease were also unable to alter their bile saturation index by adding wheat bran for a period of 12 months.[153] The lack of any change in the mean saturation index of subjects in this last study may be because their colonic disease interfered with the action of bran, which is thought to occur in the right colon.[151]

Those studies which measured the total bile acid pool size found that it was not changed by the addition of bran to the diet.[148,152] However, the proportion of the individual bile acids did change. All the studies that reported a bran-induced fall in the saturation index also reported a fall in the deoxycholate proportion of total bile acids.[148–150] Other studies have also found that bran reduced the proportion of deoxycholate.[151,153] Along with a fall in the proportion of deoxycholate with no change in the cholate proportion,[148,151] a rise in the proportion of cholate and no change in the chenodeoxycholate proportion,[153] and no change in the proportions of either cholate or chenodeoxycholate.[149,150]

The consistent finding of a bran-induced fall in the deoxycholate proportion, together with a lowering of the saturation index (in those with cholesterol-supersaturated bile) as described above, suggests that bran may protect against gallstones by altering the metabolism of deoxycholate. It is uncertain whether the fall in the deoxycholate proportion is due to decreased formation of deoxycholate by bacteria in the colon, or due to decreased absorption of deoxycholate from the colon because of increased binding to bran. A report that the taking of metronidazole, a drug that inhibits anaerobic bacteria in the colon, lowers the deoxycholate proportion of bile as well as the saturation index suggests that bran may act by inhibiting the bacterial formation of deoxycholate.[154] Furthermore, oral ampicillin has been reported to decrease the deoxycholic acid pool and the saturation index.[155]

It has been postulated that the metabolism of bran by colonic bacteria to short-chain fatty acids lowers the colonic pH, which in turn may decrease the conversion of primary to secondary bile acids. Thornton and Heaton[156] found that the dietary addition of lactulose, which lowers the colonic pH, also lowered the percentage of deoxycholate in bile as well as the saturation index. That bran does not alter the half-life of cholate and chenodeoxycholate further supports the notion that bran does not act by binding bile acids to increase their excretion.[148]

Two studies have reported that the ingestion of other types of dietary fiber do not alter biliary cholesterol saturation. Morbidly obese subjects who were given a combination of vegetable and cereal fiber for 6 weeks slightly increased their saturation index.[157] Moreover, for both cholate and chenodeoxycholate, pool sizes decreased and turnover increased, which is in contrast to the effect of bran. This suggests that the absorption of bile acids from the intestine was reduced by their binding to the dietary fiber added in this study. The second study found that neither psyllium hydrocolloid nor lignin given to subjects with gallstones had any effect on the saturation index or the proportions of the major bile acids.[158]

It appears that in the same way some types of dietary fiber lower serum cholesterol and others do not, so it seems that only certain types of dietary fiber can lower the saturation index in persons with supersaturated bile. It is possible that fiber that acts by inhibiting the bacterial formation of deoxycholate (e.g., bran) is protective against the formation of gallstones, while those fibers that strongly bind bile acids may actually increase the saturation index of bile (and the risk of gallstones) by depleting the bile acid pool. The latter possibility is supported by the finding that prolonged administration of cholestyramine, which strongly binds to bile acids in the gut, induces the formation of gallstones in baboons.[159]

Refined Carbohydrates. Two mechanisms have been put forward to explain a possible association between refined carbohydrates and the risk of gallstones.

First, a diet rich in refined carbohydrates lacks the bulking and satiating effect of a fiber-replete diet, so that overconsumption, and consequently obesity, which increases the risk of gallstones, are more likely to occur. Against this argument is the fact that the other major nutrients (fat and protein) have a much higher caloric content per unit of weight than do mono- or polysaccharides. Also, the energy density (kcal/ml) for fat is about twice that for refined sugar. Thus, refined carbohydrates cannot be singled out by this mechanism in preference to fat or protein.

The second mechanism is that the rapid absorption by the gut of refined carbohydrates may stimulate the pancreas to secrete more insulin, which in turn may stimulate the liver to secrete cholesterol-saturated bile.

With respect to the effect of refined carbohydrates on bile itself, no differences in the concentrations of cholesterol, bile acids, and phospholipids were found between normolipidemic patients with gallstones on a normal or high-sucrose diet. However, patients with gallstones who had pre-beta-hyperlipoproteinemia on the high-sucrose diet had a decreased concentration of bile acids, particularly chenodeoxycholic acid.[160] There is clearly a need for further controlled trials in this area.

Alcohol. The effect of alcohol ingestion on biliary metabolism and cholesterol saturation has been little studied by clinicians or laboratory scientists. This perhaps reflects a lack of awareness of the epidemiological literature, which has shown that alcohol protects against the formation of gallstones. However, the metabolic studies of alcohol ingestion that have been carried out, as well as studies of patients with cirrhosis, appear to lend some support to the epidemiological literature.

In a sterol balance study in which alcohol was given to hyperlipidemic patients and healthy volunteers for periods of up to 48 hours, fecal acidic sterol excretion increased while neutral sterol excretion was unchanged.[133] It was concluded that the increased bile acid excretion could be due to decreased bile acid reabsorption or to increased conversion of cholesterol to bile acids. If the latter explanation is correct, then alcohol should theoretically increase bile acid secretion and lower the saturation index. In support of this conclusion, patients with alcoholic pancreatitis, but normal plasma liver enzymes, were found to have an increased secretion of bile acids (461 μmol/20 min) compared with healthy volunteers (294 μmol/20 min).[161] Thus chronic ingestion of alcohol appears to increase liver bile acid secretion. This is opposite to the effects of acute alcohol ingestion, which reduces liver bile acid secretion.[161] In another study in which alcohol was given acutely (50 ml of ethanol orally per day for 2 days), no change was observed postoperatively in the saturation index of a woman who underwent cholecystectomy.[138]

Patients with hepatic cirrhosis have been described as having an increased prevalence of pigment stones but not of cholesterol stones. It would be premature to assume that moderate intakes of alcohol not resulting in liver damage affect cholesterol and bile acid metabolism in the same way as the alcohol consumption of patients with cirrhosis. More recently, it has been shown that apolipoproteins may play an important role in cholesterol transport in bile.[162] The degree of cholesterol supersaturation, by the classical micellar solubilization (by bile salts and phospholipids) may not be the only determinants of the true cholesterol holding capacity in bile. If cholesterol in the biliary compartment bears any resemblance to the cholesterol transport in the plasma compartment, then a non-micellar component (apolipoprotein) of cholesterol transport may well be an important physiological mechanism. Along this line of reasoning, alcohol ingestion has been shown to increase the plasma apolipoprotein level (high-density lipoprotein), which is reported to have an inverse relationship with the incidence of gallstone disease.[163,164] Alcohol consumption has also been demonstrated to desaturate biliary lipids.[165]

Summary of Metabolic Studies. By and large, the results of studies that have investigated the effect of the major dietary nutrients on bile metabolism and the saturation index are inconsistent (Table 18–3). The only areas of consistency are, first, the effect of increased caloric intake in raising cholesterol saturation, and second, the lowering of a raised saturation index by bran. There is also a suggestion that dietary cholesterol increases the saturation index in patients with gallstones.

A possible reason for the inconsistency in the re-

sults of the studies listed in Table 18–3 is variation between individuals in their response to dietary variables, for which there is strong evidence contained within some of these some studies. For instance, Sarles et al.[118,119] found, for the total period of their study, that there was a significant positive correlation between mean caloric intake and mean biliary cholesterol concentration for subjects with gallstones but not for controls. Patients with hypertriglyceridemia,[122] which itself is associated with an increased risk of gallstones, respond differently to polyunsaturated fats than do healthy young volunteers.[121] The effect of dietary cholesterol on the saturation index varies between individuals within the same study,[127,137] while individual variation exists for the mechanisms used to maintain cholesterol homeostasis.[132,133] In addition, bran appears only to lower the saturation index of those whose bile is already supersaturated.

Given that there are likely to exist variations between individuals in their response to the dietary nutrients, it is possible that persons who are prone to develop gallstones respond to the nutrients differently from persons not prone to gallstones. If the latter is true, it argues in favor of a threshold concept for the dietary etiology of the disease, such that above a certain threshold or level of dietary intake, those who are susceptible, either for genetic reasons or because of others factors such as pregnancy or oral contraceptive use, will form gallstones.

Science is a dynamic process, and our thinking is continuously influenced by the new influx of knowledge and concept. For example, it is now clear that the quantitation of cholesterol saturation is insufficient to explain why gallstones form at all.[166] Other variables, such as a nucleating factor[167] or an inhibiting factor for crystal precipitation[166] may be important in determining whether gallstones occur. This may also partly explain why studies on the effect of various nutritional components that have focused on the relative lipid composition in bile produced inconsistent results. The observed effects on biliary lipids, in turn, correlated poorly with the propensity to develop gallstones.

Case-Control Studies. The importance of the case-control studies is that they comprise observations on representative samples of diseased and disease-free persons, and thus provide an empirical test for the relevance of the dietary hypothesis developed by the descriptive epidemiological and clinical metabolic studies. At least 15 case-control studies that have examined the dietary etiology of gallstones have been published. Unfortunately, a number of these studies have employed inadequate study designs with rather small sample sizes, failure to use community controls (relying solely on hospital patients), failure to use the food frequency method of dietary measurement, and failure to measure diet eaten prior to the onset of symptoms.

Scragg et al.[168] have used case-control methods

TABLE 18–3. *Summary of Studies of Effects of Increased Nutrient Intakes on Biliary Cholesterol Saturation*

Nutrient	Cholesterol Saturation		
	Increase	*No Change*	*Decrease*
Calories	117,* 118,* 120, 138*		
Fats Polyunsaturated (vs unsaturated)	120, 123*	121	124,* 125*
Total fat		126	128, 129*
Cholesterol	139,* 140,* 141*	127, 136, 137	
Fiber		151, 152, 153, 157, 158*	148,* 149,* 150
Refined carbohydrates	171*	160*	
Alcohol		172	165, 173

Numbers given are reference citations.
*Study involving subjects with gallstones.

with adequate sample size including community controls and the data have been analyzed using multiple logarithmic regression analysis. They confirmed the previous observations that the use of oral contraceptives was associated with an increased risk of developing gallstones in young women, and the risk further increases with increasing parity. Interestingly, the risk was diminished in older subjects taking oral contraceptives. In both sexes, increased intake of alcohol was associated with a decreased risk of forming gallstones, while increased intake of simple sugars, total energy, or fat was associated with an increased risk.[169] Obesity correlated with an increased risk only in young women.[169] In both sexes, increased plasma insulin levels, and in young subjects, increased plasma triglyceride concentrations correlated with an increased risk of gallstones.[170] In contrast, high concentrations of high density lipoprotein cholesterol in plasma correlated with low risk of gallstones.[170] The contributions of various nutrients, the resultant plasma variables that can be measured, and their influence on gallstone formation have been summarized in Figure 18–1.

Parenteral Nutrition

Prolonged total parenteral nutrition (TPN) has been shown to be associated with a rise in serum transaminase, alkaline phosphatase, and bilirubin levels.[12] Histologically, the liver may show steatosis and intrahepatic cholestasis. In infants and children, fibrosis and even rapid progression to cirrhosis have been described.[14,174] Hepatic steatosis is a result of an imbalance in the deposition and removal of fat from the liver. Although the equation appears simple, the cause of increased hepatic triglycerides is not well understood. Excessive glucose loading may induce fatty changes in the liver,[175] and some of these changes could be reversed by substituting some of the calories by Intralipid infusion.[18]

Conversely, excessive lipid infusion may lead to fat accumulation in the liver.[17] Other suggestions include amino-acid imbalance,[19] presence of toxic amino-acid metabolites,[12] or deficiency of protein, essential fatty acid, or choline. More recently, studies using a rat model suggested that TPN induced steatosis by enhancing hepatic synthesis of fatty acids and by reducing triglyceride secretion.[20]

Intrahepatic cholestasis is a rather common but poorly understood complication of TPN, and the mechanism is probably multifactorial. Cholestatic jaundice also occurs with a high input of lipid emulsions.[176] Biliary lithocholic acid level has been shown to be elevated in TPN patients with abnormal liver function tests. Lithocholic acid is the breakdown metabolite of chenodeoxycholic by anaerobic bacteria. Recently, Capron et al.[177] found that administration

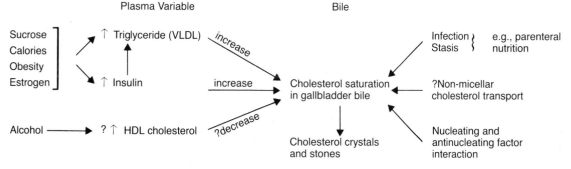

FIGURE 18–1. *Nutritional factors in gallstone formation.*

of metronidazole to TPN patients prevented the complication of cholestasis, and it was argued that metronidazole had exerted its antimicrobial effect, and had reduced the toxic effect by decreasing the lithocholic acid level.

However, before this hypothesis can be accepted unreservedly, the sequence of events should be clearly demonstrated. First, it should be shown that with TPN there is an increased anaerobic activity, and that as a result lithocholic acid is increased. Second, that the level of lithocholic acid in TPN patients is able to cause cholestasis should also be demonstrated. In this regard, the amount of sulfation and the level of conjugation of taurine and glycine may also be important, since these reactions confer unusual physical-chemical properties to the bile acid molecule that may induce cholestasis by interacting with the bile canalicular microvillous membrane[178,179] and interfering with bile secretion. Finally, it should be demonstrated that metronidazole can reduce lithocholic acid level.

Metronidazole should also be given with care to infants and young patients, since it may cause a peripheral neuropathy and induce chromosomal aberrations. Although there is no study demonstrating that there is an increased lithogenicity (cholesterol supersaturation) in bile, there are enough reports to indicate that there is an increased frequency of gallbladder abnormality in TPN patients. These include acalculous cholecystitis, the formation of biliary sludge, and gallstones.[181-183] TPN patients may also be very sick patients, often with toxemia or profound metabolic derangement. Under these conditions, acalculous cholecystitis may complicate the picture. An inflamed gallbladder with mucus hypersecretion and cell desquamation, together with gallbladder stasis during TPN, provide an environment in which the constituents in bile may precipitate in a matrix of mucus. These precipitates are composed of calcium complexes of bilirubin and cholesterol monohydrate crystals and on ultrasonography produce low-amplitude echoes without acoustic shadowing. They are known as gallbladder sludge and, especially in TPN patients, are thought to be the early stages of gallstone formation.[182] It is important to recognize these complications. They not only may add to the morbidity of the already complex clinical condition, but also not uncommonly (e.g., in acalculous cholecystitis) are the cause of death of these patients.

EFFECTS OF BILIARY TRACT DISEASE ON NUTRITION

Biliary tract disorders can affect nutrition by interfering with food intake as well as by an altered ability to mediate an adequate process of fat digestion and absorption. Patients with gallstone disease, for example, may complain of pain and dyspepsia, and consequently food intake may be diminished. It is uncommon, however, for clinical symptoms alone to reduce food intake to a level that would result in a compromised nutritional status. A high fat content in the diet has been believed to lead to more symptoms; the hypothesis is that the amount of fat would release an increased amount of cholecystokinin into the systematic circulation, increasing gallbladder contraction, which in the presence of gallstones may induce symptoms. A recent study[184] demonstrated that the amount of dietary fat did not correlate with gallbladder contraction as determined by ultrasonographic imaging. Although it used to be believed that gallstone patients have fat intolerance, this has not been backed up by objective data. The fact that patients with gallstones are unlikely to have a reduced food intake because of their symptoms is supported by the observation that obesity correlates with the prevalence of gallstones.[117,169]

More important is the effect of a reduced amount or absence of bile draining into the duodenum. Such can occur in cholestasis at the level of the hepatocytes or can result from obstruction in the extrahepatic biliary apparatus.

The amount of dietary fat intake varies greatly from community to community. For example, Japanese coal miners have a daily intake of less than 25 g (or less than 12 per cent of the total daily calories), while Los Angeles funeral directors consume approximately 160 g (or >42 per cent of total caloric intake) of fat. The intake of unsaturated fatty acids is virtually the same in these two extreme groups, indicating that in the latter group the increase in fat is due to saturated fatty acids from the use of meat and dairy fats.

In addition to being an important source of calories, fat is a major structural component of the human body. Fat, being insoluble, is a major constituent of membranes of cells and cell organelles. Without the important water:lipid interaction that lends to the rigidity of the cell membrane, the entire body would collapse.

For dietary fat to become available for use by the host, it must undergo a complex process of digestion and absorption. This has been reviewed and summarized elsewhere.[185,186] The important constituent in bile is bile salts. Bile salts are amphiphilic molecules, and above a critical micellar concentration would aggregate into macromolecular structures with the water-soluble pole oriented on the outside and the lipid-soluble pole in the inside. Therefore the entire macromolecule, or micelle, is water-soluble, whereas in the interior of the micelle fat and fat-soluble substances can be solubilized. In the intraluminal aspect of the duodenum one of the important functions of bile salts is the physical-chemical emulsification of fat. This process breaks up fat droplets into micelles that are 4 to 6 μ in diameter, or approximately one millionth the volume of fat droplets. This enormously increases the surface area and is an essential step before the chemical lipolysis by pancreatic lipases can effectively occur. At the same time, bile salts activate the pancreatic lipases. The micelles also carry the products of fat digestion, the monoglycerides and the fat-soluble vitamins A, D, E, and K, and transport the burden after diffusing through the unstirred layer, into the microvillous compartment of the enterocyte. The micelles themselves are not absorbed.

Monoglycerides and free fatty acids are absorbed mainly in the proximal small bowel, and most of the conjugated bile acids are absorbed in the terminal ileum by an active process. Since cholesterol is absorbed more slowly than are fatty acids or monoglycerides, the concentration of cholesterol in micelles rises as chyme moves down the small intestine. Some lipids that are relatively soluble in water do not require micelles. These would include short-chain and medium-chain fatty acids and they can diffuse through the unstirred layer to allow absorption without micelle formation. This led to the practical therapeutic supplementation of medium-chain triglycerides in patients with gross fat maldigestion and malabsorption.

Although bile salts and pancreatic lipases are key factors in fat digestion and absorption, some fat is absorbed in the absence of these two agents. A normal adult male can absorb 150 to 200 g of fat daily. So efficient is the digestion-absorption process that less than 4 g of fat excreted in the feces daily is of dietary origin. Intestinal secretions and desquamation as well as contribution from the colonic flora accounts for 1 to 2 g of fat in the feces. Some dietary fat is incorporated into the gut bacteria, and approximately 40 per cent of the total fecal fat is in the bodies of bacteria; the remainder is in the form of nonbacterial solids. In complete absence of bile or pancreatic drainage, fat is lost in the stool in rough proportion to the amount present in the diet. In the absence of bile salts, half of the dietary fat is not absorbed, and in the absence of pancreatic digestive enzymes two thirds escapes digestion and absorption.

The most important condition of the biliary tract affecting nutrition is obstructive jaundice. This can arise from obstruction by stones in the common bile duct, or by tumors in the pancreas or in the biliary ductal system, or from strictures within the biliary apparatus subsequent to trauma or chronic inflammation. In these conditions, in contrast to uncomplicated gallstone disease, the disease itself may commonly and profoundly affect food intake. These patients are often anorexic and they can suffer from chronic abdominal pain exacerbated by eating. In addition, eating would induce diarrhea and steatorrhea, which in itself adds to the patient's symptoms. Therefore it is common to observe a decrease in total caloric intake.

Steatorrhea is common in obstructive jaundice. The degree of steatorrhea varies with the impairment of the entry of bile into the duodenum. However, as described above, there is still absorption of fat in the complete absence of bile drainage, and gross malnutrition due to altered fat metabolism as a result of cholestasis is uncommon. However, the maldigestion and malabsorption of fat also involves other fat-soluble vitamins and thus may result in serious consequences to the host. Phylloquinones and menaquinones, which are the naturally occurring forms of vitamins K_1 and K_2, are stored in the liver in very small quantities. Their absorption is poor in the absence of bile salts. With obstructive jaundice, the endogenous store of vitamin K declines rapidly, and without replenishment hypoprothrombinemia becomes manifest quickly, often within 2 to 3 weeks. With prolonged extrabiliary obstruction, there can be secondary hepatocellular damage, and the blood coagulation profile is often complicated by an inability to synthesize prothrombin, factors VII, IX, and X. The coagulopathy associated with obstructive jaundice sometimes makes surgical procedures hazardous. When it is severe, spontaneous bleeding can occur.

Disturbances in vitamin D metabolism are less apparent, because of the relatively large stores of vitamin D in the body compared with the store of vitamin K. Much of the daily requirement of vitamin D is synthesized in the skin on exposure to ultraviolet light. In the jaundiced patient, the bilirubin in the skin may interfere with this synthetic process, and therefore the level of vitamin D_3 may be lower. However, the endogenous store of vitamin D is usually adequate to last a year. Therefore, clinical signs of vitamin D deficiency are uncommon and treatment is usually unnecessary. With chronic biliary obstruction, such as due to strictures or primary biliary cirrhosis, clinical signs of vitamin D deficiency do occur. In some patients a low vitamin D level and impaired calcium absorption combine to produce osteomalacia. However, the level of vitamin D_3 (25-hydroxycholecalciferol) correlates poorly with the degree of osteomalacia. This is probably due to the fact that there are other active metabolites of vitamin D, such as 1,25-dihydroxycholecalciferol, which is the more potent form of vitamin D. The initial hydroxylation at the 25 position takes place in the liver, whereas the 1-hydroxylation takes place in the kidney. In some cases intraluminal absorption of dietary calcium may also be impaired, thus complicating the picture of vitamin D deficiency.[67] This calcium malabsorption can be improved by treatment with 25-hydroxy vitamin D_3. With steatorrhea, poor absorption of triglycerides may result in an excessive amount of long-chain fatty acids. These can form insoluble soaps (saponification) with calcium ions and thus immobilize calcium for absorption. Medium-chain triglycerides do not form insoluble calcium soaps. Occasionally, osteoporosis occurs in patients with chronic hepatobiliary diseases. The cause is probably multifactorial, including alterations in calcium balance, and chronic generalized nutritional deficiency. Patients who are treated with corticosteroids for diseases associated with biliary tract obstruction have a higher risk of developing osteoporosis, and vertebral collapse fractures are not uncommon, especially in postmenopausal women.

Vitamin A malabsorption also occurs with steatorrhea and biliary tract obstruction. Plasma vitamin A levels are low in patients with chronic biliary tract obstruction. Retinol (vitamin A_1) is stored in the liver and is released into the plasma bound to a retinol-binding protein. Patients with chronic biliary tract obstruction often have evidence of impaired dark adaptation. The clinical signs are often unrecognized by physicians. Uncommonly, overt night blindness may be present. Vitamin A deficiency may also be manifested by keratinization of the conjunctiva and cornea, and there may be an impairment in the recognition of taste and smell.

Malabsorption of vitamin E also occurs, but again the clinical signs are often unrecognized or unrecognizable. The serum tocopherol level is decreased in patients with chronic obstructive jaundice. Vitamin E is an antioxidant; in its absence or deficient state, peroxidation of lipids occurs, and this can lead to hemolysis as well as to the accumulation of peroxidized pigments. These brown pigments (lipofuscins) sometimes accumulate in the wall of the gastrointestinal tract, giving rise to the appearance of the "brown bowel syndrome."[187,188] It is postulated that these pigmented molecules can induce abnormal function in the mitochondria of the mucosal cells, and that in itself may aggravate malabsorption. There is some evidence that treatment of the vitamin E deficiency can reverse the pigmentation of the intestines, but whether a functional improvement accompanies the disappearance of the lipofuscin granules is unproven.

NUTRITIONAL ASPECTS OF TREATMENT OF GALLSTONE DISEASE

With the controversy and confusion existing in the role of diet in the pathogenesis of gallstones as reviewed above, it is understandable that there has also been much confusion in regard to the prevention or treatment of gallstone disease by dietary means. As discussed in the review dealing with the epidemiological and metabolic studies of diet and gallstone disease, many of the claims have been neither substantiated nor confirmed. It can be accepted, however, that in the epidemiology of gallstone disease, obesity is a definite risk factor.[117,169] The data suggest that obese people have about twice the risk for gallstones,[117] and in case-control studies, obesity was associated with increased risk especially in young women.[169] A low-fat, low-cholesterol diet is usually advised, although there are no clear and convincing data that a high-fat diet has been implicated to be a

risk factor. Some physicians recommend this regimen only for those with an underlying hypertriglyceridemia or morbid obesity. It is prudent to limit total caloric intake, as increased total energy consumption is correlated with an increased risk of gallstone formation. The effect of highly refined carbohydrates and dietary fiber require further investigation, but there is some evidence to suggest that an increased amount of fiber and a reduced amount of highly refined carbohydrate may exert a beneficial effect in the prevention of gallstone disease.[190] At the same time, factors that can raise the lithogenicity of bile, such as hypocholesterolemic agents and oral contraceptive pills, should also be considered in the context of their desired therapeutic effects.

When gallstones have formed, it is highly doubtful that any change in the diet would dissolve the stones with any degree of efficacy. It has been claimed that a diet high in fiber contents assisted or enhanced medical dissolution of cholesterol gallstones using bile acid therapy.[191] However, this needs further confirmation. It used to be believed that patients with gallstones should not be given dietary fat for fear of inducing symptoms of pain and dyspepsia. The reason usually given is that fat increases cholecystokinin secretion and gallbladder contractility. The necessity of avoiding fat has never been examined critically and has been recently questioned.[184] It appears that unless fat induces symptoms in these patients, it is not necessary specifically to cut down the normal amount of dietary fat consumption.

NUTRITIONAL MANAGEMENT OF OBSTRUCTIVE JAUNDICE

For patients developing acute cessation of bile flow into the duodenum, relatively little impairment of nutritional disturbance would result and it is usually not necessary to institute any nutritional supplement. If obstruction lasts longer than 2 weeks, vitamin K deficiency may be present; in such cases it is advisable to supplement with parenteral vitamin K, especially if there are any diagnostic or surgical procedures to be done. However, the coagulopathy associated with hepatocellular damage may not be correctable with vitamin K alone, and it is also important that vitamin K should not be given excessively. A reasonable regimen would consist of 10 mg of vitamin K for a period of 5 days. Large amounts of vitamin K may even depress prothrombin levels.[192] Usually, this therapy will correct vitamin K deficiency due to straightforward biliary tract obstruction promptly.

Although there is a definite degree of fat maldigestion and malabsorption in biliary tract obstruction, this is usually not important in the total management of a patient with acute or reversible biliary tract obstruction. However, as discussed above, sometimes steatorrhea can be symptomatic, and in such a case dietary fat restriction may give symptomatic control. In contrast, patients with chronic cholestasis due to congenital or chronic inflammatory diseases, such as biliary atresia and primary biliary cirrhosis, often require more active nutritional intervention. Troublesome steatorrhea can sometimes be controlled with restriction in dietary long-chain fatty acids. Occasionally, patients with chronic cholestasis present with pruritus, and bile salt–binding resins such as cholestyramine are used to relieve the itch. It is important to bear in mind that cholestyramine would further aggravate the malabsorption by binding what little bile salts are available in the intestines, and long-term use of cholestyramine may carry an increased risk of development of cholesterol gallstones. In severe cases of steatorrhea or in young children, in whom for the purpose of growth it is necessary to increase the total caloric intake, supplementation using medium-chain triglycerides may be considered. Medium-chain triglycerides have chain lengths of 8 to 10 carbons. For example, a typical solution (Scientific Hospital Supplies Ltd.) consists of triglycerides with the following proportion of carbon chain lengths: C6 (1.1 per cent), C8 (81.1 per cent), C10 (15.7 per cent), C12 (2.1 per cent); these are relatively soluble and do not require micellar solubilization or enzymatic lipolysis before absorption. Once in the enterocytes, these triglycerides do not require re-esterification before passing to the liver in a form available for further metabolism. The solution should be introduced slowly, in increasing amounts. For a total caloric intake of 1500 kcal daily, a good target would be to have 50 g of medium-chain triglycerides, and this may be varied proportionally. Excessive use of this product may produce some ketosis and acidosis, which may require supplementation of sodium bicarbonate.

With chronic biliary obstruction, there is also malabsorption of vitamins A, D, and E. Again the degree of deficiency depends on the length of obstruction and the degree of obstruction. Many of the consequences of vitamin deficiency due to biliary tract disease are not recognized by clinicians, and the symptoms of vitamin deficiency are often attributed to the symptoms of the chronic illness itself. If obstruction is complete or nearly complete, supplementations of vitamins A, D, and K and probably E should be given on a regular and long-term basis. This can be done by giving monthly or bimonthly injections of these fat-soluble vitamins. Calcium supplements in such a case should also be considered, particularly in postmenopausal women. It is necessary to remember that vitamin D and dietary calcium supplements should not be given routinely, especially in cases in which the biliary tract obstruction is reversible. When these two compounds are given, serum calcium should be monitored to avoid the possibility of hypercalcemia.

References

1. Iber FL. Alcohol and the gastrointestinal tract. Gastroenterology 1971; 61:120–123.
2. Fallon HJ. Alcoholic Hepatitis. In Schiff L, Schiff ER (eds). Diseases of the Liver. 5th ed. Philadelphia, JB Lippincott, 1982: 693–708.
3. Lieber CS, Jones DP, DeCarli LM. Effects of prolonged ethanol intake: production of fatty liver despite adequate diets. J Clin Invest 1965; 44:1009–1021.
4. Lieber CS, DeCarli LM, Rubin E. Sequential production of fatty liver, hepatitis and cirrhosis in sub-human primates fed ethanol with adequate diets. Proc Natl Acad Sci USA 1975; 72:437–441.
5. Bebb HT, Houser HB, Witschi JC, et al. Calorie and nutrient contribution of caloric beverages to the usual diets of 155 adults. Am J Clin Nutr 1971; 24:1042–1052.
6. Westerfield WW, Schulman MP. Metabolism and caloric value of alcohol. JAMA 1959; 170:197–203.
7. Braillon A, Capron JP, Hervé MA, et al. Liver in obesity. Gut 1985; 26:133–139.
8. Miller DJ, Ishimaru K, Klatskin G. Non-alcoholic liver disease mimicking alcoholic hepatitis and cirrhosis. (Abstract.) Gastroenterology 1979; 77:27.
9. Ludwig J, Viggiano TR, McGill DB, et al. Non-alcoholic steatohepatitis. Mayo Clinic experiences with hitherto unnamed disease. Mayo Clin Proc 1980; 55:434–438.
10. Lee SP. Enhanced hepatic fibrogenesis in the cholesterol-fed mouse. Clin Sci 1981; 61:253–256.
11. Marubbio AT, Buchwald H, Schwartz MZ, et al. Hepatic lesions of central pericellular fibrosis in morbid obesity, and after jejuno-ileal bypass. Am J Clin Pathol 1976; 66:684–691.
12. Grant JP, Cox CE, Kleinman LM, et al. Serum hepatic enzyme and bilirubin elevations during parenteral nutrition. Surg Gynecol Obstet 1977; 145:573–580.
13. Benjamin DR. Hepatobiliary dysfunction in infants and children associated with longterm total parenteral nutrition. A clinicopathologic study. Am J Clin Pathol 1981; 76:276–283.
14. Dahms BB, Halpin TC. Serial liver biopsies in parenteral nutrition–associated cholestasis of early infancy. Gastroenterology 1981; 81:136–144.
15. Cohen S, Olsen MM. Pediatric total parenteral nutrition. Liver histopathology. Arch Pathol Lab Med 1981; 105:152–156.
16. Burke JF, Wolfe RR, Mullany DE, et al. Glucose requirement following burn injury. Ann Surg 1979; 190:274–285.
17. Koga Y, Ikeda K, Inokuchi K. Effect of complete parenteral nutrition using fat emulsion on liver. Ann Surg 1975; 181:186–190.
18. McDonald ATJ, Phillips MJ, Jeejeebhoy KN. Reversal of fatty liver by intralipid in patients on total parenteral nutrition. Gastroenterology 1973; 64:885.
19. Sheldon GF, Peterson SR, Sanders R. Hepatic dysfunction during hyperalimentation. Arch Surg 1978; 113:504–508.
20. Hall RI, Grant JP, Ross LH, et al. Pathogenesis of hepatic steatosis in the parenterally fed rat. J Clin Invest 1984; 74:1658–1668.
21. Charlton RW, Hawkins DM, Mavor WO, et al. Hepatic storage iron concentration in different population groups. Am J Clin Nutr 1970; 23:358–370.
22. Green R, Charlton R, Seftel H, et al. Body iron excretion in man. A collaborative study. Am J Med 1968; 45:336–353.
23. Bothwell TH. Oral iron overload. S Afr Med J 1965; 39:892–899.
24. Grace ND, Powell LW. Iron storage disorders of the liver. Gastroenterology 1974; 67:1257–1283.
25. Bothwell TH, Charlton RW. Hemochromatosis. In Schiff L, Schiff ER (eds). Diseases of the Liver. 5th ed. Philadelphia, JB Lippincott, 1982: 1003–1042.

26. Sass-Kortsak A, Bearn AG. Hereditary disorders of copper metabolism. *In* Stanbury JB, Wyngaarden JB, Frederickson DS (eds). The Metabolic Basis of Inherited Disease. 4th ed. New York, McGraw-Hill, 1978: 1098–1126.
27. Scheinberg IH, Morell AG. Ceruloplasmin. *In* Eichhorn GL (ed). Inorganic Biochemistry. Vol. I. New York, Elsevier, 1973: 306–319.
28. Frommer DJ. Defective biliary excretion of copper in Wilson's disease. Gut 1974; *15*:125–129.
29. Sternlieb I. Copper and the liver. Gastroenterology 1980; *78*:1615–1628.
30. Sternlieb I, Scheinberg IH. Wilson's disease. *In* Wright R, Alberti KGMM, Karran S, et al. (eds). Liver and Biliary Tract Disease. London, Saunders, 1979: 774–787.
31. Herbert V. Toxicity of 25,000 IU vitamin A supplements in "health" food users. Am J Clin Nutr 1982; *36*:185–186.
32. Hatoff DE. Hypervitaminosis A unmasked by acute viral hepatitis. Gastroenterology 1982; *82*:124–128.
33. Baraona, E, Pinola RC, Lieber CS. Small intestinal damage and changes in cell population produced by ethanol ingestion in the rat. Gastroenterology 1974; *66*:226–234.
34. Rubin E, Rybak BJ, Lindenbaum J, et al. Ultrastructural changes in the small intestine induced by ethanol. Gastroenterology 1972; *63*:801—814.
35. Mezey E, Jow E, Slavin RE, et al. Pancreatic function and intestinal absorption in chronic alcoholism. Gastroenterology 1970; *59*:657–664.
36. Mezey E. Intestinal function in chronic alcoholism. Ann NY Acad Sci 1975; *252*:215–227.
37. Mezey E, Potter JJ. Changes in exocrine pancreatic function produced by altered dietary protein intake in drinking alcoholics. Johns Hopkins Med J 1976; *138*:7–12.
38. Malagelada JR, Pihl O, Linscheer WG. Impaired absorption of micellar long-chain fatty acids in patients with alcoholic cirrhosis. Am J Dig Dis 1974; *19*:1016–1020.
39. Lee SP, Lai KS. Exocrine pancreatic function in hepatic cirrhosis. Am J Gastroenterol 1976; *65*:244–248.
40. Vlahcevic ZR, Buhac I, Farran JT, et al. Bile acid metabolism in patients with cirrhosis. I: Kinetic aspects of cholic acid metabolism. Gastroenterology 1971; *60*:491–498.
41. Lee SP, Nicholson GI. Ceroid enteropathy and vitamin E deficiency. NZ Med J 1976; *83*:318–320.
42. Lee SP. Vitamin E in the treatment of the brown bowel syndrome. Mayo Clin Proc 1980; *54*:752.
43. Owen OE, Reichle FA, Mozzoli MA, et al. Hepatic, gut, and renal substrate flux rates in patients with hepatic cirrhosis. J Clin Invest 1981; *68*:240–252.
44. Owen OE, Trapp VE, Reichard GA Jr, et al. Nature and quantity of fuels consumed in patients with alcoholic cirrhosis. J Clin Invest 1983; *72*:1821–1832.
45. Alberti KGMM, Record CO, Williamson DH. Metabolic changes in active chronic hepatitis. Clin Sci 1972; *42*:591–605.
46. Rothschild MA, Oratz M, Zimmon D, et al. Albumin synthesis in cirrhotic subjects with ascites studied with carbonate-[14]C. J Clin Invest 1969; *48*:344–350.
47. Kirsch R, Frith L, Black E. Regulation of albumin synthesis and catabolism by alteration of dietary protein. Nature 1968; *217*:578–579.
48. Deutsch E. Blood coagulation changes in liver diseases. *In* Popper H, Schaffner F (eds). Progress in Liver Diseases. New York, Grune & Stratton, 1965: 69–83.
49. Roberts HR, Cederbaum AI. The liver and blood coagulation: physiology and pathology. Gastroenterology 1972; *63*:287–320.
50. Rudman D, DiFulco TJ, Galambos JT, et al. Maximum rates of excretion and synthesis of mean in normal and cirrhotic subjects. J Clin Invest 1973; *52*:2241–2249.
51. Khatra BS, Smith RB III, Millikan WJ. Activities of Krebs-Henseleit enzymes in normal and cirrhotic human liver. J Lab Clin Med 1974; *84*:708–715.
52. Teng CS, Ho PWM, Yeung RTT. Down-regulation of insulin receptors in postnecrotic cirrhosis of the liver. J Clin Endocr Metab 1982; *55*:524–530.
53. Simon JB, Kepkay DL, Poon R. Serum cholesterol esterification in human liver disease: role of lecithin-cholesterol acyltransferase and cholesterol ester hydrolase. Gastroenterology 1974; *66*:539–547.
54. Sabesin SM, Bertram PD, Freeman MR. Lipoprotein metabolism in liver disease. Adv Intern Med 1980; *25*:117–146.
55. Mistillis SP, Ockner RK. Effect of ethanol on endogenous lipid and lipoprotein metabolism in small intestine. J Lab Clin Med 1972; *80*:34–36.
56. Manzato E, Fellin R, Baggio G, et al. Formation of lipoprotein-X: its relationship to bile compounds. J Clin Invest 1976; *57*:1248–1260.
57. Marco J, Diego J, Villaneuva ML, et al. Elevated plasma glucagon levels in cirrhosis of the liver. N Engl J Med 1973; *289*:1107–1111.
58. Morgan AG, Kelleher J, Walker BE, et al. Nutrition in cryptogenic cirrhosis and chronic aggressive hepatitis. Gut 1976; *17*:113–118.
59. Leevy CM, Thompson A, Baker H. Vitamin and liver injury. Am J Clin Nutr 1970; *23*:493–499.
60. Hines JD, Cowan DH. Studies on the pathogenesis of alcohol-induced sideroblastic bone marrow abnormalities. N Engl J Med 1970; *283*:441–446.
61. Lumeng L, Li TK. Vitamin B_6 metabolism in chronic alcohol abuse: pyridoxal phosphate levels in plasma and the effects of acetaldehyde on pyridoxal phosphate synthesis and degradation of human erythrocytes. J Clin Invest 1974; *53*:693–704.
62. Leevy CM, Kiernan T. Nutritional factors and liver disease. *In* Read AE (ed). Modern Trends in Gastroenterology. London, Butterworth, 1975: 250–261.
63. Eichner ER, Pierce HI, Hillman RS. Folate balance in dietary-induced megaloblastic anemia. N Engl J Med 1971; *284*:933–938.
64. Paine CJ, Eichner ER, Dickson V. Concordance of radioassay and microbiological assay in the study of ethanol-induced fall in serum folate level. Am J Med Sci 1973; *266*:135–138.
65. Smith FR, Goodman DS. The effects of diseases of the liver, thyroid and kidneys on the transport of vitamin A in human plasma. J Clin Invest 1971; *50*:2426–2436.
66. Hepner GW, Roginsky M, Moo HF. Abnormal vitamin D metabolism in patients with cirrhosis. Am J Dig Dis 1976; *21*:527–532.
67. Bengoa JM, Sitrin MD, Meredith S, et al. Intestinal calcium absorption and vitamin D status in chronic cholestatic liver disease. Hepatology 1984; *4*:261–265.
68. Mobarhan SA, Russell RM, Recker RR, et al. Metabolic bone disease in alcoholic cirrhosis: a comparison of the effect of vitamin D2, 25-hydroxyvitamin D, or supportive treatment. Hepatology 1984; *4*:266–273.
69. Reed JS, Meredith SC, Nemchansky BA, et al. Bone changes in primary biliary cirrhosis: reversal of osteomalacia with oral 25-hydroxyvitamin D. Gastroenterology 1980; *78*:512–517.
70. Herlong HF, Recker RR, Maddrey WC. Bone disease in primary biliary cirrhosis: histologic features and response to 25-hydroxyvitamin D. Gastroenterology 1982; *83*:103–108.
71. Stein JH, Smith WD, Ginn HE. Hypophosphatemia in acute alcoholism. Am J Med Sci 1966; *252*:78–83.
72. Tasman-Jones C, Kay RG, Lee SP. Zinc and copper deficiency with particular reference to parenteral nutrition. Surg Annual 1978; *10*:23–52.
73. Hoagland CL, Labby DH, Kankel HC, et al. An analysis of the effect of fat in the diet on recovery in viral hepatitis. Am J Publ Health 1946; *36*:1287–1292.
74. Chalmers TC, Eckhardt RD, Reynolds WE, et al. The treatment of acute infectious hepatitis: studies of the effect of diets, rest, and physical reconditioning on the acute course of the disease and on the incidence of relapse and residual abnormalities. J Clin Invest 1955; *34*:1163–1235.
75. Farivar M, Bucher NLR, Wands J, et al. Beneficial effect of

insulin and glucagon on fulminant murine hepatitis. Gastroenterology 1976, *70*:981.

76. Mosley JW, Galambos JT. Viral hepatitis. *In* Schiff L (ed). Diseases of the Liver. Philadelphia, JB Lippincott, 1975: 500–593.

77. Bassendine MF, Della Seta L, Salmeron J, et al. Incidence of hepatitis B viral infection in alcoholic liver disease. HBsAg negative chronic active liver disease and primary liver cell cancer in Britain. Liver 1983; *3*:65–70.

78. Zieve L. The mechanism of hepatic coma. Hepatology 1981; *1*:360–365.

79. Jones EA, Schafer DF, Ferenci P, et al. The neurobiology of hepatic encephalopathy. Hepatology 1984; *4*:1235–1242.

80. Fischer JE, Funovic JM, Aguirre A, et al. The role of plasma amino acids in hepatic encephalopathy. Surgery 1975; *78*:276–290.

81. Fischer JE, Yoshimura N, Aguirre A, et al. Plasma amino acid in patients with hepatic encephalopathy: effects of amino acid infusions. Am J Surg 1974; *127*:40–47.

82. Conn HO, Leevy CM, Vlahcevic ZR, et al. Comparison of lactulose and neomycin in the treatment of chronic portal-systemic encephalopathy. Gastroenterology 1977; *72*:573–583.

83. Rossi-Fanelli F, Riggio O, Cangiano C, et al. Branched-chain amino acids vs lactulose in the treatment of hepatic coma: a controlled study. Dig Dis Sci 1982; *27*:929–935.

84. Wahren J, Denis J, Desurmont P, et al. Is intravenous administration of branched chain amino acids effective in the treatment of hepatic encephalopathy? A multicenter study. Hepatology 1983; *3*:475–480.

84a. Cerra FB, Cheung NK, Fischer JE, et al. A multicenter trial of branch chain enriched amino acid infusion (F080) in hepatic encephalopathy. (Abstract.) Hepatology 1982; *2*:699.

85. Horst D, Grace ND, Conn HO, et al. Comparison of dietary protein with an oral branched chain–enriched amino acid supplement in chronic portal-systemic encephalopathy: a randomised trial. Hepatology 1984; *4*:279–287.

86. Freund H, Yoshimura N, Fischer JE. Chronic hepatic encephalopathy—long-term therapy with a branched-chain and amino-acid-enriched elemental diet. JAMA 1979; *242*:347–349.

87. Eriksson LS, Person A, Wahren J. Branched-chain amino acids in the treatment of chronic hepatic encephalopathy. Gut 1982; *23*:801–806.

88. McGhee A, Henderson M, Millikan W, et al. Comparison of the effects of Hepatic-Aid and a casein modular diet on encephalopathy, plasma amino acids, and nitrogen balance in cirrhotic patients. Ann Surg 1983; *197*:288–293.

89. Ingelfinger FJ. Digestive disease as a national problem. V: Gall stones. Gastroenterology 1968; *55*:102–104.

90. Almy TP. Prevalence and significance of digestive disease. Gastroenterology 1975; *68*:1351–1371.

91. Hoppe-Seyler H. Cholelithiasis. *In* Nothnagel's Encyclopaedia of Practical Medicine. American Edition. Philadelphia, WB Saunders, 1903; *6*:525–607.

92. Thudichum JLW. A treatise on gall stones; their chemistry, pathology and treatment. London, John Churchill & Sons, 1963: 37.

93. Frerichs FT. A Clinical Treatise on Diseases of the Liver. Vol. 2. London, New Sydenham Society, 1861: 510.

94. Budd G. On Diseases of the Liver. London, John Churchill & Sons. 1852: 358.

95. Lindstrom CG. Frequency of gallstone disease in a well-defined Swedish population. A prospective necropsy study. Scand J Gastroenterology 1977; *12*:341–346.

96. Sampliner RE, Bennett PH, Comers LJ, et al. Gallbladder disease in Pima Indians. Demonstration of high prevalence and early onset by cholecystography. N Engl J Med 1970; *283*:1358–1364.

97. Marinovic I, Guerra C, Larach G. Incidencia de litiasis biliar en material de autopsias y analisis de composicion de los calculos. Rev Med Chile 1972; *100*:1320–1327.

98. Zahor Z. Atherosclerosis in relation to cholelithiasis and cholesterolosis. Bull WHO 1976; *53*:531–537.

99. Doouss TW, Castleden WM. Gallstones and carcinoma of the large bowel. NZ Med J 1973; *77*:162–165.

100. Bateson MC, Bouchier IAD. Prevalence of gallstones in Dundee: a necropsy study. Br Med J 1975; *4*:427–430.

101. Torvik A, Hoivik B. Gallstones in an autopsy series. Incidence, complications and correlations with carcinoma of the gall bladder. Acta Chir Scand 1960; *120*:168–174.

102. Hogan J, Lonergan M, Holland PDJ. The incidence of cholelithiasis in an autopsy series. J Irish Med Assoc 1977; *70*:608–611.

103. Kalos A, Dalidou A, Kordosis T, et al. The incidence of gallstones in Greece: an autopsy study. Acta Hepatogastroenterol 1977; *24*:20–23.

104. Stitnimankarn T. The necroscopy incidence of gallstones in Thailand. Am J Med Sci 1960; *240*:349–352.

105. Newman HG, Northrup JD. The autopsy incidence of gallstones. Int Abstr Surg 1959; *109*:1–13.

106. Rodewald H. Zur Pathologie der Gallenblase. II: Über die Häufigkeit der Gallensteine. Zbl Allg Path 1957; *96*:301.

107. Salzer GM, Olbrich E, Kutschera H. Zur Epidemiologie der Cholelithiasis. Acta Hepatogastroenterol 1970; *17*:65–74.

108. Horn G. Observations on the aetiology of cholelithiasis. Br Med J 1956; *2*:732–737.

109. Hurang WS. Cholelithiasis in Singapore. Gut 1970; *11*:141–152.

110. Koutselinis A, Boukis D, Kalapothaki V, et al. Postmortem study of the prevalence of gallstones in Athens. Digestion 1975; *13*:304–307.

111. Miayake H. Gallstones in Orient and Occident. *In* Proceed Third World Congress Gastroenterol. Tokyo, 1966; *4*:148–155.

112. Sarles H, Gerolami A, Cros RD. Diet and cholesterol gallstones. A multicentre study. Digestion 1978; *17*:121–127.

113. Ehrstrom R. The prevalence of gallstones and the standard of living in Finland 1836–1939. Nordisk Med 1942; *14*:1559–1565.

114. Kameda H. Gallstones. Compositions, structural characteristics and geographical distribution. *In* Proceed Third World Congress Gastroenterol. Tokyo, 1966. *4*:117–124.

115. Insull W, Oiso T, Tsuchiya K. Diet and nutritional status of Japanese. Am J Clin Nutr 1968; *21*:753–777.

116. Carey MC. Biliary lipids and gallstone formation. *In* Csomós G, Thaler H (eds). Clinical Hepatology. Heidelberg, Springer-Verlag, 1983; *5*:52–69.

117. Bennion LJ, Grundy SM. Risk factors for the development of cholelithiasis in man. N Engl J Med 1978; *299*:1221–1227.

118. Sarles H, Hauton S, Lafont H, et al. Effect of diet on the biliary cholesterol concentration in normals and gallstone patients. Clin Chim Acta 1968; *19*:147–155.

119. Sarles H, Hauton S, Planche N, et al. Diet, cholesterol gallstones and composition of the bile. Am J Dig Dis 1970; *15*:251–260.

120. Bennion LJ, Grundy SM. Effect of obesity and calorie intake on biliary lipid metabolism in man. J Clin Invest 1975; *56*:996–1011.

121. Dam H, Kruse I, Jensen K, et al. Studies on human bile. II. Influence of two different fats on the composition of human bile. Scand J Clin Lab Invest 1967; *19*:367–378.

122. Grundy SM. Effects of polyunsaturated fats on lipid metabolism in patients with hypertriglyceridemia. J Clin Invest 1975; *55*:269–282.

123. Van der Linden W, Nakayam F. Effect of intravenous fat emulsion on hepatic bile. Acta Chir Scand 1976; *142*:401–406.

124. Lewis B. Effects of certain dietary oils on bile-acid secretion and serum cholesterol. Lancet 1958; *1*:1090–1092.

125. Watanabe N, Gimbel NS, Johnston CG. Effect of polyunsaturated and saturated fatty acid on the cholesterol holding capacity of human bile. Arch Surg 1962; *85*:136–141.

126. Grundy SM, Metzger AL. A physiological method for estimation of hepatic biliary lipids in man. Gastroenterology 62:1200–1217.

127. Andersen E, Hellstrom K. The effects of cholesterol feeding on bile acid kinetics and biliary lipids in normolipidemic and hypertriglyceridemic subjects. J Lipid Res 1979; 20:1020–1027.

128. Andersen E, Hellstrom K. Influence of fat-rich versus carbohydrate-rich diets on bile acid kinetics, biliary lipids, and net steroid balance in hyperlipidemic subjects. Metabolism 1980; 29:400–409.

129. Hepner GW. Effect of decreased gallbladder stimulation on enterohepatic cycling and kinetics of bile acids. Gastroenterology 1975; 68:1574–1581.

130. Aschoff G. The origin of gallstones. In Lectures on Pathology. New York, Hoeber, 1924: 206–232.

131. Bhattathing EPM, Siperstein MD. Feedback control of cholesterol synthesis in man. J Clin Invest 1963; 42:1613–1618.

132. Quintao E, Grundy SM. Arhrens EH. Effects of dietary cholesterol on the regulation of total body cholesterol in man. J Lipid Res 1971; 12:233–247.

133. Nestel PJ, Poyser A. Changes in cholesterol synthesis and excretion when cholesterol intake is increased. Metabolism 1976; 25:1591–1599.

134. Lin DS, Conner WE. The longterm effects of dietary cholesterol upon the plasma lipids, lipoprotein, cholesterol absorption and the steroid balance in man: the demonstration of feedback inhibition of cholesterol biosynthesis and increased bile acid excretion. J Lipid Res 1980; 21:1042–1052.

135. Wilson JD, Lindsey CA. Studies on the influence of dietary cholesterols on cholesterol metabolism in the isotopic steady state in man. J Clin Invest 1965; 44:1805–1814.

136. Conner WE, Lin DS. The intestinal absorption of dietary cholesterol by hypercholesterolemic (types II) and normocholesterolemic humans. J Clin Invest 1974; 53:1062–1070.

137. Dam H, Prange I, Jensen K, et al. Studies on human bile. IV. Influence of ingestion of cholesterol in the form of eggs on the composition of bile in healthy subjects. Z Ernährungswiss 1971; 10:178–187.

138. Sarles H, Crotte C, Gerolami A, et al. Influences of cholestyramine, bile salt and cholesterol feeding on the lipid composition of hepatic bile in man. Scand J Gastroenterol 1970; 5:603–608.

139. DenBesten L, Conner WE, Bell S. The effect of dietary cholesterol on the composition of human bile. Surgery 1973; 73:266–273.

140. Maudgal DP, Bird R, Blackwood WS, et al. Low-cholesterol diet: enhancement of effect of CDCA in patients with gallstones. Br Med J 1978; 2:851–853.

141. Cohen H, Marks JW, Bonorris GG. Alteration of dietary cholesterol influences biliary saturation in gallstone patients. (Abstract.) Gastroenterology 1980; 79:1010.

142. Biss K, Ho KJ, Mikkelson B. Some unique biologic characteristics of the Masai of East Africa. N Engl J Med 1971; 284:694–699.

143. Hoffman NE, Hofman AF, Thistle JL. Effect of bile acid feeding on cholesterol metabolism in gallstone patients. Mayo Clin Proc 1974; 49:236–239.

144. Pedersen L, Arnfred T, Thaysen EH. Turnover of plasma cholesterol in patients with cholesterol gallstones. Acta Med Scand 1975; 197:421–425.

145. Trowell H. The development of the concept of dietary fiber in human nutrition. Am J Clin Nutr 1978; 31:S3–S11.

146. Heaton KW. Bile Salts in Health and Disease. Edinburgh, Churchill Livingstone, 1972: 156.

147. Burkitt DP. Some diseases characteristic of modern Western civilisation. Br Med J 1973; 1:274–278.

148. Pomare EW, Heaton KW, Low-Beer TS, et al. The effect of wheat bran upon bile salt metabolism and upon the lipid composition of bile in gallstone patients. Am J Dig Dis 1976; 21:521–526.

149. McDougall RM, Yakymyshyn L, Walker K, et al. Effect of wheat bran on serum lipoproteins and biliary lipids. Can J Surg 1978; 21:433–435.

150. Watts JM, Jablonski P, Toouli J. The effect of added bran to the diet on the saturation of bile in people without gallstones. Am J Surg 1978; 135::321–324.

151. Wicks ACB, Yeates J, Heaton KW. Bran and bile: time-course of changes in normal young men given a standard dose. Scand J Gastroenterol 1978; 13:289–292.

152. Huijbregts AWM, Van Berge–Henegonwen GP, Hectors MPC, et al. Effects of a standardized wheat bran preparation on biliary lipid composition and bile acid metabolism in young healthy males. Eur J Clin Invest 1980; 10:451–458.

153. Tarpila S, Miettinen TA, Metsaranta L. Effect of bran on serum cholesterol, faecal mass, fat, bile acids and neutral sterols and biliary lipids in patients with diverticular disease of the colon. Gut 1978; 19:137–145.

154. Low-Beer TS, Nulten S. Colonic bacterial activity, biliary cholesterol saturation and pathogenesis of gallstones. Lancet 1978; 2:1063–1065.

155. Carulli N, Ponz de Leon M, Loria M, et al. Effect of the selective expansion of cholic acid pool on bile lipid composition: possible mechanism of bile acid induced biliary cholesterol saturation. Gastroenterology 1981; 81:539–546.

156. Thornton JR, Heaton KW. Do colonic bacteria contribute to cholesterol gallstone formation? Effects of lactulose on bile. Br Med J 1981; 282:1018–1020.

157. Meyer PD, DenBesten L, Mason EE. The effects of a high-fiber diet on bile acid pool size, bile acid kinetics, and biliary lipid secretory rates in the morbidly obese. Surgery 1979; 85:311–316.

158. Bryden WG, Borup-Christensen S, Van der Linden W, et al. The effect of dietary psyllium hydrocolloid and lignin on bile. Z Ernährungswiss 1979; 18:77–80.

159. Redinger RN, Grace DM. Cholestyramine induced cholesterol gallstones in the baboon. Clin Res 1976; 24:666A.

160. Chalin E, Jensson J, Nilsson S, et al. Biliary lipid composition in normolipidemic and pre-betahyperlipoproteinemic gallstone patients. Scand J Gastroenterol 1973; 8:449–456.

161. Marin GA, Ward NL, Fischer R. Effects of ethanol on pancreatic and biliary secretions in humans. Am J Dig Dis 1973; 18:825–833.

162. Sewell RB, Mao SJT, Kawamoto T, et al. Apolipoproteins of high, low, and very low density lipoproteins in human bile. J Lipid Res 1983; 24:391–401.

163. Thornton JR, Heaton KW, MacFarlane DG. A relation between high density lipoprotein cholesterol and bile cholesterol saturation. Br Med J 1981; 283:1352–1354.

164. Petitti DB, Friedman GD, Klatsky AL. Association of a history of gallbladder disease with a reduced concentration of high-density-lipoprotein cholesterol. N Engl J Med 1981; 304:1396–1398.

165. Thornton JR. Moderate alcohol intake reduces bile cholesterol saturation and raises HDL cholesterol. Lancet 1983; 2:819–822.

166. Holzbach RT, Kibe A, Thiel E, et al. Biliary proteins: unique inhibitors of cholesterol crystal nucleation in human gallbladder bile. J Clin Invest 1984; 73:35–45.

167. Lee SP, LaMont JT, Carey MC. Role of galbladder mucus hypersecretion in the evolution of cholesterol gallstones. J Clin Invest 1981; 67:1712–1723.

168. Scragg RKR, McMichael AJ, Seamark RF. Oral contraceptives, pregnancy and endogenous oestrogen in gallstone disease—a case-control study. Br Med J 1984; 288:1795–1799.

169. Scragg RKR, McMichael AJ, Borghurst PA. Diet, alcohol, and relative weight in gallstone disease: a case-control study. Br Med J 1984; 288:1113–1119.

170. Scragg RKR, Calvert GD, Oliver JR. Plasma lipids and insulin in gallstone disease: a case-control study. Br Med J 1984; 289:521–525.

171. Heaton KW. Gallstones. *In* Trowell HC, Burkitt DP (eds). Western Diseases: Their Emergence and Prevention. London, Edward Arnold, 1981: 47–59.

172. Schwartz CG, Almonde HR, Vlahcevic ZR. Bile acid metabolism in cirrhosis. V. Determination of biliary lipid secretion rates in patients with advanced cirrhosis. Gastroenterology 1979; 77:1177–1182.

173. Vlahcevic ZR, Yoshida T, Juttidjudata P, et al. Bile acid metabolism in cirrhosis. IV. Biliary lipid secretion in patients with cirrhosis and its relevance to gallstone formation. Gastroenterology 1973; 64:298–303.

174. Cohen C, Olsen MM. Pediatric total parenteral nutrition: liver histopathology. Arch Pathol Lab Med 1981; 105:152–156.

175. Stiges-Serra A. Pallares R, Jaurrieta E, et al. Clinical, biochemical and morphological studies of liver function in adult patients on total parenteral nutrition. *In* Kleinberger G, Deutsch E (eds). New Aspects of Clinical Nutrition. Basel, S Karger, 1983: 540–547.

176. Allardyce DB. Cholestasis caused by lipid emulsions. Surg Gynecol Obstet 1982; 154:641–647.

177. Capron JP, Gineston JL, Herve MA, et al. Metronidazole in prevention of cholestasis associated with total parenteral nutrition. Lancet 1983; 1:446–447.

178. Carey MC, Wu SF, Watkins JB. Solution properties of sulfated monohydroxy bile salts: relative insolubility of the disodium salt of glycolithocholate sulfate. Biochim Biophys Acta 1979; 575:16–26.

179. Toulonkian RG, Seashore JH. Hepatic secretory obstruction with total parenteral nutrition in the infant. J Pediatr Surg 1975; 10:353–360.

180. Petersen SR, Sheldon GF. Acute acalculous cholecystitis: a complication of hyperalimentation. Am J Surg 1979; 138:814–817.

181. Roslyn JJ, Pitt HA, Mann LL, et al. Gallbladder disease in patients on long-term parenteral nutrition. Gastroenterology 1983; 84:148–154.

182. Messing B, Borics C, Kunstlinger F, et al. Does total parenteral nutrition induce gallbladder sludge formation and lithiasis? Gastroenterology 1983; 84:1012–1019.

183. Pitt HA, King W, Mann LL, et al. Increased risk of cholelithiasis with prolonged total parenteral nutrition. Am J Surg 1983; 145:106–112.

184. Mogadam M, Albarelli J, Ahmed SW, et al. Gallbladder dynamics in response to various meals: is dietary fat restriction necessary in the management of gallstones? Am J Gastroenterol 1984; 79:745–747.

185. Patton JS. Gastrointestinal lipid digestion. *In* Johnson LR (ed). Physiology of the Gastrointestinal Tract. New York, Raven Press 1981: 1123–1146.

186. Thomson ABR, Dietschy JM. Intestinal lipid absorption: major extracellular and intracellular events. *In* Johnson LR (ed). Physiology of the Gastrointestinal Tract. New York, Raven Press, 1981; 46:1147–1220.

187. Lee SP, Nicholson GI. Ceroid enteropathy and vitamin E deficiency. NZ Med J 1976; 83:318–320.

188. Lee SP. Vitamin E in the treatment of the brown bowel syndrome. Mayo Clin Proc 1980; 54:752.

189. Bennion LJ, Grundy SM. Risk factors for the development of cholelithiasis in man. N Engl J Med 1978; 299:1221–1227.

190. Williams CN, Scallion SM, McCarthy SC. A diet containing highly refined carbohydrate will adversely affect bile lipid composition to that seen in cholesterol-gallstone disease. Ann R Coll Phys Surg Can 1979; 1:49.

191. Williams CN. Diet changes enhance cholesterol gallstone dissolution. *In* Paumagarten G, Stiehl A, Gerok W (eds). Bile Acids and Cholesterol in Health and Diseases. Lancaster, England, MTP Press, 1982: 381–386.

192. Cohn VH. Vitamin K and Vitamin E. *In* Goodman LS, Gillman A (eds). The Pharmacological Basis of Therapeutics. New York, MacMillan, 1975: 1591–1600.

19

ENDOCRINE DISEASES

HARVEY L. KATZEFF / RICHARD S. RIVLIN

The release of hormones from the various endocrine organs performs vital roles in the regulation of cellular metabolism. Of equal importance are the macro- and micronutrients in the diet, which regulate many intracellular functions. The goal of this chapter is to review the effects of normal and abnormal secretion of various hormones on several aspects of nutrition and metabolism: regulation of calorie expenditure, mineral balance, and the metabolism of vitamins. Since minerals and vitamins frequently serve as cofactors of the important enzyme systems, it is not surprising that hormones, such as thyroid hormones, have wide-ranging effects on nutrient metabolism.

There are numerous interrelationships among the various metabolic actions of hormones and the nutritional state of an individual. Changes in hormonal secretion may alter nutritional requirements, and alterations in nutrient intake, in turn, may alter hormonal secretion. Thus the clinical effects of an increase or decrease in hormonal secretion may be modulated by the nutritional status of the individual. One such example is the occurrence of weight loss and malnutrition in a hyperthyroid patient. Hyperthyroidism frequently produces weight loss in an individual, but in 10 to 20 per cent of those affected the increase in appetite may actually produce a weight gain.[1] This is but one example of the effect of a clinical syndrome of altered hormonal secretion on nutrition. This chapter will be devoted to elucidating the interrelationships among hormone secretion, nutritional state, and the clinical status of the individual.

PITUITARY HORMONES

Growth Hormone

Intermediary Metabolism. Growth hormone (GH) regulates nutrition and metabolism via both direct and indirect mechanisms. The main actions of growth hormone (Table 19–1) include stimulation

TABLE 19–1. *Major Actions of Growth Hormone upon Nutrients*

Intermediary Metabolism

Protein
  Stimulates cellular amino acid uptake
  Stimulates DNA and RNA synthesis
  Stimulates bone growth

Carbohydrate
  Impairs nonhepatic glucose uptake
  Decreases insulin sensitivity
  Stimulates insulin secretion

Lipid
  Stimulates adipose tissue lipolysis
  Stimulates hepatic oxidation of free fatty acids

Mineral and Vitamin Metabolism

Calcium
  Increases plasma concentrations of 1,25-dihydroxyvitamin D_3
  Increases concentration of intestinal calcium-binding protein
  Decreases renal phosphate excretion

Vitamin A
  Decreases liver stores of retinol
  Increases tissue uptake of retinol

Vitamin B_6
  Facilitates pyridoxine-induced amino acid uptake by cells

of longitudinal growth of long bones, increased protein synthesis, and increased fatty acid oxidation with suppression of peripheral glucose uptake into cells. Recent research[2] suggests that growth hormone itself probably has no direct action on bone growth but rather that it mediates this and certain other effects via stimulation of the production of the protein somatomedin C (IGF I). Growth hormone stimulates sulfate incorporation into cartilage in vivo but not in vitro, whereas somatomedin C produces a marked sulfation of chondroitin both in vivo or in vitro.[3] An increase in hepatic synthesis of somatomedin C can be observed within 1 hour after a rise in plasma growth hormone levels.[3] In addition to its ability to stimulate the growth of the chondrocytes at the epiphyseal plate, somatomedin C has several anabolic and growth-promoting properties.[4,5] It stimulates leucine incorporation into protein, synthesis of RNA and DNA, and production of collagen. Somatomedin C also produces a rise in plasma phosphorus and a net increase in calcium balance. Growth hormone stimulates the production of somatomedins A and B (IGF II and III), proteins which stimulate DNA synthesis but are not believed to be responsible for bone growth.

These findings indicate that a major portion of the growth-promoting effects of GH are coordinated via GH-stimulated synthesis of somatomedins. Nutritional factors such as level of protein and calorie intake are also extremely important in the regulation of somatomedin production. Somatomedin C concentrations in blood fall dramatically to less than 50 per cent of baseline in hospitalized malnourished patients.[6] Protein-calorie malnutrition in man and protein malnutrition in rats also produce marked

falls in serum somatomedin concentrations.[7,8] Chronic diseases that may produce growth retardation, such as Crohn's disease and poorly controlled diabetes mellitus, are also associated with low somatomedin C blood concentrations.[9] Thus, nutritionally induced decrements in somatomedin concentrations contribute to decreased growth in the presence of adequate GH concentrations in blood.

Growth hormone exerts direct effects on carbohydrate and lipid metabolism. Infusions of physiological concentrations of growth hormone during forearm perfusion studies suppress glucose uptake by muscle.[10] In addition, growth hormone lowers the rate of glucose disappearance during intravenous glucose tolerance tests. Recent studies indicate that growth hormone impairs insulin action on fat cells at the postreceptor level, possibly by opposing insulin's effect on cyclic AMP.[11] Insulin secretion is stimulated by GH, apparently both by raising blood glucose levels and by directly stimulating the beta cells of the pancreas. These effects of GH are clinically apparent as impairment of glucose tolerance during hypersecretion of GH.

Growth hormone is a potent stimulator of adipose tissue lipolysis, yet concentrations of plasma free fatty acids (FFA) in GH-deficient children are normal.[12] GH concentrations in blood rise acutely in response to underfeeding but are normal in chronic malnutrition. FFA release from adipose tissue lipolysis is a major energy source during chronic malnutrition; however, the GH concentration in blood is normal or low during chronic starvation, suggesting that other factors such as increased catecholamine sensitivity and low insulin levels can promote lipolysis.[13] In addition, GH-stimulated lipolysis is absent when glucose uptake into adipose tissue is not suppressed, as occurs in underfeeding.

Growth hormone also stimulates the oxidation of free fatty acids in liver. There are falls in both the respiratory quotient and concentrations of ketone bodies in blood and urine following intravenous administration of GH, indicating an increased efficiency of FFA oxidation in the liver. Growth hormone's ability to promote hepatic FFA oxidation may be important during chronic malnutrition. The resulting increase in hepatic ATP production stimulates hepatic gluconeogenesis and may help to prevent fasting hypoglycemia, a common occurrence in GH-deficient children. These findings suggest a role for GH-mediated FFA oxidation in the normal metabolic adaptation to undernutrition.

Obesity is associated with a lower GH concentration in blood in the postabsorptive period and a decreased GH response to insulin-induced hypoglycemia.[14] Recent data suggest that growth hormone releasing factor (GHRF) secretion is normal but that decreased pituitary responsiveness to GHRF is present in obesity.[15] Since the GH response to GHRF is normalized after weight loss, it has been suggested that the defect is secondary to the obese state. The lower concentrations of GH in obesity lead to the improper use of exogenous GH (and human chorionic gonadotropin [HCG]) to stimulate adipose tissue lipolysis and to promote fat loss. This is an inappropriate use of these hormones, since obese individuals have normal or increased plasma FFA concentrations and FFA turnover, indicating that whole-body FFA mobilization from adipose tissue is normal.

Mineral and Vitamin Metabolism. Normal skeletal growth requires positive calcium and phosphorus balance to promote skeletal ossification. It has long been known that growth hormone produces positive calcium balance in mammals. Recent studies indicate that GH may stimulate calcium absorption by increasing the renal activity of the 1 α-hydroxylase enzyme, which converts 25-hydroxyvitamin D_3 into its active derivative, 1,25-dihydroxyvitamin D_3.[16] There are conflicting data on whether GH increases plasma concentrations of 1,25-dihydroxyvitamin D_3; these levels are increased above normal in acromegaly but do not appear to rise with GH therapy in hypopituitarism.[17,18] Despite these conflicting findings, GH therapy during hypopituitarism tends to increase the concentration of the vitamin D–dependent calcium-binding protein in the intestinal mucosa, which is correlated with calcium accretion and rate of growth in young animals. The synthesis of this protein is regulated by 1,25-dihydroxyvitamin D_3.[19] GH therapy produces a positive balance of phosphate by decreasing the renal tubular clearance of phosphate, a function also thought to be regulated by vitamin D. These data suggest that GH may regulate calcium balance indirectly via control of vitamin D metabolism.

Acromegaly. Excessive growth hormone secretion has several important nutritional and metabolic effects. Glucose tolerance is impaired, and non–insulin-dependent diabetes mellitus can occur in individuals who are otherwise not at risk for this disease. Owing to the increased stimulation of collagen synthesis, there is a marked generalized increase in the formation of connective tissue, more so than of bone throughout the body. Hypercalcemia, hypercalciuria, and hyperphosphatemia have been reported in acromegaly along with an increase in concentrations of both 25-hydroxyvitamin D_3 and 1,25-dihydroxyvitamin D_3 concentrations in blood. As discussed above, both an increase in intestinal absorption of calcium and a decrease in phosphate clearance from the kidney are believed to be responsible for these electrolyte disturbances.[17] It is curious that in spite of the increase in calcium absorption, osteoporosis tends to occur in acromegaly of long duration. Clearly, the pathophysiology of osteoporosis in this disorder is not known. Growth hormone is calorigenic, but the elevated BMR that has been reported in acromegaly may be spurious in some instances, since individuals with acromegaly tend to have a relatively high proportion of lean body tissue to surface area, and correspondingly low total body fat.

Growth Hormone Deficiency. This disease presents several clinical problems due to growth retardation in children and increased susceptibility to fasting hypoglycemia. Approximately 50 per cent of GH-deficient children have episodes of hypoglycemia, presumably because of diminished gluconeogenesis in the liver. There are few, if any, metabolic abnormalities associated with GH deficiency in the adult.

Data from animal studies suggest that there is a decrease in the tissue uptake of retinol from retinol-binding protein in GH-deficient states. Vitamin A may serve as a tissue growth factor, but it is unclear whether decreased tissue levels of vitamin A have any relationship to the decreased growth rate of GH-deficient children. Growth hormone is also apparently necessary to facilitate pyridoxine-stimulated amino acid uptake by cells, but pyridoxine deficiency has not been reported in GH deficiency.

Prolactin

Interest in the metabolic and nutritional actions of prolactin has gained considerable momentum in the past decade with the development of a specific and sensitive radioimmunoassay for this hormone.[20] The major function of prolactin in females is the production of milk proteins and normal lactation postpartum.[21] Prolactin may also be necessary for pubertal breast development, but only in the presence of estrogens.

There is evidence that suggests a role for prolactin in the regulation of calcium absorption during pregnancy. Studies in animals reveal that prolactin can stimulate intestinal calcium absorption by both a direct action on intestinal mucosa and via stimulation of 1,25-dihydroxyvitamin D_3 production,[22] but the doses used were above the physiologic range. Studies in humans find no differences in serum calcium, serum PTH, or serum 1,25-dihydroxyvitamin D_3 concentrations in lactating and nonlactating women postpartum.[23] In addition, patients with hyperprolactinemia do not appear to have evidence of increased calcium absorption or serum calcium or phosphate concentrations. Further work will be required to establish a direct link between prolactin and calcium metabolism in man.

Results of experiments performed in vitro also indicate that prolactin has weak nitrogen retaining activity and produces insulin resistance, but as with calcium metabolism these findings are probably not clinically relevant since patients with hyperprolactinemia per se do not have any features of acromegaly.

Hyperprolactinemia. The major nutritional focus has been on the positive association between hyperprolactinemic states and decreased bone mass. Recently, it has been shown that women with hyperprolactinemia due to pituitary tumors have decreased vertebral bone mass.[24,25] The decrease in trabecular bone appears to be most strongly related to the duration of the hyperprolactinemic state. The rate of decline in bone mass versus age is not accelerated compared with the rate in normal women.[26] This effect of prolactin on bone mass appears in part to be independent of estrogen. Klibanski et al. found an association with serum estrogen concentrations and decreased trabecular bone mass in hyperprolactinemia; however, their study was cross-sectional rather than longitudinal over time.[24] Prolactin has direct resorptive effects on bone in vitamin D deficient animals and additionally acts to diminish ovarian estrogen production, which in turn also favors bone resorption. Sustained hyperprolactinemia decreases bone mass, probably via direct effects and secondarily via a decrease in estrogen secretion. Therapy may be required to prevent osteoporosis in later years.

THYROID HORMONES

Cellular Metabolism

Thyroid hormones, both thyroxine (T_4) and triiodothyronine (T_3), are essential for normal growth and development in children and regulate many aspects of cellular metabolism in adult humans. Thyroid hormones do not specifically control any single cellular function; rather, they act to modulate several different cellular functions which in turn regulate oxygen consumption. An example of such a system is the Na^+/K^+ ATPase enzyme; it is estimated that the maintenance of intracellular potassium concentration against the electrochemical gradient by this enzyme requires 20 to 45 per cent of the total cellular ATP production.[27] Thyroid hormones are essential for normal activity of Na^+/K^+ ATPase and therefore have an effect on basal energy expenditure, which is related in part to control of the activity of this enzyme.

Thyroid hormones, acting in conjunction with catecholamines, are major determinants of the whole-body resting metabolic rate. Thyroxine is secreted from the thyroid gland under the control of TSH stimulation. A significant portion of T_4 is deiodinated to either T_3 or reverse-T_3 in tissues containing the 5'-deiodinase enzyme system. These tissues include the liver, lung, kidney, brain, and brown adipose tissues. Approximately 85 per cent of T_3 produced is via extrathyroidal T_4 deiodination; the remainder is directly secreted from the thyroid gland. Although serum concentrations of T_4 are 40- to 60-fold greater than those of T_3, the intracellular concentrations are similar and T_3 is metabolically more active than T_4. The current thinking is that T_4 is primarily a prohormone and T_3 the active hormone intracellularly. The control of T_4 to T_3 conversion is therefore an important metabolic regulator of thyroid hormone action.

Alterations in both the level and composition of caloric intake modulate nonthyroidal production of T_3 in humans, and the level of free T_3 in blood parallels the production rate of T_3 during both over- and undernutrition.[28,29] Complete fasting produces a dramatic fall in serum T_3 within 10 days without any change in the serum T_4 concentration. Adding 500 kcal/day of carbohydrate, but neither fat nor protein, to the fast will return the serum T_3 concentration to near normal. Overfeeding 2000 kcal/day produces an 80 per cent rise in the rate of T_3 production.[28] The resting metabolic rate tends to follow the changes in serum T_3 concentrations; it falls during acute underfeeding and rises during overfeeding out of proportion to any change in body weight.[29,30] These data suggest that nutritionally induced alterations in T_3 production rate regulate a portion of resting metabolic rate that has been named adaptive thermogenesis. There are also data suggesting that certain obese humans such as the Pima Indians may have defects in adaptive thermogenesis related to abnormalities in thyroid hormone secretion and catecholamine-induced thermogenesis.[31]

Thyroid hormones have been studied as an aid to stimulating weight loss in obese individuals. The addition of less than full replacement doses of either T_4 or T_3 to an individual on a weight maintenance diet will do little to alter energy expenditure. This phenomenon is due to the suppression of TSH secretion and maintenance of the euthyroid state. Administration of T_3 during a period of feeding on a hypocaloric diet to maintain normal serum T_3 concentrations does produce an acceleration of weight loss, but the weight lost is predominantly lean body tissue, not fat.[32] This is an unsafe medical practice which can lead to myocardial fibrosis and myocardial conduction abnormalities. In addition, animal studies indicate that there is the development of resistance to the thermogenic actions of T_3 during starvation.[33] These findings indicate that there is no rationale for the use of thyroid hormones as an adjunct to dieting for the treatment of obesity.

In addition to its direct effects on energy expenditure, thyroid hormones control the body's sensitivity to the thermogenic and metabolic effects of catecholamines. This regulatory mechanism is responsible for the apparent increase in norepinephrine activity during hyperthyroidism when, in fact, secretion and plasma concentrations of norepinephrine are low. The converse is true during hypothyroidism.[34,35]

Changes in caloric intake affect the secretion of other hormones besides the thyroid hormones; insulin, somatomedins, and norepinephrine secretion in the blood are all decreased during underfeeding and rise during overfeeding. It has been hypothesized that the mechanism for the fall in these hormones during underfeeding is a compensatory effort to maintain lean body mass and decrease protein catabolism. During periods of overfeeding, an increase in lean body mass and fat synthesis are observed, coupled with an increase in resting metabolic rate which is lost as heat. This calorie wastage, which is now termed adaptive thermogenesis, was first named luxus-consumption by Neumann[36] in 1902. The metabolic processes by which overfeeding may produce an excess in heat production have not been identified, but there are several possible intracellular futile cycles that oxidize fatty acids or glucose without producing ATP. Such examples include the malate shuttle and the glycerophosphate dehydrogenase shuttle. Also, uncoupling of oxidative phosphorylation has been proved in brown adipose tissue of overfed rodents.[37] Whether this mechanism is applicable to humans is not known.

INTERMEDIARY METABOLISM

Protein Metabolism. Thyroid hormones modulate other metabolically costly processes such as protein synthesis.[38] There are receptors for T_3 on nuclear membranes, and there is strong evidence that this action, like many others of thyroid hormones, is mediated via translation and transcription of mRNA and finally via microsomal protein production.[39,40] Proteins that are increased in activity by thyroid hormones include enzymes required for glycolysis and oxidative phosphorylation, such as mitochondrial α-glycerophosphate dehydrogenase. Thyroid hormones also induce the synthesis of glycolytic enzymes, including isocitrate dehydrogenase, hexokinase, glucose-6-phosphate dehydrogenase, and 6-phosphogluconate dehydrogenase, suggesting that the capacity for glycolysis is dependent on thyroid hormone action.

Lipid Metabolism. Thyroid hormones stimulate both lipolysis and re-esterification of triglyceride in white adipose tissue, but the net effect of this stimulation is an efflux of free fatty acids into blood.[41] In smaller mammals, adaptation to chronic cold is necessary for survival. Thyroid hormones are necessary for cold acclimatization in small mammals, stimulating lipolysis and uncoupling oxidative phosphorylation in the mitochondria of brown adipocytes.[42] These specialized fat cells are abundant in small mammals and are also present in several sites in adult humans.[43] The activity of brown adipose tissue is regulated via sympathetic nervous system activity, but thyroid hormones are essential for the observed hyperplasia and hypertrophy of brown adipose tissue during cold adaptation.[44] The role of brown fat in cold acclimatization in adult humans remains controversial.

Glucose Metabolism. Thyroid hormones stimulate glucose uptake from the gut, probably by increasing the height and surface area of the villi. Glucose utilization is stimulated via increased glucose uptake in peripheral tissues and increased mitochondrial enzyme content of cells oxidizing glucose.

HYPERTHYROIDISM

Hyperthyroidism increases the activity of the Na^+/K^+ pump, but the clinical significance of this effect is uncertain.[27] Hyperthyroidism is associated with increased basal temperature, and indeed a hallmark of thyroid storm is hyperpyrexia. Abnormalities of the thermoregulatory system are the primary cause of hyperpyrexia, but increased cellular thermogenesis may also be contributory. Clinically, the increase in cellular thermogenesis translates into an increase in caloric requirements to maintain body mass. This effect frequently produces weight loss despite weight loss hyperphagia. Occasionally, however, hyperthyroid-induced hyperphagia leads to weight gain, usually in younger individuals.

The increase in substrate utilization predisposes the hyperthyroid patients toward an accelerated state of starvation. Increased free fatty acid oxidation and ketonuria are often present, but frank hypoglycemia is rare. Hyperthyroidism produces a marked increase in adipose tissue lipolysis with enhanced release of free fatty acids and glycerol into blood.[45] Although the predominance of evidence is that hyperthyroidism does not increase sympathetic nervous system activity, as measured by concentrations of catecholamines in plasma and urine, there may be a marked increase in sensitivity to both the lipolytic and thermogenic actions of norepinephrine in this disorder.[34,35] Increases in both plasma free fatty acid and glycerol concentrations and the increased energy expenditure observed during hyperthyroidism are partially abolished by administration of the beta-adrenergic blocker propranolol.[46,47] These results indicate that the changes in lipolysis and metabolic rate observed in hyperthyroidism are likely due to both direct and indirect effects of thyroid hormones.

Hyperthyroidism increases the capacity for oxidative phosphorylation and may be responsible for the increase in glucose utilization in extrahepatic tissues.[48] The rate of glucose emptying from the stomach, glucose absorption from the gut, and hepatic gluconeogenesis from both lactate and glycerol are also stimulated during hyperthyroidism. The increase in glycerol release from adipose tissue and amino acid release from muscle each promote increased hepatic gluconeogenesis.

Hypoglycemia is rare in spite of the increased glucose utilization observed in hyperthyroidism. There are often abnormalities in the oral glucose tolerance test; the early (30- and 60-minute) concentrations of blood glucose are frequently elevated secondarily to an increased rate of glucose absorption from the gut and to impairment of normal insulin suppression of hepatic gluconeogenesis.[49] Although hyperthyroid patients tend to exhibit impaired glucose tolerance to an oral glucose load, intravenous glucose tolerance tends to be relatively normal and vascular complications characteristic of diabetes have not been observed.

HYPOTHYROIDISM

Hypothyroidism decreases the activity of the Na^+/K^+ pump. This effect is believed to impair free water clearance from the kidney and to promote hyponatremia.[50] Decreased energy expenditure is present in hypothyroidism but it is not certain that decreased activity of the Na^+/K^+ pump is responsible. The weight gain that is observed in 44 to 76 per cent of individuals is due to a combination of increased fluid retention and excess adipose tissue stored with altered energy expenditure. Weight gain is rarely greater than 20 lb, since appetite is usually decreased concomitantly. During hypothyroidism there is an inability to maintain basal body temperature in response to cold and there is a decrease in the thermogenic response to norepinephrine.[51] Abnormal Na^+/K^+ pump activity may be partly responsible for the impaired thermogenic response to cold in hypothyroidism.

Hypothyroidism retards both the catabolic and synthetic rates of triglycerides to result in lower plasma FFA concentrations and suppressed lipolytic sensitivity to catecholamines. Lipoprotein lipase activity is lower and triglyceride levels in plasma are variably elevated in hypothyroidism. Low-density lipoproteins, the main carrier of cholesterol in blood, are usually elevated in blood secondary to their depressed catabolism.

Hypothyroidism decreases the tissue uptake of glucose even in the presence of high insulin concentrations.[52] It is likely that decreased glucose uptake represents a postreceptor abnormality of insulin action. In spite of this finding, hypothyroidism tends to be associated with a relatively flat glucose tolerance curve, most likely as a result of delayed glucose uptake in the gut.[53]

Calcium and Phosphate Metabolism

Hyperthyroidism. Abnormalities in thyroid hormone concentrations alter calcium and phosphate metabolism by more than a single mechanism. Hyperthyroidism is often associated with hypercalcemia, but nephrocalcinosis is relatively rare in spite of increased urinary calcium and phosphorus excretion. The source of calcium leading to hypercalcemia appears to be bone, since intestinal absorption of calcium is decreased and fecal excretion of calcium is increased in hyperthyroidism.[54] The main mechanism of hypercalcemia appears to be increased bone turnover and bone destruction, which if untreated can lead to osteoporosis and osteitis fi-

brosa.[55] Urinary hydroxyproline excretion is a specific marker for bone turnover and tends to be increased in hyperthyroidism.[56] Other methods of measuring bone turnover include determination of activity in blood, bone, and urine of radiotracer amounts of ^{45}calcium and naturally occurring strontium. Data obtained using each of these methods support the view that there is increased calcium flux in bone with relatively greater rates of resorption than formation.

The cause of the increase in bone resorption in hyperthyroidism is not completely understood. The negative nitrogen balance induced by the hyperthyroid state is one possibility, but hyperthyroid patients who have been placed in positive nitrogen balance by the addition of extra protein to the diet still exhibit negative calcium balance.[54] Although bone histology in hyperthyroidism generally is similar to that noted in hyperparathyroidism, plasma PTH levels tend to be normal or low.[57] Plasma levels of 1,25-dihydroxyvitamin D_2 in hyperthyroidism are decreased, consistent with decreased calcium absorption and normal or increased tubular phosphate reabsorption.[58] Hyperthyroidism stimulates osteoclastic activity directly in addition to possibly increasing sensitivity to the osteoclastic actions of PTH.

Hypothyroidism. There is an increase in calcium absorption from the gut and a decrease in calcium excretion in the kidney in hypothyroidism.[53,58] There is also a decrease in the pool of exchangeable calcium. These factors may occasionally produce hypercalcemia during acute calcium loading in hypothyroidism, but this finding is uncommon. The rate of bone turnover, as measured by urinary hydroxyproline excretion, is decreased, as is calcium deposition during hypothyroidism.[56] These changes in calcium flux in bone are all reversible with thyroxine treatment.

Vitamin Metabolism

Certain vitamins function as coenzymes for such important and varied cellular functions as oxidative phosphorylation, glycolysis, and hemoglobin synthesis. It would be an oversimplification to state that vitamin requirements are increased during hyperthyroidism, since thyroid hormones regulate specific and selective aspects of vitamin metabolism. Hypothyroidism is also the cause of certain vitamin deficiencies, most commonly due to decreased cellular processing of the active vitamin precursors.

VITAMIN A

Carotene is normally converted to retinyl esters in the gut prior to absorption and then stored in the liver. Vitamin A is transported to other tissues via retinol-binding protein (RBP) and prealbumin. The level of vitamin A in blood is dependent among other factors on liver synthesis of these carrier proteins. During adequate calorie intake, the level of RBP in blood is generally proportional to the vitamin stores in the liver.

Hyperthyroidism. Hyperthyroidism increases intestinal absorption and hepatic stores of vitamin A, but serum levels of vitamin A, retinol-binding protein, and prealbumin are decreased.[59-61] Thyroid hormones appear to depress the concentration of the vitamin A transport system in blood, but the clinical syndrome of night blindness due to vitamin A deficiency is rarely detected.

Hypothyroidism. In myxedema there is often a characteristic orange-yellow pigmentation of the volar surfaces of the extremities, most probably due to excessive deposition of carotene, the precursor of vitamin A. Elevated serum levels of beta carotenes may be a reflection of a generalized increase in serum lipoproteins to which carotenes are bound. In hypothyroidism, serum levels of vitamin A are increased, but concentrations of retinol-binding protein and prealbumin tend to be normal.[62] These findings suggest there are abnormalities in the tissue delivery of vitamin A. Hypothyroidism has been occasionally associated with disturbances in night vision, suggesting that a block in tissue delivery may be clinically significant.[63]

THIAMINE

Hyperthyroidism. Early experiments by Drill suggested that hyperthyroidism can provoke an acute state of thiamine deficiency.[63] Tissue levels of thiamine were low, and increased excretion of thiamine degradation products was observed. Later, more sophisticated measurements of thiamine status were performed by measuring red cell transketolase activity. This enzyme is thiamine-dependent, and the increase in enzyme activity provoked by administration of thiamine in vitro is inversely proportional to endogenous thiamine stores. During hyperthyroidism a *decrease* was noted in thiamine-augmented transketolase activity, suggesting that there is likely no deficiency of thiamine nutriture in hyperthyroid patients.[64]

Hypothyroidism. Thiamine itself may have antithyroid properties. It impairs the synthesis of iodotyrosines in tissue slices in animal studies both in vitro and in vivo.[66] The administration of large doses of thiamine does not, however, appear to lead to goiter or hypothyroidism.

Riboflavin

Hyperthyroidism. There appear to be several interactions between thyroid hormones and the metabolism of riboflavin and its coenzyme derivatives, flavin mononucleotide (FMN) and flavin adenine dinucleotide (FAD).[65] There are increases in riboflavin requirements in the hyperthyroid state, which

may be due to increases in flavin-dependent enzyme activity. This suggestion is supported by findings that hyperthyroidism induces a positive riboflavin balance in both humans and rats.[66,67] Thyroid hormones directly stimulate the conversion of riboflavin to FMN and FAD. This is shown diagrammatically below (Fig. 19–1). Hyperthyroidism increases the activity of flavokinase twofold, with a resultant increase in FMN production.[67] There are also increases in the activities of flavoprotein enzymes, such as xanthine oxidase and D-amino acid oxidase. Hepatic enzymes that require PMN or FAD as coenzymes are also dependent on the level of thyroid hormones. The activity of these enzymes, mitochondrial α-glycerophosphate dehydrogenase and glutathione reductase, is proportional to the concentration of thyroid hormones in tissues. Glutathione reductase modulates the nonthyroidal deiodination of thyroxine to triiodothyronine. The ratio of reduced to oxidized glutathione is critical for the activation of the hepatic 5'-deiodinase enzyme.[68] Thus, it is possible that riboflavin deficiency suppresses the ratio of reduced to oxidized GSH, which in turn decreases hepatic 5'-deiodinase activity and hepatic thyroxine deiodination.

Hypothyroidism. Hypothyroidism reduces hepatic FMN and FAD concentrations in part because of a decrease in flavokinase activity.[66,67] There is a secondary decline in the activity of the flavin-dependent enzymes discussed above. Thus, riboflavin deficiency and hypothyroidism each produces similar changes in hepatic enzyme activities. The reduction in flavokinase activity is similar in both riboflavin deficiency and hypothyroidism.

PYRIDOXINE (VITAMIN B6)

There appear to be increased requirements for pyridoxine during hyperthyroidism. Tissue levels of pyridoxine and activities of hepatic vitamin B5–dependent enzymes generally are decreased during hyperthyroidism and increased in the hypothyroid state.[69] Alterations of thyroid hormone production in experimental animals do not appear to affect the rate of synthesis of pyridoxal phosphate, suggesting that alterations in tissue levels of vitamin B6 are likely to be secondary to changes in rate of degradation.

Investigators have searched for clinical pyridoxine deficiency in hyperthyroidism by means of tryptophan loading tests. Xanthurenic acid is a urinary excretion product of tryptophan, and its excretion is increased during pyridoxine deficiency. In hyperthyroidism excretion of xanthurenic acid is increased, and treatment with pyridoxine reverses the abnormality.[70] This finding, taken together with the decrease in pyridoxine-dependent enzyme activities observed in hyperthyroidism, suggests that pyridoxine deficiency probably can occur during hyperthyroidism.

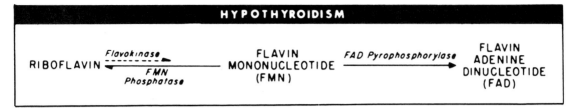

FIGURE 19–1. *Diagrammatic representation of the changes in riboflavin metabolism in hypothyroidism. Hepatic flavokinase activity is diminished, and the hepatic concentrations of the coenzymes, flavin mononucleotide (FMN) and flavin adenine dinucleotide (FAD), are reduced. The activities of the other two enzymes shown are unchanged in hypothyroidism. A fourth enzyme, FAD pyrophosphatase, degrades FAD to FMN and has not been measured in hypothyroidism. (From Rivlin RS. Medical Grand Rounds 1984; 3:74. Reproduced with permission.)*

VITAMIN B₁₂ AND FOLATE

Studies in experimental hyperthyroidism suggest that there may be abnormalities in vitamin B_{12} and folate metabolism. The administration of vitamin B_{12} to hyperthyroid rats given a constant caloric intake will improve nitrogen balance, as will other vitamins, such as thiamine and riboflavin.[71]

Macrocytic anemias are common in both hyper- and hypothyroidism, as is the incidence of pernicious anemia. Several reports indicate that vitamin B_{12} levels in the blood may be decreased in hyperthyroidism and that vitamin B_{12} retention is increased after a vitamin B_{12} loading test.[72,73] Other recent studies have found no differences in vitamin B_{12} or folate levels in blood in hyperthyroidism.[74] Further research is needed to clarify the effects of altered function in man upon vitamin B_{12} and folate metabolism.

PARATHYROID HORMONE

Normal Physiology

The secretion of parathyroid hormone (PTH) from the parathyroid glands is of major significance in regulating the blood calcium concentration. Parathyroid hormone is secreted in response to a lowering of the ionized serum calcium concentration and normally is suppressed during hypercalcemia. It was previously thought that elevations of the serum phosphate level also stimulate PTH secretion, but this hypothesis has not been substantiated. The serum level of magnesium also has an effect upon PTH secretion; an acute decrease in serum magnesium will stimulate PTH release, but this stimulatory effect is weaker than that occurring after an equivalent fall in serum calcium. Chronic magnesium depletion in man is associated with hypocalcemia and decreased PTH levels in blood, a finding consistent with results of in vitro experiments showing that intracellular magnesium is required for normal PTH release.[75,76]

Parathyroid hormone has five known distinct nutritional and metabolic actions by means of which the levels of calcium and phosphorus in blood are controlled. These actions are summarized in Table 19–2.

Parathyroid hormone reduces the reabsorption of the cations, sodium and calcium, and their anions, phosphate and bicarbonate, within the proximal tubule of the kidney.[77] There is, however, a marked increase in calcium resorption from the distal tubule, which is regulated by PTH. Although there is often an increase in calcium excretion above 150 mg/24 hours on a standard 800 mg/day calcium diet in normal individuals, it rarely rises above 500 mg/24 hours under these conditions. By contrast, experimental elevations of the serum calcium level resulting from intravenous calcium infusions produce a greater than normal increase in urinary calcium excretion.[78] Parathyroid hormone increases the urinary excretion of both phosphate and bicarbonate owing to reduced reabsorption of these anions from the distal tubule. This action of PTH produces the characteristic renal tubular acidosis that is associated with primary hyperthyroidism. The magnitude of the phosphaturic response to PTH is a linear dose-response in the normal range of PTH concentrations. This finding suggests that while PTH is not secreted in response to phosphate, nevertheless, in physiological concentrations PTH regulates the concentration of phosphorus in blood.

The regulation of calcium and phosphate absorption from the gut is probably not under the direct control of PTH. There are new and convincing data that PTH modulates the activity of 1-α-hydroxylase, the enzyme that is responsible for the conversion of 25-hydroxyvitamin D_3 to its most active form, 1,25-dihydroxyvitamin D_3. The 1-α-hydroxylase is located in the renal tubular cells. 1,25-dihydroxyvitamin D_3 is responsible for the absorption of both calcium and phosphorus from the GI tract. The

TABLE 19–2. Nutritional and Metabolic Actions of Parathyroid Hormone

Increases renal calcium retention
Increases renal phosphate excretion
Stimulates intestinal calcium absorption
Stimulates bone resorption
Stimulates bone anabolism

coefficient of calcium absorption from the GI tract has been shown to correlate directly with the level of 1,25-dihydroxyvitamin D_3 in the serum in both normal and hyperparathyroid individuals.[80]

The stimulation of bone resorption by PTH is well established but its mode of action is complex. There is an acute mobilization of calcium but not of phosphate in response to PTH that is not dependent on protein synthesis, suggesting that calcium is being mobilized from the extracellular bone fluid compartment. The hypercalcemic response to PTH is associated with osteoclast proliferation and is apparently initiated 15 to 20 hours after infusion of PTH.[81]

The anabolic effects of PTH on bone are not completely understood and in the past have been controversial. Nevertheless, data obtained both by x-ray analysis and by measurements of bone weight indicate that small doses of PTH do increase bone mass.[82] This effect is not surprising, since PTH stimulates both calcium and phosphorus absorption from the gastrointestinal tract, primarily by increasing the biosynthesis of 1,25-dihydroxyvitamin D_3. There are data indicating that low-dose infusions of PTH produce both hypercalcemia and a positive calcium balance in bone, whereas stimulation of osteoclast formation has usually been observed only at high concentrations of PTH.[83] Normal physiological concentrations of PTH in conjunction with adequate calcium intake probably act as an anabolic bone hormone. It is only with certain disorders (decreased calcium intake, renal disease, primary hyperparathyroidism) that PTH acts to promote bone catabolism, resulting in maintaining or increasing the serum calcium level.

Hyperparathyroid States

Almost all of the symptoms and nutritional complications of primary hyperparathyroidism are due ultimately to abnormal calcium and phosphate metabolism. PTH also has primary effects on the renal tubules that can produce renal tubular acidosis, renal concentrating defects, aminoaciduria, and glycosuria. Increased PTH activity promotes increased calcium retention at the distal renal tubule, as noted above, but urinary calcium excretion overall is usually increased above normal, owing to increased calcium filtration at the level of the glomerulus. This effect usually results in negative calcium balance. Early in the course of primary hyperparathyroidism, the anabolic actions of PTH may predominate, but invariably with the passage of time increased bone resorption eventually develops as a result of the negative Ca^{++} balance.

In the past osteitis fibrosa cystica was a common bone lesion observed in hyperparathyroidism, but its prevalence is now decreasing.[84] The most frequent skeletal abnormality noted at present in patients with hyperparathyroidism is diffuse osteopenia.[85] This bone abnormality is generally similar to that of postmenopausal osteoporosis, and the pathogenesis of both disorders may be similar. The reasons for this change in the character of bone pathology over time are unclear, but there are suggestions that hyperparathyroidism is now being diagnosed at an earlier stage than formerly, perhaps because of more widespread use of screening tests for serum calcium concentrations.

Nephrocalcinosis is a complication of primary hyperparathyroidism, the incidence of which is proportional to the increase in urinary calcium excretion and the serum level of 1,25-dihydroxyvitamin D_3.[80,86] This finding suggests that increased calcium absorption in response to increased vitamin D activity is the source of the hypercalcemia in these individuals and that bone tends to be relatively spared under these conditions.

There are still a significant number of individuals with excess PTH secretion who do not appear to have any manifestations of bone pathology. The type and severity of bone disease that occurs in primary hyperparathyroidism appears to be dependent not only on the duration and degree of increased PTH activity, but also on the dietary calcium intake and the concentration of vitamin D metabolites, which in turn increase intestinal calcium absorption and renal clearance of calcium. In fact, both nephrocalcinosis and PTH-induced osteopenia generally do not occur in the same individual. This finding suggests that PTH-induced bone disease may be produced when an individual does not increase absorption to maintain the hypercalcemia but rather depletes calcium from bone.

The second major manifestation of primary parathyroid hormone excess is hypophosphatemia. Calcium absorption from the intestine is very responsive to changes in serum concentrations of 1,25-dihydroxyvitamin D_3 and PTH. The status of kidney function and the limits imposed by the solubility product of calcium and phosphate in the blood are the major regulators of the blood phosphate level. Hypophosphatemia is a frequent although not invariable finding in primary PTH excess, and the chloride/phosphate ratio in the blood is usually greater than 33, indicating the presence of a renal tubular acidosis. Treatment with oral phosphate raises the blood phosphate level, which in turn decreases serum and extracellular calcium concentrations, because of the solubility product of calcium and phosphate, and will eventually increase intracellular calcium concentrations.

The renal loss of bicarbonate during hyperparathyroidism impairs the urinary secretion of other acids including sodium urate, resulting in hyperuricemia in approximately 20 per cent of affected individuals. This effect is associated with deposition of calcium and urate crystals in articular cartilages and the clinical syndromes of gout and pseudogout.

TABLE 19–3. *Mechanisms of Hypocalcemia in Hypoparathyroidism*

Decreased gastrointestinal absorption of calcium
Decreased renal tubular reabsorption of calcium
Increased serum phosphate concentrations
Decrease in the solubility constant for calcium and phosphorus in blood

Hypoparathyroidism

Parathyroid hormone deficiency, either idiopathic or surgically induced, produces biochemical changes that are related to its effects on the gut, kidney, and bone. PTH deficiency impairs the hydroxylation of 25-hydroxyvitamin D_3 to its more active metabolite, 1,25-dihydroxyvitamin D_3.[87] The deficiency of both PTH and 1,25-dihydroxyvitamin D_3 produces hypocalcemia by a number of mechanisms (Table 19–3).

The normal activity of PTH in serum raises the solubility product of calcium hydroxyapatite. In the complete absence of PTH the concentration of calcium in the blood is on the order of 5.0 mg/dl. In partial PTH deficiency states, serum calcium will be decreased when calcium intake is low and/or phosphate intake is excessive.

Hyperphosphatemia is less frequent in hypoparathyroid states than is hypocalcemia. The reason for this observation is that the renal tubule is more sensitive to the phosphaturic effect of PTH than to its hypercalcemic effect.[88] There is also a decreased phosphate load delivered to the kidney due to decreased skeletal release and intensive absorption of phosphate.

ADRENAL CORTICAL STEROIDS

Adrenal cortical steroids are commonly divided into four major categories: glucocorticoids, mineralocorticoids, androgens, and estrogens. In this section we shall discuss the nutritional and metabolic actions of glucocorticoids, the major secretory product of the adrenal cortex. Glucocorticoids are similar to the thyroid hormones in that they are responsible for long-term control of intermediary metabolism and are required for normal growth and development. The brain is dependent on glucose for normal function; thus, prevention of hypoglycemia during prolonged fasting is essential. Although a fall in insulin may delay the advent of hypoglycemia, maintenance of glucose production is required for prevention of hypoglycemia. Glucocorticoids perform this function and are thought to be long-term counterregulatory hormones to insulin in order to maintain adequate blood glucose concentrations, especially during undernutrition and stress. Although there is a circadian rhythm of ACTH and cortisol secretion, protein intake in man and rat has been shown also to stimulate cortisol secretion, indicating nutritional regulation by cortisol.[89,90] The differential activities of glucocorticoids in respect to intermediary metabolism are presented in Table 19–4.

Normal Physiology

Carbohydrate Metabolism. A major function of glucocorticoids is the prevention of hypoglycemia under varying physiological conditions. Glucose concentrations normally are maintained by a combination of increased glucose production by the liver and decreased glucose utilization by peripheral tissues. Hepatic gluconeogenesis is increased via several mechanisms. The first is an increase in gluconeogenic precursors from the catabolism of protein and triglyceride. Cortisol administration results in a marked increase in release of amino acids from peripheral tissues; its major effect is the release of alanine from muscle tissue, with resultant uptake by the liver.[91] There are also increases in liver transaminases, enzymes that deaminate amino acids and produce the 3-carbon precursors of glucose. Glycerol is another gluconeogenic precursor which normally resides in combination with free fatty acids as triglyceride. Cortisol administration stimulates adipose tissue lipolysis, with a resultant increase in both glycerol and free fatty acid concentrations in blood. Hepatic uptake of glycerol is proportional to the concentration of glycerol in blood; thus, cortisol increases the liver uptake of glycerol. There are also increases in the activity of the synthetic enzymes, phosphoenolpyruvate carboxykinase and glucose-6-phosphatase.[92]

Glucose utilization by a variety of different tissues is suppressed by cortisol administration.[93] This effect appears to be an important result of cortisol's action

TABLE 19–4. *Effects of Glucocorticoids on Intermediary Metabolism*

Carbohydrate Metabolism
Increases hepatic gluconeogenesis
Increases amino acid release from muscle to act as precursor for hepatic gluconeogenesis
Decreases glucose uptake in peripheral tissues
Increases glycerol release from adipose tissue to act as precursor for hepatic gluconeogenesis
Increases sensitivity to glucagon- and catecholamine-stimulated gluconeogenesis
Increases hepatic glycogen stores via increased glycogen synthetase activity

Protein Metabolism
Increases alanine flux from muscle to liver
Stimulates rate of protein catabolism
Decreases rate of protein synthesis

Lipid Metabolism
Stimulates lipolysis by direct action on adipose cells
Increases plasma glycerol and free fatty acid turnover
Increases sensitivity to catecholamine-induced lipolysis
Increases very low density lipoprotein (VLDL) synthesis in the liver
Increases low density lipoprotein (LDL) production in blood
Impairs hepatic endothelial lipase activity

in provoking an impairment of glucose tolerance. The decrease in glucose uptake by the periphery stimulates insulin secretion and a subsequent down regulation of insulin receptors. Adipocytes are *not* resistant to the antilipolytic effects of insulin, which then may produce increased lipogenesis. Further discussion will follow in the section on hypercortisolism.

Cortisol also stimulates hepatic glycogen storage. This action has probably evolved as protection against hypoglycemia during prolonged fasting. Glycogen storage is increased by conversion of glycogen synthetase from its inactive to its active form. A secondary increase in insulin secretion produced by cortisol also can increase glycogen stores in the body. Although insulin and cortisol usually have opposite metabolic actions, in this instance both cortisol and insulin act to maintain glycogen stores.

Protein Metabolism. Corticosteroids are required for normal growth and development, yet two major effects of cortisol are increases in protein catabolism and in whole-body nitrogen excretion.[89] There are increases in the free amino acid pool in muscle, which correspond to an increase in blood amino acid concentrations after acute cortisol administration.[91] Long-term administration of cortisol is associated with a rise in the serum alanine concentration, which is probably due to the conversion of the other amino acids to alanine in muscle. Alanine is the most important gluconeogenic amino acid; the liver's capacity to transaminate this amino acid is greater than that of other amino acids, and the activities of these transaminases are increased further with cortisol treatment.[92]

The net effect of the increase in alanine flux from muscle to liver is an increase in protein catabolism. Urinary nitrogen excretion is decreased in hypoadrenal states and increased in hypercortisolism, suggesting a direct link between the rates of protein excretion and cortisol concentration.[93] In addition, observations after administration of trace quantities of leucine indicate that cortisol stimulates leucine oxidation. On the other hand, cortisol increases liver protein synthesis, especially that of transaminases and gluconeogenic enzymes. These data indicate that muscle likely acts as a storage depot of amino acids available as gluconeogenic precursors when glycogen stores and caloric intake are inadequate to meet metabolic needs.

Cortisol also inhibits protein synthesis in peripheral tissues, but protein balance can be maintained with increased protein intake. Protein synthesis is greater than protein catabolism in the postprandial state, but acute cortisol administration decreases the rate of protein synthesis, resulting in negative nitrogen balance. Cortisol also decreases DNA synthesis and inhibits mRNA activity.

Lipid Metabolism. Cortisol is thought of as a lipogenic hormone, since hypercortisolism is associated with weight gain, but in reality cortisol is a stimulator of lipolysis. The main action of cortisol on adipose tissue is to increase the lipolytic activity of catecholamines and growth hormone. In animals that are treated with cortisol there are increases in weight gain, but pair-fed littermates have greater quantities of fat.[94] Cortisol also inhibits lipid synthesis in adipose tissue by inhibiting glucose uptake and glycerol synthesis in adipose cells. This effect produces an increase in plasma free fatty acid (FFA) concentration, but hypercortisolism does not increase FFA turnover in blood.[95] The increase in blood FFA concentration also inhibits glucose uptake by cells and produces insulin resistance.

Chronic cortisol excess increases hepatic synthesis of very low density lipoproteins (VLDL), with a resultant rise in serum VLDL concentrations, but it is unclear whether this is a primary effect of cortisol or whether it is secondary to an increase in insulin secretion.[96,97] There is no alteration in lipoprotein lipase activity, and the removal rate of VLDL from blood is normal.

Calcium Metabolism. More than 70 years ago it was discovered that the adrenal gland has an important effect on calcium metabolism. Adrenalectomy in both man and animals raises the serum calcium concentration and may produce hypercalcemia.[98] Excessive glucocorticoids are associated with negative calcium balance,[99] and a fall in the serum calcium concentration occurs in a portion of hypercalcemic individuals treated with these agents.

The major effect of glucocorticoids on calcium metabolism is to decrease intestinal calcium absorption.[100] The decrease in calcium absorption was thought to be secondary to an antagonistic effect on vitamin D action in the gut. Newer data suggest that this is not true. Glucocorticoid excess is not associated with any known alteration in the production rate or metabolic clearance of 1,25-dihydroxyvitamin D_3, and the physiological responses to 1,25-dihydroxyvitamin D_3 are normal.[101] Glucocorticoids do not impair renal 1-α-hydroxylase activity but may impair 1,25-dihydroxyvitamin D_3 production in nonrenal tissues, such as in sarcoidosis.[102] This action of glucocorticoids may be responsible for their ability to lower serum calcium concentrations in sarcoidosis.

It appears that glucocorticoids inhibit calcium absorption by a direct action on the intestinal mucosa. The exact mechanism of this effect is not known but may involve impairment of brush border function.

Another important property of glucocorticoids is their ability to increase urinary calcium excretion. Cortisol also may lower the serum calcium concentration by shifting calcium from the extracellular space to the intracellular space.

Supraphysiological concentrations of glucocorticoids frequently produce loss of bone mass in man. The loss of bone mass is due to both direct and secondary effects of glucocorticoids. Glucocorticoids decrease protein synthesis, which inhibits collagen formation and directly inhibits osteoblastic function.

Addition of cortisone to osteoblasts in culture reduces protein synthesis and prevents the recruitment of progenitor cells to mature osteoblasts. There are increased rates of bone resorption during hypercortisolism, but cortisol does not directly stimulate osteoclastic activity in vitro.[103] The fall in calcium absorption secondary to supraphysiological concentrations of glucocorticoids is associated with a rise in the serum PTH concentration. This rise in PTH is probably the cause of the increase in bone resorption, since the increase can be prevented by calcium infusion or parathyroidectomy.[101]

Cushing's Syndrome

Hypercortisolism produces important nutritional and metabolic abnormalities. Impaired glucose tolerance and diabetes mellitus are frequent complications and are probably due to a combination of the metabolic actions of cortisol and genetic factors. An increase in gluconeogenic precursors and enzyme activities promotes increased hepatic glucose output. There is also impairment of insulin-stimulated glucose uptake in muscle and adipose tissues. These effects alone probably produce impaired glucose tolerance, but it takes an abnormality of insulin secretion in addition to insulin resistance to produce overt diabetes. Whether a genetic predisposition toward diabetes mellitus is required or whether the impairment of insulin secretion can be an acquired defect is unknown. Interestingly, if diabetes mellitus occurs during hypercortisolism it may still continue after the hypercortisolism is no longer present.

Hypercortisolism stimulates protein catabolism and suppresses protein synthesis. These actions translate clinically into a loss of muscle mass. The loss of lean tissue plus the deposition of adipose tissue stores in the face, supraclavicular region, and trunk produce the classic signs of Cushing's syndrome. In hypercortisolism secondary to ectopic ACTH secretion, muscle wasting and electrolyte abnormalities are the primary clinical findings. Patients with this type of hypercortisolism are usually seriously ill and their disease progresses more rapidly. Decreased caloric intake may be present and accelerate the loss of lean body mass. Recent data suggest that high-protein diets (more than 2 gm/kg body weight/day) may prevent the loss of muscle mass during exogenous glucocorticoid administration.[104] Further supporting work will be required before this recommendation should be given to patients.

Although cortisol administration stimulates adipose tissue lipolysis, hypercortisolism is associated with excessive fat deposition on the face, supraclavicular region, and trunk. The exact cause of the selective deposition of fat is not certain. It may be due to differential sensitivity of adipose tissue sites to cortisol. In addition, there is a rise in the plasma insulin concentration in hypercortisolism which promotes triglyceride deposition in adipose tissue. The combination of effects of both excess cortisol and insulin may promote fat deposition at selective sites in the body under these conditions.

Hypercortisolism, either endogenous or exogenous, may have profound effects on calcium metabolism in man. The level of cortisol and the duration of illness are the major determinants of the extent of glucocorticoid-induced calcium depletion. Since bone is the storage organ of 99 per cent of calcium in the body, it should not be surprising that hypercortisolism also has important effects on calcium metabolism in bone. Glucocorticoid excess is associated with decreased calcium absorption from the gut. Early studies suggested that this effect was secondary to an inhibition of 25-dihydroxyvitamin D_3, but recent studies have found no defect in serum concentrations or whole body synthesis of 1,25-dihydroxyvitamin D_3, the more active metabolite.[101] The mechanism by which hypercortisolism suppresses calcium absorption is not clear, and there is no evidence for or against a direct antagonism of vitamin D activity in the intestinal cell by cortisol.

Several studies indicate that the decrease in the calcium absorption produced by hypercortisolism induces a secondary rise in PTH secretion in order to maintain a normal serum calcium concentration in blood. The increase in PTH activity increases bone resorption and promotes osteopenia. In addition, glucocorticoids decrease the synthesis of bone collagen and inhibit the transformation of progenitor cells to functioning fibroblasts.[105] These actions of glucocorticoids combined with the glucocorticoid-induced rise in PTH produce a severe form of osteopenia. The osteopenia is predominantly in the vertebrae and ribs, which are largely trabecular, as opposed to the long bones. Compression fractures of the vertebrae and rib fractures are relatively common (16 per cent of cases) and heal with abundant callus formation.[106]

Adrenal Insufficiency

Weight loss is a common sign of adrenal insufficiency. It may vary between 2 and 15 kg and increases with the severity of the disease. Anorexia and other gastrointestinal symptoms frequently accompany adrenal insufficiency and lead to decreased caloric intake and a loss of lean body tissue. The absence of both cortisol and mineralocorticoids in primary adrenal insufficiency promotes a loss of sodium frequently resulting in dehydration. In patients who have been on exogenous glucocorticoid therapy and develop symptoms of adrenal insufficiency during withdrawal of the steroids or afterward, dehydration is uncommon since mineralocorticoid secretion is intact. It is not clear whether the weight loss can be explained entirely by a decrease in caloric intake or if a minimal cortisol concentration is required for maintenance of lean body mass.

Among individuals with adrenal insufficiency, hypoglycemia is more frequent in children than adults and is provoked by stresses such as infection, nausea and vomiting, or other conditions that prevent normal intake of calories. Individuals with adrenal insufficiency are prone to fasting hypoglycemia since they are less able than normal individuals to stimulate hepatic gluconeogenesis in response to stress. They are unable to use muscle amino acids as a source of 3-carbon glucose precursors when cortisol is absent. These biochemical abnormalities may be clinically significant, especially during stress, when oxygen consumption is increased and the body's glucose utilization also rises. Hypoglycemia may be present in acute adrenal crises but is rare in chronic adrenal insufficiency because there may be sufficient cortisol secretion to maintain glucose concentrations in the basal state but not enough to stimulate an increase in glucose production during stress.

Calcium metabolism is often abnormal in adrenal insufficiency, and this abnormality is sometimes manifested as hypercalcemia.[98,107] Adrenal insufficiency appears to increase the protein-bound fraction of calcium in serum and leave the free or ionized portion of calcium relatively normal. The concentrations of serum proteins are also increased, mimicking the clinical picture of dehydration. The hypercalcemia is probably the result of several factors. Cortisol promotes the transfer of extracellular calcium to the intracellular space, and cortisol deficiency presumably reverses this process. Glucocorticoids inhibit osteoclast formation in vitro, and the absence of cortisol may promote osteoclast activity, increased bone resorption, and hypercalcemia. An increase in tubular reabsorption of calcium in the kidney is present in adrenal insufficiency and can contribute to the hypercalcemia.

SYMPATHOADRENAL SYSTEM

Intermediary Metabolism

The sympathoadrenal axis consists of the adrenal medulla and the postganglionic receptors of the peripheral sympathetic nervous system. The adrenal medulla secretes epinephrine (EPI) into the blood as an immediate response to stresses, such as acute fasting, exercise, or hypoglycemia. In contrast, the peripheral sympathetic nervous system (SNS) secretes norepinephrine (NE) on a relatively continuous basis. The rate of NE release from the postganglionic synapses reflects the level of SNS activity. In response to an acute stress, there is an activation of both the adrenal medulla and the peripheral sympthetic nervous system. Under certain conditions, such as long-term underfeeding, there is a differential stimulation of the peripheral SNS and the release of EPI from the adrenal medulla.[108] This differential has important implications for the adaptation to chronic underfeeding and will be discussed below.

Catecholamines increase whole-body oxygen consumption and substrate utilization.[109] They perform these functions by several of the mechanisms illustrated in Figure 19–2. Although catecholamines exert their effects on various tissues such as muscle and adipose tissue, their main function is to maintain blood glucose concentrations by increasing hepatic glucose output. An increase of catecholamines results in glycogenolysis via beta receptor–stimulated cAMP production and activation of glycogen phosphorylase. Hepatic gluconeogenesis is stimulated directly by an increase in the formation of gluconeogenic precursors, such as alanine and glycerol, and indirectly by suppression of insulin release and an increase in glucagon release from the pancreas.[110] Catecholamines provide the body acutely with a rapid infusion of glucose from the liver.

The stores of triglyceride in adipose tissue serve as the major energy reserve for the body. Catecholamines, via the beta$_1$ receptor, are potent stimulators of adipose tissue lipolysis both in vivo and in vitro. Catecholamines also stimulate FFA oxidation and ketogenesis in the liver, which produces a fall in the respiratory quotient. Thus, catecholamines have the capability to hydrolyze triglyceride rapidly, and then to oxidize the FFA that are released into the circulation in response to an acute stress.

Catecholamines stimulate glycogenolysis and lipolysis in muscle in a similar manner as in other organs. The increase in intracellular glucose pro-

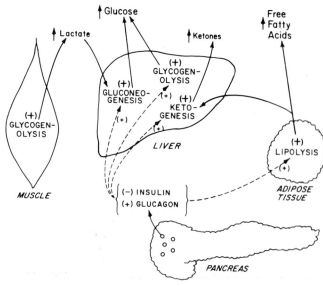

FIGURE 19–2. Effects of catecholamines on generation of utilizable substrates from stored fuels. Indirect effects of catecholamines mediated through changes in insulin and glucagon secretion augment the direct catecholamine effects. (+) indicates stimulation; (−) indicates inhibition. (From Young JB, Landsberg L. Clin Endocrinol Metab 1977; 6:599–631. Reproduced with permission.)

motes the synthesis of lactate, which is then transported to the liver as a precursor for gluconeogenesis. Epinephrine and norepinephrine both suppress proteolysis in muscle.[111] No alterations in serum alanine concentrations have been observed during either EPI or NE infusions in man.[112,113] The overall effects of catecholamines on muscle are to increase substrate utilization and hepatic output of glucose.

Cold Adaptation. The release of epinephrine from the adrenal medulla is important in conditions in which rapid substrate mobilization is required. These conditions include the acute response to cold, first recognized by Cannon[114] over 50 years ago. Tachycardia, increased cardiac output, increased glucose and FFA mobilization and oxidation, and increased muscle contraction (shivering) are all secondary to EPI release. These actions have the net effect of increasing oxygen consumption and heat production, which results in raising the core temperature. In chronic cold adaptation, EPI secretion is normal but there is an increase in peripheral SNS activity and release of NE. NE is responsible for nonshivering thermogenesis in mammals during cold adaptation.[115]

As discussed in the section on thyroid hormones, brown adipose tissue (BAT) is the site of nonshivering thermogenesis in mammals.[116] NE induces the hydrolysis of triglycerides within these cells for mitochondrial oxidation. These mitochondria are capable of uncoupling oxidative phosphorylation and producing heat without increasing ATP production.[37] Cold adaptation is possible only when an animal is given unlimited access to greater quantities of food than that required to maintain its body mass; otherwise the lipid stores in BAT would shrink and the tissue would be unable to fulfill its normal function.[117]

Food Intake. Epinephrine secretion is increased in the first 72 to 96 hours of starvation in man and then declines to normal levels. This rise may be helpful in initiating the increases in glycolysis, lipolysis, and gluconeogenesis that are observed in early starvation. Chronic starvation, however, is characterized by a relative decrease in energy expenditure, which involves decreases in FFA oxidation and in glucose utilization. In chronic starvation there are decreases in both urinary EPI and NE secretion in humans and a decrease in NE release from tissues in rodents.[118] Although data obtained from experiments performed in vitro suggest a decrease in the lipolytic sensitivity to NE during underfeeding, data obtained in vivo indicate an increase in the lipolytic response to NE, independent of a fall in the serum insulin concentration.[13,29] Therefore, the physiological role of SNS activity in maintaining substrate utilization during chronic underfeeding remains uncertain.

As described above, chronic underfeeding decreases SNS activity. There are also new data that indicate a role for nutritional regulation of SNS activity during both weight maintenance and overfeeding. Plasma NE concentrations, an indirect measure of SNS activity, increase in response to either an intravenous or oral carbohydrate load, but not to either protein or fat.[119,120] Chronic overfeeding also increases the plasma level of NE.[121] These data combined with the results of underfeeding studies indicate that the SNS is regulated, in part, by both the magnitude of calorie intake and the type of calories ingested.

Nutritionally induced alterations in SNS activity may therefore be responsible, at least in part, for a portion of the acute thermic effect of glucose and the more chronic alterations in energy expenditure observed during both over- and underfeeding. The results of animal experiments indicate that chronic overfeeding induces changes in SNS activity and in BAT function similar to those of cold adaptation and suggest a common central regulation for both cold-induced and nutritionally induced alterations in energy expenditure.

Obesity and non–insulin-dependent diabetes mellitus are both associated with insulin resistance. Experiments in humans utilizing combined glucose-insulin infusion suggest that insulin resistance impairs carbohydrate stimulation of the SNS and the thermic effect of glucose. Treatment by weight reduction improves both the insulin resistance and the thermic response to glucose.[122] These data also suggest that insulin-resistant individuals may be less able to "waste" excess calories than normal individuals ingesting a similar number of calories.

Exercise. Catecholamines are also important in the metabolic adaptation to exercise. Although exercise has been described as an accelerated state of starvation, there are major differences between the two conditions. In exercise, unlike in starvation, energy expenditure is increased, not decreased, and there is activation, not suppression, of the SNS. During chronic aerobic exercise there are increases in the rates of both glucose and FFA oxidation. There is a rise in the plasma NE concentration that parallels the increase in work load. When the anaerobic threshold is achieved, epinephrine is secreted and lactate production is increased.[123] It was originally thought that catecholamines were responsible for the increase in FFA production and transport from adipose tissue to muscle. Steinberg[124] then administered nicotinic acid to runners before a race. Nicotinic acid suppressed NE-stimulated lipolysis but did not affect the cardiovascular effects of NE. No differences in the runner's ability to complete the race were observed, although the respiratory quotient increased. This paper suggests that regulation of transport of FFA to muscle from adipose tissue during exercise is not physiologically critical. Propranolol, a complete beta-adrenergic blocker, does impair endurance work capacity, however, indicating that the cardiovascular effects of catecholamines are important for work capacity.

Pheochromocytoma

The clinical findings observed in patients with pheochromocytoma, especially those related to the cardiovascular system, may vary greatly from one individual to another. The reasons for this may be that secretion of EPI and NE by each tumor is also very variable and that each kind of catecholamine has its own distinctive effects. The metabolic and nutritional findings in patients with pheochromocytoma are more consistent because EPI and NE have similar metabolic effects. Increases of energy expenditure up to 30 to 40 per cent above normal have been recorded, and in one study the rise in energy expenditure was related to the fasting FFA concentration in blood.[125] The rise in energy expenditure was suppressed by beta blockade, as was the plasma FFA concentration. Since plasma FFA concentrations are correlated to FFA turnover, this finding suggests that patients with increased triglyceride hydrolysis provide greater substrate loads (FFA), thus resulting in an increase in oxidative phosphorylation and in energy expenditure. This rise in energy expenditure is clinically corroborated by a significant weight loss.

Catecholamines also increase the rate of glucose oxidation and suppress insulin secretion. Impaired glucose tolerance and a secondary form of diabetes mellitus have been observed in patients with pheochromocytomas. One may hypothesize that the decrease in insulin secretion may also promote weight loss by allowing catecholamine-stimulated lipolysis to continue at an increased rate.

Acknowledgment

Supported by grants 5P01 CA 29502, 5T32 CA 09427 and CA 08748 from the National Institutes of Health and by grants from the Stella and Charles Guttman Foundation, the William H. Donner Foundation, Inc., the Alcoholic Beverage Medical Research Foundation, the Richard Molin Memorial Foundation, the Loet A. Velmans Fund, and the General Foods Fund. This research was performed in the Sperry Corporation Nutrition Research Laboratory. Dr. Katzeff is the recipient of a New Investigator Award, NIADDK, NIH.

References

1. Means JH. The Thyroid and its Diseases. 2nd ed. Philadelphia, JB Lippincott, 1948: 319–320.
2. Van Wyck J, Underwood LE, Hintz RL, et al. The somatomedins: a family of insulin-like hormones under growth hormone control. Rec Prog Horm Res 1974; 30:259–275.
3. Hall K. Effect of intravenous administration of human growth hormone on sulfation factor activity in serum of hypopituitary subjects. Acta Endocrinol (Copenh) 1971; 66:491–498.
4. Salmon WD Jr, DuVall MR. A serum factor with sulfation factor activity stimulates in vitro incorporation of leucine and sulfate into protein polysaccharide complexes, uridine into RNA and thymidine into DNA of costal cartilages from hypophysectomized rats in vitro. Endocrinology 1970; 86:721–727.
5. Hall K, Uthne K. Some biological properties of purified sulfation factor from human plasma. Acta Med Scand 1971; 190:137–144.
6. Unterman TG, Vazquez RM, Slas AJ, et al. Nutrition and somatomedin. XIII. Usefulness of somatomedin-C in nutritional assessment. Am J Med 1985; 78:228–232.
7. Grant DB, Hambley J, Becker D, et al. Reduced sulfation factor in undernourished children. Arch Dis Child 1973; 48:596–600.
8. Price DA, Wit JM, van Buul-Offers S, et al. Serum somatomedin activity and cartilage metabolism in acutely fasted, chronically malnourished and refed rats. Endocrinology 1979; 105:851–861.
9. Kelts DG, Grand RF, Shen G, et al. Nutritional basis of growth failure in children and adolescents with Crohn's disease. Gastroenterology 1979; 76:720–727.
10. Fineberg SE, Merimee TJ. Acute metabolic actions of human growth hormone. Diabetes 1974; 23:499–504.
11. Fain JN, Dodd A, Novak L. Relationship of protein synthesis and cyclic AMP to the lipolytic action of growth hormone and glucocorticoids. Metabolism 1971; 20:109–118.
12. Raben MS, Hollenberg CH. Effect of growth hormone on free fatty acids. J Clin Invest 1959; 38:484–492.
13. Arner P, Engfeldt P, Nowak J. In vivo observations on the lipolytic effect of noradrenaline during therapeutic fasting. J Clin Endocrinol Metab 1981; 53:1207–1212.
14. Tchobroutsky G, Rosselin G, et al. Growth hormone secretion in obese subjects with and without diabetes mellitus. In Vague J (ed). Pathophysiology of Adipose Tissue. New York, Excerpta Medica, 1969: 269–288.
15. Williams T, Berelowitz M, Joffe SN, et al. Impaired growth hormone responses to growth hormone–releasing factor in obesity: a pituitary defect reversed with weight reduction. N Engl J Med 1984; 311:1403–1407.
16. Brown DJ, Spanos E, MacIntyre I. Role of pituitary hormones in regulating renal vitamin D metabolism in man. Br Med J 1980; 280:272–278.
17. Lund B, Eskilden PC, Lund B, et al. Calcium and vitamin D metabolism in acromegaly. Acta Endocrinol (Copenh) 1981; 96:444–448.
18. Gertner JM, Tamborlane WV, Hintz RL, et al. The effects on mineral metabolism of overnight growth hormone infusion in growth hormone deficiency. J Clin Endocrinol Metab 1981; 53:818–822.
19. Bruns EH, Vollmer SS, Bruns DE, et al. Human growth hormone increases intestinal vitamin D–dependent calcium-binding protein in hypophysectomized rats. Endocrinology 1983; 113:1387–1390.
20. Hwang P, Guyda H, Friesen HA. A radioimmunoassay for human prolactin. Proc Natl Acad Sci USA 1970; 68:1902–1905.
21. Lyons WR, Li CH, Johnson RE. The hormonal control of mammary growth and lactation. Rec Prog Horm Res 1968; 14:219–227.
22. Pahuja DN, DeLuca HF. Stimulation of intestinal calcium transport and bone calcium mobilization by prolactin in vitamin D–deficient rats. Science 1981; 214:1037–1038.
23. Spanos E, Colston KW, Evans IMF, et al. Effect of prolactin on vitamin D metabolism. Mol Cell 1976; 5:163–167.
24. Klibanski AK, Neer RM, Beitins IZ, et al. Decreased bone density in hyperprolactinemic women. N Engl J Med 1980; 303:1511–1514.
25. Schlechte JA, Sherman B, Martin R. Bone density in amenorrheic women with and without hyperprolactinemia. J Clin Endocrinol Metab 1983; 56:1120–1123.
26. Koppelman MCS, Kurtz DW, Morrish KA, et al. Vertebral body bone mineral content in hyperprolactinemic women. J Clin Endocrinol Metab 1984; 59:1050–1054.

27. Ismail-Beigi F, Edelman IS. The mechanism of the calorigenic action of thyroid hormones. Stimulation of NA$^+$ + K$^+$ activated adenosine triphosphatase activity. J Gen Physiol 1971; 57:710–722.

28. Danforth E Jr, Horton ES, O'Connell M, et al. Dietary-induced alterations in thyroid hormone metabolism during overnutrition. J Clin Invest 1979; 64:1336–1347.

29. Katzeff HL, O'Connell M, Horton ES, et al. Metabolic studies in human obesity during overnutrition and undernutrition: thermogenic and hormonal responses to norepinephrine. Metabolism 1986; 35:166–175.

30. Keys A, Brozek J, Henschel A, et al. The Biology of Human Starvation. Minneapolis, University of Minnesota, 1950.

31. Katzeff HL, Daniels RJ. The sympathetic nervous system in human obesity. Int J Obesity 1985; 9(Suppl 2):131–137.

32. Bray GA, Raben MS, Londono J, et al. Effect of triiodothyronine, growth hormone, and anabolic steroids on nitrogen excretion and oxygen consumption of obese patients. J Clin Endocrinol Metab 1971; 33:293–299.

33. Wimpheimer C, Saville E, Viriol MJ, et al. Starvation-induced decreased sensitivity of resting metabolic rate to triiodothyronine. Science 1979; 205:1272–1273.

34. Bayliss RIS, Edwards OM. Urinary excretion of free catecholamines in Graves' disease. Endocrinology 1971; 49:167–169.

35. Aoki VS, Wilson WR, Theilen EO: Studies of the reputed augmentation of the cardiovascular effects of catecholamines in patients with spontaneous hyperthyroidism. J Pharmacol Exp Therap 1972; 181:362–369.

36. Neumann RO. Experimentelle Beitrage zur Lahre von dem taschlichen Narungsbedarf des Menschen unter besondere. Beruksichtigung der notwendigen Eiwessmenge. Arch Hyg 1902; 45:1–22.

37. Nicholl DG. Hamster brown adipose tissue mitochondria. Purine nucleotide control of the ion conductance of the inner membrane, the nature of the nucleotide binding site. Eur J Biochem 1976; 62:223–228.

38. Tata JR, Widnell CC. Ribonucleic acid synthesis during the early actions of thyroid hormones. Biochem J 1966; 98:604–620.

39. Oppenheimer JH, Koerner D, Schwartz AL, et al. Specific nuclear triiodothyronine binding sites in rat liver and kidney. J Clin Endocrinol Metab 1972; 35:330–333.

40. Bronk JR. Thyroid hormone: effects on electron transport. Science 1966; 153:638–639.

41. Fisher JN, Ball EG. Studies on the metabolism of adipose tissue. XX. The effect of thyroid status on oxygen consumption and lipolysis. Biochemistry 1967; 6:637–641.

42. Tulp OL, Frink R, Danforth E Jr. Effect of cafeteria overfeeding on brown and white tissue cellularity, thermogenesis and body composition in rats. J Nutr 1982; 112:2250–2260.

43. Heaton JM. The distribution of brown adipose tissue in the human. J Anat 1972; 112:35–39.

44. Sellers EA, You SS. The role of thyroid hormone in the metabolic response to a cold environment. Am J Physiol 1950; 163:145–158.

45. Nikkila EA, Kekki M. Plasma triglyceride metabolism in thyroid disease. J Clin Invest 1972; 51:2103–2106.

46. Steinberg D, Nestel PJ, Buskirk ER, et al. Calorigenic effect of norepinephrine correlated with free fatty acid turnover and oxidation. J Clin Invest 1964; 43:167–176.

47. Ortigosa JL, Mendoza F, Argote RM, et al. Propranolol effect on plasma glucose, free fatty acid insulin and growth hormone in Graves' disease. Metabolism 1976; 25:1201–1207.

48. Marecek RL, Feldman JM. Effect of hyperthyroidism on insulin and glucose dynamics in rabbits. Endocrinology 1973; 92:1604–1608.

49. Hales CN, Hyams CE. Plasma concentrations of glucose, non-esterified fatty acid, and insulin during glucose-tolerance tests in thyrotoxicosis. Lancet 1964; 2:69–71.

50. Ismail-Beigi F, Edelman I. Effects of thyroid status on electrolyte distribution in rat tissues. Am J Physiol 1973; 225:1175–1179.

51. Hsieh ACL, Carlson LD. Role of thyroid in the metabolic response to low temperature. Am J Physiol 1957; 188:40–44.

52. Elrick H, Hlad CJ, Arai Y. Influence of thyroid function on carbohydrate metabolism and a new method for assessing response to insulin. J Clin Endocrinol Metab 1961; 21:387–392.

53. Althausen TL, Stockholm M. Influence of the thyroid gland on absorption in the digestive tract. Am J Physiol 1938; 123:577–580.

54. Cook PB, Nassim JR, Collins J. The effects of thyrotoxicosis upon the metabolism of calcium, nitrogen and phosphorus. Q J Med 1959; 28:505–512.

55. Mundy GR, Shapiro JL, Bandelin JG, et al. Direct stimulation of bone resorption by thyroid hormones. J Clin Invest 1976; 58:529–536.

56. Kivirikko KI, Laitinen O, Lamberg BA. Value of urine and serum hydroxyproline in the diagnosis of thyroid disease. J Clin Endocrinol Metab 1965; 25:1347–1381.

57. Bouillon R, DeMoor P. Parathyroid function in patients with hyper- or hypothyroidism. J Clin Endocrinol Metab 1974; 38:999–1003.

58. Aub JC, Bauer W, Heath C, et al. Studies of calcium and phosphorus metabolism. II. The effects of thyroid hormones and thyroid disease. J Clin Invest 1929; 7:97–104.

59. Ascarelli I, Budowski P, Nir I, et al. The influence of thyroid status on the utilization of vitamin A and carotene by chickens. Poult Sci 1964; 43:370–374.

60. Cama HR, Goodwin TW. Studies in vitamin A. The role of thyroid in carotene and vitamin A metabolism. Biochem J 1949; 45:236–239.

61. Smith FR, Goodman DS. The effects of diseases of the liver, thyroid and kidneys on the transport of vitamin A in human plasma. J Clin Invest 1971; 50:2426–2432.

62. Walton KW, Campell DA, Tonks EL. The significance of alterations in serum lipids in thyroid dysfunction. I. The relationship between serum lipoproteins, carotenoids and vitamin A in hypothyroidism and thyrotoxicosis. Clin Sci 1965; 29:199–203.

63. Drill VA. The effect of experimental hyperthyroidism on the vitamin B$_1$ content of some rat tissues. Am J Physiol 1938; 122:486–491.

64. Kontinnen A, Viherkoski M. Blood transketolase and erythrocyte glucose-6-phosphate dehydrogenase activities on thyrotoxicosis. Clin Chim Acta 1968; 22:145–147.

65. Rivlin RS: Medical progress: riboflavin metabolism. N Engl J Med 1970; 283:463–466.

66. Rivlin RS, Fazekas AG, Huang YP, et al. Flavin metabolism and its control by thyroid hormone. In Singer T (ed). Flavins and Flavoproteins. Amsterdam, Elsevier Press, 1976:747–753.

67. Palagiano V: La riboflavinemia nel morbo di Basedow prima e dopo l'intervento chirurgico. Acta Chir Ital 1961; 17:273–277.

68. Sato KS, Mimura H, Wakai K, et al. Modulating effect of glutathione disulfide on thyroxine 5'-deiodination by rat hepatocytes in primary culture: effect of glucose. Endocrinology 1983; 13:878–886.

69. Labousse J, Chatagner F, Jolles-Bereget B. Dosage de phosphate de pyridoxal dans le foie du rat normal, du rat thyrotoxique, et du rat thyroidectomise. Biochim Biophys Acta 1960; 39:372–376.

70. Wohl MG, Levy HA, Szutka A, et al. Pyridoxine deficiency in hyperthyroidism. Proc Soc Exp Biol Med 1960; 105:523–526.

71. Rupp J, Paschkis KE, Cantarow A. Influence of vitamin B$_{12}$ and liver extract on nitrogen balance of normal and hyperthyroid rats. Proc Soc Exp Biol Med 1951; 76:432–436.

72. Alperin JB, Haggard ME, Haynie TP. A study of vitamin B$_{12}$ requirements in a patient with pernicious anemia and thyrotoxicosis: evidence of an increased need for vitamin

B_{12} in the presence of hyperthyroidism. Blood 1970; *36*:632–637.

73. Ziffer H, Guttman A, Pasher I, et al. Vitamin B_{12} in thyrotoxicosis and myxedema. Proc Soc Exp Biol Med 1957; *96*:229–233.

74. Caplan RH, Davis K, Bengston B, et al. Serum folate and vitamin B_{12} levels in hypothyroid and hyperthyroid patients. Arch Intern Med 1975; *135*:701–703.

75. Targovnik JH, Rodman JS, Sherwood LM: Regulation of parathyroid hormone secretion *in vitro*: quantitative aspects of calcium and magnesium ion control. Endocrinology 1971; *88*:1477–1480.

76. Anast CS, Mohs JM, Kaplan SL, et al. Evidence for parathyroid failure in magnesium deficiency. Science 1972; *177*:606–609.

77. Hellman D, Au WYW, Bartter FC. Evidence for a direct effect of parathyroid hormone on urinary acidification. Am J Physiol 1965; *209*:643–650.

78. Peacock M, Robertson WG, Nordin BEC. Relation between serum and urinary calcium with particular reference to parathyroid activity. Lancet 1969; *1*:384–386.

79. Garabedian M, Holick MF, DeLuca HF, et al. Control of 25-hydroxycholecalciferol metabolism by the parathyroid gland. Proc Natl Acad Sci USA 1972; *69*:1673–1677.

80. Broadus AE, Horst RL, Lang R, et al. The importance of circulating 1,25-dihydroxyvitamin D in the pathogenesis of hypercalciuria and renal-stone formation in primary hyperparathyroidism. N Engl J Med 1980; *302*:421–426.

81. Talmage RV. Effect of fasting and parathyroid hormone injection on plasma ^{45}Ca concentration in rats. Calcif Tiss Res 1975; *17*:103–112.

82. Seyle H. On the stimulation of new bone formation with parathyroid extract and irradiated ergosterol. Endocrinology 1932; *16*:547–558.

83. Parsons JA, Reit B. Chronic response of dogs to parathyroid hormone infusion. Nature 1974; *250*:254–257.

84. Aurbach GD, Mallette LE, Patten BM, et al. Hyperparathyroidism: recent studies. Ann Intern Med 1973; *79*:566–573.

85. Genant HK, Baron JM, Straus FH II, et al. Osteosclerosis in primary hyperparathyroidism. Am J Med 1975; *59*:104–110.

86. Peacock M: Renal stone disease and bone disease in primary hyperparathyroidism and their relationship to the action of parathyroid hormone on calcium absorption. *In* RV Talmage, M Owen, JA Parsons (eds). Calcium-Regulating Hormones. Amsterdam, Excerpta Medica, 1975: 78–81.

87. Kooh SW, Fraser D, DeLuca HL, et al. Treatment of hypoparathyroidism and pseudohypoparathyroidism with metabolites of vitamin D: evidence for impaired conversion of 25-hydroxyvitamin D to 1,25-dihydroxyvitamin D. N Engl J Med 1975; *293*:840–847.

88. Parfitt AM: The spectrum of hypoparathyroidism. J Clin Endocrinol Metab 1972; *34*:152–159.

89. McCallister B, Millere BM, Lacy WW, et al. The effect of acute and chronic glucocorticoid excess on leucine kinetics and protein turnover in vivo. J Surg Res 1983; *35*:426–432.

90. Slag MF, Admed M, Gannon MC, et al. Meal stimulation of cortisol secretion: a protein induced effect. Metabolism 1981; *30*:1104–1108.

91. Wise JK, Hendler R, Felig P. Influences of glucocorticoids on glucagon and plasma amino acid concentrations in man. J Clin Invest 1973; *52*:2774–2782.

92. Stalmans W, Laloux M. Glucocorticoids and hepatic glycogen metabolism. *In* Baxter JD, Rousseau GG (eds). Glucocorticoid Hormone Action. New York, Springer-Verlag, 1979: 517–533.

93. David DS, Grieco MH, Cushman P. Adrenal glucocorticoids after 20 years. A review of their clinically relevant consequences. J Chron Dis 1970; *22*:637–651.

94. Hausberger FX, Hausberger BC. Effects of insulin and cortisone on weight gain, protein and fat content of rats. Am J Physiol 1958; *193*:455–465.

95. Birkenhager JC, Timmermans HAT, Lamberts SWJ. Depressed plasma FFA turnover rate in Cushing's syndrome. J Clin Endocrinol Metab 1976; *42*:28–37.

96. Rizza RA, Mandarino LJ, Gerich JE. Cortisol-induced insulin resistance in man: impaired suppression of glucose production and stimulation of glucose utilization due to a post-receptor defect. J Clin Endocrinol Metab 1982; *54*:131–138.

97. Taskinen, MR, Nikkila, EA, Pelkonen R, et al. Plasma lipoproteins, lipolytic enzymes, and very low density lipoprotein triglyceride turnover in Cushing's syndrome. J Clin Endocrinol Metab 1983; *57*:619–626.

98. Walser M, Duckett J Jr. The hypercalcemia of adrenal insufficiency. J Clin Invest 1983; *42*:456–465.

99. Lukert BP, Adams JS. Calcium and phosphorus homeostasis in man: effect of corticosteroids. Arch Intern Med 1976; *136*:1249–1252.

100. Kimberg, DV, Baerg, RD, Gershon E, et al. Effect of cortisone treatment on the active transport of calcium by the small intestine. J Clin Invest 1971; *50*:1309–1326.

101. Seeman E, Kumar R, Hunder GG, et al. Production, degradation, and circulating levels of 1,25-dihydroxyvitamin D in health and in chronic glucocorticoid excess. J Clin Invest 1980; *66*:664–669.

102. Papapoulos SE, Fraher LJ, Sandler LM, et al. 1,25-Dihydroxycholecalciferol in the pathogenesis of the hypercalcemia of sarcoidosis. Lancet 1979; *1*:627–628.

103. Wong GL. Basal activities and hormone responsiveness of osteoclast-like and osteoblast-like bone cells are regulated by glucocorticoids. J Biol Chem 1979; *254*:6337–6340.

104. Motil KJ, Grand RJ, Maletskos CJ, et al. The effect of disease, drug, and diet on whole body protein metabolism with Crohn disease and growth failure. J Pediatr 1982; *101*:345–351.

105. Jowsey J, Riggs BL. Bone formation in hypercortisolism. Acta Endocrinol (Copenh) 1970; *63*:21–29.

106. Hough S, Teitelbaum SL, Gergefeld MA, et al: Isolated skeletal involvement in Cushing's syndrome: response to therapy. J Clin Endocrinol Metab 1981; *52*:1033–1038.

107. Jorgensen H. Hypercalcemia in adrenocortical insufficiency. Acta Med Scand 1973: *193*:175–179.

108. Young JB, Landsberg L. Suppression of the sympathetic nervous system during fasting. Science 1977; *196*:1473–1475.

109. Young JB, Landsberg L. Catecholamines and intermediary metabolism. Clin Endocrinol Metab 1977; *6*:599–632.

110. Himms-Hagen J. Effects of catecholamines on metabolism. *In* Blashko H, Muscholl E (eds). Handbook of Experimental Pharmacology. Vol. 33. Catecholamines. Berlin, Springer-Verlag, 1976: 363–462.

111. Garber AJ, Karl IE, Kipnis DM. Alanine and glutamine synthesis and release from skeletal muscle. IV. Beta-adrenergic inhibition of amino acid release. J Biol Chem 1976; *251*:851–857.

112. Silverberg AB, Shah SD, Haymond MW, et al. Norepinephrine: hormone and transmitter. Am J Physiol 1978; *234*:252–253.

113. Leblanc J, Pouloit M. Importance of noradrenaline in cold adaptation. Am J Physiol 1964; *207*:853–856.

114. Cannon WB, McIver MA, Bliss SW. Studies on the conditions of activity in endocrine glands. XIII. A sympathetic and adrenal mechanism for mobilizing sugar in hypoglycemia. Am J Physiol 1924; *69*:46–66.

115. Leblanc J, Pouloit M. Importance of noradrenaline in cold adaptation. Am J Physiol 1964; *207*:853–856.

116. Foster DO. Calorigenic potential of rat brown adipose tissue and muscle reevaluated from blood flow measurements with tracer microspheres. Physiologist 1976; *19*:194–199.

117. Hardman MJ, Hull D. The effect of environmental conditions on the growth and function of brown adipose tissue. J Physiol 1971; *214*:191–199.

118. Landsberg L, Young JB. Fasting, feeding and the regulation of sympathetic activity. N Engl J Med 1978; *298*:1295–1301.

119. Welle S, Lilavivathana U, Campbell RG. Increased plasma norepinephrine concentrations and metabolic rates following glucose ingestion in man. Metabolism 1980; *29*:806–809.

120. Galbo H, Holst J, Christensen NJ, et al. Glucagon and plasma catecholamines during beta-receptor blockade in exercising man. J Appl Physiol 1976; *40*:855–863.

121. Engelman K, Mueller PS, Sjoerdsma A. Elevated plasma free fatty acid concentrations in patients with pheochromocytoma. N Engl J Med 1964; *270*:865–870.

122. Kimberg DV, Schachter D, Schenker H. Active transport of calcium by intestine: effects of dietary calcium. Am J Physiol 1961; *200*:1256–1262.

123. Lukert BP, Stanbury SW, Mawer EB. Vitamin D and intestinal transport of calcium: effects of prednisolone. Endocrinology 1973; *93*:718–722.

124. Steinberg D, Nestel PJ, Buskirk ER, et al. Calorigenic effect of norepinephrine correlated with free fatty acid turnover. J Clin Invest 1965; *43*:167–168.

125. Engelman K, Mueller PS, Sjoerdsma A. Elevated plasma free fatty acid concentrations in patients with pheochromocytoma. N Engl J Med 1964; *270*:865–870.

20

DIABETES MELLITUS

CHARLES R. SHUMAN

Regulation of nutrient metabolism in diabetes mellitus is reviewed in Chapter 2. The purpose of this chapter is to outline the dietary management of patients with this disease.

Before the discovery of insulin, there was little to offer the diabetic patient other than dietary advice. Among the earliest recommendations were the feeding of sugars and starches to replace urinary loss of glucose. Subsequently the intake of carbohydrate foods was restricted, with meats and fats favored as the principal dietary sources.[1] None of these regimens received satisfactory evaluation until the studies of Allen were begun in 1914.[2] Based on observations made on pancreatectomized dogs, a regimen was devised for treatment of diabetic patients providing 1500 to 2000 kcal in which protein and fat were given at relatively high quantities with carbohydrate added in quantities short of that causing glycosuria.[2] This calorically deficient diet was successful in prolonging the lives of many patients.

After the development of insulin treatment, although liberated from the rigors of undernutrition, diabetic patients continued to receive diets restricted in carbohydrates until modified insulin preparations became available. With the introduction of long-acting insulin preparations a trend toward less restrictive diets gained in popularity. This move toward liberalization of dietary management was moderated by the development of the Food Exchange System adopted by the American Diabetes Association and the American Dietetic Association.[3]

Current programs of diabetic management continue to emphasize the fundamental role of diet in the regulation of blood glucose.[4] Basic nutritional requirements for diabetic patients are essentially the same as those established for the general population, and the objective of dietary therapy is to achieve a normal pattern of food consumption. Dietary choices have been made sufficiently flexible to provide customary selections of foods according to taste and eating habits, although the intake of sugar is limited. In addition, the trend to a general reduction in fat and cholesterol intake in Western countries has been strongly advocated for the diabetic population. In general, the goal of the dietary treatment is to promote uniformity of food intake at levels providing energy requirements to achieve and maintain ideal body weight (IBW) in nutritious and appealing meal planning programs.[4]

Planning for the diet requires consideration of the type of diabetes and the caloric needs of the individual based on age, activities, cultural and psychosocial aspects, and the presence of complications of diabetes or associated illness.

DIAGNOSTIC CRITERIA AND CLASSIFICATION CRITERIA OF DIABETES

Diabetes mellitus is identified by the presence of an elevation of blood glucose concentrations in the fasting state, after meals, or following a standard oral glucose load. Hyperglycemia and other biochemical derangements are the consequence of diminished secretion or activity of insulin, the key hormone in the regulation of glucose, lipid, and protein metabolism. The degree of insulin deprivation determines the severity of symptoms of the disease, which vary from an absence of complaints in mild insulin deficiency to extreme thirst, weight loss, polyuria, dehydration, coma, and death in severe, untreated cases of insulin deficiency. In the chronic diabetic state, there are progressive and characteristic changes in the retina, kidneys, peripheral nerves, and connective tissue, and accelerated arteriosclerotic disease of coronary, cerebral, and lower extremity vessels.

Classifications of diabetes proposed by an International Work Group sponsored by the National Diabetes Data Group (NDDG), National Institutes of Health,[5] and by the World Health Organization (WHO) Expert Committee on Diabetes Mellitus[6] in 1980 have been given general acceptance. The major subclasses of clinical diabetes, insulin-dependent diabetes mellitus and non–insulin-dependent diabetes mellitus, have been expanded by the addition of malnutrition-related diabetes mellitus by WHO in 1985[7] because of the high prevalence of this disorder in tropical and developing countries. The clinical categories of diabetes and glucose intolerance as revised in the WHO Technical Report 727 of 1985 are shown in Table 20–1.

In the developed countries, the major subclasses of diabetes are insulin-dependent diabetes mellitus (IDDM) and non–insulin-dependent diabetes mellitus (NIDDM), with the latter accounting for nearly 85 per cent of their diabetic populations. The term Type I diabetes has been used interchangeably with IDDM and bears the connotation of autoimmunity in its pathogenesis and the presence of genetic markers such as islet cell antibody and certain HLA groups (DR3/DR4). Insulin deprivation causes marked hyperglycemia and the presence of ketone bodies in blood and urine in the basal state; the ke-

TABLE 20–1. Classification of Diabetes Mellitus and Glucose Intolerance

Diabetes Mellitus (DM)
  Insulin-dependent diabetes mellitus (IDDM)
  Non–insulin-dependent diabetes mellitus (NIDDM)
   a) Non-obese
   b) Obese
  Malnutrition-related diabetes mellitus (MRDM)
  Other types associated with certain conditions or syndromes
   a) Pancreatic disease
   b) Hormonal etiology
   c) Drug- or chemical-induced
   d) Abnormalities related to insulin or its receptors
   e) Certain genetic syndromes
   f) Miscellaneous
Impaired Glucose Tolerance (IGT)
   a) Non-obese
   b) Obese
   c) Association with certain conditions
Gestational Diabetes (GD)

tone bodies represent reliable clinical markers of IDDM. Type II diabetes is an alternative designation for NIDDM and includes those patients not requiring insulin therapy for survival and who are ketosis-resistant under basal and non-gravid states. A subgroup of patients within the Type II category has been identified as having latent Type I disease. These patients may be identified by the presence of islet cell antibodies and manifest slowly progressive beta cell loss and a long latency period.[8] The distinctions between these two major clinical groups are shown in Table 20–2.

Diagnostic criteria for diabetes mellitus were proposed in 1979 by the NDDG based upon epidemiological studies of several large populations.[5] These criteria have been accorded broad acceptance. They have been modified and simplified in reports of a WHO Study Group in 1985.[7] In the latter method, blood glucose determinations are obtained after overnight fast and at 2 hours following a 75 gm oral glucose load (OGTT). The $\frac{1}{2}$, 1, $1\frac{1}{2}$ hour samples used in the NDDG criteria are not required since these values have not been shown to have significance in the interpretation of the OGTT. The diagnostic criteria are shown in Table 20–3.

For purposes of screening for diabetes, a single blood sample obtained 2 hours after a 75 g glucose load may provide the most definitive data provided certain precautions are met. The patient is prepared with a 3-day period of normal diet including a minimum of 150 g of carbohydrate during which normal activities are maintained. The presence of infection, stress, and medications known to affect glucose tolerance should be noted as factors influencing the blood glucose concentrations. Screening for diabetes is indicated in those at risk for the disease, including persons with close relatives having diabetes, the obese, the elderly, pregnant females, and patients with arteriosclerosis, heart disease, and hypertension.

TABLE 20–2. Comparison between IDDM and NIDDM

	IDDM	NIDDM
Former names	Juvenile, growth onset Ketosis-prone	Adult, maturity onset Ketosis resistant
Age of onset	Usually under 30; occurs at any age	Peak incidence—5th decade May occur at younger ages
Symptoms	Usually abrupt Thirst, polyuria, weight loss	Frequently none; or thirst, fatigue, visual blurring; or symptoms of vascular or neural complications
Nutritional status	Usually thin	60 to 80% are obese
Coma syndrome	Diabetic ketoacidosis	Hyperosmolar state Ketosis rarely with infection or stress
Endogenous insulin and C-peptide	Negligible to absent	Normal levels, but low in re- lation to blood sugar
Lipid abnormalities	Frequent cholesterol and LDL elevations Hyperlipidemia in ke- toacidosis	Triglyceride (VLDL) and LDL cholesterol increased
Insulin	All patients dependent upon insulin	Required for 20–30%
Sulfonylurea	No response	Effective for majority
Diet	Mandatory	Mandatory; diet alone may control blood sugar

INDIVIDUALIZING THE DIET

Despite controversy concerning dietary policies in the management of diabetes, it is now clear that a properly devised diet is an essential component in the control of the disease. Physicians involved in the treatment of diabetes must be familiar with the methods used for the determination of daily caloric requirements and the partitioning of calories into the dietary content of carbohydrate, protein, and fat for the meal planning program.[3] Although these fundamental concepts of nutritional components are known to most physicians, the services of a registered dietician or nutritionist are usually required to translate the calculated diet into food selections and structured meals for the patient. Trained personnel are available in most communities and hospitals to provide the essential services for circulating knowledge of the composition of foods, basic nutritional needs, and the practical aspects of meal planning. While there is no single food plan suitable for all diabetic patients, preplanned diets are available that can be readily personalized for patients by physicians and health care professionals (Table 20–4).

TABLE 20–3. Criteria for Diagnosis of Diabetes Mellitus and Impaired Glucose Tolerance

	Plasma		Whole Blood	
	Venous	*Capillary*	*Venous*	*Capillary*
Diabetes mellitus				
Fasting glucose*	≥140 (7.8)	≥140 (7.8)	≥120 (6.7)	≥120 (6.7)
2 hr post glucose†	≥200 (11.1)	≥220 (12.2)	≥180 (10.0)	≥200 (12.2)
Impaired Glucose Tolerance				
Fasting glucose*	<140 (7.8)	<140 (7.8)	<120 (6.7)	<120 (6.7)
2 hr post glucose†	140–200 (7.8–11.1)	160–220 (8.9–12.2)	120–180 (6.7–10.0)	140–200 (7.8–11.1)

Gestational Diabetes
(1) W.H.O. criteria are the same as those given for diabetes mellitus.
(2) O'Sullivan and Mahan criteria: using a 100 g glucose load, two or more of the following values must be met or exceeded.
*Venous Plasma Glucose**

Fasting—105 (5.8)	1 hr—190 (10.6)	2 hr—165 (9.2)	3 hr—145 (8.1)

*mg/100 ml (mmol/L)
†Oral glucose challenge is 75 g for adults and 1.75 g/kg to 75 g for children.
Diagnostic criteria for children are same as those for adults.

TABLE 20–4. *Dietary Strategies in Diabetic Management*

	IDDM	NIDDM
Effect of diet	Essential for glycemic control with insulin	May suffice for control as sole therapy
Calories	Increased to reverse undernutrition and achieve IBW	Reduced caloric intake to correct obesity and aid in glycemic control
Consistency of food intake	Necessary for control and for correlation with insulin action	Desirable for weight reduction, avoid gorging
Caloric distribution	Carbohydrate equally distributed in meals or adjusted for insulin timing	Equal distribution of CHO not essential
Timing of meals	Regularity of meals needed for intermediate insulin Flexibility permitted with regular insulin	Desirable but not crucial on diet alone Necessary if receiving insulin
Interval snack	Frequently required are 3:00 P.M. and bedtime snacks	Not recommended
Food supplement for exercise	CHO—20 g/hr for moderate physical activity	Necessary if controlled on insulin or sulfonylurea

CALORIC DISTRIBUTION

Determination of caloric requirements is the initial and dominant factor in dietary planning for the patient with diabetes. The energy sources and nutritional components must fulfill the objective of attaining and maintaining ideal body weight and meet energy demands for graded levels of physical activity and for the repair and growth of tissues.[4] The earlier focus on carbohydrates and fat distribution assumes a secondary role following observations that increased carbohydrate and lower fat intakes provide a palatable diet without significantly altering the plasma glucose concentration when compared with isocaloric diets of restricted carbohydrate content.

Excessive caloric intake associated with weight gain has been shown to promote an increase in circulating insulin concentrations in nondiabetic patients.[9] Despite incremental plasma insulin concentrations, glucose tolerance tends to decrease with advancing adiposity. Resistance to insulin activity in obese patients has been related to alterations in insulin receptor function in skeletal muscle, liver, and adipose tissue. A decrease in the number of receptors (down-regulation) associated with increased circulating insulin and a decrease in responsiveness to insulin, a post-receptor defect, have been implicated as causes of insulin resistance.[10]

Obese patients are treated with hypocaloric diets, which lower plasma glucose concentrations and improve the sensitivity of the tissue to insulin.[11] Resistance to insulin action, whether related to a post-receptor defect or to reduced receptor populations on cell membrane, is decreased by caloric restriction in the obese diabetic patient. These improvements in insulin sensitivity are observed even before significant losses of stored adipose tissue are achieved.

In general, the average daily negative energy balance rather than the dietary composition is the major factor in improving the carbohydrate and lipid homeostasis of these overweight diabetic patients.[11]

For nonobese patients and those engaged in increased activity, the level of caloric intake is increased. Their daily caloric requirement does not differ from that of the nondiabetic population and will be dependent upon age, sex, and degree of energy expenditure as outlined by the Food and Nutrition Board of the National Research Council.[12] The underweight patient will require an increased daily caloric intake to achieve nutritional rehabilitation. This condition is encountered most frequently in the catabolic insulin-deficient Type I patient who has lost tissue protein and fat during periods of unrecognized or poorly treated diabetes.

Children with diabetes require adequate calories to maintain normal growth and maturation. Prepubertal children receive a caloric intake of 1000 kcal plus an additional 100 kcal for each year of age until puberty is reached. This approximates 90 kcal/kg in the age range 4 to 6 years and 80 kcal/kg in the 7 to 11 age range.[12] During puberty, the caloric allowance for males rises to 3200 to 3600 daily and for females, 2400 to 2800 calories daily. These young patients are monitored on growth charts to maintain normal developmental curves.

DIETARY DETERMINATION OF MAJOR NUTRIENTS

Carbohydrate Intake

Several lines of evidence have led to the liberalization of the carbohydrate content of the diabetic diet. Recent research has implicated serum lipid disturbances, particularly hypercholesterolemia, as an important risk factor in the pathogenesis of atherosclerosis.[13-15] This had led to the recommendation that dietary fat intake be reduced with replacement of these calories as carbohydrate. Evidence that an increase in dietary carbohydrate is associated with improved glucose tolerance was demonstrated initially by Himsworth using normal subjects.[16] These observations were confirmed in patients with NIDDM[17] and have been expanded by the work of Kiehm and coworkers[18] in diabetic patients treated with a high-carbohydrate, high-fiber diet. Reductions in plasma glucose and of low-density-lipoprotein (LDL) cholesterol concentration were observed in both IDDM and poorly controlled NIDDM patients during treatment with increased carbohydrate intake of high fiber content. Improvement in plasma glucose concentration with fiber-enriched diets is independent of alterations in insulin availability and appears to be associated with an increase in tissue insulin sensitivity and a decrease in rates of glucose absorption.[19,20] In IDDM patients receiving a high-carbohydrate diet, however, a deterioration in postprandial glycemia is observed if no increase in dietary fiber is provided.[21] Epidemiological studies demonstrate that diabetic patients consuming diets increased in carbohydrate and reduced in fat content have a low incidence of coronary heart disease compared with those receiving the diets of higher fat content.[13]

Current recommendations by authoritative diabetes associations have endorsed the provision of dietary carbohydrate intake of 50 per cent of total calories with a corresponding reduction of fats to approximately 30 to 35 per cent, and protein, 15 to 20 per cent[22-24] (Table 20–5). Thus, the consensus is that the intake of carbohydrate-containing foods for diabetic patients should equal that found in the typical nondiabetic diet. The sources of dietary carbohydrate are mainly complex starches, legumes, fruits, and vegetables, with approximately 10 to 15 per cent of the carbohydrate calories provided as sugars derived from natural sources such as fruits and milk. Diets of increased carbohydrate and fiber

content have been associated with a decrease in plasma lipid levels.[19] Isocaloric substitution of physiological amounts of simple sugars, sucrose or fructose, has not altered the plasma lipid, glucose, or fasting insulin concentrations in the diet of normal[25] and diabetic subjects.[26,27] While some diabetic patients have manifested transitory rises in triglyceride levels with increased carbohydrate diets,[28] this is usually reversed with continued control of plasma glucose. Patients with sustained carbohydrate-induced hypertriglyceridemia may require reduced amounts of dietary carbohydrate or the use of lipid lowering agents if a response is not seen with adjustments in the diet.[29]

Dietary Fiber and the Glycemic Response

Studies by Burkett and Trowell[30] have related the influence of refinement of dietary carbohydrate to the rising incidence of diabetes in several populations, an observation which supported the hypothesis that fiber-depleted refined foods constituted a risk factor in diabetes and that dietary fiber enrichment was protective. Subsequently, numerous investigators have examined the effects of increased dietary fiber and unrefined carbohydrates on plasma glucose, lipid, and insulin responses in normal and diabetic subjects.[19,20,31,32] The initial clinical studies reported by Anderson's group on 12 diabetic patients treated first with a control diet followed by an isocaloric high-carbohydrate (70 per cent), high-fiber (65 g) diet daily (HCF diet) manifested greatly improved diabetic control on the latter program with reduction in dosage or elimination of sulfonylurea or insulin therapy.[18] Numerous observations have confirmed the improvement in glucose tolerance and insulin requirements together with a decrease in plasma cholesterol and triglyceride concentrations during fiber enrichment of meals in both IDDM and NIDDM patients. For the obese patient, the increased fiber content may enhance satiety as a salutary factor in weight reduction.

Dietary fibers are found in food sources such as whole-grain products, fruits, legumes, vegetables, and nuts in which they serve as structural, reparative, or storage components of the cells.[32] They are classified as viscous or nonviscous depending on their respective properties of water solubility or insolubility. Soluble fibers, including pectins, polysaccharide, gum, mucilage, and some hemicelluloses, form gels which influence transit time and absorption of digested food from the gastrointestinal lumen. Insoluble fibers, including cellulose, lignins, and other hemicelluloses, increase the fecal bulk since they are not digested significantly in the colon as are the soluble components when subjected to bacterial action (Table 20–6).

Food exchange groups containing dietary fiber are bread exchanges, whole fruits, and vegetables. The

TABLE 20–5. Caloric Components of the Diabetic Diet

Carbohydrate	50% of total calories
	Starches, vegetables, fruit, milk
	Natural sugars and sucrose 15%
Protein	15 to 20% of total calories
	20% for children, pregnancy, lactation
	0.5 g per pound minimum for adults
Fat	30–35% of total calories
	$\dfrac{\text{Polyunsaturated}}{\text{Saturated}}$ (P/S ratio)
	$= \dfrac{<10\%}{>10\%}$ of total calories
	Cholesterol: 300 mg

TABLE 20–6. Dietary Fiber: Plant Constituents Not Metabolized in Small Intestine

Sources	Whole grain products, vegetables, legumes, fruits with edible skins and seeds, nuts
Types	Viscous, water-soluble: pectin, gums, mucilages, polysaccharides, some hemicelluloses
	Nonviscous, water-insoluble: cellulose, lignins, bran, most hemicelluloses
Effects	Form gels (soluble) or increase bulk (insoluble) in gastrointestinal lumen
	Delay gastric emptying, alter intestinal transit time
	Reduce plasma glucose, cholesterol, triglyceride
	Reduce plasma insulin levels (NIDDM)
	Decrease insulin or sulfonylurea requirements
Adverse effects	Flatulence, abdominal discomfort
	Increased defecation, diarrhea
	Phytobezoar formation
	Potential for vitamin/mineral losses

remaining exchange groups, meat, milk, and fats (except nuts and seeds), do not contain fiber. Acceptable purified fiber preparations have not yet become widely available, so that the current method to increase dietary fiber to levels of 30 to 40 g daily is to emphasize inclusion of whole-grain products, legumes, vegetables, whole fruits, and nuts in the diet. While studies are under way to define specific amounts and types of fiber to be recommended, the use of natural foods containing unrefined carbohydrate sources of high fiber content should be planned for the diet of all diabetic patients because of beneficial effects on plasma glucose and lipid concentrations.[33] Side effects of such diets have included flatulence (sometimes intolerable), colic, and increased frequency of bowel movements. Phytobezoar has occurred in patients with autonomic neuropathy and gastric hypotony. Studies on vitamin and mineral metabolism have shown no evidence of deficiencies with dietary fiber enrichment in long-term studies during which serum levels of micronutrients remained normal.[34]

Until recently, complex carbohydrate foods have been considered to be equivalent in their effects upon the blood glucose concentration. Evidence has now accumulated demonstrating that various foods in this category affect blood glucose concentrations differently.[35,36] Some starches will cause a rapid rise in blood glucose, while equivalent amounts of other starches result in a significantly lower glycemic response.

Recent scientific reports by Crapo and Olefsky[37] and others[38,39] have delineated significant differences in the responses of plasma glucose to chemically similar foods. Equivalent portions of complex carbohydrates or starches such as potatoes or white bread elicited higher plasma glucose responses than does rice or pasta. The data show that fiber is not the sole determinant of the glycemic response, since the wheat in pasta and cereals yields lower glycemic responses than that in breads. Similar divergent glucose responses occur comparing rice flour and whole rice or with whole apples versus apple puree. The

rate of release of products of carbohydrate digestion differ depending upon characteristics such as particle size, structural integrity, and rates of hydrolysis by gastrointestinal enzymes.[39,40]

Among the factors influencing the glycemic response of foods are the modes of preparation and processing, the fiber content, the type of starch, intrinsic antienzyme properties, and the digestive processes. While many studies have been performed on individual foods, the content of fat and protein in mixed meals introduces another important variable in the glycemic response.[41,42] These observations have raised questions concerning the reliability of the present system of meal planning, and nutritionists are considering the advisability of classifying carbohydrate based on its effect on plasma glucose responses. In this context, the foods producing a reduced glycemic response may be given preference in meal planning with the objective of improving the control of blood glucose concentrations without compromising overall nutrition and health.

Jenkins has devised the "glycemic index" based on studies conducted on a large number of commonly used carbohydrates.[36,38,40] Differences in the 2-hour glucose response area for different foods given alone were compared to that obtained after ingestion of an equivalent amount of glucose. Subsequently, the pooled data were revised using white bread as the standard.[38] Glycemic index values are expressed as a percentage of that for white bread. For example, the value of 66 for pasta indicates a blood glucose response in one observation which is 66 per cent of that obtained when white bread of equivalent amount is consumed. In general, the lower glycemic index foods are legumes, beans, and rice, while the higher responses occur with potatoes, breads, and cereals. This type of information may provide a useful basis for meal planning for control of postprandial hyperglycemia in the diabetic patient. Until concrete data using mixed meals are available, patients are encouraged to test the effects of various carbohydrate foods with self-monitoring of blood glucose following meals to evolve a palatable diet with a predictable beneficial response (Table 20–7).

Nutritional counseling has emphasized restriction of sugars in favor of slowly digested complex carbohydrates in the diabetic diet. In recent studies, however, sucrose substituted isocalorically for a portion of dietary carbohydrate produced no change in diurnal glucose profile, plasma lipids, or glycosylated hemoglobin in either insulin-dependent or non–insulin-dependent patients consuming high-fiber, low-fat diets.[27] However, caution is required in the use of sugar-containing foods since standardization of these sweetened foods and drinks has not been defined and the ingestion of these confections will undoubtedly lead to excesses.

Protein Intake

As an index of diabetic control, the plasma concentration of branched-chain amino acids is equiv-

TABLE 20–7.   Mean Glycemic Index (GI) of Some Foods Proportionally Adjusted So White Bread = 100

Food	Mean GI	Food	Mean GI
Bread:		Dried legumes:	
Rye crisp	95	Baked beans (canned)	60
White (wheat)	100	Butter beans	52
Wholegrain rye	58	Haricot beans	45
Wholemeal (wheat)	99	Kidney beans	54
		Soy beans (dried)	22
Cereal products:		Soy beans (canned)	20
Buckwheat	74	Chick peas	49
Millet	103	Dried green peas	56
Rice (brown)	96	Red lentils	43
Rice (white)	83		
Spaghetti (white)	66	Fruit:	
Spaghetti (whole wheat)	61	Apple	53
Sweet corn	87	Banana	79
		Cherries	32
Breakfast cereals:		Grapefruit	36
All-Bran	73	Grapes	62
Cornflakes	119	Orange	66
Muesli	96	Orange juice	67
Porridge oats	85	Peach	40
Shredded wheat	97	Pear	47
Weetabix	109	Plum	34
		Raisins	93
Biscuits:			
Digestive	82	Sugars:	
Oatmeal	78	Fructose	30
Rich tea	80	Glucose	138
Water	91	Honey	126
		Maltose	152
Vegetables:		Sucrose	86
Frozen peas	74		
		Dairy products:	
Root vegetables:		Ice cream	52
Potato (instant)	116	Skim milk	46
Potato (new, boiled)	81	Whole milk	49
Potato (russet, baked)	135	Yogurt	52
Potato (sweet)	70		
Yam	74		

This chart compares equal amounts of carbohydrate, not equal caloric or serving portions. Although some of the data come from nondiabetic individuals, the same foods tested in diabetic individuals have similar glycemic indexes even though the absolute incremental area responses are greater. The chart is meant to illustrate the wide variety in glycemic effects between different carbohydrate-containing foods.

Adapted from Jenkins DJA, et al. Lancet 1984; 2:388–391.

alent to the plasma glucose concentration.[43] Decreased insulin activity diverts amino acids from protein synthesis and leads to nitrogen losses through gluconeogenesis.[44] The protein allotment of 15 to 20 per cent of total calories exceeds that required to preserve endogenous protein stores and to maintain proteogenesis. This level of protein intake is consistent with that consumed in most developed countries and is greater than the recommended daily allowance of 0.8 g/kg of ideal body weight.[12] To assure a balanced amino acid profile for protein biosynthesis, it is advisable to provide 50 per cent of dietary protein of high biological value from the meat exchange lists. Lacto-ovovegetarian diets can be nutritionally satisfactory with respect to protein and amino acid requirements. Modification of the protein intake to lower levels may be required for patients with renal insufficiency commonly seen in diabetes. Food sources such as milk, egg albumin, and meats can provide high biological value protein,

permitting a reduction of total protein intake to 40 to 60 g daily. This adjustment decreases nitrogen retention and may delay the progress of renal disease.[45] During dialysis programs, an increase in the protein ration to 0.8 g/kg of body weight is permitted because amino acids are lost into the dialysate. Dietary restrictions for the diabetic patient with renal insufficiency can be liberalized with careful monitoring during hemodialysis or continuous ambulatory peritoneal dialysis.

Fat Intake

A major clinical problem and leading cause of mortality in the diabetic population is the occurrence of arteriosclerotic disease attributed in part to elevated lipid concentrations.[46,47] A direct relationship has been demonstrated between atherosclerosis and increased serum cholesterol levels.[15] Based on data from epidemiological, experimental, and clinical trial investigations,[13,15,47,48] it is prudent to utilize dietary measures as a primary therapeutic modality for improving the frequently encountered disturbances in the lipid profile of diabetic patients. Current recommendations include a reduction in the daily fat intake to 30 per cent of total calories with emphasis on selections of polyunsaturated fats as an effective method for lowering plasma cholesterol and triglyceride levels. Revised listings of food exchanges identify items containing mono- and polyunsaturated fats to facilitate selections of appropriate meats and fats for meal planning.

Beneficial affects of marine lipids, omega-3 unsaturated fatty acids, have been demonstrated in epidemiological and clinical studies, suggesting that the inclusion of fish in the diet or dietary enrichment with marine lipids may reduce the incidence of coronary vascular disease.[49] Lowering of daily cholesterol intake to 300 mg daily can be achieved by the selection of unsaturated fat sources. Thus, a fat-controlled, cholesterol-restricted diet with emphasis on polyunsaturated fats, including marine sources, and weight reduction for the obese patients, are the recommended dietary measures for combating hyperlipidemia. These dietary modifications together with avoidance of smoking, increased physical conditioning, and careful glycemic regulation should provide protection against the progression of diabetic macrovascular disease.

Events leading to the formation of atherosclerotic plaques result in the deposition of LDL cholesterol in areas of endothelial damage and smooth muscle cell proliferation.[50] Among the lipid derangements occurring in diabetes are increases in LDL and its precursor, very-low-density lipoprotein (VLDL).[46] Both increased production and decreased cellular uptake of LDL have been demonstrated, the latter related to reduced LDL receptor activity in insulin-deficient patients.[51] Protection against local cholesterol accumulation is afforded by the action of high-density lipoprotein (HDL), which assimilates cholesterol for transport to the liver, where it can be recycled or converted to bile salts.[52] Acceleration of atherosclerosis has been associated with low plasma concentrations of HDL, a condition observed in poorly controlled diabetes.[47] With good metabolic control and dietary fat modifications, the cellular utilization of LDL is enhanced and plasma levels of HDL are raised. Additional measures that raise plasma HDL cholesterol are physical conditioning, modest alcohol intake, and weight reduction.[47] The sum of these factors provides an effective mechanism for deterrence of atherosclerosis by elevating the ratio of plasma HDL cholesterol to total cholesterol. The role of apoproteins, the protein carriers of lipids, in the pathophysiology of atherosclerosis is an important topic for research in this field[53] (Table 20–8).

TABLE 20–8. Dietary Strategies for Diabetic Patients with Hyperlipidemia

Phase I (Prudent diet)	Hypocaloric diet for weight reduction
	Fat intake, 30% of total calories
	Polyunsaturated : saturated fat ratio of 1.0
	Cholesterol 300 g daily
	Increase fiber content of diet
Phase II	Hypocaloric or very-low-calorie diet for obese patients
	Fat intake, 25% of total calories
	Cholesterol 200 g daily
Phase III	Caloric restriction as in Phase II
	Fat intake, 20% of total calories
	Cholesterol 100 g daily
	Pharmacological intervention may be needed
Insulin-dependent diabetes—glycemic stabilization with insulin and weight maintenance, fat-controlled diet	

Dietary Sweeteners in Diabetes

Provision of acceptable sweeteners for the diet is regarded as an important factor in improving dietary compliance. Limitations are recommended on the amounts of sucrose, glucose, lactose, and fructose, each of which can elevate plasma glucose concentrations if not substituted for carbohydrate. However, when these sugars are given in restricted quantities with mixed meals as part of the carbohydrate ration, the effect on plasma glucose is blunted. This is apparent for lactose as a component of milk.

A number of alternative sweeteners are available,[54] classified as (1) nutritive (sorbitol, mannitol, fructose, xylitol, and aspartame) and (2) non-nutritive (saccharin and cyclamate). Fructose is the only one of the nutritive sweeteners having caloric significance in the diabetic diet. It occurs in the normal diet in honey and fruits and is now available in pure crystalline form or as high-fructose corn syrup (HFCS) for general use. The latter product contains as much as 58 per cent glucose, which is a major concern in its use by diabetic patients. Although fructose and glucose have the same caloric value (4 kcal/g) fructose is more slowly absorbed from the gastrointestinal tract than glucose and is metabolized by the liver, forming glycogen or glucose.[55] The caloric value of fructose additives should be calculated as carbohydrate in the diabetic diet. In poorly regulated diabetes, fructose is associated with a prompt rise in the blood sugar.[56] The American Diabetes Association has warned that foods sweetened with fructose should be used with caution.[54]

Sorbitol, mannitol, and xylitol are sugar alcohols that have attributes of sweetness but have little effect on plasma glucose or insulin. These chemicals are poorly absorbed from the bowel and are associated with diarrhea when consumed in daily quantities of 30 g or more. Xylitol production has been curtailed because of animal studies linking it to tumor induction.[57]

Aspartame, approved for use in 1981, is the newest alternative sweetener prepared as the dipeptide of L-phenylalanine and L-aspartic acid. It is classified as a nutritive sweetener but, being 120 to 280 times sweeter than sugar, it contributes little to the caloric intake because of the small quantities required to attain a sweet taste. (One commercial preparation is buffered with lactose, yielding 4 calories for the equivalent sweetness of 1 teaspoon of sugar.) Aspartame cannot be used in cooking because of molecular disruption and loss of sweetness. No recognizable adverse effects have been noted at levels likely to be ingested, and extensive studies have shown that it is not cariogenic.[59] Reports of seizure disorders induced by this agent[60] have not been confirmed. Aspartame should not be used in patients with phenylketonuria (PKU), but is safe for use by diabetic patients, lactating women, healthy adults, and children.

Saccharin is the only non-nutritive sweetener used in the United States. It is 300 to 400 times sweeter than sucrose but has the disadvantage of a metallic or bitter aftertaste. Although it is purported to be carcinogenic, the evidence for this effect has been questioned. Based on current investigations, the American Diabetes Association has approved the use of saccharin pending further studies.[61] The proposed restrictions on the use of this agent appear to have little justification.

Cyclamate is a nonnutritive sweetener that was banned in the United States in 1970; it is being reviewed by the Cancer Assessment Committee of the Food and Drug Administration.

Alcohol and Diabetes

Although there is no useful purpose served by alcohol in the diabetic diet, these beverages are often consumed in a social setting. For this reason, it is necessary for the patient to understand that limited quantities of alcohol may be used in substitution for an equivalent caloric intake of dietary fat. The caloric value of alcohol is 7 kcal/g. The calculations of calories derived from alcohol can be determined by the following calculations.[62]

Kilocalories = 0.8 × proof × ounces consumed
(proof = 2 × percentage of alcohol by volume)

Thus, 5 ounces of wine (12 per cent alcohol) provides 0.8 × 24 × 5 = 96 kcal. Consumption of 5 ounces of wine requires elimination of 2 fat exchanges. Similar calculations can be used for spiritous liquors or other alcoholic beverages.

Alcohol is not permitted for diabetic patients with neuropathy, hypertriglyceridemia, impotence, gastrointestinal disorders including pancreatitis, or unstable diabetes or for those with a history of alcohol abuse. The prudent use of alcohol requires that careful instructions be provided concerning substitution of alcohol-derived calories in the diet, potential problems with weight reduction, and strict avoidance of excessive ingestion of alcohol-containing beverages.

Hyperglycemia may occur in diabetic patients during intemperate alcohol ingestion because of inability to maintain dietary restraints. The counter-regulatory hormones, epinephrine and glucagon, are released during alcohol ingestion resulting in the augmentation of hepatic glycogenolysis and glucose output.[63–65] Current research (Boden)[66] demonstrates an inhibitory effect of alcohol and its congener, acetate, on peripheral glucose uptake. While these factors contribute to hyperglycemia in conditions of high ethanol intake, the modest use of alcohol is not accompanied by a rise in blood sugar and is permitted by many physicians for diabetic patients.

Alcohol-induced hypoglycemia occurs in 2 to 3 day fasted individuals within hours after the consumption of moderately large amounts of alcohol-containing beverages.[67] The principal mechanism involved is the inhibition of hepatic gluconeogenesis by ethanol in the absence of ingested carbohydrate foods.[67,68] Hypoglycemic symptoms vary from tremulousness and sweating to severe neuroglucopenic manifestations culminating in coma with blood glucose concentrations usually below 40 mg/dl.[64] In sulfonylurea-treated patients, the hypoglycemic effect of alcohol is particularly hazardous and may lead to irreversible coma. The ingestion of wine or other sources of alcohol may induce disulfiram-like reactions in patients treated with sulfonylurea agents.

In discussing the inclusion of alcohol in the diet with the patient, health professionals should emphasize the hazards associated with the effects of high levels of alcohol on body metabolism. For social or gustatory purposes, the sources of alcohol should be those of low carbohydrate content. Unsweetened mixers or dilution with water is advocated. Dry wines, light beer, or unsweetened spirits should be selected with exclusion of cordials, sweet wines, and regular beer. Alcoholic intake should be limited to one or two conventional portions. The prescribed diet is consumed, except for the fat exchanges replaced by alcohol. The health professional will discourage the use of alcohol by patients for whom it represents a risk and will provide information concerning its use in a social manner in the management of appropriately selected patients[69,70] (Table 20–9).

TABLE 20–9. Alcoholic Beverages Equivalent to Two Fat Exchanges

	Calories
Regular beer, 12 oz (+1 bread exchange)	151
Light beer, 12 oz	97
Dry wine, 5 oz	80
Sweet wine, 4 oz (+⅓ bread exchange)	102
Champagne, 4 oz	98
Spirits, 86 proof, 1½ oz (whiskey, gin, vodka, rum)	107

MODIFICATIONS OF THE DIABETIC DIET

Sodium Restriction

Hypertension, renal disease, and congestive heart failure are conditions frequently encountered in the diabetic population which require a reduction in the sodium in the diet. Management of hypertension is usually initiated with sodium restriction and weight control followed by, or in association with, diuretic therapy and the use of other antihypertensive medications.[71] Renal disease associated with edema and hypertension is treated with reduced dietary sodium. Patients with congestive heart failure caused by decreased cardiac output require sodium control to lessen cardiac work. For these conditions, the dietary sodium intake is restricted to the level of 1 to 2 g (43 to 87 mEq) daily. Some diuretic drugs may affect diabetes adversely. Therefore, the use of dietary sodium restriction is advisable as the primary measure in the management of sodium retaining states.[72] The usual intake of sodium, not salt (sodium chloride), in the United States is 4 to 7 g daily.

Reduction of sodium intake requires the elimination of many convenience foods and sodium-containing staples. Canned and prepared foods and soups, cold meats, and frozen foods are avoided. Many foods, breads, soups, and special food items are now available in low sodium and salt-free form. The desired level of sodium intake, 500 to 4000 mg daily, can be achieved with selections of foods of low sodium content from the Food Exchange Lists (see Table 20–18).

Potassium Restriction

A reduction in potassium intake may be required for diabetic patients in renal failure and for those manifesting hyperkalemia with the hyporeninemic, hypoaldosterone syndrome.[73] The potassium content of the diet can conveniently be lowered to 60 to 80 mEq daily from the usual intake of approximately 100 mEq. Foods of low potassium content can be found in standard food tables.

Potassium Supplementation

Diuretic medications, thiazides or loop diuretics prescribed for alleviation of fluid retention and hypertension, frequently result in the loss of potassium from body fluids and tissues.[71,72] An increase in dietary potassium, while not effective in correcting established hypokalemia, may offset the increase in primary potassium excretion induced by diuretic therapy (Table 20–10). The high-potassium diet should not be used in patients with renal failure or in patients receiving potassium-sparing diuretics

TABLE 20–10. High-Potassium Diet

		Potassium (mEq)
Milk	3 cups	27
Meats	7 oz	30
Bread exchange	6 exchanges	16
Vegetables*	4 exchanges	30
Fruits	6 exchanges	55
Fats, beverages		7
		165

*Potatoes, beans, peas, legumes, vegetables.
Exchange lists: Table 20–20.

such as spironolactone or triamterine. Salt substitutes contain variable amounts of potassium: 12 to 16 mEq per 1/4 teaspoon. Monitoring of serum potassium concentrations is required for all patients in whom dietary potassium modifications have been prescribed.

Potatoes, orange juice and whole oranges, bananas, and melons are among the higher sources of potassium. Standard food tables provide complete lists of dietary sources rich in potassium.

Gastrointestinal Disorders in Diabetic Patients

Diseases of the gastrointestinal tract such as cholecystitis, pancreatitis, and malabsorption states are frequently observed in diabetic patients. These conditions and the hyperlipoproteinemias of diabetes require the use of fat-restricted diets. Current dietary recommendations for the management of diabetes include reduction in fat intake so that minor modifications will achieve a level of 50 g of fat per day to conform with the low-fat diet. For patients with cholecystic disease, strongly flavored foods and certain vegetables (cabbage, onions, cucumbers) may not be tolerated. Following cholecystectomy, the dietary modifications are not required.

During the acute phases of enteritis, colitis, or diverticulitis, a fiber-restricted or bland type of diet may be required to facilitate recovery of the inflamed bowel. A reduction in dietary fiber is achieved with refined cereal products, fruits, and vegetables of low fiber content. The long-term use of the low-fiber diet is not advocated. Following recovery from acute inflammation, a normal diet is resumed. An increase in dietary fiber content is recommended for patients with diverticulosis and irritable bowel conditions unless luminal stenosis is present.

Protein Restrictions

Patients in renal failure and those with the encephalopathy of hepatic failure require restriction of dietary protein. Chronic renal failure patients (creatinine clearance < 30 ml/min) are usually given diets of 40 to 60 g of protein daily, to which may be added the daily urinary protein loss.[45] The caloric intake is maintained at optimal levels by increasing the carbohydrate and fat allowances. Dietary protein supplied as cereals and vegetables is of low biological value, so that the limited number of meat exchanges must be of high biological value to supply essential amino acids.

Very-Low-Calorie Diet

Achievement of weight reduction for the obese NIDDM patient has been an elusive goal. A genetic factor has been demonstrated in obesity that may be operative in frustrating efforts for weight loss. Recent improvements in the composition of liquid diets containing 600 to 800 kcal daily has permitted their use in those patients without the hazards formerly associated with these products.[74,75] The very-low-calorie diet is employed for those requiring a carefully structured program for weight loss.

In this group of patients, these dietary preparations have been well tolerated when supplemented with vitamins and minerals and administered for periods of 8 to 12 weeks. The loss of weight is rapid and is accompanied by impressive improvement in the metabolic derangements of hyperglycemia and hyperlipidemia.[75] Insulin or sulfonylurea therapy is usually discontinued or sharply curtailed at the outset of treatment. With the restoration of metabolic regulation, there is the gradual resumption of food intake at a low caloric level combined with behavioral modification to maintain weight control at the desired level. With expanding experience and further investigation, the very-low-calorie programs may become an important adjunct in the management of obese patients.

DIETARY ADJUSTMENTS FOR SICK DAYS

Insulin-requiring patients are advised to continue treatment with insulin during periods of acute illness. The dosage of insulin may be decreased if vomiting or diarrhea is present, but the stress of infection may require supplementary regular insulin to prevent symptomatic hyperglycemia. These conditions may necessitate the use of insulin, de novo, in patients who are usually managed without it. Self-monitoring of blood glucose and the urinary testing for ketone bodies are important procedures for treating diabetes with supplementry regular insulin during illness. Carbohydrate intake must be maintained to prevent hypoglycemia and to provide the glucose sources for the impedance of ketone body production. Dietary protein and fats are ignored in favor of easily assimilable carbohydrate-containing liquids and soft foods, such as soups, juices, custards, ice cream, and sweetened beverages (Table 20–11). These foods are used to replace the carbohydrate

TABLE 20–11. Carbohydrate Content of Foods for Sick Days

10 g	
Juices: apple, orange, grapefruit, grape	List 2*
Fruits: applesauce, banana, prunes	List 2
Colas, ginger ale, Gatorade	4 oz
Jello, sweetened	¼ cup
12 g	
Milk, yogurt	1 cup
15g	
Egg nog	½ cup
Custard, puddings	½ cup
Toast	1
Crackers	List 4
Cereals	List 4
Potatoes, rice	List 4
Creamed soup	1 cup

*See Table 20–20.

allowances for each meal and may be consumed slowly over longer periods than the customary feedings.

ADDITIONAL DIETARY CONTROL MEASURES

1. A nutritional history provides an insight into the nutritive adequacy of the antecedent diet and assists in arranging a dietary program consistent with established eating habits. For some patients, it is feasible to utilize the accustomed diet as a basis for the diabetic meal-planning recommendations with modifications to accommodate the appropriate division of foods within the major meals and snacks.

2. Variations in the daily caloric consumption of about 15 per cent occur in all dietary programs, whether self-selected or structured on the Food Exchange System. Inaccuracies in measurement, glycemic response to different starches, and the differences in protein, fat, and carbohydrate content of foods are responsible for daily caloric variations.

3. Reinforcement of the dietary treatment by follow-up review of the program is required. An effective method is the maintenance of a diary of foods consumed during a typical day for review by the dietitian or physician. Weight curve measurements are required for all patients, particularly for obese patients for whom predetermined goals of weight loss have been described.

4. "Eating out" requires the ability to select menu items that are consistent with the prescribed diet, avoiding creamed or breaded foods unless appropriate adjustments in the total composition of the meal are made.

5. Convenience foods or frozen meals can often be adapted to the diabetic diet. Many of these have the nutrient content on the package. Special diet foods are not recommended.

6. During sick days, patients must maintain an adequate level of carbohydrate derived from easily assimilable foods and beverages. In general, the ill

patient can substitute sweetened beverages, juices, custards, sherbets, and puddings for the usual diet without consideration of protein or fat content of the diet. Similar substitutions of unconsumed foods are required for hospitalized patients to maintain glycemic control during illness.

7. Exercise or unexpected strenuous exertion should be covered by supplementary feedings (20 to 30 g carbohydrate per hour) to avoid hypoglycemia induced by rapid utilization of circulatory glucose by the exercising muscle tissue and to compensate for increased rates of insulin absorption during activities.

8. The changes in blood glucose concentrations during illness or exercise or in response to various foodstuffs can be readily ascertained by self-monitoring of blood glucose. This important adjunct for glycemic control should be made available to all diabetic patients for the improvement in daily glucose regulation and to protect them from hyperglycemia and hypoglycemia during illness, stress, or increased exertion.

DIET FOR PREGNANT OR LACTATING DIABETIC PATIENTS

Gestational diabetes is defined as the occurrence of hyperglycemia within ranges established as criteria for the diagnosis of this condition that has its onset or initial recognition during pregnancy.[76] Because this condition is seen in 2 per cent of pregnancies and has adverse effects upon the fetus, it is recommended that all pregnant women be screened for hyperglycemia when seen initially and again at 24 to 26 weeks of pregnancy if the initial screening is negative and the index of suspicion is high. The screening test recommended for detection of patients who are glucose-intolerant during pregnancy uses 50 g of oral glucose given after an overnight fast with determination of plasma glucose at 1 hour. A 1-hour plasma glucose of greater than or equal to 150 mg/dl is an indication for performance of a glucose tolerance test using either 75 g of glucose for the WHO criteria or 100 g for the O'Sullivan criteria.[77] Women predisposed to this condition are obese patients or those with a family history of diabetes or a personal history of large babies, spontaneous abortion, hydramnios, or glycosuria.[77] Following parturition, the metabolic abnormalities of gestational diabetes usually disappear, although some patients continue to manifest impaired glucose tolerance or overt diabetes mellitus. Of those who return to normal, 40 per cent will develop diabetes within 10 years following from gestational diabetes.[5]

Pregestational diabetes mellitus is present in 1 per 1000 pregnant patients. Careful regulation of the diabetic state is required because of the increased risk of hyperglycemia for the mother and infant.[78–80] There is an increased incidence of fetal and neonatal mortality and morbidity, caused by prematurity, macrosomia, congenital defects, respiratory distress syndrome, and hyperbilirubinemia; these effects are attributed to fetal hyperinsulinemia and associated metabolic perturbations.[80] The diabetic mother may experience the risks of diabetic ketoacidosis, hypoglycemia, infection, hydramnios, and acceleration of microvascular complications, particularly diabetic retinopathy.[80] The presence of hypertension aggravates these maternal complications.

During recent years, the outcome of the diabetic pregnancy has improved remarkably with advances in fetal monitoring and with improved techniques for diabetic control using intensive insulin therapy and self-monitoring of blood glucose. Planning for pregnancy is advocated for the known diabetic to provide euglycemia at conception, since hyperglycemia during the first weeks of pregnancy is associated with a high risk for congenital anomalies during early embryogenesis.[81] With improved methods of management of the pregnant diabetic, the principal cause of fetal loss is now the occurrence of birth defects.

Dietary Management During Pregnancy

Determination of the caloric intake is based on the need for 30 kcal/kg/day for the usual patient,[78] to which is added 300 kcal required for the developing conceptus. The basal caloric level is increased if the level of physical activity is high or if the patient is undernourished. The caloric intake is not lowered for the obese patient since weight reduction will introduce the hazards of ketonemia or nutritional inadequacy, both of which are dangerous for the fetus. During the first trimester, the extra caloric needs may be less than 300 kcal rising to 300 kcal or more during the second and third trimesters. The determination of caloric requirements is based on biweekly measurements of body weight.

Weight gain during pregnancy should follow a pattern of 1 to 2 kg (2.5 to 4.5 lb) during the first trimester. The optimal gain during the second and third trimesters is 350 to 400 g (0.8 to 0.9 lb) weekly, with a total gain during pregnancy of 1ʊ to 12 kg (22 to 26 lb).[78,80] Adjustment of the caloric intake may be required during the course of pregnancy to achieve these levels. Evaluation of fluid retention and hydramnios is required to assess their effect on the weight curve. If body weight increases rapidly, without evidence of fluid retention, fat exchanges may be reduced to slow the gain of body weight.

During lactation, the extra caloric requirements rise to 600 to 800 kcal above the basal maintenance level. For the obese patient or those with excessive weight gain, the increase may be limited to 400 to 500 kcal.

The carbohydrate, protein, and fat apportionment is essentially the same as that for the nongravid female.[80] Approximately 50 per cent of total calories are provided as carbohydrate sources with emphasis on food providing an increased fiber/energy ratio. A desirable level of fiber intake is approximately 30 to 40 g daily to improve glucose tolerance and to reduce insulin requirements. It should be remembered that the fetus requires about 50 g of glucose daily and that an inadequate carbohydrate intake or the "accelerated starvation" of pregnancy may induce maternal ketonemia.

Protein intake is calculated at 20 per cent of total calories, which includes the vegetable sources of protein as well as meat exchanges. In order to obtain fully balanced amino acid intake, one half of the protein should be provided from meat exchanges since vegetable protein is lacking in adequate supplies of certain essential amino acids such as lysine and methionine. The protein requirements ranging from 1.25 g/kg for mature women to 1.7 g/kg for younger girls are achieved at this level of protein feeding.

Fat comprises 30 per cent of the caloric intake to complete the caloric prescription. The use of lean meats and other products of low fat content will permit the inclusion of fat exchanges to provide palatability in the meal-planning program. The same recommendations are made concerning the division of fat sources between polyunsaturated and saturated fats as for nongravid patients.

Caloric distribution is arranged to provide carbohydrate, protein, and fat in each of three feedings, with smaller rations of carbohydrate and protein for a bedtime snack. For some patients, a mid-afternoon snack is included in the dietary planning. The consistency and uniformity of meal timing and the ratios of food components in each feeding should equilibrate with the time-activity course if insulin for optimal control of plasma glucose and utilization of substrates derived from the diet.

Standards for glycemic regulation during pregnancy are rigorous but can be achieved by the majority of motivated patients. Fasting plasma glucose, 60 to 90 mg/dl; and postprandial plasma glucose, 120 to 140 mg/dl, are recommended levels of control.[78,79] For some gestational diabetic patients, diet therapy alone may suffice during the early months of pregnancy. With increasing diabetogenicity of the advancing pregnancy, insulin will usually be required in the late second trimester. A reduction in the caloric level is not used as a method of improving glucose regulation. The diets recommended for the pregnant diabetic patient are nutritionally adequate with respect to vitamin and mineral content; nevertheless, it is customary to prescribe a multivitamin and mineral supplement to assure an adequate intake of nutrients, particularly iron and folic acid.

MEAL PLANNING PROCEDURES

A practical and effective scheme for translating the dietary prescription into a planned program of meals and snacks is the Food Exchange System as modified by the American Diabetes Association in 1977.[3] The Food Exchanges consist of six categories of foods including milk products, vegetables, fruits, bread and its equivalents, meats, and fats. Within each category, the individual foods have approximately the same caloric value and comparable amounts of carbohydrate, protein, and fat. As experience is gained, the patient can use household measurements, including teaspoon, tablespoon, and measuring cup, to achieve a consistent caloric and nutrient intake in meal planning programs providing a wide selection of food choices. Meal planning programs are devised as specific numbers of food exchanges arranged into meals and snacks approximating the patient's usual eating habits.

Exchange lists have been revised to emphasize foods low in cholesterol and saturated fats. This is achieved by listing the preferred foods in heavy print so that their selection may aid in improvement in the lipid profile which is needed for many diabetic patients. Information concerning the fiber content of various foods is also available to assist in enrichment of this aspect of the diet, a measure useful in reducing plasma glucose and lipid concentrations.[32] An initial period of weighing of certain items with a food scale is useful in demonstrating the size of representative servings. With brief periods of instruction by an experienced dietician, the details of selection and amounts of food recommended can be mastered; it is often helpful, however, to provide sample menus in addition to the meal planning program to facilitate cooperation and understanding of the diet. An important but often neglected feature of dietary education is *reinforcement* accomplished by follow-up appointments at 3- to 6-month intervals with the dietician. The use of computer-based techniques for dietary instruction of diabetic patients has been applied successfully and will receive further attention as experience is gained in this area.[82]

As discussed previously, there is new awareness of the significant variations in glycemic responses to different foods containing equivalent amounts of carbohydrate and to the same food prepared in various forms. The classification of carbohydrate foods according to their glycemic indices provides recognition of the wide range of blood glucose responses to various types of dietary carbohydrate as compared with that following ingestion of white bread. While many factors are involved in the glycemic response, it is noteworthy that foods of the highest fiber content are among those with the lowest glycemic index. Further research is needed to develop a practical system by which these differences in glycemic response can be applied to meal planning for the diabetic population.

STEPS IN PREPARING DIET PRESCRIPTION

1. Determine standard weight of patient using conventional height or weight tables or the rule of

"5's and 6's" when tables are not available (Tables 20–12 and 20–13).

2. Calculate the total daily caloric requirement based on standard weight and activity factors shown in Tables 20–14 and 20–15.

3. Total daily calories are converted into grams of carbohydrate, protein, and fat based on the percentages of these components in the diet (Table 20–16).

4. The grams of carbohydrate, protein, and fat are converted into servings of foods using the exchange lists. Each list indicates the grams of carbohydrate, protein, and/or fat provided in the food within the respective category (Table 20–17).

5. The number of daily food servings within each group is then distributed among the three major meals and snacks to provide the recommended meal planning program for the patient. The distribution of food items is based on the eating habits, the time-activity of insulin or sulfonylurea, and the patient's work schedule (Table 20–18).

6. Insulin-dependent patients and those receiving diets of higher caloric content will usually receive intermeal and bedtime snacks. For obese patients, intermeal snacks are usually omitted (Table 20–19).

7. Once the diet prescription is established, individual meals can be planned by selecting servings of appropriate foods from the Food Exchange Lists (Table 20–20).

TABLE 20–12. Determination of Standard Weight (Rule of 5's and 6's)

Frame Size	Male	Female
Medium	For first 5 feet, 106 lb	For first 5 feet, 100 lb
	For each additional inch, add 6 lb	For each additional inch, add 5 lb
Small	Subtract 5–10 lb	Subtract 5–10 lb
Large	Add 10-15 lb	Add 10–15 lb

TABLE 20–13. 1983 Metropolitan Height and Weight Tables

MEN					WOMEN				
Height Feet	Height Inches	Small Frame	Medium Frame	Large Frame	Height Feet	Height Inches	Small Frame	Medium Frame	Large Frame
5	2	128–134	131–141	138–150	4	10	102–111	109–121	118–131
5	3	130–136	133–143	140–153	4	11	103–113	111–123	120–134
5	4	132–138	135–145	142–156	5	0	104–115	113–126	122–137
5	5	134–140	137–148	144–160	5	1	106–118	115–129	125–140
5	6	136–142	139–151	146–164	5	2	108–121	118–132	128–143
5	7	138–145	142–154	149–168	5	3	111–124	121–135	131–147
5	8	140–148	145–157	152–172	5	4	114–127	124–138	134–151
5	9	142–151	148–160	155–176	5	5	117–130	127–141	137–155
5	10	144–154	151–163	158–180	5	6	120–133	130–144	140–159
5	11	146–157	154–166	161–184	5	7	123–136	133–147	143–163
6	0	149–160	157–170	164–188	5	8	126–139	136–150	146–167
6	1	152–164	160–174	168–192	5	9	129–142	139–153	149–170
6	2	155–168	164–178	172–197	5	10	132–145	142–156	152–173
6	3	158–172	167–182	176–202	5	11	135–148	145–159	155–176
6	4	162–176	171–187	181–207	6	0	138–151	148–162	158–179

Courtesy of Statistical Bulletin, Metropolitan Life Insurance Co. Source of basic data 1979 Build Study, Society of Actuaries and Association of Life Insurance Medical Directors of America, 1980.

TABLE 20–14. Calculation of Daily Caloric Requirement

Adult
  Basal calories: ideal body weight (IBW) (lb) × 10
  Calories added for activity level
    Sedentary: IBW (lb) × 3
    Moderate: IBW (lb) × 5
    Strenuous: IBW (lb) × 10
  Add 300 to 500 calories: weight gain, pregnancy, lactation
  Subtract 500 calories for weight loss in obesity
Child
  1000 calories + 100 calories per year to puberty
  Puberty: Females 2400–2800
         Males 2600–3400
  Caloric needs vary with rate of growth and activity
  Adjust calories to maintain normal growth
    (Wetzel, Iowa, or Stuart graphs)

TABLE 20–15. Mean Heights, Weights, and Recommended Energy Intakes for Adults

| | Age, yr* | Weight, kg | Height, cm | Caloric Requirements† | |
				Mean, kcal	*Range, kcal*
Male	23–50	70	178	2700	2300–3100
	51–75	70	178	2400	2000–2800
	76+	70	178	2050	1650–2450
Female	23–50	55	163	2000	1600–2400
	51–75	55	163	2000	1400–2200
	76+	55	163	1600	1200–2000

*Body composition change with aging: lean body mass is reduced and body fat is increased; caloric requirements decrease.
†Mean values for light activity: range varies from sedentary to strenuous exertion.
From Recommended Dietary Allowances, 9th revised edition. Washington, National Research Council—National Academy of Sciences, Food and Nutrition Board, Committee on Dietary Allowances, 1980.

TABLE 20–16. Distribution of Calories as Carbohydrate, Protein, and Fat: Method for Calculating Diet

Example: Female diabetic patient, 42 years old, is a housewife, 5 feet, 4 inches in height, weighing 123 pounds. Two children attend high school and her husband works in a bank.
  Diet for this patient:
    Ideal body weight calculation
          For 5 feet   100
          For 4 inches   20
                        120 lb
    Her actual weight approximates ideal weight.
  Calculation of caloric requirement for weight maintenance:
          120 lb × 10 = 1200 kcal
          120 lb × 5 = 600 kcal
                        1800 calories for diet
  Divide calories into grams of carbohydrate (50%), protein (20%), and fat (30%)
      Carbohydrate: 1800 × 0.50 = 900 kcal ÷ 4 = 225 g
      Protein: 1800 × 0.20 = 360 kcal ÷ 4 = 90 g
      Fat: 1800 × 0.30 = 540 kcal ÷ 9 = 60 g
      Diet prescription: kcal 1800, CHO 225 g, P 90 g, F 60 g

TABLE 20–17. *Method for Conversion of Diet Prescription into Food Exchange*

Exchange Group	Grams per Exchange			No. of Exchanges	Total Amount in Grams		
	CHO	*P*	*F*		CHO	P	F
Milk	12	8	0				
	12	8	5	2	24	16	10
	12	8	10				
Vegetable	5	2	0	2	10	4	0
Fruit	10	0	0	5	50	0	0

Total CHO from sources other than Bread Exchange					84		

1. Subtract g CHO other than bread exchanges from total g CHO
2. Divide by 15 g CHO for each bread exchange = number of bread exchanges

$$225 - 84 = 141 \div 15 = 9 \text{ bread exchanges}$$

Bread	15	2	0	9	135	18	0

Total P from sources other than Meat Exchange						38	

3. Subtract g P other than meat exchanges from total g P
4. Divide by 7 g P for each meat exchange = number of meat exchanges

$$90 - 38 = 52 \div 7 = 8 \text{ meat exchanges}$$

Meat	0	7	3	7	0	49	21
	0	7	5.5	1	0	7	5.5
	0	7	8	0			

Total F from sources other than Fat Exchange							36.5

5. Subtract g F in milk and meat from total g F
6. Divide by 5 g F for each fat exchange = number of fat exchanges

$$60 - 36.5 = 23.5 \div 5 = 5 \text{ fat exchanges}$$
(All values are rounded off to nearest 5)

Fat	0	0	5	5	0	0	25

Total g: CHO, P, F					219	94	61.5
Total calories: CHO, P, F					×4 876	×4 376	×9 553.5

Total calories: 1806

Diet Plan	Number of Exchanges	Approximate Distribution of CHO (220 g)			
		Breakfast	*Lunch*	*Dinner*	*Bedtime*
Milk	2				
Vegetable	2	2/10	3/10	4/10	1/10
Fruit	5	44	66	88	22
Bread	9				
Meat, lean	7				
medium	1				
Fat	5				

TABLE 20–18. Sample Meal Plan with Food Exchanges for 1800 kcal Diet

Meals	Exchanges	Food Choices	Portions
Breakfast			
Fruit	1	Orange juice	½ cup
Bread	2	Oatmeal	½ cup
		Whole wheat toast	1
Meat	1	Poached egg	1
(Medium fat)			
Milk	1	Milk, 2%	1 cup
Fat	1	Margarine	1 teaspoon
Free	—	Coffee or tea, sugar substitute, diet jelly	
Lunch			
Meat (lean)	3	Hamburger (lean)	3 ounces
Bread	3	Roll, hamburger	1
		Pretzels, 3-ring	5
Vegetable	1	Tomato with lettuce	1
Fat	1	Salad dressing	1 tablespoon
Fruit	1	Pear	1 small
Free	—	Diet beverage, sugar-free	
Dinner			
Meat (lean)	4	Chicken breast	4 ounces
Bread	3	Potato, baked	1 small
Vegetable	1	Carrots, lettuce wedge	
			½ cup
Fat	2	Margarine	2 teaspoons
Fruit	2	Fruit cup: grapes,	12
		orange slices	½ cup
Milk	½	Milk, 2%	½ cup
Free	—	Coffee or tea, sugar substitute	
Evening snack			
Fruit	1	Apple	1 small
Bread	1	Graham crackers	2
Milk	½	Milk, 2%	½ cup

If nonfat milk is used, 2 fat exchanges are added to the diet.

A copy of Exchange Lists is given to patient. The dietician should supervise the preparation or sample meal plans by the patient for one day's meals.

TABLE 20–19. Division of Carbohydrate (CHO) into Meals and Snacks

Adjust to usual activity, eating habits, and work schedule
Dividing total CHO into tenths gives good flexibility
NIDDM—3 meals and bedtime snack
IDDM—3 meals and 2 or 3 snacks

	Breakfast	A.M. Snack	Lunch	P.M. Snack	Dinner	Bedtime Snack
NIDDM	2/10		4/10		4/10	
	2/10		3/10		4/10	1/10
IDDM	2/10		3/10	1/10	3/10	1/10
	2/10	1/10	2/10	1/10	3/10	1/10

TABLE 20–20. Food Exchange Lists for Diabetes

Each list of food exchange consists of items having similar nutritive value. Measured amounts of foods within the group may be used as "substitutes" for one another in planning meals. A single exchange provides equal amounts of calories, carbohydrates, proteins, and fats. Dietary fiber content follows portion size in parentheses.

Exchange List	Measurement	Carbohydrate*	Protein*	Fat*	Calories†
Milk, skim	1 cup	12	8	0	80
2%	1 cup	12	8	5	125
Whole	1 cup	12	8	10	150
Vegetable	½ cup cooked	5	2		25
Fruit	see list	10	0	0	40
Bread	see list	15	2	0	70
Meat‡	1 ounce				
Lean		0	7	3	55
Medium		0	7	5.5	78
Fat		0	7	8	100
Fat	see list	0	0	5	45

LIST I   MILK EXCHANGES

This list shows the kinds and amounts of milk or milk products to be used for one Milk Exchange. Those which appear in BOLD TYPE are NON-FAT. Estimates of dietary fiber in grams appear in (   ).

NON-FAT FORTIFIED MILK (one exchange contains 8 grams protein, 12 grams carbohydrate, a trace of fat and 80 calories)

SKIM OR NON-FAT MILK	1 CUP	(0)
POWDERED (NON-FAT DRY, BEFORE ADDING LIQUID)	1/2 CUP	(0)
CANNED, EVAPORATED-SKIM MILK	1/2 CUP	(0)
BUTTERMILK MADE FROM SKIM MILK	1 CUP	(0)
YOGURT MADE FROM SKIM MILK (PLAIN, UNFLAVORED)	1 CUP	(0)

LOW-FAT FORTIFIED MILK (one exchange contains 8 grams proteins, 12 grams carbohydrate, 5 grams of fat and 125 calories)

2% fat fortified milk (omit 1 Fat Exchange)	1 cup	(0)
Yogurt made from 2% fortified milk (plain, unflavored) (omit 1 Fat Exchange)	1 cup	(0)

WHOLE MILK (Omit 2 Fat Exchanges) (one exchange contains 8 grams protein, 12 grams carbohydrate, 10 grams fat and 170 calories)

Whole Milk	1 cup	(0)
Canned, evaporated whole milk	1/2 cup	(0)
Buttermilk made from whole milk	1 cup	(0)
Yogurt made from whole milk (plain, unflavored)	1 cup	(0)

TABLE 20–20. *Food Exchange Lists for Diabetes* **Continued**

<u>LIST 2</u> <u>VEGETABLE EXCHANGES</u> (one exchange of vegetable contains about 5 grams of carbohydrate, 2 grams of protein and 25 calories). Estimates of dietary fiber in grams appear in ( ).

This list shows the kinds of vegetables to use for one Vegetable Exchange. One Exchange is 1/2 cup cooked, unless otherwise indicated.

Asparagus (1.3)
Bean sprouts (1.5)
Beets (2.1)
Broccoli (3.5)
Brussel sprouts (2.3)
Cabbage, raw (1.2) cooked (2.1)
Carrots, raw (1.8) cooked (2.4)
Cauliflower, raw (1.1) cooked (1.6)
Celery, raw (1.1)
Cucumbers, raw (1.1)
Eggplant
Green pepper, raw (1.0)
Greens:
    Beets
    Chards
    Collards
    Dandelion
    Kale (1.3)

Greens:
    Mustard, raw (2.0)
    Spinach, raw (0.2)
        cooked (6.5)
    Turnip (1.6)
Mushrooms, raw (0.9)
Okra
Onions, raw (1.2)
    cooked (1.4)
Rhubarb
Rutabaga, raw (1.7)
Sauerkraut
String beans, green or
    yellow, raw (1.9)
Summer squash (2.0)
Tomatoes, raw (1.5)
    cooked (1.5)
Tomato juice
Turnips (1.6)
Vegetable juice cocktail
Zucchini, raw (2.0)

The following raw vegetables may be used as desired: (Fiber per 1/2 cup)

Chicory
Chinese Cabbage
Endive
Escarole

Lettuce (0.4)
Parsley
Radishes (1.3)
Watercress (1.0)

Starchy Vegetables are found in the Bread Exchange List.

<u>LIST 3</u> <u>FRUIT EXCHANGES</u> (One Exchange of fruit contains 10 grams of carbohydrate and 40 calories)

This list shows the kinds and amounts of fruits to use for one Fruit Exchange.

Apple, 1 small (2.0)
Apple juice 1/3 cup (0)
Applesauce (unsweetened) 1/2 cup (2.6)
Apricots, fresh 2 medium (1.4)
Apricots, dried 4 halves
Banana, 1/2 small (1.5)
Berries
    Blackberries, 1/2 cup (4.5)
    Blueberries, 1/2 cup
    Raspberries, 1/2 cup (4.6)
    Strawberries, 3/4 cup (2.3)

Cherries, 10 large (1.1)
Cider, 1/3 cup (0)
Dates, 2 (1.6)
Figs, fresh, 1
Figs, dried, 1 (3.7)
Grapefruit, 1/2 (0.8)
Grapefruit juice 1/2
Grapes, 12 (0.5)
Grape juice, 1/4 cup (0)

TABLE 20-20. Food Exchange Lists for Diabetes Continued

Mango 1/2 small
Melon
    Cantaloupe, 1/4 small (1.0)
    Honeydew, 1/8 medium (0.4)
    Watermelon, 1 cup (1.4)
Nectarine, 1 small (1.5)
Orange, 1 small (1.6)
Orange juice, 1/2 cup (0)
Papaya, 3/4 cup
Peach, 1 medium (2.3); 1.2 C cooked (1.8)
Pear, 1 small (2.0); 1/2 C cooked (2.0)
Persimmon, native, 1 medium
Pineapple, raw, 1/2 cup (0.8)
Pineapple juice, 1/3 cup
Plums, 2 medium (1.8)
Prunes, 2 medium (2.4)
Prune juice, 1/4 cup
Raisins, 2 tbsp. (1.3)
Tangerine, 1 medium (2.0)

Cranberries may be used as desired if no sugar is added

LIST 4 BREAD EXCHANGES (one exchange of bread contains 15 grams of carbohydrate, 2 grams of protein and 70 calories). Estimates of dietary fiber in grams appear in ( ).

This list shows the kinds and amounts of Breads, Cereals, Starchy Vegetables and Prepared Foods to use for one Bread Exchange. Those which appear in BOLD TYPE are LOW-FAT.

BREAD
WHITE (INCLUDING FRENCH AND ITALIAN)	1 SLICE (.7)
WHOLE WHEAT	1 SLICE (1.3)
RYE OR PUMPERNICKEL	1 SLICE (.8)
RAISIN	1 SLICE
BAGEL, SMALL	1/2
ENGLISH MUFFIN, SMALL	1/2
PLAIN ROLL, BREAD	1 (0.8)
FRANKFURTER ROLL	1/2
HAMBURGER BUN	1/2
DRIED BREAD CRUMBS	3 TBSP.
TORTILLA, 6"	1

CEREAL (See Supplementary list of fiber content at end of section)
BRAN FLAKES	1/2 cup (3.0)
OTHER READY-TO-EAT UNSWEETENED CEREAL	3/4 cup
PUFFED CEREAL (UNFROSTED)	1 cup (23)
CEREAL (COOKED)	1/2 cup
GRITS (COOKED)	1/2 cup (1.8 dry)
RICE OR BARLEY (COOKED) (0.8)	1/2 cup (3.2)
PASTA (COOKED)	1/2 cup
SPAGHETTI, NOODLES, (0.8)	
MACARONI (0.6)	
POPCORN (POPPED, NO FAT ADDED)	3 cups (6.9)
CORNMEAL (DRY)	2 Tbs. (1.0)
FLOUR	2½ Tbs. (0.3)
WHEAT GERM	1/4 cup (3.8)

TABLE 20–20. Food Exchange Lists for Diabetes Continued

CRACKERS
ARROWROOT	3
GRAHAM	2 (1.4)
MATZOTH	1/2
OYSTER	20
PRETZELS	25
RYE WAFERS	3 (2.3)
SALTINES	6 (0.7)
SODA	4

DRIED BEANS, PEAS AND LENTILS
BEANS, PEAS, LENTILS (DRIED AND COOKED)	1/2 cup
KIDNEY (9.7)	
PINTOS (8.9)	
LENTILS (3.7)	
WHITE (7.9)	
BAKED BEANS, NO PORK (CANNED)	1/4 cup

STARCHY VEGETABLES
CORN	1/3 small (4.7)
CORN ON COB	1 small
LIMA BEANS	1/2 cup (8.3)
PARSNIPS	2/3 cup (4.0)
PEAS, GREEN (CANNED OR FROZEN) (6.7 raw)	1/2 cup
POTATO, WHITE	1 small (3.1)
POTATO (MASHED)	1/2 cup
PUMPKIN	3/4 cup
WINTER SQUASH, ACORN OR BUTTERNUT	1/2 cup (3.5)
YAM OR SWEET POTATO	1/4 cup (1.7)

Prepared Foods
Biscuit 2" dia. (omit 1 Fat Exchange)	1 (0.7)
Corn Bread, 2" x 2" x 1" (omit 1 Fat Exchange)	1 (0.8)
Corn muffin, 2" dia. (omit 1 Fat Exchange)	1
Crackers, round butter type (omit 1 Fat Exchange)	5 (0.6)
Muffin, plain small (omit 1 Fat Exchange)	1
Potatoes, French Fried, length 2" to 3½" (omit 1 Fat Exchange)	8
Potato or Corn Chips (omit 2 Fat Exchange)	15
Pancake, 5" x 1/2" (omit 1 Fat Exchange)	1 (0.6)
Waffle, 5" x 1/2" (omit 1 Fat Exchange)	1 (1.1)

LIST 5   MEAT EXCHANGES (one exchange of lean meat (1 oz.) contains
Lean Meat   7 grams of protein, 3 grams of fat and
     55 calories)

This list shows the kinds and amounts of Lean Meat and other Protein-Rich Foods to use for one Low-Fat Meat Exchange.

Beef   :   Baby Beef (very lean), Chipped Beef, Chuck, Flank Steak, Tenderloin, Plate Ribs, Plate Skirt Steak, Round.   1 oz.

Lamb   :   Leg, Rib, Sirloin, Loin (roast and chops), Shank, Shoulder.   1 oz.

TABLE 20–20. Food Exchange Lists for Diabetes Continued

```
Pork    :  Leg (Whole Rump, Center Shank), Ham, Smoked
           (center slices).                           1 oz.

Veal    :  Leg, Loin, Rib, Shank, Shoulder, Cutlets   1 oz.

Poultry :  Meat without skin of chicken, Turkey, Cornish hen,
           Guinea Hen, Pheasant.                       1 oz.

Fish    :  Any fresh or frozen                         1 oz.
           Canned Salmon, Tuna, Mackerel, Crab and
                        Lobster                        1/4 cup
           Clams, Oysters, Scallops, Shrimp            5 or 1 oz.
           Sardines                                    3
```

```
Cheeses containing less than 5% butterfat
Cottage cheese, dry and 2% butterfat
Dried Beans and Peas (omit 1 Bread Exchange)           1/2 cup
```

LIST 5   MEAT EXCHANGES   (For each Exchange of Medium-Fat Meat
         Medium-Fat Meat   omit 1/2 Fat Exchange)

   This list shows the kinds and amounts of Medium-Fat Meat
and other Protein-Rich Foods to be used for one Medium-Fat
Meat Exchange.

```
Beef:      Ground (15% fat), Corned Beef (canned), Rib Eye,
           Round (ground commercial)                   1 oz.

Pork:      Loin (all cuts Tenderloin), Shoulder Arm (picnic),
           Shoulder Blade, Boston Butt, Canadian Bacon,
           Boiled Ham.                                 1 oz.

Liver, Heart, Kidney and Sweetbreads (these are high in
    cholesterol)                                       1 oz.

Cottage Cheese, creamed                                1/4 cup

Cheese:  Mozzarella, Ricotta, Farmer's cheese,
         Neufchaterl, Parmesan                         1 tbsp.

Egg (high in cholesterol)                              1

PEANUT BUTTER (omit 2 additional Fat Exchanges) (2.2)  2 tbsp.
```

LIST 5   MEAT EXCHANGES (For each Exchange of High-Fat Meat and
         High-Fat Meat   other Exchange)

   This list shows the kinds and amounts of High-Fat Meat and
other Protein-Rich Foods to be used for one High-Fat Meat
Exchange.

```
Beef:      Brisket, Corned Beef (Brisket), Ground Beef
           (more than 20% fat), Hamburger (commercial),
           Chuck (ground commercial), Roasts (Rib),
           Steaks (Club and Rib)                       1 oz.

Lamb:    Breast                                        1 oz.
```

***TABLE 20–20. Food Exchange Lists for Diabetes* Continued**

Pork:	Spare Ribs, Loin (Back Ribs), Pork (ground), Country style, Ham, Deviled Ham	1 oz.
Veal:	Breast	1 oz.
Poultry:	Capon, Duck (domestic), Goose	1 oz.
Cheese:	Cheddar Types	1 oz.
Cold Cuts		1 slice
Frankfurter		1 small

LIST 6   FAT EXCHANGES   (one exchange of fat contains 5 grams of fat and 45 calories)

This list shows the kinds and amounts of Fat-Containing Foods to be used for one Fat Exchange. To plan a diet low in Saturated Fat select only those Exchanges which appear in BOLD TYPE. They are POLYUNSATURATED or MONOUNSATURATED.

MARGARINE, SOFT, TUB OR STICK*	**1 teaspoon**
AVOCADO (4" IN DIAMETER)** (0.5)	**1/8**
OIL, CORN, COTTONSEED, SAFFLOWER,	
** SOY, SUNFLOWER**	**1 teaspoon**
OIL, OLIVE**	**1 teaspoon**
OIL, PEANUT**	**1 teaspoon**
OLIVES** (1.3)	**5 small**
ALMONDS** (1.3)	**10 whole**
PECANS** (0.5)	**2 large whole**
PEANUTS**	
** SPANISH**	**20 whole**
** VIRGINIA** (1.)	**10 whole**
WALNUTS (0.4)	**6 small**
NUTS, OTHER**	**6 small**
Margarine, regular stick	1 teaspoon
Butter	1 teaspoon
Bacon fat	1 teaspoon
Bacon, crisp	1 strip
Cream, light	2 tablespoons
Cream, sour	2 tablespoons
Cream, heavy	1 tablespoon
Cream cheese	1 tablespoon
French dressing***	1 tablespoon
Italian dressing***	1 tablespoon
Lard	1 teaspoon
Mayonnaise***	1 teaspoon
Salad dressing, mayonnaise type***	2 teaspoons
Salt Pork	3/4 inch cube

---

*   Made with corn, cottonseed, safflower, soy or sunflower oil only.
**   Fat content is primarily monounsaturated.
*** If made with corn, cottonseed, safflower, soy or sunflower oil can be used on fat modified diet.

TABLE 20–20. *Food Exchange Lists for Diabetes* Continued

FOODS ALLOWED	FOODS TO AVOID
Diet beverages	Sugar
Coffee	Candy
Tea	Honey
Bouillon without Fat	Jam
Unsweetened Gelatin	Jelly
Unsweetened Pickles	Cookies
	Syrup
Salt	Condensed Milk
Pepper	Chewing Gum
Paprika	Soft Drinks
Garlic	Pies
Celery Salt	Cakes
Parsley	
Nutmeg	
Lemon	
Mustard	
Chili Powder	
Onion Salt or Powder	
Horseradish	
Vinegar	
Mint	
Cinnamon	
Lime	

SUPPLEMENTARY LIST

CEREAL FIBER CONTENT

Cereal	Fiber	Measure
All (100%) Bran	8.4	1/3 cup
BranChex	4.1	1/2 cup
CornChex	2.6	3/4 cup
Corn Bran	4.4	1/2 cup
Corn Flakes	2.6	3/4 cup
Farina or Cream of Wheat	0.6	1/2 cup
Grapenut Flakes	2.5	2/3 cup
Grapenuts	2.7	3 Tbsp.
Oatmeal, instant, dry	2.5	3/4 package
Rice Krispies	0.9	3/4 cup
Total	2.5	3/4 cup
Wheaties	2.6	3/4 cup
Shredded Wheat	3.3	1/2 cup

*Amounts of carbohydrate, protein, and fat in grams.
†Calories: Carbohydrate 1 g = 4 kcal
　　Protein 1 g = 4 kcal
　　Fat 1 g = 9 kcal
‡Dried beans and peas count as 1 meat and 1 bread exchange.
Exchange lists from Major S (ed). Temple University Hospital Diet Manual. Philadelphia, Temple University Hospital, Department of Dietetics and Food Service, 1984.

References

1. Rollo J. In Cases of the Diabetes Mellitus. 2nd ed. London, Dilly, 1798.
2. Allen FM. Studies concerning diabetes. JAMA 1914; 63:939–943.
3. American Diabetes Association and American Dietetic Association. A Guide for Professionals: The Effective Application of Exchange Lists for Meal Planning. New York, 1977.
4. American Diabetes Association. Principles of nutrition and dietary recommendations for individuals with diabetes mellitus. Diabetes 1979; 28:1027–1030.
5. National Diabetes Data Group. Classifications and diagnosis of diabetes mellitus and other categories of glucose intolerance. Diabetes 1979; 28:1039–1057.
6. WHO Expert Committee on Diabetes Mellitus. Geneva, World Health Organization, 1980.
7. Report of a WHO Study Group. Diabetes Mellitus. Technical Report Series 727. Geneva, World Health Organization, 1985.
8. Groop LC, Bottazzo GJ, Doniach D. Islet cell antibodies identify latent Type I diabetes in patients age 35–75 years at diagnosis. Diabetes 1986; 35:237–241.
9. Horton, ES, Danforth E Jr, Sims EAH, et al. Endocrine and metabolic alterations in spontaneous and experimental obesity. In Bray GA (ed). Obesity in Perspective. Washington, U.S. Government Printing Office, 1975: 323–340.
10. Olefsky JM. Insulin resistance and insulin action. An in vitro and in vivo perspective. Diabetes 1981; 30:148–162.
11. Genuth SM. Insulin secretion in obesity and diabetes, an illustrative case. Ann Intern Med 1977; 87:714–716.
12. Food and Nutrition Board. Recommended Dietary Allowances. Washington, National Academy of Sciences, 1980.
13. West KM. Epidemiology of Diabetes and Its Vascular Lesions. New York, Elsevier, 1978.
14. Gotto AM Jr, Bierman EL, Connor WE, et al. Recommendations for treatment of hyperlipidemia in adults: a joint statement of the AHA Nutrition Committee and the Council on Arteriosclerosis. Circulation 1984; 69:1065A–1090A.
15. Consensus Conference. Lowering blood cholesterol to prevent heart disease. JAMA 1985; 253:2080–2086.
16. Himsworth HP. The dietetic factor determining glucose tolerance and sensitivity to insulin in healthy man. Clin Sci 1935; 2:67–94.
17. Bagdade JD, Bierman EL, Porte D Jr. Significance of basal insulin levels in the evaluation of the insulin response to glucose in diabetic and non-diabetic subjects. J Clin Invest 1967; 46:1549–1557.
18. Kiehm TG, Anderson JW, Ward K. Beneficial effects of a high carbohydrate, high fiber diet on hyperglycemic diabetic men. Am J Clin Nutr 1976; 29:895–899.
19. Anderson JW, Ward K. Long-term effects of high carbohydrate, high fiber diets on glucose and lipid metabolism. A preliminary report on patients with diabetes. Diabetes Care 1978; 1:77–80.
20. Ray TK, Mansell KM, Knight LC, et al. Long-term effects of dietary fiber on glucose tolerance and gastric emptying in non–insulin-dependent diabetic patients. Am J Clin Nutr 1983; 37:376–380.
21. Perrotti N, Santoro D, Genovese S, et al. Effects of digestible carbohydrates on glucose control in insulin-dependent diabetic patients. Diabetes Care 1984; 7:354–359.
22. American Diabetes Association. Principles of nutrition and dietary recommendations for individuals with diabetes mellitus. Diabetes 1979; 28:1027–1030.
23. Nutrition Subcommittee of the British Diabetes Association's Medical Advisory Committee. Dietary recommendations for diabetics for the 1980's. Human Nutr Appl Nutr 1982; 36:378–386.
24. Canadian Diabetes Association. 1980 Guidelines for the nutritional management of diabetes mellitus. J Can Diabetes Assoc 1981; 421:110–118.
25. Bossetti BM, Kocher LM, Moranz JF, et al. The effects of physiological amounts of simple sugars on lipoprotein, glucose and insulin levels in normal subjects. Diabetes Care 1984; 7:309–312.
26. Bantle JP, Laine DC, Castle GW, et al. Postprandial glucose and insulin responses to meals containing different carbohydrates in normal and diabetic subjects. N Engl J Med 1983; 309:7–12.
27. Peterson DB, Lambert J, Gerring S, et al. Sucrose in the diet of diabetic patients—just another carbohydrate? Diabetologia 1986; 29:216–220.
28. Reaven G. How high the carbohydrate? Diabetologia 1985; 19:409–413.
29. Lipid Research Clinics Program. The Lipid Research Clinics Coronary Primary Prevention Trial Results, I and II. JAMA 1984; 251:351–374.
30. Burkett DP, Trowell HC (eds). Refined Carbohydrate Foods and Disease: Some Implications of Dietary Fiber. New York, Academic Press, 1975.
31. Miranda PM, Horwitz DL. High fiber diets in the treatment of diabetes mellitus. Ann Intern Med 1978; 88:482–486.
32. Anderson JW, Sieling E. HCF Diets: A Professional Guide to High-Carbohydrate, High-Fiber Diets. Lexington, KY, University of Kentucky Diabetes Fund, 1979.
33. Goulder TJ, Alberti KGMM, Kenkins DA. Effects of added fiber on the glucose and metabolic responses to a mixed meal in normal and diabetic subjects. Diabetes Care 1978; 1:351–355.
34. Anderson JW, Ferguson SK, Karonnos D, et al. Mineral and vitamin status of high fiber diets: long-term studies of diabetic patients. Diabetes Care 1980; 3:38–40.
35. Crapo PA, Reaven G, Olefsky J. Postprandial plasma glucose and insulin responses to different complex carbohydrates. Diabetes 1977; 26:1178–1183.
36. Jenkins DJA, Wolever TMS, Taylor RH, et al. Glycemic index of foods: a physiologic basis for carbohydrate exchange. Am J Clin Nutr 1981; 34:362–366.
37. Crapo PA, Olefsky JM. Food fallacies and blood sugar. N Engl J Med 1983; 309:44–45.
38. Jenkins DJA, Wolever TM, Jenkins AL, et al. The glycaemic response to carbohydrate foods. Lancet 1984; 2:388–391.
39. Collier G, O'Dea K. Effect of physical form of carbohydrate on the postprandial glucose insulin, and gastric inhibitory polypeptide responses in Type II diabetes. Am J Clin Nutr 1982; 36:10–14.
40. Jenkins DJA. Lente carbohydrate: a newer approach to dietary management of diabetes. Diabetes Care 1982; 5:634–641.
41. Collier G, McLean A, O'Dea K. Effect of co-ingestion of fat on the metabolic responses to slowly and rapidly absorbed carbohydrates. Diabetologia 1984; 26:50–54.
42. Nuthall FQ, Arskaj D, Mooradian AD, et al. Effects of protein ingestion on the glucose and insulin response to a standardized glucose load. Diabetes Care 1984; 7:465–470.
43. Cahill GF Jr. Physiology of insulin in man. Diabetes 1971; 20:785–789.
44. Owen OE, Block BSB, Patel M, et al. Human splanchnic metabolism during diabetic ketoacidosis. Metabolism 1977; 26:381–384.
45. Kopple JD. Nutritional therapy in renal failure. Nutrition 1981; 39:193–206.
46. Colwell J, Lopes-Virella M, Halushka P. Pathogenesis of atherosclerosis in diabetes mellitus. Diabetes Care 1981; 4:121–133.
47. Brown WV. Diabetes mellitus and atherosclerosis; risk factors, mechanisms and management. In Peterson C (ed). Diabetes Management in the 80's. New York, Praeger, 1982: 40–55.
48. Hjermann I, Holmi I, Byre KV, et al. Effect of diet and smoking intervention in the incidence of coronary heart disease. Lancet 1985; 2:1303–1310.
49. Kromhout D, Bosscheiter FB, Coulander CD. The inverse relationship between fish consumption and 20-year mor-

tality from coronary heart disease. N Engl J Med 1985; *312*:811–817.

50. Ross R. The pathogenesis of atherosclerosis—an update. N Engl J Med 1986; *314*:488–500.

51. Chait A, Beirman EL, Albers JJ. Regulatory role of insulin in the degradation of low density lipoprotein by cultured human fibroblasts. Biochim Biophys Acta 1978; *529*:292–299.

52. Gordon T, Castelli WP, Hjortlund MC, et al. High density lipoprotein as a protective factor against coronary heart disease. The Framingham Study. Am J Med 1977; *62*:707–714.

53. Eckel RH, McLean JJ, Albers MC, et al. Plasma lipids and microangiopathy in insulin-dependent diabetes mellitus. Diabetes Care 1981; *4*:447–453.

54. American Diabetes Association. Statement on Sweeteners. Diabetes Care 1987; *3*:2390.

55. Crapo PA, Kolterman OG. The metabolic effects of 2-week fructose feeding in normal subjects. Am J Clin Nutr 1984; *39*:525–534.

56. Olefsky J, Crapo P. Fructose, xylitol, or sorbitol as a sweetener in diabetes mellitus. Diabetes Care 1980; *3*:390–393.

57. Smith RJ. Xylitol: another sweetener turns sour. Science 1978; *199*:670–671.

58. U.S. Food and Drug Administration. Food additives permitted for direct addition to food for human consumption: aspartame. Fed Reg 1984; *49*:6672–6682.

59. Horwitz DL, Bauer-Nehrling JK. Can aspartame meet our expectations? J Am Diet Assoc 1983; *83*:142.

60. Wurtman RJ. Neurochemical changes following high-dose aspartame with dietary carbohydrate. (Letter). N Engl J Med 1983; *309*:429.

61. Select Committee on Sugar Substitutes. American Diabetes Association Policy Statement: saccharin. Diabetes Care 1978; *1*:209–210.

62. Gastineau CF. Nutrition note: alcohol and calories. Mayo Clin Proc 1976; *51*:86–87.

63. McMonagle J, Felig P. Effects of ethanol ingestion on glucose tolerance and insulin secretion in normal and diabetic subjects. Metabolism 1975; *24*:625–632.

64. Lieber CS. The effects of alcohol and alcoholic liver disease on the endocrine system and intermediary metabolism. *In* Metabolic Disorders of Alcoholism. Pathogenesis and Treatment. Philadelphia, WB Saunders, 1982: 140.

65. Noth R, Walter R. The effects of alcohol on the endocrine system. Med Clin North Am 1984; *68*:133–146.

66. Boden G. In press.

67. Arky RA, Freinkel N. Alcohol hypoglycemia: V. Alcohol in-

fusion to test gluconeogenesis in starvation, with special reference to obesity. N Engl J Med 1966; *274*:426–433.

68. Arky RA, Veverbrants E, Abramson EA. Irreversible hypoglycemia: a complication of alcohol and insulin. JAMA 1968; *206*:554.

69. Franz MJ. Diabetes mellitus: considerations in the development of guidelines for the occasional use of alcohol. J Am Diet Asssoc 1983; *83*:147–152.

70. Guandiani L, Feingold KR. Alcohol and diabetes: mix with caution. Clin Diabetes 1984; *2*:121–132.

71. Cristlieb AR. Treating hypertension in the patient with diabetes. Med Clin North Am 1982; *66*:1373–1388.

72. Seltzer HS. Diagnosis of Diabetes. *In* Ellenberg M, Rifkin E (eds). Diabetes Mellitus: Theory and Practice. 3rd ed. New Hyde Park, NY, Medical Examination Publishing Co., 1983: 433.

73. Sunderlin FS Jr, Anderson GH Jr, Streeten DHP, et al. The renin-angiotensin-aldosterone system in diabetic patients with hyperkalemia. Diabetes 1981; *30*:335–341.

74. Genuth S. Supplemented fasting in the treatment of obesity and diabetes. Am J Clin Nutr 1979; *32*:2579–2586.

75. Henry RR, Weist-Kent TA, Schaeffer L, et al. Metabolic consequences of very low calorie diet therapy in obese non–insulin-dependent diabetic and nondiabetic subjects. Diabetes 1986; *35*:155–164.

76. American Diabetes Association Workshop. Conference on Gestational Diabetes, Summary and Recommendations. Diabetes Care 1980; *3*:499–501.

77. O'Sullivan JB, Mahon CM. Criteria for the oral glucose tolerance test in pregnancy. Diabetes 1964; *13*:278.

78. Jovanovic L, Braun CB, Druzin ML, et al. The management of diabetes and pregnancy. *In* Peterson CM (ed). Diabetes Management in the 80's. New York, Praeger, 1982: 248–266.

79. Murphy J, Peters J, Morris P, et al. Conservative management of pregnancy in diabetic women. Br Med J 1984; *288*:1203–1205.

80. Freinkel N, Dooley SL, Metzger BE. Care of the pregnant woman with insulin-dependent diabetes mellitus. N Engl J Med 1985; *313*:95–101.

81. Miller E, Hare JW, Cloherty JP, et al. Elevated maternal hemoglobin A$_{1c}$ in early pregnancy and major congenital anomalies in infants of diabetic mothers. N Engl J Med 1981; *304*:1331.

82. Wheeler LA, Wheeler ML, Ours P, et al. Evaluation of computer-based diet education in persons with diabetes mellitus and limited educational background. Diabetes Care 1985; *8*:537–544.

83. Major S (ed). Temple University Hospital Diet Manual. Philadelphia, Temple University Hospital, Department of Dietetics and Food Service, 1984.

21

DISEASES OF THE EXOCRINE PANCREAS

MICHAEL J. McMAHON

The pancreas is a relatively small organ which lies in a concealed and guarded position draped across the posterior wall of the upper abdomen. It weighs 85 g in women and 90 g in men, but has manufacturing (exocrine) and control (endocrine) functions that give it a key role in nutrition and metabolism. Between 700 and 2500 ml of pancreatic juice are produced by the cells of the exocrine pancreas each day. The juice contains bicarbonate, electrolytes, and a daily output of about 7.5 g of protein, 90 per cent of which is made up of digestive enzymes. Although some enzymes are secreted into the juice in an active form (amylase, lipase, phospholipase), others are secreted as inactive zymogens. Activation of zymogens normally occurs when pancreatic juice mixes with enterokinase within the lumen of the duodenum; activation of juice within the pancreas is prevented by the presence of protease inhibitors within the acinar cells and in the pancreatic juice. Because it is quantitatively the most important source of digestive enzymes, disease or malfunction of the exocrine pancreas may have major implications upon nutrition. In addition, the inappropriate activation of pancreatic enzymes can lead to other clinical sequelae. Enzymes stored within the pancreas and present in the pancreatic juice have considerable digestive power, and if this is released within the gland itself, in the peripancreatic tissues or within the peritoneal cavity, catastrophic consequences can result.

The pancreas develops from ventral and dorsal endodermal outgrowths that originate from the foregut in the abdomen during the fifth week of intrauterine life. The pancreatic juice normally drains via a combination of the dorsal duct (duct of Santorini) in the body and tail of the gland and the ventral duct (duct of Wirsung) in the head of the gland. The latter opens into the duodenum with the common bile duct at the ampulla of Vater. Occasionally, the pancreas may drain through the dorsal duct, which opens directly into the duodenum through the more proximally placed accessory ampulla. During development of the foregut, the duodenum takes up a position that is principally to the right of the midline, and the pancreas becomes draped across the posterior abdominal wall to occupy a transverse position.

The duct system of the pancreas develops from the foregut as an arrangement of tubules that branch from the main duct and are lined by columnar or cuboidal epithelium. These primitive ducts terminate in clumps of cells known as cell buds, from which the acini develop. It has been suggested that the endocrine cells of the pancreas develop from migrating ectoderm of the neural crest, but the weight of evidence favors pluripotentiality of the cell buds leading to the development of both endocrine and exocrine components of the pancreas. The exocrine pancreas consists of the acini and duct systems; the endocrine pancreas consists of highly vascularized clusters of cells embedded within the lobules of acinar tissue. A type of portal venous system appears to exist by which arterial blood passes to the endocrine islets, breaks up into a network of capillaries, and then passes into a further capillary network around adjacent acini. The exocrine and endocrine components of the pancreas thus have close morphological, embryological, and vascular relationships, and there is accumulating evidence that they are functionally interdependent. It is clearly artificial to consider the exocrine pancreas as a separate entity, but convenient to do so for clinical purposes.

The exocrine secretion of the pancreas is especially important to normal growth and development during childhood. Cystic fibrosis, the principal disease entity related to pancreatic failure in children, will form the subject of a separate chapter. The current chapter is concerned with nutritional causes of pancreatic disease, and with the management of nutritional problems that occur in patients suffering from pancreatic diseases.

EXOCRINE PANCREATIC PHYSIOLOGY

Endocrine cells found in the wall of the gastrointestinal tract and in the pancreas itself produce peptide hormones, which appear to be able to exert their effects by the usual blood-borne route and also by diffusing locally in the extracellular fluid (paracrine effects). It has been traditional to attempt to segregate the neural and hormonal influences upon pancreatic secretion, but the identification of central neurotransmitters with immunochemical resemblances to gastrointestinal peptides suggests that the two influences may not be truly separable.[1]

The pancreas is innervated by efferents from the dorsal vagal nucleus, which pass via the posterior vagal trunk to the celiac plexus. The majority of the fibers pass through the plexus without synapse, the cell bodies of peripheral neurons being found within the pancreas itself. Vagal afferents pass centrally from the pancreas. Branches from sympathetic roots T5 to T10 pass via the lower sixth thoracic and upper two lumbar ganglia and the greater splanchnic nerve into the celiac plexus and superior mesenteric plexus. From here, postganglionic fibers are distributed to the pancreas with its arterial blood supply. Whereas vagal stimulation results in pancreatic secretion, sympathetic stimulation causes modification of the distribution of blood to the exocrine and endocrine pancreas and may serve to inhibit pancreatic secretion.

Pancreatic juice is approximately isotonic with plasma, and is variable in flow rate, concentration of bicarbonate (total anion concentration being maintained by reciprocation with chloride), and concentration of enzymes. Although the secretion rate is low under basal conditions, a small amount of juice is constantly secreted in the interdigestive period and it contains both bicarbonate and enzymes.

The digestive period of pancreatic secretion is conventionally subdivided into three phases, although the interrelationships between the phases are so complex that the distinction is more important to the physiologist than to the clinician. The anticipation, sight, smell, and taste of attractive food constitutes the cephalic phase of pancreatic secretion, which results in the stimulation of both bicarbonate and pancreatic enzymes. The mechanism is believed to operate through the stimulation of vagal efferents by afferent stimuli resulting from the perception or anticipation of food. The response of the pancreas is rapid, suggesting the importance of direct vagal stimulation of pancreatic secretion, but vagal effects may also be mediated through the release of gastrin, which stimulates pancreatic enzyme output in man. Although the exact magnitude of the pancreatic response to the cephalic phase is unclear, it may be an important initiator of pancreatic secretion, contributing perhaps more than 10 per cent of the total output of pancreatic juice in response to a meal.

The gastric phase of pancreatic secretion is due to the stimulatory effect upon the pancreas of food within the stomach. Gastric distention stimulates the secretion of pancreatic juice. The effect is probably mediated by both vagal stimulation and the release of gastrin from the antrum. The stomach has further profound influences upon pancreatic secretion mediated by the extent to which it permits partial digestion of protein and fat prior to gastric emptying, by the magnitude of gastric acid secretion, and by the rate of release of chyme into the duodenum.

The intestinal phase of pancreatic secretion is the most potent. The presence of acid in the duodenum stimulates the release of secretin from the upper small bowel (principally the duodenum).[2] Secretin is a powerful stimulant of fluid and bicarbonate secretion from the pancreas. The presence of the products of fat and protein digestion in the duodenum and jejunum liberates pancreozymin, which in turn stimulates enzyme output from the pancreas. Undigested proteins have little or no stimulatory effect upon pancreatic secretion,[3] but polypeptides, oligopeptides, and mixtures of amino acids have a strong stimulatory effect. Individual amino acids have less stimulatory effect than combined amino acid solutions, and are somewhat variable in their effect; phenylalanine, valine, and tryptophan are the most powerful. Enzyme output from the pancreas is also stimulated by calcium in the duodenal lumen,[4] and there is evidence that bile salts may stimulate both enzyme and bicarbonate output.[5] The interrelationships of secretin and pancreozymin have been controversial, but there is evidence that protein digestion augments acid-induced pancreatic secretion.[6]

Inhibition of Pancreatic Secretion

Food and the products of digestion play a stimulatory role in pancreatic regulation, which is followed by inhibition of pancreatic secretion as gastric emptying becomes complete. This aspect of pancreatic regulation has received relatively little attention, but it has recently become apparent that dietary influences that hamper the physiological shutdown of pancreatic secretion during digestion might be of relevance to the genesis of pancreatic disease. Moreover, the induction of pancreatic "rest" by the oral administration of inhibitors of pancreatic secretion has a potential role in the therapy of pancreatic disease.

The consumption of hypertonic glucose solutions has been shown to inhibit pancreatic secretion in man, and the instillation of oleic acid in the distal small bowel and colon of animals has been shown to have a similar effect, probably mediated by a hormone to which the name pancreatone has been given.[7–9] A similar mechanism has recently been demonstrated in man by the infusion of oleic acid into the right colon through an orally introduced catheter.[10] There is evidence to suggest that the sympathetic nervous system has an inhibitory effect upon pancreatic secretion mediated by the splanchnic nerves and also by circulating catecholamines. Other intestinal polypeptides that have a candidate role as inhibitory hormones (chalones) with an influence upon the pancreas are glucagon,[11] somatostatin,[12,13] and pancreatic polypeptide.[14]

In the rat, the administration of dietary trypsin inhibitors enhances pancreatic enzyme output[15] and increases both the size and protein content of the pancreas.[16] Duodenojejunal resection abolishes this effect.[17] Conversely, infusion of trypsin or chymotrypsin into the duodenum of the rat inhibits pancreatic enzyme secretion.[18] Support for the existence of similar mechanisms in man comes from the study of a patient with a pancreatic fistula[19] and from duodenal intubation studies in normal volunteers.[20] The effect of trypsin is mediated hormonally rather than

via cholinergic nerves.[21] The existence of inhibition of pancreatic secretion by luminal trypsin has been disputed on the basis of experiments carried out in normal volunteers in whom balloon catheters were used to aspirate duodenal contents.[22] The fact that intraluminal balloons themselves influence pancreatic secretion[23] might partially explain this apparent discrepancy. Slaff et al.[24] demonstrated that the addition of trypsin (10 g/L) to an amino acid solution that was used to perfuse the duodenum resulted in a lower level of chymotrypsin output in normal subjects, and to a lesser extent, patients with chronic pancreatitis. A dose-response curve was demonstrated in one patient; the lowest level of trypsin to influence chymotrypsin output was 0.9 g/L, and the maximum effect was observed at 2.5 g/L. The inhibiting effect of intraduodenal trypsin was abolished when the active site of the enzyme was blocked.

Adaptation to Diet and Parallelism of Pancreatic Enzyme Secretion

In 1943, Grossman et al.[25] showed that when rats were fed a diet rich in casein, there was an increase in the proteolytic enzyme content of the gland, and when they were given a diet rich in starch, the amylase content of the gland increased. Subsequent studies have confirmed these findings, showing that in rats a starch-rich diet induces a threefold to fourfold greater amylase concentration than in rats fed a diet rich in casein (70 per cent) and low in starch (20 per cent).[26] In the "high casein" rats chymotrypsinogen concentration was two to three times higher than in the "low casein" rats (15 per cent casein in diet), but increases in trypsinogen were not as marked. Adaptation required a period of dietary stability of 5 to 28 days to become maximal, the time required being dependent upon the magnitude and direction of change of the diet. The relative proportions of enzymes in the pancreatic juice reflect the adaptive changes found in the gland itself.[27] Adaptation of lipase and co-lipase to lipid-rich foods has also been demonstrated.[28] The mechanism of adaptation appears to be a change in the rate of biosynthesis of the enzyme, and the stimulus for its occurrence is the intraduodenal or intravenous presence of dietary substrates or their digestion products. Adaptation of proteolytic enzymes appears to occur in response to intraduodenal proteins, peptides, or amino acids. Cholecystokinin has been proposed as a mechanism, but subcutaneous administration of this hormone induces an increase not only of proteolytic enzymes, but also of amylase,[29] suggesting that an alternative hormonal pathway may be responsible. The amylase content of the pancreas adapts to either oral or intravenous glucose. The possibility that insulin may be implicated in the mechanism has been suggested.[30] Similarly, adaptation of lipase appears to occur in response to both oral and intravenous lipid administration.

Parallelism of enzyme secretion implies that within the short term, and thus independent of more chronic changes due to dietary adaptation, the same relative proportions of enzymes are secreted in response to a variety of stimuli of pancreatic exocrine function. The concept of parallelism, which may be explained as the idea that all enzymes are present within the zymogen granule and are thus discharged as a "packet" into the lumen of the acinus, was first proposed by Babkin in 1906. Although there is evidence to support parallelism,[31] other studies suggest that it does not occur in normal individuals,[32,33] but that the ability to modify the enzyme proportions within pancreatic juice in response to different stimuli is lost when diseases such as chronic pancreatitis or carcinoma of the pancreas become advanced.[34] Specific stimuli may exist for individual pancreatic enzymes, and a polypeptide has been isolated from the porcine small intestine that is capable of specifically stimulating chymotrypsinogen when injected intravenously.[35] The mechanism of nonparallel secretion has been explained by the existence of more than one type of acinar cell[36] and by differences in the rate of synthesis of different enzymes.[37] Recent evidence suggests that in man, intravenously infused cholecystokinin favors the secretion of lipase and chymotrypsinogen rather than secretion of amylase.[38] Similar data have emerged from studies in rabbits, suggesting that nonparallelism may be due to distinct protein synthetic and secretory pathways within the acinar cell.[39]

The concept that absorption of carbohydrates from a starch-containing meal can be "blocked" by ingestion of an amylase inhibitor was developed in an attempt to treat or prevent obesity. The presence of alpha-amylase inhibitors in wheat and kidney beans was recognized more than 40 years ago. Phaseolamin, a kidney bean amylase inhibitor, was characterized and purified in 1975; since then numerous commerical preparations have become available. Evidence for the efficacy of amylase inhibitors came from experiments in rats, in which impaired weight gain and a rise in fecal starch excretion were found, and from studies in man that demonstrated a reduction in the postprandial blood glucose response to a starch meal. More recently, however, evidence has accumulated to suggest that amylase inhibitors do not lead to carbohydrate malabsorption in man.[40,41] The cause of failure may be in part that the preparations that are currently available contain inadequate amounts of amylase inhibitor[42] and in part that the undigested starch is fermented to fatty acids in the colon.[43] Adaptation may also play a part in the defeat of this attractive carbohydrate "carte blanche"; low amylase levels (due to inhibition) and high starch levels may lead to progressively greater amylase outputs from the pancreas. Because of doubts concerning the safety and efficacy of amylase

inhibitors, they have now been classified as drugs by the Food and Drug Administration, and thus removed from the counters of health food shops in the United States.

NUTRITION AND THE ETIOLOGY OF PANCREATIC DISEASE

An interesting paradox exists in the relationship between nutrition and pancreatic disease, in that histologically similar forms of chronic pancreatitis appear to result from both dietary excesses and dietary deficiencies. Our knowledge of the details of these relationships is scant, a fact that should not occasion surprise in view of the multivariate nature of the problem and of the difficulties associated with the collection of precise epidemiological data.

Pancreatitis and the Westernized Diet

The commonest causes of acute pancreatitis in developed countries are gallstones and excessive alcohol consumption. It is generally considered that the former plays a very minor role in the etiology of chronic pancreatitis, and that the latter almost invariably indicates the presence of chronic pancreatic damage. It is generally accepted that alcohol abuse is the most common cause of chronic pancreatitis, and it is doubtful whether occasional heavy indulgence in alcohol causes either form of the disease. There appears to be an increase in frequency of both acute and chronic pancreatitis in many Westernized countries (Figs. 21–1 and 21–2), the main reason for which is increasing consumption of alcohol.[44,45] In contrast to alcohol-related cirrhosis, pancreatitis caused by alcohol abuse appears to be associated with a diet that is rich in protein and fat.[46,49] However, in a careful comparison of alco-

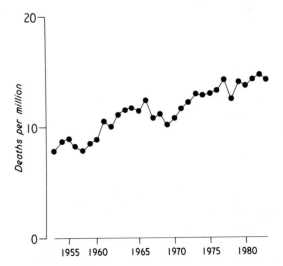

FIGURE 21–1. Mortality rate (deaths per million) of acute pancreatitis in England and Wales, 1953 to 1983.

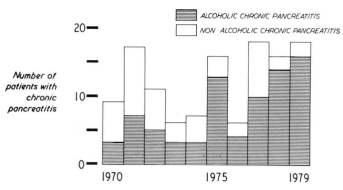

FIGURE 21–2. *Increasing frequency of chronic pancreatitis in Copenhagen, 1970 to 1979. (From Nyboe Andersen B, Thorsgaard Pedersen N, Scheel J, et al. Scand J Gastroenterol 1982; 17:249. Reproduced with permission.)*

holic pancreatitis and alcoholic cirrhosis in New York City, Pitchumoni et al.[50] found that the protein and fat content of the diet of patients with pancreatitis was higher than that of patients with cirrhosis, but was nevertheless lower than the average intake in the population. The dietary intake of protein and fat of the New York patients was approximately half that of patients with chronic pancreatitis in France and Germany. The association between increased ethanol consumption and chronic pancreatitis is well established in men but weaker in women.[51,52] No clear-cut relationship has emerged to implicate specific types of alcoholic beverage in the causation of pancreatitis.[49] There is evidence that there is a linear relationship between the logarithm of the risk of development of chronic pancreatitis and the mean daily consumption of alcohol. Moreover, the risk is increased by high levels of fat and protein in the diet.[53] Yen et al.,[52] in a careful epidemiological study, found a strong association between chronic pancreatitis and smoking in men and a weak association in women.

There is an association between acute pancreatitis and hyperlipidemia, although ethanol is also generally implicated,[54] hyperlipidemia being uncommon in patients with acute pancreatitis resulting from other causes.[55] Acute pancreatitis has been shown to be induced more readily in dogs given a high-fat diet,[56] and the perfusion of the isolated canine pancreas with fluid containing triglycerides results in formation of edema and hemorrhage.[57] Postoperative acute pancreatitis has been recorded in children after colonic resection for ulcerative colitis when intravenous fat emulsion was used as part of the preoperative nutritional regimen.[58] Whether the fat emulsion was directly related to the pancreatitis in these and other patients is difficult to establish, however.[59] Mechanisms relating excessive circulating lipid to the etiology of acute pancreatitis remain obscure. It has been suggested that under the influence of pancreatic lipase, free fatty acids are released that

are toxic to the pancreas,[57] toxicity being mediated by the production of oxygen-derived free radicals.[60] Stimulating the pancreas after the induction of experimental pancreatitis worsens the prognosis in the rat, although in the isolated canine pancreas the secretory state of the gland appeared to be without influence upon the severity of pancreatitis induced by infusion of free fatty acids.[61]

It was originally suggested that ethanol induced pancreatic damage by stimulating secretion,[62] but recent studies suggest that ethanol has various morphological and biochemical effects upon the gland (Table 21–1). The response of the pancreas to ethanol is probably dependent not only upon the amount and type of alcohol consumed but also upon factors such as diet, the relationship between eating and drinking, and the presence of alcohol-related gastric mucosal changes. Nevertheless, the exact mechanisms that lead to the characteristic morphological and function manifestations of chronic pancreatitis remain obscure.[63]

A unifying concept has been proposed by Sarles[64] that hinges upon changes in a secretory protein termed pancreatic stone protein (PSP). This protein, which has a molecular weight of 13,500 daltons, is distributed within the endoplasmic reticulum and zymogen granules of the pancreatic cell and is secreted into the juice, contributing about 14 per cent of the pancreatic juice protein. PSP appears to prevent precipitation of calcium carbonate, which is normally present in the juice as a supersaturated solution. Under the influence of chronic alcohol abuse, there is a reduction in the concentration of PSP, often combined with an increase in the total protein concentration of pancreatic juice and a decrease in juice volume. These circumstances permit the aggregation of protein into "plugs" which block small duct radicles and also allow precipitation of calcium carbonate, the latter being further facilitated by a reduction in the citrate concentration of the juice. Obstruction of the small duct radicles, perhaps

TABLE 21–1.   Effects of Ethanol upon the Pancreas

Morphological changes within acinar and duct cells
  Mitochondrial swelling
  Appearance of lipid droplets
  Focal cytoplasmic degeneration

Biochemical changes within acinar cells
  Reduced oxidation of fatty acids
  Increased biosynthesis of lipids
  Reduced protein synthesis
  Reduced concentration of nonsecretory phospholipase

Changes in pancreatic juice
  Increased protein concentration
  Decreased volume of juice
  Increased viscosity
  Reduced concentration of pancreatic stone protein
  Reduced citrate concentration
  Reduced concentration of protease inhibitor
  Reduced concentration of bicarbonate

Other changes
  Increased tone in sphincter of Oddi

by damaging the acinar cells or by allowing enzymes to pass into the periacinar spaces, leads to a combination of acute and chronic inflammation and eventually the characteristic changes of chronic pancreatitis. This hypothesis is the subject of considerable controversy at the present time, and would appear to relate to the mechanism that is specific to the genesis of chronic calcifying pancreatitis.

An alternative unifying concept, which has applicability to both acute and chronic pancreatitis, suggests that under the influence of alcohol excess, and in other situations that lead to pancreatitis, zymogen is activated within the acinar cells of the pancreas by lysosomal hydrolases.[65] Activation is normally prevented by the segregation of secretory and nonsecretory enzymes within zymogen granules and lysosomes, respectively, but may occur if abnormal vacuoles containing both types of enzyme are produced or if secretory and nonsecretory vacuoles fuse.

The suggestion that acute pancreatitis follows a heavy meal or an alcoholic debauch has been a feature of many accounts of the disease. White[66] provides a characteristic example: "The first symptom is usually abdominal pain, sometimes mild, occasionally prostrating, with the majority of attacks, in obese people, following over-indulgence of food and drink." Paxton and Payne[67] also commented on the relationship between pancreatitis and a large meal and also failed to provide data. Shallenberger and Kapp[68] in a review of 72 attacks of acute pancreatitis in 54 patients admitted to a hospital in Sayre, Pennsylvania, considered that a heavy or fatty meal was a precipitating cause of 44 per cent of the attacks, and that 22 per cent of them followed a drinking spree. Others authors, however, have failed to find an association between acute pancreatitis and a recent heavy intake of food or drink.[69,70]

Nutrition and Pancreatitis in Developing Countries

A variant of chronic pancreatitis which bears strong morphological similarities to alcohol-induced chronic pancreatitis was first described by Zuidema in Indonesia in 1959[71] and shortly afterwards in Uganda and India. Although alcohol appears to play at most a minor role in the etiology (many of the patients were total abstainers), the pathological appearances of the lesion are very similar to those of chronic calcifying pancreatitis in heavy drinkers. Fibrosis is a major feature, and ductal irregularities and stone formation are common. There is widespread acinar and islet destruction. The clinical features of the disease differentiate it from alcoholic pancreatitis.[72] The usual presentation is with intermittent and perhaps rather low-grade pain in childhood and adolescence, which progresses to diabetes mellitus, which usually becomes overt before the age

of 30. As with alcohol-related pancreatitis, pain may disappear in the later stages. The diabetes is characteristically brittle, and hypoglycemic attacks are common. In Kerala, Southern India, diabetic ketoacidosis was recorded in 18 per cent of the patients, which is similar to an incidence of 20 per cent observed in the Congo. A marked deficit of pancreatic exocrine function has been demonstrated by secretory studies[73] and is further confirmed by the 70 per cent incidence of a subnormal plasma amylase. Perhaps because of the low fat content of the diet, steatorrhea is not a common clinical problem. Death ensues between the ages of 20 and 40 years, and is usually due to hypoglycemia, infection, renal failure, or hepatic failure.

There is no doubt that nutritional pancreatitis occurs in parts of the world where malnutrition is common. In India, a relationship appears to exist between the incidence of calcifying pancreatitis in the hospital population and the daily intake of protein and fat[74] (Table 21–2). Severe protein malnutrition causes impairment of pancreatic function,[75] which is largely reversible upon resumption of an adequate diet.[76] A marked but reversible decline in pancreatic secretory function has also been demonstrated in a patient who received long-term total parenteral nutrition.[77] It has been suggested that nutritional pancreatitis is caused by effects of severe malnutrition upon pancreatic secretion with blockage of ducts by laminated secretions and mucous plugs,[78] but there is evidence that other factors are also important. The pancreatic lesions which occur in patients with kwashiorkor do not usually lead to calcification and necrosis. Moreover, patients with nutritional pancreatitis do not usually have a history of kwashiorkor and, despite the high incidence of nutritional pancreatitis in Kerala in India, the disease is quite uncommon in the neighboring state of Tamil Nadu, which has an equal if not higher incidence of kwashiorkor.[72] It has been suggested that nutritional pancreatitis might be related to the consumption of cassava (*Manihot esculenta*), which is a staple food in Kerala and in parts of Nigeria where there is also a high incidence of nutritional pancreatitis. Cassava contains the cyanogenic glycosides linamarin and linamarase, and the combination of these toxins and a diet that is poor in sulfur-containing amino acids might play a central role in the etiology of nutritional pancreatitis in man. In animals, dietary deficiencies of zinc, selenium, and copper have been shown to cause pancreatic damage,[79] but the importance of micronutrient deficiencies to the human pancreas is unclear.

Chronic pancreatitis is also common in parts of South America and in the black population of South Africa, but mainly in areas where alcohol consumption is high.[49] There has been a recent change in the pattern of pancreatitis in the black population of South Africa.[80] Traditionally alcohol was consumed as home-brewed beer with an alcohol concentration

TABLE 21–2. *Relationship between Hospital Incidence of Calcifying Pancreatitis and Dietary Intake in India*

State	Hospital Incidence of Calcifying Pancreatitis (%)	Daily Protein Intake (g)	Daily Fat Intake (g)
Kerala	1–1.7	26	20
Maharashtra	0.2	53	26
Punjab	0.05	62	25

Data from Vakil.[74]

of only 3 per cent. Chronic pancreatitis was an uncommon disease, but iron overload was a common problem owing to absorption of iron from the utensils used to make the beer. In 1962 the Pass Laws were modified and members of the black population of South Africa were able to purchase spirits and fortified wines, thus assuming a Western style of alcohol consumption. Chronic pancreatitis is now a common problem among the black population. The delay between the change in the law on drinking and the emergence of higher rates of pancreatitis was approximately 16 years.

Recent studies in Japan, where there is a low alcohol consumption and a low fat consumption and where pancreatitis is less frequent than in countries where a Western diet is common, have suggested that susceptibility to pancreatitis might be increased by essential fatty acid deficiency.[81] In the hamster, an additive effect of essential fatty acid deficiency and vitamin E deficiency upon the severity of the pancreatitis produced by infusing a solution of taurocholate, trypsin, and cephalothin into the pancreatic duct has been demonstrated (Fig. 21–3). Cases of acute pancreatitis treated with vitamin E analogues and fat emulsions rich in linoleic acid have been described[81]; however, it is difficult to evaluate such anecdotal data, and the role of essential fatty acid deficiency and vitamin E deficiency in the etiology and treatment of acute pancreatitis remains unclear.

Nutrition and the Etiology of Pancreatic Cancer

The incidence of adenocarcinoma of the pancreas has been increasing in most Westernized communities, and this disease now accounts for more than 20,000 deaths annually in the United States. Incidence rates vary considerably from one country to another and also among different ethnic groups.[82] The most clearly established risk factor for pancreatic cancer is cigarette smoking, but dietary factors are probably of importance. Some studies have not demonstrated any association between alcohol consumption and pancreatic cancer,[82] although a recent case control study from France suggested that the relative risk of pancreatic cancer rose with increasing alcohol consumption[83] (Fig. 21–4).

The prevalence of pancreatic cancer appears to be related to the fat content of the diet.[84] In a case-control study that included 69 patients with pancreatic cancer and 199 controls, fat intake emerged as one of the strongest differences between the two groups. An association between butter consumption and pancreatic cancer emerged from a case-control study in Baltimore.[85] Support for the association has also emerged from studies in animals. The induction of pancreatic cancers in rats by azaserine was shown to be enhanced by a diet that contained 20 per cent corn oil, but not by a diet containing a similar amount of saturated fat,[86] and a lower than expected number of tumors was found in rats fed a low-fat diet. Enhancement of pancreatic carcinogenesis by increasing dietary polyunsaturated fat has also been demonstrated in the Syrian hamster.[87] Recently polyunsaturated fat has been shown to promote pancreatic cancer in rats given injections of N-nitroso(2-hydroxypropyl)(2-oxypropyl)amine (HPOP) and also to promote the development of atypical acinar cells, and even cancer, in rats that were given injections of saline instead of HPOP.[88]

Results obtained from a study conducted in Japan suggest that dietary protein is also related to the incidence of pancreatic cancer. Individuals who ate meat daily had 1.5 times the pancreatic cancer risk of those who ate it less frequently.[89] However, other

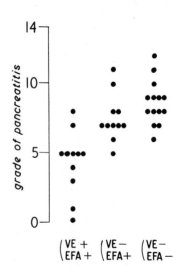

FIGURE 21–3. *Severity of acute pancreatitis in hamster according to dietary content of essential fatty acids (EFA) and vitamin E (VE). (From Tanimura H, Kato H, Hikasa Y. Ann NY Acad Sci 1982; 393:215. Reproduced with permission.)*

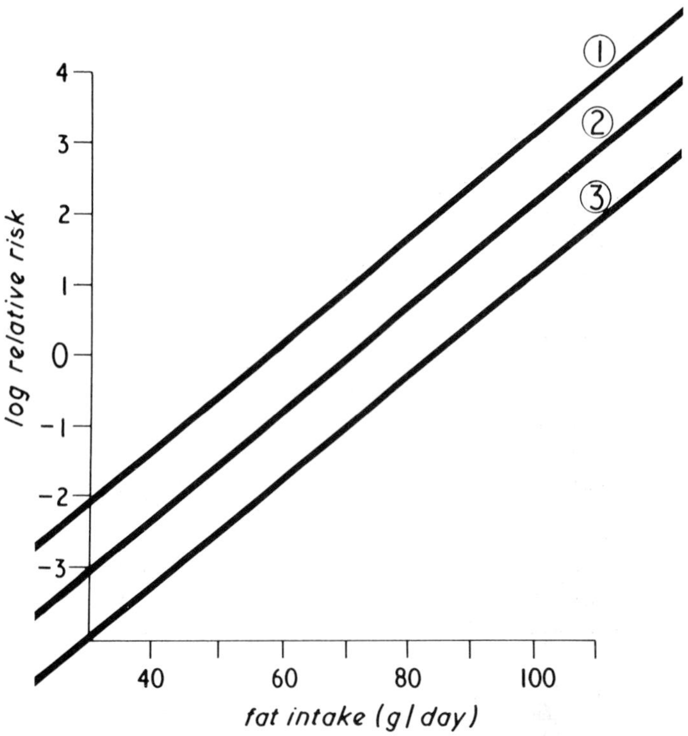

FIGURE 21–4. Relationship between daily fat intake, daily alcohol consumption, and risk of carcinoma of the pancreas. Alcohol consumption: (1) 40 g/day, (2) 80 g/day, (3) 120 g/day. (From Durbec JP, Chevilotte G, Bidart JM. Br J Cancer 1983; 47:468. Reproduced with permission.)

studies have failed to correlate protein intake or protein-rich foods with pancreatic cancer.[80,86] Although the provision of a protein-free diet to Syrian hamsters during the initiation stage of carcinogenesis with BOP led to the development of fewer pancreatic cancers than in control animals,[90] a low-protein diet given to rats during the initiation stage of tumor induction by azaserine had no demonstrable effect.[91] A high-protein diet given to rats did not increase the number of tumors that resulted from azaserine treatment; unexpectedly a lower number was found.[86]

The oral administration of protease inhibitors to rats induces an increase in the size and protein content of the pancreas.[16] A similar effect is observed after raw soya flour (which contains an inhibitor of trypsin and chymotrypsin) is given to rats for a period of 10 to 20 days.[92] In a carefully controlled series of experiments, McGuinness et al.[93] showed that if a diet containing raw soya flour is administered to rats for a year or more, pancreatic cancers then develop. Moreover, the soya flour was able to potentiate the action of subthreshold amounts of known pancreatic carcinogens. Soya milk powder as well as cow's milk powder contains inhibitors of human trypsin, although human breast milk does not (Fig. 21–5). The relevance of these data to the widespread use of soya products by food faddists, patients with hyperlipoproteinemia, and infants who are allergic to cow's milk indicates the need for further studies.

Based on epidemiological data, it has been suggested that coffee drinking may increase the risk of pancreatic cancer.[94] There is some support for this contention[85,95] as well as some disagreement.[96–100] The difficulties involved in trying to establish a link between coffee and pancreatic cancer are formidable, as has been acknowledged in the literature.

INFLUENCE OF ELEMENTAL DIETS AND INTRAVENOUS NUTRITION UPON PANCREATIC SECRETION

The principal indications for the use of enteral and parenteral nutrition in the management of patients with pancreatic disease are severe or complicated attacks of pancreatitis and operations for pancreatic cancer. It is generally accepted that a desirable aim of therapy for inflammatory pancreatic disease is that it should "rest" the pancreas by minimizing the stimulation of exocrine or endocrine function. There is no evidence that nutritional treatment can inhibit pancreatic secretion and thus provide sub-basal levels of enzyme secretion. Indeed, most forms of nutrition stimulate the gland, and thus a compromise is sometimes necessary in order to use a form of nutritional support that is appropriate to the patient's clinical condition and to the facilities available, while at the same time aiming to minimize the stimulation of pancreatic function.

Elemental Diets

Under similar circumstances, elemental diets generally cause less stimulation of pancreatic exocrine

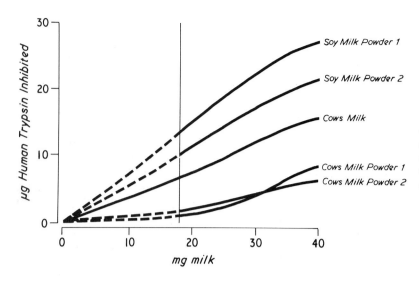

FIGURE 21–5. Trypsin inhibitory capacity of soy milk powder (two preparations), cow's milk powder (two preparations) and cow's milk. Human breast milk did not show inhibitory capacity. (From McGuinness E, Morgan RGH, Wormsley KG. Environ Health Perspect 1984; 56:210. Reproduced with permission.)

secretion than a full diet. In dogs, oral elemental diets lead to a reduction in the volume of pancreatic juice and the secretion of amylase, lipase, and trypsinogen compared with that stimulated by regular dog chow.[101,102] In part, these effects may be due to differences in the composition of the diets and in the willingness of the dogs to consume as much of the elemental diet as of their regular chow. Cassim and Allardyce[103] investigated the effect of an infusion of an elemental diet or a blenderized ward diet into the proximal jejunum of dogs in which 50 per cent of maximum pancreatic secretion had been induced by an intravenous infusion of secretin and cholecystokinin. A brisk volume response was induced by both diets, but whereas the blenderized diet produced a rise in the protein concentration of pancreatic juice, the elemental diet resulted in a more dilute juice (Fig. 21–6). Although the authors designed their experiments carefully in order to provide infusion rates that gave the same caloric load, the nitrogen-to-calorie ratio was almost twice as great in the ward diet, which may have profoundly influenced the results. In dogs in which a chronic pancreatic fistula had been established, the infusion of

a full liquid diet to the distal duodenum stimulated greater pancreatic secretion than the infusion of an elemental diet (Vivonex), particularly with respect to protein output.[104] Despite the absence of protein from the elemental diet, the nitrogen concentration (6.7 g/L as amino acid) was greater than that of the full liquid diet (5.3 g/L). Both diets were infused at isocaloric rates, but the fat content of the full diet (40 g/L) was greater than that of the elemental diet (1 g/L).

In addition to the type of diet, the site at which it is administered or infused may have a large influence upon the pancreatic response. Clearly, an infusion into the stomach or small bowel potentially eliminates the cephalic phase of pancreatic secretion. Kelly and Nahrwold[105] found that when an elemental diet was infused intraduodenally into dogs, stimulation of pancreatic secretion was less than when the same diet was given orally. Infusion of an elemental diet into the proximal jejunum resulted in a pancreatic juice that was very "enzyme poor."[104] The acidity of the infused diet may be a further factor of importance to the pancreatic response. By infusing an amino acid solution similar to that found in

FIGURE 21–6. Protein concentration in duodenal juice in response to intraduodenal infusion of an elemental diet or a blenderized ward diet. (From Cassim MM, Allerdyce DB. Ann Surg 1974; 180:230. Reproduced with permission.)

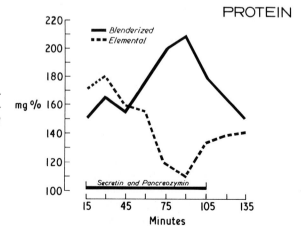

elemental diets (pH 5.4) into Thiry-Vella loops in dogs, Ragins et al.[106] recorded no stimulation of pancreatic secretion above that induced by secretin (0.5 GIH units/kg/hr), but when the same solution was infused at a pH of 3.5, strong pancreatic stimulation was recorded.

It is clear that use of the gastrointestinal tract to provide nutritional supports always induces some degree of pancreatic stimulation. Experimental data suggest that this might be minimized, while acceptable nutrition is still provided, by the infusion of an elemental diet at neutral pH into the proximal jejunum. These conclusions are based upon observations of responses in dogs, and neither in normal humans nor in subjects with pancreatic disease. However, Vidon et al. have confirmed that in normal human volunteers, intrajejunal perfusion of a crushed food homogenate induces greater stimulation of pancreatic enzyme secretion than an elemental diet.[107] Similar findings were obtained in three patients with chronic pancreatitis in whom an indwelling silicone rubber T-tube had been placed in the pancreatic duct at the time of pancreatojejunostomy. Compared with a normal oral diet, intragastric Vivonex HN induced smaller volumes of pancreatic juice.[108] An intraduodenal elemental diet had previously been shown to induce similar degrees of pancreatic secretion in response to an infusion of cholecystokinin at 2 units/kg/hr.[109]

Not only is enteral feeding a less potent stimulus to the exocrine pancreas than regular oral intake, but it has a smaller trophic effect upon the gland. This was demonstrated by Callegari et al. in the rat.[110] After 20 days of a partially hydrolyzed diet or an elemental diet, pancreatic weight and DNA content were less than in animals given normal chow. The elemental diet resulted in the most marked reduction in pancreatic weight and DNA content.

Intravenous Nutrition

Nakajima and Magee[111] showed that an intravenous infusion of 40 per cent glucose inhibited the pancreatic secretory output of fluid, protein, amylase, and lipase in dogs after pancreatic function had been stimulated by secretin. Hamilton et al.[112] confirmed that similar effects were observed when a solution consisting of 20 per cent dextrose and 5 per cent amino acids was infused intravenously into dogs with gastric and duodenal cannulas in which pancreatic secretion had been induced by secretin and cholecystokinin. They also observed an increase in the bicarbonate concentrations of duodenal fluid. Without the stimulus of secretin or cholecystokinin, basal levels of secretion from the pancreas measured during an infusion of intravenous physiological saline were marginally increased when an intravenous infusion of amino acids and 50 per cent glucose was commenced, although in the same animals a much

greater pancreatic response was seen to intraduodenal or intragastric elemental diet.[105] Further support for these findings has come from the dose-response studies carried out in dogs by Stabile et al.,[104] who demonstrated that the pancreatic response to the intraduodenal administration of an elemental diet or a full liquid diet was not observed after intravenous hyperalimentation with amino acids and glucose (Fig. 21–7). In other experiments carried out in a canine model, Towne et al.[113] showed that when pancreatic exocrine secretion was stimulated by secretin and cholecystokinin, the inhibitory effect caused by an intravenous infusion of 20 per cent glucose and 5 per cent amino acids appeared to be due principally to the glucose and not the amino acid component, although the latter alone did produce significant inhibition. Stabile and Debas[114] showed that in dogs intravenous fat emulsion (2.5 to 20 per cent; 100 ml/hr), amino acid (1.25 to 10 per cent; 100 ml/hr), and glucose (6.25 to 50 per cent; 100 ml/hr) all failed to stimulate pancreatic secretion when given individually. Basal secretion in the dog was stimulated with respect to volume of pancreatic juice, protein, and bicarbonate output by both a full liquid and elemental diet, but no stimulation was observed in response to graded doses of an intravenous solution consisting of 10 per cent amino acid and 50 per cent glucose.[104] Konturek et al.[115] reported a series of experiments carried out in dogs with chronic pancreatic fistulas. Both an amino acid mixture and fat emulsion infused intravenously in graded doses produce a dose-dependent rise in pancreatic protein secretion that reached about 40 per cent of the maximal response observed in response to CCK. The data are in apparent conflict with those of Fried et al.,[116] who also studied dogs with chronic pancreatic fistulas, but found that neither an intravenous solution of amino acids (4.5 per cent) nor of fat emulsion (10 per cent) stimulated pancreatic juice volume or protein output. In addition, this study demonstrated that neither infusion stimulated a change in the plasma concentration of CCK or PP. Other experiments in dogs with chronic pancreatic fistulas have demonstrated that an inhibitory effect of intravenous glucose upon pancreatic secretion stimulated by secretin and CCK became significant only when plasma glucose levels rose above 100 mg/dl, perhaps owing in part to an osmotic effect.[117] This suggestion is supported by the observation that 20 per cent mannitol also suppressed pancreatic secretion.

A reduction in the drainage of fluid from patients with pancreatic or duodenal fistulas has been noted in several reports.[118–122] An interesting feature common to many of these observations is that with the commencement of intravenous nutrition there was a reduction of the fistula fluid output to a lower level than that observed when the patient was receiving 5 per cent dextrose or physiological saline (Fig. 21–8). This suggests that in the presence of a fistula,

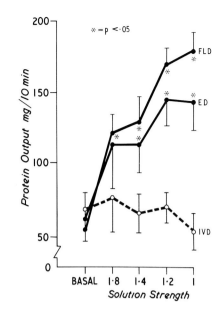

FIGURE 21-7. Pancreatic protein output from pancreatic fistula in dogs fed with increasing doses of intraduodenal full liquid diet (FLD), enteral diet (ED), and intravenous nutrition (IVD). (From Stabile BE, Borzatta M, Stubbs RS. JPEN 1984; 8:379. Reproduced with permission.)

pancreatic exocrine secretion may be suprabasal, and thus susceptible to inhibition by intravenous nutrition.

Digestion of intravenously administered protein inhibits the hormonally stimulated pancreatic secretion of normal subjects,[123] a finding that is consistent with many of the studies carried out in dogs. In a patient with a pancreatic fistula, the inhibition of volume and protein output from the fistula that was achieved by an intravenous infusion of 25 per cent glucose and 3.5 per cent amino acids was apparently uninfluenced by the addition of intravenous lipid emulsion (Fig. 21–8).[122] The lack of influence of intravenous fat emulsion upon pancreatic secretion in man, with or without the presence of a secretin in-

fusion, was confirmed in studies upon normal subjects in whom duodenal juice was aspirated via a double lumen tube,[124] and in other studies carried out in patients with pancreatic fistulas.[125]

In summary, the available evidence suggests that although there is wide variation among different formulations, enteral diets frequently induce less pancreatic stimulation than a full oral diet, but are, nonetheless, considerably more potent in their stimulatory effect than intravenous nutrition. Although in some respects data concerning the effects of intravenous nutrition upon pancreatic secretion are apparently in conflict, there is sufficient consistency to conclude that intravenous nutrition is probably the optimal nutritional technique to support patients in whom the avoidance of pancreatic secretion is considered to be important.

NUTRITIONAL MANAGEMENT OF PATIENTS WITH CHRONIC PANCREATITIS

A patient with chronic pancreatitis may develop a complication, such as an abscess or pseudocyst of the pancreas, that superimposes an acute event with potential nutritional consequences upon a disease that may include significant pancreatic insufficiency among its clinical manifestations. The nutritional management of the acute episodes is more appropriately considered within the section concerned with acute pancreatitis (see below). The existence of chronic pancreatitis implies a subnormal capacity to secrete pancreatic enzymes into the duodenum, but exocrine insufficiency must be of marked degree before it becomes symptomatic. DiMagno et al.[126] showed that significant steatorrhea occurs only when the pancreatic enzyme output falls to less than 10 per cent of normal (Fig. 21–9). In the majority of patients, even with this degree of pancreatic secre-

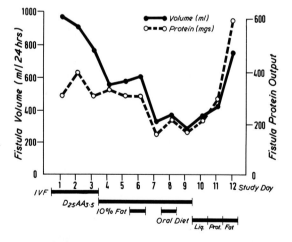

FIGURE 21-8. Fluid volume and protein output from a chronic pancreatic fistula in response to intravenous dextrose/saline (IVF), glucose-based intravenous nutrition providing 8 to 17 g N/24 hr (D_{25} $AA_{3.5}$), intravenous lipid emulsion (400 to 450 ml/24 hr; 10 per cent fat), and an oral liquid diet (Oral Diet). (From Bivins BA, Bell RM, Rapp RP, et al. JPEN 1984; 8:35. Reproduced with permission.)

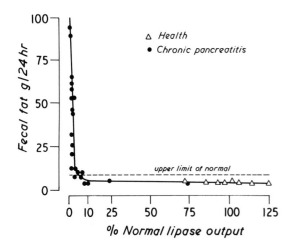

FIGURE 21–9. *Relationship between pancreatic lipase output and fecal fat excretion in patients with chronic pancreatitis and normal subjects. Enzyme secretion was stimulated by intraduodenal infusion of essential amino acids and by intravenous infusion of cholecystokinin-pancreozymin. Values of fecal fat above the dashed line denote steatorrhea. (From DiMagno EP, Go VLW, Summerskill WHJ. N Engl J Med 1973; 288:814. Reproduced with permission.)*

tory impairment, limitation of dietary fat intake is usually sufficient to prevent symptoms of steatorrhea. In a small proportion of patients other nutritional problems may emerge; these may be due to the lack of pancreatic secretion or to poor eating habits imposed by pancreatic pain, or associated with the excessive alcohol intake, which is so frequently a factor in patients with chronic pancreatitis. In particular, deficiencies of fat-soluble vitamins and of vitamin B_{12} may arise,[127–129] as may deficiencies of minerals, particularly of calcium, magnesium, zinc, and trace elements.[130–133] It is clearly important to ensure that the diet of patients with chronic pancreatitis contains adequate amounts of vitamins, minerals, and trace elements.

Apart from problems consequent upon alcohol abuse and a disordered lifestyle, the essential lesion creating malabsorption in patients with chronic pancreatitis is failure of production of sufficient enzymes to bring about normal digestion of food. The logical remedy to this problem is to supplement food with an enzyme preparation. This has been shown in practice to have two advantages, one being symptomatic and the other nutritional. Pain is a disabling symptom to many patients with chronic pancreatitis. The exact mechanism of production of the pain is unclear, but one possibility is overstimulation of the gland by the presence of undigested or partially digested products of food in the small bowel. The pancreatic secretion that results is partially from acini that drain into ducts blocked by strictures or protein plugs. Continuing secretion behind the obstruction leads to raised pressure within the duct segment and hence to retrograde diffusion of pancreatic enzymes

into the interstitium of the gland, with consequent inflammation and stimulation of pain afferents. Under normal circumstances, the drive to exocrine secretion would be inhibited by the presence of free protease enzymes within the duodenal lumen (see Inhibition of Pancreatic Secretion, above). On the basis of this hypothesis, it is interesting to note that Sarles[134] records that two tablets of a preparation of bovine pancreatic extract (pancreatin) taken three times a day with meals resulted in a reduction in the pain of chronic pancreatitis. The ability of effective enzyme supplementation to reduce pancreatic pain was also demonstrated by a double-blind crossover study carried out in Sweden.[135] The patients were given 7.5 ml of a granular preparation of pancreatin (Pankreon) five times daily for 1 week compared with a 1-week course of treatment with heat-inactivated granules. The active preparation significantly reduced pain (Fig. 21–10). Slaff et al.[24] recently showed that the pancreatic exocrine response to an intraduodenal infusion of amino acids in patients with chronic pancreatitis could be reduced by adding trypsin or chymotrypsin to the infusate. It was also confirmed, using a double-blind crossover technique, that supplementation with pancreatin in tablet form (Ilozyme) significantly reduced the pain of chronic pancreatitis.

Pancreatin has been available for many years and has been used extensively for the treatment of steatorrhea in children with cystic fibrosis. It is probably necessary in only a minority of patients with chronic pancreatitis to provide enzyme supplementation in order to control steatorrhea or maintain nutrition. Pancreatin is available as powder, which can be sprinkled on the food, in tablet form, or in capsules. It has an unpleasant taste and smell, which limits compliance for preparations without an enteric coat. There has been considerable controversy over the merits of different preparations and whether or not pancreatin should be combined with an antacid or

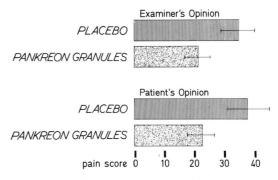

FIGURE 21–10. *Effect of granular pancreatin (Pankreon granules) versus placebo (heat-inactivated granules) on pain in patients with chronic pancreatitis. Data represent mean ± standard error of mean and significance levels refer to Student's t test. Data are from a double blind crossover study in which each treatment was administered for 1 week. (From Isaksson G, Ihse I. Dig Dis Sci 1983; 28:99. Reproduced with permission.)*

H_2-receptor antagonist.[136] Duodenal pH may be lower than normal in patients with chronic pancreatitis,[137] and there is probably a case for using a combination of pancreatin with an H_2-receptor antagonist (cimetidine or ranitidine) when acid output from the stomach is high.[138] Recently, microspheres or coated pancreatin granules have become available that are designed to release their contained enzymes when the pH rises towards neutrality (Creon, Pancrease, Pancreatin granules). Compared with more traditional pancreatin preparations, which are frequently without noticeable effect, granular preparations have been shown to increase enzyme levels in the duodenum, and to diminish steatorrhea in patients with chronic pancreatitis.[139–141] Effects were seen when 10 to 20 ml of granules (Pankreon, or Pancreatin granules) were taken with each meal or when three capsules of Pancrease (containing 1.5 g of granular pancreatin) were taken with each meal. Long-term use of Pancrease capsules (containing the granules) was shown to lead to weight gain in patients with chronic pancreatitis[141] (Fig. 21–11). Thus enzyme supplementation appears to bring both symptomatic and nutritional benefits to patients with chronic pancreatitis, and is probably indicated in patients with pain, steatorrhea, or overt undernutrition. The cost of the enteric-coated granular preparations is a significant consideration, and it remains unclear if supplementation therapy is justifiable in patients with less severe symptoms. Dosage remains unclear, but it is my present practice to commence with two capsules of granular pancreatin taken immediately before or just after the start of a meal. The dose can be increased or reduced as necessary to meet individual needs.

The most important dietary recommendation for patients with chronic pancreatitis is complete abstinence from alcohol. This alone can lead to relief of pancreatic pain in half those who suffer from it.[134] Dietary fat should be reduced to less than 25 per cent of total calories in order to avert steatorrhea and avoid undue stimulation of the gland. In patients with severe exocrine insufficiency, it may be necessary to increase dietary protein intake. Diabetes complicates chronic pancreatitis in a small proportion of patients, and appropriate dietary measures should be undertaken. Even if steatorrhea is controlled, there may be deficiency of fat-soluble vitamins,[129] and supplementation is advised.

NUTRITIONAL MANAGEMENT OF PATIENTS WITH ACUTE PANCREATITIS AND ACUTE COMPLICATIONS OF CHRONIC PANCREATITIS

As a result of changes in dietary habits and alcohol consumption in the community, acute pancreatitis is becoming increasingly common in Westernized countries (Fig. 21–1). Not only is the prevalence changing, but so are the problems facing the clinician concerned with the management of pancreatitis.

It is convenient to regard acute pancreatitis as a disease with two components. Patients initially experience an acute systemic illness that can be of sufficient severity to result in death from shock and multi-organ failure. It is generally considered that this systemic response is due to the release of pancreatic enzymes or their bioactive digestion products into the tissues around the pancreas, the peritoneal cavity, or the blood stream. If the patient survives the first few days of the attack, the lesions within the pancreas itself may give rise to local complications such as pseudocyst, abscess, or pancreatic necrosis, which may themselves lead to death. Fortunately, in the majority of attacks, the patient survives the initial systemic illness without the need for more intensive therapeutic measures than analgesia, nasogastric suction, and intravenous fluid, and then proceeds to an uneventful recovery without the development of local complications.

Whereas it was common for death from acute pancreatitis to occur within the first week of the attack, largely as a result of the effects of the initial systemic illness,[142] contemporary techniques of intensive therapy frequently secure survival from this component

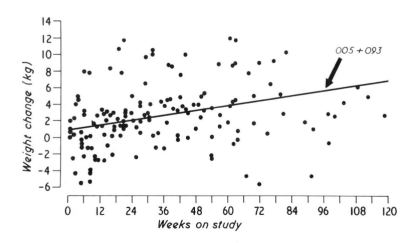

FIGURE 21–11. Plot of weight changes against time for 22 patients with chronic pancreatitis who were receiving granular pancreatin (Pancrease capsules). Mean weight gain was 4.0 ± 1.1 kg over an average of 54 weeks. (From Valerio D, White EHA, Schlamm HT. JPEN 1981; 5:112. Reproduced with permission.)

of the illness, although the patient may succumb from later complications. In northern Europe and North America, it is generally accepted that the initial management of acute pancreatitis is conservative, operative intervention being reserved for those patients in whom conservative management is clearly failing to achieve success. If abscess, pseudocyst, or pancreatic necrosis supervenes, it is a general principle of management to refrain from operative intervention, if possible, for 4 to 6 weeks in order that granulation tissue and fibrous tissue can mature around the cavity and thus enable surgical drainage to be undertaken safely. While this plan of management can be followed in many patients, in others evidence of severe sepsis develops and urgent surgical intervention is necessary. From the commencement of the attack of pancreatitis to the point when the patient is able to return to normal food consumption, there is a nutritional risk. This time interval may extend to several months, during which sepsis may be a recurring problem, rendering nutritional considerations crucial to survival. Other patients do not require surgery to drain a necrotic pancreas or a cystic collection but are unable to tolerate food for as long as many weeks because of the swollen and inflamed pancreas. In such patients, survival may also depend upon the provision of adequate nutritional support. Patients who develop acute complications of chronic pancreatitis such as pseudocyst or abscess formation face similar nutritional risks, rendered more acute if they were previously malnourished as a result of pancreatic exocrine insufficiency.

Severe acute pancreatitis produces a systemic illness not dissimilar in its metabolic effects to severe sepsis or burn injury, and results in rapid loss of body weight, fat, and protein.[143-145] In a study from the Boston City Hospital[145] a mean weight loss of 24 per cent of body weight was recorded in eleven patients with severe pancreatitis. The nutritional status of the patients was compared with a large body of data relating to nutritional status in patients with a spectrum of different diseases. Severe pancreatitis was one of the most potent causes of malnutrition and appeared to result in a more specific depletion of muscle bulk than other gastrointestinal diseases. In view of the severity of the catabolic response, it is probably reasonable practice to commence nutritional support for patients with severe pancreatitis within a week of admission to the hospital. Patients with severe pancreatitis develop reduced plasma and muscle levels of glutamine, and increased levels of branched-chain amino acids in muscle.[146] Abnormally high peripheral resistance to insulin is present with an overall correlation between the magnitude of the disturbance of amino acid metabolism and the severity of the pancreatitis. Data we have recorded in Leeds (unpublished) suggest that patients with severe acute pancreatitis may exhibit an elevation of resting energy expenditure similar to that seen in patients with severe sepsis or severe burns. In the acute, fulminant stage of pancreatitis, intravenous nutrition appears to be the most practicable way to provide nutritional support. Later in the course of the attack, when paralytic ileus and other manifestations of the acute toxic illness have subsided, enteral nutrition may be appropriate to bridge the gap between intravenous nutrition and the resumption of an oral diet.

On the basis of clinical evidence, it has been suggested that premature return to an oral diet might increase the incidence of pancreatic abscess in patients with acute pancreatitis,[147,148] but this view is not universally accepted. Most clinicians allow the patient to eat when he is able to do so without pain or discomfort, but it is usual to allow a gradual transition from nil orally, through clear fluids and then nutritious fluids such as soup, to solid food. Failure to tolerate food can be a sign of a developing abscess or pseudocyst. Pancreatic enzyme secretion may remain abnormally low for weeks or months after acute pancreatitis.[149] Recent evidence suggests that granular pancreatin can "rest" the gland during convalescence from acute pancreatitis,[150] but it remains to be shown whether benefit accrues to the patient.

Intravenous nutrition has two potential roles in the management of patients with acute pancreatitis. First, by virtue of its ability to inhibit stimulation of pancreatic exocrine function, intravenous nutrition may possess the potential to modify the natural history of acute pancreatitis. Techniques designed to "rest" the pancreas have become routine in the management of acute pancreatitis, the two most widely adopted being the use of nasogastric aspiration and atropine-like drugs. Can intravenous nutrition provide an alternative and effective method of resting the pancreas and thus hastening recovery from acute pancreatitis? The second potential use for intravenous nutrition in patients with acute pancreatitis, which is less controversial, is to provide nutritional support to enable the patient to survive until eating can be resumed.

Can Intravenous Nutrition Influence the Natural History of Acute Pancreatitis?

If the continued production of pancreatic enzymes during acute pancreatitis is responsible for increased severity of the systemic component of the attack or the development of later complications, then suppression of the synthesis or secretion of enzymes has the potential to ameliorate the severity of the attack. Counter to this concept is the finding that in rats, the induction of pancreatitis causes a marked reduction in the volume and protein output of the pancreatic juice.[151] Earlier studies suggested rapid normalization of pancreatic exocrine function after an attack of acute pancreatitis in man,[152] but more recent work suggests that it may be impaired for weeks or months after the attack.[149]

Kawaura et al.[153] investigated the effect of 5 per cent glucose (supplemented with vitamins), 21 per cent glucose, fat, and amino acids, and 21 per cent glucose and fat but no amino acids, given intravenously to dogs in which pancreatitis had been induced by injection of bile into the pancreatic duct. The treatment was continued for 1 month. The two dogs allocated to the 5 per cent glucose group both died within 10 days, but the other four remained alive. Data were presented that suggested that plasma protein levels were maintained in the four animals that received the 21 per cent glucose. In addition to these experiments, the authors described four patients with acute pancreatitis who had been treated with intravenous nutrition with fat emulsion and glucose as the calorie source. The authors concluded, "In the treatment of acute pancreatitis intravenous hyperalimentation (IVH) is the ideal therapy. . . . The most important thing is to give fat emulsion intravenously." From the data presented, however, it is difficult to accept such firm conclusions.

In a small randomized study, patients with acute pancreatitis were given standard conservative management with no specific nutritional support or Intralipid 1.5 g/24 hr commencing on the second day in the hospital. There was no apparent benefit accruing to the use of Intralipid, but the general spectrum of pancreatitis was mild, and only 31 attacks were included in the study.[154] In another small randomized study, patients with acute pancreatitis received a solution of glucose (1.7 g/kg/24 hr), a glucose solution plus an amino acid preparation supplying 1 g/kg/24 hr of "protein" or a solution of glucose, amino acids, and 10 per cent lipid emulsion. The clinical outcome was apparently uninfluenced by the intravenous regimen, though the patients who received glucose alone had a marked negative nitrogen balance compared with the other two groups. Two of the patients who received lipid emulsion developed modest hypertriglyceridemia.[155] We have recently calculated that in order to show the clinical effect of a therapeutic manipulation in patients with acute pancreatitis it is probably necessary to include a minimum of 50 patients with a severe attack in each group. In view of the fact that only about one fifth of attacks of acute pancreatitis can be classified as severe, it is probable that none of these studies were large enough to demonstrate clinical differences between the regimens that were employed.

A retrospective study of patients with pancreatitis admitted to the Massachusetts General Hospital was undertaken in order to examine the influence of intravenous nutrition upon the development of complications of acute pancreatitis.[156] Data from 46 admissions among 44 patients were included in the study and represented 11 per cent of the total number of patients admitted to the hospital with acute pancreatitis during the 36-month period chosen for the study. Eighty-eight per cent of the patients underwent operative treatment, and there was a 20 per cent mortality rate. Incidences of renal failure, respiratory failure, and the need to intervene surgically were similar to those reported in other published series of patients with severe pancreatitis, and thus the authors drew the conclusion that intravenous nutrition had not significantly altered the natural history of the attack. While this was a detailed and clearly documented account of the difficulties associated with the use of intravenous nutrition in patients with severe pancreatitis, there must be reservations concerning the ability of such a retrospective study to address its central theme. The time interval between the onset of symptoms and the commencement of intravenous nutrition was not detailed. There is evidence that pancreatic collections begin to develop early in the course of acute pancreatitis,[157] and therapeutic measures designed to influence them should be similarly timed. Similar conclusions regarding the lack of impact of intravenous nutrition upon the course of acute pancreatitis were drawn from a retrospective study from Duke University Medical Center, Durham, North Carolina,[158] but similar criticism regarding the validity of the conclusion must apply. It is probable that the only way to resolve the question of whether intravenous nutrition can influence the natural history of acute pancreatitis is through a carefully planned randomized prospective study. This poses a daunting prospect, and it is doubtful whether the theoretical basis for the use of intravenous nutrition in this context justifies such extensive effort. At the present time, therefore, the administration of intravenous nutrition to patients with acute pancreatitis in order to attempt to prevent the onset of complications is difficult to justify.

Nutritional Support in the Patient with Severe Acute Pancreatitis

One of the conclusions from a review of 200 attacks of acute pancreatitis that were treated at the Montreal General Hospital was that "profound nutritional depletion" was a feature of 40 per cent of the attacks.[144] The report suggested that both intravenous and enteral nutrition played a valuable role in the management of the nutritional depletion, but detailed data were provided from only 2 of the patients. In another report[145] full intravenous nutrition was used in the management of 4 patients with acute pancreatitis, peripheral amino acid therapy (3 per cent) was used in 7 patients, and enteral nutrition with a defined-formula diet was used in 9 patients of a total experience of 77 patients with acute pancreatitis. Nutritional support was thought to be particularly appropriate for patients with severe protracted pancreatitis (an attack that was initially severe according to an objective grading system and in which evidence of pancreatic inflammation persisted for more than 14 days). This report drew attention to the length of time for which nutritional support may be necessary in patients with severe acute pancreatitis. When patients who died or who developed an abscess were excluded, nutritional support was given for a mean of 63 days.

White and Heimbach[159] described 30 patients with hemorrhagic pancreatitis, in the majority of whom a laparotomy was carried out owing to failure of medical treatment 10 or more days after the onset of the attack. Patients were maintained using intravenous nutrition before and after surgery, and in many of them a feeding jejunostomy was used to continue nutritional support via the enteral route. This was also a retrospective report, but the 80 per cent survival rate, which is high for such severely ill patients, was probably due in part to the careful nutritional support that was provided. Another factor that may have been important was that the mean age of the patients was 43 years.

Although Goodgame and Fisher[156] and Grant et al.[158] failed to provide evidence to support the use of intravenous nutrition as a therapy to prevent the emergence of complications of acute pancreatitis, both reports gave a detailed analysis of the practical difficulties encountered in the provision of intravenous nutrition to patients with severe pancreatitis. Catheter-related sepsis emerged as a particular problem. Glucose intolerance was frequently observed when intravenous nutrition was commenced, and many patients required additional insulin. Metabolic complications were otherwise uncommon. Despite anecdotal reports that lipid emulsion may precipitate pancreatitis, no disadvantage to its use in their patients was observed by Grant et al.[158] This observation was consistent with the conclusion of a previous report.[160]

Other reports suggest that acute pancreatitis and its sequelae can be adequately managed postoperatively using an enteral diet delivered nasogastrically, via a gastrostomy or via a jejunostomy.[101,143]

In summary, patients with severe acute pancreatitis rapidly develop nutritional depletion, and it is probably expedient to commence nutritional therapy within a week of the onset of the attack if the patient's return to a normal diet is not considered imminent. The patients may become markedly toxic and intolerant of high rates of glucose infusion. Although clearance of lipid emulsion may be impaired under these circumstances, a clinical problem infrequently arises. In the first instance, while gastrointestinal function is compromised, nutritional support is most appropriately provided intravenously, although there is evidence to suggest that at later stages enteral nutrition may suffice. The great value of nutritional therapy is that it enables the physician to play a waiting game because both the return of adequate alimentary function and recovery from the complications of acute pancreatitis may take weeks or months.

References

1. Grossman MI. Neural and hormonal regulation of gastrointestinal function: an overview. Ann Rev Physiol 1979; 41:27–33.
2. Schaffalitzky de Muckadell OB, Fahrenkrug J. Role of secretin in man. In Bloom SR (ed). Gut Hormones. Edinburgh, Churchill Livingstone, 1978: 197–201.
3. Meyer JH. Release of secretin and cholecystokinin. In Thompson JC (ed). Gastrointestinal Hormones. Austin, University of Texas Press, 1975: 475–489.
4. Holtermuller KH, Malagelada JR, McCall JT, et al. Pancreatic, gallbladder and gastric responses to intraduodenal calcium perfusion in man. Gastroenterology 1976; 70:693–696.
5. Wormsley KG. Stimulation of pancreatic secretion by intraduodenal infusion of bile salts. Lancet 1970; 2:586–588.
6. Fink AS, Miller JC, Jehn DW, et al. Digests of protein augment acid induced canine pancreatic secretion. Am J Physiol 1982; 242:G634–G641.
7. Hage G, Tiscornia O, Palasciano G, et al. Inhibition of pancreatic exocrine secretion by intracolonic oleic acid infusion in the dog. Biomedicine 1974; 21:263–267.
8. Laugier R, Sarles H. Action of oleic acid on the exocrine pancreatic secretion of the conscious rat: evidence for an anticholecystokinin-pancreozymin factor. J Physiol 1977; 271:81–92.
9. Harper AA, Hood AJC, Mushen J, et al. Inhibition of external pancreatic secretion by intracolonic and intraileal infusions in the cat. J Physiol 1979; 292:445–454.
10. Owyang C, Green L, Radar D. Colonic inhibition of pancreatic and biliary secretion. Gastroenterology 1983; 84:470–475.
11. Dyck WP, Texter EC, Lasater JM, et al. Influence of glucagon on pancreatic exocrine secretion in man. Gastroenterology 1970; 58:532–539.
12. Hanssen LE, Hanssen KF, Myren J. Inhibition of secretin release and pancreatic bicarbonate secretion by somatostatin infusion in man. Scand J Gastroenterol 1977; 12:391–394.
13. Holtermuller KH, Schittelkop G, Schulmeric H. Somatostatin (SRIF) inhibits pancreatic enzyme secretion and gallbladder emptying caused by intraluminal digestive products and exogenous cholecystokinin (CCK) in man. Irish J Med Sci 1977; 146:Suppl 14.
14. Konturek SJ, Meyers CA, Kwiecien N, et al. Effect of human pancreatic polypeptide and its C-terminal hexapeptide on pancreatic secretion in man and in the dog. Scand J Gastroenterol 1982; 17:395–399.
15. Lyman RL, Wilcox JS, Monsen RE. Pancreatic enzyme secretion produced in the rat by trypsin inhibitors. Am J Physiol 1962; 202:1077–1082.
16. Arnesjo B, Ihse I, Lundquist I, et al. Effects on exocrine and endocrine pancreatic functions by bovine lung trypsin inhibitor administered perorally. Scand J Gastroenterol 1973; 8:545–554.
17. Ihse I. Abolishment of oral trypsin inhibitor stimulation of the rat exocrine pancreas after duodeno-jejunal resection. Scand J Gastroenterol 1976; 11:11–15.
18. Green GM, Lyman RL. Feedback regulation of pancreatic enzyme secretion as a mechanism for trypsin inhibitor-induced hypersecretion in rats. Proc Soc Exp Biol Med 1972; 140:6–12.
19. Ihse I, Lilja P, Lundquist I. Feedback regulation of pancreatic enzyme secretion by intestinal trypsin in man. Digestion 1977; 15:303–308.
20. Owyang C, Leksell K, May D, et al. Intraduodenal trypsin inhibits cholecystokinin release and pancreatic enzyme secretion in man. Gastroenterology 1983; 84:1268.
21. Owyang C, Dismond S, May D. Feedback regulation of pancreatic enzyme secretion in man is stimulus specific. Gastroenterology 1984; 86:1205.
22. Hotz J, Ho VLW, et al. Short-term inhibition of duodenal

tryptic activity does not affect human pancreatic biliary or gastric functions. J Lab Clin Med 1983; 101:488–495.

23. Lambert JR, Hansky J. Effect of intraluminal small intestine distension on canine pancreatic secretion. Gastroenterology 1984; 86:1150.

24. Slaff J, Jacobson D, Tillman CR, et al. Protease-specific suppression of pancreatic exocrine secretion. Gastroenterology 1984; 87:44–52.

25. Grossman MJ, Greengard H, Ivy AC. The effect of dietary composition on pancreatic enzymes. Am J Physiol 1943; 138:676–682.

26. Desnuelle P, Reboud JP, Ben Abdeljlil A. Influence of the composition of the diet on the enzyme content of rat pancreas. In Reuck AVS, Cameron MP (eds). The Exocrine Pancreas. Normal and Abnormal Function. London, CIBA, 1962: 90–114.

27. Ben Abdeljlil A, Desnuelle P. Sur l'adaptation des enzymes exocrine du pancreas a la composition du regime. Biochim Biophys Acta 1964; 81:136–149.

28. Gidez LL. Effect of dietary fat on pancreatic lipase level in the rat. J Lipid Res 1973; 14:169–177.

29. Barrowman JA, Mayston PD. The trophic influence of cholecystokinin on the rat pancreas. J Physiol 1974; 238:73–75.

30. Palla JC, Ben Abdeljlil A, Desnuelle P. Action de l'insuline sur la biosynthese de l'amylase et de quelques autres enzymes due pancreas de rat. Biochim Biophys Acta 1968; 158:25–35.

31. Wormsley KG, Goldberg DM. The inter-relationships of the pancreatic enzymes. Gut 1972; 13:398–412.

32. Dagorn JC. Non-parallel enzyme secretion from rat pancreas. In vivo studies. J Physiol 1978; 280:435–448.

33. Dagorn JC, Sahel J, Sarles H. Nonparallel secretion of enzymes in human duodenal juice and pure pancreatic juice collected by endoscopic retrograde catheterization of the papilla. Gastroenterology 1977; 73:42–45.

34. Minaire Y, Descos L, Dacy JP, et al. The inter-relationships of pancreatic enzymes in health and disease under cholecystokinin stimulation. Digestion 1973; 9:8–20.

35. Adelson JW, Rothman SS. Selective pancreatic enzyme secretion due to a new peptide called chymodinin. Science 1974; 183:1087–1089.

36. Malaisse-Lagae F, Ravazzola M, Robberecht P, et al. Exocrine pancreas: evidence for topographic partition of secretory function. Science 1975; 190:795–797.

37. Dagorn JC, Mongeau R. Different action of hormonal stimulation on the biosynthesis of three pancreatic enzymes. Biochim Biophys Acta 1977; 498:76–82.

38. Sommer H, Schrezenmeir J, Kasper H. Protein output dependent non-parallelism in pancreatic secretion of enzymes in man. Gastroenterology 1984; 86:1260.

39. Adelson JW, Miller PE, Thesee G. Pancreatic secretion by "non-parallel exocytosis" resolution of a major controversy. Gastroenterology 1984; 86:1012.

40. Bo-Linn GW, Santa Ana CA, Morawski SG, et al. Starch blockers—their effect on calorie absorption from a high starch meal. N Engl J Med 1982; 307:1413–1416.

41. Carlson GL, Li BUK, Bass P, et al. A bean α-amylase inhibitor formulation (starch blocker) is ineffective in man. Science 1983; 219:393–395.

42. Digno EP, George L, Gores A. Why don't amylase inhibitors cause carbohydrate malabsorption in humans? Gastroenterology 1983; 84:1137.

43. Li BUK. Starch blockers. (Letter.) N Engl J Med 1983; 308:902–903.

44. Svensson J-O, Norback B, Bokey EL, et al. Changing pattern in aetiology of pancreatitis in an urban Swedish area. Br J Surg 1979; 66:159–161.

45. Nyboe Andersen B, Thorsgaard Pedersen N, Scheel J, et al. Incidence of alcoholic chronic pancreatitis in Copenhagen. Scand J Gastroenterol 1982; 17:247–252.

46. Sarles H. An international survey on nutrition and pancreatitis. Digestion 1973; 9:389–403.

47. Gastard J, Lubaud F, Farbost T, et al. Etiology and course of primary chronic pancreatitis in western France. Digestion 1973; 9:416–428.

48. Goebel H, Hotz J. Nutritional aspects of chronic pancreatitis in Germany. Biol Gastroenterol 1975; 8:365.

49. Sarles H, Cros RC, Bidart JM. A multicenter inquiry into the etiology of pancreatic diseases. Digestion 1979; 19:110–125.

50. Pitchumoni GS, Sonnenshein M, Candido FM, et al. Nutrition in the pathogenesis of alcoholic pancreatitis. Am J Clin Nutr 1980; 33:631–636.

51. Voirol M, Infante F, Brahime-Reteno O, et al. Consommation d'alcool, de tabac et de nutriments dans les affections pancreatiques. Schweiz Med Wochenschr 1980; 110:854–855.

52. Yen S, Hsieh CC, MacMahon B. Consumption of alcohol and tobacco and other risk factors for pancreatitis. Am J Epidemiol 1982; 116:407–414.

53. Durbec JP, Bidart JM, Sarles H. Interaction between alcohol and other foodstuffs: epidemiological aspects. Colloques Inserm 1980: 95:33–52.

54. Cameron JL, Zuidema GD, Margolis S. A pathogenesis for alcoholic pancreatitis. Surgery 1975; 77:754–763.

55. Dickson AP, O'Neill J, Imrie CW. Hyperlipidemia, alcohol abuse and acute pancreatitis. Br J Surg 1984; 71:685–688.

56. Haig THB. Experimental pancreatitis intensified by a high fat diet. Surg Gynecol Obstet 1970; 131:914–918.

57. Saharia P, Margolis S, Zuidema GD, et al. Acute pancreatitis with hyperlipaemia: studies with an isolated perfused canine pancreas. Surgery 1977; 82:60–67.

58. Noseworthy J, Colodny AH, Eraklis AJ. Pancreatitis and intravenous fat: an association in patients with inflammatory bowel disease. J Pediatr Surg 1983; 18:269–272.

59. Raasch RH, Hak LJ, Benaim V, et al. Effects of intravenous fat emulsion on experimental acute pancreatitis. JPEN 1983; 7:254–256.

60. Sanfey H, Bulkley BG, Cameron JL. The role of oxygen-derived free radicals in the pathogenesis of acute pancreatitis. Ann Surg 1984; 200:405–413.

61. Kimura T, Zuidema GD, Cameron JL. Experimental pancreatitis: influence of secretory state of the pancreas. Surgery 1980; 88:661–666.

62. Schapiro H, Wruble LD, Britt LG. The possible mechanism of alcohol in the production of acute pancreatitis. Surgery 1966; 60:1108–1111.

63. Geokas MC, Lieber CS, French S, Halsted CH. Ethanol, the liver and the gastrointestinal tract. Ann Intern Med 1981; 95:198–211.

64. Sarles H. Epidemiology and physiopathology of chronic pancreatitis and the role of the pancreatic stone protein. Clin Gastroenterol 1984; 13:895–912.

65. Steer ML, Meldolesi J, Figarella C. Pancreatitis. The role of lysosomes. Dig Dis Sci 1984; 29:934–938.

66. White TT. Pancreatitis. London: Arnold, 1966.

67. Paxton JR, Payne JH. Acute pancreatitis. A statistical review of 307 established cases of acute pancreatitis. Surg Gynecol Obstet 1948; 86:69–75.

68. Shallenbergr PL, Kapp DF. Acute pancreatitis: a clinical review of 72 attacks occurring in 54 patients. Ann Intern Med 1958; 48:1185–1191.

69. Pollock AV. Acute pancreatitis. Analysis of 100 patients. Br Med J 1959; 1:6–14.

70. Foster PD, Ziffren SE. Severe acute pancreatitis. Arch Surg 1962; 85:252–259.

71. Zuidema PJ. Cirrhosis and disseminated calcification of the pancreas in patients with malnutrition. Trop Geogr Med 1959; 11:70–74.

72. Pitchumoni CS. Special problems of tropical pancreatitis. Clin Gastroenterol 1984; 13:941–959.

73. George PK, Banks PS, Pai KN, et al. Exocrine pancreatic function in calcific pancreatitis in India. Gastroenterology 1971; 60:858–863.

74. Vakil BJ. Chronische Pankreatitis in Indien. Leber Magen Darm 1976; 6:276–281.

75. Tandon BN, Banks PA, George PK, et al. Recovery of exocrine pancreatic function in adult protein-calorie malnutrition. Gastroenterology 1970; 58:358–362.

76. Banwell JG, Hutt MRS, Leonard PJ, et al. Exocrine pancreatic disease and the malabsorption syndrome. Gut 1967; 8:388–401.

77. Kotler DP, Levine GM. Reversible gastric and pancreatic hyposecretion after long-term total parenteral nutrition. N Engl J Med 1979; 300:241–242.

78. Nwokolo C, Oli J. Pathogenesis of juvenile tropical pancreatitis syndrome. Lancet 1980; 1:456–458.

79. Koo SI, Turk DE. Effect of zinc deficiency on the ultrastructure of the pancreatic acinar cell and intestinal epithelium in the rat. J Nutr 1977; 107:896–908.

80. Segal I, Lerios M, Grieve T. The emergence of chronic calcific pancreatitis in a developing country. In Gyr KE, Singer MV, Sarles H (eds). Pancreatitis: Concepts and Classification. Amsterdam, Excerpta Medica, 1984: 417–420.

81. Tanimura H, Kato H, Hikasa Y. The role of vitamin E in the etiology and treatment of pancreatitis. Ann NY Acad Sci 1982; 393:214–216.

82. MacMahon B. Risk factors for cancer of the pancreas. Cancer 1982; 50:2676–2680.

83. Durbec JP, Chevillotte G, Bidart JM. Diet, alcohol, tobacco and risk of cancer of the pancreas. A case-control study. Br J Cancer 1983; 47:463–470.

84. Wynder EL. An epidemiological evaluation of the causes of cancer of the pancreas. Cancer Res 1975; 35:2228–2233.

85. Gold EB, Gordis L, Drener MD, et al. Diet and other risk factors for cancer of the pancreas. Cancer 1985; 55:460–467.

86. Roebuck BD, Yager JD, Longnecker DS. Dietary modulation of azaserine-induced pancreatic carcinogenesis in the rat. Cancer Res 1981; 41:888–893.

87. Birt DF, Salmasi S, Pour PM. Enhancement of experimental pancreatic cancer in Syrian golden hamsters by dietary fat. J Natl Cancer Inst 1981; 67:1327–1332.

88. Longnecker DS, Roebuck BD, Kuhlman ET. Enhancement of pancreatic carcinogenesis by a dietary unsaturated fat in rats treated with saline or N-nitroso(2-hydroxypropyl)(2-oxypropyly)amine. J Natl Cancer Inst 1985; 74:219–222.

89. Hirayama T. A large-scale cohort study on the relationship between diet and selected cancers of digestive organs. In Bruce WR, Correa P, Lipkin S, et al. (eds). Banbury Report No. 7. Gastrointestinal Cancer: Endogenous Factors. Cold Spring Harbor, NY, Cold Spring Harbor Laboratory, 1981.

90. Pour PM, Birt DF, Salmasi SZ, et al. Modifying factors in pancreatic carcinogenesis in the hamster model. 1. Effect of protein-free diet fed during the early stages of carcinogenesis. 1983; 70:141–146.

91. Roebuck BD, Yager JD, Longnecker DS, et al. Promotion by unsaturated fat of azaserine-induced pancreatic carcinogenesis in the rat. Cancer Res 1981; 41:3961–3966.

92. Rackis JJ. Physiological properties of soybean trypsin inhibitors and their relationship to pancreatic hypertrophy and growth inhibition of rats. Fed Proc 1965; 24:1488–1493.

93. McGuinness E, Morgan RGH, Wormsley KG. Effects of soybean flour on the pancreas of rats. Environ Health Perspect 1984; 56:205–212.

94. MacMahon B, Yen S, Trichopoulos D, et al. Coffee and cancer of the pancreas. N Engl J Med 1981; 304:630–633.

95. Nomura A, Stemmerman GM, Heilbrun LK. Coffee and pancreatic cancer. Lancet 1981; 2:415.

96. Jick H, Dinan BJ. Coffee and pancreatic cancer. Lancet 1981; 2:92.

97. Goldstein HR. No association between coffee and cancer of the pancreas. N Engl J Med 1982; 306:997.

98. Elinder CG, Millquist K, Floderus-Myrhed B. Swedish studies fail to support the hypothesis on the relationship between coffee and pancreatic cancer. Lakartidningen 1981; 78:3676–3677.

99. Severson RK, Davis S, Polissar L. Smoking, coffee and cancer of the pancreas. Br Med J 1982; 285:214.

100. Wynder EL, Hall NEL, Polansky M. Epidemiology of coffee and pancreatic cancer. Cancer Res 1983; 43:3900–3906.

101. McArdle AH, Echave W, Brown RA, et al. Effect of elemental diet on pancreatic secretion. Am J Surg 1974; 128:690–692.

102. Neviackas JA, Kestein MD. Pancreatic enzyme response with an elemental diet. Surg Gynecol Obstet 1976; 142:71–74.

103. Cassim MM, Allardyce DB. Pancreatic secretion in response to jejunal feeding of elemental diet. Ann Surg 1974; 180:228–231.

104. Stabile BE, Borzatta M, Stubbs RS. Pancreatic secretory responses to intravenous hyperalimentation and intraduodenal elemental and full liquid diets. JPEN 1984; 8:377–380.

105. Kelly GA, Nahrwold DL. Pancreatic secretion in response to an elemental diet and intravenous hyperalimentation. Surg Gynecol Obstet 1976; 143:87–91.

106. Ragins H, Levenson SM, Signer R, et al. Intrajejunal administration of an elemental diet at neutral pH avoids pancreatic stimulation. Am J Surg 1973; 126:606–614.

107. Vidon N, Hecketsweiler P, Butel J, et al. Effect of continuous jejunal perfusion of elemental diet and complex nutritional solutions on pancreatic enzyme secretion in human subjects. Gut 1978; 19:194–198.

108. Keith RG. Effect of a low fat elemental diet on pancreatic secretion during pancreatitis. Surg Gynecol Obstet 1980; 151:337–343.

109. Wolfe BM, Keltner RM, Kaminski DL. The effect of an intraduodenal elemental diet on pancreatic secretion. Surg Gynecol Obstet 1975; 140:241–245.

110. Callegari C, Lami F, Cornia GL, et al. Effect of chemically defined formula diet on pancreatic mass in the rat. JPEN 1985; 9:334–338.

111. Nakajima S, Magee DF. Inhibition of exocrine pancreatitis secretion by glucagon and D-glucose given intravenously. Can J Physiol Pharmacol 1970; 48:299–305.

112. Hamilton RF, Davis WC, Stephenson DV, et al. Effects of parenteral hyperalimentation on upper gastrointestinal tract secretions. Arch Surg 1971; 102:348–352.

113. Towne JB, Hamilton RF, Stephenson DV. Mechanism of hyperalimentation in the suppression of upper gastrointestinal secretions. Am J Surg 1973; 126:714–716.

114. Stabile BE, Debas HT. Intravenous versus intraduodenal amino acids, fats and glucose as stimulants of pancreatic secretion. Surg Forum 1981; 32:224–226.

115. Konturek SJ, Tasler J, Cieszkowski M, et al. Intravenous amino acids and fat stimulate pancreatic secretion. Am J Physiol 1979; 236:E678–E684.

116. Fried GM, Odgen WD, Rhea A, et al. Pancreatic protein secretion and gastrointestinal hormone release in response to parenteral amino acids and lipids in dogs. Surgery 1982; 92:902–905.

117. Adler M, Pieroni PL, Takeshimat T, et al. Effects of parenteral hyperalimentation on pancreatic and biliary secretion. Surg Forum 1975; 26:445–446.

118. Thomas PO, Ross CA. Effect of exclusive parenteral feeding on the closure of a pancreatic fistula. Arch Surg 1948; 57:104–112.

119. Hull HC, Barnes TG. Total intravenous alimentation in the treatment of small bowel fistulas. Ann Surg 1951; 133:644–650.

120. Zajtchuk R, Amato JC, Shoemaker WC. The relationship between blood glucose levels and external pancreatic secretion in man. J Trauma 1969; 9:629–637.

121. Dudrick SJ, Wilmore DW, Steiger E. Spontaneous closure of traumatic pancreatoduodenal fistulas with total intravenous nutrition. J Trauma 1970; 10:542–553.

122. Bivins BA, Bell RM, Rapp RP, et al. Pancreatic exocrine response to parenteral nutrition. JPEN 1984; 8:34–36.

123. DiMagno EP, Go VLW, Summerskill WHJ. Intraluminal and post-operative effects of amino acids on pancreatic enzyme secretion. J Lab Clin Med 1973; 82:241.

124. Edelman K, Valenzuela GE. Effect of intravenous lipid on human pancreatic secretion. Gastroenterology 1983; 85:1063–1066.

125. Grundfest S, Steiger E, Selinkoff MD, et al. Effect of intravenous fat emulsions in patients with pancreatic fistula. JPEN 1980; 4:27–31.

126. DiMagno EP, Go VLW, Summerskill WHJ. Relations between pancreatic enzyme outputs and malabsorption in severe pancreatitic insufficiency. N Engl J Med 1973; 288:813–815.

127. Toskes PP, Dawson W, Curington C, et al. Non-diabetic retinal abnormalities in chronic pancreatitis. N Engl J Med 1979; 300:942–946.

128. Allen RH. Cobalamin (vitamin B$_{12}$) absorption and malabsorption. Dig Dis Sci 1982; 14:17–20.

129. Dutta SK, Bustin MP, Russell RM, et al. Deficiency of fat soluble vitamins in treated patients with pancreatic insufficiency. Ann Intern Med 1982; 97:549–552.

130. D'Souza A, Floch MH. Calcium metabolism in pancreatic disease. Am J Clin Nutr 1973; 26:352–361.

131. Hersh T, Siddigui DA. Magnesium and the pancreas. Am J Clin Nutr 1973; 26:362–366.

132. Aggett DJ, Thorn HT, Dalves JT, et al. Trace element malabsorption in exocrine pancreatic insufficiency. Monogr Paediatr 1979; 10:8–11.

133. Williams RB, Russell RM, Dutta SK, et al. Alcoholic pancreatitis: patients at high risk of acute zinc deficiency. Am J Med 1979; 66:889–893.

134. Sarles H, Sahel J, Staub JL, et al. Chronic pancreatitis. In Howat HT, Sarles H (eds). The exocrine pancreas. London, WB Saunders, 1979: 402–439.

135. Isaksson G, Ihse I. Pain reduction by oral pancreatic enzyme preparation in chronic pancreatitis. Dig Dis Sci 1983; 28:97–102.

136. Grendell JH. Nutrition and absorption in diseases of the pancreas. Clin Gastroenterol 1982; 12:551–562.

137. DiMagno EP, Malagelada JR, Go VLW, et al. Fate of orally ingested enzymes in pancreatic insufficiency. N Engl J Med 1977; 296:1318–1322.

138. DiMagno EP. Controversies in the treatment of exocrine pancreatic insufficiency. Dig Dis Sci 1982; 27:481–484.

139. Ihse I, Lilja P, Lundquist I. Intestinal concentrations of pancreatic enzymes following pancreatic replacement therapy. Scand J Gastroenterol 1980; 15:137–144.

140. Worning H. The effect of enzyme substitution in patients with pancreatic insufficiency. Scand J Gastroenterol 1980; 15:529–533.

141. Valerio D, Whyte EHA, Schlamm HT. Clinical effectiveness of a pancreatic enzyme supplement. JPEN 1981; 5:110–114.

142. Storck G, Petterson G, Edlund Y. A study of autopsies upon 116 patients with acute pancreatitis. Surg Gynecol Obstet 1976; 143:241–245.

143. Voitk A, Brown RA, Echave V, et al. Use of an elemental diet in the treatment of complicated pancreatitis. Am J Surg 1973; 125:223–227.

144. Feller JH, Brown RA, Toussaint GPM, et al. Changing methods in the treatment of severe pancreatitis. Am J Surg 1974; 127:196–201.

145. Blackburn GL, Williams LF, Bistrian BR, et al: New approaches to the management of severe acute pancreatitis. Am J Surg 1976; 131:114–124.

146. Holbling N, Funovics J, Roth E, et al. Amino acid metabolism in acute necrotising pancreatitis. Aspects of parenteral nutrition. In Hollender LF (ed). Controversies in Acute Pancreatitis. Berlin, Springer-Verlag, 1982: 297–301.

147. Ranson JGC. Acute pancreatitis. Curr Probl Surg 1979; 16:1–84.

148. Rose DM, Ranson JHC, Cunningham JN Jr, et al. Patterns of severe pancreatic injury following cardio-pulmonary bypass. Ann Surg 1984; 199:168–172.

149. Mitchell CJ, Playforth MJ, Kelleher J, et al. Functional recovery of the exocrine pancreas after acute pancreatitis. Scand J Gastroenterol 1983; 18:5–8.

150. McMahon MJ, Airey M, Mayer AD. Influence of granular pancreatin upon pancreatic function during convalescence from acute pancreatitis. Br J Surg 1986; 73:496.

151. Evander A, Hederstrom E, Hultberg B, et al. Exocrine pancreatic secretion in acute experimental pancreatitis. Digestion 1982; 24:159–167.

152. Gullo L, Sarles H, Mott CB. Functional investigation of the exocrine pancreas following acute pancreatitis. Rendic Gastroenterol 1972; 4:18–21.

153. Kawaura Y, Sato H, Fukatani G, et al. The therapy of acute pancreatitis through intravenous hyperalimentation with fat emulsion. Proceedings of the Fifth Asian Pacific Congress of Gastroenterology, 1976: 682–695.

154. Durr GHK, Schaefers A, Marosked D, et al. A controlled study of the use of intravenous fat in patients suffering from acute attacks of pancreatitis. Infusionsther Klin Ernahr 1985; 12(3):128–133.

155. Hyde D, Floch MH. The effect of peripheral nutritional support and nitrogen balance in acute pancreatitis. Gastroenterology 1984; 86:1119.

156. Goodgame JT, Fischer JE. Parenteral nutrition in the treatment of acute pancreatitis. Ann Surg 1977; 186:651–658.

157. Mayer AD, McMahon MJ, Bowen M, et al. C-reactive protein: an aid to assessment and monitoring of acute pancreatitis. J Clin Pathol 1984; 37:207–211.

158. Grant JP, James S, Grabowski V, et al. Total parenteral nutrition in pancreatic disease. Ann Surg 1984; 200:627–631.

159. White TT, Heimbach DM. Sequestrectomy and hyperalimentation in the treatment of haemorrhagic pancreatitis. Am J Surg 1976; 132:270–275.

160. Silberman H, Dixon NP, Eisenberg D. The safety and efficacy of a lipid-based system of parenteral nutrition in acute pancreatitis. Am J Gastroenterol 1982; 77:494–497.

22

CYSTIC FIBROSIS

NANCY N. HUANG / DANIEL V. SCHIDLOW / JUDY PALMER
MICHAEL R. BYE / DONNA MULLER

Cystic fibrosis (CF) is the most common lethal genetic disorder in the white population, with an incidence of approximately 1 in 2000 live births. It is inherited as an autosomal recessive trait. The gene frequency is approximately 1 in 20 whites. The incidence of disease is about 1 in 17,000 in the American black population, and approximately 1 in 90,000 among Asians.[1]

Descriptions of the pathological and clinical findings of CF date back to 1857, but the entity was not named *cystic fibrosis* until 1938, by Andersen.[2] In 1944 Farber[3] suggested the term *mucoviscidosis*, since much of the pathology seemed to derive from obstruction of exocrine glands and ducts by an abnormally viscid secretion; but the still unidentified underlying metabolic abnormality affects many areas of the body, and the term most commonly used for the disease is cystic fibrosis.

Clinically, CF is characterized by chronic pulmonary infection (in 99 to 100 per cent of patients), pancreatic insufficiency (in 85 to 90 per cent), elevated sweat electrolyte levels (sweat chloride greater than 60 mEq/L in > 99 per cent), a positive family history (in 30 to 50 per cent), and male sterility (in 99 per cent). The diagnosis of cystic fibrosis is established by the findings of repeatedly positive sweat tests by quantitative pilocarpine iontophoresis[4] and one or two of the other manifestations.

One of the hallmarks of CF is poor weight gain or "failure to thrive" during infancy. Before effective modes of nutritional supplementation and nutritional and pulmonary therapy became available, the overwhelming majority of patients died within the first few years of life.[5–7] Death was usually from progressive pulmonary disease and its complications. Malnutrition and its consequences play an important role in the course of this disease. Since more effective therapy became available, longevity in patients with CF has improved markedly; now more than 30 per cent of patients with CF are adults. The earlier the diagnosis is made, the better opportunity there is[8] to focus attention on the patient's nutritional status during the critical formative years. Early institution of prophylactic therapy may also enable CF caregivers to foster improved nutritional habits in the patient and family.[9] It has been shown that those patients with less pancreatic disease and/or better nutritional states have better pulmonary function than those who are more severely malnourished.[10]

In this presentation we intend to review the pathogenesis and pathophysiology of the nutritional disorders associated with CF, with clinical and therapeutic considerations.

PATHOPHYSIOLOGY AND PATHOGENESIS OF MALNUTRITION IN CYSTIC FIBROSIS

In general, malnutrition is a result of poor nutrient intake, poor nutrient absorption, and/or increased calorie/nutrient expenditure due to chronic pulmonary infection.

Decreased Nutrient Intake

Older medical textbooks and parents of infants and children with CF have often reported voracious appetites prior to the time that the definitive diagnosis was made and therapy begun. More recently however, studies using a 3-day analysis of diet have shown that affected patients actually took in only 80 to 89 per cent of the recommended daily energy intake.[11] When these data are viewed in the light of decreased absorption of whatever nutrients are taken in, with the possibility of higher oxygen consumption because of an increased work of breathing,[12] it can be seen that the effective intake in such patients is quite suboptimal, and that the amounts of calories and nutrients available for growth and development are limited.

The reasons for the decreased intake are unclear, but may in part be related to the cramping, bloating, and diarrhea that may accompany intake of food. In addition, patients with elevated respiratory rates and chronic cough do not have good appetites for food.

Maldigestion and Malabsorption

As mentioned above, the combination of chronic pulmonary infection and decreased absorption of nutrients accounts for most of the nutritional disorders in CF. The major cause of the decrease in absorption is pancreatic exocrine insufficiency; however, pathology throughout the digestive system increases the degree of malabsorption. A reasonable approach to the pathophysiology of maldigestion and malabsorption in CF is to see how each component part of the gastrointestinal tract contributes to this malnutrition.

MOUTH

In the absence of any other disorders, CF patients have normal sucking, chewing, and swallowing functions. Significant nasal obstruction, as can occur with large nasal polyps[13] or sinusitis,[14] may result in decreased ability to take in food and to spend the proper time chewing. Older patients may have tooth discoloration, but no increased incidence of dental abnormalities has been described. Salivary glands have been shown to have their ducts plugged with eosinophilic mucus, but salivary amylase levels have been found to be normal or elevated.[15] Although this may be a compensation for decreased pancreatic amylase secretion, there was no correlation between salivary amylase levels and the presence or degree of clinical pancreatic insufficiency; the elevated levels may be a result of heightened autonomic function. Lingual gland lipase activity has also been shown to be normal to slightly elevated.[16]

ESOPHAGUS

No evidence for abnormal motility in the esophagus has been described. There are, however, several recent reports of an increased incidence of gastroesophageal reflux (GER) in patients[17] with CF. The vomiting that accompanies the GER decreases the nutrients available for absorption. Pain associated with reflux esophagitis may decrease a patient's food intake, and the increased pulmonary disease that accompanies the GER may elevate the patient's basal caloric expenditure, making weight gain more difficult. In some infants with CF and GER significant degrees of respiratory difficulty have shown marked improvement after surgical repair of the GER.

STOMACH

The gastric emptying time is normal in CF and intragastric lipolysis is increased, especially with regard to the production of triglycerides and diglycerides.[18] No other gastric abnormalities have been described. Gastric acid secretion seems normal, and no abnormalities have been noted in motility or hormone secretion.

PANCREAS

Approximately 85 to 90 per cent of CF patients have clinical and laboratory evidence of exocrine pancreatic insufficiency.[19,20] Since it is estimated that 90 per cent of the pancreatic function must be lost before there is evidence of pancreatic insufficiency, the incidence of pancreatic involvement (including subclinical involvement) may actually be higher.

The earliest pathological findings are obstruction of the acinar and duct lumens by intraluminal eosinophilic concretions.[21] Moreover, recent studies of autopsy findings in patients with minimal pancreatic disease have shown reduced numbers of acini.[22] Another early finding is distention of the acini and ductules, presumably as a result of the inspissated intraluminal secretions. As this distention continues, there may be disruption, with release of proteolytic enzymes into the parenchyma. This release may be followed by parenchymal destruction and an inflammatory response, which lead eventually to fibrosis. The changes are initially focal and later diffuse. The islets of Langerhans tend to be spared until late in the course of CF.

The pathological changes described above lead to insufficient pancreatic secretion in the duodenum. The lack of bicarbonate secretion results in an overly acidic bolus of food in the duodenum and intestines.[23] The lack of such pancreatic enzymes as amylase, lipase, trypsin, and chymotrypsin results in significant maldigestion.[24]

The digestion of fats is most affected by pancreatic insufficiency because lipolysis of triglycerides requires pancreatic lipase, bile salts, and a relatively alkaline pH (greater than 6), all of which are deficient in 90 per cent of patients with CF. In untreated patients up to 80 per cent of ingested fat will be excreted in the stool.[19] This steatorrhea results in greasy, foul-smelling stools, a common manifestation of CF. The presence of maldigested fat in the intestine can also predispose to bloating, excessive flatus, crampy abdominal pain, and intermittent episodes of partial bowel obstruction; the last is known as the *distal intestinal obstruction syndrome*, or *meconium ileus equivalent*.[25] Other complications of the inspissation of bowel contents can include intussusception or volvulus.[26,27] The degree of fat absorption varies considerably. The pancreatic insufficiency is at least partly compensated by increased lipolysis in the stomach by lingual lipase.[16]

Protein digestion is also affected in CF. The lack of pancreatic trypsin and chymotrypsin impairs the digestion of protein into peptides and amino acids. Patients with CF excrete 2 to 3 times as much ingested nitrogen as do normal subjects. Over time, this may lead to hypoproteinemia and hypoalbuminemia significant enough to cause peripheral edema and anemia.[22,28]

Pancreatic amylase is usually deficient in patients with CF, but carbohydrate digestion and absorption are minimally impaired, probably owing to the normal or increased salivary amylase, to some hydrolysis in the stomach, and to a lesser extent to the enzymes in the brush border of the intestines.

Along with the fat maldigestion and malabsorption there is poor absorption of the fat-soluble vitamins A, D, E, and K.[29–33] Clinical findings due to lack of vitamin A (mucosal abnormalities, visual impairment, pseudotumor cerebri) and vitamin K (hemorrhage from hypoprothrombinemia) are more commonly seen, usually in the first year of life. Vitamin E–deficient hemolytic anemia is rarely seen in CF, but intermittent muscle cramps have been ascribed to a lack of vitamin E. In the absence of significant liver or renal disease, overt vitamin D–deficient rickets is very rare in CF, but recent studies have found decreased blood levels of 25-hydroxy vitamin D levels, and decreased bone mineralization.[34–36]

With the exception of vitamin B_{12},[37] the water-soluble vitamins are well absorbed. The absorption of vitamin B_{12} depends on its linkage to the intrinsic factor. In the absence of pancreatic proteases there may be proteins in the intestinal lumen that will competitively inhibit this linkage and decrease the patient's ability to absorb the vitamin.

It has been shown that CF patients have deficiencies in absorption of essential fatty acids.[38–40] This has been documented by the finding of low serum and tissue levels of linoleic acid. Low levels of linoleic acid will result in altered prostaglandin synthesis, and this has been postulated to worsen the pulmonary disease in CF. One study found that patients with low serum linoleic acid levels had elevated prostaglandin $F_{2\alpha}$,[39,40] which is a potent bronchoconstrictor and causes marked pulmonary vasoconstriction. With supplementation of the essential fatty acids, the prostaglandin $F_{2\alpha}$ levels returned to normal. Although data on pulmonary functions or pulmonary arterial pressures were not reported, there is a suggestion that such prostaglandin abnormalities may lead to increased pulmonary disease and/or cor pulmonale.

With progressive fibrosis of the exocrine pancreas, the endocrine pancreas may become involved as well. When patients with CF develop diabetes mellitus,[41] they have decreased glucose uptake at the cellular level, and poorer weight gain because of the calories wasted in the urine.

LIVER

The liver is involved with steatosis in 30 per cent of patients with CF, with focal biliary cirrhosis in 20 per cent of patients, and with multilobular cirrhosis with portal hypertension in 2 to 5 per cent of patients.[42,43] In the few patients with advanced cirrhosis of the liver, hepatic dysfunction may contribute to hypoproteinemia and edema, as well as to hypoprothrombinemia. In infants, before a diagnosis is made, fatty infiltration of the liver causing hepatomegaly is sometimes observed[44]; this is reversible after treatment is instituted.

DUODENUM

Typical roentgenographic findings in the duodenum have been described, but it has been difficult to correlate these with biopsy findings. The roentgenographic findings include thickened mucosal folds, mucosal smudging, and nodular filling defects.[45] It is possible that these findings are a result of contraction of smooth muscle and epithelial thickening in response to gastric acids unopposed by pancreatic bicarbonate secretion. The same mechanism may produce a higher incidence of duodenal ulcers in patients with CF.[46]

SMALL INTESTINE

The small intestine has typical pathological findings in CF, with increased mucus, and inspissated secretions in the intestinal glands and in the lumen. Although the architecture of the villi and microvilli is usually normal, there may be deficiencies in enzyme release, increasing the maldigestion of proteins and fats. In addition, the increased intestinal mucus may serve as a mechanical barrier to the absorption of nutrients. A selective abnormality in the mucosal transport systems has also been observed in CF.[47] The incidence of lactase deficiency is probably no higher in the CF population than in the general population. The pathological findings are typical enough so that the experienced pathologist can make a diagnosis of CF on the basis of removed specimens (e.g., from the appendix).[48] The diagnosis has on occasion been made in this way before the clinical diagnosis was made.

The diagnosis of meconium ileus (which produces a pattern of small bowel obstruction in the newborn period) is more closely associated with the pathological changes in small bowel than with those of exocrine pancreatic insufficiency.[49,50] Patients with meconium ileus often require surgery; they used to have a prolonged recuperative phase, but modern surgical technique has greatly shortened the postoperative course. Patients with meconium ileus with a diagnosis of CF confirmed must have an evaluation of their pancreatic function. They should not be automatically assumed to have pancreatic insufficiency.

The findings in the small bowel lead not only to maldigestion and probably to meconium ileus, but also to other gastrointestinal complications. The accumulated secretions and mucus, mixed with unabsorbed food, cause crampy abdominal pain, bloating, the distal intestinal obstruction syndrome, intussusception, and volvulus.

LARGE INTESTINE

Rectal biopsies in CF patients have shown dilated crypts but normal intracellular mucus and normal goblet cell numbers. Other findings have included accumulation of lipid droplets in absorptive cells. Neutra and Trier[51] felt that these droplets were more relative to altered metabolism of the absorptive cells and/or their cell membranes than to deposition of nonabsorbed fats from above.

Increased Nutrient Utilization

The third very important cause for poor weight gain or weight loss is increased substrate utilization.

Adeniyi-Jones et al.[52] showed that their CF population had higher basal energy requirements, measured both as basal metabolic rate and basal oxygen consumption. Cropp et al.[53] showed that the increase in basal oxygen consumption varied inversely with the severity of the pulmonary disease. Cropp et al.[54] found that with more severe pulmonary disease (FEV_1 <50 per cent of predicted value) the energy cost of breathing is increased 3.8-fold. Thus, any conditions that increase respiration in such patients (fever, pulmonary infection, exercise, heat) will result in higher energy expenditures than would be produced in normal subjects. An acute exacerbation in pulmonary disease in CF will increase oxygen consumption, in addition to causing a decrease in appetite.

In summary, patients with CF suffer from malnutrition for a variety of reasons. They take in less calories than needed. They absorb foodstuffs poorly. Finally, they have higher energy requirements than expected, especially with progression of their pulmonary disease. This latter factor underscores the importance of the first two factors, and reflects the interrelationship of all of the pathophysiological mechanisms in the production of malnutrition in patients with CF.

ASSESSMENT OF NUTRITION

Assessment of the nutritional status of each patient with CF is extremely important and can be achieved by use of various methods described below:

Medical History

In the patient with CF a complete history will reveal weight loss or poor weight gain in spite of a "voracious appetite" as reported by parents. We routinely obtain a dietary history by asking the mother to recall the items of food eaten by the child within the last 24 hours. A method of better accuracy is the recording of 3-day dietary intake. The child's food intake is also compared with that of an age-matched sibling or that of a playmate. This method is subject to errors but is the easiest way to assess dietary intake. Inquiry must be made regarding bowel movements. Most patients with CF have frequent, bulky, foul-smelling, and greasy bowel movements indicative of excessive fecal loss of nutrients. Others have an additional history of repeated vomiting, often due to severe coughing spells or to the presence of gastroesophageal reflux. Patients with persistent pulmonary infection may run a low-grade fever, with tachypnea and increases in work of breathing and in energy consumption. The presence of infection is often associated with anorexia, which precipitates rapid weight loss during acute exacerbations. Such patients require both control of infection and increase of nutrient intake by oral or other route.

Physical Examination

Special attention should be given to the patient's general condition, behavior, skin, hair, nails, subcutaneous tissue, eyes, upper respiratory tract, musculoskeletal system, lower respiratory system, cardiovascular system, abdominal organs, and reproductive system. Children with mild pulmonary involvement and good nutritional status are generally happy and cooperative; the malnourished tend to be irritable and noncompliant. Skin must be examined for edema, rashes, dryness, and possible follicular hyperkeratosis. The hair of malnourished children lacks normal luster and is usually thin and sparse, which is not a common finding in adequately nourished patients with CF. Fingers must be inspected for clubbing, which is indicative of a generalized pulmonary involvement and is found in most patients with CF. Nail changes in the form of koilonychia and brittleness are extremely rare. Untreated patients and treated patients with advanced pulmonary involvement are often thin and lack subcutaneous fat tissue, with loose skin folds and increase of wrinkles (Fig. 22–1).

Pale conjunctiva is an important sign of anemia. We have not encountered such overt signs of vitamin A deficiency as Bitot spots or conjunctival or corneal xerosis.[55] Bulging of the fontanelle[56] is not uncommon in newly diagnosed infants with CF. The oral cavity must be carefully inspected to detect signs of nutrition deficiency. Pallor of lips and mucous membrane is associated with anemia. The lips may be dry and chapped, with excoriations at the angles of the mouth indicative of riboflavin deficiency. Cheilosis is a common finding in patients receiving long-term administration of antibiotic therapy, especially with chloramphenicol. Angular fissures may extend into buccal mucosa. The tongue is often red and smooth or has patchy areas of smoothness alternating with patchy thick white coating. Changes in gums are not striking in our experience. The incidence of dental caries is not different from that in normal children. Most of the older patients who have taken tetracycline at an early age have pigmentation of teeth, and some have abnormal enamel.

Poor muscle strength, kyphoscoliosis, and barrel chest deformity are common in older patients and especially in patients with advanced pulmonary involvement. Coughing, tachypnea, and dyspnea, with retraction of the chest wall and abnormal chest physical findings, are characteristic of pulmonary infection, which calls for a course of intensive therapy. Such patients with advanced disease may develop tachycardia with accentuation of the pulmonic component of the second sound at the base of the heart. Roentgenologic evidence of an enlarged heart, along with other signs of right heart failure, is sometimes found in very sick patients.

Hepatosplenomegaly signifies the development of biliary cirrhosis, which occurs in about 2 per cent of patients with CF. Tenderness in the right upper quadrant of the abdomen calls for evaluation for the

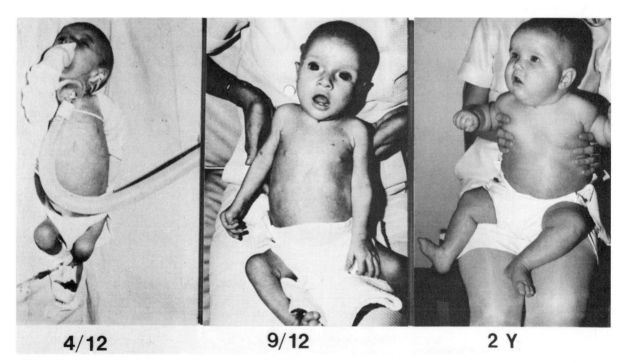

4/12   **9/12**   **2 Y**

FIGURE 22–1. BF was admitted at 4 months of age in respiratory failure, with a history of cough, tachypnea, and failure to thrive since 4 weeks of age. Diagnosis of cystic fibrosis was made on finding sweat chloride of 105 mEq/L and undetectable enzyme levels in duodenal secretion. Birth weight, 6 lb 14 oz; weight at 4 months of age, 6 lb 8 oz; weight at 9 months, 18 lb; weight at 2 years, 27 lb (50th percentile).

presence of gallstones, which are not uncommon in older patients. A palpable fecal mass in the right lower quadrant and multiple fecal masses in the left lower abdomen are common manifestations of meconium ileus equivalent. Prolapse of the rectum has the incidence of 20 to 30 per cent in infants and young children.[57] It is attributed to multiple factors, including excessive cough, bulky bowel movements, and lack of perirectal fat tissue.

Examination of the reproductive system often shows delayed onset of puberty, which is related to the severity of pulmonary involvement and to the state of nutrition. Menarche may be delayed for 3 to 4 years,[58] and menstruation is often irregular, with frequent missed periods.

Anthropometric Measurements

HEIGHT AND WEIGHT

Measurement of weight and height is an important part of the assessment of nutritional status, and is the simplest and most practical method of monitoring the clinical progress of the patient. Serial measurements of skinfold thickness and midarm circumference give additional information about total fat and muscle mass and are valuable in monitoring the course of CF. Two decades ago, Sproul and Huang[59] reported the growth patterns of 50 children with CF from infancy to adolescence. They found that the 50th percentile among patients with CF was equivalent to the 3rd to 10th percentile of a comparable normal group. The deficit in weight and height became very marked in preadolescence, with absence of the preadolescent growth spurt. The growth deficiency for height and weight correlated significantly with the severity of pulmonary involvement, without demonstrable relationship with the degree of pancreatic insufficiency. Huang et al.[60] reported improvement in the weight and height measurements of infants and children followed in the period of 1962 to 1967 over those of patients reported earlier. Berry et al.[61] in 1975 reported growth patterns in her patients with CF to be similar to those found earlier by Sproul and Huang. In the above two reports the numbers of adolescents studied were very small.

In 1979 di Sant'Agnese and Davis[62] reviewed 75 cases of adults with CF ranging in age from 18 to 47 years, with 7 patients over 30 years of age. Their data for height and weight showed that some patients with CF, and particularly males, were quite tall. The heights of 60 per cent of the men and 83 per cent of the women were below the 50th percentile; only 7 per cent of the men and women had heights below the 3rd percentile. Five patients in this series were overweight; all of these patients had mild pulmonary disease, and all had pancreatic insufficiency.

In 1987 Huang et al.[63] reported 142 patients with cystic fibrosis who had survived to age 18 years and beyond. They found low clinical scores, low weight percentile, and *Pseudomonas cepacia* colonization of the lower respiratory tract at the age of 18 years to indicate a poor prognosis. The graphic presentations of the height and weight data on 68 males and 54 females are shown in Figure 22–2. The median values for the height of males and females at each age ranged from close to the 10th percentile to the 25th percentile. The median weights for females at each age ranged from just above the 5th percentile to close to the 25th percentile, while those for males ranged from below the 5th percentile to the 10th percentile.

MIDARM CIRCUMFERENCE AND TRICEPS SKINFOLD MEASUREMENTS

Since these measurements may not be carried out routinely in CF clinics, the technical aspect is described below.

The mass of the upper arm is composed primarily of bone, muscle, and fat. Since bone mass is relatively constant, the simultaneous measurements of midarm circumference and triceps skinfold thickness provide a means of evaluating the relative proportions of muscle and fat respectively. Measured values may be used for serial assessment or compared with tables of normal values for children.[64] Estimates of total body fat and muscle derived from these measurements correlate well with those made by other methods.

Midarm circumference is measured on the right arm with a ¼-inch steel tape. The arm should hang loosely at the side of the standing subject. The midpoint of the upper arm is determined by holding the end of the tape at the acromion process, allowing the weighted end of the tape to hang freely over the side of the arm. The midpoint between the acromion process and olecranon process is marked lightly on the skin. For infants, the midpoint is approximated. The tape is then wrapped gently around the arm at the midpoint, with care taken neither to compress the tissues nor to leave gaps between tape and skin. Each measurement should be made two or three times and mean value reported.

The triceps skinfold thickness is measured at the midpoint of the right upper arm with the arm in relaxed position. The examiner stands behind the subject and uses thumb and forefinger of the left hand (thumb medial to skin fold) to grasp a fold of skin and subcutaneous tissue. One must be careful not to include muscle in the fold; asking the subject to flex the elbow while holding the skin fold will aid in making sure this is not the case. While the examiner holds the fold, calipers held in the horizontal plane are applied to the fold just below the examiner's fingers. To ensure a uniform degree of tissue compression with each measurement, the examiner

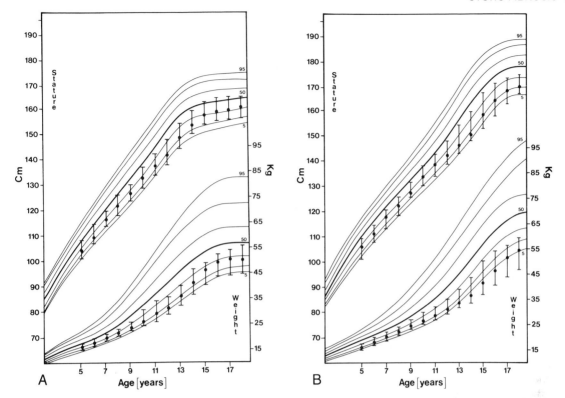

FIGURE 22–2. Height and weight graphs of 68 males (A) and 54 females (B) with cystic fibrosis who lived to age 18 years. Patients entered the sample at any age between 5 and 18 years. Bars show 25th percentile, median, and 75th percentile. (Unpublished data from Cystic Fibrosis Center, St. Christopher's Hospital for Children, Philadelphia, PA.)

should count to three before reading the dial. The fold should be released and regrasped for the next measurement.

Figure 22–3 illustrates the techniques used for measurement of midarm circumference and of triceps skinfold thickness.

We have obtained measurements of triceps skinfold thickness and midarm circumference on 50 young adult patients with CF (24 women and 26 men). These patients were randomly selected from our clinic population and were all in stable clinical condition at the time of assessment. The results of these measurements are given in Table 22–1.

Our results showed that these measurements varied widely in both males and females, with the majority being lower than 100 per cent of mean for age for both triceps skinfold thickness and midarm circumference. The median percentage of mean for age is lower in females than in males, and more female measurements fall below 100 per cent of mean for age than do measurements for males. The differences between sexes do not reach statistical significance (p > 0.05). Serial measurements of these indices are useful in following of the courses of individual patients with CF.

Laboratory Assessment

In CF centers routine laboratory assessment of nutrition consists of determinations of fecal fat content, serum albumin, triglycerides, cholesterol, and iron and a complete blood count, including differential white cell count. Measurements have been reported of all nutritional components, including essential fatty acid concentrations, nitrogen balance, vitamin levels, and trace metals.

LIPIDS

Quantitative analysis of a 3-day collection of feces for fat content is a routine test in most CF centers. It is a satisfactory test for assessment of fecal loss of nutrients and for evaluation of pancreatic function. In order to obtain valid results the patient must ingest a high-fat diet, containing at least 100 g of fat in 24 hours. Our results, as well as that of others, have shown marked variations in the severity of steatorrhea among individual patients. Fecal fat loss ranges from 5 to 6 per cent of that ingested to 75 per cent, with mean stool fat loss of close to 40 per cent (this compares with the less than 5 per cent found in normal persons).[19,20]

Kuo et al.[65] compared the means and ranges of serum lipid levels of 20 children with CF with those of 20 aged-matched control subjects. The ranges are large for all the serum lipid fractions in both groups of subjects, but the mean value of each lipid fraction from children with CF was lower than the respective value in the controls. The results are tabulated in Table 22–2. Huang et al. reviewed serum cholesterol levels of 96 young adults with cystic fibrosis at a mean age of 21.5 years. The results showed mean serum

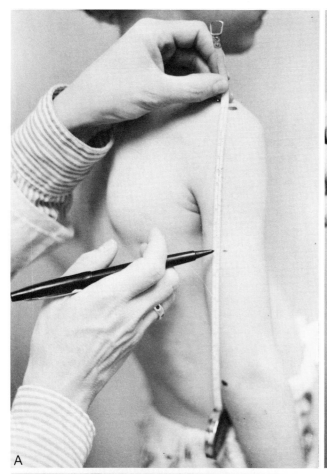

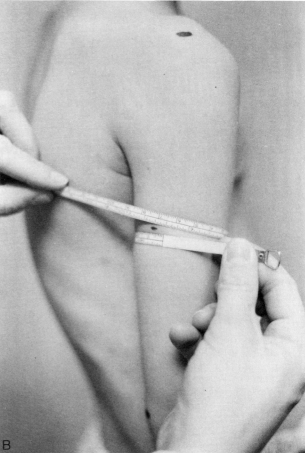

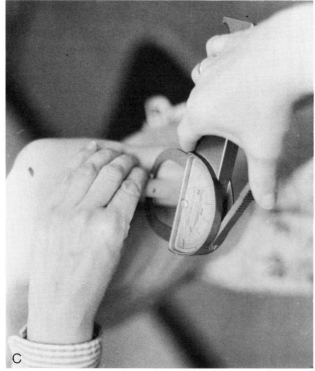

FIGURE 22–3. Technique used for measurement of mid-arm circumference and triceps skinfold thickness. A, Determination of the midpoint of the upper arm. B, Measurement of midarm circumference. C, Measurement of triceps skinfold thickness. (Refer to text for details.)

TABLE 22–1. Measurements of Triceps Skinfold Thickness and Midarm Circumference in 50 Adolescents and Young Adults with Cystic Fibrosis

Subjects			Triceps Skinfold Thickness (As % of Mean for Age)		Midarm Circumference (As % of Mean for Age)	
No.	Sex	Age (Yr)	Range	Median	Range	Median
24	F	10–24	50–125	82	60–115	80
26	M	9.7–30	60–110	90	40–120	85

cholesterol level of 120.4 ± 33.9 mg/dl (range 66–293; control 163 ± 24–40) (unpublished data).

Serum chylomicron composition was studied by Kuo et al.[65] The results showed that children with CF showed higher concentrations of palmitoleic acid (16:1) and oleic acid (18:1) and lower concentrations of palmitic (16:0), stearic (18:0), and linoleic (18:2) acids than are found in normal children. These differences in serum chylomicron composition between the two groups of children are in agreement with the findings of Chase and Dupont,[66] who measured plasma and red blood cell linoleic acid levels in patients with CF and found values 2 standard deviations below those of normal subjects in more than half of their patients with CF. Essential fatty acid deficiency may lead to an increase in prostaglandin $F_{2\alpha}$, which can cause bronchoconstriction and possible aggravation of chronic pulmonary disease in patients with CF. The fatty acid composition of plasma and red blood cells in CF without pancreatic insufficiency is the same as that of normal persons. Fatty acid abnormalities, therefore, cannot be responsible for the pathophysiology of the clinical manifestations of CF. We have not found essential fatty acid (EFA) deficiency to be associated with such classic clinical abnormalities as dry, scaly skin progressing to exofoliative dermatitis. Others, however, have observed EFA deficiency syndrome in infants with desquamative skin lesions, diarrhea, and weight loss. The diagnosis of EFA deficiency is established by determining fasting plasma linoleic acid levels using gas chromatography.

BILE

Roy et al. studied biliary composition in patients with CF.[68,69] The fasting bile from patients with CF contains a high molar percentage of cholesterol. It provides a physicochemical explanation of the increased incidence of gallstones associated with CF. Patients who have CF with pancreatic insufficiency and receive no pancreatic enzyme supplementation excrete large amounts of bile acids in their stools. The bile acid pool is, therefore, decreased in the duodenum; this adversely affects micelle formation, the essential function of bile acids in fat digestion. Pancreatic enzyme supplementation has an important added role in maintaining normal biliary composition and preventing gallstones.

PROTEIN

In spite of the fact that pancreatic insufficiency involves lack of trypsin, chymotrypsin, and carboxypeptidases for hydrolysis of protein and peptides, it is rare to find low serum protein levels in patients so long as pancreatic enzyme is given.

We found serum albumin concentrations of 19 infants and young children (0.4 to 4.5 years) with CF who were receiving pancreatic enzyme supplement and an adequate diet to have a mean value of 4.4 g/dl (range 4.0 to 4.9) and the mean serum albumin levels of 96 young adults with cystic fibrosis at a mean age of 21.5 years to be 4.1 gm/dl (range 2.7–5.1, control 3.5–5.0). Three patients with low serum albumin levels all had cirrhosis of liver (unpublished data).

Fleisher et al.[70] reviewed case reports of 22 young infants with CF whose first major recognized problem was hypoproteinemia and edema at less than 6 months of age. They added 4 cases from the Philadelphia area. Most of those infants had been fed with soybean formula[71] and some human milk. Anemia was a frequent finding in these infants. Their total serum protein levels ranged from 1.9 to 4.9 g/dl, serum albumin from 0.8 to 3.3 g/dl, and hemoglobin concentration from 7.1 to 9.1 g/dl. Hypoproteinemia in such cases is attributed to the poor qual-

TABLE 22–2. Plasma Lipid Levels of Children with CF Compared with Those of Controls

	No. of Subjects	Plasma Lipids (mg/dl)		
		Cholesterol	Phospholipid	Triglyceride
Controls without steatorrhea	12	150* (118–179)†	191 (115–255)	81 (41–126)
Cystic fibrosis patients on pancreatic enzyme supplementation	15	115 (59–156)	152 (90–225)	63 (37–116)

*Mean
†Range

ity of protein in soybean milk and/or the low quantity of protein in human milk. A high mortality rate was reported in the early cases. Institution of cow's milk feeding with pancreatic enzyme supplements induced prompt improvement in serum albumin levels with disappearance of edema and anemia. Metabolic balance studies in 5 infants with CF receiving soybean formula showed negative nitrogen balances, whereas nitrogen retention was significantly higher in infants fed a cow's milk formula.

The evaluation of protein nutrition in children with CF followed in our center consists of periodic dietary evaluation and measurements of total serum protein and albumin levels

Lapey et al.[20] studied fecal nitrogen excretion in 20 patients with CF ranging from 12 to 17 years of age. Fecal nitrogen averaged 21 per cent of intake, ranging from 11 to 50.9 per cent (Lapey's own range of normal values is 7.1 ± 2.9 per cent). Fecal nitrogen excretion showed a significant but not dramatic decrease with pancreatic enzyme supplement.

CARBOHYDRATE

In spite of the lack of pancreatic amylase, carbohydrate metabolism is not affected in CF. Antonowicz et al.[78] found a significant decrease in lactase level of small intestinal mucosal biopsies in 7 out of 21 patients. In these patients oral lactose tolerance tests showed flat curves. Five of the 7 patients with lactase deficiency could tolerate some intake of lactose, whereas 2 others could not.

Diabetes mellitus (DM)[79,80] and glucose intolerance are relatively common among patients with CF. Various reports have estimated the incidence of DM among CF patients to be from 1 to 2 per cent in childhood to as high as 14 per cent in young adults.[63] Glucose intolerance without DM has been reported in 17 to 63 per cent of CF patients evaluated.[41,81–83] Patients with CF have also been shown to have a delayed and diminished insulin response to a glucose load, and to have abnormally low serum levels of glucagon.[83,84] DM in patients with CF is further characterized by the less frequent occurrence of ketoacidosis,[85,86] the older age of onset (typically older child or adolescent), and lower insulin requirements than are seen in juvenile diabetics.[87]

Anatomical abnormalities with progressive "strangulation" of islet tissue by the pancreatic fibrosis has been suggested as a mechanism of the glucose intolerance.[41] The relative mildness of the carbohydrate intolerance may be explained in part by enhanced peripheral tissue sensitivity to insulin,[83] owing possibly to increased numbers and enhanced sensitivity of insulin receptors.[88]

The onset of DM in the patient with CF may be gradual or sudden. Hyperglycemia after meals or hypoglycemia 3 to 5 hours after eating may be the initial manifestation. Occasionally, hyperglycemia may develop rather suddenly during an acute exacerbation of respiratory disease. Diabetes mellitus should be suspected in the patient with CF who has unexplained acute weight loss.

VITAMINS

Pancreatic insufficiency leads to malabsorption of fat and fat-soluble vitamins, principally vitamins A, D, E, and K. If untreated, vitamin deficiency syndromes may develop.

Vitamin A. It is a routine practice to give double doses of a multiple vitamin preparation to all patients with CF, and to give pancreatic enzyme supplementation to those with pancreatic insufficiency. Treated patients rarely show clinical manifestations of vitamin A deficiency. Littlewood et al.[32] studied serum carotene, vitamin A, and retinol-binding protein of patients with CF receiving pancreatic enzyme supplementation and the usual double dose of multiple vitamin preparations. Their results showed low carotene levels in 27 of 28 patients studied. In spite of the administration of 4000 IU of vitamin A (contained in double dose of multiple vitamins), the authors found 13 of the 30 patients studied (43 per cent) to have serum vitamin A levels below the range of control children without gastrointestinal or pancreatic disorders. Eighteen of 27 CF patients also had significantly low levels of retinol-binding protein. There was a significant correlation between serum vitamin A and retinol-binding protein. Both of these factors varied with the clinical status of the patients. On the other hand, Hubbard et al.[34] found normal serum vitamin A levels in 17 treated patients with CF with pancreatic insufficiency. Vitamin A is essential for prevention of night blindness and maintains the structure and biochemical integrity of epithelial cells and may play a role in the synthesis of glucocorticoids and act as a precursor of a nonhormonal growth-promoting factor. Serum vitamin A levels should be periodically monitored.

Vitamin D. Clinical evidence of rickets in patients with CF is very rare. Recently Hahn et al.[33] found that in spite of standard multivitamin supplements plus pancreatic enzyme replacement, 21 adolescents and young adults had a 36 per cent reduction in serum 25-hydroxyvitamin D concentration and a 14 per cent decrease in bone mass as measured by the photon absorption technique. Hubbard et al.[34] studied 17 patients with CF with pancreatic insufficiency and 2 patients with CF with normal pancreatic activity. Their results showed that the majority of the patients with CF with pancreatic insufficiency receiving pancreatic enzyme supplementation had serum concentrations of 25-hydroxyvitamin D within the normal range. One patient had a higher than normal level of 25-OH-D, and 3 had slightly lower than normal levels. All 17 CF patients with pancreatic insufficiency had serum vitamin A levels within the normal range. The authors concluded that CF patients receiving supplements of pancreatic enzyme and vitamin D can maintain normal levels of vitamin D through intestinal absorption and endogenous production. It is important to monitor serum vitamin D activity of individual patients in order to detect subclinical deficiency states, because additional vitamin D supplementation may be necessary in certain patients.

With the administration of vitamin D in multiple vitamin preparations plus pancreatic enzyme supplements and a diet rich in dairy products, we have not found abnormal levels of calcium and phosphorus in our patients with CF.

Vitamin E. Most of the patients with CF who have pancreatic insufficiency have very low serum tocopherol levels.[89–91] Some complain of leg cramps, which can be promptly relieved by vitamin E supplementation. Huang et al.[30] determined serum tocopherol by the method of Quaife et el.[92] on (1) 16 patients with CF who had frequent leg cramps, (2) 19 who had pancreatic insufficiency without leg cramps, and (3) 18 age-matched control subjects. Muscle biopsy of one patient with severe leg cramps failed to show the muscle necrosis reported by Oppenheiner.[31] The mean serum tocopherol of group (1) was found to be 0.19 mg/dl ± 0.10, that of group (2) 0.36 mg/dl ± 0.21, and that of group (3) 0.75 mg/dl ± 0.26. The differences between groups 1 and 2, 1 and 3, and 2 and 3 were significant on statistical analysis. The range of levels in the normal control group (3) was 0.52 to 1.53 mg/dl. We also administered a vitamin E loading test to 19 patients with CF with pancreatic insufficiency (PI) without enzyme supplementation, and to the same 19 patients while they were receiving pancreatic enzyme supplementation, as well as to 2 patients with CF without PI and to 8 control subjects without digestive problems. Serum tocopherol levels were measured before and 4, 8, 24, and 48 hours after oral administration of a loading dose of 10 mg/kg of alpha-tocopherol. Results are given in Table 22–3 and showed increases of serum tocopherol levels up to 0.50 mg/dl in patients with CF without pancreatic enzyme administration, and up to 0.86 ± 0.58 at 4 hr and to 1.03 ± 0.52 at 8 hr, with enzyme supplementation. The serum to-

copherol levels of CF patients without PI and those of control subjects were not notably different before or after the loading dose. We conclude that a daily dose of Aquasol E of 10 mg/kg is adequate to correct vitamin E deficiency in patients with CF who have PI. The amount of vitamin E present in the usual multiple vitamin preparations is inadequate to achieve normal serum tocopherol levels in children with CF with PI.

Vitamin E is a strong antioxidant, and vitamin E deficiency is found to cause hemolytic anemia and edema in premature infants.[93] The anemia that we often see in untreated infants with CF is frequently associated with hypoproteinemia. Whether increased hemolysis secondary to vitamin E deficiency also contributes to the development of anemia requires further investigation.

Vitamin E is believed to protect polyunsaturated fatty acids from oxidation.[29] The vitamin E requirement may, therefore, be higher with increased intakes of essential fatty acids. Vitamin E also plays a role in controlling the rate of prostaglandin synthesis.[66] Prostaglandin $F_{2\alpha}$ levels in blood are elevated in children with vitamin E deficiency; the levels may be lowered with vitamin E supplementation.

Vitamin E has been demonstrated to have multiple effects in laboratory animals, such as enhancement of the humoral immune responses to infections. Whether vitamin E deficiency is of any importance to the pulmonary involvement of patients with CF requires further study. In any case, CF patients with below-normal serum tocopherol levels should receive vitamin E supplementation.

Vitamin K. Infants with undiagnosed CF occasionally have massive hemorrhage from rectum or from an injection site as the first sign leading to the diagnosis of CF. After diagnosis, infants who do not receive vitamin K in addition to multivitamin therapy may also bleed as a result of vitamin K deficiency. In older children with cirrhosis of the liver, with pulmonary hemorrhage, or with prolonged antibiotic therapy, prothrombin times should be monitored.

Water-Soluble Vitamins. Littlewood et al.[32] stud-

TABLE 22–3. *Serum Tocopherol Levels of Patients with CF and Control Subjects Before and After Single Oral Vitamin E Loading Dose of 10 mg/kg*

	Number of Subjects	Mean Age (Yr)	Serum Tocopherol Level (mg/dl)				
			Before Administration	*After Administration*			
				4 hr	*8 hr*	*24 hr*	*48 hr*
CF patients with PI without enzyme	19	6.1	0.31 (±0.13)	0.55 (±0.22)	0.68 (±0.31)	0.54 (±0.22)	0.43 (±0.15)
CF patients with PI with enzyme	19	6.1	0.36 (±0.16)	0.86 (±0.58)	1.03 (±0.52)	0.73 (±0.26)	0.54 (±0.20)
CF patients without PI	2	6.5	0.80	1.37	1.61	1.19	1.13
Control subjects	8	8.0	0.64 (±0.16)	1.35 (±0.49)	1.19 (±0.45)	1.25 (±0.56)	0.97 (±0.52)

PI, pancreatic insufficiency.

ied the vitamin status of 36 patients with CF aged 10 months to 16 years (19 female, 17 male). Most of the study subjects were receiving pancreatic enzyme and multivitamin supplements. Except for some patients with minor abnormalities, most had normal serum levels of vitamins B_1, B_2, and B_6. Vitamin B_{12} absorption in patients with CF was found by Deren et al.[37] to be decreased and to be corrected by pancreatic enzyme administration. Rucker and Harrison[95] reported a case of macrocytic anemia with abnormal Schilling test in a 16-year-old patient with CF who responded to intramuscular injections of vitamin B_{12}. The B_{12} malabsorption is probably due partly to pancreatic insufficiency and partly to lack of resorption of bile acids in the small intestine, with excessive loss of B_{12} in stools. Vitamin B_{12} is present in milk, eggs, and other animal products, which are main dietary components of CF patients. Clinical evidence of vitamin B_{12} deficiency is very rare in patients with CF.

IRON

Patients with newly diagnosed CF usually have normal serum iron levels. Following the administration of pancreatic enzyme, the serum iron levels become reduced. Wang et al.[96] evaluated the serum iron, total iron-binding capacity, and hemogram profile in 170 patients with CF. They found that 60 per cent of their patients had serum iron levels below 60 μg/dl. The total iron-binding capacity was either normal or increased. The mean corpuscular hemoglobin and the mean corpuscular volume were below normal, while the hemoglobin and hematocrit levels were within normal range. The red blood cells were frequently hypochromic and microcytic, with the polychromasia and anisocytosis characteristic of iron deficiency. Recently, Ater et al.[97] evaluated hematological function in 39 stable patients with CF ranging in age from 1½ years to 22 years (19 males and 20 females). They found hemoglobin concentrations below the 50th percentile for age in 90 per cent of the patients studied, and serum ferritin levels below the normal value of 12 μg/ml in 33 per cent of these patients. Serum vitamin E levels less than 0.005 mg/dl were found in 33 per cent. They found that combined administration of iron and vitamin E was effective in elevating the mean hemoglobin concentration from 13.87 to 14.50 g/dl, with a significant rise of serum ferritin levels. This study helps to explain the lack of polycythemia in patients with CF who have severe hypoxemia.

TRACE METALS

The role of trace metals in patients with CF has not been extensively investigated. Several years ago, selenium deficiency was proposed as the underlying factor responsible for cystic fibrosis, a notion that received widespread publicity in lay literature. Dietary supplementation of selenium was adopted by some patients themselves. Thereafter, occasional patients developed selenium toxicity, as reported by Snodgrass et al.[98] Lloyd-Still et al.[99] measured whole blood selenium and erythrocyte glutathione peroxidase levels of 20 patients with CF (aged 6 months to 15 years). Glutathione peroxidase was found to be a selenoprotein, with its activity highly correlated with selenium concentration. Their results showed mean whole blood selenium levels to be 0.112 μg/g (ppm) in patients with CF, which contrasted with a mean value of 0.2 ppm for normal children and adults in the United States. It should be noted that normal values of 0.055 ppm for children and 0.070 ppm for adults have been reported in New Zealand. The whole blood selenium levels in patients with CF were comparable to those of children with phenylketonuria receiving a low-phenylalanine diet. Glutathione peroxidase levels were normal in patients with CF. The relatively low blood levels of selenium associated with CF were not considered to represent deficiency. This study does not support the hypothesis that selenium deficiency is the basic defect leading to the manifestations of CF. Cox et al.[100] reported selenium deficiency in a 19-year-old woman with CF who after 3 months of total parenteral nutrition (TPN) developed a selenium-responsive myositis with a marked rise of serum creatine kinase level. The patient's serum selenium level dropped to 0.02 μg/ml (normal 0.1 to 0.17 μg/ml). The patient responded promptly in both clinical and laboratory findings to oral supplementation with selenium (200 μg/day). Patients with advanced disease whose nutritional intake is dependent on the parenteral route must have measurements of serum or whole blood selenium.[101] Patients receiving a regular diet with pancreatic enzyme supplement rarely develop selenium deficiency.

Zinc. Zinc is an important component of a group of enzymes (metalloenzymes) that require a specific number of zinc atoms for activation of the molecule.[102] Zinc is important in maintaining the integrity of cellular membrane and intracellular compartments, and in stabilizing nucleic acid in protein synthesis, cell division, and growth of cells, tissues, and organs. Clinical features of zinc deficiency include anorexia, hypogeusia, failure to thrive in infants, growth retardation in older children, delayed sexual maturation, and delayed wound healing. Patients on total parenteral nutrition without zinc supplements develop skin lesions around the mouth resembling those of patients with acrodermatitis enteropathica. The perioral lesions may be present with reddened ichthyosiform plaques. Diagnosis of zinc deficiency is based on a high degree of suspicion from clinical manifestations and laboratory studies. Affected patients have low levels of plasma zinc (< 70 μg/dl), low content of zinc in hair (if hair growth is decreased, hair zinc levels may be normal), low levels of zinc in urine, and low activities of zinc metalloenzymes.

Plasma zinc levels have been reported to be low in children with CF with severe growth retardation and normal in those with normal growth. Others have reported normal zinc levels in 36 patients with CF,[104] and other investigations have reported plasma zinc levels to be correlated with plasma retinol-binding protein, vitamin A, and albumin in 18 children with CF but not in controls.[105]

Recently, most milk formulas for infant feeding have been supplemented with zinc. For parenteral nutrition we add to the infusate to provide a total of 150 to 300 µg/kg of zinc as RDA for infants and children. Meats, poultry, crabs, oysters, and precooked dry cereals are rich in zinc.

Copper. Copper is essential for the production of red blood cells (serving as a catalyst in hemoglobin formation) and for the absorption of iron, and is associated with the activities of many enzymes.[106] The anemia of copper deficiency is partly due to deficiency of ceruloplasmin and other ferroxidases. These enzymes are required for the oxidation of ferrous iron to the ferric state, and for binding to transferrin and subsequent transport to bone marrow.

Solomons et al.[107] measured plasma copper and ceruloplasmin in treated patients with CF and found significantly increased levels in the patients studied. Copper is mainly excreted in bile, and patients with biliary stasis conceivably have defective excretion. Further investigation is needed to verify the above observations.

MANAGEMENT OF NUTRITIONAL DEFICIENCIES

It has been repeatedly observed that patients with CF who have a mild pulmonary involvement grow better than those with severe involvement. When pulmonary infection is under control, most patients have a good appetite and take sufficient nutrients to compensate for the fecal loss. Those in good nutritional status can combat pulmonary infection far better than malnourished patients. Management of nutritional disorders therefore begins with control of pulmonary infections, and is supplemented by dietary therapy (administration of pancreatic enzyme, vitamins, electrolytes, and trace metals).

Control of Pulmonary Infection

The pathogenesis of the pulmonary infections associated with CF is not fully understood. Patients with CF have normal lungs at birth. Shortly thereafter infections begin, with dilatation and hypertrophy of bronchial glands and with goblet cell metaplasia of the bronchiolar epithelium. Mucous plugging of peripheral airways precipitates bronchiolitis and pneumonia. The earliest and most sensitive sign of pulmonary infection is increased cough with sputum production. If intervention is not instituted, the patient will develop tachypnea, anorexia, sometimes low-grade fever, weight loss, and abnormal physical findings on examination of the chest. The latter consist of increased anteroposterior diameter of the chest with localized or generalized moist rales on auscultation, with suprasternal retraction in older patients, and with subcostal and intercostal as well as suprasternal retractions in infants and young children. Chest roentgenograms show overaeration, increased lung markings, and mucous plugging, with or without atelectasis, bronchiectasis, or areas of confluent density. The white blood cell count is often increased, with an increase of polymorphonuclear neutrophils.

There is a marked variability among patients in the severity and natural course of the pulmonary involvement. In the acute and chronic phases of pulmonary infection antibiotic therapy, bronchial drainage, and other supportive and prophylactic measures are the major determinants of the morbidity and mortality of CF. Patients with a mild pulmonary disability status are usually in a better nutritional state than those with advanced disease. Acute pulmonary exacerbations are often associated with a significant weight loss, which is regained upon recovery from these episodes. Weight gain is an important measure both of therapeutic efficacy and of the severity of the disease. Accordingly, whenever there is an acute weight loss, with or without overt symptoms or signs of pulmonary infection, an in-depth clinical evaluation should be carried out.

It is extremely important to obtain adequate sputum samples for culture for bacterial pathogens. Older patients can expectorate sputum without difficulty, especially following a series of deep breaths during chest physical examination. It is important to obtain a mucus plug in the sputum for culture. Infants and young children can be induced to cough with insertion of a cotton swab deep into the pharynx to pick up a drop of mucus for culture. In young children the respiratory pathogens consist of *Staphylococcus aureus*, *Haemophilus influenzae*, and *Escherichia coli*. Patients who have had repeated hospitalizations and those with advanced disease are most often colonized predominantly with *Pseudomonas aeruginosa*. The mucoid variety is most prevalent in older children and young adults. Recently, *Pseudomonas cepacia* resistant to most of the conventional antibiotics has been isolated in the sputum of as many as 10 to 20 per cent of older children and young adults with CF and in lung cultures of postmortem samples. The epidemiology and pathogenesis of *P. cepacia* infection in CF patients warrants intensive investigation.[111]

Antibiotic therapy combined with bronchial drainage is indicated in all patients who have a productive cough. The most frequently used antibiotic agents are the semisynthetic penicillins, cephalosporins, and aminoglycosides. Oxacillin, cloxacillin, and dicloxacillin have, in the order given, increasing in vitro activity against penicillin-resistant staphylococci and higher blood levels after oral administration. Clinically, no substantial differences can be detected among these agents. A newer cephalosporin, cefaclor,[112] which is similar to cephalexin and cephradine[113] in its activity against *Staphylococcus aureus*, is more active against *Haemophilus influenzae*. It is favored by most physicians for oral therapy of patients with a cough without acute exacerbations. Other oral antibiotics consist of amoxicillin, ampicillin, erythromycin, chloramphenicol, and trimethoprim-sulfamethoxazole. Tetracycline is occasionally used in children over 8 years of age.

During acute exacerbations, patients are hospitalized for intensive antibiotic therapy using intermittent intravenous infusions. Combinations of a broad-spectrum anti-*Pseudomonas* penicillin or a cephalosporin and an aminoglycoside are most commonly employed. Methicillin or nafcillin is also frequently added to the therapeutic regimen when there is coexistent *Staphylococcus aureus*. Carbenicillin, followed by ticarcillin, and recently the ureidopenicillins, azlocillin and piperacillin,[114–116] have been used with success. Newer cephalosporins—ceftazidime, cefoperazone, and cefsulodin—with high in vitro and in vivo activity against *Pseudomonas* species are or will soon be released for clinical use. Several other related agents are also under study. Aminoglycosides including gentamicin, tobramycin, and amikacin are the most active agents against *Pseudomonas aeruginosa* and other gram-negative organisms. The choice of antibiotic agents is based on the minimal inhibitory concentration (MIC) of the antibiotic against the pathogens. The choices of dosage adequate to achieve serum concentrations higher than the MIC of the antibiotic agent against the organism is very important. Peak and trough serum levels must be obtained in order to ensure high therapeutic efficacy with minimal toxicity. Ototoxic and renal toxic effects of the aminoglycosides are of great concern.[118,119] Bleeding tendency due to platelet dysfunction and a hepatotoxic effect of the broad-spectrum penicillins have been problems.[120] The duration of each course of intensive antibiotic treatment ranges from 10 days to 3 weeks. Some patients with good home care may be treated initially in hospital, with therapy continued at home. This approach has financial, emotional, and medical advantages. Many adult patients with advanced disease requiring prolonged or repeated courses of treatment are greatly benefitted by intensive care carried out at home.

The concurrent use of aerosol antibiotics with parenteral therapy has been found efficacious in treatment of exacerbations.[121]

Following each course of intensive antibiotic therapy during acute exacerbations, it is of utmost importance to continue long-term home care with emphasis on bronchial drainage, antibiotic therapy, nutritional care, and emotional care. Periodic follow-up in a CF center clinic provides reassurance as to the patient's condition.

DIETARY CONSIDERATIONS

NUTRITION EDUCATION AND DIETARY COUNSELING

The focus of nutrition education and dietary therapy has remained the same since cystic fibrosis was first identified. Because of the maldigestion present, attention must be paid to the correction of the digestive manifestations. Complicating this feature of CF is the energy depletion from the increased energy demands of pulmonary infections. There are also nutritional side effects from drug therapy, for example, depression of appetite and interference with the metabolism of nutrients.

The techniques for obtaining the optimal nutritional status of patients have changed dramatically over the past several years. The availability of enteric-coated enzyme preparations has permitted the liberalization of dietary recommendations. Current practice is to recommend the ingestion of a wide variety of nourishing foods and beverages. Attention is concentrated on promoting the total nutritional well-being of the patient, given the constraints of the family's lifestyle and the patient's disease process. Moreover, the attempt is made to offer concrete suggestions regarding the times for meals and snacks and the kinds of foods and beverages that are best to include. Anticipatory guidance is important in fostering an awareness on the part of patients and their families of potential trouble areas. Another major advance has been the introduction of main-frame and interactive microcomputers into the health care setting. These have altered the quality and quantity of nutritional data available to clinicians and to patients and their families. Great possibilities currently exist for the immediate clinical correlation of food intake with indices of nutritional status, such as anthropometric and laboratory measurements. Computers offer the potential for dramatic changes in the kinds of methods used in, and in the precision of, educating and counseling patients and their families.

At the Time of Diagnosis. Although the family is distraught at the time of the diagnosis of CF in one or more of their children, a nutrition education and dietary counseling program should be included as one of the initial teaching sessions. Rapport must be established, reading materials available to laymen must be verbally updated, and fears must be alleviated. Positive steps the family can take in choosing foods and feeding their child are important components of fostering improved emotional attitudes and in providing a renewed sense of control over their daily lives. During the counseling session, the patient's and family's past and current food intakes, their beliefs about food (however nebulous), and their economic situations are determined. Balanced meal and snack patterns are clearly described within the context of the family's daily routines and food preferences. The rationale for and administration of pancreatic enzymes and vitamin/mineral supplements are explained. A typical day's schedule written out and specifying the times for physical therapy, administration of medication, and food intake is helpful to many families.

Since height and weight are closely monitored, a demonstration of the use of the standard growth chart and a discussion of expected short-term and long-term gains are other helpful educational techniques at the time of diagnosis.

In Infancy. The decision as to what formula is suitable to the age and medical condition of the baby is paramount in obtaining immediate success in correcting the nutritional deficiencies and feeding difficulties usually present. If the formula requires fortification of its caloric and nutrient levels, the exact preparation should be demonstrated to the family. Explanation of developmental milestones and their implications for food and feeding techniques should be provided to parents. Because the sodium chloride content has been reduced in most commercial infant and toddler foods, parents need to be instructed to add salt to formula or foods. All instructions must be individualized and must be provided in written form with the inclusion of appropriate illustrations.

In the Preschool Child. During the preschool years, after the critical period of diagnosis has passed and the child usually is seemingly doing well, the health care team and the family often diminish their attention to the nutritional needs of a child with CF. Food preferences and habits are established during the preschool years, however. The frequent restatement of ideas of balanced meal and snack menus, the close observation of growth patterns, and the judicious introduction of powdered and liquid proprietary nutritional supplements are mandatory steps for the continued nutritional well-being of the child. For example, caffeine- and sucrose-containing beverages like soda, iced tea, and "ades" devoid of protein, fat, vitamins, and minerals are often substituted (frequently without realization) for high-calorie, nutrient-dense liquids like whole milk, milkshakes, or other proprietary beverages. Once the teeth erupt, close inspection of the oral cavity is necessary in order to prevent dental decay with its resultant detrimental effects on the chewing and eating abilities of the child.

In the School-Aged Child. Whenever the child enters day-care programs or school, the adults subsequently responsible for the preparation of foods and feeding need to be included in dietary counseling sessions. Sometimes telephone consultations with school officials regarding the individual child's nutritional needs and the latest nutritional therapies make the difference in whether or not the child receives optimal nutritional support away from home. For example, some school districts require all medications to be dispensed by the nurse or teacher. In the case of pancreatic enzyme replacement, the capsules are to be swallowed immediately prior to food consumption. Considerable delay often occurs in school settings between the administration of the enzyme preparation in the nurse's office and the actual ingestion of the school lunch by the child.

Generally, as the child grows older, he or she should be involved as much as possible in counseling sessions. Simplified nutrition facts can be taught by games, paper-and-pencil activity sheets, actual food preparation experiences, and interaction with microcomputers using appropriate software packages.

In Adolescence. The growing need of teenagers for independence requires recognition by the family, by the health care team, and often, by the teenagers themselves. Frequently, the teenager can enter the dietary counseling sessions held separately from the previously held joint sessions. Devising socially acceptable nourishing meal and snack ideas often, however, requires creativity on everyone's part. Assistance to teenagers is helpful (if not always appreciated) as they attempt to develop individualized methods for obtaining the increased requirements for energy and nutrients.

In Adults. Reinforcement of balanced menu planning continues from infancy into adulthood. As medical and nutritional treatments advance and create changes in the methods by which people with CF achieve their nutritional goals, updated information must be continually supplied to patients, to their families and friends, and to health care practitioners. Adults with CF must examine their own lifestyles, such as plans for college, employment, marriage, and parenthood. Demands of schedules, including time allocated for physical exercise, must be interwoven with constantly increasing caloric requirements. In addition, adults need to learn skills in food purchasing and preparation when they become responsible for these activities.

DIETARY THERAPY

Although patients with CF have traditionally been described as having voracious appetites, when actual dietary records are obtained from parents or from a summer camp study, the caloric intake of most patients amounts to only 80 to 90 per cent of the recommended daily allowance. In consideration of the increased work of breathing and the excessive fecal loss of nutrients, the recommended daily allowance (RDA) for the child with CF is estimated to be 150 per cent of RDA for age.[122] General principles of dietary therapy consist of a diet high in calories, high in protein, adequate in carbohydrate, and liberal in fat. With the recent availability of enteric-coated microspheres of pancreatic enzyme preparations, fat restriction is no longer emphasized, but treated patients still have variable degrees of steatorrhea. The type and quantity of fat must be individualized according to the tolerance and symptoms of each patient. Protein and carbohydrates are well tolerated. Simple sugars, the monosaccharides or disaccharides, are absorbed with ease, causing less flatulence than complex carbohydrates. Lactase deficiency is occasionally present and may cause intolerance to lactose. In such instances, lactose should be eliminated from diet.

It is far easier to control the feeding of infants than that of older children, adolescents, and young adults. Infants without severe pulmonary infections generally do well on pancreatic enzyme supplement and conventional infant feedings such as evaporated milk or commercial formulas derived from cow's milk (such ad Enfamil or Similac). Older infants can take whole cow's milk with pancreatic enzyme supplements. Newly diagnosed young infants with failure to thrive, neonates in a postoperative state following meconium ileus, and infants who fail to gain weight in spite of adequate caloric intake are often fed with formulas containing predigested proteins and medium-chain triglycerides (MCT). Table 22–4 lists the composition of presently available infant formulas, and Table 22–5 shows the composition of fats in common infant formulas. Casein hydrolysates are predigested proteins containing peptides and amino acids; these are well tolerated by patients with CF and are associated with increase in weight gain. MCT oil, derived from coconut oil, is composed mainly of the triglycerides of C8 and C10 saturated fatty acids. Unlike long-chain fats, MCT can be easily absorbed in pancreatic deficiency states. In practice we have used pancreatic enzyme supplementation along with MCT feeding. Kuo and Huang[124] reported benefit in the use of MCT feeding in infants and children with CF. They observed marked reduction of steatorrhea and increased weight gain during the use of MCT. Gracey et al.[125] also found reduction of steatorrhea with MCT feedings in their patients but without weight gain. MCT have been incorporated in infant formulas such as Pregestimil and Portagen and in certain special high-calorie artificial diets described below. MCT oil has also been employed in cooking for patients with CF. An MCT oil recipe book is available from Mead Johnson & Company. The high osmolarity of MCT oil often causes abdominal pain and diarrhea. Accordingly, in order to avoid intolerance, Pregestimil and Portagen should be introduced at half strength initially, with gradual increase to full strength. These formulas should be given to infants with a problem of weight gain throughout the first year of life.

Older patients with CF can tolerate regular diets with pancreatic enzyme supplementation without any difficulty. Teenagers and adults with CF should be free to adjust their diets, and they usually know how much fat and what combination of foods are most comfortable for their gastrointestinal tracts. Table 22–6 lists the protein and caloric requirements of normal children and children with CF. It is extremely important that patients from infancy to adulthood all adhere to the calorie and nutrient intake as prescribed.

Prophylaxis against deficiency of essential fatty acids is regularly carried out by advising patients to use corn oil or soy oil for salads and vegetables, which is very well tolerated. Rosenlund et al.[126] gave corn oil orally to her patients, with clinical improvement. Others have used safflower oil and linoleic acid monoglyceride without definitive conclusions as to their value. Chase et al.[11] carried out a double-blind study on the efficacy of intravenous adminis-

TABLE 22–4. Natural and Prepared Milks for Infants with Cystic Fibrosis

Formula	Kcal/oz	Approximate Percentage Composition in Normal Dilution (g/dl)			Sources		
		Protein	Carbohydrate	Fat	Protein	Carbohydrate	Fat
Similac 20	20	1.8	7.0	3.6	Casein 82% Whey 18%	Lactose	Corn oil Coconut oil
Enfamil 24	24	1.8	8.5	4.5	Skim milk	Lactose	Soy oil 80% Coconut oil 20%
Nutramigen	20	2.2	8.6	2.6	Casein Hydrolysate	Sucrose Tapioca starch	Corn oil
Probana	20	4.2	7.9	2.2	Cow's milk Casein	Lactose Dextrose Banana powder	Milk fat 76% Corn oil 24%
Portagen*	20	2.7	7.7	3.2	Caseinate	Sucrose	MCT† 88% Corn oil 12%
Pregestimil*	20	1.8	8.6	2.6	Casein Hydrolysate Amino acids	Dextrose Tapioca starch	MCT† 88% Corn oil 12%

*Also contains vitamins and minerals.
†Medium-chain triglycerides.

TABLE 22–5. *Composition of Fats Used in Common Infant Formulas for Infants with Cystic Fibrosis*

Source	Saturated Fatty Acids (%)							Unsaturated Fatty Acids (%)				
	*8:0**	*10:0*	*12:0*	*14:0*	*16:0*	*18:0*	*20:0*	*16:1*	*18:1*	*18:2*	*18:3*	*18:4*
Corn oil					13	4	Trace		29	54		
Coconut oil		6	49.5	19.5	8.5	2.0	Trace		6	1.5		
Soy				Trace	11	4	Trace		25	51	9	
Oleomargarine			0.2	3.3	26	20			45.5	3	0.5	
MCT	68	24	Larger than C10: <5%									

*Length of carbon chain: number of double bonds.

tration of Intralipid compared with dextrose in 10 children with CF. Five children received 20 ml/kg of 10 per cent Intralipid intravenously over a 4-hour period at intervals of 2 weeks for a total of 52 weeks; the other five were given equivalent volume of 10 per cent dextrose in 0.2 per cent NaCl in the same manner as the above group. The group receiving Intralipid gained significantly more in height and weight during the study period than during the year prior to the study. On the other hand, statistically significant differences in individual tests such as weight gain and pulmonary function tests were not found between the two groups. The general improvement in both groups was attributed to the improved medical care and continued reinforcement of home care.

The recommended dosage of Intralipid is 1 g/kg, which is devoid of adverse effect. Higher dosage may cause fatty liver, reticuloendothelial fat infiltration, and increase of fatty acid levels in plasma.

Chase and Dupont[128] advised oral administration of one tablespoon of safflower oil once or twice daily along with pancreatic enzymes. The long-term effect of oral administration of essential fatty acids as dietary supplementation requires further investigation.

Artificial Diet. About 15 years ago an artificial diet was proposed by Allan et al.[129] that consisted of a mixture of beef serum hydrolysate, a glucose polymer (Caloreen) MCT oil, margarine or egg yolk,

additional minerals, vitamins, and essential fatty acids. This diet provided 6 to 10 per cent of total calorie intake from protein, 75 to 85 per cent from carbohydrate, and 10 to 15 per cent from MCT and margarine or egg yolk. Allan et al.[129] observed significant improvement in weight gain during the period of consumption of this "elemental" diet. Barclay and Shannon[130] in a controlled study of 12 patients with CF observed evidence of improved growth in mildly affected patients and in those who tolerated the special dietary therapy. The commercially available elemental diet marketed as Flexical (Mead Johnson) is of a composition similar to but modified from the above, containing MCT oil and soy oil plus sucrose and dextrin, providing 1.5 per cent protein, 2.3 per cent fat, 17.1 per cent carbohydrate, and 30 cal/oz. Vitamins and minerals in amounts of 100 to 500 per cent of US RDA for adults and older children are incorporated in this diet. Another marketed elemental high-nitrogen diet, Vivonex (Norwich Eaton Laboratories, Norwich, CT), is quite popular. It is made up of essential and nonessential amino acids, simple carbohydrates, essential fatty acids, vitamins, minerals, and trace metals. It provides 30 cal/oz., 8.2 per cent amino acids, 1.3 per cent fat, and 90.5 per cent carbohydrate. Vivonex differs from Flexical in its high nitrogen and low fat content. Sustacal (Mead Johnson), a palatable nutritionally complete food, is available in the form of liquid, powder, or pudding ready to use as a dietary supplement. It is quite popular among our patients.

TABLE 22–6. *Protein and Calorie Requirements of Normal Children and Children with Cystic Fibrosis*

Age (yr)		Wt (kg)	Kcal Required		Protein Required	
			*Normal**	*Patients with CF*	*Normal*	*Patients with CF*
0–0.5		4–6	115/kg	150/kg	2.2/kg	4.4/kg
0.5–1.0		7–10	105/kg	140/kg	2.0/kg	4.0/kg
1.0–3.0		13–15	100/kg	125/kg	1.8/kg	3.5/kg
4.0–6.0		20	80/kg	120/kg	1.5/kg	3.0/kg
7.0–10.0		24–28	2400	3600	1.5/kg	3.0/kg
11.0–14.0	(F)	35	2250	3375	50	100
11.0–14.0	(M)	35	2700	4050	45	90
15.0–18.0	(F)	40–55	2100	3150	46	90
15.0–18.0	(M)	45–66	2800	4200	56	112
>18	(F)	55	2100	3150	44	88
>18	(M)	70	2900	4350	56	112

*Recommended Dietary Allowances, 9th Edition. National Research Council, National Academy of Sciences, Washington, DC, 1980.

These elemental diets are most effective in promoting weight gain in mildly affected patients, less so in those with advanced pulmonary involvement. These diets are not very palatable and are best administered as nocturnal nasogastric infusions as a supplement to regular diet for patients with insufficient intake and poor weight gain. This form of feeding is discussed further below.

NASOGASTRIC FEEDING

In order to provide a high-caloric intake without causing extra effort on the part of the patient, other feeding methods in addition to oral intake have been tried in CF centers. One of these methods is nasogastric or nasojejunal feeding. Nasogastric feeding has been used with success in patients during acute exacerbations and in those with a poor appetite and unable to take a high-calorie diet. The intranasal insertion of a Silastic tube into the stomach or jejunum permits continuous delivery of a high-calorie liquid enteral feeding (Vivonex), given at a constant rate of 1 ml per minute for 12 hours a day from 8:00 p.m. to 8:00 a.m. This method gives the patients an additional 720 kcal per day. During daytime, the patients continue to eat regular meals and snacks, with pancreatic enzyme and vitamin supplementation. Patients who cooperate in this regimen usually gain weight dramatically. Unfortunately, not all patients can tolerate the Silastic tube. Complications consist of regurgitation, vomiting, blockage, leakage, or collapse of the tube and occasionally excessive coughing and possible aspiration. All patients who can tolerate this regimen gain weight, with improvement in their general condition. Bertrand et al.[131] studied 10 children with CF in stable condition ranging in age from 3.5 to 12 years, whose weights were lower than 90 per cent of the expected weight for height. These patients were given continuous enteral alimentation of Vivonex for 4 weeks using an IVAC pump (IVAC-530, IVAC Corporation, La Jolla, CA) through a silicone nasogastric tube for at least 16 hours a day with the exclusion of other food and without pancreatic enzyme supplementation. The same patients were also given 2 mg/kg of fat emulsion (from Nutralipid 1090, Pharmacia, Montreal) by the intravenous route at weekly intervals in order to supply essential fatty acids. Evaluation of these patients before and at the end of this treatment and 2 months later showed dramatic increases in weight gain during and shortly after the period of enteral alimentation. The weight gain was directly due to an increase of adipose tissue. The weight gain was not, however, accompanied by improvement in chest roentgenograms or pulmonary function.

Pencharz et al.[132] claimed success with nocturnal supplementation (1200 kcal) of an elemental diet delivered via a gastrostomy tube. The tube was inserted into the stomach with use of local anesthesia and without a laparotomy. Whether this method serves as an alternative to nasogastric tube feeding requires further study.

If dietary intake plus pancreatic enzyme and high-calorie supplemental feeding using a frequent feeding method cannot fulfill the nutritional requirements of the patient with CF, the next step is undoubtedly nasogastric or gastric feeding.

The patient's acceptance of nasogastric feeding will be greatly improved if such feeding is introduced during infancy and carried out on long-term basis. A long-term controlled study will generate useful information on the effect of adequate nutrition on infection, growth and development, and pulmonary status of patients with CF.

INTRAVENOUS FEEDING

Intravenous feeding has been used with increased frequency in the management of patients with CF in recent years. There has been progressive advancement in the technology of this procedure. The infusion solution now used consists of essential and nonessential amino acids, dextrose, vitamins, electrolytes, and trace minerals. It is supplemented by the intravenous administration of Intralipid to provide triglycerides of predominantly unsaturated fatty acids. The combined use of these solutions provides adequate amounts of all nutrients to meet the needs of patients with CF from infancy to adolescence. For peripheral venous alimentation glucose concentration should not exceed 10 per cent. For central venous feeding concentrations of glucose should start at 10 per cent, with a gradual increase to achieve 20 to 25 per cent concentration. This stepwise increase of glucose will enhance the tolerance of glucose load and minimize hyperglycemia, glucosuria, and osmotic diuresis. Intravenous feeding calls for teamwork involving the surgeon, physician, pharmacist, nurse, social worker, and family members. Strict asepsis is mandatory in preparing and mixing the alimentation solutions and in caring for the intravenous catheter. Many complications are related to the insertion of the catheter. Infection and metabolic disturbances are preventable if one follows scrupulously the details described in the Parenteral Nutrition Guide of St. Christopher's Hospital for Children.[137] These guidelines have been so well worked out that intravenous feeding is now quite safe and practical for both in-hospital and home usage. Occasionally a patient continues the regimen at home for long-term therapy.

Indications for intravenous feeding in the management of patients with CF are as follows:

1. Newborns with meconium ileus with extensive resection of the small intestine. These patients are greatly benefitted by short-term intravenous feeding to reduce the length of hospitalization and hasten convalescence from surgery. Total parenteral nutrition (TPN) may cause cholestatic jaundice in small infants. Discontinuation of TPN may be necessary in cases of persistent jaundice.

2. Pre- and postoperative care of patients for thoracic or abdominal surgery such as lobectomy (or occasionally pneumonectomy) and laparotomy for surgical complications.

3. Acutely ill, untreated, and newly diagnosed patients with severe malnutrition in whom nutritional support is life-saving.

4. Patients with advanced pulmonary involvement with severe anorexia.

5. Acute weight loss due to pulmonary exacerbation requiring immediate nutritional support in addition to the control of pulmonary infections.

6. Patients in whom dietary therapy has failed to provide sufficient nutrients to meet their needs and in whom nasogastric feeding is not feasible.

7. Patients with acute pancreatitis. This complication is not uncommon in patients with CF who have pancreatic function.[138] It is usually precipitated by a fatty meal and manifested by severe abdominal pain and a rise of serum amylase. In severe cases total parenteral nutrition may be necessary to provide the patient's nutritional needs.

Pancreatic Enzyme Supplementation

Pancreatic enzyme deficiency with markedly reduced or nondetectable levels of trypsin, chymotrypsin, amylase, and lipase in the duodenal secretions is found in about 90 per cent of patients with CF. This deficiency results in variable degrees of maldigestion and malabsorption of fats, proteins, carbohydrates, and fat-soluble vitamins. Supplementation of diet with pancreatic enzyme preparations partly corrects the deficiency. Most of the commercially available forms of pancreatic enzymes are of porcine origin. Non–enteric-coated pancrelipase had been used for years. Enormous doses had been employed in an attempt to enhance digestion, but the result did not prove completely satisfactory. These large doses have led to the development of hyperuricuria.

Two newer preparations (Pancrease, Cotazym-S) consist of enteric-coated microspheres of porcine pancreatic enzyme (Table 22–7). These enzyme microspheres are protected by an enteric coat that begins to disintegrate when the environment achieves a pH of 6 or greater.[139–143] Following oral administration, predictable levels of highly active enzymes are found in the duodenum or jejunum. These preparations are more efficient in combating steatorrhea and are popular among our patients. Several controlled studies showed that the new microspheres have the following advantages over the conventional non–enteric-coated preparations: (1) smaller dosages—approximately half the dosage of the conventional form is required to achieve the same results in controlling steatorrhea; (2) reduced intake of nucleoprotein lessens the danger of hyperuricuria; (3) intake of dietary fat can be more liberalized; and (4) abdominal cramping, bloating, and discomfort have been greatly reduced. The dosage depends upon the extent of steatorrhea, the age of the patient, and the dietary fat content and must be tailored to the individual patient's condition. Infants are given a quarter of a capsule of Pancrease or Cotazym-S mixed in applesauce or mashed banana before feeding. Older children swallow capsules before each meal or snack. For older children, a reasonable starting dose is one capsule of Pancrease or Cotazym-S with each meal and about half that dose with each snack. Subsequent dosage changes depend upon the character, frequency, and size of the stools and upon abdominal symptoms. With the use of the new pancreatic enzyme preparations, steatorrhea is reduced by 50 per cent or more, but digestion cannot be restored to normal. The use of L-arginine, sodium bicarbonate, and cimetidine has not been found effective in reducing fat or nitrogen excretion in feces.

Vitamin Administration

A multiple vitamin preparation containing water-miscible forms of the fat-soluble vitamins A and D

Preparation and Manufacturer	Potency			How Supplied	Dosage	Remarks
	Lipase	Amylase	Protease			
Cotazym-S capsule Enteric-coated microspheres (porcine) Organon, 5 Mt. Pleasant Ave., Orange, NJ 07052	5000 U/cap	2000 U/cap	2000 U/cap	100 cap/bottle	1–3 cap per meal and 1 cap per snack	Older children swallow capsules with meal Infants take microspheres with applesauce and swallow it without chewing
Pancrease Enteric-coated microspheres in capsules (porcine) McNeil Lab., Inc., Springhouse, PA 19477	4000 U/cap	2000 U/cap	2500 U/cap	100, 250 cap/bottle	1–3 cap per meal less per snack	Same as above If patient is allergic to pork, use beef product
Viokase Tablet	1950/tab	4000	16,250	100, 500 tab/bottle	8–10 tab	Avoid inhalation of powder, which may precipitate an asthmatic attack
Powder	13,500/tsp	28,125	112,500	4 oz, 8 oz/bottle	2–3 tsp	

TABLE 22–7. Pancreatic Enzymes: Recommended Dosages and How Supplied

and other vitamins in double the daily recommended dosage for age is routinely administered to all patients with CF. The vitamin A–deficient patient should receive 5000 to 10,000 IU of Aquasol A as a supplement to assure that serum vitamin A levels are in the range of 50 to 120 mg/dl.

Vitamin K is routinely given to infants with CF up to 1 year of age to prevent hypoprothrombinemia. It is also indicated in older patients with cirrhosis of the liver who have prolonged prothrombin times with active bleeding. Vitamin K administration is indicated when prolonged oral antibiotic therapy has altered intestinal flora, causing impairment of bacterial synthesis of vitamin K. Synkayvite, a water-soluble synthetic vitamin K analogue administered in 5-mg tablets at weekly intervals, is effective prophylaxis against vitamin K deficiency in most patients with CF. In instances of active bleeding, phytonadione (as Aquamephyton, a solubilized injectable form of vitamin K, 1 mg per 0.5 ml) can be given intramuscularly for rapid action in 1 or 2 doses followed by oral therapy to maintain normal prothrombin time.

Vitamin E supplementation is recommended for all patients with pancreatic insufficiency with low serum tocopherol levels. We give a daily dose of approximately 10 IU/kg up to a maximum dose of 400 IU daily. Aquasol E drops contain 15 IU per 0.3 ml, and are available in 12-ml and 30-ml bottles. Capsules contain 100 IU, 100 per bottle, or 400 IU, 30 per bottle.

If symptoms of vitamin B_{12} should develop, intramuscular administration of B_{12} is indicated.

Vitamin B complex and vitamin C supplementation is generally carried out in patients with moderate to advanced disease and those receiving continuous administration of antibiotics. We have found that many patients receiving long-term treatment with chloramphenicol develop cheilosis during the course of treatment, which responds readily to riboflavin supplementation. The dosage of riboflavin ranges from 5 mg daily to 5 mg t.i.d. or more. The etiology of riboflavin deficiency associated with chloramphenicol is unclear.

In places where fluoride is not added to local drinking water, we recommend that our patients each day take one multivitamin tablet containing fluoride and another plain multivitamin tablet; in this way they meet the daily requirement for fluoride without mottling of teeth due to excessive fluoride.

Salt Administration

Elevated sodium and chloride levels in the sweat of patients with CF often lead to significant depletion of these electrolytes.[144,145] During hot weather, with strenuous physical exercise, and in the event of gastroenteritis and dehydration, the patient with CF is at increased risk of developing hyponatremia and hypochloremia, which can be life-threatening. Orenstein et al.[146] studied the thermoregulatory responses of eight patients with CF and five normal controls during 90 minutes of exposure to exercise and heat stress. They found that the responses of patients with CF were similar to those of their normal counterparts except that the patients lost significantly more sodium and chloride than the controls. As soon as the diagnosis of CF is made, therefore, the patient and his or her family are advised to increase the patient's salt intake with the addition of ¼ to 1 teaspoon daily, which is mixed with food at each meal. During hot weather, patients with CF are advised to take 1 to 2 g of salt tablets before engaging in outdoor activities, and to avoid exposure to peak levels of sunshine. In patients with advanced pulmonary involvement and cor pulmonale, however, salt should be administered with caution.

Minerals

IRON

It is important to evaluate patient's serum iron level and iron-binding capacity. Iron deficiency is indicated by low levels of serum iron and persistent hypochromasia and anisocytosis of the red blood cells in the blood smear. Affected patients should receive iron supplementation according to the schedule given in Table 22–8. Iron supplementation should be continued until serum iron reaches a normal level.

TRACE METALS

Patients with advanced cystic fibrosis who are dependent on parenteral hyperalimentation are at risk for development of selenium deficiency unless selenium is added to the solution. Treatment consists of oral administration of selenium (available as 200-μg kelp-bound tablets, Vitaline), 1 tablet daily.

Children with zinc deficiency should receive 15 mg of elemental zinc daily (75 mg $ZnSO_4$). Meat, grains, nuts, and cheese are rich in zinc. High-potency preparations of multivitamins with minerals are very useful for older patients and for those with advanced disease.

SUMMARY AND CONCLUSION

In spite of recent advances in diagnosis and management of cystic fibrosis, the majority of patients with CF have some degree of nutritional disorder; most evident are their low levels of achievement of height and weight, their below-normal levels of exercise tolerance, and their blood biochemical abnormalities. In order to achieve optimal growth, it is of utmost importance to prevent or minimize pulmo-

TABLE 22–8. Iron Supplementation in Cystic Fibrosis

Weight	Fer-In-Sol* Preparation	Iron Content	Dosage†
Up to 20 kg	Drops	15 mg/0.6 ml	0.6 mg b.i.d.
20–30 kg	Syrup	30 mg/tsp	1 tsp b.i.d
Over 30 kg	Capsules	60 mg/cap	1 capsule daily or b.i.d.

Schedule recommended by Wang.[96]
*Fer-In-Sol: ferrous sulfate, Mead Johnson & Company.
†To be taken between meals.

nary infections by immunizations and environmental controls and by intensive therapy of acute exacerbations, using potent antibiotics and facilitation of bronchial drainage. In addition, these patients must receive a high energy intake to offset energy loss in feces and the increased energy consumption due to rapid breathing and high metabolic rates associated with chronic infection.

In order to achieve our ultimate goals in treating patients with CF, the following questions must be answered:

1. Is it possible to achieve normal weight gain and positive nitrogen balance in all patients with CF by dietary measures?

2. How critical is essential fatty acid deficiency, and how should diet be modified or supplemented in order to achieve normal blood and tissue levels?

3. How much of the fat-soluble vitamins is required in excess of that provided by the double daily dosage of multivitamin preparations in order to prevent deficiencies?

4. Would routine administration of high-potency multivitamin/mineral preparations prevent vitamin and mineral deficiencies?

5. What are the minimal standards for periodic clinical, anthropometric, and laboratory assessments necessary for delineation of the nutritional status of patients with CF?

Answers to the above questions must be provided for patients from infancy to adulthood, and for patients with mild to advanced pulmonary involvement. While waiting for the answers, all CF centers should make a special effort to ensure that all patients with CF are given the recommended daily requirements of caloric and nutrient intake, which range from 120 to 150 per cent of normal intake for age and sex. The following steps should be carried out:

1. Intensive nutritional counseling for parents of patients with CF, and for older patients and their spouses should be conducted at frequent intervals.

2. Nutritional monitoring must be performed on a regular basis. It should include accurate estimation of daily caloric intake and weight, height, skinfold thickness, midarm circumference, exercise tolerance, and serum concentrations of albumin, lipids, glucose, electrolytes, and iron.

3. Supplementary feeding by the oral route with or without nasogastric or gastric feeding is often nec-

essary to make up deficiencies in calories, proteins, essential fatty acids, vitamins, and minerals.

4. During acute exacerbations with severe anorexia, total or supplementary parenteral nutrition should be instituted in order to provide optimal energy intake.

5. Patients who are severely malnourished and those who are refractory to nutritional therapy should have their blood monitored for vitamins and trace metal concentrations in order to pinpoint specific deficiencies. All physicians, nutritionists, family members, and patients must make a special effort and commitment to carry out intensive nutritional care to achieve optimal growth and development in all patients with CF. Hopefully, these measures will further enhance the lifespan of these patients.

References

1. Wood RE, Boat TF, Doershuk CF. Cystic fibrosis, state of art. Am Rev Respir Dis 1976; *113*:833.
2. Andersen DH. Cystic fibrosis of the pancreas and its relation to celiac disease: a clinical and pathologic study. Am J Dis Child 1938; *56*:344.
3. Farber S. Pancreatic function and disease in early life. V. Pathologic changes associated with pancreatic insufficiency in early life. Arch Pathol 1944; *37*:238–250.
4. Gibson LE, Cooke RE. A test for concentration of electrolytes in sweat in cystic fibrosis of the pancreas utilizing pilocarpine iontophoresis. Pediatrics 1959; *23*:545.
5. Guide to Diagnosis and Management of Cystic Fibrosis. Atlanta, Cystic Fibrosis Foundation, 1971.
6. Warwick WJ, Monson S. Life table studies of mortality. Modern Probl Pediatr 1967; *10*:353–367.
7. Young WF, Jackon AD. The prognosis of cystic fibrosis. Modern Probl Pediatr 1967; *10*:350–352.
8. Shwachman H, Kowalski M, Khaw KT. Cystic fibrosis: a new outlook. Medicine 1977; *56*:129–149.
9. Doershuk CF, Matthews LW, Tucker AS, et al. A five year clinical evaluation of a therapeutic program for patients with cystic fibrosis. J Pediatr 1964; *75*:677–693.
10. Gaskin K, Gurwitz D, Durie P, et al. Improved respiratory prognosis in patients with cystic fibrosis with normal fat absorption. J Pediatr 1982; *100*:857.
11. Chase HP, Cotten E, Elliott RB. Intravenous linoleic acid supplementation in children with cystic fibrosis. Pediatrics 1979; *64*:207.
12. Levison H, Godfrey S. Pulmonary aspects of cystic fibrosis. *In* Mangos JA, Talamo RC (eds). Cystic Fibrosis: Projections into the Future. New York, Intercontinental Medical Book Corp, 1976: 3.
13. Shwachman H, Kulczycki LL, Mueller HL, et al. Nasal polyps in patients with CF. Pediatrics 1962; *30*:389.
14. Ledesman-Medina J, Osman MZ, Girdany BR: Abnormal

paranasal sinuses in patients with cystic fibrosis of the pancreas. Pediatr Radiol 1980; *9*:61–64.

15. Davidson GP, Koheil A, Forstner GG. Salivary amylase in cystic fibrosis: a marker of disordered autonomic function. Pediatr Res 1978; *12*:967–970.

16. Abrams CK, Hamosh M, Hubbard VS, et al. Lingual lipase in cystic fibrosis. J Clin Invest 1984; *72*:374–382.

17. Bendig DW, Seilheimer DK, Wagner ML, et al. Complications of gastroesophageal reflux in patients with cystic fibrosis. J Pediatr 1982; *100*:536.

18. Roult M, Weber AM, Roy CC, et al. Increased gastric lipolytic activity in cystic fibrosis. *In* Sturgess JM (ed). Perspectives in Cystic Fibrosis. Proceedings of the 8th International Cystic Fibrosis Congress, Toronto, 1980. Missanga, Ontario, Imperial Press Limited, 1980: 172.

19. Forstner G, Gall G, Corey M, et al. Digestion and absorption of nutrients in cystic fibrosis. *In* Sturgess JM (ed). Perspectives in Cystic Fibrosis. Proceedings of the 8th International Cystic Fibrosis Congress, Toronto, 1980. Missanga, Ontario, Imperial Press Limited, 1980: 137.

20. Lapey A, Kattwinkel J, di Sant'Agnese PA: Steatorrhea and azotorrhea and their relation to growth and nutrition in adolescents and young adults with cystic fibrosis. J Pediatr 1974; *84*:328–334.

21. Oppenheimer EH, Esterly JR: Pathology of cystic fibrosis: review of the literature and comparison with 146 autopsied cases. Perspect Pediatr Pathol 1975; *2*:241–278.

22. Esterly JR, Oppenheimer EH, Lauding BH. Pathology of cystic fibrosis. *In* Mangos JA, Talamo RC (eds). Cystic Fibrosis: Projection into the Future. New York, Stratton Intercontinental, 1976: 115.

23. Zoppi G, Shmerling DH, Gaburro D, et al. The electrolyte and protein contents and outputs in duodenal juice after pancreozymin and secretion stimulation in normal children and in patients with cystic fibrosis. Acta Paediatr Scand 1970; *59*:692.

24. Hadoin B, Zoppi G, Shmerling DH, et al. Quantitative assessment of exocrine pancreatic function in infants and children. J Pediatr 1968; *73*:39.

25. Hunton DB, Long WK, Tsumagari HY: Meconium ileus equivalent: an adult complication of fibrocystic disease. Gastroenterology, 1966; *50*:99–106.

26. Brown PM, Hallenbeck GA, Soule SH, et al. Cystic fibrosis with fecal retention and intussusception in late stages. Report of three cases. N Engl J Med 1960; *262*:544.

27. Holsclaw DS, Rocmaus C, Shwachman H. Intussusception in patients with cystic fibrosis. Pediatrics 1971; *48*:51.

28. Lee PA, Roloff DW, Howatt WF. Hypoproteinemia and anemia in infants with cystic fibrosis. JAMA 1974; *228*:585.

29. Underwood BA, Denning CR. Blood and liver concentrations of vitamin A and E in children with cystic fibrosis. Pediatr Res 1974; *6*:26.

30. Huang N, Sheng KT, Basavanand V. Unpublished data on vitamin E in patients with cystic fibrosis.

31. Oppenheimer EH. Focal necrosis of striated muscle in an infant with cystic fibrosis of the pancreas and evidence of lack of absorption of fat-soluble vitamins: Bull Johns Hopkins Hosp 1956; *98*:353.

32. Littlewood JM, Congdon PJ, Bruce G, et al. Vitamin status in treated cystic fibrosis. *In* Sturgess JM (ed). Perspectives in Cystic Fibrosis. Proceedings of the 8th International Cystic Fibrosis Congress, Toronto, 1980. Missanga, Ontario, Imperial Press Limited, 1980: 166.

33. Hahn TJ, Squires AE, Halstead LR, et al. Reduced serum 25-hydroxyvitamin D concentration and disordered mineral metabolism in patients with cystic fibrosis. J Pediatr 1979; *94*:38.

34. Hubbard VS, Farrel PM, di Sant'Agnese PA. Serum 25-hydroxycholecalciferol levels in patients with cystic fibrosis. J Pediatr 1979; *94*:84.

35. Scott J, Elias E, Moult P, et al. Rickets in adults with cystic fibrosis with myopathy, pancreatic insufficiency and proximal renal tubular dysfunction. Am J Med 1977; *63*:488.

36. Walter TR, Kach HF. Hemorrhagic diathesis in cystic fibrosis in infancy. Am J Dis Child 1972; *124*:641.

37. Deren JJ, Arora B, Toskes PP, et al. Malabsorption of crystalline vitamin B_{12} in cystic fibrosis. N Engl J Med 1973; *288*:949.

38. Rosenlund ML, Kim HK, Kritchevsky D, et al. Essential fatty acids in cystic fibrosis. Nature 1974; *251*:719.

39. Chase HP. Fatty acids, prostaglandins and cystic fibrosis. Pediatrics 1976; *57*:441–442.

40. Hubbard VS, Dewey DG, di Sant'Agnese PA, et al. Abnormal fatty acid composition of plasma lipids in cystic fibrosis. A primary or secondary effect. Lancet 1977; *2*:1302.

41. Handwerger S, Roth J, Gordon P, et al. Glucose intolerance in cystic fibrosis. N Engl J Med 1969; *281*:451–461.

42. Craig MM, Haddad H, Shwachman H. The pathological changes in the liver in cystic fibrosis of the pancreas. Am J Dis Child 1957; *93*:357–369.

43. Di Sant'Agnese PA, Blanc W. A distinctive type of biliary cirrhosis of the liver in patients with cystic fibrosis of the pancreas. Pediatrics 1956; *3*:787.

44. Oppenheimer EH, Esterly JR. Hepatic changes in young infants with cystic fibrosis: possible relation to focal biliary cirrhosis. J Pediatr 1975; *86*:683.

45. Taussig LM, Saldino RM, di Sant'Agnese PA. Radiographic abnormalities of the duodenum and small bowel in cystic fibrosis of the pancreas (mucoviscidosis). Radiology 1973; *106*:369.

46. Aterman K. Duodenal ulceration and fibrocystic disease. Am J Dis Child 1961; *101*:210–215.

47. Morin CL, Roy CC, Lasalle R, et al. Small bowel mucosal dysfunction in patients with cystic fibrosis. J Pediatr 1976; *88*:213.

48. Shwachman H, Holsclaw DS: Examination of the appendix at laparotomy as a diagnostic clue in cystic fibrosis. N Engl J Med 1972; *286*:1300.

49. Oppenheimer EH, Esterly JR. Pathological evidence of cystic fibrosis in patients with meconium ileus. Pediatr Res 1973; *7*:339.

50. Thomaidis TS, Arey JB. The intestinal lesion in cystic fibrosis of the pancreas. J Pediatr 1963; *63*:444–453.

51. Neutra M, Trier J. Rectal mucosa in cystic fibrosis, morphological features before and after short-term organ culture. Gastroenterology 1978; *75*:701–710.

52. Adeniyi-Jones SK, Suskind R, Klan B, et al. Growth, energy metabolism and T_3 levels in malnutrition in cystic fibrosis. Cystic Fibrosis Club Abstracts, April, 1979: 22.

53. Cropp GJ, Pullano TP, Cerny FJ, et al. Exercise tolerance and cardiorespiratory adjustments to peak work capacity in CF. Am Rev Respir Dis 1982; *126*:211–216.

54. Cropp GJ, Aneja SK, Bye MR. Oxygen cost of breathing and CO_2 responses in cystic fibrosis. (Abstract.) Chest 1982; *82*:242.

55. Peterson RA, Peterson VS, Robb RM. Vitamin A deficiency with xerophthalmia and night blindness in cystic fibrosis. Am J Dis Child 1968; *116*:662.

56. Abernathy RS. Bulging fontanelle as presenting sign in cystic fibrosis. Am J Dis Child 1976; *130*:1360.

57. Kulczycki LL, Swachman H: Studies in cystic fibrosis of the pancreas. Occurrence of rectal prolapse. N Engl J Med 1958; *259*:409.

58. Moshang T, Holsclaw DS. Menarchal determinants in cystic fibrosis. Am J Dis Child 1980; *134*:1139–1142.

59. Sproul A, Huang NN. Growth patterns in children with cystic fibrosis. J Pediatr 1964; *65*:664.

60. Huang NN, Macri CN, Girone J, et al. Survival of patients with cystic fibrosis. Am J Dis Child 1970; *120*:289.

61. Berry HK, Kellogg FW, Hunt MM, et al. Dietary supplement and nutrition in children with cystic fibrosis. Am J Dis Child 1975; *129*:165–171.

62. Di Sant'Agnese PA, Davis PB. Cystic fibrosis in adults. Am J Med 1979; *64*:121.

63. Huang NN, Schidlow DV, Szatrowski TH, et al. Clinical

features, survival rate and prognostic factors in young adults with cystic fibrosis. Am J Med 1987; *82*:871–879.

64. Frisancho A: Triceps skin fold and upper arm muscle size norms for assessment of nutritional status. Am J Clin Nutr 1974; *27*:1052.

65. Kuo PT, Huang NN, Bassett DR. Effect of impaired fat absorption upon the fatty acid composition of serum chylomicra and adipose tissue in cystic fibrosis of the pancreas. Trans Assoc Am Phys 1961; *74*:147–162.

66. Chase HP, Dupont J. Abnormal levels of prostaglandins and fatty acids in blood of children with cystic fibrosis. Lancet 1978; *2*:236–238.

67. Dodge JA, Salter DC, Yassa JG. Essential fatty acid deficiency due to artificial diet in cystic fibrosis. Br Med J 1975; *2*:192–193.

68. Roy CC, Weber AM, Moim CL, et al. Abnormal biliary lipid composition in cystic fibrosis. N Engl J Med 1977; *297*:1301.

69. Roy CC, Delage G, Fontaine A, et al. The fecal microflora and bile acids in children with cystic fibrosis. Am J Clin Nutr 1979; *32*:2404–2409.

70. Fleisher DS, Di George AM, Barness LA, et al. Hyproproteinemia and edema in infants with cystic fibrosis of the pancreas. J Pediatr 1964; *64*:341.

71. Fleisher DS, Di George AM, Auerbach VH, et al. Protein metabolism in cystic fibrosis of the pancreas. J Pediatr 1964; *56*:349.

72. Shahidi NT, Diamond LK, Shwachman H: Anemia associated with protein deficiency: a study of two cases with cystic fibrosis. J Pediatr 1961; *59*:533.

73. Strober W, Georges P, Schwartz RH. Albumin metabolism in cystic fibrosis. Pediatrics 1969; *43*:416.

74. Nebert DW, Curtis DD. Hypoproteinemia and cystic fibrosis. Calif Med 1966; *104*:57.

75. Anderson C. Fibrocystic disease of the pancreas presenting with edema and hypoproteinemia. Med J Aust 1966; *2*:195.

76. Lock J. Breast milk–induced hypoproteinemic shock, coagulopathy, and siderocytic anemia in cystic fibrosis. J Pediatr 1974; *84*:912.

77. Walker WA, Ulstrom RA, Lowman JT. Albumin synthesis rates in patients with hypoproteinemia. J Pediatr 1971; *78*:812.

78. Antonowicz I, Reddy V, Khaw KT, et al. Lactase deficiency in patients with cystic fibrosis. Pediatrics 1968; *42*:492.

79. Rosan RC, Shwachman H, Kulcyzcki LL. Diabetes mellitus and cystic fibrosis of the pancreas. Am J Dis Child 1962; *104*:625–634.

80. Kaiser G, Zuppinger K, Joss E. Mucoviscidosis and diabetes mellitus. Helv Paediatr Acta 1970; *25*:135–146.

81. Holsclaw DS, Ruskin T, Soeldner SJ, et al. The development and characterization of diabetes mellitus in cystic fibrosis. Soc Pediatr Res Abst 1970; *74*:456.

82. Wilmshurst EG, Soeldner JS, Holsclaw DS, et al. Endogenous and exogenous insulin responses in patients with cystic fibrosis. Pediatrics 1975; *55*:75–82.

83. Lippe BM, Sperling MA, Dooley RR. Pancreatic alpha and beta cell function in cystic fibrosis. J Pediatr 1977; *90*:751–755.

84. Stahl M, Girard J, Rutishauser M, et al. Endocrine foundation of the pancreas in cystic fibrosis: evidence for an impaired glucagon and insulin response following arginine infusion. J Pediatr 1974; *84*:821–824.

85. Rosan RC, Kayne HL, Neiland ML, et al. Some metabolic responses to intravenous tolbutamide in patients with cystic fibrosis of the pancreas. Metabolism 1964; *13*:480–485.

86. Poncher JR, Rowley WF, Traisman HS. Cystic fibrosis and juvenile diabetes mellitus: a case report. J Indiana State Med Assoc 1967; *60*:907–909.

87. Schwachman H, Holsclaw DS. Complications of cystic fibrosis. N Engl J Med 1969; *281*:500–501.

88. Lippe BM, Kaplan SA, Neufeld ND, et al. Insulin receptors in cystic fibrosis: increased receptor number and altered affinity. Pediatrics 1980; *65*:1018–1022.

89. Darby CW, Davidson AGF, Desai ID: Muscular performance in cystic fibrosis patients and its relation to vitamin E. Arch Dis Child 1973; *48*:72.

90. Harris JT, Muller DPR. Absorption of different doses of fat soluble and water miscible preparations of vitamin E in children with cystic fibrosis. Arch Dis Child 1971; *46*:341.

91. Blanc WA, Reid JD, Andersen DH. Avitaminosis E in cystic fibrosis of the pancreas. Pediatrics 1958; *22*:494.

92. Quaife ML, Scrimshaw NS, Lowry OH. Micromethod for assay of total tocopherol in blood serum. J Biol Chem 1949; *180*:1229.

93. Gross S. Hemolytic anemia in premature infants: relationship to vitamin E, selenium, glutathione peroxidase and erythrocyte lipids. Semin Hematol 1976; *13*:187.

94. Tortenson OL, Humphrey GB, Edison JR, et al. Cystic fibrosis presenting with severe hemorrhage due to vitamin K malabsorption: a report of three cases. Pediatrics 1970; *45*:857.

95. Rucker RW, Harrison GM. Vitamin B_{12} deficiency in CF. N Engl J Med 1973; *289*:329.

96. Wang CI. Iron deficiency. *In* Huang N (ed). Guide to Drug Therapy in Patients with Cystic Fibrosis. Atlanta, Cystic Fibrosis Foundation, 1972, revised 1974: 124.

97. Ater AL, Herbst JJ, Landau SA, et al. Relative anemia and iron deficiency in CF. Pediatrics 1983; *71*:810.

98. Snodgrass W, Rumack BH, Sullivan JB, et al. Selenium: childhood poisoning and cystic fibrosis. Clin Toxicol 1981; *18*:211–220.

99. Lloyd-Still JD, Gauther HE. Selenium and glutathione peroxidase levels in cystic fibrosis. Pediatrics 1980; *65*:1010–1012.

100. Cox K, Cannon R, Watson R, et al. Selenium-responsive myositis during prolonged home total parenteral nutrition for cystic fibrosis. CF Abstracts 1983; *24*:106.

101. Van Rij AM. Selenium supplementation in total parenteral nutrition. JPEN 1981; *5*:120–124.

102. Gordon EF, Gordon RC, Passal DB. Zinc metabolism: basic, clinical and behavioral aspects. J Pediatr 1981; *99*:341–349.

103. Palin HO, Underwood BA, Denning CR. The effect of oral zinc supplementation on plasma levels of vitamin A and retinol-binding protein in cystic fibrosis. Pediatr Res 1976; *10*:358.

104. Jacob RA, Sanstead HH, Solomons NW, et al. Zinc status and vitamin A transport in cystic fibrosis. Am J Clin Nutr 1978; *31*:638.

105. Hambridge KM. The role of zinc and other trace metals in pediatric nutrition and health. Pediatr Clin North Am 1977; *24*:95.

106. Heller RM, Kirchner SG, O'Neill JA Jr, et al. Skeletal changes of copper deficiency in infants receiving prolonged total parenteral nutrition. J Pediatr 1978; *92*:947.

107. Solomons NW, Wagonfeld JB, Bieger C, et al. Some biochemical indices of nutrition in treated patients with cystic fibrosis. Am J Clin Nutr 1981; *34*:462.

108. Harper TB. Relationship of nutrition and pulmonary function in cystic fibrosis. (Letter.) J Pediatr 1983; *103*:164–165.

109. Huang NN, Van Loon EG, Sheng KT. The flora of the respiratory tract of patients with cystic fibrosis of the pancreas. J Pediatr 1961; *59*:512.

110. Mearns MB, Hunt GH, Rushwroth R. Bacterial flora of the respiratory tract of patients with cystic fibrosis. Arch Dis Child 1972; *47*:902.

111. Isles A, Maclusky I, Corey M, et al. *Pseudomonas cepacia* infection in cystic fibrosis: an emerging problem. J Pediatr 1984; *104*:206.

112. Ginsberg CM, McCracken GH. Cefaclor and cefadroxil: a commentary on their properties and possible indication for use in pediatrics. J Pediatr 1980; *96*:340.

113. Loeinging-Baucke VA, Mischler E, Myers MG. Placebo-controlled trial of cephalexin therapy in the ambulatory man-

agement of patients with cystic fibrosis. J Pediatr 1979; 95:630.

114. Huang NN, Palmer J, Keith H, et al. Comparative efficacy and tolerance study of azlocillin and carbenicillin in patients with cystic fibrosis: a double blind study. J Antimicrob Chemother 1983; 11(Suppl B):205–214.

115. McLaughlin FJ, Matthews WJ Jr, Strieder DJ, et al. Clinical and bacteriological responses to three antibiotic regimens for acute exacerbations of cystic fibrosis: ticarcillin-tobramycin, azlocillin-tobramycin, and azlocillin-placebo. J Infect Dis 1983; 147:559–567.

116. Prince AS, Neu HC. Use of piperacillin, a semi-synthetic penicillin, in the therapy of acute exacerbations of pulmonary disease in patients with cystic fibrosis. J Pediatr 1980; 97:148.

117. Padoan R, Brienza A, Crossingnani RM, et al. Ceftazidine in treatment of patients with cystic fibrosis. J Pediatr 1983; 103:320.

118. Meyers RM. Ototoxic effects of gentamicin. Arch Otolaryngol 1970; 92:160–162.

119. Kossek JC, Mazze RL, Cousins MJ. Nephrotoxicity of gentamicin. J Lab Invest 1974; 30:48–57.

120. Drouet FH, Davies T, Lederer DA, et al. The effect of ticarcillin on the hemostatic mechanism. J Pharm Pharmacol 1975; 27:964–966.

121. Stephens D, Garey N, Isles A, et al. Efficacy of inhaled tobramycin in the treatment of pulmonary exacerbations in children with cystic fibrosis. Pediatr Infect Dis 1983; 2:209–211.

122. Parson HG, Beaudry A, Dumas A, et al. Energy needs and growth in children with cystic fibrosis. J Pediatr Gastroenterol Nutr 1983; 2:44–49.

123. Waring WW. Current management of cystic fibrosis. Adv Pediatr 1976; 23:401–438.

124. Kao PT, Huang NN. The effect of medium chain triglyceride feeding on the fat metabolism of children with cystic fibrosis. J Clin Invest 1965; 44:1924–1933.

125. Gracey M, Burke V, Anderson CM. Assessment of medium-chain triglyceride feeding in infants with cystic fibrosis. Arch Dis Child 1969; 44:401–403.

126. Rosenlund ML, Selekam JA, Kim HK, et al. Dietary essential fatty acids in cystic fibrosis. Pediatrics 1977; 59:428–432.

127. Lloyd-Still JD, Johnson SB, Johnson RT, et al. Essential fatty acid status in cystic fibrosis and the effects of safflower oil supplementation. Am J Clin Nutr 1981; 34:1–7.

128. Chase HP, Dupont J: Abnormal levels of prostaglandins and fatty acids in blood of children with cystic fibrosis. Lancet 1978; 2:236–238.

129. Allan JD, Mason A, Moss AD. Nutritional supplementation in treatment of cystic fibrosis of the pancreas. Am J Dis Child 1973; 126:22–26.

130. Barclay RPC, Shannon RS. Trial of artificial diet in treatment of cystic fibrosis of the pancreas. Arch Dis Child 1975; 50:490–493.

131. Bertrand JM, Morin LC, Lasalle R, et al. Short-term clinical nutritional and functional effects of continuous elemental enteral alimentation in children with cystic fibrosis. J Pediatr 1984; 104:41.

132. Pencharz P, Levy L, Durie P. Nutritional rehabilitation of malnourished cystic fibrosis patient by supplemental nocturnal gastrostomy feeding. Cystic Fibrosis Club Abstract 1984: 11.

133. Smith JL, Arteaga C, Heymsfield SB. Increased ureagenesis and impaired nitrogen use durng infusion of a synthetic amino acid formula: a controlled trial. N Engl J Med 1982; 306:1013.

134. Rudman D, Milikan WT, Richardson TJ, et al. Elemental balances during intravenous hyperalimentation of underweight adult subjects. J Clin Invest 1975; 55:94.

135. Heird WC, Winters RW. Total parenteral nutrition—the state of the art. J Pediatr 1975; 86:2–16.

136. Copeland EM Jr, Dudrick SJ: Intravenous hyperalimentation as adjunctive treatment in the cancer patient. Clin Digest 1976; 5:1.

137. Goldberg M, Tyrala EE. Parenteral Nutrition Guide. Philadelphia, St. Christopher's Hospital for Children, Temple University School of Medicine, 1982.

138. Shwachman H, Lebenthal E, Khaw KT. Recurrent acute pancreatitis in patients with cystic fibrosis with normal pancreatic enzymes. Pediatrics 1975; 55:86.

139. Graham DY: Enzyme replacement therapy of exocrine pancreatic insufficiency in man. N Engl J Med 1977; 296:1314.

140. DiMagno EP, Malagelada JR, Go VL, et al. Fate of orally ingested enzymes in pancreatic insufficiency: comparison of two dosage schedules. N Engl J Med 1977; 296:1318.

141. Graham DY. An enteric coated pancreatic enzyme preparation that works. Dig Dis Sci 1979; 24:906.

142. Khaw KT, Adeniyi S, Gordon D, et al. Efficacy of pancreatic preparations on fat and nitrogen absorptions in cystic fibrosis patients. Pediatr Res 1978; 12:444.

143. Warwick WJ, Budd JR. Comparison of 2 forms of enteric coated pancrelipase in 6 teenagers with cystic fibrosis. Clin Ther 1982; 5:15–20.

144. Finber L, Bernstein J. Acute hyponatremic dehydration. J Pediatr 1971; 79:499–503.

145. Douglas WAC. Acute salt depletion in fibrocystic disease of the pancreas. Med J Aust 1959; 46:962.

146. Orenstein DM, Henke KG, Costil DL, et al. Exercise and heat stress in cystic fibrosis patients. Pediatr Res 1983; 17:267.

23

ALCOHOL-ASSOCIATED DISEASES

FRANK L. IBER

Ethyl alcohol is the only habit-forming substance used in sufficient quantity to substitute as a macronutrient. It is totally absorbed and subsequently oxidized and produces 7.1 kcal/g. A standard portion of wine, beer, or distilled liquor contains 10 to 15 g of alcohol but is fairly naked of other known nutrients. Alcohol is used socially at least once a month by at least 85 per cent of North American adults. Social drinking with no identifiable adverse consequences to nutrition or health consists of 1 to 3 portions of alcohol on the average each day (10 to 45 g). Levels substantially in excess of these produce organ damage and behavioral changes that are associated with dependency and are called alcoholism. Alcoholism usually means that 20 to 75 per cent of the basal caloric intake is in the form of beverage alcohol, which is nearly empty of other nutrients.[1]

A small fraction of alcohol users, about 10 per cent, become dependent upon sustained intake of alcohol. These persons use alcohol continually throughout the day and evening, taking an initial amount sufficient to raise the blood level to 100 to 250 mg/dl and repeated portions each 1 or 2 hours to maintain the blood level. These alcoholics may consume 100 to 300 g of alcohol each day and develop impressive metabolic and neurological tolerance;[2] such tolerance prevents them from appearing drunk. By metabolic tolerance we mean the rate of conversion of ethanol to acetaldehyde and acetate is increased from the normal of approximately 10 g/hr at blood levels of about 100 mg/dl to two or even three times this level.[3] By neurological tolerance we mean that neurological and psychological processes are less impaired at a given blood level.[4,5] Both tolerances develop in alcoholics, permitting them to function in job, family, and society to a reasonable degree. Subjects with milder degrees of alcoholism drink continually for 6 to 12 hours each day, or in binges. Both develop tolerance, but manifest intoxication is infrequent.

The requirement for frequent and large portions of alcohol to support alcoholic drinking leads to certain stereotyped behavior patterns that influence health and nutritional intervention. The behaviors include denial of the need for alcohol to self and others, secretiveness in drinking, and a covert resistance to all forces to change their drinking pattern. Alcoholics develop major *self-denial* about the problem, its influence on their lives, and the lives of others. This constitutes genuine inner belief, not just a front that is presented to the therapist; all health treatment or treatment designed in one way or another to alter lifestyle must deal with this incessantly and repeatedly. To "trust" a person with alcoholism to be fully compliant with a sobriety program featuring abstinence, diet, and other treatment measures represents extreme naiveté on the part of the therapist, unless coupled with careful confirmatory checks to assist in overcoming denial. Many alcoholics become effective in their denial by making all therapeutic shortcomings the fault of the therapist, with no role for themselves. This skill is often not dealt with by physicians, nutritionists, or other health professionals caring for one aspect of the person's problem.[6,7]

Alcoholism is a chronic disease with remissions and relapses. Effective treatment increases the duration of remissions and renders the relapses shorter and less destructive. Almost all subjects will experience relapse, and the therapist needs to learn how to deal with it. The successful management of alcoholism follows measures that increase compliance with almost any change in habits. The involvement of family, friends, and employers in the process is useful, as are frequent contact with therapy of one form or another and use of self-help groups (such as Alcoholics Anonymous). All forms of health care in which the patient will participate are beneficial to control the alcoholism. Often nutritional counseling will be accepted and slowly influence the patient's health behavior in unrelated ways. Table 23–1 lists some features of the alcoholic patient that should be understood by all health professionals attempting to assist these people.

The widespread reversible injury to many organ systems in alcoholics is not widely appreciated. The injuries to the thought processes, to the peripheral nerves, and to the liver are often those most recognized by health workers, but inability to perform sexually is often of more concern to the subject. The brain is regularly shown impaired by psychological testing of memory, abstract reasoning, complex mental motor coordination, or reaction time in the chronic alcoholic. The lesions are reversible and usually return to normal by the third week after drinking ceases. Therefore, patients receiving instructions

during this period are less likely to remember directions and less able to participate in educational programs than they will be a few weeks later.[8]

Damage to sensory nerves, skeletal musculature, or occasionally motor nerves is present in at least 20 per cent of all alcoholic patients, with the less affluent usually showing more marked changes.[9] Return to physical labor is often not feasible because of these changes; they seem slowly reversible. The small intestine is uniformly injured in alcoholics in a manner interfering with active transport.[10,11]

The complex aspects of perception and performance involved in a healthy, fulfilling sex life can be impaired by alterations of the behavioral, hormonal, or neurological pathways, so many alcoholics have sexual performance problems. Alcohol is injurious to the testis,[12] alcohol ingestion alters the synthesis and release of peptide and steroid hormones, and the alcoholic has emotional pressures producing anxiety; all of these factors impact on sexuality. Fortunately, the majority of the changes are sufficiently reversible that sexual perception and performance may improve, but this may require several years.[13]

Specific or generalized nutrient depletion is common and occasionally reaches sufficient degree to cause symptoms or even pathology. Most important in impaired nutrition is an inadequate diet during drinking. Neville and coworkers recorded total intake in a group of male construction laborers during a drinking period and during one in which they were not drinking.[14] They found that while drinking these men met caloric requirements with almost half coming from alcohol, but fell below the RDA for protein, magnesium, iron, calcium, thiamine, riboflavin, folate, and vitamins A and D. Studies conducted in drinking alcoholics or alcoholics immediately after drinking ceases have demonstrated impairment in the absorption of thiamine, riboflavin, pyridoxine, folate, and vitamins A, D, and C. Calcium, magnesium, zinc, and selenium are malabsorbed. Absorption of all of these nutrients is restored to normal in 1 or 2 weeks after drinking stops.[10,11] Other factors contributing to malnutrition are noted in Table 23–2.

Alcoholic patients often eat where they drink, increasing the availability of snack foods and lessening

TABLE 23–1. General Aspects of Alcoholism

Chronic disease—relapses occur
Denial and poor compliance continue
A withdrawal syndrome occurs each time drinking stops
Injury to most organ systems occurs with drinking
Specific or general malnutrition is common
Trauma and suicide as sequelae

TABLE 23–2. Factors Contributing to Macro- and Micronutrient Deficiency in Drinking Alcoholics

Major Factors
Impaired dietary intake of nutrients
Intestinal injury blocking active transport

Minor Factors
Distorted diet other than beverages
  Food availability
  Poor dentition
  Smoking
Increased requirements or body losses
Disease
  Pancreatitis
  Liver disease

the intake of fruits, vegetables, and proteins. Alcoholic patients from age 20 to 50 lose teeth at approximately three times the rate of the nonalcoholic population and often have problems with mastication or are edentulous.[15] Almost all alcoholic patients smoke cigarettes, and this changes the taste of many foods. The metabolism of alcohol increases the requirement for certain B vitamins, including folate and pyridoxine. Alcohol produces an increased urinary loss of magnesium, zinc, potassium, and phosphorus. If there is diarrhea in the alcoholic, depletions of these materials as well as calcium and selenium may be prominent. If there is pancreatic insufficiency associated with acute or chronic pancreatitis, fat malabsorption may be prominent and many nutrients may be altered in absorption or lost from the body. Liver disease destroys the ability of the liver to store trace nutrients and releases them to the body at times of inadequate intake.

Finally, accidental injury in the home, in the workplace, or on the roads is more common in alcoholics than in other persons. Alcohol impairs both reaction time and judgment, and by these means may lead to more risk-taking with less capability. Almost one third of all suicides are by alcoholics, emphasizing the serious depression that may accompany this condition. Persons dealing with alcoholics need some knowledge of these things in order to assist alcoholic patients.

LIVER METABOLISM OF ALCOHOL

The regular consumption and metabolism of ethanol in amounts from 10 to 70 per cent of the total ingested calories alters the metabolism of *nearly all substances*, and as might be expected, has profound influences on the intermediary metabolism of many nutrients.[16] Ethanol is produced by gut organisms in all humans, and these small amounts (or larger beverage amounts) are eliminated by oxidation, the initial steps of which occur in the liver.[17] Absorption is total, but is somewhat slower from the stomach than from the small intestine.[18] The ingestion of alcohol with foods that retard gastric emptying slow the entry into the blood stream; drinking on an empty stomach or following any form of stomach surgery increases the rate of entry.[19] Absorption is into the portal vein, and the liver normally clears the alcohol until its metabolism is saturated. The hepatocyte contains two important pathways for ethanol metabolism. The alcohol dehydrogenase (ADH) pathway is the most important in social drinkers and is located in the cytosol. There is also a microsomal ethanol-oxidizing system (MEOS) located in the endoplasmic reticulum; a third system, catalase, located in peroxisomes, is quite unimportant in man. Alcoholics approximately double their alcohol-oxidizing capacity, mostly by increasing the MEOS pathway.[20]

The alcohol dehydrogenase pathway reduces one molecule of nicotinamide adenine dinucleotide (NAD) to form NADH and produces one mole of acetaldehyde, and the rate-limiting step is the dissociation of the NADH-enzyme complex.

$$CH_3CH_2OH + NAD \xrightarrow{ADH} CH_3CHO + NADH^+ + H$$

Two important metabolic consequences of this reaction occur: (1) excess reducing equivalents are produced in the liver cell, and (2) acetaldehyde is produced. The nearly obligate removal from the liver cytosol of NAD and its replacement with NADH during alcohol oxidation alters every liver reaction that depends upon NAD concentration. Table 23–3 lists some of the consequences that are important in clinical medicine or nutrition. These changes and those of acetaldehyde injury will be discussed below. There is a great deal of variability in humans in the genetic makeup of alcohol dehydrogenase,[32] and the total amount of enzyme diminishes with prolonged starvation and is lowered in alcoholics.[33,34] Although excesses of the enzyme do not seem to be associated with increased rates of ethanol metabolism, owing to limitations in NAD regeneration, diminished amounts seem to be associated with slow alcohol metabolism.[33]

Alternative pathways for ethanol metabolism are clearly present and function to metabolize significant amounts of alcohol. Complete inhibition of ADH

TABLE 23–3. Consequences of an Increased NADH+/ NAD Ratio in Liver Cells—Changed Redox Potential

Increased lactate/pyruvate ratio
  Associated with a metabolic acidosis
  Increased serum lactate[21]
  Elevated serum uric acid[22]

Citric acid cycle slowed[23]
  Increased 2,3-diglycerophosphate[23]
  Altered oxygen dissociation from hemoglobin

Decreased hepatic lipid oxidation and increased hepatic lipid storage
  Increased VLDL synthesis and release[24]
  Serum hyperlipemia[25]
  Fatty liver[26]
  Elevated cholesterol[26]

Altered mitochondrial redox state[21]
  Increased ketogenesis
  Increased blood beta-hydroxybutyrate/acetoacetate ratio

Impaired metabolism
  Galactose[27]
  Serotonin
  Impaired glutathione synthesis[28]
  Impaired glucuronide synthesis
  Steroids[29]

Impaired movement of folate into and out of liver storage
  Impaired liver uptake from diet[30]
  Lowered serum folate[31]
  Lowered bile folate

with pyrazinamide in animals slows alcohol oxidation by about 50 per cent;[35] radioisotopic tracer experiments indicate that acetaldehyde made from labeled ethanol arises from pathways other than ADH.[36] Furthermore, a strain of deer mice has been discovered that totally lack the ADH enzyme,[37] and their MEOS increases following alcohol ingestion or the ingestion of other agents that increase the endoplasmic reticulum of the liver.[38] This enzyme requires NAD and molecular oxygen.

$$CH_3CH_2OH + 1/2\ O_2 \xrightarrow[\text{MEOS}]{\text{NADP}} CH_3CHO + H_2O$$

The enzyme in man is of particular importance when alcohol is consumed in excess of 50 g/day and probably alone accounts for increased alcohol metabolism at blood levels that saturate ADH. The major nutritional consequence of the MEOS is that it is wasteful of energy.[39] Its resulting cofactor NADPH cannot be coupled with oxidative phosphorylation, and, therefore, produces heat. The ADH pathway produces NADH, which is efficiently coupled with oxidative phosphorylation and produces useful energy.

Thus, in rats, there is a rise in body temperature in animals fed large amounts of alcohol;[40] growth is less when alcohol is substituted in large amounts isocalorically for carbohydrate,[41] and studies in humans indicate that the addition of 2000 excess kilocalories as ethanol does not result in the expected weight gain.[39] The studies of Mendenhall and coworkers[42] in patients with liver disease suggest that the alcohol energy in the diet did not produce the weight gain that would be expected with excess energy intake from other sources.

Consequences of increased MEOS pathway include hypertrophy of the endoplasmic reticulum[38] and acceleration of most of the enzymes residing there. This increase in the activity of drug-metabolizing enzymes adequately accounts for the increased rate of drug clearance in humans.[43] In humans, the clearance rates of barbiturate,[44] propranolol,[45] warfarin, phenytoin, tolbutamide,[43] and isoniazid[46] have all been reported accelerated, a 50 per cent shorter clearance time being typical.[43] A further consequence of this increased metabolism in the endoplasmic reticulum is the enhanced toxicity of drugs that become toxic only when oxidized. Carbon tetrachloride was observed to be more toxic in alcoholics.[47] It is to be emphasized that alcohol is capable of increasing metabolism in the endoplasmic reticulum in animals, but the congeners (higher alcohols and other aromatics present in beverages) are probably even more potent in this effect and may be responsible for many of the changes observed in man.[48]

Acetaldehyde and its oxidation product acetate may contribute to metabolic changes. The chronic ingestion of alcohol leads to increased levels of acetaldehyde, and this becomes even more marked if there is liver damage.[49,50] Acetaldehyde seems responsible for the flush in some Japanese who develop marked plethora after one or two drinks.[51] Acetaldehyde interferes with pyridoxal phosphate metabolism by displacing it from its binding protein, and thus results in increased breakdown.[52] Acetaldehyde has been incriminated in production of tissue damage in many sites in the alcoholic.[53] Reasonable but unproven hypotheses implicate this molecule in cardiomyopathy and addiction.[54]

An intermediate product of all alcohol metabolism is acetate. The presence of more acetate causes the body to increase many reactions that are stimulated by two carbon substances. The synthesis of lipids, cholesterol, alanine, and taurine, and the use of acetate in conjugation reactions are all increased when alcohol is utilized.[55]

The many changes in Table 23–3 need to be at least partially comprehended by those working with the alcoholic in order to develop some sense of the broad disruption of ordinary metabolism by continual alcohol abuse. The items in Table 23–3 are those that have been directly proved or hypothesized to be related to temporary reduction of available cofactor NAD, by the oxidation of alcohol. Oxidations, such as that of galactose, requiring NAD, totally stop; glucose utilization slows markedly in the liver because NAD is needed to accept hydrogen removed from the substrate. In contrast, the monophosphate shunt and fructose metabolism are unchanged. Alcohol produces activated two-carbon fragments that stop the oxidation of long-chain fatty acids and increase hepatic lipid syntheses, storage, and release. A variety of intermediates are altered in their availability, and pathways of drug and hormone metabolism are changed because of altered redox pathways.[22]

Changes in hepatocyte lipid metabolism are illustrative of what occurs in all animals and in man.[56,57] The oxidation of fatty acids nearly ceases when the energy requirements of the cell are derived almost exclusively from alcohol. Hepatocytes make increased amounts of acylglycerols and store fatty acids reaching the liver. In addition, hepatocytes synthesize and release more triglycerides and cholesterol into the blood as VLDL than do livers not exposed to ethanol excess. There is increased fat content of the liver during times of no fat ingestion, the composition of which reflects endogenous hepatic lipogenesis.[25] The increased release of these fats into the blood accounts for alcoholic hyperlipemia, often sufficiently prominent to make the serum lactescent. Approximately 25 per cent of all regular users of alcohol have sufficiently elevated serum lipids to be classified as having Type IV hyperlipidemia.[58] It is uncertain whether part of the alcoholic hyperlipidemia is genetically determined. In addition to increased VLDL serum concentration, alcoholic patients also have augmented concentrations of the so-called atherosclerosis protective serum factor; this may be responsible for the beneficial effect of 1 to 4 drinks per day in preventing male coronary artery disease. This explanation has been expanded by a recent study.[59]

COMMON FORMS OF MALNUTRITION IN THE ALCOHOLIC

Total Calories and Protein

Changes in energy balance are most readily suspected based on a history of weight loss in the recent past and measurement of the height and weight for comparison with standards. Further information is obtained from measurement of the triceps skinfold thickness to estimate depot fat and of the arm muscle circumference to estimate skeletal muscle mass. Estimation of the visceral protein stores is obtained from the serum albumin and the transferrin values. Very infrequently, the creatinine-height index as an indicator of lean body mass, estimation of the nitrogen balance from the nitrogen intake and the urinary excretion, and assessment of the cellular immune function by skin testing are used to clarify nutritional status.[60] A trained person conscious of nutrition needs and estimations is essentially as good in recognition of calorie and protein problems as a less trained person utilizing the measurements noted above, but nearly all surveys emphasize that severe malnutrition affecting recovery from disease is widely under-recognized.

Malnutrition, as estimated from weight loss or protein changes, is most severe in the very heavy drinkers, subjects without regular households, and those with liver disease. A recent study[42] surveying 293 veterans entering the hospital with liver disease who consumed 228 g (1600 kcal) of alcohol per day found clinically significant weight loss in 16 to 30 per cent, depending upon criteria, but the mean weight of the group was not significantly reduced. These patients were consuming in excess of 1500 kcal in nonalcoholic foods. However, the creatinine-height index was 84 per cent of standard in patients with no liver disease and 63 per cent in those with moderate or severe liver injury. The triceps skinfold was 73 per cent of standard in those with no liver disease and 60 per cent in those with the most severe disease. Of this group, 30 to 64 per cent were anergic to at least one skin test. On the basis of this study, 42 per cent of the patients free from cirrhosis on biopsy, but with alcoholic liver damage, were rated as having marasmus (low lean body weight and below the ideal body weight) compared with 48 per cent of those who had cirrhosis. In contrast, only patients with cirrhosis showed a kwashiorkor syndrome, with 8 per cent showing low visceral proteins and markedly decreased skin sensitivity. All of these groups improved on subsequent follow-up with abstinence

from alcohol and a diet at home or in the hospital. A working understanding of energy metabolism in alcoholics therefore is that most alcoholics do not lose weight, but in those few patients who have lost weight during the previous 3 months, or those in whom the lean body mass or the height-weight index is below 80 per cent of standard, one should suspect severe disease in some organ or a specific nutrient deficiency. The weight loss of the alcoholic patient free of other disease can be regained within 1 or 2 months of abstinence and good nutrition.

Goldsmith and colleagues[9] investigated the force required to pluck hairs from the head. The pulling force diminishes in protein malnutrition and returns to normal in most alcoholics over several weeks of normal dietary intake. They also found that the epilation force, as well as the midarm muscle circumference and the hematocrit, were significantly lower in low-income alcoholics, as contrasted with medium-income ones.[9,61]

The protein ingestion of alcoholic patients[14,61] is nearly always below the RDA, but often is in the range of 0.2 g/kg, an amount eaten regularly by some healthy populations. In acute experiments in man and animals, impaired amino acid active transport by the small intestine is observed at levels of alcohol often attained in drinking persons. Furthermore, alcohol present in the range of 230 mg/dl impairs the hepatic uptake of absorbed amino acids. Although digestion and absorption of proteins and amino acids is retarded, excretion of increased nitrogen in the stool is infrequent, suggesting this slowing is of no practical importance.

Numerous changes in the plasma amino acid profile have been noted in alcoholics as compared with normal persons. There is a selective increase in the plasma branched-chain amino acids and in alpha-amino-n-butyric acid in the absence of any liver disease,[63] and a similar change has been noted in the baboon model.[64] If there is dietary protein deficiency, then the branched-chain amino acids fall to normal or are depressed.[65] The finding of depressed branched-chain amino acids is the most common one in patients entering inner-city alcoholism treatment programs, suggesting that these subjects are protein-depleted.[63,66] When liver disease develops with portal systemic shunting, there is prominent hyperglucagonemia[67] and often hyperinsulinemia.[68] These changes of insulin and glucagon further diminish the branched-chain amino acids. If there is liver disease, the levels of tyrosine and phenylalanine and the sulfur-containing amino acids are elevated.[69] Alpha-amino-n-butyric acid is a product of methionine and threonine metabolism, and increases after 4 or more weeks of steady alcohol ingestion.[70] This has been utilized as a marker of continued alcoholism and is quite valuable in studies using inner-city patients, but does not seem applicable in private patient referral studies.[70]

Protein malnutrition is common in alcoholics.

Modest reductions in forearm muscle circumference and lean body mass often lead to major underestimation of the severe reduction in visceral protein; measurements of serum albumin and transferrin, as well as lymphocyte counts, should be performed in every hospitalized patient. In a stress situation, such as trauma, infection, or emergency surgery, the alcoholic may need parenteral repletion of proteins. A trial of parenteral amino acid administration to patients with alcoholic liver disease has demonstrated a beneficial effect on survival and recovery.[71] The optimal method of treating the widespread visceral protein depletion has not been clearly addressed by careful study.

Specific Micronutrients

Water-Soluble Vitamins

Folate, thiamine, riboflavin, and pyridoxine seem more severely impaired in the alcoholic than other water-soluble vitamins.[72] Alcohol interferes with the metabolism of these substances at fairly specific sites in their complex absorption, storage, and utilization. Deficiencies of ascorbic acid and nicotinic acid occur more commonly in alcoholics than in populations at large, but this may be related solely to impaired intake and absorption. Though vitamin B_{12} levels are low, B_{12} deficiency is extremely rare in alcoholics.

Folic Acid. Folate occurs in the diet as complex polyglutamates that must be hydrolyzed for absorption. This hydrolysis is impaired in the alcoholic patient, leading to less absorption.[73,74] Absorption of folate in simple form has been shown to be impaired in the advanced alcoholic with damage to the small intestine, as noted by other measures of absorption. Folate is stored in the liver and is released to maintain the serum level. Some folate is constantly excreted into the bile to protect the small intestinal mucosa. The acute administration of alcohol to man diminishes hepatic release of folate[75] with a fall in the serum level,[30] an increased excretion into the urine,[31] a fall in biliary level,[75] and a failure to incorporate labeled folate into the marrow.[76] Sullivan and Herbert[77] demonstrated that the folate requirement in drinking alcoholics was more than twice that of a nondrinking person.[78] It is clear that alcohol interferes with folate absorption, storage, and utilization in a variety of specific ways not applicable to other trace nutrients, and, in part, explaining why this is one of the most prevalent trace nutrient deficiencies.

Measurement of serum folate is a valuable screening method for folate deficiency when the patient is not drinking,[79] but may be erroneously low, not reflecting body stores, when the person is drinking alcohol. In practice, it is the custom to give 1 to 5 mg of parenteral folate to nearly all patients drinking heavily. If granulocytopenia or macrocytic anemia is present, the same dose of folate will usually correct the anemia if secondary to folate deficiency. The cellular resistance to infection and the maintenance of tissue healing make the availability of folic acid urgent, and it is one of several vitamins that should be used liberally. A drinking alcoholic would probably require in excess of 120 μg daily to assure no folate deficiency if the drinking were to continue. Thus, 1 mg weekly should be sufficient.

Thiamine. Thiamine is absorbed from the diet by an active alcohol-sensitive and a passive alcohol-insensitive process. The simultaneous ingestion of thiamine in food with alcohol diminishes thiamine absorption by as much as 70 per cent and would be of importance in subjects ingesting marginal diet.[80,81] There do not appear to be other mechanisms by which alcohol interferes with thiamine metabolism. Once liver disease intervenes, the activation of thiamine pyrophosphate and the storage of excess thiamine are impaired.[82] Thiamine status can best be assessed by the direct measurement of thiamine or thiamine pyrophosphate in the serum, by bioassay using the microorganism *Ochronas danica*, by high-pressure liquid chromatography (HPLC) assay, or by assay of the red cell transketolase. None of these assays are widely available, but studies by Frank and Baker[83] show low levels in 40 to 80 per cent of inner-city patients; Neville and associates,[14] in contrast, found normal levels in a group of middle-class patients studied in Pittsburgh.

The severe mental changes noted in Wernicke-Korsakov syndrome[84,85] can be permanent or fatal; the known peripheral nerve injuries associated with thiamine deficiency, and the common occurrence of thiamine deficiency in alcoholics, has led to widespread treatment with thiamine supplements, usually without establishing that the deficiency exists; the syndrome is under-recognized. We recommend giving initially 100 mg parenterally to correct body stores. Daily ingestion of 10 mg or more is sufficient to maintain repletion.

Pyridoxine. The acetaldehyde produced by the oxidation of alcohol displaces pyridoxal phosphate from hepatic cytosol-binding protein leading to its more rapid hydrolysis and loss from the body. This probably is responsible for the apparent increase in pyridoxine requirements and in the widespread finding of reduced levels of this material in alcoholic patients.[72] The most sensitive measure is the serum pyridoxal phosphate, but in practice this measurement is not commonly available. Although studies in man frequently demonstrate deficiency, and approximately 50 per cent of poorer inner-city alcoholic patients have this problem, there are few clinical concomitants of this.[9] Recent studies have shown that the serum alanine aminotransferase in the liver and in the serum requires pyridoxine as a cofactor; the provision of pyridoxine supplements to patients with liver disease is associated with a rise of the enzyme in the serum and in the liver.

Riboflavin. Inner-city alcoholic persons with peripheral neuritis had reduced serum levels of riboflavin.[86] Approximately one quarter of patients with cirrhosis from a similar study also had low serum levels. A sensitive assay has been developed in red cells of the enzyme glutathione reductase studied before and after the additions of its cofactor NAD.[87] Using this assay, Rosenthal and coworkers[87] found riboflavin deficiency in half the chronic alcoholics studied from New York City. Although these chemical deficiencies have been prominent, syndromes related to them have been less clearly described.

Other Water-Soluble Vitamins. Pellagra with its three D's (dementia, dermatitis, diarrhea) is more common in alcoholics than in a general population, because of nicotinic acid deficiency; however, recognition of this disease is often difficult.[85] Most alcoholics have modest impairment of mental function not related to nicotinic acid deficiency, bowel disturbances are not uncommon, and the dermatitis is typical and diagnostic only when the patient has had a great deal of exposure to the sun. The observation of three or four classic cases each year in Baltimore when the spring sun becomes very prominent suggests that we miss the atypical cases the rest of the year. Direct assays of serum and red cells are available.

Scurvy, due to ascorbic acid deficiency, is rarely seen in our population. Vitamin B_{12} serum levels are often elevated, even though measurement of B_{12} absorption is impaired. A deficiency is almost never encountered.

FAT-SOLUBLE VITAMINS

Vitamin A. Vitamin A nutriture is occasionally impaired in alcoholics, and almost always impaired in those who develop cirrhosis or pancreatitis and continue to drink.[88,89] Vitamin A occurs in the diet as retinyl esters or as beta-carotene; both must be converted to retinol in order to enter the intestinal cells. In the mucosa, retinol is esterified to retinyl palmitate and absorbed in the chylomicrons. The circulating chylomicrons progressively lose their triglyceride load by interaction with lipoprotein lipase throughout the body; the retinyl palmitate remains with the chylomicron remnants and is taken up by a specific receptor on the surface of the hepatocytes. On entering the liver it is hydrolyzed, but storage occurs in the form of retinyl palmitate. Vitamin A is released from the liver as retinol tightly bound to a hepatically produced transport protein called retinol-binding protein (RBP) which is capable of transporting retinol to all of the cells of the body that require it. Once in the final cell, it is oxidized to retinal by zinc-containing enzymes. In the serum, vitamin A is found as retinyl palmitate tightly bound to chylomicrons or as retinol tightly bound to RBP, free retinyl esters are not found normally.[90] Retinyl esters occur after liver damage, in vitamin A toxicity,

and in a few alcoholic patients with cirrhosis. The functional availability of vitamin A in the eye can be measured by the level of dark adaptation.

In alcoholic patients, the serum concentrations of vitamin A (measuring all forms, retinol-RBP, retinyl esters) are frequently in the low-normal range and absorption tests show impairment.[89] About 2 per cent of alcoholics have impaired dark adaptation that is corrected by treatment with vitamin A despite marginally low levels in the serum. In contrast, about 40 per cent of drinking alcoholic cirrhotic patients will show impaired dark adaptation, which can be corrected by vitamin A.[89] The liver in alcoholic patients is less able to take up chylomicron remnants, resulting in persistence of chylomicron remnants in the circulation longer than normal. This is strikingly abnormal in cirrhosis, with some cirrhotic patients unable to clear the serum of remnants in 24 hours, in contrast to the normal clearance in 2 to 3 hours. Further, in severe cirrhosis, there is an inability to release retinol from the liver because of limited manufacture of retinol-binding protein. Liver stores of vitamin A are reduced in all forms of alcoholic liver injury, with cirrhosis showing the greatest reduction.[91]

In practice, specific clinical disease due to vitamin A deficiency is very infrequent in the alcoholic free of liver disease, and the deficiency is corrected by normal dietary intake. The cirrhotic deficiency is common and infrequently associated with mild skin changes and visual impairment. If pancreatic insufficiency is present, the damage is even more marked and may result in severe retinal injury. The status is readily estimated by measurement of the serum vitamin A level, and if this is low, a vitamin A supplement should be administered. If there is no jaundice, 25,000 IU is needed daily for 1 or 2 months. After this interval, serum levels should be remeasured.

Vitamin D. Vitamin D arises from both the diet and direct manufacture in the skin from sunlight exposure. Alcoholics often have limited exposure to sunlight, and their dietary intake of vitamin D is usually low. The absorption is impaired with heavy intake of alcohol, not unlike absorption of vitamin A.[92] Once vitamin D is in the body, two hydroxylations occur—the first in the liver, the second in the kidney—to form the active vitamin that causes the synthesis of a protein in the intestinal mucosa that increases calcium absorption. The measurement of 25-hydroxycholecalciferol is an excellent assessment of vitamin D status. This was found diminished in 8 of 112 severe alcoholics surveyed in our unit, but promptly rose to normal with supplementation. Low serum levels of 25-hydroxy vitamin D are even more common in alcoholic patients with cirrhosis, but can also be corrected with supplementation.[94] Since alcohol could affect calcium absorption, as well as vitamin D absorption or intermediary metabolism, it is appropriate to consider the effects of chronic alcoholism on bone calcium stores. In our studies of alcoholic males without cirrhosis in Baltimore, using the photon absorption of the radius and ulna, we found no difference between 108 men drinking alcohol for a mean of 14 years and free-living controls. Others using similar or different techniques have found similar changes.[94,95] It is our view that vitamin D nutriture in the alcoholic human is not usually clinically important. In alcoholic cirrhosis, there is no clear evidence that bone disease is accelerated.

Vitamins E and K. Although the absorption of these vitamins in the small intestine may be impaired, there is little evidence that clinical deficiency results from either in the alcoholic person. The manufacture and absorption of vitamin K in the colon probably is responsible for the lack of vitamin K deficiency in alcoholism. Vitamin E deficiency has been reported in severe chronic jaundice but not in alcoholic patients.[96] When liver disease occurs, deficiency in absorption and utilization of vitamin K are often present, resulting in clinically apparent bleeding problems.

MINERALS

The person exposed to alcohol over many months is often depleted in magnesium, zinc, potassium, and phosphate. Each of these can be sufficiently severe to produce symptoms, and these may infrequently be life-threatening. Chronic alcoholism produces urinary losses of magnesium, zinc, and potassium, and this, coupled with impaired intake, is probably responsible for the depletions. The serum levels of all of these are reasonable assays of the depletion. Potassium deficiency is often associated with muscular weakness and increased confusion. Levels of serum phosphate less than 1 mg/dl have been associated with paralysis. Low serum magnesium has been associated with tetany, muscular weakness, and hypocalcemia. Zinc deficiency may produce dermatitis, impaired dark adaptation, or apparent inability to overcome minor infections. All of these materials are depleted; if there is prominent diarrhea, supplements are usually required.[97–99]

Although calcium, iron, and selenium[100] are also lost from the body during drinking, it is unusual to have symptomatic depletion. Iron deficiency anemia, when present, is usually caused by bleeding.

DISEASES COMMON IN ALCOHOLICS AND THEIR SPECIAL NUTRITIONAL PROBLEMS

Skin and Mucous Membrane Disease

Table 23–4 lists common skin and mucous membrane conditions to be searched for in alcoholic patients. Recognition of the vitamin deficiencies requires usually only the consideration of the possibility. Confirmatory tests are often available, but

TABLE 23–4. Skin and Mucous Membrane Disorders to be Considered in Alcoholic Patients

Deficiency disease
  Riboflavin deficiency—cheilosis, sore tongue
  Pellagra—scaly, hyperpigmented, erythema, symmetrical in sun-exposed areas
  Vitamin A deficiency—dry, scaly skin
  Zinc deficiency—perioral, perianal crusting

Cancers
  Lip
  Mouth
  Nasopharynx

Disease of neglect
  Scabies
  Pediculosis

Rare
  Porphyria cutanea tarda

a therapeutic trial will correct deficiencies of water-soluble nutrients in 1 week and fat-soluble ones in 3 weeks.

Musculoskeletal Disease

Table 23–5 lists several categories of musculoskeletal disorders commonly occurring in alcoholic patients. Wasting of muscles, associated with protein malnutrition and disuse atrophy, is the most common cause of weakness in the alcoholic, but several forms of myopathy are also known.[101] Trauma, often not recalled by the patient in giving the history, is sufficiently common to enter all differential diagnoses. The use of muscle enzymes, such as creatine phosphokinase and aldolase, aids recognition of the myopathy. Only rarely are electromyographic studies required for diagnosis. Treatment with removal of all alcohol, with good nutrition, and with increased physical activity is usually satisfactory. Trauma appears to be the major cause of bone injury in the alcoholic patient. Aseptic necrosis of the femoral head occurs in alcoholic patients far more frequently than chance alone should dictate.

Neurological Disease

Alcohol is used socially for its central nervous system effect, and the development of tolerance occurs

TABLE 23–5. Muscle and Bone Disorders in Alcoholic Patients

Muscle problems
  Trauma—asymmetrical
  Acute myositis—pain and cramps in multiple muscles, myoglobinuria
  Subacute myositis—weakness, serum enzymes elevated
  Chronic—symmetrical, weakness

Skeletal problems
  Trauma
  Poor healing of wounds
  Aseptic necrosis of hip

in any person who uses five or more portions daily for a long period of time. Although neurology texts detail many syndromes found in advanced derelict alcoholics, we will consider only five general conditions in this section. These are the CNS damage widely prevalent in heavy drinkers of alcohol, the even more advanced and often permanent phase of CNS damage (called Wernicke-Korsakov syndrome),[102,103] the alcohol withdrawal syndrome, cerebellar disease, and peripheral neuritis.

Alcohol withdrawal syndrome[104] occurs only after tolerance develops and the alcohol intake is diminished. Tolerance is best explained by a change in structure in synaptic and neuron membranes, compensating in part for the increased membrane viscosity that accompanies chronic alcohol use. This structural adaptation, partially offsetting the impairment brought about by alcohol, is the basis of both neurological tolerance and withdrawal. In practice, withdrawal can occur only after weeks of continuous alcohol use; the longer and more intense the uninterrupted use, the more likely withdrawal is to occur and to be severe. The syndrome is an orderly progressive one in a given patient that takes 12 to 30 hours to proceed from the earliest recognizable signals to the advanced, life-threatening, and highly disruptive stage. Early recognition allows ample time to administer safe treatment that will reverse the problem. Late recognition often leads to treatments that aggravate some of the problem, such as restraints and intravenous fluids.

Alcohol withdrawal syndrome should be considered in anyone drinking alcohol heavily for months and in any patient entering a hospital, nursing home, or controlled environment facility (such as prison) where the supply of large quantities of beverage alcohol may be limited. The timing of the syndrome is remarkably stereotyped, beginning 6 to 16 hours after the last drink or substituted sedation medication, progressing in the subsequent 12 to 30 hours to peak severity, and then getting better. Agitation,

hyperactivity, and autonomic hyperactivity are the keys to recognition of the syndrome and starting of therapy. Intoxication with alcohol or other agents, head trauma, and liver encephalopathy should enter the differential diagnosis, but all of these feature depression rather than hyperactivity. Withdrawal from illicit drugs or activation of an underlying psychosis can appear identical to alcohol withdrawal, but the difference is apparent in the different time of improvement; treatment of these conditions for a day or two as alcohol withdrawal does not produce harm. Table 23–6 indicates some of the stages of alcohol withdrawal that are useful for recognition. All symptoms are masked or altered by any form of CNS-active medication, including morphine-type analgesics, anesthesia, benzodiazepines, or sedatives.

Once a consciousness of the syndrome is present and treatment is started, it is rare for the more advanced stages to occur in the hospital; they are seen only in patients who have had treatment delayed. There are many similarities in the presentation and treatment of alcohol withdrawal syndrome and sensory deprivation syndrome of psychology. Both include hyperactivity, confusion, hallucination, and acute psychosis. To the degree that the patient can be kept in familiar surroundings (his clothes vs. hospital ones, armchair vs. bed, familiar friendly people vs. hospital garbed attendants), many of the more alarming symptoms can be dissipated. The enforcement of bed rest, intravenous infusions, and exposure to shadows and hospital noise occasionally convert a manageable patient to an unmanageable one. Medications in safe dosage (10 mg diazepam or 100 mg chlordiazepoxide every 2 hours orally) until the process stops worsening and improves, will effectively control all patients in whom the treatment is started before stage 3. Patients who may require anesthesia, or who have had injury, may need shorter-acting treatment, such as ethanol intravenously (30 to 100 g), or very-short-acting barbiturates. When the patient is stable, treatment with the

TABLE 23–6. Alcohol Withdrawal Symptoms and Signs—A Progression for Recognition

Stage	Time After Last Drink	Symptoms and Signs
0	4–6 hr	Uneasiness, a consciousness of visceral signals. No signs visible to examiner.
1	6–12 hr	Restless, wants sedation or drink. Purposeless movements and nervous activity prominent.
2	8–20 hr	Severe uneasiness, insomnia, hyperactivity. Pulse over 100, respiration over 20, usually sweaty and may be red-faced. Mentally quite clear.
3	16–30 hr	Mental lapses, anguished, pleads for relief. Severe agitation. Severe restlessness, possibly severe tremulousness, seems very frightened, autonomic hyperactivity prominent.
4	24–36 hr	Hallucinations. Acute psychosis, convulsions. Extreme fright, severe autonomic hyperactivity. May be quite noncommunicative.

longer-acting benzodiazepines may be safely used, once sufficient medication is present to arrest the progression and no further doses need to be given. Phenytoin 300 mg q.d. for 5 to 7 days is recommended to avoid convulsions in patients with a history of convulsions. Those who enter the hospital in stage 3 or 4 of withdrawal usually require large parenteral doses of both haloperidol (to control psychosis) and diazepam.

BRAIN DAMAGE IN THE ALCOHOLIC AND THE WERNICKE-KORSAKOV SYNDROME

Quantitative assessment of the memory, reasoning, and learning abilities of the alcoholic indicates a wide prevalence of impairment,[102,103] which in nearly all cases improves slowly with time. There are some analogies between the changes found in alcoholism and those of aging, but there are also prominent differences. Serial CT scans of the brain, or serial psychological tests, indicate diminished cortical volume and function with prolonged drinking. With cessation of drinking, improvement continuing at least 3 to 5 years has been observed. Even the volume of the brain increases on CT scan; this finding probably is similar to nutritional diminution in the brain size of patients with anorexia nervosa, which can increase with parenteral hyperalimentation.

The implications to the therapist are several. First, the learning ability of the recovered alcoholic patient is on the average less than in other patients, and they need more reinforcement and repetition in any treatment regimen. Second, the fear of "loss of mind" and the associated loss of power over one's own life are often sufficient to focus the person on therapy. Finally, all studies show improvement over time with abstinence and an adequate diet, suggesting hope for the patient. In practice, at least 80 per cent of the improvement is apparent in the first 3 to 6 months.

Late in the 19th century, Wernicke described alcoholic patients with global confusion, peripheral neuritis, and cerebral palsies and correlated the lesions of the mammillary bodies at death with this syndrome. Korsakov very soon thereafter described global confusion associated with loss of acute memory, and both syndromes were subsequently found to be common in alcoholic patients. Victor and coworkers[103] have clarified the clinical and anatomical findings in this syndrome, and the term Wernicke-Korsakov syndrome has come to mean the more severe degrees of alcoholism-associated central nervous system disease, usually that which does not clear up sufficiently for the person to function in an unsupervised fashion in society. It seems that this is only the extreme clinical degree (tip of the iceberg) of a widespread phenomenon that occurs in the alcoholic or other malnourished patients. The prominent features are a loss of acute memory, usually peripheral neuritis, often sixth cranial nerve palsies, nystagmus, and a global confusional state. Some features of this disease are reproduced entirely by thiamine deficiency and are corrected by the administration of thiamine. The sixth nerve ophthalmoplegia usually disappears completely within 24 hours of administration of as little as 2 mg of thiamine, but the other features resolve much more slowly, if at all. Gibson and Blass have proposed that patients who manifest the thiamine-responsive Wernicke-Korsakov syndrome have an inherited defect in all of the cells of the body that renders them more sensitive to thiamine deficiency.[85]

In practice, all patients with central nervous system impairment should have repletion of B vitamins (including thiamine) sufficient to treat any deficiency and should be given an opportunity to demonstrate recoverability for 60 to 90 days before being declared permanently nonfunctional. Since the recognition of minor memory or ophthalmoplegia is not always possible, in my practice all severe alcoholic patients are given thiamine supplementation (100 mg intramuscularly) upon entry into treatment programs.

PERIPHERAL NEURITIS

In human malnutrition, pure single vitamin deprivations are infrequent. Thiamine, pyridoxine, riboflavin, and nicotinic acid deficiencies are capable of producing damage to the peripheral nerves, but in the alcoholic, it is not clear whether these are direct toxicities from alcohol or its metabolites or deficiency. Clinically, at least 20 per cent of inner-city alcoholic patients have a symmetrical loss of sensation in their feet and occasionally in their fingers. Nerve conduction studies indicate the prevalence to be at least twice as high. This form of neuropathy is readily reversible with slow return of sensation when alcohol use ceases; the provision of vitamin supplements does not clearly affect this disease. When motor paralysis is present, the prognosis for recovery is less clear. Asymmetrical damage to motor nerves is probably related to trauma.

CEREBELLAR INJURY

Intense alcoholism associated with severe malnutrition can lead to permanent injury to the cerebellum, most marked in those regions controlling the trunk musculature. There does not seem to be any recovery, and the cause is unknown.

Heart and Lung Disease

Cardiomyopathy is well known in beri beri and in intense chronic alcoholism. Alcohol has many reversible injurious effects on the myocardium.[101] There is no clear method to differentiate alcoholic myocardiopathy from idiopathic varieties in the alcoholic drinking person. About 99 per cent of alcoholic patients are also heavy tobacco smokers, and smoking accounts for the majority of the lung injury.

Liver Damage and Cirrhosis

Almost all heavy consumers of alcohol develop some indications of liver injury, manifested by abnormal hepatic function tests, by hepatic enlargement, and by fatty increases and cellular injury seen in hepatic tissue biopsy. The development of alcoholic hepatitis and cirrhosis is distinctly less frequent. Table 23–7 indicates a consensus on the importance of nutrition and alcohol ingestion in the development of these lesions. This emphasizes that alcohol ingestion alone is most important in the nonspecific changes and in the development of fatty liver, but that alcoholic hepatitis and cirrhosis have increasing roles in malnutrition.[62]

A large multicenter Veterans Administration study of alcoholic liver disease showed clearly that cirrhosis occurred in the most malnourished patients; particular emphasis was placed on visceral protein impairment as reflected by low serum albumin concentrations. In addition, malnutrition was reflected by decreased muscle mass and diminished skin hypersensitivity.[42]

From studies of populations, it is clear that among persons with comparably heavy intake of alcohol, some develop cirrhosis and some remain free of significant liver disease. No single theory of the pathogenesis of alcoholic liver damage adequately accounts for the differences in susceptibility between persons. However, there are a variety of situations in man in which the susceptibility to liver damage from alcohol seems to be increased. Table 23–8 lists some of these.

These observations suggest that there are persons who by reasons of genetic makeup or exposure are more susceptible to the permanent liver damage of alcohol. Efforts to diminish alcohol intake or improve nutrition may be beneficial in such persons.

The liver is central in the metabolism and/or storage of many trace nutrients. Because of this central role, nutritional problems arise in liver disease in alcoholic patients that are somewhat different from those found in other patients with liver disease and involve special considerations.

TABLE 23–7. *The Importance of Alcohol Ingestion and Malnutrition in the Development of Liver Disease*

Stage	Alcohol Ingestion	Malnutrition
Nonspecific injury	+ + + +	0
Fatty liver	+ + + +	0
Alcoholic hepatitis	+ + + +	+ + +
Cirrhosis	+ +	+ +

TABLE 23–8. *Conditions Increasing the Prevalence of Alcohol Injury to the Liver and Cirrhosis*

Genetic
  Females
Anatomical
  Following subtotal gastrectomy
  Following jejunoileal bypass
Concomitant injury
  Chronic hepatitis B carriers
  Chronic use of certain drugs
    Methyltrexate for psoriasis
    Isoniazid for tuberculosis

Energy requirements are usually increased in liver disease because there are impairments in digestion and storage of energy and there is the need for energy for tissue repair and inflammation. In cirrhotic patients with jaundice, there is substantial malabsorption of fat, and losses in the stool of 20 per cent of the dietary fat are not uncommon. Bacterial overgrowth in the gut may compete for certain trace nutrients. In general, feeding 25 per cent excess calories will overcome these problems. Carbohydrate metabolism is altered when portal hypertension is present; as much as 50 per cent of the intestinal blood is shunted past the liver. Insulin and glucagon released by the pancreas reach the peripheral circulation in higher than normal concentrations, and the liver in much lower than normal concentrations. As a result, there may be postprandial hyperglycemia, and occasionally there is loss of glucose in the urine.

Protein synthesis by the liver is usually retarded in proportion to the amount of liver damage. Poor protein nutriture can make this worse, but excess feeding will not effect an improvement. The profile of individual amino acids in the serum is distorted, probably making protein synthesis a little more difficult; amino acids with high serum concentrations are often lost in the urine of patients with severe liver disease. Improvement in alcoholic liver disease in many cases may reflect restoration of adequate protein to the diet. In many forms of liver injury, regeneration can be substantially enhanced by increased protein in the diet. Limited studies in alcoholic cirrhosis are consistent with this view. There is a great deal of clinical evidence to support the giving of sufficient protein in the diet to permit liver healing. If there is hepatic encephalopathy, protein can usually be given parenterally with impunity. A few days after antibiotics are initiated to alter intestinal flora, one can usually return to oral feeding. In practice, a minimum of 50 per cent above normal protein requirements should be given.

Trace nutrients, particularly the fat-soluble vitamins, B vitamins, iron, zinc, copper, and selenium, are stored in the liver. Liver disease seems to reduce the storage capacity as well as the ease with which these substances are moved into and out of storage form. In alcoholic liver disease iron often increases in the liver, but the reasons are not clear. Removal of this excess iron does not appear to have a beneficial role. The provision of adequate amounts of the vitamins occasionally leads to dramatic clinical improvement. Clear advantages are associated with efforts to replete vitamin K. Laboratory improvement has followed administration of vitamins A and D and zinc, but the clinical need for other substances in cirrhosis is less clear.

The provision of restricted sodium diets when ascites and edema are present and of restricted protein diets when encephalopathy is present are discussed in other chapters.

Alcoholic Pancreatitis

Injury to the pancreas in alcoholics[105,106] occurs first in the small ductules of the gland, and at least half of the time is clinically silent. When large amounts of injury occur simultaneously, pancreatitis is recognized by its associated syndrome of pain, inflammation in the abdomen, and hyperamylasemia. Many alcoholics have an impaired production of pancreatic enzymes and pancreatic bicarbonate due to silent disease. Although some of this deficiency can be corrected with proper nutriture, interference with digestion and assimilation of fats is frequent in inner-city alcoholics. This process will usually correct itself partially within a few weeks of normal diet and abstinence from alcohol.

Infrequently, pancreatic insufficiency is observed in which the total function of the pancreas is less than 5 per cent of normal. In this circumstance, severe fat malabsorption is present, with its associated severe diarrhea. Such patients usually have caloric and protein deficits and specific deficiencies of the fat-soluble vitamins, calcium, and magnesium and often of iron and zinc. If the patient is drinking alcohol, the deficiencies are even more severe.

Nearly all drinking alcoholic patients with any degree of pancreatic injury will show improvement in the first month or two of abstinence. As protein repletion occurs, the functioning remnant of pancreas will usually produce more digestive ferments; often supplements required initially to regain lost weight are not required to maintain the new weight. Depletions are predictable on the basis of the clinical history and physical examination, but often specific levels of nutrients must be measured to make certain that repletion is adequate. Diabetes mellitus is often a concomitant of pancreatic insufficiency. Management with insulin is taxing to the physician and the patient, with frequent measurements of blood glucose levels needed for reasonable regulation. Damage to the salivary glands is frequent in alcoholic subjects and may elevate the serum amylase.[107]

Alcohol Damage to the Reproductive System and Fetal Alcohol Syndrome

Although feminization of male cirrhotic patients with gynecomastia and loss of sexual hair have been prominently described in cirrhosis, only in the past decade has injury to the testis been clearly studied and correctly attributed to a direct toxic effect of alcohol.[108]

After only 6 weeks of study, testicular atrophy, decrease in the weight of the prostate and seminal vesicles, and diminution in the serum testosterone levels are found in pair fed rats given alcohol. The loss of testicular tissue is greatest in the Leydig cells, but there is loss also in the seminiferous tubules. In addition to the direct effect on the testis, the trophic hormone, luteinizing hormone (LH), is decreased. Similar findings are noted in humans with lowered plasma testosterone levels and a fall in levels of LH. Diminution in testicular size is noted in chronic alcoholic patients. In cirrhosis, this process is even more advanced. There is an increased conversion of androgen precursors to estrogen. These changes account fairly well for the fall in libido, diminished sperm counts, loss of testicular size, and feminization of cirrhotic males. Although libido may improve with prolonged sobriety, low testicular size or low testosterone levels do not change. Treatment trials with testosterone and clomiphene citrate have not led to impressive improvement.

Changes in women are less thoroughly studied. The secretion of LH and follicle-stimulating hormone (FSH) seems impaired in all chronic alcoholic women. Disorders of menstruation are common in alcoholic women, and it is rare for patients with cirrhosis to have a child. Loss of female sex characteristics and low estrogens are common in cirrhotic females.

Lemoine and colleagues[109] and later Jones and associates[110] brought to attention brain and growth retardation of infants born from alcoholic mothers. This disorder became known as the fetal alcohol syndrome (FAS).[111] It occurs with increasing frequency in women using more than 50 g of alcohol each day throughout pregnancy. FAS has occurred at alcohol levels of two drinks per day, but is most prominent in very heavy drinkers. Fetal wastage is certainly increased with any amount of drinking. The brain and growth retardation is irreversible, and FAS may be one of the three major causes of mental retardation in the United States.

Hematological Disorders

The multiple nutritional deficiencies and widespread impairment of protein synthesis and cellular turnover can produce anemia, leukopenia, lymphopenia, and low platelets. Anemia is often megaloblastic in the marrow, and these are invariably folate deficiency. One to 5 mg of folate will usually rapidly correct them. Sideroblastic anemia is recognized by iron stains of the bone marrow, demonstrating the iron-containing sideroblasts. This anemia seems to be a direct toxic effect of alcohol, possibly augmented by a marginal diet. Rarer types of anemia include those associated with clear vacuolization in marrow erythroid precursors, and the hemolytic anemia often associated with Zieve's syndrome. Clear vacuoles in the pronormoblasts can be produced by the ingestion of alcohol and are frequently found in marrow samples from alcoholic patients with anemia. This is mostly related to direct alcohol toxicity and disappears within 2 weeks of abstinence. The anemia, however, may have many components; it does not respond nearly as rapidly as the disappearance of the vacuoles.

In Zieve's syndrome, there is a prominent hemolytic anemia with a rapid symptomatic fall in the hematocrit, disappearance of haptoglobin from the circulation, and marrow evidence of a reaction to the sudden anemia. Hyperlipidemia and fatty liver were associated with the original syndrome, but it is apparent that the triad of hemolytic anemia, hyperlipidemia, and fatty liver is little more than a chance occurrence in a severe alcoholic patient. Thus, each of the components may occur without the other. There is no specific etiology, and the syndrome is self-limiting.

Severe hypophosphatemia produces hemolysis, and is sometimes observed in chronic alcoholic patients.

The mean corpuscular volume (MCV) of the red blood cells in alcoholic patients is often mildly elevated and may or may not be associated with anemia. This has been proposed as a marker of alcoholism. The cause is uncertain, but it is not corrected or prevented by folate administration. It usually disappears in a few weeks of abstinence if there is no other disease. Should cirrhosis occur, many new forms of anemia characteristic of cirrhosis may occur. These include hemolysis of hypersplenism, spur cell anemia related to elevated bile salts, and bleeding. White cell problems are often prominent. Folate deficiency is often responsible for the failure to have a leukocytosis with infection. Lymphocytes are often below 1500/μl, visceral proteins are depleted, and skin anergy to standard antigens occurs in the malnourished alcoholic patient. Zinc deficiency is known to inhibit the function of leukocytes, but not their numbers. Studies of the responses in skin chambers in the intoxicated subject indicate clearly that alcohol impairs mobilization of granulocytes. In vitro specific studies indicate decreased responsiveness of "drunk" granulocytes in clearance or phagocytic function.

Thrombocytopenia is occasionally life-threatening in the alcoholic patient. Although this problem occurs repeatedly in sensitized subjects, other factors, such as infection or decreased formation of platelets, may account for the deficit state. Bleeding from thrombocytopenia is very common in cirrhosis when hypersplenism and activated coagulation occur in concert.

Trauma with tissue injury, infection with altera-

tions of marrow function and coagulation, and organ injury also occur commonly and account for many of the moderate changes in the alcoholic.

Other Organs

Alcoholic patients lose their teeth at an accelerated rate.[15] Taste and smell[112] seem changed mostly by zinc and vitamin A deficiency. A toxic amblyopia may occur, and with abstinence this disorder is resolved.[113] Vagal injury occurs in advanced alcoholics.[114] Cancers of the mouth and lip, esophagus, and stomach seem to be increased in alcoholism and increased even further if there is smoking.[115]

Summary

Nearly all organs are damaged by alcohol, but most of the damage is reversible. Organs with rapid turnover of cells recover rapidly when the alcohol consumption is stopped, and the macro- and micronutrient deficiencies are repleted. Thus, with many injuries to the brain, intestine, marrow, and liver there may be a return nearly to normal in 1 or 2 weeks. Recovery from other reparable injuries often associated with protein deficiency occurs more slowly, requiring 3 to 6 weeks. The injuries to the brain, eye, fine sensory nerves, muscle, and severe injuries of the liver and pancreas seem to require this time for recovery. A few lesions seem much more permanent; these include cerebellar disease, motor neuron damage, symmetrical myopathy, and severe testicular damage.

In practice, since many nutritional depletions may be present, repletion with vitamin and mineral supplements and a highly nutritious diet along with enforced abstinence from alcohol are offered to all patients. In the majority, substantial recovery will occur.

SPECIAL PROBLEMS OF ALCOHOLICS IN MEDICAL TREATMENT

The Unsuspected Alcoholic Discovered Postoperatively or in the Coronary Care Unit

Denial of alcoholism is widespread. Most physicians and surgeons will encounter the totally unsuspected alcoholic patient whose disease usually becomes manifest by a profound and symptomatic depletion or by severe withdrawal symptoms. The depletions that may produce problems are usually related to very low blood phosphate, magnesium, or potassium concentrations or leukopenia. The agitation that heralds early withdrawal in the known alcohol drinker is usually dismissed in the acute care situation, when hallucination or acute psychosis may be the predominant presentation.

The management of such patients is the same with or without correct diagnosis. The recognized depletions should be repleted. The patient must be heavily sedated to become manageable. Short-acting barbiturates often bring about control acutely, while proper dosage of benzodiazepines (such as diazepam) can be administered to achieve necessary sedation. If the patient is heavily sedated, appropriate pulmonary and skin care must be given.

The Alcoholic with Major Trauma to Head, Abdomen, or Major Bones

Alcoholism contributes heavily to vehicular accidents, and the associated trauma is frequently seen in active emergency rooms. Repletion of vitamins, minerals, and protein should be administered almost without concern for diagnosis, and the methods used in total parenteral nutrition are applicable. Folate, thiamine, pyridoxine, and riboflavin and probably vitamin K should be given parenterally. If the patient cannot be fed, which is usually the case, intravenous nutrients, including trace minerals (most importantly magnesium and zinc) and adequate potassium and phosphate, should be given. Intravenous amino acids are indicated in the usual amounts.

Sedation may interfere with subsequent surgery, but short-acting sedatives that clear rapidly can be used if indicated. Intravenous alcohol in doses of 20 to 40 g each hour provides both calories and sedation and will manage the patient until further surgery is not needed and longer-acting agents can be given. With intramuscular magnesium sulfate, it is possible to maintain sedation, but the average dose to control alcohol withdrawal is of the order of fifteen 2-ml ampules of 50 per cent magnesium sulfate solution. Willingness to use these large amounts usually requires familiarity with this form of treatment.

The Alcoholic As an Outpatient Who is Believed to be Drinking

Testing for alcohol in biological media is the most direct approach to overcome this form of uncertainty. Blood, saliva, urine, and any other body fluids have about the same alcohol concentration. Most alcoholic patients cannot limit alcohol use sufficiently long to be regularly free of alcohol in their body fluids during visits to the doctor; therefore, high concentrations of ethanol are often present in biological fluids. If alcohol testing is positive, the positive test should be presented to the patient as a part of the disease, alcoholism; it should not be the basis to reject the patient from further treatment. Careful study has found that alcohol use occurs in more than half of alcoholic patients undergoing medical therapy.[116]

References

1. Shaw S, Lieber CS. Alcoholism. *In* Schneider HA, Anderson CE, Coursin DB (eds). Nutritional Support of Medical Practice. 2nd ed. Philadelphia, Harper & Row, 1985.
2. Leevy CM, Zetterman RK. Malnutrition and alcoholism: an overview. *In* Rothschild MA, Oritz M, Schreiber S (eds). Alcohol and Abnormal Protein Biosynthesis, Biochemical and Clinical. Vol 1. New York, Pergamon Press, 1975: 3–15.
3. Kater RMH, Roggin G, Tobon F, et al. Increased rate of clearance of drugs from the circulation of alcoholics. Am J Med Sci 1969; *258*:35–39.
4. Isbell H, Fraser HF, Wikler A, et al. An experimental study of the etiology of "rum fits" and delirium tremens. Q J Stud Alcohol 1955; *16*:1–33.
5. Kalant H, LeBlanc AE, Gibbs RJ. Tolerance to, and dependence on, some non-opiate psychotropic drugs. Pharmacol Rev 1971; *23*:135–191.
6. Chappel NJ. Attitudinal barriers to physician involvement with drug abusers. JAMA 1973; *224*:1011.
7. American Medical Association Manual on Alcoholism. Chicago, American Medical Association, 1978: 6.
8. Begleiter H, Platz A. The effects of alcohol on the central nervous system in humans. *In* Kisin B, Begleiter H (eds). The Biology of Alcoholism. Vol 2. New York, Plenum, 1971.
9. Goldsmith RH, Iber FL, Miller PA. Nutritional status of alcoholics of different socioeconomic class. J Am Coll Nutr 1983; *2*:215–220.
10. Roggin GM, Iber FL, Kater RMH, et al. Malabsorption in the chronic alcoholic. Johns Hopkins Med J 1969; *125*:321–330.
11. Bjarnason I, Ward K, Peters TJ. Leaky gut of alcoholism. Possible route of entry for toxic compounds. Lancet 1984; *2*:179–182.
12. Van Thiel DH, Gavaler JS, Lester R, et al. Alcohol-induced testicular atrophy: an experimental model for hypogonadism occurring in chronic alcoholic men. Gastroenterology 1975; *69*:326–332.
13. Wright JW, Fry D, Merry J, et al. Abnormal hypothalamic-pituitary-gonadal function in chronic alcoholics. Br J Addict 1976; *71*:211–215.
14. Neville JN, Eagles JA, Samson G, et al. Nutritional status of alcoholics. Am J Clin Nutr 1968; *21*:1329–1340.
15. King WH, Tucker TM. Dental problems of alcohol and non-alcoholic psychiatric patients. Q J Stud Alcohol 1973; *34*:1208–1211.
16. Lieber CS. Hepatic and metabolic effects of alcohol (1966–1973). Gastroenterology 1973; *65*:821—846.
17. Krebs HA, Perkins JR. The physiological role of liver alcohol dehydrogenase. Biochem J 1970; *118*:635–644.
18. Elmslie RG, Davis RA, Magee DF, et al. Absorption of alcohol after gastrectomy. Surg Gynecol Obstet 1965; *119*:1256.
19. Hanzlick PJ, Collins RJ. Quantitative studies on the gastrointestinal absorption of drugs. III. The absorption of alcohol. J Pharmacol Exp Ther 1983; *5*:185.
20. Teschke R, Hasumura Y, Lieber CS. Hepatic microsomal ethanol oxidizing system: Solubilization, isolation and characterization. Arch Biochem Biophys 1974; *163*:404–415.
21. Domschke S, Domschke W, Lieber CS. Hepatic redox state: attenuation of the acute effects of ethanol induced by chronic ethanol consumption. Life Sci 1974; *15*:1327–1334.
22. Lieber CS. Alcohol, protein metabolism, and liver injury. Gastroenterology 1980; *79*:373–390.
23. Nikkila EA, Ojala K. Role of hepatic L-α-glycerophosphate and triglyceride synthesis in production of fatty liver by ethanol. Proc Soc Exp Biol Med 1963; *113*:814–817.
24. Klatsy AL, Friedman GD, Siegelaub AB. Alcohol consumption before myocardial infarction: results from the Kai-

ser-Permanente epidemiologic study of myocardial infarction. Ann Intern Med 1974; *81*:294–301.

25. Jones DP, Losowsky MS, Davidson CS, et al. Effects of ethanol on plasma lipids in man. J Lab Clin Med 1963; *62*:675–682.

26. Lieber CS, Jones DP, Mendelson J, et al. Fatty liver, hyperlipemia and hyperuricemia produced by prolonged alcohol consumption, despite adequate dietary intake. Trans Assoc Am Phys 1963; *76*:289–300.

27. Lieber CS. Metabolic effects produced by alcohol in the liver and other tissues. Adv Intern Med 1968; *14*:151–199.

28. Wendel A, Fenerstein S, Konz KH. Acute paracetamol intoxication of starved mice leads to lipid peroxidation in vivo. Biochem Phys 1979; *28*:2051–2055.

29. Cronholm T, Sjovall J. Effect of ethanol metabolism on redox state of steroid sulphates in man. Eur J Biochem 1970; *13*:124–131.

30. Eichner ER, Hillman RS. Effect of alcohol on serum folate level. J Clin Invest 1973; *52*:584–591.

31. Russell RM, Ismail-Beigi F, Afrasiabi K, et al. Folate levels among various populations in central Iran. Am J Clin Nutr 1976; *29*:794–798.

32. Smith M, Hopkinson DA, Harris H. Studies on the subunit structure and molecular size of the human alcohol dehydrogenase isozymes determined by the different loci ADH1, ADH2, and ADH3. Ann Hum Genet 1973; *36*:401–404.

33. Bode C, Goebell H, Stahler M. Anderunger der Alkohol-dehydrogenase-Aktivität in der Rattenleber durch Eiweissmangel und Athanol. Gesamte Exp Med 1970; *152*:111–124.

34. Horn RS, Manthei RW. Ethanol metabolism in chronic protein deficiency. J Pharmacol Exp Ther 1965; *147*:385–390.

35. Papenberg J, Von Wartburg JP, Aebi H. Metabolism of ethanol and fructose in the perfused rat liver. Enzym Biol Clin 1970; *11*:237–250.

36. Rognstad R, Clark DG. Tritium as a tracer for reducing equivalents in isolated liver cells. Eur J Biochem 1974; *42*:51–60.

37. Burnett KG, Felder MR. Ethanol metabolism in *Peromyscus* genetically deficient in alcohol dehydrogenase. Biochem Pharmacol 1980; *28*:1–8.

38. Sato C, Matsuda Y, Lieber CS. Increased hepatotoxicity of acetaminophen after chronic ethanol consumption in the rat. Gastroenterology 1981; *80*:140–148.

39. Pirola RC, Lieber CS. The energy cost of the metabolism of drugs, including ethanol. Pharmacology 1972; *7*:185–196.

40. Hosein EA, Bexton B. Protective action of carnitine on liver lipid metabolism after ethanol administration to rats. Biochem Pharmacol 1975; *24*:1859–1863.

41. Saville PD, Lieber CS. Effect of alcohol on growth bone density and muscle magnesium in the rat. J Nutr 1965; *87*:477–488.

42. Mendenhall CL, Anderson S, Weesner RE, et al. Protein-calorie malnutrition associated with alcoholic hepatitis. Veterans Administration Cooperative Study Group on Alcoholic Hepatitis. Am J Med 1984; *76*:211–222.

43. Sato C, Hasumura Y, Takeuchi J. Interaction of ethanol with drugs and xenobiotics. *In* Seitz HK, Kommerell B. Alcohol-Related Diseases in Gastroenterology. Berlin, Springer-Verlag, 1985:172–184.

44. Misra PS, Lefevre A, Ishii H, et al. Increase of alcohol meprobamate and phenobarbital metabolism after chronic ethanol administration in man and rats. Am J Med 1971; *51*:346–351.

45. Pritchard JF, Schneck DW. Effects of ethanol and phenobarbital on the metabolism of propranolol by 9000 g rat liver supernatant. Biochem Pharmacol 1977; *26*:2453–2454.

46. Martin EW. Hazards of Medications. Philadelphia, JB Lippincott, 1971: 435.

47. Hasumaur Y, Teschke R, Lieber CS. Increased carbon tetrachloride hepatotoxicity, and its mechanism, after chronic ethanol consumption. Gastroenterology 1974; *66*:415–422.

48. Auty RM, Branch RA. Proceedings: The metabolism of ethyl, n-propyl, n-butyl and iso-amyl alcohol by the isolated perfused rat liver. Br J Pharmacol 1974; *53*:443P.

49. Pikkarainen PH, Gordon ER, Lebsack ME. Determinants of plasma free acetaldehyde level during the steady state of oxidation of ethanol: effects of chronic ethanol feeding. Biochem Pharmacol 1981; *30*:799–802.

50. Lindros KO, Stowell A, Pikkarainen P, et al. Elevated blood acetaldehyde in alcoholics with accelerated ethanol elimination. Pharmacol Biochem Behav 1980; *13*:119–124.

51. Wolff H. Vasomotor sensitivity to alcohol in diverse mongoloid populations. Am J Hum Genet 1973; *25*:193–199.

52. Veitch RL, Lumeng L, Li T-K. Vitamin B-6 metabolism in chronic alcohol abuse: the effect of ethanol oxidation on hepatic pyridoxal 5-phosphate metabolism. J Clin Invest 1975; *55*:1026–1032.

53. Walsh MJ. Role of acetaldehyde in the interactions of ethanol with neuroamines. *In* Roach MK, McIsaac WM, Creaven PJ (eds). Biological Aspects of Alcohol. Austin, University of Texas Press, 1971: 233.

54. Schreiber SS, Oratz M, Rothschild MA, et al. Alcoholic cardiomyopathy. II. The inhibition of cardiac microsomal protein synthesis by acetaldehyde. J Molec Cell Cardiol 1974; *6*:207–213.

55. Crouse JR, Gerson CD, DeCarli LM, et al. Role of acetate in the reduction of plasma free fatty acids produced by ethanol in man. J Lipid Res 1968; *9*:509–512.

56. Lieber CS, DeCarli LM. Quantitative relationship between the amount of dietary fat and the severity of the alcoholic fatty liver. Am J Clin Nutr 1970; *23*:474–478.

57. Lieber CS, Teschke R, Hasumura Y, et al. Differences in hepatic and metabolic changes after acute and chronic alcohol consumption. Fed Proc 1975; *34*:2060–2074.

58. Kudzma DJ, Schonfeld G. Alcohol hyperlipidemia: induction by alcohol but not by carbohydrate. J Lab Clin Med 1971; *77*:384–395.

59. Haskell WL, Camargo C Jr, Williams PT, et al. The effect of cessation and resumption of moderate alcohol intake on serum high-density-lipoprotein subfractions: a controlled study. N Engl J Med 1984; *310*:805–810.

60. Blackburn GL, Bistrain BR, Maini BS, et al. Nutritional and metabolic assessment of the hospitalized patient. JPEN 1977; *1*:11–22.

61. Tomaiolo PP, Kraus V. Nutritional status of hospitalized alcoholic patient. JPEN 1980; *4*:1–3.

62. Patek AJ Jr. Alcohol, malnutrition, and alcoholic cirrhosis. Am J Clin Nutr 1979; *32*:1304–1312.

63. Siegel FL, Roach MK, Pomero LR. Plasma amino acid patterns in alcoholism: the effects of ethanol loading. Proc Natl Acad Sci USA 1964; *51*:605–611.

64. Shaw S, Lue SL, Lieber CS. Biochemical tests for the detection of alcoholism: comparison of alpha-amino-n-butyric acid with other available tests. Alcoholism 1978; *2*:3–7.

65. Swendseid ME, Yamada C, Vinyard E, et al. Plasma amino acid levels in young subjects receiving diets containing 14 or 3.5 grams nitrogen per day. Am J Clin Nutr 1968; *21*:1381–1383.

66. Zinneman HH, Seal US, Doe RP. Plasma and urinary amino acids in Laennec's cirrhosis. Am J Dig Dis 1969; *14*:118–126.

67. Morgan MY, Milsolm JP, Sherlock S. Plasma ratio of valine, leucine, and isoleucine to phenylalanine and tyrosine in liver disease. Gut 1978; *19*:1068–1073.

68. Iwasaki Y, Sato H, Ohkubo A, et al. Effect of spontaneous portal-systemic shunting on plasma insulin and amino acid concentrations. Gastroenterology 1980; *78*:677–683.

69. Iob V, Coon WW, Sloan M. Altered clearance of free amino acids from plasma of patients with cirrhosis of the liver. J Surg Res 1966; *6*:233–239.

70. Shaw S, Worner TM, Borysow MF, et al. Detection of al-

coholism relapse: comparative diagnostic value of MCV, GGTP and AANB. Alcoholism 1979; 4:297–301.

71. Nasrallah SM, Galambos JT. Amino acid therapy of alcoholic hepatitis. Lancet 1980; 2:1276–1277.

72. Leevy CM, Baker H, Ten Hove W, et al. B-complex vitamins in liver disease of the alcoholic. Am J Clin Nutr 1965; 16:858–874.

73. Halsted CH. Folate deficiency in alcoholism. Am J Clin Nutr 1980; 33:2736–2744.

74. Halsted CH, Robles EA, Mezey E. Decreased jejunal uptake of labeled folic acid (3H-PGA) in alcoholic patients: roles of alcohol and nutrition. N Engl J Med 1971; 285:701–706.

75. Alcohol and the enterohepatic circulation of folate. Nutr Rev 1980; 38:220–223.

76. Brown JP, Davidson GE, Scott JM. Effect of diphenylhydantoin and ethanol feeding on the synthesis of rat liver folates from exogenous pteroyl-glutamate (3H). Biochem Pharmacol 1973; 22:3287–3289.

77. Sullivan LW, Herbert V. Suppression of hematopoiesis by ethanol. J Clin Invest 1964; 43:2048–2061.

78. Lindenbaum J, Lieber CS. Hematologic effects of alcohol in man in the absence of nutritional deficiency. N Engl J Med 1969; 281:333–338.

79. Klipstein FA, Lindenbaum J. Folate deficiency in chronic liver disease. Blood 1965; 25:443–456.

80. Tomasulo PA, Kater RMN, Iber FL. Impairment of thiamine absorption in alcoholism. Am J Clin Nutr 1968; 21:1340–1344.

81. Thomson AD, Levy CM. Observations on the mechanism of thiamine hydrochloride. Clin Sci 1972; 43:153–158.

82. Cole M, Turner A, Frank O, et al. Extraocular palsy and thiamine therapy in Wernicke's encephalopathy. Am J Clin Nutr 1969; 22:44–51.

83. Frank O, Baker H. Vitamin profile in rats fed stock or liquid ethanolic diets. Am J Clin Nutr 1980; 33:221–226.

84. Iber FL, Blass JP, Brin M, et al. Thiamine in the elderly—relation to alcoholism and to neurological degenerative disease. Am J Clin Nutr 1982; 36:1067–1082.

85. Blass JP, Gibson GE. Abnormality of a thiamine-requiring enzyme in patients with Wernicke-Korsakoff syndrome. N Engl J Med 1977; 297:1367–1370.

86. Fennelly J, Frank O, Baker H, et al. Peripheral neuropathy of the alcoholic: I. Etiological role of aneurin and the other B-complex vitamins. Br Med J 1964; 2:1290–1293.

87. Rosenthal WS, Adham NF, Lopez R, et al. Riboflavin deficiency in complicated chronic alcoholism. Am J Clin Nutr 1973; 26:858–860.

88. Van Thiel DH, Gavaler J, Lester R. Ethanol inhibition of vitamin A metabolism in the testes: possible mechanism for sterility in alcoholics. Science 1974; 186:941–942.

89. Morrison SA, Russell RM, Carney EA, et al. Failure of cirrhotics with hypovitaminosis A to achieve normal dark adaptation performance on vitamin A replacement. Gastroenterology 1976; 71:922–928.

90. Russell RM. Vitamin A and zinc metabolism in alcoholism. Am J Clin Nutr 1980; 33:2741–2748.

91. Leo MA, Arai M, Sato M, et al. Hepatotoxicity of moderate vitamin A supplementation in the rat. Gastroenterology 1982; 82:194–205.

92. Avioli LV, Haddad JG. Vitamin D: current concepts. Metabolism 1979; 22:507–528.

93. Posner D, Russell R, Absood S, et al. Effective hydroxylation of vitamin D-2 in advanced alcoholic cirrhosis. Gastroenterology 1977; 72:1113–1117.

94. Nilsson BE, Westlin NE. Changes in bone mass in alcoholics. Clin Orthop 1973; 90:229–232.

95. Roginsky MS, Zanzi I, Cohn SH. Skeletal and lean body mass in alcoholics with and without cirrhosis. Calcif Tissue Res 1976; 21:386–391.

96. Phillips RS, Iber FL, Shamszad M, et al. Subclinical vitamin K deficiency among severe alcoholics without liver disease. Hepatology 1983; 3:832.

97. Sargent WQ, Simpson JR, Beard JD. The effects of acute and chronic ethanol administration in divalent cation excretion. J Pharmacol Exp Ther 1974; 190:507–514.

98. Sullivan JF, Heaney RP. Zinc metabolism in alcoholic liver disease. Am J Clin Nutr 1970; 23:170–177.

99. Sullivan JF, Lankford HB. Zinc metabolism and chronic alcoholism. Am J Clin Nutr 1965; 17:57–63.

100. Dutta SK, Miller PA, Greenberg LB, Levander OH. Selenium and acute alcoholism. Am J Clin Nutr 1983; 38:713–718.

101. Van Thiel DH, Gavalier JS. Myocardial effects of alcohol abuse: clinical and physiological changes. In Galanter M (ed). Recent Advances in Alcoholism. Vol 3. New York, Plenum, 1985:181–200.

102. Butters N, Cermak LS. Alcoholic Korsakoff's syndrome. An information-processing approach to amnesia. New York, Academic Press, 1980.

103. Victor M, Adams RD, Collins GH. The Wernicke-Korsakoff syndrome. Philadelphia, FA Davis, 1971.

104. Baum RA, Iber FL. Initial treatment of the alcoholic patient. In Gitlow SE, Peyser HS (eds). Alcoholism: A Practical Treatment Guide. New York, Grune & Stratton, 1980: 73–87.

105. Banks PA. Pancreatitis. New York, Plenum Medical, 1979.

106. Singer MV, Goebell H. Acute and chronic actions of alcohol on pancreatic exocrine secretion in humans and animals. In Seitz HK, Kommerell B (eds). Gastroenterology. Berlin, Springer-Verlag, 1985.

107. Narang A, Dutta SK, Smalls U, et al. Abnormal parotid gland function in patients with stable alcoholic cirrhosis. Gastroenterology 1982; 82:1238.

108. Van Thiel DH, Cavalier JS, Cobb CF, et al. Alcohol-induced testicular atrophy in adult male rats. Endocrinology 1979; 105:888–895.

109. Lemoine P, Haroussean H, Borteyrl JP, et al. Les enfantes de parents alcooliques: Anomalies observees a propos de 127 cas. Quest Medical 1968; 25:476–482.

110. Jones KL, Smith DW, Hanson JW. The fetal alcohol syndrome: clinical delineation. Ann NY Acad Sci 1976; 273:130–137.

111. Iber FL. Fetal alcohol syndrome. A teaching aid. Nutrition Today 1980; Sept-Oct, 4–11.

112. Garrett MS, Russell RM. Abnormal taste and olfactory threshold in alcoholic cirrhosis. Clin Res 1980; 29:602.

113. Adams V, Mancall EL, Dreyfus PM. Deficiency amblyopia in alcoholic patient: a clinical pathological study. Arch Ophthalmol 1960; 64:1.

114. Tan ETH, Lambie DG, Johnson RH, et al. Release of glucagon in male alcoholics with vagal neuropathy. Alcoholism 1983; 7:416–419.

115. Rothman E, Keller AZ. The effect of joint exposure to alcohol and tobacco on risk of cancer of the mouth and pharynx. J Chronic Dis 1972; 25:711–716.

116. Helzer JE, Robins LN, Taylor JR, et al. The extent of long-term moderate drinking among alcoholics discharged from medical and psychiatric inpatient facilities. N Engl J Med 1985; 312:1678–1682.

24

EDEMA AND HYPERTENSION

E. VICTOR ADLIN

Edema and hypertension are disorders related to the accumulation and circulation of body fluids. Edema most commonly is a secondary manifestation of systemic disease; if severe, it can cause marked discomfort and disability. The underlying cause of the edema, however, be it heart failure, nephrosis, cirrhosis, or a less serious disorder, is likely to determine the outlook for survival and recovery.

Hypertension, on the other hand, is usually a primary disorder, without discernible cause. It seldom causes symptoms or disability in its early stages, but leads to greatly increased risk, over a period of years, of major complications: strokes, heart failure, heart attacks, and renal failure.

Both disorders are affected by nutritional and metabolic factors. Whatever the primary cause of edema, it may be made worse by the increased fluid retention that follows excessive sodium intake, or by the decrease in intravascular osmotic pressure that results from hypoalbuminemia. While the cause (or causes) of essential hypertension are unknown, the possible roles of dietary sodium, potassium, and calcium intake, and of obesity, are widely discussed; interest is heightened by evidence that modification of these factors through changes in diet may affect the blood pressure of patients with hypertension.

EDEMA

Pathophysiology

STARLING'S FORCES AND THE CAUSES OF EDEMA

Edema is an abnormal increase in the volume of interstitial fluid, the extravascular component of the extracellular fluid. When this increase exceeds about 2 L in an adult, swelling of soft tissues becomes evident, especially in dependent parts of the body, and clinical edema is present.

The movement of fluid between the vascular and interstitial compartments depends on the forces described by Starling: the hydrostatic pressure within the capillaries and the interstitial colloid osmotic pressure, which tend to move fluid from the vascular to the interstitial space, and the colloid osmotic pressure of the plasma proteins, which has the opposite effect.[1,2] At the arterial end of the capillary bed the balance of forces favors movement of fluid into the interstitial space, and at the venous end the forces favor movement into the vascular space. Lymphatic drainage contributes to the removal of interstitial fluid.

Generalized edema may be caused by primary retention of salt and water by the kidneys, as in acute tubular necrosis or acute glomerulonephritis. The fluid retention leads to expansion of the extracellular fluid volume and increased transudation of fluid into the interstitial compartment (Fig. 24–1).

A different sequence of events leads to the edema of congestive heart failure, hepatic cirrhosis, and the nephrotic syndrome. Anatomical and physiological abnormalities related to these conditions cause contraction of the effective arterial blood volume, and this in turn leads to secondary retention of salt and water by the kidneys, through a number of mechanisms that regulate the renal handling of sodium.[3]

Localized edema may result from an increase in capillary hydrostatic pressure caused by obstruction of the venous or lymphatic drainage of a region of the body. Also, localized injury to the capillary endothelium may be caused by allergic reactions, infection, or trauma, and the loss of plasma proteins into the interstitial space may cause local edema through an increase in the interstitial colloid osmotic pressure.

REGULATION OF RENAL SODIUM EXCRETION

In generalized edema, renal excretion of sodium and water is diminished, either primarily, as a result of renal disease, or secondarily, as a physiologic homeostatic response to a fall in effective arterial blood volume.[2,3] The effective circulating arterial volume is determined by a number of factors: blood volume, blood viscosity, cardiac output, arterial resistance, and the distribution of blood within the vascular tree.[1] Homeostatic mechanisms enable the kidneys to recognize and respond to changes in the effective arterial blood volume, and return this volume to a normal level by adjustments of renal excretion or retention of sodium and water. Some of these mechanisms are well-established, while others are incompletely understood or controversial. But whatever the exact means by which it is accomplished, the retention of sodium and water by the kidneys when effective arterial circulation is diminished is a major factor in the formation of edema.

Glomerular Filtration Rate and Renal Hemodynamics. When effective arterial blood volume is reduced, renal blood flow tends to fall. This results from a decrease in renal artery perfusion pressure, and also from constriction of the renal arterioles caused by angiotensin II and sympathetic neural stimulation.[4] The glomerular filtration rate (GFR) falls less than the renal plasma flow (RPF), largely because the renal arteriolar constriction is more intense in the efferent arterioles distal to the glomeruli than in the afferent arterioles, tending to maintain the GFR. The filtration fraction, which is the ratio

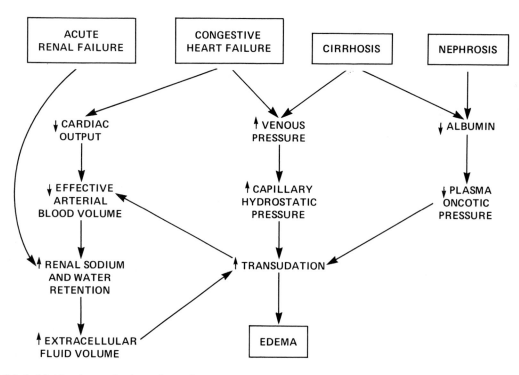

FIGURE 24–1. Mechanisms of edema formation.

of GFR to RPF, therefore tends to rise. A higher filtration fraction leads to an increase in postglomerular capillary protein concentration, and therefore an increase in the plasma oncotic pressure. The higher filtration fraction also decreases the postglomerular capillary hydrostatic pressure. Both the raised oncotic pressure and lowered hydrostatic pressure in the peritubular capillaries favor an increase in reabsorption of sodium and water in the proximal tubule.

Although the GFR may be maintained when effective arterial blood volume is mildly reduced, with greater reduction in renal perfusion pressure the renal arteriolar constriction becomes more intense and involves the afferent as well as efferent arterioles;[4] GFR falls, and the decrease in filtered load of sodium may further lower sodium excretion.

Renin-Angiotensin-Aldosterone System. Aldosterone is the principal mineralocorticoid, or sodium-retaining hormone, produced by the outer zone (zona glomerulosa) of the adrenal cortex. Its main site of action is the distal renal tubule, where it causes reabsorption of sodium ions in exchange for potassium or hydrogen ions. It therefore contributes to the ability of the kidney to conserve sodium.

The main factor controlling the secretion of aldosterone is the production of renin by the juxtaglomerular cells of the kidney. Renin is an enzyme that acts on an alpha-2 globulin of hepatic origin, renin substrate (angiotensinogen), to release a decapeptide, angiotensin I. This is inert, but it is converted to the potent octapeptide, angiotensin II, by angiotensin converting enzyme. Angiotensin II has two principal actions: It is a potent vasoconstrictor, and it is the main hormonal stimulus for adrenal production of aldosterone.

There are several mechanisms through which a fall in extracellular volume leads to stimulation of the renin-angiotensin-aldosterone system, with consequent increase in sodium reabsorption, and volume expansion.[5] Vascular receptors in the renal afferent arterioles sense a fall in renal perfusion pressure or wall tension, and stimulate the release of renin by the juxtaglomerular cells. The macula densa, a group of specialized cells in the distal tubule, is anatomically associated with the juxtaglomerular cells of the afferent arteriole, and is believed to increase renin release in response to a fall in the delivery of sodium to the distal tubule. The juxtaglomerular apparatus has a rich supply of sympathetic nerve endings, and renal adrenergic stimulation increases in response to volume depletion, exercise, or upright posture, causing renin release.

Natriuretic Hormone. In animal experiments designed to prevent changes in GFR and aldosterone levels, plasma expansion has nevertheless resulted in a rise in sodium excretion, suggesting the existence of a "third factor" that is neither GFR nor aldosterone.[6] Extensive search for such a factor has been inconclusive, but there is much evidence favoring the existence of a humoral substance in the blood of volume-expanded animals and humans that decreases distal tubular reabsorption of sodium by ouabain-like inhibition of the Na^+-K^+ pump.[7] This hormone is thought to originate in the central nervous system, in response to volume expansion, and to aid in the restoration of normal extracellular volume by its natriuretic action.

Other Factors. Renal sympathetic nerve stimulation and circulating catecholamines may increase sodium reabsorption by direct as well as indirect hemodynamic mechanisms.[8,9] Angiotensin II, when renal perfusion pressure is low, may maintain a state of increased renal vascular resistance through constriction of the efferent arteriole; this helps to maintain the GFR, and may increase sodium reabsorption by causing a decrease in postglomerular capillary hydrostatic pressure and an increase in postglomerular oncotic pressure.[1,10] Renal prostaglandins increase sodium excretion, both through direct effects on the renal tubule and through the indirect effects of renal vasodilatation.[11,12]

Conditions Associated with Edema

RENAL FAILURE

The most direct chain of events leading to expansion of the extracellular fluid volume and edema is seen in patients with renal failure. In acute renal failure, caused by acute glomerulonephritis or oliguric acute tubular necrosis, the ability of the kidneys to excrete sodium and water is impaired. Unless the intake of salt and water is sharply curtailed there may be rapid fluid accumulation and edema. In chronic renal failure the GFR falls more gradually, but when it is severely reduced the kidneys may be unable to maintain sodium balance unless sodium intake is markedly restricted.[1]

CONGESTIVE HEART FAILURE

Failure of the heart to maintain sufficient output for the needs of peripheral tissues leads to fluid retention and edema through several mechanisms.[4] Impaired systolic emptying of the ventricles causes an increase in the filling pressure in the atria and large veins, and increased venous hydrostatic pressure promotes transudation of fluid from the intravascular to the interstitial space. In addition to this "backward failure," the lowered cardiac output causes a reduction in arterial filling, or "forward failure"; the loss of plasma volume due to the increased venous hydrostatic pressure combines with the fall in cardiac output to produce a reduction in the effective arterial blood volume.

The kidneys respond to this decrease in effective arterial blood volume by retaining sodium and water, through the mechanisms outlined above. An additional factor in patients with congestive heart failure is a decrease in the metabolic clearance rate of aldosterone,[13] caused by a reduction in hepatic blood flow; this enhances the elevation in aldosterone levels brought about by the stimulation of renin production.

NEPHROTIC SYNDROME

The urinary protein loss characteristic of the nephrotic syndrome leads to severe hypoalbuminemia, with reduction in colloid oncotic pressure within the capillary bed. The consequent transudation of fluid from the intravascular to the interstitial space results in edema and a fall in effective arterial blood volume. The latter change activates the renal sodium-reabsorbing mechanisms that lead to fluid retention. Because of the continued hypoalbuminemia the additional fluid cannot be retained within the vascular compartment in sufficient quantity to correct the deficit in effective arterial blood volume, and the stimulus to renal sodium retention continues to be present.

CIRRHOSIS

The mechanisms of edema formation in hepatic cirrhosis are less clearly defined. The traditional view that a decrease in effective arterial blood volume is the cause of renal sodium retention has been challenged by the "overflow" theory; this theory claims that sodium retention is the primary event, somehow caused by the liver disease, and ascites and edema result from the effects of volume overload on the splanchnic and peripheral circulations.

In the classic scheme, both hypoalbuminemia, as in the nephrotic syndrome, and hemodynamic changes, as in congestive heart failure, lead to a decrease in the effective arterial blood volume. The hypoalbuminemia is a consequence of decreased production of albumin by the damaged liver, and leads to a fall in capillary colloid oncotic pressure and loss of fluid from the vascular compartment. Inflammatory and fibrotic changes in the liver produce increased pressure in the hepatic and portal veins, splanchnic pooling of blood, and the transudation of fluid into the abdominal cavity. Also, the presence of arteriovenous shunting in cirrhosis reduces peripheral resistance and further decreases the effective circulating blood volume. Decreased ability of the damaged liver to inactivate aldosterone may further contribute to the sodium retention that occurs in response to these circulatory changes. The "underfilling" theory thus holds that renal sodium retention in cirrhosis occurs as a response to a reduction in effective arterial blood volume.

The "overflow" theory is based on the observation that total plasma volume in cirrhosis is normal or increased, rather than low.[14] In experimental cirrhosis in dogs, renal sodium retention occurred before a change in cardiac output or peripheral resistance could be demonstrated.[15] However, a specific mechanism by which liver damage might directly cause renal salt retention has not been shown.

There is evidence against the "overflow" theory. When central blood volume is expanded by the use of a peritoneovenous shunt[16] or by immersion of cirrhotic patients in water,[17] the abnormal retention of salt and water is corrected; this would seem to be better explained if volume contraction, rather than primary renal dysfunction, were the initiating event. Also, the hormonal changes associated with volume depletion, not volume expansion, are present in cirrhosis: elevated levels of vasopressin,[18] renin,[18] aldosterone,[18] and norepinephrine.[19] It seems most likely that the classic explanation of edema formation in cirrhosis is correct, and the failure to demonstrate volume contraction by direct measurement is attributable to the ability of the multiple compensatory mechanisms to maintain circulating volume within narrow limits.[20]

IDIOPATHIC EDEMA

Although primarily a diagnosis of exclusion, as the name implies, idiopathic edema tends to affect a particular group of patients and to present a clinical picture that is sufficiently characteristic to suggest the diagnosis.[21,22] This condition is seen almost exclusively in women, usually in their reproductive years, although it may persist after menopause. The edema is most marked in dependent areas, but affects the face, upper extremities, and trunk more frequently than does edema of other causes. Fluid retention tends to be accompanied by emotional changes such as depression and irritability, as well as aching and discomfort in the swollen areas. Because the excessive interstitial fluid may have a relatively high protein content and be widely distributed, pitting edema may not be obvious to the physician, but fluid retention can easily be documented by the marked gain in weight that these patients experience each day while they are up and about.[23]

The most often proposed explanation of idiopathic edema places the primary defect in the capillary wall. Increased vascular permeability leads to transudation of plasma protein and water into the interstitial space, especially in dependent parts of the body, when capillary hydrostatic pressure is increased by upright posture. The movement of protein into the interstitial space increases the interstitial colloid oncotic pressure, further favoring the movement of fluid out of the vessels. Decreased intravascular volume activates renal sodium retention, replenishing intravascular volume and allowing further movement of fluid into the interstitial space.

Direct evidence for this defect is limited to a few studies. Sims and co-workers[24] found thickening and irregularity in the basement membranes of 11 women with idiopathic edema, 7 of whom had positive family histories of diabetes mellitus. Several studies have shown an increased rate of loss of radiolabeled albumin from the vascular compartment[25,26] and a high protein level in edema fluid[25] in this syndrome. Other evidence for increased vascular permeability is indirect: The application of external pressure to the lower half of the body by means of a G-suit prevents not only the edema but also the abnormalities in water excretion associated with upright posture.[21]

Many investigators have found exaggerated aldosterone responses to upright posture in idiopathic edema, and measures that prevent aldosterone from acting, such as adrenalectomy[21] or the use of the aldosterone antagonist spironolactone, have at least a partial beneficial effect on the edema. Some have suggested that the control of aldosterone secretion is abnormal in idiopathic edema; for example, there is evidence for a decrease in dopaminergic inhibition of aldosterone production.[27] But there is no evidence that aldosterone plays a primary role in this syndrome rather than a secondary role in response to effective arterial blood volume depletion.

Nutritional Aspects of Management

SODIUM INTAKE

Total body sodium is the main determinant of extracellular fluid volume. Sodium and its anions, chloride and bicarbonate, make up more than 90 per cent of the total solute in the extracellular fluid.[1] Cell membranes retain potassium and other solutes within the cell while extruding sodium by active transport mechanisms. Since cell membranes are freely permeable to water, the osmolality of intracellular and extracellular fluid must be equal. Therefore the addition of sodium to the extracellular fluid compartment will temporarily result in an osmotic gradient, and intracellular water will move across the cell membrane, increasing the extracellular fluid volume. Other mechanisms by which extracellular fluid osmolality is maintained will also contribute to expansion of this compartment: Stimulation of the hypothalamic thirst center by the increased osmolality will bring about water ingestion, and stimulation of vasopressin release will lead to decreased free water clearance. Sodium balance, therefore, plays a crucial role in the regulation of extracellular fluid volume. In edematous states a negative sodium balance will produce a fall in extracellular fluid volume, which should affect both the vascular and interstitial compartments, although the balance of Starling forces in the capillary bed may profoundly affect the ability to mobilize edema fluid.

One of the mainstays of treatment in patients with edema of any cause, therefore, is dietary restriction of sodium.[28,29] A severely edematous patient is likely to have marked sodium retention, with excretion rates below 20 mEq daily. If the usual dietary intake of 100 to 200 mEq of sodium is maintained, sodium balance will remain markedly positive and fluid retention will continue. If sodium intake can be restricted to 10 to 20 mEq daily, it is not likely that a significantly negative balance can be achieved, but at least the progressive salt and water accumulation and edema formation will be interrupted.

The other measures of greatest importance in the treatment of edema, in addition to any steps that can be taken to lessen the severity of the underlying disease, are the enforcement of bed rest and the use of diuretics. Bed rest decreases the pooling of blood in the veins of the lower extremities, leading to expansion of the effective arterial blood volume and an increase in renal perfusion; this fluid shift may lessen or correct the deficit in circulating volume that is responsible for the sodium retention. Natriuresis and mobilization of edema fluid frequently occur promptly after a patient is hospitalized, even when the only changes in management are a stricter enforcement of salt restriction and bed rest.

If these measures are inadequate to control edema, the use of diuretics may be considered. These drugs will induce negative sodium balance with less need for rigid dietary salt restriction. However, if other factors are equal, a lower sodium intake will be associated with a more negative sodium balance in a diuretic-treated patient, and more rapid loss of edema.

In the early stages of heart failure, cirrhosis, and nephrosis, sodium and water are retained isosmotically, and serum sodium levels are usually normal. In the more severe, later stages of these diseases, there is a tendency for water to be retained in excess of sodium, leading to hyponatremia. The causes of this are not completely understood, but it seems likely that nonosmotic stimulation of ADH by a very severely diminished effective arterial blood volume,[18] a decrease in sodium available for reabsorption at the renal tubular diluting sites, and the effects of angiotensin II in stimulating thirst and ADH[30] lead to increased water retention. It is important to remember that the cause of the hyponatremia is likely to be water excess, not sodium depletion; fluid restriction, not sodium loading, is the appropriate dietary treatment. The restriction of fluid intake to 500 to 1000 ml/day should help to raise the level of serum sodium.

Care must be taken to avoid the induction of excessively negative sodium balance with the use of salt restriction and diuretics. Some believe that in idiopathic edema further stimulation of the renin-angiotensin-aldosterone system by too vigorous sodium depletion may worsen the edema. MacGregor and co-workers[31] have shown that levels of renin and aldosterone that are increased by salt restriction and diuretics remain elevated for up to 10 days after the treatment is discontinued. They speculate that some patients who restrict dietary sodium irregularly might have marked sodium retention during times when high aldosterone levels persist following prior salt restriction, but when the effects of the increased aldosterone are not counterbalanced by current diuretic use or salt restriction.

In cirrhosis, nephrosis, or heart failure, sodium and water should not be removed by salt restriction and diuresis at a faster rate than edema fluid can be mobilized, which will seldom exceed 1 L/day. Too rapid contraction of the vascular space, with inadequate shifting of fluid from the interstitial to the vascular compartment, may lead to circulatory impairment and prerenal azotemia. In cases of intractable edema the potency of the Starling forces that prevent return of interstitial fluid into the circulation may be the limiting factor in treatment.

Protein Intake

While sodium is of primary importance in the control of extracellular fluid volume, serum albumin plays a similar dominant role in the partitioning of extracellular fluid between the vascular and interstitial compartments. Human albumin is a small protein, with a molecular weight of about 66,000,[32] that accounts for 80 per cent of the colloid osmotic pressure of the blood. The molecule is large enough to be retained within the vascular space by the capillary walls, except for small quantities that escape into the interstitial space and are returned to the bloodstream by the lymphatics. Because of the higher concentration of albumin within the vessels, the osmotic pressure of the plasma is about 28 mm Hg, compared with 10 mm Hg in the interstitial fluid. The difference, or 18 mm Hg, is the effective osmotic pressure of the plasma proteins, or the "oncotic" pressure.[33] When serum albumin falls the oncotic pressure is reduced, and the balance of Starling forces shifts in the direction favoring edema formation.

Approximately 40 per cent of the albumin in the body is in the circulation, and the rest is distributed widely among the other organs and tissues.[32] Albumin is synthesized in the liver, and degraded in many organs, in particular the liver and kidneys. It has a half-life of 19 days,[32] and a daily synthesis rate in adults of 14 to 23 g.[34] Hepatic synthesis of albumin is regulated by the supply of amino acids to the liver, and by the colloid osmotic pressure of the plasma; a fall in amino acids or an increase in osmotic pressure decreases albumin synthesis.

Hypoalbuminemia is a major factor in the production of edema in patients with hepatic cirrhosis and patients with the nephrotic syndrome. In cirrhosis a number of derangements may contribute to the low albumin:[32,35,36] poor nutrition, with decreased protein intake; direct toxic effects of ethanol on hepatic synthesis of albumin; destruction of liver cells; and direct loss of newly synthesized albumin

into ascitic fluid. In the nephrotic syndrome, the main cause of decreased serum albumin is the loss of small proteins in the urine because of the defect in glomerular permeability. An additional factor is an increase in the catabolism of albumin by the kidney. Albumin in tubular fluid may be taken up by the tubular epithelial cells and degraded to free amino acids, which are returned to the circulation. In the absence of abnormal glomerular permeability to small proteins, only minimal amounts of albumin enter the tubular fluid and are exposed to the renal tubular catabolic sites. But in a nephrotic patient, whose glomeruli allow large quantities of protein to enter the tubular fluid, significant renal degradation of albumin may occur.[37,38]

Protein-losing enteropathy includes a number of diseases of the gastrointestinal mucosa or lymphatics in which large quantities of protein are lost into the bowel, with or without malabsorption of fat or other nutrients.[39] Hypoalbuminemia, with fluid retention and edema, may be a prominent manifestation.

In the management of patients with edema caused wholly or partially by hypoalbuminemia, several measures may help to restore the circulating albumin pool toward normal. The first consideration should be treatment of the underlying disease; other approaches are the use of human serum albumin and an increase in dietary protein intake.

Normal human serum albumin, manufactured from the plasma of volunteer donors, is available in units containing 12.5 g of albumin, either as a 5 per cent (250 ml) or a 25 per cent (50 ml) solution. These preparations are useful chiefly in acute hypovolemia associated with surgery, trauma, or hemorrhage.[34] Albumin infusions are seldom indicated in chronic edematous states with hypoalbuminemia, such as cirrhosis and nephrosis, since this form of treatment is expensive and of limited efficacy in these conditions. In cirrhosis, some patients may have a decrease in edema if large quantities of albumin are given, but others may have increased fluid accumulation owing to passage of the added albumin into the ascitic fluid.[40] Long-term albumin administration does not seem to prolong life or favorably affect the course of the disease.[40] In the nephrotic syndrome the volume expansion produced by an infusion of albumin leads to increased glomerular permeability to albumin,[41] and the administered albumin is rapidly lost in the urine. However, in cases of severe fluid retention unresponsive to diuretics and other measures, especially if the disorder is relatively acute, administration of human serum albumin for several days may be of value. The rapid (although transient) expansion of plasma volume may restore the patient's responsiveness to diuretics, with subsequent natriuresis and clinical improvement. Twenty-five to 50 g of albumin should be given daily for a period of 3 to 10 days.[34,42]

Dietary protein intake has a major effect on hepatic synthesis of albumin. Starvation or a low protein intake results in a rapid fall in albumin synthesis to less than 50 per cent of the original rate.[35,43–45] This is presumed to be caused by the decreased availability of amino acids for protein synthesis.[32,44] The rate of catabolism of albumin also falls, but not enough to compensate for the decreased synthesis.[45] The intravascular albumin pool is reduced to a lesser degree than the extravascular pool, because of transfer of extravascular albumin to the bloodstream,[46,47] but the net result of these changes is a fall in plasma albumin concentration. A high protein intake can produce a positive nitrogen balance in patients with nephrosis[48] and can promptly reverse the hypoalbuminemia produced by starvation in animals.[49]

It it therefore important to maintain a high protein intake in patients with edema related to hypoalbuminemia. Poor nutrition in anorexic patients with cirrhosis or nephrosis will worsen the hypoalbuminemia that is already a major factor in the disease. Ideally these patients should receive 50 to 60 kcal/kg of ideal body weight, and 1.5 g/kg of high-quality protein.[50,51]

In patients with nephrosis a high protein intake may cause increased proteinuria; this is expected if serum protein levels are raised, and does not indicate worsening of the kidney disease.[51] If the blood urea nitrogen rises when the protein intake is increased, a balance must be reached between the benefits of protein repletion and the risk of urea retention.[51] In cirrhosis, hepatic encephalopathy may be the factor that limits protein intake. If symptoms of encephalopathy progress despite antibiotic treatment, protein intake must be decreased or stopped, but should be resumed as soon as possible.[52]

CALORIE INTAKE

In patients with hepatic cirrhosis or the nephrotic syndrome, calorie intake must be adequate to ensure that protein and amino acids are utilized to maintain the visceral protein stores and serum albumin, rather than to provide energy. However, in patients with idiopathic edema, who tend to be overweight,[21,22,53] dietary management has different goals. Obese patients with idiopathic edema often have marked lessening of fluid retention if they lose weight; Streeten has documented the disappearance of edema with weight reduction in two such patients[21] (Fig. 24–2). The cause of edema associated with obesity, and the frequency of this association, are not known. A low-calorie diet, perhaps with a high protein and low carbohydrate content,[53] as well as sodium restriction, is indicated in overweight patients with idiopathic edema.

NUTRITIONAL EDEMA

In developed countries generalized edema is most commonly related to primary disease of the heart, liver, or kidneys, and therapeutic alteration of the dietary intake of sodium, protein, and calories is an attempt to favorably affect certain secondary manifestations of the disease. In many parts of the world, however, edema is a common manifestation of primary nutritional deficiency, especially kwashiorkor, a form of starvation in which protein intake is low in relation to energy intake.

The edema of chronic starvation is probably caused by several factors.[54,55] Hypoalbuminemia results from the lack of amino acids available for hepatic synthesis of albumin.[56] Circulatory failure occurs, with a marked fall in cardiac output.[57] Renal function may be decreased because of direct effects of starvation, and because of a decrease in renal perfusion caused by circulatory failure.[55] Careful refeeding should be followed by disappearance of the edema.

HYPERTENSION

Pathogenesis

Hypertension has been called mankind's most common disease, affecting 15 to 20 per cent of all adults.[58] In a few cases, probably in less than 3 per cent of patients with hypertension, a specific cause can be found, such as renovascular disease, primary aldosteronism, or pheochromocytoma. In most cases, those that we consider "primary" or "essential" hypertension, the cause is unknown.

A great deal is known, however, about the physiological changes and environmental factors associated with hypertension, and many experimental procedures have induced blood pressure elevation in animals. To understand the role that changes in dietary intake of various nutrients may play in the etiology and management of hypertension, one must understand the many interrelated forces that control arterial pressure (Fig. 24–3).

Blood pressure is determined by cardiac output and peripheral resistance; if either increases, without a compensating fall in the other, the blood pressure will rise. The events that cause an increase in blood pressure through an increase in cardiac output are those that cause salt and water retention, with consequent expansion of the extracellular and plasma volume; such causes include renal disease, excessive levels of sodium-retaining hormones, and perhaps excessive dietary sodium intake. The factors that raise peripheral resistance are those that cause increased vascular constriction and narrowing of the arterial lumen, such as increased sympathetic nervous system activity and increased levels of vasoconstrictors like angiotensin II and norepinephrine. The events leading to increased cardiac output may interact with those that raise peripheral resistance. For example, sodium retention may lead to an increase in sodium content of the arterial walls, in-

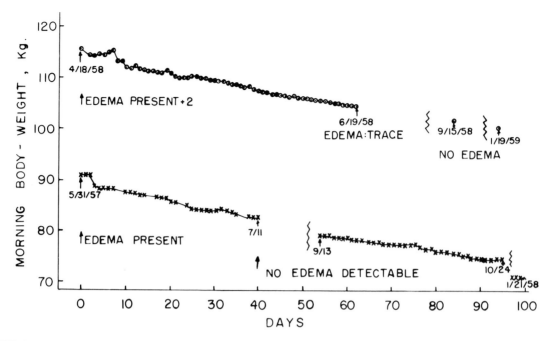

FIGURE 24–2. Disappearance of edema with weight loss in two women with severe obesity. (From Streeten DHP. Metabolism 1978; 27:353–383. Reproduced with permission.)

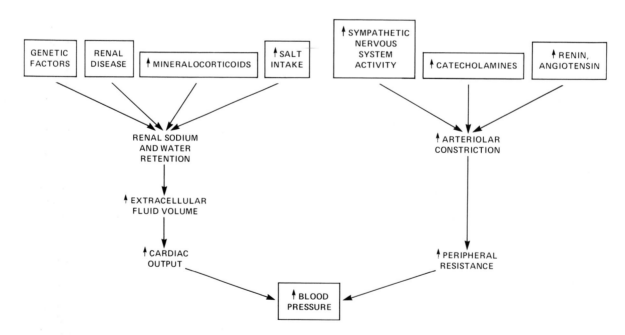

FIGURE 24–3. Some of the factors that may cause or contribute to hypertension, and their roles in its pathogenesis.

creasing the vascular reactivity to pressor stimuli. Also, prolonged excessive blood flow through the tissues, as a result of increased cardiac output, may bring about an autoregulatory response in which the local tissue resistance is increased, raising the total peripheral resistance. Whatever the initiating event, renal control of salt and water balance might be expected to return pressure to normal unless the abnormal process somehow affects the kidneys.[59] Although renal excretion of salt and water seems normal in hypertension, it is postulated that the normal output is achieved only through the elevation in arterial pressure; that is, a renal abnormality allows adequate excretory function only at the expense of increased renal perfusion pressure.[59]

The conditions that cause secondary hypertension affect blood pressure through one or more of the pathways described above. In renovascular hypertension the stenotic renal arterial lesion decreases the perfusion pressure in the afferent renal arterioles, stimulating renin production by the juxtaglomerular cells; angiotensin II is increased, causing arteriolar vasoconstriction, and increased adrenal production of aldosterone, with consequent sodium retention. Renal functional impairment may hinder sodium and water excretion, further expanding plasma volume. In primary aldosteronism the increased circulating levels of aldosterone cause sodium retention and volume expansion. The norepinephrine and epinephrine produced by a pheochromocytoma raise blood pressure by increasing peripheral vasoconstriction and cardiac output.

Which of these or other mechanisms is responsible for essential hypertension is not known. In fact, the observation that some hypertensive patients have low plasma renin activity, suggesting volume expansion,[60] while others have high renin levels, suggesting peripheral vasoconstriction,[61] contributes to the impression that essential hypertension is a heterogeneous condition with multiple causes. Also, the fairly simple pathogenetic scheme outlined above does not take into account a great many factors that are of potential importance in blood pressure regulation and that are being extensively investigated, such as prostaglandins, kinins, and cation transport across cell membranes.

Nutritional Aspects of Etiology and Management

Hypertension is associated with a greatly increased risk of cerebrovascular disease, congestive heart failure, coronary artery disease, and renal failure. Fortunately, drugs are available that can lower blood pressure to normal in a large proportion of hypertensive patients, with marked reduction in the risk of cardiovascular and other complications. But many patients are unwilling to take a lifelong course of medication, which sometimes causes unpleasant side effects, for an asymptomatic condition. It is no wonder, then, that there is great interest in the idea that dietary factors may be important in the etiology of hypertension. A link between a specific nutrient and hypertension, if proved, not only would further our understanding of the causes of the disease but could also provide a means to lower pressure without the use of drugs, through dietary modification. A number of specific dietary factors have been studied as possible contributing causes of hypertension.

Sodium Intake

The theory that salt ingestion is a major factor in the etiology of hypertension is the most widely known of the postulated links between nutrition and high blood pressure. The importance of salt intake was suggested in the 1940's by the success of extreme sodium restriction in the reduction of elevated blood pressure, and subsequent animal studies, epidemiological surveys, and dietary trials have both supported and contradicted this view.

The Rice Diet. Kempner treated 500 patients with severe hypertension, averaging 199/117 mm Hg, with a diet that consisted of rice, fruit, and sugar and contained about 2000 kcal, 15 to 25 g of protein, 4 to 6 g of fat, and less than 150 mg (7 mEq) of sodium.[62] Two thirds of his patients showed a fall in mean blood pressure of 20 mm Hg or more. The original rationale for this diet was the belief that the low protein intake reduced blood pressure by decreasing the work of the kidneys,[62,63] but later studies pointed to the very low sodium content of the diet as the important factor.[64,65]

This work can be justly criticized because the effects of hospitalization, weight loss, and the placebo effect of the diet were not taken into account.[66] Nevertheless, the success of the rice diet in lowering blood pressure in a group of patients with severe, previously intractable hypertension, at a time when effective drugs were not available, is striking, and must be counted among the observations favoring a role for sodium restriction in the treatment of high blood pressure.

Experimental Observations. A large body of experimental data, collected over the past 3 decades, links sodium and hypertension. People with essential hypertension[67] and animals with renovascular and mineralocorticoid hypertension[68] have increased concentrations of sodium in their arterial walls. Most forms of experimental hypertension are more readily induced and of greater magnitude if the salt intake of the animal is raised, and can often be prevented by salt restriction.[69] By selectively inbreeding rats according to their tendency to develop higher blood pressure when fed salt, Dahl was able to produce two strains, one very sensitive and one very resistant to sodium.[70] On a low salt intake both the salt-sensitive and salt-resistant animals have normal blood pressure, but when salt intake is raised, the sensitive rats retain sodium and develop hypertension, while the resistant rats excrete the additional sodium and remain normotensive.

Increased sodium intake raises the blood pressure of normal human volunteers, but only if high quantities, in the range of 800 to 1500 mEq daily, are consumed.[71] Studies suggest, however, that genetic factors may make some people less able to handle a salt load than others. Similarities in the rate of renal excretion of sodium are greater in monozygotic twins than in dizygotic twins.[72] Normotensive young people with positive family histories of hypertension have shown an increased stress-induced blood pressure rise after salt loading, compared with subjects with negative family histories.[73] Normal white subjects may excrete a sodium load more rapidly than normal black subjects[74] or white subjects with hypertensive first-degree relatives.

Epidemiological Studies. In many societies throughout the world the average blood pressure is low and does not rise with age, and hypertension is rare. These societies are mainly primitive tribal groups whose diet is low in sodium and high in potassium.[75–77] The Yanomamo Indians of northern Brazil and southern Venezuela, for example, eat bananas, supplemented by game, fish, and wild vegetables; their urine contains 152 mEq of potassium and only 1 mEq of sodium in 24 hours.[78] Although they have levels of renin activity and aldosterone that are extremely high compared with the levels in normal North Americans or Europeans, their blood pressure averages only 98 to 108 mm Hg systolic and 62 to 69 diastolic, and does not increase with age. Hypertension is unknown.

Other populations with low salt intake and low blood pressure have been described in Africa, Australia, New Guinea, the Solomon Islands, Polynesia, and elsewhere.[75,77] In some cases it has been possible to compare two genetically related populations with dissimilar diets; in each case the population with the higher blood pressure had a higher level of salt consumption.[79–81] When certain members of a low blood pressure population have raised their salt intake, as in the case of Samburu nomads of East Africa who joined the British Army, their blood pressure has risen.[82]

An analysis of 27 studies of individual populations, including groups with low and high salt intake, revealed a highly significant positive correlation between average blood pressure and salt consumption;[79] correlation coefficients for diastolic blood pressure and salt intake were 0.63 for women and 0.66 for men. The relationship between salt intake and blood pressure, based on data from 30 population surveys, is shown in Figure 24–4.[83] One cannot conclude with certainty, however, that the level of salt intake is causally related to the level of blood pressure, since other environmental changes often accompany the acculturation and urbanization associated with increased salt consumption. Increased

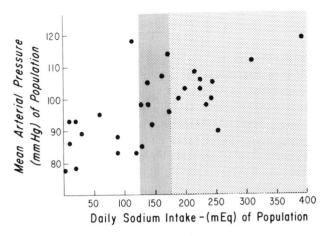

FIGURE 24–4. Mean arterial pressure and dietary sodium intake in 30 populations. (From McCarron DA, Henry HJ, Morris CD. Hypertension 1982; 4[Suppl III]:2–13. Reproduced with permission.)

psychological stress, decreased physical activity, greater dietary fat intake, higher calorie intake, and increased prevalence of obesity tend to go along with a more "civilized" way of life, and these changes, rather than (or in addition to) the increase in salt consumption, may affect blood pressure levels.

Although high sodium intake is unquestionably associated with higher blood pressure when separate populations are compared, studies are almost as consistent in failing to reveal a relation between sodium intake and blood pressure within individual societies. Studies of 24-hour urine sodium excretion,[84,85] studies of sodium excretion in morning urine samples,[86] and dietary surveys in large samples of the U.S. population[87,88] have shown no relation between blood pressure and sodium intake or excretion. In the occasional study that has found an association between blood pressure and salt intake, the correlation has been very weak and has explained only a small percentage of the variance in blood pressure.[89,90]

How can one reconcile the strong evidence for an association between dietary sodium and blood pressure levels between populations with the consistent failure to find such an association within individual populations? Several explanations have been offered. If salt has a blood pressure–raising effect in only a specific small segment of the population, as suggested by some studies,[91] this relation might be obscured by the lack of association of salt and blood pressure in the rest of the population.[69,92] Also, the range of sodium intake within a population might be too narrow to reveal an association with blood pressure levels. Finally, because of the sigmoid shape of the curve that describes the relation between salt intake and hypertension[93] (Fig. 24–5), the rise in prevalence of hypertension may be very slight as salt intake increases above 100 mEq daily; that is, within the range of daily sodium intake of 100 to 300 mEq

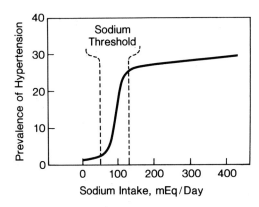

FIGURE 24–5. The probable association between usual dietary sodium intake and the prevalence of hypertension in large populations. (From Kaplan NM. JAMA 1984; 251:1429–1430. Reproduced with permission.)

that is common in Western societies, a relation between salt intake and blood pressure might not be evident.

Effects of Moderate Salt Restriction. Limitation of daily sodium intake to levels of 20 to 40 mEq or less leads to a fall in blood pressure in hypertensive patients, and a very low incidence of hypertension within a population. Such severe salt restriction is possible, however, only if one adheres strictly to a diet that is drastically different from usual Western fare, for example the rice-fruit diet, or if one lives in a society in which such a diet is the norm. The crucial question, then, is whether a less strict limitation of salt intake that could be adhered to without undue difficulty by the typical patient is of benefit in the management of hypertension.

In a number of studies, some well controlled, patients with mild to moderate hypertension have followed moderately salt-restricted diets, with daily sodium intake (or urine sodium excretion) between 40 and 120 mEq. These studies have tended to show a fall in blood pressure of about 8/5 mm Hg (Table 24–1, Fig. 24–6).[94–99] In one study a marked decrease in antihypertensive medication was possible in salt-restricted patients.[97] Variability in response to sodium restriction was marked, with some patients

actually experiencing an increase in blood pressure.[99]

The Role of Sodium Restriction in the Management of Hypertension. A view can be arrived at that is consistent with most of the observations summarized above concerning the role of sodium intake in hypertension. This view holds that about 10 to 20 per cent of individuals have a genetically related tendency to develop high blood pressure. If sodium intake is below a minimum level, which has been estimated to be about 70 mEq daily,[77] this hypertension-prone subgroup will not experience an increase in blood pressure. In most societies, however, sodium intake is higher than this threshold, that is, high enough to allow the development of hypertension in susceptible persons. The other 80 or 90 per cent will not become hypertensive, even with high salt consumption, and their blood pressure will not be related to their individual levels of salt intake.

In accord with this view, there is no evidence that people who do not have a tendency to develop high blood pressure are benefitted in any way by a decrease in their salt consumption. The popular notion that eating less salt will prevent hypertension may be true in many cases, especially in patients with borderline hypertension, but careful monitoring of blood pressure and the recommendation of salt reduction in appropriate instances seems preferable to the indiscriminate curtailment of dietary salt. On the other hand, patients who have a tendency to develop hypertension are likely to benefit from salt restriction.

If reduction of sodium intake to 70 to 100 mEq daily will lower the blood pressure of the average patient by 7 to 10 mm Hg systolic and 4 to 6 mm Hg diastolic, as studies suggest, this dietary change would be of value: Some patients with mild hypertension would become normotensive with reduced salt intake alone and not require medication, while others would be able to take less medication, with fewer side effects and less expense. The factor limiting the usefulness of dietary modification is patient compliance. Even mild restriction of salt requires the avoidance of many foods and a decrease in the palatability of many others. A patient who is highly

TABLE 24–1. Controlled Studies of Moderate Sodium Restriction in Patients with Mild to Moderate Hypertension

Study	Number of Subjects	Sodium in Diet or 24-Hour Urine During Treatment (mEq)	Duration of Study	Fall in Blood Pressure (mm Hg) Compared with Control Group
Parijs[94]	22	93 (urine)	1 month	8/4
Morgan[95]	48	70 (diet)	8 weeks	13/7
MacGregor[96]	19	86 (urine)	4 weeks	10/5
Beard[97]	90	37 (urine)	12 weeks	5/3*
Silman[98]	12	117 (urine)	12 months	9/6
Richards[99]	12	80 (diet)	4–6 weeks	4/3

*Antihypertensive medication was decreased as blood pressure fell; this may have lessened the difference between the diet and control groups.

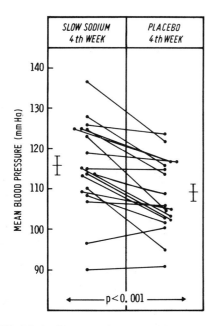

FIGURE 24–6. Changes in mean blood pressure between the fourth week of a low-sodium diet plus an oral sodium supplement, Slow Sodium (urine sodium 162 mEq/24 hours) and the fourth week of a low-sodium diet plus placebo (urine sodium 86 mEq/24 hours). Nineteen patients were studied in an 8-week double-blind randomized crossover trial. (From MacGregor GA, Markandu ND, Best FE, et al. Lancet 1982; 1:351–355. Reproduced with permission.)

motivated to control his or her blood pressure by nonpharmacological means, and willing to endure the inconvenience of long-term dietary alteration, may benefit from salt restriction. Other patients, probably a substantial majority, would prefer to decrease their total body sodium by the use of diuretics rather than diet. This is a less physiologic approach, and may subject the patient to the risk of long-term undesirable effects of diuretics, such as an increase in low-density lipoproteins. While the benefits of blood-pressure reduction clearly outweigh the slight risks of diuretic use in patients with moderate and severe hypertension, the risk-benefit ratio in patients with mild hypertension is much less clear.[100] Although some have stressed the potential dangers of salt restriction, such as hyponatremia and volume depletion,[66,101] these would be a risk only under extreme climatic conditions or in patients with concurrent diuretic use or gastrointestinal disease.

A reasonable approach, then, would be to strongly encourage salt restriction in patients who are motivated to control their hypertension by dietary means and in patients in whom drug therapy alone has provided unsatisfactory control. Other patients should be advised that salt restriction is of value, but a realistic approach will focus more on drug therapy than on diet.

POTASSIUM INTAKE

The evidence linking potassium intake to hypertension, though not as extensive as the evidence implicating sodium, is based on similar observations: dietary patterns in hypertension-free societies, the relation between potassium ingestion and blood pressure, the physiological effects of potassium, and blood pressure changes induced by potassium in hypertensive patients. But potassium differs from sodium in that it is suspected of playing a protective rather than a causative role in the development of hypertension.

The natural diet of primitive societies consists largely of fruit, vegetables, and wild game, and is low in sodium and high in potassium. Civilization brings the use of salt as a preservative and condiment, and the practice of cooking, which removes potassium from foods.[102] The unacculturated, hypertension-free societies that have low sodium consumption tend also to have high dietary levels of potassium, which must be considered as a factor that may contribute to the low blood pressure. Studies that compare potassium excretion with blood pressure are suggestive. Black subjects in Evans County, Georgia, who had a much higher prevalence of hypertension than whites, had no greater intake of sodium, but their potassium intake was only half the potassium intake of the white subjects.[103] Although studies within populations have usually failed to find a positive correlation between sodium excretion and blood pressure, several such studies have found a negative correlation between urinary potassium and blood pressure[86] or a positive correlation between the urinary sodium:potassium ratio and blood pressure.[89,90] Even when significant, however, these correlations have been weak, accounting for no more than 5 per cent of the variance in blood pressure.[86]

There are several physiological actions of potassium that might contribute to the lowering of blood pressure. Potassium has a natriuretic effect, inhibiting renal sodium reabsorption; it inhibits renin production by a direct effect on the kidneys; and it causes vasodilatation, perhaps through stimulation of the Na^+-K^+ pump.[102,104] But potassium has other effects that may oppose its blood pressure–lowering actions, such as a secondary stimulation of renin production because of potassium's natriuretic effect, and a direct stimulatory effect on adrenal production of aldosterone.[102,104]

Several studies have examined the effect of increased potassium intake on the blood pressure of hypertensive patients (Table 24–2). The oral administration of 100 mEq daily of additional potassium was followed by a fall in mean arterial pressure of 11 mm Hg in a 10-day study,[105] and a 3-mm Hg fall in a trial lasting 12 weeks.[106] In another carefully controlled study, the addition to the diet of 60 mEq of potassium per day was associated with a 4-mm Hg fall in mean arterial pressure over a 4-week period.[107] In patients with a high sodium intake, 260

TABLE 24–2. *Effect of Increased Potassium Intake on Blood Pressure in Patients with Essential Hypertension*

Study	Number of Subjects	Potassium in Diet (mEq/Day)	Duration of Study	Fall in Mean Arterial Pressure (mm Hg)
Iimura[105]	20	175	10 days	11
Parfrey[106]	15	120*	12 wks	3
MacGregor[107]	23	120	4 wks	4

*Patients were also mildly sodium-restricted: urine sodium 123 mEq/24 hr.

mEq daily, the fall in blood pressure with added potassium was accompanied by natriuresis and weight loss,[105] but in patients with lower sodium intakes, 120 to 170 mEq, blood pressure reduction occurred without a loss of weight.[106,107]

Because the data on the antihypertensive effect of added potassium are limited, and the results modest, and because a high potassium intake could be hazardous in patients with renal insufficiency, potassium supplementation is not recommended as antihypertensive therapy at this time.[104] The effect of potassium on elevated blood pressure is, however, a promising subject for investigation, suggesting a nutritional intervention that may prove to be useful in the management of hypertension.

OBESITY

Hypertension is more common in people who are overweight, and the degree of blood pressure elevation is related to the degree of obesity. Sixty per cent of the patients studied in the Hypertension Detection and Follow-up Program were more than 20 per cent above ideal weight, compared with 24 per cent of all American women and 14 per cent of American men.[108] In the Framingham study of 5127 men and women,[109] the prevalence of hypertension rose sharply as relative weight increased (Table 24–3). The correlation coefficient between systolic blood pressure and relative weight was 0.3; similar correlations have been found in other large epidemiological surveys.[110–112] The Framingham data predict that a 10 per cent rise or fall in weight would result in a rise or fall in systolic blood pressure of 6.6 mm Hg in men and 4.5 mm Hg in women.[113]

TABLE 24–3. *Prevalence of Hypertension by Sex and Age, According to Framingham Relative Weight*

	Percent Hypertensive (BP 160/95 or Higher)			
	Relative Weight*			
	<85	85–99	100–114	>114
Men, 30–39	3	5	14	27
Men, 50–59	13	22	26	47
Women, 30–39	1	1	5	17
Women, 50–59	18	27	26	46

Adapted from Kannel et al.[109]
*Relative weight: Percentage of the median weight of all subjects of the same height and sex.

The correlation between blood pressure and weight is stronger in whites than in blacks; one study suggested that control of obesity could potentially prevent 28 per cent of new cases of hypertension in blacks and 48 per cent in whites.[114]

Support for a cause-and-effect relationship between obesity and hypertension is provided by studies that demonstrate a fall in blood pressure coincident with caloric restriction and weight loss. A review of older reports concluded that weight loss was followed by a reduction in blood pressure in a large percentage of obese hypertensive patients.[111] Recent studies, in which weight losses of 8 to 21 kg have been achieved through the use of low-calorie diets, with or without salt restriction, have produced blood pressure reductions of 10 to 22 mm Hg (Table 24–4).[115–119]

The reasons for the association between obesity and hypertension are not known. It has been thought that blood volume and cardiac output are elevated in obesity,[120,121] but when these measurements in moderately obese hypertensive subjects are corrected for body surface area they are no higher than in nonobese hypertensive individuals and slightly lower than in normal subjects;[122] this question is unresolved. Insulin is suspected of playing a role in volume regulation in overweight subjects, since it is elevated in obesity, and has been shown to cause renal sodium retention.[123] DeFronzo and co-workers[124] demonstrated a prompt fall in urine sodium after insulin infusion in normal subjects whose blood glucose, renal blood flow, and glomerular filtration rate were kept constant. An antinatriuretic action of insulin is supported by other observations, and is consistent with the sodium loss that occurs with fasting, a state in which insulin is low, and the sodium retention that occurs with carbohydrate refeeding, a state in which insulin is stimulated. Interestingly, a physical training program in obese women that caused a fall in insulin and glucose levels produced a fall in blood pressure, even though the subjects did not lose weight.[125]

Changes in sympathetic nervous system activity and catecholamine levels may be involved in the blood pressure changes of obesity and weight loss. Fasting suppresses and overfeeding stimulates the sympathetic nervous system in animals.[126] A fall in norepinephrine levels has been shown to accompany the reduction in blood pressure that occurs with caloric restriction.[117,118,127] Decreased sympathetic ac-

TABLE 24–4. Studies of Blood Pressure Response to Weight Reduction in Normotensive and Hypertensive Obese Patients

Study	Unrestricted Sodium Diet			Low-Sodium Diet		
	Weight Loss (kg)	Fall in MAP* (mm Hg)	Sodium Intake or Excretion (mEq/24 hr)	Weight Loss (kg)	Fall in MAP (mm Hg)	Sodium Intake or Excretion (mEq/24 hr)
Reisin[115]	8.8	22	165	—	—	—
Tuck[116]	20.2	16	120	20.2	19	40
Sowers[117]	—	—	—	21	21	40
Reisin[118]	10	10	176	—	—	—
Fagerberg[119]	8	4	195	9	12	96

*Mean arterial pressure.

tivity may lower blood pressure not only through a decrease in arteriolar constriction, but also through a reduced adrenergic effect on renal sodium reabsorption[8,9] and a reduced adrenergic stimulation of renin production.[117]

Many have suspected that the blood pressure fall accompanying weight loss was largely the result of a reduction in salt intake. The study of Reisin and co-workers challenged this view.[115] These investigators produced weight loss in obese hypertensive patients with a low-calorie diet that was unrestricted in salt, and found a marked fall in blood pressure despite continued urinary excretion of more than 150 mEq of sodium daily. Fagerberg and co-workers,[119] on the other hand, observed a marked fall in blood pressure only in patients treated with salt restriction as well as caloric restriction, although patients with only caloric restriction lost an equal amount of weight (Table 24–4).

Whatever the mechanism, loss of weight in obese hypertensive patients is commonly accompanied by a substantial decrease in blood pressure, often into the normal range. Unlike other measures that lower blood pressure, such as salt restriction and antihypertensive drugs, weight loss lowers pressure in normal as well as hypertensive subjects.[108,116] The success of weight reduction in lowering blood pressure in recent clinical studies suggests that weight loss should be a prime goal of any treatment program in hypertension.

Calcium Intake

Epidemiological studies have suggested that cardiovascular mortality and blood pressure levels are higher in localities with soft drinking water, and lower in areas with hard water.[128,129] Since hardness of water depends largely on the concentration of calcium salts, these studies have raised the possibility that calcium is protective against hypertension.

Although recent reviews have emphasized the uncertainty of the association between soft water and cardiovascular disease,[130,131] other findings have provoked renewed interest in calcium as a factor in blood pressure regulation. The dietary intake of calcium appears to be lower in people with hyperten-

sion.[132–136] Twenty-four-hour dietary recall showed a daily calcium intake of 668 mg in 46 hypertensive patients, compared with 886 mg in matched control subjects.[132] Similar differences were detected in a large dietary study, the Health and Nutrition Examination Survey I of 1971 to 1974.[133] Confounding factors, particularly age and alcohol intake, must be considered, since calcium intake is lower in the elderly and in alcoholics, while hypertension increases with age and alcohol intake. A study in which age, obesity, and alcohol intake were controlled statistically showed a significant, but very small, negative correlation between blood pressure and calcium intake in men, but not in women.[135]

Studies of blood calcium levels in hypertension are few, and the results inconsistent. McCarron[137] found a lower serum ionized calcium level (2.07 mEq/L) in 23 untreated hypertensive patients than in matched controls (2.17 mEq/L), while total calcium levels were not different. Large population surveys, on the other hand, have shown positive correlations between total serum calcium and blood pressure.[138,139] Serum albumin is slightly higher in patients with hypertension,[140,141] which may account for the higher total calcium levels, but the lower ionized calcium is more difficult to explain, since ionized calcium is thought to be regulated by a feedback mechanism involving parathyroid hormone and perhaps calcitonin, independent of serum albumin.[142] In a study of ionized calcium levels in 98 hypertensive patients, Resnick and co-workers[143] confirmed low levels in patients with low plasma renin activity (2.09 mEq/L compared with 2.20 mEq/L in normal subjects), but found elevated levels (2.34 mEq/L) in hypertensive patients with high plasma renin activity.

How might calcium protect against hypertension? The simplest explanation would be a direct effect of calcium in causing relaxation of vascular smooth muscle cells,[133] which occurs under certain conditions in vitro.[144] However, hypercalcemia has been observed to cause an increase rather than a decrease in blood pressure in some clinical situations.[145,146] Also, the observation that hypercalcemic patients with primary hyperparathyroidism have elevated rather than decreased blood pressure[147,148] suggests that factors in addition to blood calcium must be considered. Parathyroid hormone (PTH) increases intracellular calcium levels in kidney cells[149] and liver cells;[150] similar changes in vascular smooth muscle cells are known to cause vasoconstriction, and so might raise blood pressure. A deficient calcium intake might promote hypertension by leading to higher blood levels of PTH;[151] the finding of increased PTH levels in patients with hypertension[152] supports this idea.

Of greatest interest is the possibility that increased dietary calcium might favorably affect hypertension. Spontaneously hypertensive rats had less severe blood pressure elevations when calcium intake was increased.[153] Treatment of 57 normal young people with 1 g of elemental calcium daily, in addition to their regular diet, led to a fall in diastolic blood pressure of 5 per cent in women and 9 per cent in men.[151] The response of 48 hypertensive patients to supplementation with 1 g of calcium daily for 8 weeks varied widely, but systolic blood pressure fell an average of 3.8 mm Hg and diastolic an average of 5.6 mm Hg.[154]

The available evidence that calcium intake may affect blood pressure is provocative, but one cannot yet draw definite conclusions. Certainly no recommendations can be made concerning alterations of dietary calcium. It would seem prudent, however, to avoid a dietary deficiency of calcium, such as might occur if a desire to lower blood cholesterol leads to avoidance of dairy products. Calcium intake should be maintained at least at the recommended daily level of 800 to 1000 mg, especially among groups, such as blacks and elderly persons, who tend to have low calcium intakes and a high prevalence of hypertension.[133]

ALCOHOL

Many studies of large populations have shown a relationship between alcohol consumption and blood pressure.[155–162] Both an increase in blood pressure levels with alcohol use and a higher prevalence of hypertension in heavy drinkers have been observed. (Heavy alcohol intake is generally considered to be more than 4 or 5 drinks a day; a "drink" is typically considered to contain 13 g of ethanol, the approximate amount in 12 ounces of beer, 4 ounces of wine, or 1.25 ounces of 80-proof whiskey.[163]) Some studies describe a threshold effect: Heavy alcohol consumption is associated with elevated blood pressure, but no effect is noted among those who take fewer than 3 to 5 drinks daily.[156,158] Other reports describe a linear increase in pressure with rising alcohol intake.[157,160] In one study blood pressure was actually lower in people with low levels of alcohol intake than in teetotalers.[159] The reported average increase in systolic and diastolic blood pressure in heavy drinkers ranges from 2 to 11 mm Hg. The prevalence of hypertension, defined as blood pressure higher than 160/95 mm Hg, increased twofold

in heavy drinkers.[159] The relation between alcohol intake and blood pressure is not explained by the potentially confounding factors of age, obesity, smoking habits, coffee consumption, or social class.[156,161]

A cause-and-effect relation between alcohol and hypertension is suggested by the observation that blood pressure falls to normal in heavy drinkers who abstain from alcohol for prolonged periods, and returns to hypertensive levels when drinking is resumed.[160,164] But an experimental basis for the understanding of alcohol-induced hypertension is lacking. The acute administration of ethanol to normal subjects does not consistently raise blood pressure;[159] large quantities of ethanol, in fact, depress blood pressure as well as heart rate and respiratory rate.[165] Recent studies, however, in hypertensive[166] and normotensive men[167,168] have suggested a direct pressor effect of ethanol. Blood pressure is, moreover, commonly elevated during withdrawal from alcohol, and is higher in patients with more severe withdrawal symptoms.[164] Norepinephrine levels are elevated 13 to 24 hours after cessation of ethanol intake,[169] and increased sympathoadrenal activity is thought to contribute to the blood pressure elevation. Other causes of ethanol-induced hypertension have been considered, such as increased levels of cortisol, aldosterone, and plasma renin activity,[163] and a direct effect of ethanol on the N^+-K^+ pump,[170] but there is little evidence to support an important role for these factors.

Some have suggested that the hypertension associated with alcohol is caused in large part by recurring ethanol-withdrawal manifestations.[159,171,172] A heavy drinker who intentionally avoids alcohol for 12 to 24 hours before a visit to the physician may have a higher-than-usual blood pressure at that visit; the possibility of transient hypertension related to recent ethanol ingestion must be kept in mind by the physician.

Although its etiological relation to high blood pressure is not understood, alcohol abuse, because of its prevalence in Western society, may be an important cause of curable hypertension. If estimates are correct that alcohol is responsible for 10 per cent or more of cases of hypertension,[155,157] it is a far more common cause than renal artery stenosis and other surgically curable lesions. Evaluation of the hypertensive patient must include a detailed history of alcohol intake, including the temporal relation between elevated blood pressure readings and recent alcohol consumption. Although experience suggests that it is easier for physicians to convince patients to take pills than to decrease their alcohol intake, the latter intervention is obviously more physiologic, may be equally (or more) effective, may have additional benefits besides the effect on blood pressure, and should be strongly advised.

TRACE ELEMENTS

A relation between cadmium ingestion and hypertension has been proposed.[173] This is largely based on experiments in which cadmium administration to rats, in quantities not far different from levels of human intake, caused blood pressure elevation.[174,175] Also, soft water, which may be associated with an increased cardiovascular mortality rate, contains increased concentrations of cadmium; a blood pressure–raising effect of cadmium in soft water, rather than an antihypertensive effect of the calcium in hard water, could account for the differences in cardiovascular mortality.[130] Mechanisms proposed include renal effects of cadmium, causing sodium retention, and a direct vasoconstrictor effect of cadmium on peripheral arterioles.[176]

However, the hypertension produced in rats by cadmium administration is not dose-related, and does not occur with high doses.[177] Autopsy studies and levels of urinary cadmium excretion in humans have failed to prove higher levels in persons with hypertension.[177] A role for cadmium in the etiology of human hypertension is not supported by extensive evidence at this time.

Isolated observations have suggested abnormalities of other trace elements in hypertension. For example, red blood cell levels of zinc were found to be about 30 per cent higher in patients with high blood pressure.[178] Some patients with hypertension and renal failure had increased lead excretion after EDTA administration, suggesting an increase in lead absorption.[179] Hypertension is one of the manifestations of poisoning with mercury or thallium.[177] However, more evidence will be needed before trace elements can be implicated in the etiology of hypertension.

CAFFEINE

When the amount of caffeine in about two cups of coffee, 250 mg, was administered to non–coffee drinkers, it caused a rise in blood pressure of 14/10 mm Hg in 1 hour, along with an increase in plasma renin activity and epinephrine and norepinephrine levels.[180] However, when the regular ingestion of 150 mg of caffeine with each meal was continued for 1 to 4 days, nearly complete tolerance developed to the blood pressure–raising effects of caffeine.[181]

The absence of a long-term effect of caffeine on blood pressure levels has been borne out by epidemiological studies. The Framingham study[182] and a survey of 72,000 company employees[183] found no relation between the number of cups of coffee drunk each day and blood pressure levels. Although a recent report describes an acute blood pressure elevation caused by caffeine in hypertensive patients after overnight abstinence,[184] the bulk of evidence suggests that coffee drinking is not a significant factor in most cases of hypertension.

DIETARY FAT

The unacculturated populations that have little hypertension, discussed above in connection with their low sodium intake, also consume lower quantities of other dietary components, such as animal fats. Epidemiological studies of blood pressure levels in populations with differing dietary customs, and studies of the effect of alterations in fat intake on the blood pressure of animals and humans, have suggested that lower consumption of saturated fat and cholesterol, and a higher polyunsaturated:saturated fat ratio, are associated with lower blood pressure.[185,186]

In a well-controlled study, a reduction of the percentage of energy intake derived from fat from 39 to 23 per cent, and an increase in the polyunsaturated:saturated fat ratio from 0.27 to 0.98, led to a fall in blood pressure of 8/8 mm Hg during a 6-week period.[187] Similarly, normal persons randomly assigned to a vegetarian diet for 6 weeks had a fall in blood pressure of 5 to 6/2 to 3 mm Hg, with a return to their original pressure levels when they resumed meat consumption.[188] In both these studies the fall in blood pressure was not explained by changes in sodium or calorie intake.

It is postulated that an increase in linoleic acid intake leads to greater production of blood pressure–lowering prostaglandins.[185,189] However, not all studies have shown a fall in blood pressure with dietary restriction of saturated fat.[190] Much more must be learned about the effects on blood pressure of changes in specific components of dietary lipids before changes in dietary fat intake can be recommended for patients with hypertension.

CONCLUSIONS

Of the many nutritional factors that may affect blood pressure, several are closely enough linked to hypertension that their modification may benefit patients with this disease. Weight loss in an obese hypertensive patient is likely to result in a substantial fall in blood pressure. Abstinence from alcohol is likely to lower the blood pressure of a heavy drinker. Severe salt restriction is often effective, and moderate salt restriction is sometimes effective, in lowering blood pressure. It seems reasonable, therefore, to consider weight control, moderation in alcohol intake, and, in some cases, salt restriction as worthwhile goals in the management of hypertension.

Other nutritional factors, such as potassium, calcium, lipids, and several minerals and trace elements, have provoked wide interest, but their role in hypertension is not yet sufficiently established to warrant widespread modification of their dietary intake.

References

1. Schrier RW, Anderson RJ. Renal sodium excretion, edematous disorders, and diuretic use. *In* Schrier RW (ed).

Renal and Electrolyte Disorders. 2nd ed. Boston, Little, Brown, 1980: 65–114.

2. Levy M, Seely JF. Pathophysiology of edema formation. *In* Brenner BM, Rector FC Jr (eds). The Kidney. 2nd ed. Philadelphia, WB Saunders, 1981: 723–776.

3. Kurtzman NA, Martinez-Maldonado M. Pathophysiology of edema. *In* Kurtzman NA, Martinez-Maldonado M (eds). Pathophysiology of the Kidney. Springfield, IL, Charles C Thomas, 1977: 1029–1043.

4. Cannon PJ. The kidney in heart failure. N Engl J Med 1977; *296*:26–32.

5. Davis JO. What signals the kidney to release renin? Circ Res 1971; *28*:301–306.

6. DeWardener HE, Mills IH, Clapham WF, et al. Studies on the efferent mechanism of the sodium diuresis which follows the administration of intravenous saline in the dog. Clin Sci 1961; *21*:249–258.

7. Gruber KA, Whitaker JM, Buckalew VM Jr. Endogenous digitalis-like substance in plasma of volume-expanded dogs. Nature 1980; *287*:743–745.

8. DiBona GF. Neurogenic regulation of renal tubular sodium reabsorption. Am J Physiol 1977; *233*:F73–F81.

9. Besarab A, Silva P, Landsberg L, et al. Effect of catecholamines on tubular function in the isolated perfused rat kidney. Am J Physiol 1977; *233*:F39–F45.

10. Hall JE, Guyton AC, Jackson TE, et al. Control of glomerular filtration rate by renin-angiotensin system. Am J Physiol 1977; *233*:F366–F372.

11. Anderson RJ, Berl T, McDonald KM, et al. Prostaglandins: effects on blood pressure, renal blood flow, sodium and water excretion. Kidney Int 1976; *10*:205–215.

12. Altsheler P, Klahr S, Rosenbaum R, et al. Effects of inhibitors of prostaglandin synthesis on renal sodium excretion in normal dogs and dogs with decreased renal mass. Am J Physiol 1978; *235*:F338–F344.

13. Tait JF, Bougas J, Little B, et al. Splanchnic extraction and clearance of aldosterone in subjects with minimal and marked cardiac dysfunction. J Clin Endocrinol Metab 1965; *25*:219–228.

14. Lieberman FL, Denison EK, Reynolds TB. The relationship of plasma volume, portal hypertension, ascites, and renal sodium retention in cirrhosis: the overflow theory of ascites formation. Ann NY Acad Sci 1970; *170*:202–206.

15. Levy M. Sodium retention and ascites formation in dogs with experimental portal cirrhosis. Am J Physiol 1977; *233*:F572–F585.

16. Blendis LM, Greig PD, Langer B, et al. The renal and hemodynamic effects of the peritoneovenous shunt for intractable hepatic ascites. Gastroenterology 1979; *77*:250–257.

17. Epstein M. Renal effects of head-out water immersion in man: implications for an understanding of volume homeostasis. Physiol Rev 1978; *58*:529–581.

18. Bichet D, Szatalowicz V, Chaimovitz C, et al. Role of vasopressin in abnormal water excretion in cirrhotic patients. Ann Intern Med 1982; *96*:413–417.

19. Bichet DG, Van Putten VJ, Schrier RW. Potential role of increased sympathetic activity in impaired sodium and water excretion in cirrhosis. N Engl J Med 1982; *307*:1552–1557.

20. Epstein FH. Underfilling versus overflow in hepatic ascites. N Engl J Med 1982; *307*:1577–1578.

21. Streeten DHP. Idiopathic edema: pathogenesis, clinical features, and treatment. Metabolism 1978; *27*:353–383.

22. Ferris TF, Bay WH. Idiopathic edema. *In* Brenner BM, Stein JH (eds). Sodium and Water Homeostasis. New York, Churchill Livingstone, 1978: 131–153.

23. Kuchel O, Horky K, Gregorova I, et al. Inappropriate response to upright posture: a precipitating factor in the pathogenesis of idiopathic edema. Ann Intern Med 1970; *73*:245–252.

24. Sims EAH, MacKay BR, Shirai T. The relation of capillary angiopathy and diabetes mellitus to idiopathic edema. Ann Intern Med 1965; *63*:972–987.

25. Coleman M, Horwith M, Brown JL. Idiopathic edema: studies demonstrating protein-lacking angiopathy. Am J Med 1970; *49*:106–113.

26. Gill JR Jr, Waldmann TA, Bartter FC. Idiopathic edema: 1. The occurrence of hypoalbuminemia and abnormal albumin metabolism in women with unexplained edema. Am J Med 1972; *52*:444–451.

27. Sowers J, Catania R, Paris J, et al. Effects of bromocriptine on renin, aldosterone, and responses to posture and metoclopramide in idiopathic edema: possible therapeutic approach. J Clin Endocrinol Metab 1982; *54*:510–516.

28. Schroeder HA. Studies on congestive heart failure. 1. The importance of restriction of salt as compared to water. Am Heart J 1941; *22*:141–153.

29. Eisenmenger WJ, Ahrens EH Jr, Blondheim SH, et al. The effect of rigid sodium restriction in patients with cirrhosis of the liver and ascites. J Lab Clin Med 1949; *34*:1029–1038.

30. Packer M, Medina N, Yushak M. Correction of dilutional hyponatremia in severe chronic heart failure by converting-enzyme inhibition. Ann Intern Med 1984; *100*:782–789.

31. MacGregor GA, Markandu ND, Roulston JE, et al. Is "idiopathic" edema idiopathic? Lancet 1979; *1*:397–400.

32. Peters T Jr. Serum albumin. *In* Putnam FW (ed). The Plasma Proteins. 2nd ed. New York, Academic Press, 1975: 133–181.

33. Frisell WR. Human Biochemistry. New York, Macmillan, 1982: 428.

34. Tullis JL. Albumin. JAMA 1977; *237*:355–360, 460–462.

35. Rothschild MA, Oratz M, Mongelli J, et al. Effects of a short-term fast on albumin synthesis studied in vivo, in the perfused liver, and on amino acid incorporation by hepatic microsomes. J Clin Invest 1968; *47*:2591–2599.

36. Rothschild MA, Oratz M, Schreiber SS. Alcohol, amino acids, and albumin synthesis. Gastroenterology 1974; *67*:1200–1213.

37. Sellers AL, Katz J, Rosenfeld S. Plasma albumin catabolism in experimental nephrosis. Nature 1961; *192*:562–563.

38. Strober V, Waldmann TA. The role of the kidney in the metabolism of plasma proteins. Nephron 1974; *13*:35–66.

39. Jeffries GH. Protein-losing gastroenteropathy. *In* Sleisenger MH, Fordtran JS (eds). Gastrointestinal Disease. 3rd ed. Philadelphia, WB Saunders, 1983: 280–288.

40. Wilkinson P, Sherlock S. The effect of repeated albumin infusions in patients with cirrhosis. Lancet 1962; *2*:1125–1129.

41. Malmendier C, DeKoster JP, Lambert PP. Effects of an increase in plasma volume on glomerular permeability to albumin in proteinuric patients. Clin Sci 1960; *19*:605–617.

42. Lambert PP. Major syndromes. *In* Hamburger J, Crosnier J, Grunfeld J-P (eds). Nephrology. New York, John Wiley & Sons, 1979: 157–183.

43. Rothschild MA, Oratz M, Schreiber SS. Albumin synthesis. N Engl J Med 1972: *286*:748–757, 816–821.

44. Kirsch R, Frith L, Black E, et al. Regulation of albumin synthesis and catabolism by alteration of dietary protein. Nature 1968; *217*:578–579.

45. Kelman L, Saunders SJ, Frith L, et al. Effects of dietary protein restriction on albumin synthesis, albumin catabolism, and the plasma aminogram. Am J Clin Nutr 1972; *25*:1174–1178.

46. Hoffenberg R, Black E, Brock JF. Albumin and gamma globulin tracer studies in protein depletion states. J Clin Invest 1966; *45*:143–152.

47. Waterlow JC. Observations on the mechanisms of adaptation to low protein intakes. Lancet 1968; *2*:1091–1097.

48. Blainey JD. High protein diets in the treatment of the nephrotic syndrome. Clin Sci 1954; *13*:567–581.

49. Elman R, Brown FA Jr, Wolf H. Studies on hypoalbuminemia produced by protein-deficient diets. II. Rapid correction of hypoalbuminemia with an ad libitum meat diet. J Exp Med 1942; *75*:461–464.

50. Kopple JD. Nutritional therapy in kidney failure. Nutr Rev 1981; 39:193–206.

51. Kark RM, Oyama JH. Nutrition, hypertension, and kidney disease. In Goodhart RS, Shils ME (eds). Modern Nutrition in Health and Disease. 6th ed. Philadelphia, Lea & Febiger, 1980: 998–1044.

52. Davidson CS. Nutrition in diseases of the liver. In Goodhart RS, Shils ME (eds). Modern Nutrition in Health and Disease. 6th ed. Philadelphia, Lea and Febiger, 1980: 962–976.

53. Lau K, McCurdy DK. Disorders of fluid and electrolyte balance. In Spittell JA Jr (ed). Clinical Medicine. Vol 7. Philadelphia, Harper & Row, 1981: 1–37.

54. Scrimshaw NS. Undernutrition, starvation, and hunger edema. In Wyngaarden JB, Smith LH Jr (eds). Cecil Textbook of Medicine. 16th ed. Philadelphia, WB Saunders, 1982: 1365–1366.

55. Viteri FE, Torun B. Protein-calorie malnutrition. In Goodhart RS, Shils ME (eds). Modern Nutrition in Health and Disease. 6th ed. Philadelphia, Lea & Febiger, 1980: 697–720.

56. Cohen S, Hansen JDL. Metabolism of albumin and gamma globulin in kwashiorkor. Clin Sci 1962; 23:352–359.

57. Viart P. Hemodynamic findings in severe protein-calorie malnutrition. Am J Clin Nutr 1977; 30:334–348.

58. Kaplan NM. Clinical Hypertension. 3rd ed. Baltimore; Williams & Wilkins, 1982: 6.

59. Guyton AC, Coleman TG, Cowley AW Jr, et al. Arterial pressure regulation: overriding dominance of the kidneys in long-term regulation and in hypertension. Am J Med 1972; 52:584–594.

60. Channick BJ, Adlin EV, Marks AD. Suppressed plasma renin activity in hypertension. Arch Intern Med 1969; 123:131–140.

61. Laragh JH. Vasoconstrictor-volume analysis for understanding and treating hypertension. Am J Med 1973; 55:261–274.

62. Kempner W. Treatment of hypertensive vascular disease with rice diet. Am J Med 1948; 4:545–577.

63. Chapman CB, Gibbons TB. The diet and hypertension. Medicine 1950; 29:29–69.

64. Watkin DM, Froeb HF, Hatch FT, et al. Effects of diet in essential hypertension: results with unmodified Kempner rice diet in fifty hospitalized patients. Am J Med 1950; 9:441–493.

65. Dole VP, Dahl LK, Cotzias GC, et al. Dietary treatment of hypertension. Clinical and metabolic studies of patients on the rice-fruit diet. J Clin Invest 1950; 29:1189–1206.

66. Laragh JH, Pecker MS. Dietary sodium and essential hypertension: some myths, hopes, and truths. Ann Intern Med 1983; 98(Part 2):735–743.

67. Tobian L Jr, Binion JT. Tissue cations and water in arterial hypertension. Circulation 1952; 5:754–758.

68. Tobian L Jr, Binnion J. Arterial wall electrolytes in renal and DCA hypertension. J Clin Invest 1954; 33: 1407–1414.

69. Tobian L. Human essential hypertension: implications of animal studies. Ann Intern Med 1983; 98(Part 2):729–734.

70. Dahl LK, Heine M, Tassinari L. Effects of chronic excess salt ingestion: evidence that genetic factors play an important role in susceptibility to experimental hypertension. J Exp Med 1962; 115:1173–1190.

71. Murray RH, Luft FC, Bloch R, et al. Blood pressure responses to extremes of sodium intake in normal man. Proc Soc Exp Biol Med 1978; 159:432–436.

72. Grim CE, Miller JZ, Luft FC, et al. Genetic influences on renin, aldosterone, and the renal excretion of sodium and potassium following volume expansion and contraction in normal man. Hypertension 1979; 1:583–590.

73. Falkner B, Onesti G, Hayes P. The role of sodium in essential hypertension in genetically hypertensive adolescents. In Onesti G, Kim KE (eds). Hypertension in the Young and the Old. New York, Grune & Stratton, 1981: 29–35.

74. Luft FC, Weinberger MH, Grim CE, et al. Sodium sensitivity in normotensive human subjects. Ann Intern Med 1983; 98:(Part 2):758–762.

75. Shaper AG. Cardiovascular disease in the tropics. III: Blood pressure and hypertension. Br Med J 1972; 3:805–807.

76. Page LB, Damon A, Moellering RC Jr. Antecedents of cardiovascular disease in six Solomon Islands societies. Circulation 1974; 49:1132–1146.

77. Freis ED. Salt, volume, and the prevention of hypertension. Circulation 1976; 53:589–595.

78. Oliver WJ, Cohen EL, Neel JV. Blood pressure, sodium intake and sodium related hormones in the Yanomamo Indians, a "no-salt" culture. Circulation 1975; 52:146–151.

79. Gliebermann L. Blood pressure and dietary salt in human populations. Ecology of Food and Nutrition 1973; 2:143–156.

80. Sever PS, Gordon D, Peart WS, et al. Blood-pressure and its correlates in urban and tribal Africa. Lancet 1980; 2:60–64.

81. Prior IAM, Evans JG, Harvey HPB, et al. Sodium intake and blood pressure in two Polynesian populations. N Engl J Med 1968; 279:515–520.

82. Shaper AG, Leonard PJ, Jones KW, et al. Environmental effects on the body build, blood pressure and blood chemistry of nomadic warriors serving in the army in Kenya. East Afr Med J 1969; 46:282–289.

83. McCarron DA, Henry HJ, Morris CD. Human nutrition and blood pressure regulation: an integrated approach. Hypertension 1982; 4(Suppl III):2–13.

84. Dawber TR, Kannel WB, Kagan A, et al. Environmental factors in hypertension. In Stamler J, Stamler R, Pullman T (eds). The Epidemiology of Hypertension. New York, Grune & Stratton, 1967: 255–288.

85. Simpson FO, Waal-Manning HJ, Bolli P, et al. Relationship of blood pressure to sodium excretion in a population survey. Clin Sci Mol Med 1978; 55(Suppl 4):373s–375s.

86. Walker WG, Whelton PK, Saito H, et al. Relation between blood pressure and renin, renin substrate, angiotensin II, aldosterone and urinary sodium and potassium in 574 ambulatory subjects. Hypertension 1979; 1:287–291.

87. Holden RA, Ostfeld AM, Freeman DH Jr, et al. Dietary salt intake and blood pressure. JAMA 1983; 250:365–369.

88. Stanton JL, Braitman LE, Riley AM Jr, et al. Demographic, dietary, life style and anthropometric correlates of blood pressure. Hypertension 1982; 4(Suppl III):135–142.

89. Miller GD. Relationship between urinary sodium and potassium, and arterial blood pressure: an epidemiologic study. J Nat Med Assoc 1984; 76:47–52.

90. Watson RL, Langford HG, Abernethy J, et al. Urinary electrolytes, body weight, and blood pressure: pooled cross-sectional results among four groups of adolescent females. Hypertension 1980; 2(Suppl I):93–98.

91. Kawasaki T, Delea CS, Bartter FC, et al. The effect of high-sodium and low-sodium intakes on blood pressure and other related variables in human subjects with idiopathic hypertension. Am J Med 1978; 64:193–198.

92. Luft FC, Weinberger MH. Sodium intake and essential hypertension. Hypertension 1982; 4(Suppl III):14–19.

93. Kaplan NM. Dietary salt intake and blood pressure. (Letter.) JAMA 1984; 251:1429–1430.

94. Parijs J, Joossens JV, Van der Linden L, et al. Moderate sodium restriction and diuretics in the treatment of hypertension. Am Heart J 1973; 85:22–34.

95. Morgan TO, Myers JB. Hypertension treated by sodium restriction. Med J Aust 1981; 2:396–397.

96. MacGregor GA, Markandu ND, Best FE, et al. Double-blind randomised crossover trial of moderate sodium restriction in essential hypertension. Lancet 1982; 1:351–355.

97. Beard TC, Cooke HM, Gray WR, et al. Randomised controlled trial of a no-added-sodium diet for mild hypertension. Lancet 1982; 2:455–458.

98. Silman AJ, Locke C, Mitchell P, et al. Evaluation of the effectiveness of a low sodium diet in the treatment of mild to moderate hypertension. Lancet 1983; 1:1179–1182.

99. Richards AM, Nicholls MG, Espiner EA, et al. Blood-pressure response to moderate sodium restriction and to potassium supplementation in mild essential hypertension. Lancet 1984; 1:757–761.

100. Freis ED. Should mild hypertension be treated? N Engl J Med 1982; 307:306–309.

101. Swales JD. Dietary salt and hypertension. Lancet 1980; 1:1177–1179.

102. Treasure J, Ploth D. Role of dietary potassium in the treatment of hypertension. Hypertension 1983; 5:864–872.

103. Grim CE, Luft FC, Miller JZ, et al. Racial differences in blood pressure in Evans County, Georgia: relationship to sodium and potassium intake and plasma renin activity. J Chron Dis 1980; 33:87–94.

104. Tannen RL. Effects of potassium on blood pressure control. Ann Intern Med 1983; 98(Part 2):773–780.

105. Iimura O, Kijima T, Kikuchi K, et al. Studies on the hypertensive effect of high potassium intake in patients with essential hypertension. Clin Sci 1981; 61:77s–80s.

106. Parfrey PS, Vandenburg MJ, Wright P, et al. Blood pressure and hormonal changes following alteration in dietary sodium and potassium in mild essential hypertension. Lancet 1981; 1:59–63.

107. MacGregor GA, Smith SJ, Markandu ND, et al. Moderate potassium supplementation in essential hypertension. Lancet 1982; 2:567–570.

108. Dustan HP. Mechanisms of hypertension associated with obesity. Ann Intern Med 1983; 98(Part 2):860–864.

109. Kannel WB, Brand N, Skinner JJ Jr, et al. The relation of adiposity to blood pressure and development of hypertension. Ann Intern Med 1967; 67:48–59.

110. Epstein FH, Francis T Jr, Hayner NS, et al. Prevalence of chronic diseases and distribution of selected physiologic variables in a total community, Tecumseh, Michigan. Am J Epidemiol 1965; 81:307–322.

111. Chiang BN, Perlman LV, Epstein FH. Overweight and hypertension. Circulation 1969; 39:403–421.

112. Havlik RJ, Hubert WB, Fabsitz RR, et al. Weight and hypertension. Ann Intern Med 1983; 98(Part 2):855–859.

113. Ashley FW Jr, Kannel WB. Relation of weight change to changes in atherogenic traits: the Framingham study. J Chron Dis 1974; 27:103–114.

114. Tyroler HA, Heyden S, Hames CG. Weight and hypertension: Evans County studies of blacks and whites. In Paul O (ed). Epidemiology and Control of Hypertension. New York, Stratton, 1975: 177–205.

115. Reisin E, Abel R, Modan M, et al. Effect of weight loss without salt restriction on the reduction of blood pressure in overweight hypertensive patients. N Engl J Med 1978; 298:1–6.

116. Tuck ML, Sowers J, Dornfeld L, et al. The effect of weight reduction on blood pressure, plasma renin activity, and plasma aldosterone levels in obese patients. N Engl J Med 1981; 304:930–933.

117. Sowers JR, Nyby M, Stern N, et al. Blood pressure and hormone changes associated with weight reduction in the obese. Hypertension 1982; 4:686–691.

118. Reisin E, Frohlich ED, Messerli FH, et al. Cardiovascular changes after weight reduction in obesity hypertension. Ann Intern Med 1983; 98:315–319.

119. Fagerberg B, Andersson OK, Isaksson B, et al. Blood pressure control during weight reduction in obese hypertensive men: separate effects of sodium and energy restriction. Br Med J 1984; 288:11–14.

120. Alexander JK. Obesity and the circulation. Mod Conc Cardiov Dis 1963; 32:799–803.

121. Messerli FH, Christie B, DeCarvalho JGR, et al. Obesity and essential hypertension: hemodynamics, intravascular volume, sodium excretion, and plasma renin activity. Arch Intern Med 1981; 141:81–85.

122. Mujais SK, Tarazi RC, Dustan HP, et al. Hypertension in obese patients: hemodynamic and volume studies. Hypertension 1982; 4:84–92.

123. Sims EA. Mechanisms of hypertension in the overweight. Hypertension 1982; 4(Suppl III):43–49.

124. DeFronzo RA, Cooke CR, Andres R, et al. The effect of insulin on renal handling of sodium, potassium, calcium, and phosphate in man. J Clin Invest 1975; 55:845–855.

125. Krotkiewski M, Mandroukas K, Sjostrom L, et al. Effects of long-term physical training on body fat, metabolism, and blood pressure in obesity. Metabolism 1979; 28:650–658.

126. Landsberg L, Young JB. Fasting, feeding and regulation of the sympathetic nervous system. N Engl J Med 1978; 298:1295–1301.

127. Jung RT, Shetty PS, Barrand M, et al. Role of catecholamines in hypotensive response to dieting. Br Med J 1979; 1:12–13.

128. Neri LC, Mandel JS, Hewitt D. Relation between mortality and water hardness in Canada. Lancet 1972; 1:931–934.

129. Stitt FW, Clayton DG, Crawford MD, et al. Clinical and biochemical indicators of cardiovascular disease among men living in hard and soft water areas. Lancet 1973; 1:122–126.

130. Neri LC, Johansen HL. Water hardness and cardiovascular mortality. Ann NY Acad Sci 1978; 304:203–219.

131. Comstock GW. Water hardness and cardiovascular diseases. Am J Epidemiol 1979; 110:375–400.

132. McCarron DA, Morris CD, Cole C. Dietary calcium in human hypertension. Science 1982; 217:267–269.

133. McCarron DA. Calcium and magnesium nutrition in human hypertension. Ann Intern Med 1983; 98(Part 2): 800–805.

134. Langford HG, Watson RL. Electrolytes, environment and blood pressure. Clin Sci Mol Med 1973; 45:111s–113s.

135. Ackley S, Barrett-Connor E, Suarez L. Dairy products, calcium, and blood pressure. Am J Clin Nutr 1983; 38:457–461.

136. Garcia-Palmieri MR, Costas R Jr, Cruz-Vidal M, et al. Milk consumption, calcium intake, and decreased hypertension in Puerto Rico: Puerto Rico Heart Health Program study. Hypertension 1984; 6:322–328.

137. McCarron DA. Low serum concentrations of ionized calcium in patients with hypertension. N Engl J Med 1982; 307:226–228.

138. Kesteloot H, Geboers J. Calcium and blood pressure. Lancet 1982; 1:813–815.

139. Kotchen TA, Kotchen JM, Guthrie GP Jr, et al. Serum calcium and hypertension. (Letter.) N Engl J Med 1982; 307:1525.

140. Tibblin G, Bergentz S-E, Bjure J, et al. Hematocrit, plasma protein, plasma volume, and viscosity in early hypertensive disease. Am Heart J 1966; 72:165–176.

141. Ohlsson O, Henningsen NC, Malmquist I. Blood pressure, heart rate and plasma albumin in relatives of hypertensive patients. Acta Med Scand 1981; 209:445–450.

142. Aurbach GD, Marx SJ, Spiegel AM. Parathyroid hormone, calcitonin, and the calciferols. In Williams RH (ed). Textbook of Endocrinology. 6th ed. Philadelphia, WB Saunders, 1981: 922–1031.

143. Resnick LM, Laragh JH, Sealey JE, et al. Divalent cations in essential hypertension: relations between serum ionized calcium, magnesium, and plasma renin activity. N Engl J Med 1983; 309:888–891.

144. Bohr DF. Vascular smooth muscle: dual effect of calcium. Science 1963; 139:597–599.

145. Blum M, Kirsten M, Worth MH Jr. Reversible hypertension, caused by the hypercalcemia of hyperparathyroidism, vitamin D toxicity, and calcium infusion. JAMA 1977; 237:262–263.

146. Weidmann P, Massry SG, Coburn JW, et al. Blood pressure effects of acute hypercalcemia: studies in patients with chronic renal failure. Ann Intern Med 1972; 76:741–745.

147. Rosenthal FD, Roy S. Hypertension and hyperparathyroidism. Br Med J 1972; 4:396–397.

148. Heath H III, Hodgson SF, Kennedy MA. Primary hyperparathyroidism: incidence, morbidity, and potential economic impact in a community. N Engl J Med 1980; 302:189–193.

149. Borle AB, Uchikawa T. Effects of parathyroid hormone on the distribution and transport of calcium in cultured kidney cells. Endocrinology 1978; 102:1725–1732.

150. Chausmer AB, Sherman BS, Wallach S. The effect of parathyroid hormone on hepatic cell transport of calcium. Endocrinology 1972; 90:663–672.

151. Belizan JM, Villar J, Pineda O, et al. Reduction of blood pressure with calcium supplementation in young adults. JAMA 1983; 249:1161–1165.

152. McCarron DA, Pingree PA, Rubin RJ, et al. Enhanced parathyroid function in essential hypertension: a homeostatic response to a urinary calcium leak. Hypertension 1980; 2:162–168.

153. Ayachi S. Increased dietary calcium lowers blood pressure in the spontaneously hypertensive rat. Metabolism 1979; 28:1234–1238.

154. McCarron DA, Morris CD. Blood pressure response to oral calcium in persons with mild to moderate hypertension. Ann Intern Med 1985; 103:825–831.

155. Mathews JD. Alcohol use, hypertension and coronary heart disease. Clin Sci Mol Med 1976; 51(Suppl):661s–663s.

156. Klatsky AL, Friedman GD, Siegelaub AB, et al. Alcohol consumption and blood pressure: Kaiser-Permanente multiphasic health examination data. N Engl J Med 1977; 296:1194–1200.

157. Mitchell PI, Morgan MJ, Boadle DJ, et al. Role of alcohol in the aetiology of hypertension. Med J Aust 1980; 2:198–200.

158. Dyer AR, Stamler J, Paul O, et al. Alcohol, cardiovascular risk factors and mortality: the Chicago experience. Circulation 1981; 64(Suppl III):20–27.

159. Wallace RB, Lynch CF, Pomrehn PR, et al. Alcohol and hypertension: epidemiologic and experimental considerations. The Lipid Research Clinics program. Circulation 1981; 64(Suppl III):41–47.

160. Arkwright PD, Beilin LJ, Rouse I, et al. Effects of alcohol use and other aspects of lifestyle on blood pressure levels and prevalence of hypertension in a working population. Circulation 1982; 66:60–66.

161. Cooke KM, Frost GW, Thornell IR, et al. Alcohol consumption and blood pressure: survey of the relationship at a health-screening clinic. Med J Aust 1982; 1:65–69.

162. Cairns V, Keil U, Kleinbaum D, et al. Alcohol consumption as a risk factor for high blood pressure: Munich blood pressure study. Hypertension 1984; 6:124–131.

163. Larbi EB, Copper RS, Stamler J. Alcohol and hypertension. Arch Intern Med 1983; 143:28–29.

164. Saunders JB, Beevers DG, Paton A. Alcohol-induced hypertension. Lancet 1981; 2:653–656.

165. Friedman GD, Klatsky AL, Siegelaub AB. Alcohol, tobacco, and hypertension. Hypertension 1982; 4(Suppl III):143–150.

166. Potter JF, Beevers DG. Pressor effect of alcohol in hypertension. Lancet 1984; 1:119–122.

167. Puddey IB, Beilin LJ, Vandongen R, et al. Evidence for a direct effect of alcohol consumption on blood pressure in normotensive men: randomized controlled trial. Hypertension 1985; 7:707–713.

168. Potter JF, Watson RDS, Skan W, et al. The pressor and metabolic effects of alcohol in normotensive subjects. Hypertension 1986; 8:625–631.

169. Carlsson C, Haggendal J. Arterial noradrenaline levels after ethanol withdrawal. (Letter.) Lancet 1967; 2:889.

170. Knochel JP. Cardiovascular effects of alcohol. Ann Intern Med 1983; 98(Part 2):849–854.

171. Saunders JB, Beevers DG, Paton A. Factors influencing blood pressure in chronic alcoholics. Clin Sci 1979; 57:295s–298s.

172. Friedman GD, Klatsky AL, Siegelaub AB. Alcohol intake and hypertension. Ann Intern Med 1983; 98(Part 2):846–849.

173. Schroeder HA. Cadmium, chromium, and cardiovascular disease. Circulation 1967; 35:570–582.

174. Schroeder HA. Cadmium hypertension in rats. Am J Physiol 1964; 207:62–66.

175. Kopp SJ, Glonek T, Perry HM Jr, et al. Cardiovascular actions of cadmium at environmental exposure levels. Science 1982; 217:837–839.

176. Perry HM Jr. Water hardness and cardiovascular mortality: discussion. Ann NY Acad Sci 1978; 304:220–221.

177. Saltman P. Trace elements and blood pressure. Ann Intern Med 1983; 98(Part 2):823–827.

178. Frithz G, Ronquist G. Increased red cell content of Zn^{++} in essential hypertension. Acta Med Scand 1979; 205:647–649.

179. Batuman V, Landy E, Maesaka JK, et al. Contribution of lead to hypertension with renal impairment. N Engl J Med 1983; 309:17–21.

180. Robertson D, Frolich JC, Carr RK, et al. Effects of caffeine on plasma renin activity, catecholamines and blood pressure. N Engl J Med 1978; 298:181–186.

181. Robertson D, Wade D, Workman R, et al. Tolerance to the humoral and hemodynamic effects of caffeine in man. J Clin Invest 1981; 67:1111–1117.

182. Dawber TR, Kannel WB, Gordon T. Coffee and cardiovascular disease: observations from the Framingham study. N Engl J Med 1974; 291:871–874.

183. Bertrand CA, Pomper I, Hillman G, et al. No relation between coffee and blood pressure. (Letter.) N Engl J Med 1978; 299:315–316.

184. Freestone S, Ramsay LE. Effect of coffee and cigarette smoking on the blood pressure of untreated and diuretic-treated hypertensive patients. Am J Med 1982; 73:348–353.

185. Iacono JM, Dougherty RM, Puska P. Reduction of blood pressure associated with dietary polyunsaturated fat. Hypertension 1982; 4(Suppl III):34–42.

186. Smith-Barbaro PA, Pucak GJ. Dietary fat and blood pressure. Ann Intern Med 1983; 98(Part 2):828–831.

187. Puska P, Iacono JM, Nissinen A, et al. Controlled, randomised trial of the effect of dietary fat on blood pressure. Lancet 1983; 1:1–5.

188. Rouse IL, Beilin LJ, Armstrong BK, et al. Blood-pressure–lowering effect of a vegetarian diet: controlled trial in normotensive subjects. Lancet 1983; 1:5–10.

189. Galli C, Agradi E, Petroni A, et al. Modulation of prostaglandin production in tissues by dietary essential fatty acids. Acta Med Scand (Suppl) 1980; 642:171–179.

190. Sacks FM, Marias GE, Handysides G, et al. Lack of an effect of dietary saturated fat and cholesterol on blood pressure in normotensives. Hypertension 1984; 6:193–198.

25

HYPERLIPOPROTEINEMIA

R. PHILIP EATON

The dietary strategies of the management of hyperlipidemia have evolved as the key studies and intervention trials of Helsinki, Finland,[1] the Western Electric study,[2] Veterans Administration in Los Angeles,[3] Oslo, Norway,[4] Multiple Risk Factor Intervention Trial (MRFIT),[5] and the Lipid Research Clinics (Coronary Primary Prevention Trial [LRC-CPPT])[6] have been evaluated; as thoughtful positions have been taken by the Research Committee of the American Heart Association,[7] the Research Committee of the Medical Research Council,[8,9] and the Council on Scientific Affairs of the AMA;[10] and from particularly incisive reviews by eminent academicians.[11–16] While this review does not represent any of these sources in their entirety, it draws significantly from each in philosophy, perspective, and concept. Total caloric content, total cholesterol content, total carbohydrate content, substitution of unsaturated fat for saturated fat, and increased soluble fiber content of the diet represent the major clinical variables that have been shown to influence lipoprotein metabolism.

The clinical response to these nutritional strategies is apparently independent of the type of hyperlipoproteinemia, so that precision in diagnosis of the classical "hyperlipoproteinemia" states contributes little to dietary recommendations. Patient populations must be designated as demonstrating endogenous hypercholesterolemia, endogenous hypertriglyceridemia, or exogenous hypertriglyceridemia, but further separation into Types I, II, III, IV, and V, mixed hyperlipemia, familial hyperlipemia, familial hypercholesterolemia, and so forth have little relevance to the available decisions of nutritional management.

The degree of clinical improvement in any hyperlipemic state with dietary therapy will be directly related to the severity of the underlying lipemia. The same diet will produce a much greater lipid-lowering response in those patients with higher initial blood levels of lipoproteins than it will in less lipemic patients. Moreover, normal subjects need not respond with any reduction in plasma cholesterol, triglyceride, or lipoprotein.

GOALS OF THERAPY

The goals of management of hyperlipidemia have evolved as understanding of lipoprotein metabolism has expanded and the clinical potential for regression of coronary artery disease has become recognized. The first goal was originally defined as any degree of lowering of total plasma cholesterol concentration, which later evolved to the goal of the "normal" value corrected for age and sex. Table 25–1 provides plasma cholesterol values in the white population of the United States obtained by the NIH–Lipid Research Clinics Survey,[17] which demonstrate the variation with age and sex. It was the recommendation of the Advisory Panel to the Council on Scientific Affairs of the American Medical Association that the 90th percentile for a patient's age and sex be defined as the lower limit for "overt hypercholesterolemia."[10] As an alternative goal, it has been suggested that treatment should be directed to achieving that threshold region for cholesterol concentration above which, based on epidemiological studies, risk for coronary artery disease accelerates with increasing plasma cholesterol concentration. The National Cooperative Pooling Project[18] has suggested that this threshold is 200 to 250 mg/dl, while others have suggested that it may be as low as 130 mg/dl. More recently, it has been recognized that total plasma cholesterol includes not only low-density lipoprotein cholesterol (LDL-C) as the major cholesterol transport lipoprotein, but also very-low-density lipoprotein cholesterol (VLDL-C), intermediate-density lipoprotein cholesterol (IDL-C), and high-density lipoprotein cholesterol (HDL-C), which may not participate in the risk for increased coronary artery disease. Thus an alternate goal may be to reduce the plasma LDL-C. Unfortunately, the precise value that might correlate with no vascular disease remains to be defined. Table 25–2 gives the plasma LDL-cholesterol values in the white population of the United States obtained by the NIH–Lipid Research Clinics Survey.[17] It would be reasonable to define the 90th percentile as overt clinical hypercholesterolemia, and to use the 50th percentile as a goal of management. For men, this guideline would make an LDL-C of 140 mg/dl the "normal" maximum, while for women a value up to 150 mg/dl might be selected. It is of interest that the LRC-CPPT intervention study recruited hypercholesterolemic men for treatment defined by a plasma cholesterol level of 265 mg/dl or greater (the 95th percentile for 40 to 49 years) who also had an LDL-C level of 190 mg/dl or greater.[6] During the initial diet phase of the study, those subjects who were responsive demonstrated a reduction in LDL-C to less than 175 mg/dl and thus were not further treated with drugs.[6] Subjects with genetic deficiency in LDL-C have levels of 46 ± 3 mg/dl and are reported to demonstrate significant longevity and reduced coronary artery vascular disease.[12]

A second goal of management of hyperlipidemia, which has evolved from clinical observation, is to maximize the concentration of plasma HDL. Values for normal HDL concentrations in the white populations of the United States, as obtained by the NIH–Lipid Research Clinics Survey,[17] are given in Table 25–3. This goal derives from epidemiological observations that demonstrate a striking correlation between low concentrations of plasma HDL and increased incidence of coronary artery disease.[19–23] Patients with familial elevations in HDL in the range of 81 ± 1 mg/dl of HDL-C are reported to dem-

TABLE 25–1. Plasma Total Cholesterol (mg/dl) (Population Distribution)

Age (Years)	White Males Percentiles							White Females Percentiles						
	5	10	25	50	75	90	95	5	10	25	50	75	90	95
0–4	—	—	—	—	—	—	—	—	—	—	—	—	—	—
5–9	125	131	141	153	168	183	189	131	136	151	164	176	190	197
10–14	124	131	144	160	173	188	202	125	131	142	159	171	191	205
15–19	118	123	136	152	168	183	191	118	126	140	157	176	198	207
20–24	118	126	142	159	179	197	212	121	132	147	165	186	220	237
25–29	130	137	154	176	199	223	234	130	142	158	178	198	217	231
30–34	142	152	171	190	213	237	258	133	141	158	178	199	215	228
35–39	147	157	176	195	222	248	267	139	149	165	186	209	233	249
40–44	150	160	179	204	229	251	260	146	156	172	193	220	241	259
45–49	163	171	188	210	235	258	275	148	162	182	204	231	256	268
50–54	156	168	189	211	237	263	274	163	171	188	214	240	267	281
55–59	161	172	188	214	236	260	280	167	182	201	229	251	278	294
60–64	163	170	191	215	237	262	287	172	186	207	226	251	282	300
65–69	166	174	192	213	250	275	288	167	179	212	233	259	282	291
70+	144	160	185	214	236	253	265	173	181	196	226	249	268	280

Adapted from Rifkind BM, Segal P. Lipid Research Clinics Program reference values for hyperlipidemia and hypolipidemia. *In* Lipid Research Clinics Population Studies Data Book. Vol 1, The Prevalence Study. 1980, NIH Publication No. 80–1527.

TABLE 25–2. Plasma LDL-Cholesterol (mg/dl) (Population Distribution)

Age (Years)	White Males Percentiles							White Females Percentiles						
	5	10	25	50	75	90	95	5	10	25	50	75	90	95
0–4	—	—	—	—	—	—	—	—	—	—	—	—	—	—
5–9	63	69	80	90	103	117	129	68	73	88	98	115	125	140
10–14	64	72	81	94	109	122	132	68	73	81	94	110	126	136
15–19	62	68	80	93	109	123	130	59	65	78	93	111	129	137
20–24	66	73	85	101	118	138	147	57	65	82	102	118	141	159
25–29	70	75	96	116	138	157	165	71	75	90	108	126	148	164
30–34	78	88	107	124	144	166	185	70	77	91	109	128	147	156
35–39	81	92	110	131	154	176	189	75	81	96	116	139	161	172
40–44	87	98	115	135	157	173	186	74	84	104	122	146	165	174
45–49	98	106	120	141	163	186	202	79	89	105	127	150	173	186
50–54	89	102	118	143	162	185	197	88	94	111	134	160	186	201
55–59	88	103	123	145	168	191	203	89	97	120	145	168	199	210
60–64	83	106	121	143	165	188	210	100	105	126	149	168	191	224
65–69	98	104	125	146	170	199	210	92	99	125	151	184	205	221
70+	88	100	119	142	164	182	186	96	108	127	147	170	189	206

Adapted from Rifkind BM, Segal P. Lipid Research Clinics Program reference values for hyperlipidemia and hypolipidemia. *In* Lipid Research Clinics Population Studies Data Book. Vol 1, The Prevalence Study. 1980, NIH Publication No. 80–1527.

onstrate increased longevity in comparison with control populations with normal HDL-C levels of 53 ± 5 mg/dl.[12] This longevity occurs even in the presence of "normal" levels of plasma LDL-C of 105 ± 5 mg/dl. HDL-C less than 30 mg/dl is considered as a high risk for vascular disease, and correction to higher levels may be viewed as a primary goal of management independent of the total plasma cholesterol or LDL-C concentrations. Similarly, values above the level of 80 mg/dl are considered to confer a low risk for vascular disease, and may in fact balance a simultaneous slight elevation in total plasma cholesterol and/or LDL-C. In familial hypercholes-

terolemia the HDL-cholesterol level is reported to be an independent predictor of atherosclerosis.[19]

A third goal of management of hyperlipidemia is the reduction of plasma triglyceride concentration to less than the 95th percentile for plasma triglycerides; in adults this is about 250 mg/dl. This goal is controversial, as the relationship between plasma triglycerides and vascular disease remains unclear, particularly as an independent risk factor.[24] The frequent association of hypertriglyceridemia with a parallel reduction in HDL concentration has suggested to some investigators that the low HDL confers the dominant risk. Moreover, the rise in plasma HDL

TABLE 25–3. Plasma HDL-Cholesterol (mg/dl) (Population Distribution)

Age (Years)	White Males Percentiles							White Females Percentiles						
	5	10	25	50	75	90	95	5	10	25	50	75	90	95
0–4	—	—	—	—	—	—	—	—	—	—	—	—	—	—
5–9	38	42	49	54	63	70	74	36	38	47	52	61	67	73
10–14	37	40	46	55	61	71	74	37	40	45	52	58	64	70
15–19	30	34	39	46	52	59	63	35	38	43	51	61	68	74
20–24	30	32	38	45	51	57	63	33	37	44	51	62	72	79
25–29	31	32	37	44	50	58	63	37	39	47	55	63	74	83
30–34	28	32	38	45	52	59	63	36	40	46	55	64	73	77
35–39	29	31	36	43	49	58	62	34	38	44	53	64	74	82
40–44	27	31	36	43	51	60	67	34	39	48	56	65	79	88
45–49	30	33	38	45	52	60	64	34	41	47	58	68	82	87
50–54	28	31	36	44	51	58	63	37	41	50	62	71	84	92
55–59	28	31	38	46	55	64	71	37	41	50	60	73	85	91
60–64	30	34	41	49	61	69	74	38	44	51	61	75	87	92
65–69	30	33	39	49	62	74	78	35	38	49	62	73	85	98
70+	31	33	40	48	56	70	75	33	38	48	60	71	82	92

Adapted from Rifkind BM, Segal P. Lipid Research Clinics Program reference values for hyperlipidemia and hypolipidemia. *In* Lipid Research Clinics Population Studies Data Book. Vol 1, The Prevalence Study. 1980, NIH Publication No. 80–1527.

that commonly occurs with reduction of the concentration of triglycerides may also mediate any vascular benefit arising from treatment of the hypertriglyceridemia. While controversy exists regarding the role of triglyceride in vascular disease, the relationship to pancreatitis seems more secure, though mechanisms remain unclear. Thus, treatment of hypertriglyceridemia that exceeds 2000 mg/dl seems clinically indicated independent of coronary artery considerations.

DIETARY CHOLESTEROL

The contribution of dietary cholesterol to plasma lipoprotein cholesterol has been the basis of enormous numbers of conflicting investigations and controversy. In general, very-low-density lipoprotein cholesterol (VLDL-C) as well as low-density lipoprotein cholesterol (LDL-C) concentrations are decreased in individuals who respond to dietary cholesterol intake.[25–28] It would appear that the high-density lipoprotein cholesterol (HDL-C) concentration remains relatively unaffected by changes in dietary cholesterol,[25–28] though a change in HDL apoprotein subunit composition may occur.[29]

Therapy with liquid diets containing total cholesterol restriction has been reported to provide a significant reduction in total plasma cholesterol. However, in studies of patients' responses to solid diets in which cholesterol has been removed, more variable results have been reported.[30–37] The variability of response has been attributed to the simultaneous variations in cholesterol-restricted diets, including saturated/unsaturated fatty acid composition, mineral content, total caloric exposure, and changes in patient behavior including exercise, smoking, weight loss, and the introduction of medications. Moreover, patient populations have been diverse in the various studies, particularly with regard to initial plasma levels of cholesterol and/or triglyceride.

Table 25–4 summarizes selected investigations of the influence of dietary cholesterol restriction, usually in conjunction with substitution of polyunsaturated fat for saturated fat. It can be appreciated that

restriction of dietary cholesterol intake to less than 300 mg/day is associated with a 10 to 15 per cent reduction in total plasma cholesterol concentration. This level of cholesterol intake has been selected as a dietary goal for the United States by the Select Committee on Nutrition and Human Needs of the United States Senate.[38] In the population of patients with elevated plasma cholesterol concentrations in the range of 260 mg/dl (90th percentile), this type of dietary restriction may be predicted to reduce the plasma cholesterol concentration by 25 to 35 mg/dl. Much lesser degrees of cholesterol lowering may be expected in subjects who initially have a "normal" total plasma cholesterol level. Similarly, patients who initially demonstrate plasma cholesterol levels of 350 mg/dl may demonstrate a reduction to 280 to 300 mg/dl, but rarely more than this 50 to 70 mg/dl fall in concentration.

Similar degrees of reduction in plasma cholesterol have been observed in vegetarians within the United States. As reported from a group designated "The Farm" in Tennessee,[39] reduced levels of both total plasma cholesterol as well as LDL-cholesterol were observed in men and women in comparison with a parallel population in St. Louis, Missouri. Confirmation of such a role for dietary restriction of cholesterol has also been noted in evaluation of the Tarahumara Indians of Mexico.[40] In this population, the daily ingestion of cholesterol rarely exceeds 300 mg/day, and often is less than 50 mg/day. A linear relationship between plasma cholesterol concentration and dietary cholesterol intake is reported for this population, in which the average cholesterol intake is only 71 mg/day and the mean plasma cholesterol concentration is 120 ± 52 mg/dl.[40] Below 400 mg intake of cholesterol per day, dietary cholesterol is an important determinant of plasma cholesterol. In diet studies employing different quantities of cholesterol ranging from 0 to 317 mg/1000 kcal of food, Mattson et al. demonstrated a linear elevation of serum cholesterol over the entire range of cholesterol feeding.[31] Each 100 mg of cholesterol in the diet resulted in a 12 mg/dl increase in serum cholesterol concentration. Subjects ingesting a 317 mg cholesterol/1000 kcal diet, similar to that of the

TABLE 25–4. Change in Plasma Cholesterol in Major Dietary Intervention Trials

	Years of Follow-up	Mean Cholesterol of Treated Subjects	
		Initial	Final
Medical Research Council (MRC) of London low-fat[8]	3	240 mg/dl	219 mg/dl
Medical Research Council (MRC) of London soybean oil[9]	4	258 mg/dl	224 mg/dl
New Jersey Diet[46]	5	260 mg/dl	234 mg/dl
Oslo Diet[4]	5	284 mg/dl	243 mg/dl
Los Angeles Veterans Administration[3]	8	233 mg/dl	186 mg/dl
Helsinki Diet[1]	12	235 mg/dl	211 mg/dl

United States norm, demonstrated a 40 mg/dl rise in serum cholesterol. Finally, it has been shown that the movement of populations with natural cholesterol restriction, such as the Eskimo or Japanese, to socioeconomic areas with normally greater cholesterol content of the diet, such as from Greenland to Sweden or from Japan to California,[11] results in increased concentrations of cholesterol in the plasma. This increase seems to be roughly 25 to 35 mg/dl, which is comparable to the reduction observed with imposed limitations in dietary cholesterol.

Central to the consideration of dietary cholesterol limitation with such a minimal improvement of only 25 mg/dl in plasma cholesterol is the issue of benefit to the patient. The epidemiology of this relationship has recently been confirmed in the Western Electric study reporting a 2-year follow-up of the risk of coronary death in middle-aged American men.[2] Based upon the diet analysis at entry into the study, there was a highly significant relationship between the intake "score" of cholesterol and polyunsaturated fatty acids, and the serum cholesterol concentration. Moreover, there was a positive association between the baseline diet score and the 19-year risk of death from coronary artery disease. A large number of similar epidemiological and cross-cultured studies have been performed.[7,41] While not all have observed significant correlations between dietary cholesterol, serum cholesterol, and the risk of coronary heart disease, the genetic heterogeneity and dietary homogeneity limitations of design may have obscured correlations noted elsewhere. Familial hypobetalipoproteinemia (low LDL) is characterized by reduced levels of plasma cholesterol and LDL, and men and women from such kindreds have reported life expectancies 6 to 7 years longer than white populations in the United States.[12] Combined morbidity and mortality of myocardial infarction is fivefold less than in normolipemic controls, and reduced vascular disease has been confirmed in postmortem study of such subjects.[42]

Extrapolation to the response to dietary treatment of hypercholesterolemic populations has been the subject of considerable controversy, and several prospective studies have attempted to illuminate the issue. Foremost of these are the Oslo study,[4,43–45] the Seymore Dayton VA study,[3] the Montclair, New Jersey, study,[46] the MRFIT study,[5] and most recently the LRC collaborative study.[6] In each case, dietary limitation of cholesterol with conservative considerations given to increasing unsaturated fat and limiting saturated fat, controlling for smoking, and generally focusing on remaining "healthy" was pursued. A reduction in coronary events, coronary death, or other hard cardiovascular endpoints occurred in each study, but could not always be attributed to an effect of lowering cholesterol levels. For example, the MRFIT study achieved too small a difference between the cholesterol levels of the two treatment groups (2 per cent) to assess the contributions of

lowering cholesterol levels.[5] Table 25–5 shows the cholesterol content of foods typically eaten in the United States. It can be appreciated that 300 mg of cholesterol in the diet of a given day is easily achieved. Complete substitution of soybean protein in the diet has been shown to achieve a 0 mg cholesterol intake and reduce the plasma cholesterol concentration.[47] The diet for the management of hypercholesterolemia that has been proposed by the American Heart Association includes a daily intake of 300 mg of cholesterol, with no more than 10 per cent of calories derived from saturated animal fats, and 10 per cent of calories derived from fats and oils rich in polyunsaturated fatty acids.[10] If a satisfactory response is not achieved, then a progressive reduction in cholesterol intake to less than 100 mg/day is recommended.

Dietary limitation of cholesterol must also be considered as nutritional therapy for pediatric familial hypercholesterolemia. The incidence of this entity is approximately 1 in 150 live births.[48] It is associated with severe premature coronary and peripheral vascular atherosclerosis.[49] Dietary limitation of cholesterol and increased unsaturated fatty acid intake can be initiated in the neonatal period following cessation of breast feeding. Such therapy has been shown to be effective in reducing plasma cholesterol to normal levels by 6 to 23 months of age.[50] Moreover, such alterations in the diet are feasible and can be maintained in children below the age of 10 years with appropriate compliance and normalization of plasma cholesterol.[51,52] Longitudinal data referable to amelioration of atherosclerosis by long-term cholesterol lowering in these children have not yet been reported.

TABLE 25–5. Cholesterol Content of Popular American Foods

Food	Serving Size	Cholesterol (mg per serving)
Meats		
Liver	4 oz	497
Tuna	4 oz	171
Shrimp	4 oz	117
Crab	4 oz	114
Veal	4 oz	114
Beef	4 oz	107
Chicken	4 oz	103
Pork	4 oz	101
Lobster	4 oz	96
Dairy Products		
Whole egg	1 egg	252
Cheddar cheese	4 oz	112
Swiss cheese	4 oz	112
Condensed milk	8 oz	105
Ice cream	1 cup	86
Sour cream	½ cup	76
Butter	1 oz	71
Cottage cheese	4 oz	48
Whole milk	8 oz	34

DIETARY CARBOHYDRATE

Beginning with the description of "carbohydrate-induced hyperlipemia" by Ahrens et al. in 1961,[53] it has been recognized that the ingestion of carbohydrate can induce an elevation in plasma triglyceride concentration.[54,55] In a normal person, this phenomenon spontaneously resolves in approximately 2 weeks and may be related to the concomitant insulin secretion and reduced glucagon secretion resulting from the carbohydrate in the diet.[56,57] However, the observation by DenBesten et al.[58] that a high-carbohydrate diet given intravenously does not cause triglyceridemia, in spite of insulin excess, suggests an important role of the intestinal mucosa in the etiology of carbohydrate-induced lipemia. In patients with pre-existing endogenous hypertriglyceridemia, carbohydrate in the diet aggravates the degree of hyperlipoproteinemia in a sustained fashion. For this reason, any patient with endogenous hypertriglyceridemia may benefit from restriction in the carbohydrate content of the diet, with calories provided from protein and fat.

The basis for this response appears to relate to the metabolic effects of dietary carbohydrate upon hepatic lipoprotein production. The resulting secretion of very-low-density lipoproteins (VLDL) releases into the blood a family of lipoproteins that contain a cargo of triglyceride and cholesterol in a ratio of 5:1. This endogenous hypertriglyceridemia of excessive production of VLDL occurs to a sustained degree only in a patient with abnormal metabolism of VLDL, who may be classified by the clinician as having Type IV hyperlipoproteinemia. Some of these patients may have a further genetically determined defect in the metabolism of VLDL, such that they also accumulate a degradation production of VLDL metabolism, termed intermediate-density-lipoprotein (IDL). This predominant IDL abnormality may be classified as Type III hyperlipoproteinemia, and is characterized by excessive IDL circulation in the plasma with a triglyceride and cholesterol content in the ratio of 1:1. In these patients excessive production of hepatic triglyceride-bearing lipoprotein remains the functional disorder, and restriction of carbohydrate in the diet may result in a clinically significant reduction in the degree of hypertriglyceridemia. A further group of patients may be found to demonstrate excessive production of VLDL, accumulation of IDL, and excessive circulating concentrations of LDL from a primary abnormality in LDL cholesterol metabolism. While classified formally as Type IIb lipoproteinemia, from the standpoint of nutritional therapy, this entity represents a carbohydrate-sensitive form of endogenous hypertriglyceridemia.

Regardless of the clinical classification, all patients with endogenous hypertriglyceridemia with excessive production of hepatic lipoproteins may respond clinically to restriction of dietary carbohydrate. Usually, the greater the compliance of the patient to extensive restriction of carbohydrate, the greater will be the reduction in plasma triglyceride-bearing lipoproteins. In this context, nutritional advice requires education of the patient as to those foodstuffs rich in carbohydrate content, and a plan to substitute protein and/or fat calories in their place. Sufficient carbohydrate is required to permit taste to be satisfied.

It has been generally observed that with reduction in the concentration of plasma triglycerides, a parallel rise in concentration of HDL may occur in some[59] but not all[60] subjects. The mechanisms mediating this response are not established, but it has been reported that the change is predominantly in the HDL_2 subclass and is associated with an elevation in the apoC apoprotein content.[61] Other investigators have reported that a low plasma level of HDL-cholesterol in hypertriglyceridemia patients may reflect decreased binding of cholesterol by normal plasma concentrations of the HDL apoprotein (apoA-I and apoA-II)[62] resulting from abnormalities in lipoprotein lipase. Such patients may face no additional risk for coronary artery disease.[62]

Unlike the studies of dietary cholesterol restriction, there are no convincing studies relating clinical benefits to carbohydrate restriction in the diet in patients with endogenous hyperlipoproteinemia. Indeed, there remains considerable controversy as to the cardiovascular risk imposed by endogenous hyperlipoproteinemia. If extrapolation from studies of drug therapy directed toward reducing VLDL and IDL in the plasma can be considered as evidence that a similar reduction in VLDL and IDL induced by carbohydrate restriction would be beneficial, then some support for nutritional therapy may be obtained. A number of studies utilizing fibric acid–related drugs have reported clinical benefits in terms of cardiovascular endpoints from pharmacological reduction in endogenous hypertriglyceridemia.[63–65] Detailed analysis and/or interpretation of these conclusions is beyond the scope of this discussion, but when a similar degree of improvement in endogenous triglyceridemia is achieved by dietary carbohydrate restriction, a comparable clinical benefit may be anticipated.

Concern is often expressed over the response to the fat ingestion imposed by a diet in which carbohydrate has been significantly removed. Ordinarily, in a patient with no disturbance in exogenous chylomicron disposal, increasing the dietary content of fat does not affect the concentration of endogenous lipoproteins, or of fasting total plasma triglyceride content. This is because the mechanisms responsible for exogenous fat removal are distinct from those responsible for endogenous (VLDL, IDL) fat production. However, as discussed below, if the clinical picture is mixed endogenous and exogenous hypertriglyceridemia in which dietary chylomicrons persist in the plasma in the fasting state, then simple carbohydrate restriction with excessive fat calories ingested may lead to an aggravation of the total lipemia. This condition is usually clinically classified as having Type V hyperlipoproteinemia, which implies a combination of endogenous Type IV disease with exogenous Type I chylomicronemia. In this setting, it may be necessary to impose fat restriction as well, making dietary management of both endogenous and exogenous hypertriglyceridemia unachievable. In this setting, drug therapy may be obligatory to achieve normalization of the hyperlipoproteinemia.

DIETARY CALORIES

Obesity is often associated with endogenous hypertriglyceridemia of the clinical classification Type IV, characterized by excessive plasma concentrations of VLDL. Weight reduction accomplished by caloric restriction is clearly recognized to lead to a reduction in both plasma triglyceride and cholesterol concentrations.[66–73] It has been observed in both animals and humans that there exists a linear correlation between body weight and hepatic VLDL production.[70,74]

Because of this recognized association between body weight and hepatic endogenous triglyceride-bearing lipoprotein overproduction, caloric restriction to achieve normalization of body weight is an appropriate nutritional strategy. The nutritional management of obesity is discussed in detail in Chapter 8, but suffice it to say that restriction in total protein, total fat, and total carbohydrate constitutes appropriate nutritional caloric restriction for obese patients, in whom endogenous hypertriglyceridemia may appear. Curiously, not all obese subjects demonstrate clinical hypertriglyceridemia, suggesting that other aspects of peripheral VLDL and IDL metabolism and disposal must compensate for hepatic overproduction of these lipoproteins. It is also observed that complete normalization to ideal body weight may not be necessary to correct the hypertriglyceridemia significantly, though rigorous definition of these responses remains to be established. Finally, some but not all patients demonstrate a rise in HDL levels,[69–71,75] and some patients respond with an unexpected rise in LDL.[69] Variable response to weight reduction secondary to caloric restriction may relate to differences in the degree of obesity, underlying associated defects in lipoprotein removal mechanisms, and genetic differences in lipoprotein regulation. The clinical response must thus be monitored in individual patients.

SUBSTITUTION OF UNSATURATED FOR SATURATED FAT

The role of increased unsaturated fatty acids relative to saturated fatty acid in the regulation of plasma cholesterol concentration has been of great interest as a nutritional strategy since the 1950's.[13,76,77] With the availability of unsaturated fatty acid oils to the general public in such products as corn oil, soybean oil, and filled milk products for infant nutrition in which unsaturated fat is substituted for milk fat, dietary emphasis upon unsaturated fatty acid intake has been achievable. Studies with experimental formula diets have unequivocally demonstrated a cholesterol-lowering effect, but the mechanisms remain undetermined.[78] Recent investigations have reported a reduction in hepatic production of LDL in association with increased fractional metabolic clearance of LDL as participating in the observed lowering in LDL-cholesterol concentration.[79] Other reports suggest that fecal neutral steroid and perhaps bile acid secretion are increased, resulting in a negative steroid balance.[80,81]

The nutritional recommendation is not to add polyunsaturated fat to the diet, but to substitute polyunsaturated fat in place of saturated fat intake. The average American diet contains approximately 40 per cent of the total calories as fat. Of these calories, perhaps 17 per cent are derived from saturated fats of animal origin, or vegetable oils including palm oil, coconut oil, cocoa butter, and hydrogenated margarines. Only approximately 6 per cent of dietary calories are derived from polyunsaturated fats. The American Heart Association has recommended a reduction in saturated fats to 10 per cent of total calories, and the substitution of polyunsaturated fats[7] for additional fat calories to a total of 20 to 30 per cent of total dietary calories from fat. Since the total nutritional impact of high intake of polyunsaturated fats is not known, most nutritionists suggest only doubling the polyunsaturated fat intake to no more than 10 per cent of total calories, consistent with American Heart Association guidelines. Polyunsaturated fats have been implicated in increased risk for gallstone formation[82] and may have cocarcinogenic potential in animals.[83]

Within the last decade there has been increasing interest in the polyunsaturated ω-fatty acids present in fish oils. Like the ω-6 fatty acids present in vegetable oils, of which linoleic acid is the principal fatty acid, the ω-3 fatty acids also lead to hypocholesterolemia when substituted for saturated fatty acids in the diet.[84] Certain population groups, including the British Columbian coastal Indians and Greenland Eskimos, consume large amounts of ω-3 oils derived from seals, whales, and fish,[85] and this diet has been associated with reduced rates of atherosclerotic disease.[86] For this reason, inclusion of fish and/or fish oil to the diet in substitution for saturated fat holds clinical attraction. As summarized by Oliver,[13] for any level of dietary polyunsaturated fat intake, the greater the ω-3/ω-6 ratio, the less the risk of coronary heart disease. It seems likely that the clinical benefits of ω-3 fatty acids must derive from factors other than cholesterol lowering, such as their effect upon platelet function.[84]

The clinical application of substitution of unsaturated fatty acids for saturated fat in the diet has been difficult to realize, and efficacy remains to be demonstrated. Investigations utilizing increased polyunsaturated fatty acid usually also include cholesterol restriction, so that outpatient ambulatory studies concerning compliance and clinical effect are elusive. In the Dayton VA study, patients were fed in restricted dining areas, and biopsies of their buttocks fat were utilized to confirm that a change in unsaturated fatty acid content had been achieved.[3] In this study (see Table 25–4), a reduction in cholesterol content of the plasma was observed with dietary unsaturated fatty acid excess and cholesterol restriction. As previously discussed, drawing upon all types of cholesterol-lowering management, it may be concluded that the cholesterol reduction achieved with polyunsaturated fatty acid substitution may also confer clinical benefit in terms of cardiovascular endpoints.

DIETARY FIBER

Studies of fiber in the diet have suggested that ingestion of excess mucilaginous fiber may be associated with lower levels of plasma cholesterol-bearing lipoproteins[87] and less vascular atherogenesis in humans[88–94] and laboratory animals.[95] In some reports it has been suggested that plasma high-density lipoprotein (HDL) may increase in concentration, though this response seems variable. Much of the available data is consistent with the concept that plasma low-density lipoprotein may be reduced by the dietary addition of pectin fiber, which contains soluble components.[95] When fiber is provided in the form of a totally insoluble cellulose, the hypocholesterolemic effect is lacking. It thus appears that those fibers which are predominantly soluble (such as pectin, gum guar, carrageenan, or oat bran) are regularly associated with a reduction in plasma cholesterol concentration and a rise in plasma HDL. In contrast, those studies using predominantly insoluble fibers (such as alfalfa, wheat bran, or cellulose) show no reduction in plasma cholesterol concentration. The chemical nature of soluble pectin, galacturonic acid units, is distinct from other plant fiber structures and could be critical to this metabolic response observed with the mucilaginous fibers.[96]

The mechanisms involved in the reduction in plasma LDL and elevation in HDL in fiber-fed animals are not established. Lymphatic absorption of cholesterol in the rat is reduced by dietary fiber,[97] which may explain the observation that the greatest hypocholesterolemic effects of fiber occur with high-cholesterol diets. Ingestion of fiber also results in an increased fecal loss of endogenous neutral sterols and of bile acids.[98] Such a fecal loss of endogenous

cholesterol would be compatible with increased hepatic conversion of cholesterol to bile acids, leading to a reduction in both plasma LDL cholesterol and hepatic cholesterol availability.[99] Such a response may be similar to that observed clinically with cholesterol-binding resins, which have been shown in the LRC collaborative study to reduce both plasma cholesterol concentration and the risk of cardiovascular events.[6]

Burkitt[100] and Trowell[101] proposed that many diseases of the Western world are associated with diets high in refined carbohydrates and low in fiber. This concept is based upon the fact that the average intake of dietary fiber in the United Kingdom is 20 g/person/day,[102] whereas that in rural Africa may be 100 to 170 g/day.[102] While it may be premature to identify dietary recommendations for fiber intake, and specifically for soluble fiber in the diet, it is provocative to anticipate that such considerations may become appropriate.

FUTURE CHALLENGE

There is no question that prevention of coronary heart disease through the identification of hyperlipoproteinemia and modification of diet to correct this problem is a responsibility for today's medical profession. The problem of compliance for a lifetime presents almost insurmountable obstacles for many patients who would otherwise benefit from dietary management,[103] but they can be overcome.[104,105] In the clinical arena, it is not so much proof of efficacy that the patient requires, but assistance in changing a life's pattern of dietary intake. To achieve this goal, the profession requires maximum support from dieticians, nutritionists, psychologists, nurse assistants, physician assistants, and educational specialists.

A major step in quantitative support of dietary management of hyperlipemia has been the use of computer-assisted nutrient analysis of a 3-day diet history.[106–109] An example of such an evaluation is shown in Figure 25–1. In this procedure the patient will review dietary goals with a dietician, monitor and record his or her dietary intake for 3 days, and have the opportunity to review concepts such as cholesterol, unsaturated and saturated fatty acid, carbohydrate, fiber, and total calories with the physician. This quantitative effort can be repeated at appropriate intervals, and the results compared to monitor compliance and reinforce the instruction.[109] The probability of physician-patient-dietician interaction is enhanced by this effort, and this may improve the clinical response.

Thus, while advances in understanding pathophysiology and mechanisms of action will undoubtedly clarify our understanding of hyperlipoproteinemia and diet management, the challenge will remain at the level of persuasion and compliance if a successful outcome is to emerge.

Diet Record

Name: JOE SAMPLE   Date: Mon, 2 Apr 1984   ID: CNP 001 01

Quan Meas Code	Item #	Description	Kcal	T-Fat Gm	A-Fat Gm	P-Fat Gm	Chol mG	Fiber Gm	Caff mG	Na mG
7:30 Breakfast at Home										
2 Large (12)	16-0060	EGG WHOLE, FRIED IN BUTTER	166	12.8	12.8	0.0	491	0.		288
2 Slice (44)	50-2010	BACON (ANY) COOKED	92	7.8	7.8	0.0		0.		153
2 Slice (44)	57-0450	WHOLE WHEAT TOAST	110	1.4	0.0	1.4		0.722		238
0.5 Tbsp (05)	70-2030	JAM, ASSORTED	27	0.0	0.0	0.0	0	0.1		1
2 Pat (36)	50-0015	BUTTER REGULAR	72	8.1	8.1	0.0	22	0.	0.	83
6 Vol Oz(01)	45-1250	ORANGE JUICE UNSW, FROZEN CONC. DILUTED W/ 3 PARTS WATER	92	0.2	0.0	0.2	0	.1867	0.	2
10:00 Morning snack at Company Cafeteria										
1 Cup (02)	01-0050	COFFEE, BREWED BEVERAGE	7	0.2	0.0	0.2		0.	134.8	2
1 Pkg (35)	70-0040	SUGAR GRANULATED WHITE	17	0.0	0.0	0.0	0	0.		0
1 Pkg (35)	09-6060	COFFEE WHITENER, NON-DAIRY POWDERED	16	1.1	0.0	1.1	0	0.		5
12:30 Lunch at Restaurant										
0.25 Pound (74)	20-2370	BEEF ROUND GROUND LMF COOKED, RAW WT	205	12.1	12.1	0.0	74	0.		47
1 Avg (16)	57-1040	HAMBURGER BUN	119	2.2			0	0.08		202
1 Slice (44)	48-4840	ONION (DRY YELLOW) RAW, WHOLE	4	0.0	0.0	0.0	0	0.06	0.	1
15 Strip (48)	47-0270	POTATO FRENCH FRIED	226	10.9	0.0	10.9	0	0.825	0.	5
12 Vol Oz(01)	01-0330	COLA TYPE BEVERAGE, CARBONATED	144	0.0	0.0	0.0	0	0.	59.88	1
2 Pkg (35)	75-0110	CATSUP REGULAR	30	0.1	0.0	0.1		.1402		292
15:30 Afternoon snack at Company Cafeteria										
1.5 Medium(11)	58-1060	DOUGHNUT/FRYCAKE CAKE TYPE ICING/SUGAR	275	11.9	1.0	10.9		Trace		338
1 Cup (02)	01-0050	COFFEE, BREWED BEVERAGE	7	0.2	0.0	0.2		0.	134.8	2
1 Pkg (35)	09-6060	COFFEE WHITENER, NON-DAIRY POWDERED	16	1.1	0.0	1.1	0	0.		5
1 Pkg (35)	70-0040	SUGAR GRANULATED WHITE	17	0.0	0.0	0.0	0	0.		0
17:30 Afternoon snack at Home										
1 Bt/Can(18)	03-0030	BEER, 4.5% ALCOHOL BY VOLUME	151	0.0	0.0	0.0		0.		25
0.25 Cup (02)	81-0650	PEANUTS DRY ROASTED, PLANTERS	217	17.0	0.0	17.0	0			434
18:00 Dinner at Home										
0.33 Cup (02)	48-1440	PEAS GREEN IMMATURE FROZEN COOKED, BOILED DRAINED	36	0.2	0.0	0.2	0	1.003	0.	61
0.5 Cup (02)	47-0645	POTATO MASHED, DEHYDRAT GRANULES MADE W/WATER MILK MARGARINE	101	3.8				0.21	0.	269
3 Teasp (06)	50-0015	BUTTER REGULAR	101	11.4	11.4	0.0	31	0.	0.	116
1 Medium(11)	25-1270	CHICKEN (FRYER) THIGH FRIED IN VEGETABLE FAT	122	5.9	4.4	1.4	47			44
1 Medium(11)	25-1080	CHICKEN (FRYER) BREAST HALF FRIED IN VEGETABLE FAT	160	5.1	3.0	2.1	63			51
0.5 Cup (02)	48-1080	LETTUCE ICEBERG RAW, CHUNKS	5	0.0	0.0	0.0	0	.1875	0.	3
2 Medium(11)	48-2070	TOMATO RAW, SLICE/WEDGE	9	0.1	0.0	0.1	0	0.205	0.	1
1 Tbsp (05)	50-3230	ITALIAN DRESSING	68	7.2	0.0	7.1	Trace	.0292	0.	115
1 Cup (02)	09-0340	WHOLE MILK, FLUID, 3.3% FAT, FORT W/D	149	8.1	8.1	0.0	34	0.		120
21:00 Evening snack at Home										
0.5 Cup (02)	66-0120	VANILLA ICE CREAM, REGULAR (10% FAT) HARDENED	134	7.2	7.2	0.0	30	0.		58
2 Tbsp (05)	70-2620	SIRUP CHOCOLATE, THIN TYPE	98	0.8	0.0	0.8		0.24		21
4 Medium(11)	62-0120	CHOCOLATE CHIP COOKIE	138	6.1	0.2	5.9		.1168		117

Diet Record Processing

Nutrient Summary			RDA	% Cal
Kilocalories	3130		115 %	
Total Protein	125.9	Gm	225 %	16 %
Animal Protein	90.8	Gm *		
Plant Protein	24.9	Gm *		
Total Fat	142.8	Gm		41 %
Animal Fat	76.1	Gm *		
Plant Fat	60.6	Gm *		
Total Carb	322.7	Gm		41 %
Refined Carb	88.4	Gm *		
Natural Carb	192.4	Gm *		
Alcohol	13.0	Gm *		3 %
Tot Polyunsat FA	12.6	Gm *		
Total Sat FA	49.88	Gm *		
Cholesterol	792	mG *		
Total Vitamin A	3941	IU *	79 %	
Total Tocoph	5.5	mG *	51 %	
Ascorbic Acid	136.7	mG *	228 %	
Thiamin	1.403	mG *	90 %	
Niacin	35.18	mG *	301 %	
Riboflavin	2.246	mG *	120 %	
Pyridoxal B6	988.6	uG *	45 %	
Vitamin B12	3.444	uG *	115 %	
Folic Acid	.3694	mG *	92 %	
Iron	16.13	mG *	161 %	
Calcium	710.6	mG *	89 %	
Phosphorus	1692	mG *	212 %	
Sodium	3102	mG	A	
Potassium	4387	mG	A	
Magnesium	274.8	mG *	79 %	
Zinc	13.11	mG *	87 %	

ID: CNP 001 01
Date: Mon, 2 Apr 1984   Ideal Wt: 70.0 Kg
Name: JOE SAMPLE   28 Yr Male Ht: 180 cm Wt: 0.0 Kg

FIGURE 25–1. *A computer printout of diet intake for one day, nutrient analysis of food ingested, and summary of nutrient intake with attention to cholesterol, unsaturated fat, saturated fat, carbohydrate, protein, vitamins, and trace metals. Data processed on an IBM 360 computer, accessed via a remote Decwriter terminal, using the Case Western Reserve Nutrient Analysis Program Release #4 at the University of New Mexico.*

References

1. Miettinen M, Turpeinen O, Darvonen JJ, et al. Effect of cholesterol-lowering diet on mortality from coronary heart disease and other causes—12 year clinical trial in men and women. Lancet 1972; 2:835–838.
2. Shekelle RB, Shryrock AM, Oglesby P, et al. Diet, serum cholesterol, and death from coronary heart disease. The Western Electric Study. N Engl J Med 1981; 304:65–70.
3. Dayton S, Pearce ML, Hashimoto S, et al. A controlled clinical trial of a diet high in unsaturated fat in preventing complications of atherosclerosis. Circulation 1969; 40(Suppl 2):1–63.
4. Leren P. The Oslo Diet Heart Study: eleven year report. Circulation 1970; 42:935–942.
5. Multiple Risk Factor Intervention Trial: (MRFIT): Risk factor changes and mortality results. JAMA 1982; 248:1465–1477.
6. Lipid Research Clinics Program: The Lipid Research Clinics Coronary Primary Prevention Trial results. JAMA 1984; 251:351–374.
7. Grundy SM, Bilheimer D, Blackburn H, et al. Rationale of the Diet-Heart Statement of the American Heart Association. Report of Nutrition Committee. Circulation 1982; 65:839A–854A.
8. Research Committee to the Medical Research Council: Low-fat diet in myocardial infarction—a controlled trial. Lancet 1965; 2:501–504, 1965.
9. Research Committee to the Medical Research Council: Controlled trial of soy-bean oil in myocardial infarction. Lancet 1968; 2:693–700.
10. Council on Scientific Affairs. Dietary and pharmacologic therapy for the lipid risk factors. JAMA 1983; 250:1873–1882.
11. Keys A, Kimura N, Kusukawa A, et al. Lessons from serum cholesterol studies in Japan, Hawaii, and Los Angeles. Ann Intern Med 1958; 48:83–94.
12. Glueck CJ, Gartside P, Fallat RW, et al. Longevity syndromes: familial hypobeta and familial hyperalpha lipoproteinemia. J Lab Clin Med 1976; 88:941–957.
13. Oliver MF. Dietary prevention of coronary heart disease: the role of essential fatty acids. *In* Grotto AM Jr, Smith LC, Allen B (eds). Atherosclerosis V. New York, Springer-Verlag, 1980: 235–244.
14. Glueck CJ, Connor WE. Diet–coronary heart disease relationships reconnoitered. Am J Clin Nutr 1978; 31:727–737.
15. Connor WE, Connor SL. The key role of nutritional factors in the prevention of coronary heart disease. Prev Med 1972; 1:49–83.
16. Stamler J. Public health aspects of optimal serum lipid-lipoprotein levels. Prev Med 1979; 8:733–766.
17. Rifkind BM, Segal P. Lipid Research Clinics Program reference values for hyperlipidemia and hypolipidemia. *In* Lipid Research Clinics Population Studies Data Book. Vol 1, The Prevalence Study. 1980. NIH Publication No. 80–1527.
18. Primary prevention of the atherosclerotic diseases: National Cooperative Pooling Project of the American Heart Association. Circulation 1970; 42:A55–A94.
19. Streja D, Steiner G, Kwiterovich PO. Plasma high density lipoprotein and other lipids and lipoproteins and ischemic heart disease in a large Newfoundland pedigree with familial hypercholesterolemia. Ann Intern Med 1978; 87:871–880.
20. DeBacker G, Rossenau M, Deslypere JP. Discriminative value of lipids and apoproteins in coronary heart disease. Atherosclerosis 1982; 42:197–203.
21. Albert JJ, Wahl PW, Cabana VG, et al. Quantitation of apolipoprotein A-1 of human plasma high density lipoprotein. Metabolism 1976; 25:633–644.
22. Ishikawa T, Fidge N, Thelle DS, et al. The Tromso Heart Study: serum apolipoprotein A-1 concentration in relation to future coronary heart disease. Eur J Clin Invest 1978; 8:179–182.
23. Fager G, Wiklund O, Olofsson S-O, et al. Serum apolipoprotein levels in relation to acute myocardial infarction and its risk factors. Determination of polypeptide A-II. Artery 1979; 6:188–204.
24. Lippel K, Tyroler HA, Eder H, et al. Meeting summary: relationship of hypertriglyceridemia to atherosclerosis. Arteriosclerosis 1981; 1:406–417.
25. Nestle PH, Poyser A. Changes in cholesterol synthesis and excretion when cholesterol intake is increased. Metabolism 1976; 25:1591–1599.
26. Applebaum D, Cahn J, Hazzard W, et al. Short term cholesterol feeding in humans: failure to induce B-migrating very low density lipoproteins (B-VLDL). (Abstract.) Clin Res 1977; 25:158A.
27. Flaim E, Ferreri LF, Thye FS, et al. Plasma lipid and lipoprotein cholesterol concentrations in adult males consuming normal and high cholesterol diets under controlled conditions. Am J Clin Nutr 1981; 34:1103–1108.
28. Schonfeld G, Patsch W, Rudel LL, et al. Effects of dietary cholesterol and fatty acids on plasma lipoproteins. J Clin Invest 1982; 69:1072–1080.
29. Mahley RW, Innerarity TL, Bersot TP, et al. Alterations in human high-density lipoproteins, with or without increased plasma cholesterol, induced by diets high in cholesterol. Lancet 1978; 2:807–809.
30. Connor WE, Hodges RE, Bleiker RE. The serum lipids in men receiving high cholesterol and cholestrol-free diets. J Clin Invest 1961; 40:894–900.
31. Mattson FH, Erickson BA, Kligman AM. Effect of dietary cholesterol on serum cholesterol in man. Am J Clin Nutr 1972; 25:589–594.
32. Beveridge JMR, Connell WF, Mayaer GH, et al. The response of man to dietary cholesterol. J Nutr 1960; 71:61–65.
33. Keys A, Anderson JT, Mickelsen O, et al. Diet and serum cholesterol in man: lack of effect of dietary cholesterol. J Nutr 1956; 59:39–56.
34. Keys A, Anderson JT, Grande F. Serum cholesterol response to changes in the diet. II. The effect of cholesterol in the diet. Metabolism 1965; 14:759–765.
35. Mistry P, Miller NE, Laker M, et al. Individual variation in the effects of dietary cholesterol on plasma lipoproteins and cellular cholesterol homeostasis in man. J Clin Invest 1981; 67:493–502.
36. Quig DS, Thye FW, Ritchey SJ, et al. Effects of short-term aerobic conditioning and high cholesterol feeding on plasma total and lipoprotein cholesterol levels in sedentary young men. Am J Clin Nutr 1983; 38:825–834.
37. Ginsberg H, Le NA, Mays C, et al. Lipoprotein metabolism in nonresponders to increased dietary cholesterol. Arteriosclerosis 1981; 1:463–470.
38. Dietary Goals for the United States. Prepared by Select Committee on Nutrition and Human Needs, United States Senate. Washington, U.S. Govt. Printing Office, 1977. Cat. No. Y 4.N95:D 63/3.
39. Burslem J, Schonfeld G, Howald MA, et al. Plasma apoprotein and lipoprotein lipid levels in vegetarians. Metabolism 1978; 27:711–719.
40. Connor WE, Cerqueira MT, Connor RW, et al. The plasma lipids, lipoproteins, and diet of the Tarahumara Indians of Mexico. Am J Clin Nutr 1978; 31:1131–1142.
41. Keys A (ed). Coronary Heart Disease in Seven Countries. American Heart Association Monograph No. 29. Circulation 1970; 21(Suppl 1):I1–I199.
42. Kahn JA, Glueck CJ. Familial hypobetalipoproteinemia: absence of atherosclerosis in a postmortem study. JAMA 1978; 240:47–48.
43. Hjermann I, Holme I, Velve Byre K, et al. Effect of diet and smoking intervention on the incidence of coronary heart disease. Lancet 1981; 2:1304–1311.
44. Holme I. On the separation of the intervention effects of diet and anti-smoking advice on the incidence of major

coronary events in coronary high risk men. The Oslo Study. J Oslo City Hospital 1982; *32*:31–54.

45. Jacobsen BK, Tyrgg K, Hjermann I, et al. Acyl pattern of adipose tissue triglycerides, plasma free fatty acids, and diet of a group of men participating in a primary coronary prevention program. (The Oslo Study). Am J Clin Nutr 1983; *38*:906–913.

46. Bierenbaum ML, Fleischmann AI, Green DP, et al. The 5-year experience of modified diet on younger men with coronary heart disease. Circulation 1970; *92*:943–952.

47. Sirtori CR, Agradi E, Conti F, et al. Soybean-protein diet in the treatment of type II hyperlipoproteinemia. Lancet 1977; *1*:275–277.

48. Glueck CJ, Heckman F, Schoenfeld M, et al. Neonatal familial type II hyperlipoproteinemia: cord blood cholesterol in 1,800 births. Metabolism 1971; *20*:597–608.

49. Slack J. Risks of ischaemic heart disease in familial hyperlipoproteinemia states. Lancet 1969; *2*:1380–1382.

50. Glueck CJ, Tsang RC. Pediatric familial type II hyperlipoproteinemia: effects of diet on plasma cholesterol in the first year of life. Am J Clin Nutr 1972; *25*:224–230.

51. Glueck CJ, Tsang RC, Fallat R, et al. Diet in children heterozygous for familial hypercholesterolemia. Am J Dis Child 1977; *131*:162–166.

52. Larsen R, Glueck CJ, Tsang RC. Special diet for familial type II hyperlipoproteinemia. Am J Dis Child 1974; *128*:67–72.

53. Ahrens EH Jr, Hirsch J, Oette K, et al. Carbohydrate-induced and fat-induced lipemia. Trans Assoc Am Phys 1961; *74*:134–136.

54. Beveridge JMR, Jagannathan SN, Connell WR. The effect of the type and amount of dietary fat on the level of plasma triglycerides in human subjects in the postabsorptive state. Can J Biochem 1964; *42*:999–1005.

55. Farquhar JW, Grank A, Gross RC, et al. Glucose, insulin and triglyceride responses to high and low carbohydrate diets in man. J Clin Invest 1966; *45*:1648–1653.

56. Reaven GM, Lerner RL, Stern MP, et al. Role of insulin in endogenous hypertriglyceridemia. J Clin Invest 1967; *46*:1756–1759.

57. Eaton RP, Nye WHR. The relationship between insulin secretion and triglyceride concentration in endogenous lipemia. J Lab Clin Med 1973; *81*:682–695.

58. DenBesten L, Reyna RH, Connor WE, et al. The different effects on the serum lipids and fecal steroids of high carbohydrate diets given orally or intravenously. J Clin Invest 1973; *52*:1384–1393.

59. Eaton RP, Allen RC, Koopmans LH, et al. Overview of lipoprotein metabolism: perspectives in a free-living Southwest population in Bernalillo County, New Mexico. *In* Garry PJ (ed). Human Nutrition—Clinical and Biochemical Aspects. Washington, DC, American Association for Clinical Chemistry, 1981: 109–120.

60. Witztum JL, Dillingham MA, Giese W, et al. Normalization of triglycerides in type IV hyperlipoproteinemia fails to correct low levels of high-density-lipoprotein cholesterol. N Engl J Med 1980; *303*:907–914.

61. Kashyap ML, Barnhart RL, Srivastava LS. Effects of dietary carbohydrate and fat on plasma lipoproteins and apolipoproteins C-II and C-III in healthy men. J Lipid Res 1982; *23*:877–886.

62. Brunzell JD, Schrott HG, Motulsky AG, et al. Myocardial infarction in the familial forms of hypertriglyceridemia. Metabolism 1976; *25*:313–320.

63. Group of Physicians of the Newcastle-Upon-Tyne Region: Trial of clofibrate in the treatment of ischaemic heart disease. Br Med J 1971; *4*:767–775.

64. Research Committee of the Scottish Society of Physicians: Ischaemic heart disease: a secondary prevention trial using clofibrate. Br Med J 1971; *4*:775–784.

65. Coronary Drug Project Research Group: Clofibrate and niacin in coronary heart disease. JAMA 1975; *231*:360–381.

66. Galbraith WB, Connor WE, Stone DB. Weight loss and serum lipid changes in obese subjects given low calorie diets of varied cholesterol content. Ann Intern Med 1966; *64*:268–275.

67. Jackson IMD: Effect of prolonged starvation on blood lipid levels of obese subjects. Metabolism 1969; *18*:13–17.

68. Jackson RA, Moloney M, Lowy C, et al. Differences between metabolic responses to fasting in obese diabetic and obese nondiabetic subjects. Diabetes 1971; *20*:214–227.

69. Wilson DE, Lees RS. Metabolic relationships among the plasma lipoproteins—reciprocal changes in the concentrations of very low and low density lipoproteins in man. J Clin Invest 1972; *51*:1051–1057.

70. Olefsky J, Reaven GM, Farquhar JW. Effects of weight reduction on obesity—studies of lipid and carbohydrate metabolism in normal and hyperlipoproteinemic subjects. J Clin Invest 1974; *53*:64–76.

71. Jourdan M, Margen S, Bradfield RB. Turnover rate of serum glycerides in the lipoproteins of fasting obese women during weight loss. Am J Clin Nutr 1974; *27*:850–858.

72. Blacket RB, Woodhill JM, Leelarthaepin B, et al. Type-IV hyperlipidemia and weight gain after maturity. Lancet 1975; *2*:517–520.

73. Kudchodkar BJ, Sodhi HS, Mason DT, et al. Effects of acute caloric restriction on cholesterol metabolism in man. Am J Clin Nutr 1977; *30*:1135–1146.

74. Robertson RP, Garaveski DJ, Henderson JD, et al. Accelerated triglyceride secretion: a metabolic consequence of obesity. J Clin Invest 1973; *52*:1620–1626.

75. Taskinen MR, Nikkila EA. Effect of caloric restrictions on lipid metabolism in man. Atherosclerosis 1979; *32*:289–299.

76. Kinsell LW, Partridge J, Boling L, et al. Dietary modification of serum cholesterol and phospholipid levels. J Clin Endocrinol 1952; *12*:909–913.

77. Ahrens EH Jr, Hirsch J, Insull W Jr, et al. The influence of dietary fats on serum lipid levels in man. Lancet 1957; *1*:943–950.

78. Horrobin DF, Manku MS. How do polyunsaturated fatty acids lower plasma cholesterol levels? Lipids 1983; *18*:558–562.

79. Shepherd J, Packard CH, Grundy SM, et al. Effects of saturated and polyunsaturated fat diets on the chemical composition and metabolism of low density lipoproteins in man. J Lipid Res 1980; *21*:91–99.

80. Moore RB, Anderson JT, Taylor HL, et al. Effect of dietary fat on the fecal excretion of cholesterol and its degradation products in man. J Clin Invest 1968; *47*:1517–1534.

81. Nestel PH, Havenstein N, Homma Y, et al. Increased sterol excretion with polyunsaturated fat high-cholesterol diets. Metabolism 1975; *24*:189–198.

82. Strudevant RAL, Pearce ML, Dayton S. Increased prevalence of cholelithiasis in man ingesting a serum-cholesterol-lowering diet. N Engl J Med 1973; *288*:24–27.

83. Carroll KK, Khor HT. Effects of level and type of dietary fat on incidence of mammary tumors induced in female Sprague-Dawley rats by 7,12-dimethylbenz anthracene. Lipids 1971; *6*:415–420.

84. Harris WS, Connor WE, Goodnight SH Jr. Dietary fish oils, plasma lipids and platelets in man. Prog Lipid Res 1981; *20*:75–79.

85. Bang HO, Dyerberg J, Hyorne N. The composition of food consumed by Greenland Eskimos. Acta Med Scand 1976; *200*:69–73.

86. Dyerberg J, Bang HO, Stoffersen E, et al. Eicosapentaenoic acid and prevention of thrombosis and atherosclerosis. Lancet 1978; *2*:117–119.

87. Behall KM, Lee KH, Moser PB. Blood lipids and lipoproteins in adult men fed four refined fibers. Am J Clin Nutr 1984; *39*:209–214.

88. Morris JN, Marr JW, Clayton DG. Diet and heart: a postscript. Br Med J 1977; *2*:1307–1314.

89. Phillips RL, Leman FR, Beeson WL, et al. Coronary heart disease mortality among Seventh-Day Adventists with dif-

fering dietary habits: a preliminary report. Am J Clin Nutr 1978; *31*:S191–S198.

90. Jenkins DJA, Leeds AR, Slavin B, et al. Dietary fiber and blood lipids: reduction of serum cholesterol in type II hyperlipidemia by guar gum. Am J Clin Nutr 1979; *32*:16–18.

91. Anderson JW, Chen W, Sieling B. Hypolipidemic effects of high-carbohydrate high-fiber diets. Metabolism 1980; *29*:551–558.

92. Chen W, Anderson JW. Effects of plant fiber in decreasing plasma total cholesterol and increasing high-density lipoprotein cholesterol. Proc Soc Exp Biol Med 1979; *162*:310–313.

93. Kirby RW, Anderson JW, Sieling B, et al. Oat-bran intake selectively lowers serum low-density lipoprotein cholesterol concentrations of hypercholesterolemic men. Am J Clin Nutr 1981; *34*:824–829.

94. Kay RM. Dietary fiber: review. J Lipid Res 1982; *23*:221–242.

95. Wilson JM, Wilson SP, Eaton RP. Dietary fiber and lipoprotein metabolism in the genetically obese Zucker rat. Arteriosclerosis 1984; *4*:147–153.

96. Selvendran RR. The plant cell wall as a source of dietary fiber: chemistry and structure. Am J Clin Nutr 1984; *39*:320–337.

97. Vahouny FV, Timothy R, Gallo LL, et al. Dietary fibers. III. Effects of chronic intake on cholesterol absorption and metabolism in the rat. Am J Clin Nutr 1980; *33*:2182–2191.

98. Story JA, Kritchevsky D. Bile acid metabolism and fiber. Am J Clin Nutr 1978; *21*:S199–S202.

99. Kelly JJ, Tsai AC. Effect of pectin, gum arabid, and agar on cholesterol absorption, synthesis, and turnover in rats. J Nutr 1978; *108*:630–639.

100. Burkitt DP. Some diseases characteristic of modern Western civilization. Br Med J 1973; *1*:274–278.

101. Trowell H. Definition of dietary fiber and hypothesis that it is a protective factor in certain diseases. Am J Clin Nutr 1976; *29*:417–427.

102. Bingham S, Cumming JH, McNeil NI. Intakes and sources of dietary fiber in the British population. Am J Clin Nutr 1979; *32*:1313–1319.

103. West KM. Diet therapy of diabetes: an analysis of failure. Ann Intern Med 1973; *79*:425–434.

104. Luepker RV, Smith KK, Rothchild SS, et al. Management of hypercholesterolemia: evaluation of practical clinical approaches in healthy young adults. Am J Cardiol 1978; *41*:590–596.

105. Kaufmann RL, Arral JP, Soeldner JS, et al. Plasma lipid levels in diabetic children—effect of diet restricted in cholesterol and saturated fats. Diabetes 1975; *24*:677–679.

106. Danford DE. Computer applications to medical nutrition problems. JPEN 1981; *5*:441–446.

107. Stewart Kent K. Nutrient analyses of food: a review and a strategy for the future. *In* Beecher GR (ed). Human Nutrition Research. Beltsville Symposia in Agricultural Research Series, No. 4. Totowa, NJ, Allanheld, Osmun & Co, 1981: 209–220.

108. Dennis B, Ernst N, Hjortland M, et al. The NHLBI nutrition data system. J Am Diet Assoc 1980; *77*:641–647.

109. Hsu N, Gormican A. The computer in retrieving dietary history data. J Am Diet Assoc 1973; *63*:402–407.

26

HEART DISEASES

STEVEN B. HEYMSFIELD / ROBERT D. HOFF
T. FLINT GRAY / JOHN GALLOWAY / KATIE CASPER

Dietary intake, body composition, and tissue function are closely interrelated. Withdrawal of a single essential nutrient from the diet results in a depletion of body stores and a loss in one or more functions associated with the indispensable substrate. Excess intake of an essential dietary factor is coupled with an expansion of the body pool of the nutrient, and in some cases this may also cause derangements in selected metabolic pathways. Abnormally low or high body pools of any of about half of the 37 nutrients required by the adult human may cause definable cardiovascular effects. Not all of these circulatory effects are well characterized, and the information currently available for humans and animals is summarized in Table 26–1.

Of the numerous essential nutrient–cardiovascular interactions presented in Table 26–1, the most common encountered in medical practice relate to protein and energy. In the first section of the chapter we review the associations between dietary protein and energy intake, body composition, whole body metabolism, and the cardiovascular system. The two main nutritional disorders in this category are protein-energy malnutrition and obesity, and the resulting circulatory derangements are secondary to inadequate or excess dietary protein and energy, respectively. The second section is devoted to an indepth review of these two syndromes. In the third section we describe the syndrome of cardiac cachexia, a disorder in which the primary abnormality is severe congestive heart failure. Protein-energy malnutrition and other micronutrient deficiencies are a consequence of this circulatory impairment.

METABOLIC, RESPIRATORY, AND CARDIOVASCULAR INTERRELATIONS

Energy supplied in the diet replaces thermal and chemical losses of body fuels. Thermogenesis in humans can be divided into two major states: (1) fasting and (2) intra- or postprandial; heat losses related to physical activity are superimposed on these two states.

TABLE 26–1. Cardiovascular Syndromes That Develop When the Daily Intake of a Nutrient Is Persistently below or above the Daily Requirement

Essential Nutrient Imbalance	Species	Cardiac Abnormalities	Reference
Energy and protein deficiency	Human	See remaining sections in chapter	
Essential amino acid deficiency	Human,* rat	Endomyocardial and interstitial fibrosis, cardiomegaly, and congestive heart failure secondary to dietary tryptophan deficiency	2, 3
Ascorbic acid deficiency	Human	Hemorrhagic pericardium; electrocardiographic abnormalities	4
Thiamine deficiency	Human, rat	Cardiac beriberi; high-output heart failure, depressed myocardial contractility	5
Niacin deficiency	Human	Electrocardiographic abnormalities	6
Vitamin E deficiency	Rabbit	Necrosis of cardiac muscle fibers and fibrosis	7
Calcium deficiency	Human, rat	Depression of myocardial contractility, electrocardiographic changes; myofibrillar degeneration, and irreversible depression of contractility and excitability	8
Phosphorus deficiency	Human,* dog	Congestive cardiomyopathy	9, 10
Magnesium deficiency	Human, dog, rat	Predisposition to ventricular arrhythmias; focal necrosis and myocardial calcification, vascular degenerative lesions, vacuolation, and swelling of sarcosomes and mitochondria	11, 12
Copper deficiency	Swine, rat	Myocardial fibrosis and hypertrophy, sudden death, heart failure	13
Potassium deficiency	Rat, human	Loss of myofibril striation, vacuolation, and fragmentation; interstitial cellular infiltrate; myocardial necrosis; fibroblastic proliferation; electrocardiographic abnormalities	14, 15
Selenium and vitamin E deficiency	Pig	Hydropericardium, patchy necrosis of myocardium, myofibrillar degeneration and lysis, mitochondrial swelling and disruption; mild fibrosis and scattered macrophage	16
Selenium deficiency	Human	Congestive cardiomyopathy	17
Energy excess	Human	Obesity and heart disease, described in this chapter	
Calcium excess	Human	Increased myocardial contractility and decreased myocardial automaticity; electrocardiographic changes	18
Iron excess	Human	Conduction disturbances and congestive cardiac failure	19
Magnesium excess	Human	Vasodilation, electrocardiographic abnormalities, myocardial depression	20
Potassium excess	Human	Conduction abnormalities and arrhythmias	21
Cobalt excess	Human, rat	Congestive cardiomyopathy, hyaline necrosis, and dystrophic vacuolar degeneration of cardiac muscle cells	22
Vitamin D excess	Human	Metastatic calcifications	23

*Suspected relationship.
Modified from Heymsfield SB, Nutter DO. The heart in protein-calorie undernutrition. *In* Hurst JW (ed). Update I: The Heart. New York, McGraw-Hill, 1979: 191–209.

Fasting Thermogenesis

Fasting thermogenesis, often referred to as the basal or resting energy expenditure, is the thermal byproduct of fuel oxidation. These reactions are characterized by two basic equations:

$$Fuel + O_2 \rightarrow ATP + CO_2$$
$$+ H_2O + (urea) + heat \quad (Eq. 1)$$

$$ATP \rightarrow ADP + P_i + heat \quad (Eq. 2)$$

The energy contained within the chemical bonds of organic fuel is transferred to adenosine triphosphate (ATP), which in turn is the primary energy source for most cellular reactions.[24] The oxidative byproducts are carbon dioxide (CO_2), water (H_2O), urea (protein-oxidation), and heat. Utilization of ATP ultimately results in release of the stored energy with generation of adenosine diphosphate (ADP), inorganic phosphorus (P_i), and heat. The total heat generated by the complete oxidation of 1 g of fat, protein, and carbohydrate are respectively 9.4, 5.65, and 4.1 kcal. The biochemical details of these energy-generating reactions are summarized in Table 26–2. The table also provides the volume of oxygen consumed and carbon dioxide released for each kilocalorie of fuel metabolized during complete substrate oxidation. The ratio of carbon dioxide released to oxygen consumed for the three primary fuel oxidation reactions is termed the respiratory exchange ratio or respiratory quotient (RQ). The value of the RQ ranges from 0.7 for free fatty acid oxidation to 0.80 and 1.0 for amino acid and carbohydrate oxidation, respectively.

The cardiovascular system is responsible for delivering fuels and oxygen to cells and for removal of the reaction byproducts such as carbon dioxide, water, urea, and heat. The lungs are involved in transferring oxygen from air to blood and in disposal of carbon dioxide and water. The kidneys excrete water and the metabolic end-product urea.

The main determinant of fasting thermogenesis in the normal individual is body composition. Body weight can be divided into two main components, total body fat and lean or fat-free body mass. The fat-free tissues, which consist mainly of protein (19 per cent) and water (81 per cent), are the principal source of metabolic activity. The adipocytes, which store fat as triacylglycerol, have a finite but low rate of fasting thermogenesis. Fat mass becomes thermogenically significant only in extreme obesity.[26] Figure 26–1 shows the relation between fat-free body mass and the rate of oxygen consumption ($\dot{V}O_2$), carbon dioxide production ($\dot{V}CO_2$), and heat release (Q) in healthy adults within 10 per cent of ideal body weight. In addition, a linear association exists between fat-free body mass, minute ventilation ($\dot{V}_E$),

heart weight, and cardiac output.[25,29] The quantitative relationship between fat-free body mass, metabolism, and respiration is summarized in Table 26–3. Thus lean tissue mass, fuel metabolism, respiration, heart weight, and cardiac output are all highly interrelated.

In the healthy nonobese adult the rate of fasting thermogenesis per kilogram of lean tissue is largely independent of sex and age.[32] Fasting thermogenesis per kilogram of lean tissue increases in some normal physiological states and in a variety of pathological conditions; pregnancy, the luteal phase of the menstrual cycle, thyrotoxicosis, febrile states, and severe thermal or traumatic injury are a few examples. A reduction in fasting thermogenesis per kilogram of lean tissue also occurs during deep sleep, hypothermia, hyperthyroidism, and prolonged undernutrition. Hence a rise or fall in metabolic rate, and thus in respiratory and cardiovascular demands, can be brought about either by a change in lean body mass or a shift in energy expenditure per unit of fat-free tissue. Both of these effects are shown in the data from underweight subjects with anorexia nervosa presented in Table 26–4. Compared with control women at ideal body weight, the anorexic women have a marked absolute reduction in fat-free body mass, $\dot{V}O_2$, $\dot{V}CO_2$, minute ventilation ($\dot{V}_E$), and heat production (Q); $\dot{V}O_2$, $\dot{V}CO_2$, and heat production per kilogram of fat-free mass are also reduced below control levels.

Thermic Response to Food

Maintaining energy balance requires dietary replacement of fuels depleted through oxidative metabolism or lost in chemical form through skin, urine, and stool. The healthy adult accomplishes this by ingesting one to six meals per day. The metabolic-cardiovascular profile of fasting changes rapidly with ingestion of food. Vatner has shown an almost immediate cardiovascular effect in dogs with presentation of the meal.[33] Increases in cardiac output and intestinal blood flow are thought to represent the hemodynamic component of the cephalic phase of digestion. A similar state might exist under certain conditions in humans, but the topic has not yet been critically examined.

Within 15 to 30 minutes after food enters the stomach the rate of thermogenesis rises to a peak at 30 to 60 minutes, and then gradually declines over the next 2 to 10 hours.[34] This response is referred to as the thermic effect of food, and it is associated with rises in $\dot{V}O_2$, $\dot{V}CO_2$, $\dot{V}_E$, heat output, heart rate, stroke volume, cardiac output, myocardial oxygen consumption, and systolic blood pressure, a fall in peripheral vascular resistance, and no change in diastolic blood pressure.[34,35] A typical response is diagrammatically portrayed in Figure 26–2. The magnitude of the meal response is highly variable and

TABLE 26-2. Oxidative and Anabolic Fate of Metabolic Fuels

SUBSTRATE	REACTION	CALORIC VALUE OF FUEL		GAS EXCHANGE†		RQ
		kcal/g fuel§§	kcal/L O$_2$	Oxygen Consumed	Carbon Dioxide Produced	
Carbohydrate						
Glucose oxidation	$C_6H_{12}O_6 + 6O_2 \rightarrow 6CO_2 + 6H_2O$	3.74	5.01	200	200	1.00
Glycogen biosynthesis‡	Glucose + glycogen + $H_2O \rightarrow$ glycosyl-glycogen + H	3.74	5.01	10	10	1.00
Fat						
Triglyceride oxidation						
C$_{54}$ LCT§	$2C_{54}H_{101}O_6\P + 152.5O_2 \rightarrow 108CO_2 + 101H_2O$	9.11	4.51	221	157	0.71
C$_{55}$ LCT#	$C_{55}H_{104}O_6** + 78O_2 \rightarrow 55CO_2 + 52H_2O$	9.11	4.48	223	157	0.705
MCT	$C_{27}H_{53}O_6 + 37.25O_2 \rightarrow 27CO_2 + 26.5H_2O$	8.3	4.705	213	154	0.725
Triglyceride biosynthesis from glucose						
C$_{54}$ LCT§	$26C_6H_{12}O_6 + 35O_2 \rightarrow 2C_{54}H_{101}O_6†† + 48CO_2 + 55H_2O$	3.74/9.51	18.22	4.5	61.7	13.71
C$_{55}$ LCT#	$13.5C_6H_{12}O_6 + 3O_2 \rightarrow C_{55}H_{104}O_6 + 26CO_2 + 29H_2O$	3.74/9.51	13.95	7.4	63.9	8.67
Palmitic acid‡‡	$4.5C_6H_{12}O_6 + 4O_2 \rightarrow C_{16}H_{32}O_2 + 11CO_2 + 11H_2O$	9.4	7.06	29.6	81.4	2.75
Triglyceride biosynthesis from triglyceride‡	Triglyceride → free fatty acid → triglyceride	9.51	5.01	12	12	1.00
Triglyceride biosynthesis from amino acids	21 amino acids + $48.3O_2 \rightarrow$ tripalmitylglycerate + $36CO_2$ + 14.4 urea	4.34/9.51	—	82.9	61.3	0.74
Protein						
Amino acid oxidation	1 amino acid + $5.1O_2 \rightarrow 4.1CO_2 + 2.8H_2O$ + 0.7 urea	4.34	4.46	239	191	0.80
Protein biosynthesis	1 amino acid + 5 ATP → 1 peptide	—	—	—	—	—
Other						
Ethanol oxidation	$C_2H_6O + 3O_2 \rightarrow 2CO_2 + 3H_2O$	7.1	4.86	206	138	0.67
Glycerol oxidation	$C_3H_8O_3 + 7O_2 \rightarrow 6CO_2 + 8H_2O$	4.32	5.07	197	170	0.86

*Modified from Heymsfield, S. B., Head, C. A., McManus, C. B., et al.: Respiratory, cardiovascular and metabolic effects of enteral hyperalimentation: Influence of formula dose and composition. Am. J. Clin. Nutr., 40:116–130, 1984.

†Amount of oxygen consumed and carbon dioxide liberated (both in ml/min) in the reaction for each kilocalorie of reactant.

§§Glucose/triglyceride.

‡Reactions require ATP, which is assumed to originate from glucose oxidation. Actual gas exchange will vary with diet.

§From Kuksis, A. (ed.): Handbook of Lipid Research. Volume 1. Fatty Acids and Glycerides. New York, Plenum Press, 1978; and Cathcart, E. P., and Cuthbertson, D. P.: The composition and distribution of the fatty substances of the human subject. J. Physiol. (Lond.), 72:349–360, 1931.

¶Typical human liver triglyceride, analyzed by chemical means.

#From Elwyn, O. H., and Kinney, J. M.: A unique approach to measuring total energy expenditure by indirect calorimetry. In Kinney, J. M. (ed.): Report of the First Ross Conference on Medical Research. Columbus, Ohio, Ross Laboratories, 1980.

**Triglyceride containing equimolar amounts of palmitic, stearic, and oleic acids.

††Typical human adipose tissue triglyceride, analyzed by chemical means.

‡‡Suggested by Flatt, J. P.: Conversion of carbohydrate to fat in adipose tissue: An energy yielding and, therefore, self-limiting process. J. Lipid Res., 11:131–143, 1970.

RQ = respiratory quotient.
LCT = long-chain triglyceride.
MCT = medium-chain triglyceride.

From Heymsfield SB, Erbland M, Casper K, et al. Clin Chest Med 1986; 7:41–67.

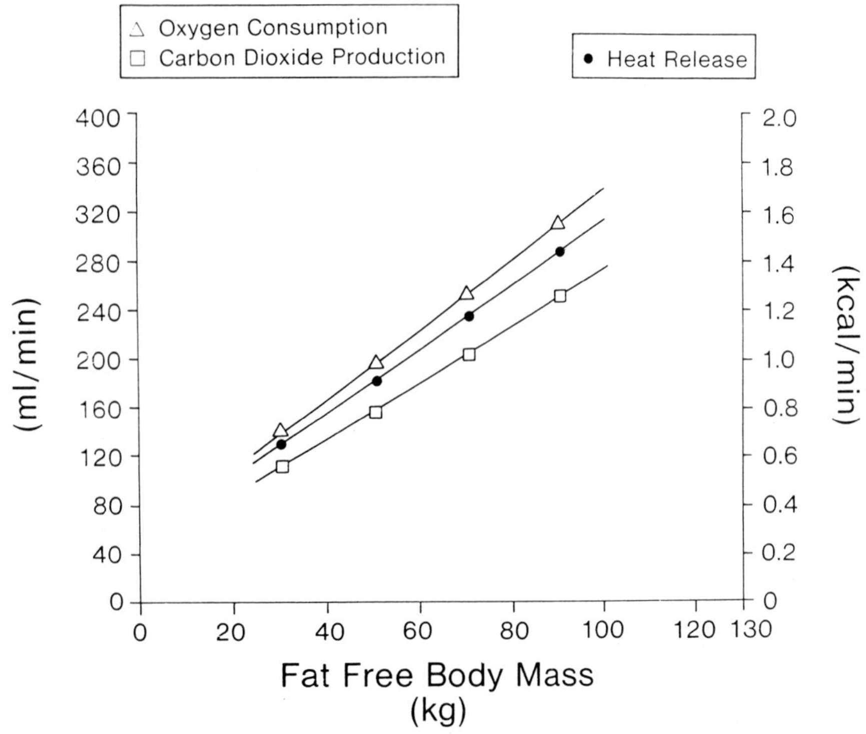

FIGURE 26–1. Correlation between fat-free body mass and metabolic indices. Corresponding regression equations are provided in Table 26–3. (From Heymsfield SB, Williams PJ. Nutritional assessment by clinical and biochemical methods. In Shils ME, Young VR [eds]. Modern Nutrition in Health and Disease. 7th ed. Philadelphia, Lea & Febiger, in press. Reproduced with permission.)

TABLE 26–3. Equations Describing the Relation between Metabolism, Respiration, and Fat-Free Body Mass (FFM)*

	Equation	r	n	p
$\dot{V}O_2$ (ml/min) =	3.09 FFM + 46.7	0.78	78	<0.001
$\dot{V}O_2$ max (L/min) =	0.13 FFM − 3.95	0.78	12	<0.01†
$\dot{V}CO_2$ (ml/min) =	2.83 FFM + 21.5	0.77	78	<0.001
$\dot{V}_E$ (L/min) =	0.049 FFM + 2.36	0.51	78	<0.001
$\dot{M}$ (kcal/min) =	0.015 FFM + 0.21	0.80	78	<0.001
Q (kcal/min) =	0.013 FFM + 0.28	0.83	78	<0.001

*FFM is in kg. Subjects were healthy men and women, and the equations depict results on the pooled groups.
†Buskirk ER, Taylor H.[31]
Abbreviations: $\dot{M}$ is the rate of free energy liberation calculated from $\dot{V}O_2$ and $\dot{V}CO_2$; Q is the rate of heat release measured by direct calorimetry; $\dot{V}CO_2$ is fasting-resting carbon dioxide production; $\dot{V}_E$ is the minute ventilation rate; $\dot{V}O_2$ and $\dot{V}O_2$ max are the fasting-resting and fasting-maximal rate of oxygen consumption.
Modified from Heymsfield SB, Head CA, McManus CB, et al. Am J Clin Nutr 1984; 40:116–130.

TABLE 26–4. Reduced Absolute and Relative Metabolic and Respiratory Indices in Semistarvation Due to Anorexia Nervosa*

	Anorexia Nervosa		Control	
	Absolute	Per kg FFM	Absolute	Per kg FFM
Weight (kg)	41.0	—	63.8	—
Height (cm)	163.8	—	163.5	—
FFM (kg)	36.0	—	42.3	—
Fat (kg)	5.0	—	21.5	—
$\dot{V}O_2$ (ml/min)	110.6	3.1	175.3	4.1
$\dot{V}CO_2$ (ml/min)	94.7	2.6	139.3	3.3
$\dot{V}_E$ (L/min)	3.2	0.09	4.4	0.10
$\dot{M}$ (kcal/hr)	32.3	0.9	50.8	1.20

*Average values for n = 4 anorexic women and n = 20 control women of similar age.
Abbreviations: FFM, fat-free body mass; M, metabolic rate (kcal/hr).

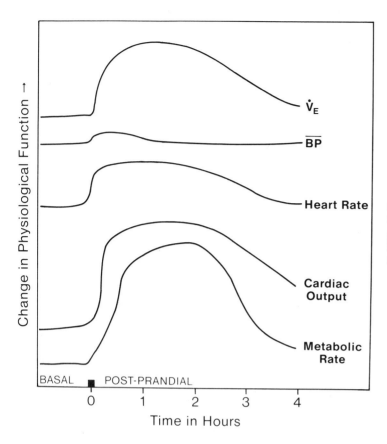

FIGURE 26–2. *Graphic representation of the changes in various physiological functions following ingestion of a meal. $\overline{BP}$, mean arterial blood pressure; $\dot{V}_E$, minute ventilation rate. (From Heymsfield SB, Erbland M, Casper K, et al. Clin Chest Med 1986; 7:41–67.)*

depends upon the nature and amount of foods ingested and the nutritional state of the subject. In a recent study Bagatell and Heymsfield showed a progressive increase in the peak metabolic and cardiovascular response following meals of increasing energy content.[34] Five meal sizes were supplied that ranged from 15 to 75 per cent of daily energy requirements, with meal composition fixed at 30 per cent fat, 15 per cent protein, and 55 per cent carbohydrate. These results showed an increase in metabolic, respiratory, and cardiovascular measurements as a function of meal energy content. The relevant regression equations are summarized in Table 26–5. These equations indicate that a large meal (50 per cent of daily energy requirements) would produce a peak rise in $\dot{V}O_2$, cardiac index, and calculated myocardial oxygen consumption (heart rate × mean blood pressure) of 30, 23, and 20 per cent, respectively.

An important conclusion of this study was that the relative demands on the cardiovascular system associated with meal ingestion were small in comparison with other daily activities. For example, physical exertion is often described in mets, where 1 met = basal $\dot{V}O_2$ in ml/min. A bed bath is 2.6 mets and a shower is 3.7 mets. Small, medium, and large meals in the Bagatell study were only 1.1, 1.2, and 1.3 mets, respectively.

The specific mechanisms involved in the physiological changes associated with meal ingestion are uncertain. The mechanical and metabolic work involved in chewing, digesting, and absorbing foods is usually considered only a minor component of the thermic response to food.[36] A portion of the rise in cardiac output is related to the increase in mesenteric blood flow associated with food ingestion.[37] The remainder must be attributed to the rise in whole body oxygen consumption. Current thought suggests that this metabolic response is largely related to the processing and storage of nutrients.[38]

While ingesting solid foods in discrete meals is the usual means of replacing nutrients, many hospitalized patients receive liquid formulas either parenterally or enterally. In most cases the solution is fed continuously over 18 to 24 hours, thereby eliminating the "peak and valley" thermic response of usual meals. The thermogenesis of continuous feeding is spread out over the feeding cycle, and this form of heat production is termed the thermic response to fuel.[39] In the resting subject receiving continuous feeding over 24 hours, the intraprandial metabolic rate varies only ±5 per cent during the awake hours. This is the same variability observed with fasting.

Three factors determine the metabolic, respiratory, and cardiovascular response to continuous feeding:[25] the rate of energy infusion, formula composition, and disease state.

The first determinant is the rate of energy infusion. As the flow rate of an enterally administered formula is increased from fasting to the maintenance

TABLE 26–5. *Correlation between Percentage Change in Hemodynamic/Metabolic Measurement and Meal Size**

Metabolic/Hemodynamic Measurements	Equation	r	p
Total-body $\dot{V}O_2$	$\%\Delta = 0.60$ (meal size)† $- 0.004$ (meal size)$^2 + 5.4$	0.59	<0.001
Cardiac index	$\%\Delta = 0.61$ (meal size) $- 7.6$	0.77	<0.001
Heart rate	$\%\Delta = 0.33$ (meal size) $- 1.5$	0.54	<0.001
Stroke volume index	$\%\Delta = 0.14$ (meal size) $- 1.8$	0.38	<0.05
Systolic pressure	$\%\Delta = 0.13$ (meal size) $- 0.0014$ (meal size)$^2 + 2.3$	0.30	NS
Diastolic pressure	$\%\Delta = 0.02$ (meal size) $+ 1.3$	0.07	NS
Heart rate × mean blood pressure‡	$\%\Delta = 0.56$ (meal size) $- 2.9$	0.51	<0.01

*Cardiac index and stroke volume were measured using echocardiographic methods.
†Meal size in percentage of daily energy requirements.
‡An index of myocardial oxygen consumption.
From Bagatell CJ, Heymsfield SB. Am J Clin Nutr 1984; *39*:421–426. ©Am J Clin Nutr, American Society for Clinical Nutrition. Reproduced with permission.

energy plane, little or no change is observed in resting energy expenditure and $\dot{V}O_2$; however, a small increase in heart rate is noted. This is shown in Table 26–6, where nine normal volunteers were subjected to a 2-day protocol.[40] The subjects began a fast the evening prior to day one, and continued this until noon on the first study day. They then were allowed to eat normally. That evening a thin nasoenteric catheter was inserted and infusion of a polymeric enteral formula (40 per cent fat, 15 per cent protein, 45 per cent carbohydrate) was begun at a rate that met 24-hour energy requirements (1.4 × average fasting metabolic rate). This feeding program was continued through day two. When compared with fasting measurements, there was no significant change with continuous feeding in $\dot{V}O_2$, $\dot{V}CO_2$, $\dot{V}_E$, and metabolic rate ($\dot{M}$); a small and significant increase in heart rate was observed.

Increasing the formula infusion rate above maintenance energy requirements results in a rise in energy expenditure and associated cardiac and respiratory changes. A typical response is shown in the healthy subject presented in Figure 26–3. The subject was first placed on continuous infusion of a polymeric formula (40 per cent fat, 15 per cent protein, 45 per cent carbohydrate) for 1 week at maintenance energy requirements. Beginning in week two the

formula infusion rate was doubled, resulting in strongly positive energy balance and weight gain. Within 3 days intraprandial $\dot{V}O_2$, $\dot{V}CO_2$, $\dot{V}_E$, $\dot{M}$, and heart rate achieved a new higher steady state. These metabolic and respiratory indices remained at this level until the seventh day of overfeeding, when the infusion rate was once again returned to the maintenance level. Within 3 days all indices decreased to the lower rates observed during the first maintenance period. While not extensively studied, the relation between formula energy infusion rate and $\dot{V}O_2$, $\dot{V}CO_2$, $\dot{V}_E$, $\dot{M}$, and heart rate appear to be linear from the maintenance plane of support into the repletion range.[30] Linear regression equations describing these relations for a high-fat formula (50 per cent fat, 15 per cent protein, 35 per cent carbohydrate) are presented in Table 26–7. Increasing the infusion rate to twice the maintenance level results in increases of approximately 23, 20, 18, and 19 per cent, respectively, in $\dot{V}O_2$, $\dot{V}CO_2$, $\dot{V}_E$, and resting $\dot{M}$. Heart rate would be increased by 8 beats/minute.

The metabolic and chronotropic response to parenteral infusion of a standard glucose–amino acid mixture (C1800) was very similar to the enteral formulas. There was no significant change in resting energy expenditure from the fasting to the maintenance level of support (Fig. 26–4A).[41] Energy in-

TABLE 26–6. *Metabolic and Cardiovascular Indices ($\overline{X} \pm SD$) during Fasting and Continuous Infusion of an Enteral Formula at Near Zero Energy Balance**

	Fasting	Maintenance
$\dot{V}O_2$ (ml/min)	193.8 ± 46.5	192.0 ± 48.5
$\dot{V}CO_2$ (ml/min)	175.9 ± 63.7	174.1 ± 64.1
$\dot{V}_E$ (L/min)	5.2 ± 2.1	5.2 ± 2.1
$\dot{M}$ (kcal/hr)	57.0 ± 14.5	56.4 ± 15.1
Heart rate (beats/min)	60.8 ± 5	65.7 ± 7.2†
Blood pressure		
Systolic (mm Hg)	112.0 ± 3.7	115.2 ± 7.8
Diastolic (mm Hg)	82.3 ± 4.5	78.4 ± 7.8

*n=9 healthy subjects. Infusion rate = 1.4 × fasting metabolic rate.
†p <0.05 compared with fasting value.
From Heymsfield SB, Hill JO, Evert M, et al. Am J Clin Nutr 1986; *45*:135–153.

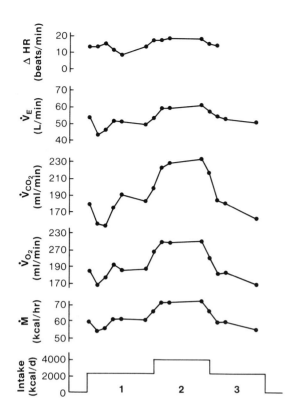

FIGURE 26–3. Changes in physiological indices when continuous nasoenteral feeding was increased from near-zero energy balance (period 1) into the repletional range (period 2). In the third period formula infusion rate was returned to the period 1 level. Each infusion period lasted 1 week. The subject was a healthy male volunteer. HR, changes in resting heart rate from fasting; Ṁ, resting metabolic rate.

TABLE 26–7. Regression Equations Describing the Correlation between Enteral Formula Infusion Rate and Metabolism, Respiration, and Heart Rate*

Formula	n	Equation	r	p	m(slope)	Slope Equality Fat vs CHO†
$\dot{V}O_2$: Oxygen consumption (ml/kg FFM/min), normal fasting value: 3.96 ± 0.6						
High fat	8	$\dot{V}O_2 = 36.5\ \text{dose} + 3.5$	0.78	<0.05	36.5	<0.21
High CHO	8	$\dot{V}O_2 = 62.0\ \text{dose} + 2.4$	0.86	<0.01	62.0	
$\dot{V}CO_2$: Carbon dioxide production (ml/kg FFM/min), normal fasting value: 3.18 ± 0.48						
High fat	8	$\dot{V}CO_2 = 29.0\ \text{dose} + 3.0$	0.78	<0.05	29.0	<0.01
High CHO	8	$\dot{V}CO_2 = 71.4\ \text{dose} + 2.0$	0.93	<0.01	71.4	
$\dot{V}_E$: Minute ventilation (L/kg FFM/min), normal fasting value: 0.10 ± 0.02						
High fat	8	$\dot{V}_E = 0.94\ \text{dose} + 0.11$	0.67	<0.05	0.94	<0.07
High CHO	8	$\dot{V}_E = 1.91\ \text{dose} + 0.09$	0.96	<0.001	1.91	
Ṁ: Rate of free energy production (kcal/kg FFM/min), normal fasting value: 0.10 ± 0.02						
High fat	8	$\dot{M} = 0.17\ \text{dose} + 0.01$	0.79	<0.05	0.17	<0.06
High CHO	8	$\dot{M} = 0.32\ \text{dose} + 0.01$	0.86	<0.01	0.32	
HR: Change in heart rate (beats/min)						
High fat	6	$\Delta HR = 336.8\ \text{dose} - 10.9$	0.77	<0.05	336.8	<0.62
High CHO	6	$\Delta HR = 249.4\ \text{dose} - 4.0$	0.73	<0.05	249.4	
Combined	12	$\Delta HR = 292.4\ \text{dose} - 7.4$	0.69	<0.01	292.4	

*Normal values derived at Emory Clinical Research Facility (n = 50). Formula dose is expressed in kcal/kg FFM/min.
†Probability of equality of slopes, high fat versus high carbohydrate. When p <0.05, slopes are significantly different.
From Heymsfield SB, Head CA, McManus CB, et al. Am J Clin Nutr 1984; 40:116–130. ©Am J Clin Nutr, American Society for Clinical Nutrition. Reproduced with permission.

fusion rates above the maintenance level resulted in linear rises in the resting energy expenditure and heart rate (Fig. 26–4B).

In terms of cardiovascular demands, the increase in $\dot{V}O_2$ and heart rate seen with advancing the formula infusion rate above the maintenance level are relatively small. When considered in terms of mets, even high levels of energy intake with formula diets are associated with a $\dot{V}O_2$ of less than 1.6 mets. Normal subjects can increase cardiac output by a factor of four to five, with trained athletes accomplishing an even greater increase in circulatory flow. This peak output in healthy individuals would correspond to about 7 mets. More relevant, however, is the limited cardiac reserve in patients with severe cardiac failure, a topic revised in detail in a later section of this chapter.

The second determinant of the physiological response to continuous feeding is composition of the diet. The two main categories relevant to clinical practice are high-carbohydrate and normal or high-fat preparations. In a recent study, our group ex-

amined the relation between formula energy infusion rate, diet composition, and changes in metabolism, respiration, and hemodynamic status for these two types of dietary solutions.[30] Both formulas were fed continuously via nasogastric tube with protein, fat, and carbohydrate set at 15, 50, and 35 per cent (high-fat), and 15, 2, and 83 per cent (high-carbohydrate) of total energy, respectively. As noted earlier, a linear increase in metabolic indices, respiration, and heart rate as a function of formula infusion rate was noted for the high-fat diet (Table 26–7). A similar increase was also observed during the high-carbohydrate formula infusion, but there were important differences. As energy infusion rate was increased from maintenance to repletion, $\dot{V}CO_2$ and $\dot{V}_E$ increased more rapidly on the high-carbohydrate formula relative to the high-fat solution. These differences are apparent in the slopes of the regression equations (Table 26–7), which provide a measure of the rate of change in $\dot{V}CO_2$ and $\dot{V}_E$ as a function of increasing energy infusion rate. For $\dot{V}CO_2$ the slopes of the regression lines for the high-carbohydrate and

FIGURE 26–4. Panel A, *Resting metabolic rate ($\dot{M}$) versus caloric infusion rate (dose) for a central intravenous hyperalimentation formula (C1800) in eight stable depleted individuals undergoing long-term balance studies. Panel B, Heart rate versus caloric infusion rate for the eight subjects presented in* panel A. *(Adapted from Galloway J, Stensby J, Heymsfield SB. Clin Res 1979; 27:226A.)*

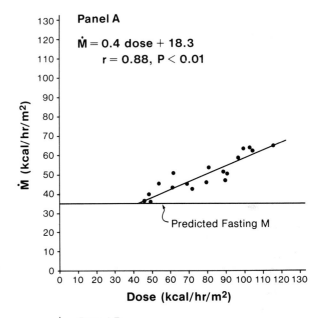

Panel A

$\dot{M} = 0.4$ dose $+ 18.3$
$r = 0.88$, $P < 0.01$

Predicted Fasting M

$\dot{M}$ (kcal/hr/m²)

Dose (kcal/hr/m²)

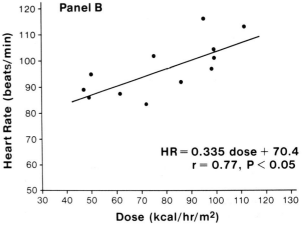

Panel B

$HR = 0.335$ dose $+ 70.4$
$r = 0.77$, $P < 0.05$

Heart Rate (beats/min)

Dose (kcal/hr/m²)

high-fat formulas were 36.5 and 15 ml/kcal (p<0.05), and for $\dot{V}_E$ slopes were 3.2 and 1.6 L/kcal (p<0.07), respectively. There were no significant differences in slope between the formulas for $\dot{V}O_2$ and heart rate.

A classic observation is that protein ingestion induces a relatively large increase in thermogenesis.[38] Our group therefore examined the effect of amino acids on the thermic response to continuous fuel infusion. While receiving a steady flow of C1800, four depleted patients underwent two 7-day metabolic balance studies: standard C1800 solution followed by a nitrogen-free C1800 solution (C1800-NF) isocaloric to the first period. The results are presented in Table 26–8 and indicate that the isocaloric switch from standard to protein-free formula caused negative nitrogen balance (ΔN) but no appreciable change in metabolic rate ($\dot{M}$) and cardiac output. These results indicate that protein per se is not responsible for the metabolic and cardiovascular effects of continuous formula infusion. One proviso is that our study was performed at energy inflow rates at or near maintenance levels. The effect of protein at repletional infusion rates needs to be examined.

What are the mechanisms involved in explaining the physiological changes observed with increasing formula infusion rate and altering nutrient composition? The changes in ventilation ($\dot{V}_E$) can be ascribed primarily to the alterations in carbon dioxide production ($\dot{V}CO_2$), and the two are highly correlated with each other.[25] Figure 26–5 illustrates that as $\dot{V}CO_2$ rises with enteral feeding, there is a corresponding increase in $\dot{V}_E$. Carbon dioxide levels in blood stimulate peripheral and central chemoreceptors, which in turn modulate ventilation through a neural reflex arc.[42] This carbon dioxide sensitivity is diminished in patients with severe lung disease who have chronic hypercapnia and hypoxia.[43] In these individuals the primary stimulus for ventilation is the arterial oxygen saturation. Changes in heart rate and cardiac output are normally correlated with fluctuations in oxygen consumption and arterial pO_2. Again, peripheral and central chemoreceptors are responsible for mediating the oxygen consumption–cardiac output reflex arc. While $\dot{V}O_2$ and $\dot{V}CO_2$ are the primary determinants of cardiac and respiratory activity, other factors are also involved. Changes in mesenteric blood flow,[37] total blood volume, and a stimulation of the sympathetic nervous system with feeding[44] are a few examples.

The fundamental questions are: (1) Why is there an increase in $\dot{V}O_2$ and $\dot{V}CO_2$ with advancing formula infusion rate? (2) What relation do these observed metabolic changes have to formula composition? During the intraprandial state characteristic of continuous feeding, two factors contribute to the observed resting thermogenesis. The first is the energy generated for maintaining the basal reactions described earlier (Table 26–2). The second thermogenic factor, superimposed upon these oxidative reactions, is the anabolic pathways that lead to the biosynthesis of glycogen, triacylglycerol, and protein. The specific pathway through which each substrate flows during the biosynthetic process determines the net use of ATP and oxygen, and generation of carbon dioxide. Table 26–2 shows some of the more widely recognized anabolic reactions and the associated $\dot{V}O_2$ and $\dot{V}CO_2$. Of relevance to this discussion are the two pathways leading to triacylglycerol biosynthesis. In the first pathway glucose is converted to triacylglycerol, with a small requirement for oxygen but a large release of carbon dioxide (RQ of between 8 and 13). In comparison,

TABLE 26–8. *Metabolic and Cardiovascular Effects of Nitrogen-Free C1800**

Subject	Infusion Rate (kcal/hr/m²)	$\dot{M}$ (kcal/hr/m²)	Cardiac Index† (L/min/m²)	ΔN (g/D)
DF				
C1800	103.8	63.4±3.5‡	3.96	1.9±0.7‡
C1800-NF	99.5	63.4±38	3.93	−1.7±0.5
EJ				
C1800	49.5	36.1±3	3.53	4.1±1.2
C1800-NF	47.1	35.1±3.7	2.83	−2.5±0.3
CC				
C1800	116	65±2.1	5.65	5.6±1.7
C1800-NF	97	58.7±5.1	5.15	−3.7±0.2
CW				
C1800	76.4	42.1±1.9	3.29	6.3±0.9
C1800-NF	69.4	44.9±1.6	4.36	−3.7±0.2
SUMMARY (n=4)				
C1800	86.4±30	51.7±14.7	4.10±1.06	4.5±1.9
C1800-NF	78.3±24.8	50.3±12.9	4.07±0.97	−2.8±0.9

*Results are expressed ±SD. C1800 is a standard 1800 mOsm central intravenous hyperalimentation mixture of glucose, free amino acids, minerals, and vitamins.

†Measured by M-mode echocardiography.

‡Average (±SD) of six measurements for that respective period. C1800-NF is the standard mixture minus nitrogen.

From Galloway J, Stensby J, Heymsfield SB. Clin Res 1979; 27:226A. Reproduced with permission.

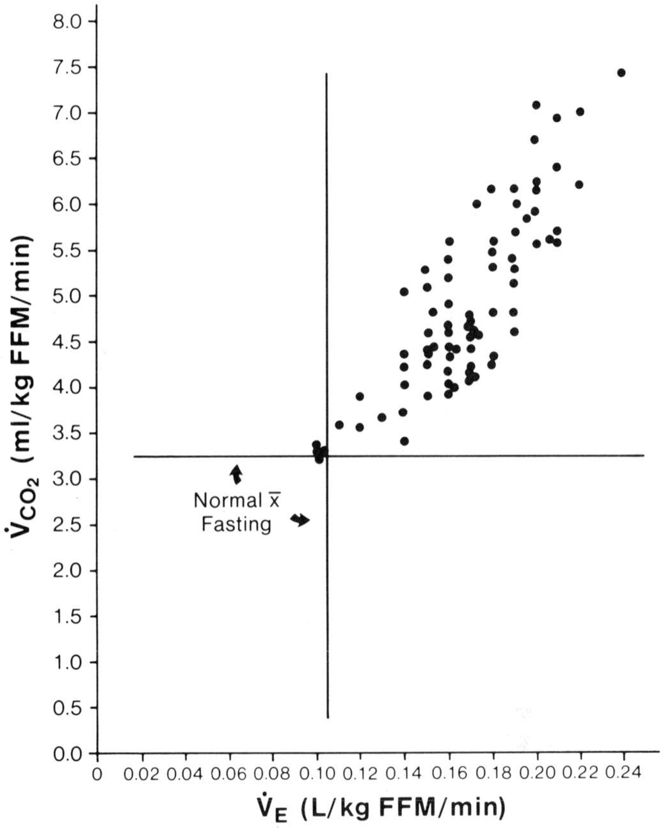

FIGURE 26–5. Relation between intraprandial carbon dioxide production ($\dot{V}_{CO_2}$) and minute ventilation ($\dot{V}_E$); the normal fasting values are noted by the solid lines. The plotted points were derived during continuous infusion of an enteral formula. Feeding increased $\dot{V}_{CO_2}$ with a corresponding increase in $\dot{V}_E$. FFM, fat-free body mass.

in the second pathway conversion of dietary triglyceride into tissue triglyceride has a slightly lower oxygen requirement, but the release of carbon dioxide is lower by a factor of 30. This may partially explain why a high-carbohydrate formula causes a marked rise in $\dot{V}CO_2$ and $\dot{V}_E$ during periods of strongly positive energy balance; the reaction dietary glucose → tissue triacylglycerol is predominant over the reaction dietary triacylglycerol → tissue triacylglycerol. The high-carbohydrate formula was also associated with a more rapid increase in $\dot{V}O_2$ with increasing energy infusion rate; however, the difference from the corresponding slope produced by the high-fat formula was not statistically significant. As noted earlier, the theoretical $\dot{V}O_2$ for the reaction glucose → triacylglycerol is larger than that for fat biosynthesis via dietary lipid, but the differences are small (Table 26–2). Note that not all of the increase in thermogenesis observed during an anabolic state can be accounted for by substrate biosynthesis.

The third determinant of the metabolic response to continuous feeding is disease state. The studies described above were conducted on depleted or normally nourished subjects, all of whom were in a stable noncatabolic state. After a major trauma (e.g., burn) there follows the acute catabolic phase of injury. As described in more detail elsewhere,[45] there occurs a variable increase per kilogram of lean tissue in resting $\dot{V}O_2$, $\dot{V}CO_2$, respiration, and cardiac demands. When hyperalimentation is superimposed on this

stress state, a marked rise is detected in $\dot{V}O_2$ and $\dot{V}CO_2$.[46] Oxygen consumption and carbon dioxide production increase in parallel, with the RQ usually remaining unchanged. A rise in catecholamine output with feeding has also been noted.[47] Even with a high-carbohydrate formula, the RQ remains below 1.0. The current assumption is that these observed changes in metabolism with feeding are greater in magnitude than those observed in the depleted eumetabolic patient relative to the rate of caloric infusion. The working hypothesis is that lipolysis is not suppressed by exogenous carbohydrate, and this abnormality leads to an unusually high rate of glycogen formation.[47] The important implication from the cardiovascular perspective is that the hemodynamic response to hyperalimentation may be more marked in a patient suffering from a major injury than in the nonstressed individuals described earlier. Such a patient would already have an increased cardiac output secondary to the underlying injury and associated metabolic abnormalities.

Exertional Thermogenesis

Metabolic fuel supplies the energy required for performing physical work. The rate of thermogenesis rises during exercise, with the increase related to the type and duration of work performed. Table 26–9 provides the rates of thermogenesis typical of

TABLE 26–9. Energy Cost of Physical Activities in a Hospital Environment

Activity	Kcal/min/m²*	Increase above Resting (%)	Mets
Resting supine	0.630 ± 0.028	0.0	1.0
Sitting	0.680 ± 0.033	7.9	1.1
Standing	0.749 ± 0.038	17.4	1.2
Walking (1.5 mph)	1.494 ± 0.049	137.1	2.4

*Energy cost given ± SE for n = 10.
Adapted from Long CL. The energy and protein requirements of the critically ill patient. *In* Wright RA, Heymsfield SB (eds). Nutritional Assessment. Boston, Blackwell, 1984: 15–26.

activities found in ambulatory hospitalized patients and healthy adults.

Metabolic, hemodynamic, and respiratory changes parallel the exercise-induced rise in thermogenesis.[49] Whole-body $\dot{V}O_2$ increases linearly with workload and reaches a maximum ($\dot{V}O_2$ max) at about 20 times the resting-fasting level. The $\dot{V}O_2$ max is determined in large part by fat-free body mass (Table 26–3), although genetic and conditioning factors account for some of the differences between individuals.[50]

In order to meet the increased oxygen needs of exercise, cardiac output and ventilation rise. A linear relation exists between $\dot{V}O_2$ and cardiac output during physical activity at levels below 80 per cent of $\dot{V}O_2$ max, and this correlation is independent of age, sex, posture, or type of dynamic work.[50] The increase in cardiac output in turn is determined by an interplay between heart rate and stroke volume. Heart rate increases linearly with total body $\dot{V}O_2$ and workload and may reach a frequency of 200 beats/minute in healthy adults. Small adjustments are also noted in stroke volume, with peak values reached at about 40 to 50 per cent of $\dot{V}O_2$ max. Systolic blood pressure increases linearly with $\dot{V}O_2$ and cardiac output, and values may reach 200 to 220 mm Hg. Diastolic blood pressure remains constant or falls near the peak of exercise capacity; therefore, mean arterial blood pressure increases to a modest degree.

Total peripheral resistance falls during exercise, a reflection of net vasodilation. Minute ventilation ($\dot{V}_E$) increases in parallel with $\dot{V}O_2$ and may reach levels 10 to 20 times the resting value. Figure 26–6 summarizes the physiological response to upright exercise.

A recent controversial observation is that the rate of the exercise-induced thermogenesis during the postprandial state is higher than the rate of energy expenditure for the same exercise during fasting.[51] Only part of this increase can be accounted for by the thermic effect of food, indicating that the various thermogenic components may not be additive. Thus eating and exercising may cause a larger cardiac response than the sum of the effects of the two activities occurring separately. Ongoing studies are examining the relation between thermogenesis, meal ingestion, physical activity, and cardiac output.

Integration of Thermogenic Determinants

An individual's metabolic rate, cardiac output, and respiration at any given moment are determined by the integration of the factors described above. From the minimal activity of these three physiological functions during fasting and sleep, each can potentially increase by a factor of 15 to 25 during normal daily activities.

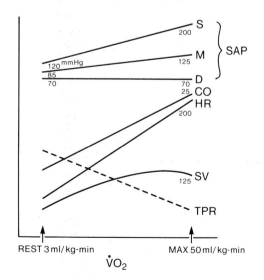

FIGURE 26–6. Schematic of hemodynamics from rest to maximal work during upright, dynamic exercise. SAP, systemic arterial pressure; S, systolic; M, mean; D, diastolic; CO, cardiac output; HR, heart rate; SV, stroke volume; TPR, total peripheral resistance. (From Nutter DO. Exercise and the heart. In Hurst JW [ed]. Update I: The Heart. New York, McGraw-Hill, 1979.)

PROTEIN-ENERGY MALNUTRITION AND OBESITY

Clinical Syndromes

A loss or gain in weight causes readjustments in the cardiovascular system. Extreme weight change in either direction is associated with classic nutritional syndromes. The genesis and cardiovascular consequences of these conditions are outlined in Figure 26–7. Consider the standard body composition in health as point A in the figure. Weight is constant and energy and nitrogen balance are zero. Disease or famine then leads to negative energy and nitrogen balance. The consequence is resorption of adipose tissue triglycerides and lean tissue protein and water. Persistent negative balance leads to ongoing weight loss and depletion of body fuels until the subject reaches the minimal tissue mass consistent with survival (point B_U). Further tissue loss results in death due to semistarvation. The more severe degrees of depletion encompass the syndromes referred to collectively as protein-energy malnutrition.

The two major subgroups of protein-energy malnutrition are marasmus and kwashiorkor.[52] Typically the marasmic patient shows extreme degrees of wasting although serum albumin levels are often remarkably normal. Edema is usually not present. The disorder evolves over prolonged periods of inadequate energy and protein intake, and characteristically infections are absent. The kwashiorkor patient presents with three cardinal signs: preservation of adipose tissue with severe lean tissue atrophy, hypoalbuminemia, and edema. The syndrome usually appears following markedly inadequate protein intake, a reduction that is out of proportion to low energy ingestion. Infection usually triggers or accompanies the acute phase of the disease.

Not all patients with protein-energy malnutrition reach point B_U without complications. Often clinical conditions develop as a result of malnutrition. These events are noted by the pathway C_U.

Our discussion in this section will focus on the cardiovascular changes that occur as patients move from health (point A) to terminal semistarvation (point B_U) and how these changes are reversed during refeeding. There are also important potential cardiac disturbances that can cause severe morbidity or death during semistarvation (point C_U), and we will also review these conditions.

The second group of disorders related to protein and energy develop following prolonged positive nutrient balance and weight gain. The result is enlargement of the adipose tissue organ and lean tissues. For simplicity, we refer to this as exogenous obesity. Profound obesity (point B_O, Figure 26–7) and related complications (point C_O) are analogous to those described for protein-energy malnutrition. Our concern with cardiovascular changes is focused on the patient moving from point A to point B_O (weight gain), point B_O to point A (weight loss), and point A to point C_O (cardiac complications of obesity). The discussion begins with the changes in cardiac output and mass that occur in protein-energy malnutrition and obesity.

Cardiac Output

Basic Physiology. The cardiovascular system is responsible for supplying tissues with metabolic fuel

FIGURE 26–7. Anatomic and functional changes in the heart with undernutrition (U) and overnutrition (O). Point A is the body composition found in lean, healthy adults; body weight is stable and energy, nitrogen, and H_2O balances (ΔE, ΔN, ΔH_2O) are zero. Positive balance leads to weight gain, and point B_O is considered massive obesity. Negative balance causes weight loss and severe protein-energy malnutrition as described by point B_U. The associated cardiac changes with over- and undernutrition are described in the figure. Cardiac complications occur in subjects moving away from or toward point A, and these are described by points C_O and C_U. These endorgan events are outlined in the figure. (Modified from Heymsfield SB, Williams PJ. Nutritional assessment by clinical and biochemical methods. In Shils ME, Young VR [eds]. Modern Nutrition in Health and Disease. 7th ed. Philadelphia, Lea & Febiger, in press. Reproduced with permission.)

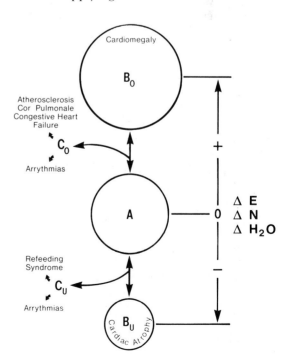

and oxygen and for removal of waste products such as carbon dioxide and urea. Recall from an earlier section that cellular metabolism varies with fasting, feeding, and exercise. Accordingly there are changes in cardiac output that match these cellular events. Four major factors combine to determine cardiac output: preload, afterload, contractile state, and heart rate.

Preload is a measure of the myocardial pressure-volume status immediately prior to ventricular contraction.[53] Preload in the intact heart is reflected by the ventricular end-diastolic volume. On an ultrastructural level this corresponds to the degree of resting sarcomere stretch. Preload determines stroke volume according to the Frank-Starling law, which states that for any given change in end-diastolic volume (or pressure), there is a corresponding change in ventricular output.[54] Hence an increase in preload results in an increase in stroke volume. Thus changes in preload help to provide a functional reserve of myocardial performance such that increases in stroke volume and ultimately cardiac output are possible in order to meet metabolic demands. This reserve capacity is available on a beat-to-beat basis, allowing the heart to continually match performance with cellular requirements. Ordinarily stroke volume is set at about two thirds of end-diastolic volume; however, this ejection fraction of 0.6 to 0.7 can increase to about 0.9.

The three main determinants of preload are total blood volume, blood volume distribution, and venous return to the heart.[53] Total blood volume in health is a function of body weight. The distribution of blood in the vascular tree is determined by intrathoracic pressure, intrapericardial pressure, venous tone, and body position.

Two key interacting factors determine venous return to the heart, the mean systemic filling pressure and total peripheral resistance.[55] The mean systemic filling pressure is the effective pressure in the peripheral circulation that pushes blood back towards the heart. When total peripheral resistance is held constant, venous return is a function of the difference between mean systemic filling pressure and right atrial pressure. The mean systemic filling pressure is largely determined by blood volume and venous tone. When mean systemic filling pressure and right atrial pressure are held constant, venous return and cardiac output are inversely proportional to total peripheral resistance. Thus, venous return to the heart, preload, and cardiac output are increased when blood volume is expanded, venous tone is heightened, and/or total peripheral resistance is lowered.

The second determinant of cardiac output is afterload. The afterload is defined as the tension, force, or stress in the ventricular wall immediately after the onset of contraction.[53,54] The ventricular wall stress is determined by ventricular volume, intracavitary pressure, and wall thickness. We noted

earlier that ventricular volume at end-diastole is the main determinant of preload. Thus, afterload is in part determined by preload. Intracavitary pressure is related to aortic impedance, which in turn is primarily determined by peripheral vascular resistance; contributing factors of less importance are blood viscosity, elasticity of the aorta, and the physical characteristics of the vascular tree.

In the clinical setting afterload is estimated from mean arterial pressure, which is equal to cardiac output divided by peripheral vascular resistance. In practical terms, peripheral vascular resistance is the major determinant of afterload. Peripheral resistance is regulated by neural, hormonal, and pharmacological mechanisms. An acute increase in peripheral vascular resistance decreases fiber shortening and thereby reduces stroke volume and cardiac output.

The concept of preload and afterload implies that the myocardium is subject to extrinsic work demands. When formulated in this fashion, preload and afterload are the end-diastolic and end-systolic wall stress or tension (Tw) as described by the Laplace equation:

$$Tw = \frac{(P)(r)}{2h} \qquad (Eq. 3)$$

where P is the ventricular end-diastolic or systolic pressure, r is the chamber radius, and h is the myocardial wall thickness.[53,54] The relevance of the interrelation described by Equation 3 is that preload and afterload are determinants of myocardial wall thickness and mass; this important relationship is reviewed in a later section.

The third factor that determines cardiac output is inotropic state or contractility of the myocardial fibers.[53,54] The classic definition of contractility is an increase in ejection while preload and afterload are held constant. Under constant loading conditions a positive inotropic effect enhances cardiac performance, whereas a negative inotropic effect reduces cardiac performance. The inotropic state of the myocardium is influenced by the neuroendocrine system, acid-base status, tissue oxygenation, and pharmacological agents. Contractility is also influenced by the rate and rhythm of cardiac contraction. For example, a ventricular extrasystole augments contractility for the next several beats. A simple increase in heart rate also increases contractility. In the failing heart a depressed inotropic state is usually the factor that limits the heart from achieving a normal output.

The fourth determinant of ventricular performance is heart rate. The intrinsic rhythmicity of the sinoatrial node, cardiovascular reflexes, and circulating neurohumoral substances control heart rate.

Thus cardiac output is determined by an interplay between preload, afterload, contractility, and heart rate. These same four factors plus heart weight also determine the myocardial oxygen consumption ($M\dot{V}O_2$), which can be divided into two components. The first is the basal $M\dot{V}O_2$, which in the arrested myocardium is 2 to 3 ml/min/100 g of heart tissue. The second component derives from the electrical and beating activity of the heart muscle; this increases $M\dot{V}O_2$ from the basal level to 8 to 9 ml/min/100 g of heart tissue. As the normal whole body resting $\dot{V}O_2$ is 200 to 250 ml/min and the normal heart is 200 to 250 g, the $M\dot{V}O_2$ repesents about 10 per cent of total resting energy expenditure.

How are cardiac output and $M\dot{V}O_2$ influenced in protein-energy malnutrition and obesity? In the previous section we reviewed the mechanisms whereby the cardiovascular system responds to acute changes in metabolic needs. The change in body mass resulting from weight loss or weight gain usually occurs over months or years, and therefore there are circulatory readjustments of a more chronic nature.

Three basic principles underlie the cardiac readjustments during chronic weight change: stroke volume changes in proportion to metabolic requirements; the myocardium remains at a relatively constant position on the myofibrillar length-tension curve, thereby preserving ejection fraction at 0.6 to 0.7; and the total myofibrillar wall tension (Equation 3) remains constant.

The first principle, described in an earlier section, is that resting stroke volume is largely determined by whole body $\dot{V}O_2$ and lean body mass. The second principle states that as stroke volume readjusts to new metabolic demands, the ejection fraction is maintained in the general range of 0.6 to 0.7; this preserves the usual ejection reserve. A corollary of this effect is that ventricular chamber volume is 1.0/0.6 to 1.0/0.7 or 1.4 to 1.7 times stroke volume. Finally, changing end-systolic and end-diastolic chamber volume alters myofibrillar wall tension and $M\dot{V}O_2$, and the latter are the key determinants of muscle growth. The third principle then implies that muscle wall thickness readjusts to preserve total wall tension constant. Thus an alteration in metabolic requirements leads to a predictable change in cardiac chamber volumes and muscle mass. This is obviously a greatly simplified scheme adapted for heuristic purposes, but the general validity of these principles is established in the following sections.

Protein-Energy Malnutrition. What alterations occur in stroke volume, heart rate, and cardiac output in protein-energy malnourished patients? In severe uncomplicated protein-energy malnutrition the stroke volume is markedly reduced.[56] Preload is lowered owing to a group of interrelated factors: reduced fat-free body mass, lowered whole-body oxygen consumption, depleted total and central blood volume, reduced circulating triiodothyronine (T_3), a slowing of sympathetic turnover, and a low core temperature. These physiological adjustments to negative energy and nitrogen balance lower venous blood return to the heart and decrease preload.

The reduced preload in chronic undernutrition is accompanied by a normal peripheral vascular resistance. Thus, the combined effect of the extracardiac determinants of ventricular output, preload, and afterload is to reduce stroke volume and $M\dot{V}O_2$ in protein-energy malnutrition.

Current information indicates that the third determinant of stroke volume, contractility, remains normal in the human or animal with the marasmic form of protein-energy malnutrition. Evidence for this is the following: normal resting echocardiographic ejection fraction and circumferential fiber shortening in undernourished adult patients with chronic wasting illnesses;[56,57] normal muscle mechanics in adult rats subjected to weight loss on a balanced diet of one third of their usual intake (Fig. 26–8);[58] and normal in situ ventricular function curves in adult protein-energy malnourished rats (Fig. 26–9).[58] While these studies indicate that cardiac contractility is preserved in the marasmic form of protein-energy malnutrition, the myocardial inotropic state may be depressed in kwashiorkor. For example, Abel and colleagues created a canine model of protein-energy malnutrition in which the animals developed myofiber atrophy and marked myocardial interstitial edema.[59] Left ventricular function was then evaluated in an isovolumic preparation during cardiopulmonary bypass. Ventricular compliance was decreased, and calculated force-velocity data suggested a depression of left ventricular contractility.

Another consideration related to cardiac contractility in humans is that micronutrient deficiencies often accompany protein energy malnutrition, and some of these abnormalities may adversely influence the inotropic state of the myocardium (Table 26–1).

Thus in the undernourished subject the reductions in stroke volume and end-diastolic volume occur largely because of a decrease in lean tissue mass and cellular metabolism. When the undernourished patient suffers from other underlying abnormalities and micronutrient deficiencies, the stroke volume and each of its determinants may be altered in an unpredictable fashion.

The total amount of blood leaving the heart per unit time, or cardiac output, is the product of heart rate and stroke volume. In classic semistarvation the heart rate declines in association with the fall in oxygen consumption and core temperature.[57,60] Profound bradycardia is sometimes noted in cases of anorexia nervosa or during famine, with observed heart rates varying between 30 and 50 beats per minute. The reduction in cardiac output is proportional to the decrease in metabolic demands.[56]

A low cardiac output, hypertension, and cool cyanotic extremities in the severely malnourished subject do not necessarily reflect cardiovascular dysfunction. These clinical findings are the systemic manifestations of an adaptive hypometabolic state.

A classic feature of semistarvation is low blood

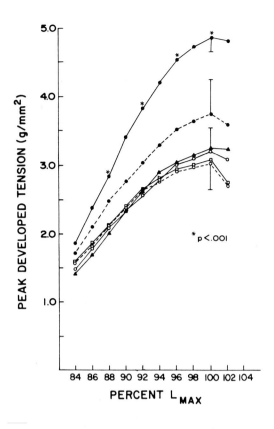

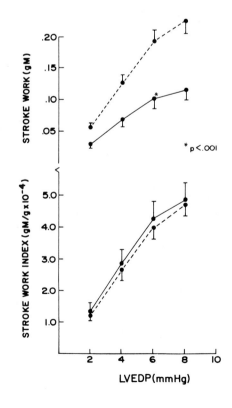

pressure. As blood pressure is the product of cardiac output and peripheral vascular resistance, most of the decrease in blood pressure can be attributed to the low stroke volume and heart rate.

Obesity. The stroke volume and end-diastolic volume are increased in obesity, and in many respects this occurs in a fashion almost exactly opposite to that observed in protein-energy malnutrition. Preload is augmented owing to the collective effects of an increase in fat-free body mass, a higher whole body oxygen consumption,[61] and an expanded total and central blood volume.[62] An additional factor is the added metabolic load and vascular perfusion needs of adipose tissue, which may contribute significantly to the requirements for cardiac output in severe obesity.[63]

Afterload is variably affected in obesity.[64,65] Expansion of the ventricular end-diastolic volume and a higher preload causes an increase in systolic wall tension and afterload per se. Peripheral vascular resistance remains normal or may even decrease in many subjects with moderate and severe obesity. On the other hand, an increase in peripheral vascular resistance and high blood pressure are commonplace in the obese population. While an acute increase in afterload reduces ventricular ejection and decreases venous return to the heart, this effect is overcome in the chronically obese state and stroke volume remains elevated.

The effect of obesity on myocardial contractility is not precisely defined. Mild to moderate obesity leads to cardiac hypertrophy, and there are apparently no derangements in ventricular function in this setting. For example, Messerli and colleagues demonstrated normal systolic ejection indices in normotensive obese subjects weighing an average of 94 to 110 kg.[64,65]

With increasing severity and chronicity of obesity the situation is clearly different. De Divitiis and co-workers detected abnormal left ventricular function, compliance, and end-diastolic pressure in obese patients whose average weight was 124 kg.[66] Reduced ventricular performance was noted by Alexander and Pettigrove in patients with morbid obesity.[67] These studies must be interpreted with caution, as subjects often suffered from both obesity and high blood pressure.

Stroke volume thus increases in obesity in response to the augmentation in metabolic demands and intravascular volume. As obese patients have no appreciable difference in heart rate relative to normal subjects, the observed increase in cardiac output occurs primarily as a function of enhanced stroke volume.

As noted earlier, circulatory dysfunction is not usually seen in mild or moderate obesity. On the other hand, cardiac dysfunction and congestive heart failure are clearly recognized in severe obesity. Smith and Willius first described congestive heart failure in obese subjects who had no other apparent cause of heart disease.[68] While the exact pathophysiology of this congestive state is unknown, the following constellation of factors must be considered in each case: a marked increase in the requirements for ventricular output; ventricular hypertrophy and abnormal myocardial function; associated hypoventilation syndrome and cor pulmonale; systemic arterial hypertension; and atherosclerotic cardiovascular disease. Symptoms of a congestive state are often present for many years, and cardiac failure is a well-recognized component of the terminal phase of massive obesity.[69]

Obesity therefore leads to an increase in stroke volume and cardiac output caused primarily by an increase in lean and adipose tissue mass, an expansion in circulating fluid volume, and an elevation in whole-body oxygen consumption. Congestive heart failure may occur in the individual with severe obesity; although the pathophysiology of this state is not clearly defined, it no doubt results from an interplay between the increased requirements for cardiac output and an abnormal myocardium.

Myocardial Mass

Basic Physiology. The change in demands for cardiac output associated with protein-energy malnutrition and obesity has a direct effect on the myocardial mass. A fundamental principle is that myocardial muscle tissue grows or atrophies to match the applied workload and wall stress.[70] Once again the main determinants of ventricular wall stress and myocardial oxygen consumption are described by the Laplace relation (Equation 3). Wall stress varies throughout the cardiac cycle, and the absolute amount of myofibrillar tension is determined by an interplay between intraventricular pressure, cavity radius, and myocardial wall thickness. The peak systolic wall stress is normally about 8 to 9 times higher than the end-diastolic wall stress.

When the myofibrillar wall tension is chronically augmented because of an increase in either intraventricular pressure or radius, the myocardium responds by a thickening of the ventricular wall; the accretion of fibers has the net effect of normalizing the total wall tension.[71] The current consensus is that the peak systolic wall stress is the main determinant of ventricular muscle hypertrophy and myocardial mass.[71]

The process begins when cardiac work is increased due to a volume or pressure load. With volume loading the stroke volume and end-diastolic volume increase, as described earlier. The expanded chamber volume increases diastolic wall stress, and this is hypothesized to stimulate series replication of cardiac fibers until a new optimum chamber size (1.3 to 1.4 times stroke volume) is reached.[71] An expanded chamber volume also increases systolic wall stress, and this is thought to be the main stimulus for par-

TABLE 26–10. Hypotheses Relating Hypertrophic Stimuli to Myofibrillar Growth

1. Increased work demands lead to local tissue hypoxia. Energy stores are depleted and metabolites accumulate; the latter induce or derepress the synthetic process.
2. Increased wall tension or hypoxia results in a "wear and tear effect" leading to the breakdown of macromolecules with the release of substances that stimulate growth.
3. Stretch of the muscle cell secondary to enhanced preload or afterload results in the augmented synthesis.
4. Humoral or hormonal factors initiate the hypertrophy.

Adapted from Zak R. Cardiac hypertrophy and atrophy. *In* Opie L (ed). The Heart: Physiology, Metabolism, Pharmacology, Therapy. London, Grune & Stratton, 1984: 198–209.

allel replication of sarcomeres and ventricular wall thickening.[71] The hypertrophy of the myocardial wall then normalizes both systolic wall stress and the tension developed in each myofibril. When volume loading is the only stimulus to increased cardiac work, the heart grows larger in a proportional manner. Hence, the relation between wall thickness and ventricular radius (h/r) remains unchanged. Referred to as magnification hypertrophy, the ventricular cavity enlarges laterally in the chest and becomes eccentric in relation to its normal position. Thus, this form of cardiac enlargement is sometimes described as eccentric hypertrophy.[72]

When the myocardium is subjected to an increase in pressure work there is an elevation in systolic wall stress; diastolic wall stress is largely unaffected. The result is an increase in wall thickness and a normalization of systolic wall stress; chamber size and stroke volume remain unchanged. Thus, the ratio of wall thickness to cavity radius (h/r) increases, a feature that characterizes concentric hypertrophy.

The precise biochemical mechanisms relating an increase in wall tension to myofibrillar growth are unknown. Four current hypotheses are under investigation as outlined in Table 26–10. The first three theories relate directly to changes in wall tension on muscle stretching. The fourth proposed mechanism is stimulation of myofibrillar protein synthesis and growth by humoral or hormonal factors.

While apparently not essential for cardiac growth, a permissive role is ascribed to insulin, adrenocortical, thyroid, and growth hormones (Table 26–11).[74–76] The relation between cardiac protein synthesis, circulating fuels, and hormonal substances is summarized in Figure 26–10.

Up to this point, our discussion has focused on the stimuli for cardiac chamber enlargement and muscle growth. While substantially less information is available on the mechanisms of cardiac atrophy, presumably the same or similar principles apply. The available information in this area will be reviewed in the next section.

Protein-Energy Malnutrition. The heart weight is subnormal in the undernourished subject.[56,57] The proportional loss of muscle tissue in all four chambers contributes to the total reduction in myocardial mass. Histological examination of heart tissue reveals an attenuation in myofibrillar diameter.[1] Interstitial edema occurs in about one fourth of autopsy cases. This finding is most evident in patients receiving high-sodium fluids and those with preterminal edema or ascites.[1]

The mechanisms leading to cardiac atrophy in patients with protein-energy malnutrition are not well characterized. We suggest that the pathophysiology may be as follows. Negative energy and nitrogen balance lead to a reduction in fat-free body mass, whole-body oxygen consumption, blood volume, and serum hormones such as insulin and T_3 (Table 26–11). Cardiac output decreases in proportion to the fall in metabolic demands. This is accomplished by a lowering of both stroke volume and heart rate. The ventricular end-diastolic volume gradually declines, reducing end-diastolic and end-systolic wall stress. The result is a shortening and thinning of myofibrils in a fashion that preserves end-diastolic volume at 1.4 to 1.6 times stroke volume and maintains normal systolic wall stress.

Partial support for this theorized series of events is provided by several published studies. First, the decrease in cardiac output and stroke volume in undernourished patients with anorexia nervosa occurs

TABLE 26–11. Trophic Effects of Hormones on the Heart and Relation to Nutritional Status

	General Effects on the Heart	Nutritional Interrelations
Thyroid	Probable trophic action. Indirectly increases cardiac work by modulating whole-body $\dot{V}O_2$. Also directly affects contractile sites and fiber shortening rate, tension development, myofibrillar amino acid uptake, and B-receptors.	Overfeeding and underfeeding increase and decrease the peripheral conversion of T_4 to T_3, respectively. High and low serum T_3 levels occur during overfeeding and underfeeding, respectively. Chronically undernourished subjects have reduced circulating levels of TSH, T_4, and T_3. Serum thyroid hormone levels are normal in obese subjects.
Insulin	Direct trophic effect on the heart uncertain; influences cardiac protein turnover.	Underfeeding and weight loss associated with reduced 24-hour insulin secretion. Opposite changes with overfeeding and obesity.
Growth hormone	May exert indirect trophic effect by stimulating growth of other lean tissues, thus increasing cardiac demands.	Increased in malnourished infants. Output in response to a variety of stimuli is subnormal in obesity. Normal linear growth in obesity may be secondary to normal somatomedin activity.

Data from references 74, 75, 76.

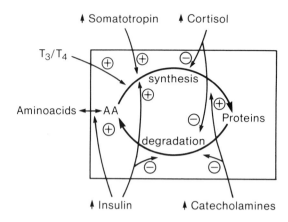

FIGURE 26–10. *Metabolic signals that can influence the rate of protein synthesis or degradation in the heart. The exact physiological role of these factors is still not known, nor is it clear which signals are involved in the enhanced protein synthesis occurring during a hemodynamic load. T_3/T_4, thyroid hormones; AA, intracellular amino acids. (Modified from Givers W. Synthesis and turnover of cardiac proteins. In Opie L [ed]. The Heart: Physiology, Metabolism, Pharmacology, Therapy. London, Grune & Stratton, 1984.)*

in proportion to the fall in whole-body $\dot{V}O_2$.[1,56,57] Since the latter decreases to a slightly greater extent than fat-free body mass, it is expected that cardiac output per unit of lean tissue is somewhat low (Fig. 26–11). Ejection fraction in the anorexia nervosa patient is preserved at 0.6 to 0.7, indicating a constant relation between stroke volume and end-diastolic volume. The reduced chamber volume is matched by a thinning of the left ventricular wall (h), and thus the ratio h/r is unchanged from normal (Fig. 26–12). This implies a form of atrophy almost exactly opposite to the concentric hypertrophy observed in obesity. Finally, there is no significant difference in systolic wall stress between undernourished anorexia nervosa patients and normal-weight controls, indicating the remodeling process maintains a normal level of myofibrillar tension.

Obesity. The heart muscle mass is increased in normotensive obese subjects, and in mild and moderate obesity this occurs in proportion to the rise in whole-body $\dot{V}O_2$ and fat-free body mass. There are corresponding changes in stroke volume and cardiac output (Fig. 26–10) with a preservation of the normal resting ejection fraction. The presumed stimulus for heart muscle growth is the increased volume demands with associated enhancement of systolic and diastolic wall stress. As the heart enlarges, the h/r remains constant, indicating magnification or eccentric hypertrophy. Microscopic examination of the myocardium in patients dying with severe obesity reveals an increase in myofibrillar diameter.[69] An abundance of epicardial fat is sometimes noted, and in rare cases massive myocardial triglyceride accumulation may be present.[79]

When peripheral resistance is increased, as occurs in both lean and obese hypertensive subjects, the augmented afterload initially causes a rise in systolic wall stress. Wall thickening then proceeds until systolic myofibrillar tension returns to normal. The resulting concentric hypertrophy, in which the h/r is increased, occurs in patients with high blood pressure (Fig. 26–11).[64,65] The added workload of systemic arterial hypertension causes only a modest ad-

ditional increase in the h/r and ventricular mass in the obese.[64,65]

The above simplified overview indicates that the human myocardium can either reduce or enlarge its volume and mass according to the applied metabolic and hemodynamic workload. In the absence of systemic arterial hypertension, cardiac output and myocardial mass are related directly to metabolic demands. Of course, other factors may be operative in either extreme undernutrition or obesity.

Recovery from Protein-Energy Malnutrition

Recall from an earlier section that uncomplicated semistarvation is accompanied by a constellation of findings: a depleted lean tissue mass, a decreased whole-body $\dot{V}O_2$, low levels of serum T_3, hypothermia, bradycardia, a reduced cardiac output, hypertension, and a small myocardial mass. When feeding is reinstated, energy and nitrogen balance return to zero or become positive; the result is an arrest in tissue losses or a regrowth of the depleted cytoplasmic mass.

The rate of weight gain during the recovery phase of protein-energy malnutrition depends upon a complex interplay of energy, nitrogen, water, and sodium balance. Two aspects of these interrelations are relevant to the cardiovascular system. First, the adaptive metabolic state of semistarvation is reversed during refeeding, and the rate and degree to which this occurs depends on the supply of energy and nitrogen.[30] A gradual return to the eumetabolic state occurs when the recovery diet consists of regular meals designed to produce increasingly positive energy and nitrogen balance over days or weeks. Rapid recovery is prompted by an accelerated feeding schedule, one that favors a strongly positive balance and rapid weight gain. Analogous to a recovery diet, the rate of continuous energy and nitrogen infusion during therapy with enteral or parenteral feeding largely determines the rate of weight gain and degree of positive energy and nitrogen balance.

The second major determinant of weight gain is

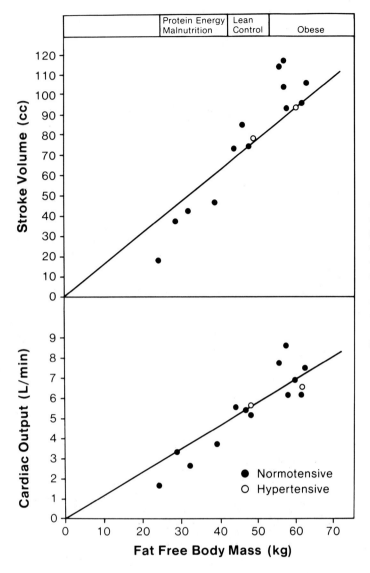

FIGURE 26–11. Stroke volume and cardiac output versus fat-free body mass. Three subject groups are depicted: protein-energy malnourished patients, lean controls, and obese individuals. The solid lines have a slope equal to the ratios of stroke volume to fat-free body mass and of cardiac output to fat-free body mass for the lean control group. The graphs show that overall ventricular output is matched to lean tissue mass, and this occurs with or without hypertension. Data derived from references 29, 56, 57, 64, 65, and 78, and applied with the assumption that fat-free body mass was 95 per cent and 55 per cent of body weight in patients with protein-energy malnutrition and obesity, respectively.

FIGURE 26–12. Relation of left ventricular diastolic wall thickness to intraventricular chamber radius in three groups of subjects. These two measurements represent the h and r of the Laplace equation, respectively. The solid line was drawn with a slope for h/r equal to that of the lean control group. Note that in normotensive undernourished, lean, and obese subjects the h/r ratio remains constant over a large heart size range. The h/r increases in the presence of hypertension, indicating concentric hypertrophy. Data derived from references 29, 56, 57, 64, 65, and 78, and applied with the assumption that fat-free body mass was 95 per cent and 55 per cent of body weight in patients with protein-energy malnutrition and obesity, respectively.

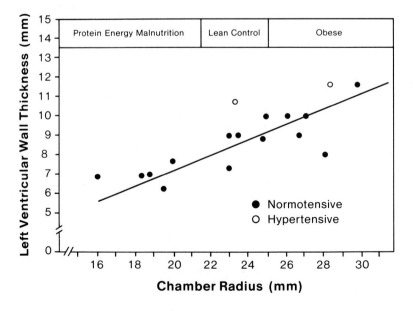

sodium intake, which strongly influences the rate of extracellular fluid expansion during the recovery period. In turn, a close relation exists between the expanding extracellular fluid space and one of its major subcompartments, plasma volume.

The combined effects of metabolic response to refeeding and enlarging plasma volume determines the cardiovascular response during the recovery period. In an earlier section we reviewed in detail how the amount, rate, and composition of dietary energy supplied to an individual influences metabolism and the cardiovascular system. The same general principles apply when undernourished subjects are refed, although qualitative differences may exist relative to normally nourished individuals. For example, the thermic response to a meal is reduced in the semistarved individual relative to a normally nourished counterpart.[80] These differences notwithstanding, the basic principle applies that a larger amount or progressively more rapid delivery rate of dietary energy will cause a correspondingly higher whole-body oxygen consumption and cardiac output.

When the semistarved patient is refed, one observes a consistent pattern of physiological changes. A representative response is provided in Figure 26–13. PD was a 22-year-old woman with moderately severe anorexia nervosa. Fat-free body mass was 27.3 kg, whereas the normal value for her age and height is 42 kg. Hypothermia and hypometabolism ($\dot{V}O_2$ = 110 ml/min; normal 164 ml/min) were present. The patient's spontaneous food intake was 700 to 800 kcal/24 hr, or 65 per cent of expected intake for her height, age, and activity level. On the second hospital day we began continuous nasoenteric infusion of a blenderized, balanced feeding solution. The full formula hourly dose of 3.0 kcal/kg fat-free body mass was reached by the third infusion day. This formula flow rate was designed to induce strongly positive energy and nitrogen balance as the hourly maintenance energy requirement for this patient was 1.4 kcal/kg fat-free body mass. Note the following response: an increase in body weight; an accretion of fat-free body mass (+ ΔN) and extracellular fluid (+ ΔNa); a marked rise in whole-body $\dot{V}O_2$ and heat release (Q, direct calorimetry); a resolution of hypothermia; a rise in serum T_3; increases in heart rate, stroke volume, and cardiac output; and little or no change in mean blood pressure. An increase in cardiac output with no change in mean blood pressure implies a corresponding decrease in peripheral vascular resistance. Ejection fraction increased slightly (0.6 to 0.7), and by the last week of therapy there was a small increase in left ventricular end-diastolic volume. This patient typifies the three main factors that alter cardiac demands during the recovery process: a resolution of the adaptive hypometabolism of semistarvation; the metabolic-hemodynamic demands imposed by feeding per se; and an expansion of the extracellular fluid compartment, which by inference indicates an increase in the circulating fluid volume.

In hemodynamic terms, the increase in cardiac output resulted from a larger stroke volume and a more rapid heart rate. The augmented stroke volume can be ascribed primarily to two factors. First, an increase in tissue oxygen consumption causes vasodilation, a fall in peripheral vascular resistance, and an increase in venous return to the heart. Second, an expanding plasma volume results in an increase in intravascular volume and mean systemic filling pressure, which in combination with a fall in peripheral vascular resistance favors an increase in venous return and preload. The result is a larger stroke volume.

An important point demonstrated by this patient is that the myocardial workload during the refeeding process is relatively small. Even though the volume output of the heart is increased, the corresponding fall in ventricular afterload (i.e., peripheral resistance) minimizes changes in myocardial wall tension and myofibrillar oxygen consumption. The reduced impedance to ventricular ejection and the adequate reserve capacity of a small but functionally normal heart prevents the development of circulatory congestion.

The quantitative aspects of the recovery response are provided in Table 26–12 for a group of six undernourished medical patients undergoing parenteral hyperalimentation. The data provided were collected at baseline (fasting) and after 15 to 20 days of continuous infusion of a standard glucose–amino acid intravenous solution (C1800). Energy intake was doubled over baseline food ingestion, causing an average increase in body weight of 10.8 per cent. The relative rate of increase in metabolic indices was more rapid than the rate of increase in body weight. The initially subnormal values for $\dot{V}O_2$ and serum T_3 showed respective increases of 50 per cent and 87 per cent. Sodium balance was positive, and plasma volume increased by 13 per cent. There were increases in heart rate (50 per cent), stroke volume (11 per cent), and cardiac output (67 per cent). No congestive heart failure was noted in any of the subjects, and ejection fraction (echocardiography) remained normal or increased slightly.

While these examples typify rapid recovery from semistarvation by means of nonvolitional feeding techniques, a similar but slower process occurs when regular meals serve as the source of renourishment. Several studies of undernourished subjects indicate that the restitution of the eumetabolic state and accretion of fat-free body mass are accompanied by an increase in heart rate, stroke volume, and cardiac output.[57,81] An interesting sidelight is the recovery phase of childhood protein-energy malnutrition. Refeeding the starved child often causes a phase of catch-up growth associated with an increase in whole-body oxygen consumption and cardiac demands.[82,84]

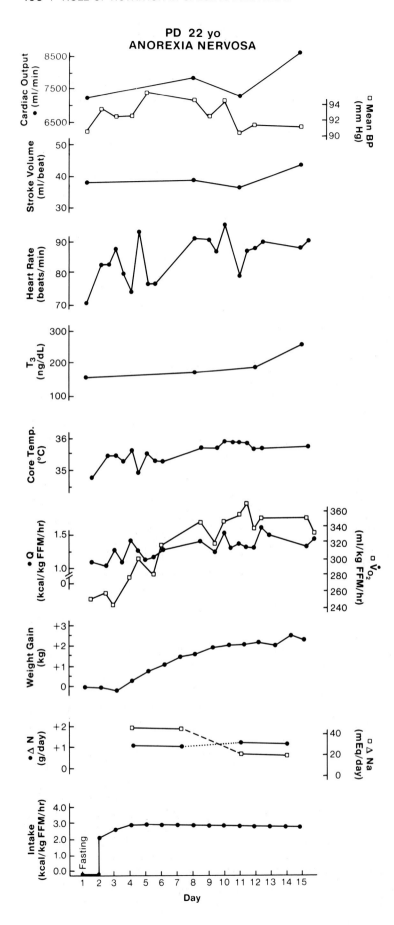

FIGURE 26–13. *Cardiovascular and metabolic response during refeeding course of a patient with undernutrition secondary to anorexia nervosa. N, nitrogen; Q, heat release measured by direct calorimetry.*

TABLE 26–12. Nutritional, Metabolic, and Cardiovascular Changes in Undernourished Patients Receiving Parenteral Nutrition*

Measurement	Units	Normal Range	Baseline	Hyperalimentation	%Δ
Nutritional:					
Body weight	kg	—	40.8 ± 8.2	45.2 ± 7.6	10.8
Intake	kcal/D	—	1822 ± 941	3527 ± 884	94
N	g/D	—	—	8.2 ± 3.2	—
Na	mEq/D	—	—	18.6 ± 6.5	—
Metabolic/Endocrine:					
$\dot{V}O_2$	ml/min/m²	115–145	99.5 ± 11.3	187.0 ± 22.5	87
TSH	IU/ml	0–6	5.8 ± 2.6	4.8 ± 4.2	−26
Total T_4	μg/dl	4.5–11.5	5.4 ± 2.7	5.1 ± 3.6	−6
Free T_4	ng/dl	1–2.3	1.4 ± 0.6	1.2 ± 0.6	−16
T_3	ng/dl	60–170	56.8 ± 10.7	73.8 ± 30.0	30
Cardiovascular					
Heart rate	beats/min	60–100	62.8 ± 16.0	94.5 ± 18.0	50
Stroke volume	cc/beat/m²	45–55	37.4 ± 6.4	41.6 ± 5.7	11
Cardiac output	L/min/m²	3.0–4.0	2.3 ± 0.8	3.9 ± 0.8	67
Ejection fraction		0.6–0.8	0.72 ± 0.06	0.80 ± 0.06	11
Plasma volume	cc	1550†	1621 ± 338	1840 ± 452	13
RBC mass	cc	1120†	943 ± 412	948 ± 468	0.5

*n = 6. Subjects studied at baseline (fasting) and during the third week of a standard glucose–amino acid parenteral formula (C1800). Results are expressed ± SD.

†Average value based upon patient's baseline body weight.

From Galloway J, Stensby J, Heymsfield SB. Clin Res 1979; 27:226A. Reproduced with permission.

While this physiological profile typifies the recovery phase of protein-energy malnutrition under strictly controlled clinical research conditions, patients in the hospital often have a far more complicated hemodynamic-metabolic state. Dehydration, diarrhea, infection, fever, anemia, and transfusion therapy may all modulate the simplified recovery response presented in the previous paragraphs. The clinician must take all of these factors into consideration when managing the recovery process.

While ventricular output promptly increases from subnormal values to normal or supranormal levels, the regrowth of heart muscle mass is a more gradual process.[56,57] Recall that an increase in cardiac work, mediated primarily through changes in ventricular wall tension, is the primary hypertrophic stimulus. With the rapid recovery process described above, the actual increase in myocardial work is rather small; preload increases on the one hand, but afterload decreases on the other. This may explain why left ventricular mass shows only a minimal increase in the initial phase of recovery from protein-energy malnutrition. Over long periods of time there occurs a series of consistent changes: left ventricular and other chamber volumes expand, the septal and left ventricular muscle walls thicken, and the total left ventricular mass enlarges.[1,56,81] Overall, the increase in heart muscle tissue occurs at the same rate as the increase in fat-free body mass. The growing heart continues to obey the Laplace principle, with wall thickness and ventricular radius maintaining the same ratio (h/r) as seen in healthy subjects.[56,57,78]

Although the usual patient experiences no cardiovascular disturbances during recovery from the undernourished state, a rare but serious complication of refeeding is congestive cardiac failure. Rec-

ognized for decades, this syndrome has led to the well-accepted dictum that states "the heart is closer to failure during recovery than in starvation."[85] The pathophysiology of this disorder, which is often described as the "refeeding syndrome," is not well defined. Three current theories attempting to explain the manifestations of this disorder include hemodynamic mechanisms, micronutrient-electrolyte disturbances,[86] and abnormal cardiac electrical activity.[87]

The hemodynamic and metabolic changes that occur during uneventful recovery from semistarvation were described in the previous section. The following three cases will highlight an abnormal recovery pattern.

Case 1. Patient WW, a 36-year-old female, suffered from severe chronic anorexia nervosa.[56] She also had a past history of chronic pyelonephritis, and her creatinine clearance was reduced to 5 ml/min. Body weight was 60 per cent of standard, and lean tissue indices showed equally severe depletion. Baseline echocardiography revealed a cardiac output of 34 and 48 per cent of respective height-matched and age-matched control values; ejection fraction was normal. A nasoenteric cannula was inserted on the second day of hospitalization, and a standard enteral formula was supplied at 3200 kcal/24 hr. She steadily gained weight, and balances of nitrogen and sodium were strongly positive. The first 18 days of repletion were uneventful except for the appearance of 1+ pedal edema on day 10. On days 19 and 20, dyspnea, tachycardia, a ventricular gallop, left pleural effusion, radiographic pulmonary edema, and pedal edema all appeared. The enlarged radiographic cardiac silhouette (Fig. 26–14) was shown by echocardiography to consist of three components: left ven-

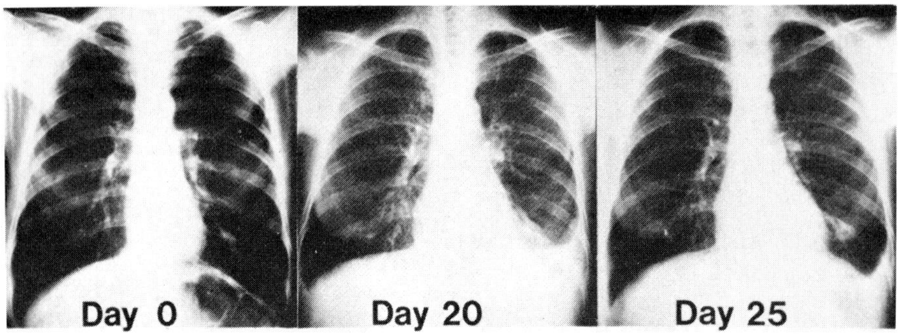

FIGURE 26–14. Radiographic changes in a patient with anorexia nervosa during a refeeding program. The small cardiac silhouette on day 0 increased markedly by day 20, and the radiographic changes were associated with symptoms and signs of cardiac failure. Reducing the feeding solution flow rate and administering a diuretic improved clinical symptoms and radiographic abnormalities by day 25. (From Heymsfield SB, Bethel R, Ansley JD, et al. Am Heart J 1978; 95:584–594. Reproduced with permission.)

tricular mass and end-diastolic volume had both increased by 50 to 60 per cent over the baseline volume, and a pericardial effusion had developed. Relative to baseline, cardiac output and whole-body $\dot{V}O_2$ had increased by 155 and 30 per cent, respectively. Ejection phase indices of left ventricular performance remained normal. Therapy with a diuretic for 3 consecutive days resolved her symptoms, and cardiac output decreased to a level 50 per cent higher than the baseline output. Her remaining hospital course was uneventful.

Case 2. CH was a 48-year-old man with short bowel syndrome secondary to a mesenteric infarction. He also had a prior history of an anterior wall myocardial infarction. A central venous line was inserted, and a standard glucose–amino acid parenteral formula was infused at a rate supplying 3000 to 3500 kcal/24 hr. Weight increased gradually, but by the third week the patient complained of late afternoon shortness of breath. Upon physical examination there was a pulse of 120 and a ventricular gallop; echocardiography revealed a large dyskinetic portion of the anterior left ventricular wall. The parenteral formula was temporarily discontinued, and within 24 hours the symptoms and physical findings resolved. Subsequent trials indicated that infusion rates supplying 2000 to 2500 kcal/24 hr were tolerated without ill effect, whereas higher infusion rates promptly restored a tachycardia and a gallop rhythm.

Case 3. LL was a 42-year-old man with severe undernutrition secondary to pancreatic insufficiency. He had a previous history of high blood pressure, although his admission blood pressure was within normal limits. Baseline echocardiography indicated a normal ejection fraction of 0.75. An elemental formula infusion was started via a nasogastric tube, and LL ultimately received between 2500 and 3000 kcal/24 hr. During the second week of therapy the patient had a marked rise in blood pressure to 170/110. He complained of shortness of breath, and a gallop rhythm was present. Echocardiography now indicated a decrease in the ejection fraction to 0.57. An-

tihypertensive therapy was initiated, but normotension was not achieved for another 5 to 10 days. No further symptoms were described by the patient, and no signs of heart failure were evident throughout the remainder of his hospitalization.

Although each of these cases is obviously complex, we can make several illustrative generalizations that provide an insight into the congestive form of the refeeding syndrome. In Case 1, WW received a large caloric and fluid load relative to her body weight that was superimposed upon moderately impaired renal function. Her congested state could be explained by the unusually large demands for ventricular output that this fluid and metabolic load placed on her relatively small heart. In Case 2, CH suffered from an intrinsic cardiac defect that became clinically significant when he was subjected to the metabolic and fluid load of parenteral hyperalimentation. In Case 3, LL developed a marked rise in blood pressure, suggesting the heart was subjected to an increase in peripheral vascular resistance and afterload. Recall that the normal refeeding response involves a reduction in peripheral vascular resistance. Hence a reasonable conclusion is that an abnormally large increase in preload, a defect in cardiac contractility, or an elevated afterload can predispose the individual to a congestive state or congestive heart failure during recovery from semistarvation.

While our focus in this section was on hemodynamic mechanisms, other factors no doubt contribute to the refeeding syndrome. Hypophosphatemia and micronutrient depletion are often cited as causative or contributing factors to myocardial failure during refeeding.[86] A rare and lethal complication during recovery from semistarvation is ventricular arrhythmia. The pathogenesis of this sudden death syndrome is unknown.[87]

A point worthy of mention in this section is that "refeeding edema" often develops during recovery from severe malnutrition. A careful history and physical examination will rule out the possibility of underlying cardiac failure. Although the specific mechanism of this syndrome is unknown, any one of a combination of three measures will promptly relieve this bothersome complication of refeeding: elastic stockings, a short period of diuretic therapy, and a low-sodium diet.

Weight Reduction in Obesity

The rate of weight reduction in obesity is related directly to the degree of negative energy and nitrogen balance. Severe nutrient restriction and rapid weight loss in obese adults results in metabolic adaptations similar to those observed in semistarvation.[88] Whole-body $\dot{V}O_2$, serum T_3, plasma insulin, and core temperature are all reduced; the proportional decrease in $\dot{V}O_2$ is greater than the relative loss in lean body mass. Accompanying these changes are reductions in cardiac output and mass.[89] With severe prolonged caloric restriction, life-threatening arrhythmias often arise. This effect of weight reduction is reviewed in detail elsewhere.[90,91]

Gradual loss of a large amount of weight results in a decrease in total body fat, fat-free body mass, and whole-body $\dot{V}O_2$. Accompanying these changes are reductions in total blood volume, mean arterial pressure, left ventricular cavity diameter, stroke volume, cardiac output, $M\dot{V}O_2$, and left ventricular mass.[69,89] It is unknown if the hypertrophied myocardium seen in obesity regresses in proportion to the reduction in body weight and metabolic demands.

While symptoms of cardiac dysfunction improve with weight loss, signs of impaired left ventricular performance may persist.[92] For example, Alexander[69] found that the elevated resting filling pressure in obese subjects decreased with weight loss to within the normal range; contrastingly, the left ventricular filling pressure with exercise remained elevated in these subjects.

CONGESTIVE HEART FAILURE

Patients with nutritional disturbances resulting from chronic congestive heart failure (CHF) can be divided into two groups.[93] The first group has "classic cardiac cachexia," a syndrome that evolves over months or years as myocardial function progressively deteriorates. Included in this category are subjects with CHF secondary to cardiomyopathy, congenital cardiac defects, and acquired valvular abnormalities. The second group of patients suffers from cardiac disease that requires corrective surgery. The preoperative state is not associated with major nutritional abnormalities. Following cardiac surgery, the postoperative course is complicated by refractory CHF, pulmonary edema, infection, or some other unfavorable condition. Nutritional disturbances similar to those observed in classic cardiac cachexia now

evolve at an accelerated rate, and this syndrome is referred to as "nosocomial cardiac cachexia." There may be an overlap between the two forms of cardiac cachexia, and the basic management principles for the two syndromes are similar.

Pathophysiology. The natural history of classic cardiac cachexia begins with an intrinsic myocardial lesion resulting in severe CHF.[94,95] The afflicted individual usually has Class IV (New York Heart Association) CHF, limited or no cardiac reserve capacity, and a markedly depressed $\dot{V}O_2$ max. Dyspnea is severe and exercise tolerance is minimal.

The physical appearance of the patient with cardiac cachexia was clearly described by Hippocrates, who stated that "the flesh is consumed and becomes water—the abdomen fills with water; the feet and legs swell, the shoulders, clavicles, chest, and thighs melt away."[94] In modern terms, there is a loss of adipose tissue and body cell mass with a corresponding enlargement of the extracellular fluid compartment. As a result, body weight may be normal or increased in the presence of skeletal muscle atrophy and a reduced total body protein mass.

The primary nutritional disturbance in cardiac cachexia is negative energy and nitrogen balance, and the causes of this abnormality are outlined in Table 26–13.[94,95] Intake is usually inadequate owing to dyspnea and "air hunger," and food ingestion is often associated with early satiety. The latter may be caused by a reduced functional gastric volume secondary to hepatomegaly and ascites. Anorexia may also be caused by pharmacological agents, especially excessive amounts of digitalis preparations. Energy and nitrogen losses are increased in the stool owing to subclinical fat and nitrogen malabsorption and protein-losing gastroenteropathy. Bowel wall edema, the intestinal cellular effects of hypoxia, and increased venous pressure are considered likely causes of the increased fecal losses.

Energy and nitrogen losses are increased in the urine when glucosuria or proteinuria is present. The excretion of other micronutrients may be increased secondary to concomitant drug therapy (Table 26–14).

Energy losses as heat may be increased secondary to hypermetabolism. Intermittent fever of uncertain cause is well described in classic cardiac cachexia.[94,95] Hypermetabolism in the absence of fever has also been documented, and this may result from an in-

---

TABLE 26–13. Nutritional Abnormalities in Cardiac Cachexia

Decreased intake secondary to hunger, early satiety, and anorectic effect of medications

Increased urinary losses secondary to generalized malassimilation, protein-losing gastroenteropathy, and possible drug effects on bowel

Hypermetabolism secondary to fever and increased cardiac and pulmonary energy requirements

Metabolic factors such as hypoxia and cardiac cirrhosis

TABLE 26–14. Drug-Nutrient Interactions Related to the Therapy of Cardiovascular Diseases

Drug	Nutrient Interaction/Systemic Effect
Alphamethyldopa (Aldomet)	Diarrhea
Digitalis preparations	Intoxication caused by these compounds results in nausea, vomiting, anorexia, diarrhea, and fatigue
Ethacrinic acid (Edecrin)	Gastrointestinal symptoms; hypokalemia; hyponatremia; hypercalciuria; hyperuricemia; hyperglycemia; azotemia
Furosemide (Lasix)	Hypokalemia; hyponatremia; hypercalciuria; hyperuricemia; hyperglycemia; azotemia
Guanethidine (Ismelin)	Diarrhea
Hydralazine (Apresoline)	Gastrointestinal symptoms recognized; vitamin B_6 and pyridoxine antagonist. Na and H_2O retention if given without diuretic
Minoxidil (Loniten)	Fluid retention if given without diuretic
Nitroprusside	Accumulation of thiocyanate with prolonged infusion is associated with nausea and weakness
Prazosin (Minipress)	Fluid retention if given without diuretic
Propranolol (Inderal)	Diarrhea
Quinidine	Diarrhea
Reserpine	Increases gastric emptying
Spironolactone	Hyperkalemia; hyperglycemia; hyperuricemia; azotemia
Thiazides	Hypokalemia; hyponatremia; magnesium depletion; hyperglycemia; azotemia; hyperuricemia

creased cardiac mass and $\dot{M}VO_2$; chronic pulmonary edema and stiff, inelastic lungs may also increase the work of breathing.

While not well documented, a current hypothesis is that the low cardiac output associated with severe CHF impairs delivery of cellular nutrients and removal of waste products.[95] This theory proposes that the lack of cellular oxygen leads to inefficient substrate oxidation and diminished synthesis of high-energy intermediary metabolites.

Thus a combination of reduced intake, increased losses, and impaired metabolism causes negative energy and nitrogen balance over months or years in the patient with severe CHF. Similar overall mechanisms operate in the patient who develops nosocomial cardiac cachexia, but the process is accelerated by the catabolic events that accompany the postoperative period.

The individual mechanisms of cardiac cachexia can be assembled into two distinct models of the syndrome (Fig. 26–15).[93] There is more than theoretical interest implied in the two models; our therapy is a direct outgrowth of the concepts developed in these pathophysiological diagrams.

The central lesion proposed in the panel on the left is low cardiac output and tissue hypoxia (pathway 1). An adaptive role is ascribed to anorexia and malabsorption, which together minimize the need for cardiac output by reducing food intake and absorption. Hence the increases in splanchnic blood flow and $\dot{V}O_2$ that follow a meal are minimal when food intake and absorption are reduced. Weight loss ultimately results in cachexia and lowering of whole-body $\dot{V}O_2$ (pathways 2 and 6). The combined effects of reduced intake and dimimished lean tissue mass

lower $\dot{V}O_2$ and the requirement for cardiac output (pathway 3). The net effect is positive in regard to the symptoms and signs of CHF. Supplying food or formula, according to this theory, would have little beneficial effect. First, efficient utilization of nutrients would be limited by the presence of tissue hypoxia. Second, the impaired myocardium may not be able to meet the increased metabolic requirements of feeding and new tissue growth. The result would be a worsening of CHF.

The panel on the right in Figure 26–15 presents a different view. Anorexia, malabsorption, and hypermetabolism are ascribed to CHF epiphenomena. An inadequate supply of energy and essential nutrients is thought to impair cardiac and noncardiac lean tissue function. Overcoming anorexia and malabsorption by specialized feeding methods theoretically would improve the functional activity of lean tissues and reduce the severity of CHF.

While the available literature[96–98] does not fully validate one or the other model, elements of both hypotheses appear correct. The currently recommended approach is the following:[93]

1. Correct micronutrient deficiencies in all CHF patients by supplying appropriate replacement therapy.

2. In patients with CHF followed long-term, prescribe a dietary plan as outlined in the following section.

3. In preoperative patients, special attention should be directed toward the evaluation of nutrient status. Most workers now agree that undernourished patients should receive a period of preoperative nutritional support. Factors of importance are the route, amount (or rate), and composition of energy

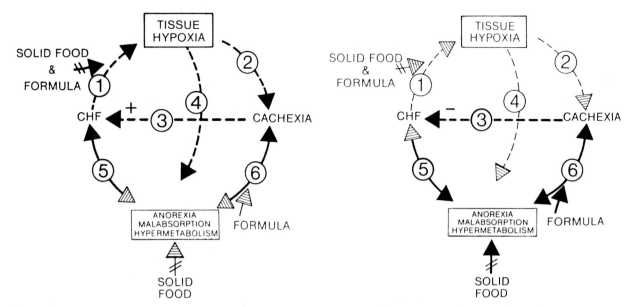

FIGURE 26–15. Proposed mechanisms and nutritional sensitivity of cardiac cachexia are shown. The panel on the left reflects the view that tissue hypoxia is central to the pathogenesis of cardiac cachexia. Tissue "stagnant anoxia" not only reduces cellular nutrient blood flow and waste removal but also purportedly causes anorexia and malabsorption. These abnormalities are considered adaptive, in that the demand for ventricular output is minimized by (1) decreasing food intake and (2) reducing the total mass of oxygen-consuming lean tissues. According to this model, hyperalimentation would be either blocked or inefficient owing to hypoxia and might adversely affect cardiac performance. The panel on the right presents an alternative view in which tissue hypoxia is considered relatively unimportant, and the cachexia-producing mechanisms anorexia, malabsorption, and hypermetabolism are now the focus. These are considered CHF epiphenomena, which hypothetically further impair cardiac function by limiting the myocardial nutrient supply required for optimum performance. Hyperalimentation using specially prepared solutions should correct lean tissue deficits in cardiac cachexia and improve CHF if this model is correct. Components of both models have been clinically validated and are discussed in the text. (From Heymsfield SB, Smith JL, Redd S, et al. Surg Clin North Am 1981; 61:636–653.)

supplied and the amount of sodium provided. Monitoring for a change in CHF status is essential. A suggested approach is provided in the next section.

4. Close monitoring of nutritional status and appropriate therapy in the postsurgical patient is essential.

Nutritional Management. Three groups of patients are targets for nutritional evaluation and therapy: those with chronic inoperable CHF, those with preoperative chronic CHF, and those who have had cardiac surgery.

Although cardiac transplantation may ultimately eliminate severe chronic CHF as a medical problem, many patients are currently under medical care for this disorder. A survey by our group at the Grady Memorial Hospital Cardiac Clinic in Atlanta indicated that about one third of patients with Class III or IV CHF were mildly or moderately undernourished.[99] A striking observation in this survey was that the undernourished state had gone undetected in most cases. Not only was there evidence of protein-energy deficiency, but patients often suffered from iron deficiency, hypomagnesemia, and a variety of other nutrition-related abnormalities. No doubt all of the factors described above were operating to produce the observed deficiencies. We recommend the following guidelines in managing outpatients with severe CHF:

1. A baseline nutritional assessment should be a component of the medical evaluation for all patients with heart disease. Details of the assessment protocol are reviewed elsewhere.[100]

2. Patients identified as being without significant nutritional problems should be re-evaluated at 6-month to 1-year intervals.

3. Overweight subjects, often with atherosclerotic cardiovascular disease, should receive counseling related to obesity, hyperlipidemia, high blood pressure, and diet.

4. Patients with protein-energy malnutrition and micronutrient deficiencies should be counseled by the dietician either every visit or every other visit. The information provided should include basic facts related to low-sodium diets, formula supplements, and mineral-vitamin preparations. The suggested cardiac diet consists of six small meals prepared from soft foods. Fat intake is limited to 30 to 40 per cent of total caloric intake. Spreading out the meals over the whole day helps to counteract the often-present early satiety and minimizes the circulatory effects of feeding described earlier. Caffeine-containing beverages should be avoided. Sodium and fluid should be restricted to 1 to 2 g and 1 to 1.5 L per day, respectively. The latter recommendations should be adjusted to the severity of CHF and diuretic sensi-

tivity. Vitamin and mineral replacement is based upon the patient's requirements. Patients who have malabsorption should receive fat-soluble vitamins in a water-miscible form.

The preoperative patient with severe chronic CHF should receive a thorough nutritional evaluation a few weeks prior to surgery. Several studies indicate that the surgical morbidity and mortality in patients with Class III or IV CHF is markedly increased in undernourished patients relative to normally nourished subjects.[101]

The immediate goals in managing the preoperative patient with CHF are similar to those enumerated earlier for managing patients with chronic heart failure. A thorough nutritional assessment, counseling on the size, frequency, and composition of meals, and mineral/vitamin supplements are all part of the program. Often intensive counseling with a nutritionist results in markedly improved nutrient intake. Diet diaries, telephone diet histories, and discussions with the family often potentiate the process.

When these simple measures fail to produce an adequate intake, the question that often arises is whether or not to apply nonvolitional feeding techniques. No firm conclusions are yet available on this important question; the practitioner must make this decision based upon a wide variety of clinical considerations. In an earlier review we provided a detailed description of the techniques used in nutritional support of the CHF patient.[93] The following is a summary of our recommended approach:

1. Apply nasoenteral feeding techniques when possible. Parenteral feeding should be used only in cases of partial or complete failure to tolerate the nasoenteral formula. Home tube-feeding[102] provides a simple, now well-established method of preoperative support.

2. Solutions used in nasoenteral feeding should provide a source of high-quality protein with a minimal amount of sodium and water. Three major categories of solutions are available: polymeric, elemental, and modular.[103] The major difference between polymeric and elemental solutions is the nature and proportion of organic fuels: elemental diets are low in fat, contain either free amino acids or predigested proteins, and supply carbohydrate as monosaccharides; polymeric formulas are usually 30 to 40 per cent fat, contain intact proteins, and provide carbohydrate as polysaccharides. These categories are not firm, with many solutions having the qualities of both an elemental and a polymeric formula.

The decision of which formula to administer is based upon the patient's gastrointestinal function and fluid status. Elemental formulas are indicated in the CHF patient with moderate or severe malabsorption. However, most elemental solutions are hyperosmolar and provide 1 ml of water per kcal. Hence with severe fluid restriction a high-caloric-density (>1.5 kcal/ml) polymeric formula should be considered. Polymeric solutions are used in patients requiring tube feeding who have normal or only mildly impaired gastrointestinal function.

The third category of solution, the modular formulas, are created from individual nutrient components.[104] Modular formulas are supplied to patients who have special nutrient requirements. These solutions are often used in patients with hyperkalemia, hypercalcemia, hyperglycemia, or nitrogen intolerance.

Table 26–15 presents a representative sample of available elemental and polymeric formulas with information relevant to the CHF patient. Table 26–16 describes available modular components.

3. The parenteral formulas can be supplied either through a peripheral or central vein cannula. The appropriate selection of parenteral access is based upon the status of the patient's peripheral veins, the duration of planned treatment, and the patient's nutrient requirements. Central intravenous feeding is generally reserved for patients who have poor peripheral venous access, who require parenteral feeding for more than a week, and who require repletional levels of nutrient intake.

Peripheral solutions can now be prepared in most American hospitals. Several premixed peripheral intravenous formulas are now available. The composition of a fluid-restricted central vein cardiac formula is presented in Table 26–17. This formula offers the advantage of a high caloric density (1.5 kcal/ml) compared with the standard parenteral formula (1.0 kcal/ml).

4. When considering the potential cardiopulmonary complications of continuous nutrient infusion, we return to the basic concepts developed earlier in the chapter. First, recall that cardiac cachexia may be hemodynamically adaptive by diminishing total-body oxygen consumption, lowering blood pressure, and reducing the cardiac demands associated with meal ingestion. Second, the rate and composition of the formula supplied directly determines the change from fasting energy expenditure, gas exchange, ventilation, and cardiac output. Hence a slow, steady infusion rate of a low-sodium formula should not lead to CHF. Close monitoring of the patient for an S3 gallop, rales, and dependent edema provides the physician with an early warning of worsening CHF. Reducing the formula infusion rate and increasing diuretic therapy will promptly relieve hyperalimentation-associated cardiovascular effects.

A second and related consideration in monitoring the patient is evaluation of hydration status. This assumes particular importance in the patient receiving minimal fluid and sodium intake who also is receiving diuretic therapy. Close attention should be directed toward measuring fluid intake and output, body weight, blood urea nitrogen levels, and urine specific gravity.

The third group of CHF patients requiring nutritional management are those in the postoperative

TABLE 26–15. Elemental and Polymeric Enteral Formulas

PRODUCT/ MANUFACTURER	CALORIC DENSITY (kcal/ml)	KCAL:N RATIO	H₂O (%)	OSMOLALITY (mosm/kg)	VOLUME FOR 100% RDAs (ml)	K (mEq/l)	Na (mEq/l)	P (mg/L)	PROTEIN (%)*	PROTEIN (g/L)	CHO (%)*	CHO (g/L)	FAT LCT (%)*	FAT LCT (g/L)	FAT MCT (%)*	FAT MCT (g/L)	COMMENTS
Elemental																	
Travasorb-HN (Travenol)	1.00	140:1	86	450	2000	30	40	500	18	45	70	175	12	13.3	—	—	Hydrolyzed lactalbumin
Vital High Nitrogen (Ross)	1.00	150:1	84	460	1500	34.1	20.3	667	16.7	41.7	73.9	185	5.2	5.9	4.2	4.86	70% protein as short-chain peptides
Vivonex TEN (Norwich-Eaton)	1.00	163:1	83	630	2000	20	20	500	15.3	38.3	82.2	206	2.5	2.8	—	—	High branched-chain amino acids
Criticare HN (Mead Johnson)	1.06	173:1	83	1060	1887	33.8	27.6	528	14	38	83	222	3	3.4	—	—	70% free amino acids; 30% short-chain peptides
Polymeric																	
Entrition/Entripak (Biosearch)	1.00	178:1	83	300	2000	30.7	30.5	500	14	35	54.5	136	31.5	35	—	—	Ready-to-feed isotonic formula
Sustacal (Mead Johnson)	1.01	104:1	84	625	1080	53.3	40.8	930	24	61.3	55	140	21	23.1	—	—	High protein
Osmolite (Ross)	1.06	178:1	84	300	1887	25.9	23.9	549	14	37.2	54.6	145	15.7	19.25	15.7	19.25	Isotonic; unpalatable for oral use
Osmolite HN (Ross)	1.06	150:1	84	310	1321	40	40.5	761	16.7	44.4	53.3	141	15	18.4	15	18.4	—
Isocal (Mead Johnson)	1.06	192:1	84	300	1887	33.7	23	528	13	34.2	50	133	29.6	35.5	7.4	9	Isotonic; unpalatable for oral use
Susta II (Mead Johnson)	1.06	147:1	84	450	1420	36.2	30.7	707	17	45.1	53	140.5	30	35.3	—	—	Added soy polysaccharide
Compleat Modified (Sandoz)	1.07	156:1	84	300	1495	35.8	55.7	1320	16	42.8	54	140	30	36.8	—	—	Blenderized; contains dietary fiber
Enrich (Ross)	1.10	173:1	83	480	1391	40	36.8	719	14.5	39.7	55	162	30.5	37.2	—	—	Added soy polysaccharide
Precision Isotein HN (Sandoz)	1.20	112:1	85	300	1750	21.7	29.5	576	23	67.8	52	156	18.8	25	6.3	8.3	High-protein isotonic formula powder
Sustacal HC (Mead Johnson)	1.50	160:1	78	650	1800	37.8	36.8	845	16	60.9	50	190	34	57.5	—	—	High-caloric-density formula
Ensure Plus (Ross)	1.50	171:1	77	600	1600	59.5	49.6	634	14.7	54.9	53.3	200	32	53.3	—	—	High-caloric-density formula
Pulmocare (Ross)	1.50	150:1	77.4	490	1000	48.8	56.9	1020	16.7	62.6	28.1	105.4	55.2	92	—	—	High-fat, low-carbohydrate formula
Traumacal (Mead Johnson)	1.50	115:1	78	490	2000	35.7	51.5	748	22	82.4	38	142	28	48	12	20.6	High-caloric-density formula
Isocal HCN (Mead Johnson)	2.00	170:1	71	690	1500	35.8	34.7	668	15	74.8	45	225	28	63.6	12	27.3	High-caloric-density formula

*Percentage of total kilocalories.
RDAs = Recommended Dietary Allowances.
CHO = carbohydrate.
LCT = long-chain triglyceride.
MCT = medium-chain triglyceride.

From Heymsfield SB, Erbland M, Casper K, et al. Clin Chest Med 1986; 7:41–67.

TABLE 26–16. Modular Formula Components

PRODUCT/MANUFACTURER	SOURCE	CALORIC DENSITY	OSMOLALITY (mosm/kg)	PROTEIN (%)*	CHO (%)*	FAT (%)*	Na (mEq/g)	K (mEq/g)	Ca (mEq/g)	P (mg/g)
Protein										
ProPac (Biosearch)	Whey protein (19.5 g/packet)	4.0 kcal/g		77		8	0.10	0.13	6.0	3.1
Pro-Mix R.D. (Navaco)	Whey protein (18.7 g/packet)	3.85 kcal/g		80	5	4	0.11	0.22	3.94	3.4
Nutrisource Protein (Sandoz)	Lactalbumin, egg albumin (19.8 g/packet)	4.04 kcal/g		76	9	7	0.12	0.15	3.54	3.03
Nutrisource Amino Acids (Sandoz)	Amino acids (15.4 g/packet)	3.90 kcal/g		97						
Nutrisource BCAA (Sandoz)	Amino acids with 6.6 g of 15.4 g/packet as BCAAs	3.90 kcal/g		97						
Casec (Mead Johnson)	Calcium caseinate powder	3.70 kcal/g		88		2	0.07	0.003	16	8.0
Fat										
Microlipid (Biosearch)	Safflower oil emulsion	4.5 kcal/ml								
MCT Oil (Mead Johnson)	MCTs; fractionated coconut oil	7.7 kcal/ml								
Nutrisource LCT (Sandoz)	Soybean oil emulsion	2.2 kcal/ml								
Nutrisource MCT (Sandoz)	Deionized corn syrup solids; MCTs	2.0 kcal/ml								
Carbohydrate										
Moducal (Mead Johnson)	Maltodextrin powder	3.8 kcal/g								
Sumacal (Biosearch)	Maltodextrin powder	3.8 kcal/g								
Polycose (Ross)	Glucose polymer of hydrolyzed cornstarch	2 kcal/ml	900							
Pro-Mix (Navaco)	Glucose polymer of hydrolyzed cornstarch	2.5 kcal/ml	315							
Nutrisource Carbohydrate (Sandoz)	Deionized corn syrup solids	3.2 kcal/g	2000							

*Percentage of total kilocalories.
CHO = carbohydrate.
BCAAs = branched-chain amino acids.
From Heymsfield SB, Erbland M, Casper K, et al. Clin Chest Med 1986; 7:41–67.

TABLE 26–17. *2172 mOsm/Liter Central Vein Cardiac Formula*

	Ml	Kcal	CHO (g)	Protein (g)
Freamine 8.5%	360	98		28
Dextrose 70%	500	1190	350	
Total	860	1288	350	28

MVI-12, vitamin K, and trace elements added daily.

Electrolytes adjusted to patient's requirements; does not contain essential fatty acids; fat emulsion can be added.

From Heymsfield SB, Smith JL, Redd S. Surg Clin North Am 1981; *61*:636–653.

period. The major focus in this period are the patients who develop postoperative complications that delay their normal resumption of food intake. This includes subjects whose intake remains inadequate for more than 3 to 5 days. When substandard intake is prolonged for weeks or months, this group of individuals develops "nosocomial cardiac cachexia." All of the same considerations related to the selection of the route, rate, and composition of formula described earlier apply to this group of patients.

References

1. Heymsfield SB, Nutter DO. The heart in protein-calorie undernutrition. *In* Hurst JW (ed). Update I: The Heart. New York, McGraw-Hill, 1979: 191–209.
2. Higginson J, Gillanders AD, Murray JF. The heart in chronic malnutrition. Br Heart J 1951; *13*:177–185.
3. Reid JVO, Berjak P. Dietary production of myocardial fibrosis in the rat. Am Heart J 1966; *71*:240–250.
4. Samen SC. Cardiac disorders in scurvy. N Engl J Med 1970; *282*:282–283.
5. Akbarian M, Yankopoulos NA, Abelmann WH. Hemodynamic studies in beriberi heart disease. Am J Med 1966; *41*:197–212.
6. Rachmilewitz M, Braun K. Electrocardiographic changes and the effect of niacin therapy in pellagra. Br Heart J 1945; 7:72–85.
7. Bragdon JH, Levine HD. Myocarditis in vitamin E deficient rabbits. Am J Pathol 1949; *25*:265–273.
8. Weiss DL, Surawicz B, Rubenstein I. Myocardial lesions of calcium deficiency causing irreversible myocardial failure. Am J Pathol 1949; *25*:265–278.
9. O'Connor LR, Wheeler WS, Bethune JE. Effect of hypophosphatemia on myocardial performance. N Engl J Med 1977; *297*:901–903.
10. Fuller TJ, Nichols WW, Brenner BJ, et al. Reversible depression in myocardial contractility in the dog with experimental phosphorous deficiency. Clin Res 1978; *26*:33A.
11. Chipperfield B, Chipperfield JR, Behr G, et al. Magnesium content of normal heart muscle in areas of hard and soft water. Lancet 1976; *1*:121–122.
12. Dyckner T, Wester P-O. Magnesium deficiency contributing to ventricular tachycardia. Acta Med Scand 1982; *212*:89–91.
13. Klevay LM. The influence of copper and zinc on the occurrence of ischemic heart disease. J Environ Pathol Toxicol 1980; 4:281–287.
14. Coni NK. The myocardium in periodic paralysis. Postgrad Med J 1969; *45*:691–694.
15. Weaver WF, Burchell HB. Serum potassium and the electrocardiogram in hypokalemia. Circulation 1960; *21*:505–521.
16. VanFleet JF, Ferrans VJ, Ruth GR. Ultrastructural altera-

tions in nutritional cardiomyopathy of selenium–vitamin E deficient swine. Lab Invest 1977; *37*:188–200.
17. Collipp PJ, Chen ST. Cardiomyopathy and selenium deficiency in a two-year-old girl. N Engl J Med 1981; *304*(21):1304–1305.
18. Harrison DC, Nelson D. The effects of calcium on isometric tension in isolated heart muscle during coupled pacing. Am Heart J 1967; *74*:663–666.
19. Skinner C, Kenmure ACF. Haemochromatosis presenting as congestive cardiomyopathy and responding to venesection. Br Heart J 1973; *35*:466–468.
20. Wacker WEC, Parisi AF. Magnesium metabolism. N Engl J Med 1968; *278*:772–776.
21. Surawicz B. Relationship between electrocardiogram and electrolytes. Am Heart J 1967; *73*:814–834.
22. Rona G. Experimental aspects of cobalt cardiomyopathy. Br Heart J 1971 (Suppl); *33*:171–174.
23. Boner JM, Freyberg RH. Vitamin D intoxication with metastatic calcification. JAMA 1946; *130*:1208–1210.
24. Mahler HR, Cordes EH. Biological Chemistry. New York, Harper and Row, 1974.
25. Heymsfield SB, Erbland M, Casper K, et al. Enteral nutritional support: metabolic, cardiovascular and pulmonary interrelations. Clin Chest Med 1986; 7:41–67.
26. Bernstein RS, Redmond A, Van Itallie TB. Prevalence and interrelationship of metabolic abnormalities in obese patients. *In* Howard A, Baird IM (eds). Recent Advances in Clinical Nutrition. London, John Libbey, 1981: 191–201.
27. Heymsfield SB, Williams PJ. Nutritional assessment by clinical and biochemical methods. *In* Shils ME, Young VR (eds). Modern Nutrition in Health and Disease. 7th ed. Philadelphia, Lea & Febiger, in press.
28. No entry.
29. Devereux RB, Lutas EM, Casale PN, et al. Standardization of M-mode echocardiographic left ventricular anatomic measurements. Am J Cardiol, in press.
30. Heymsfield SB, Head CA, McManus CB, et al. Respiratory, cardiovascular, and metabolic effects on enteral formulas: influence of formula dose and composition. Am J Clin Nutr 1984; *40*:116–130.
31. Buskirk ER, Taylor H. Relationships between maximal oxygen intake and components of body composition. Fed Proc 1954; *13*:21.
32. Letner C. Geigy scientific tables. Basel, Switzerland, Ciba Geigy, Ltd, 1981: *1*:(8).
33. Vatner SF, Franklin D, Van Citters RL. Coronary and visceral vasoactivity associated with eating and digestion in the conscious dog. Am J Physiol 1970; *219*:1380–1385.
34. Bagatell CJ, Heymsfield SB. Effect of meal size on myocardial oxygen requirements: implications for post–myocardial infarction diet. Am J Clin Nutr 1984; *39*:421–426.
35. Fagan TC, Gourley LA, Sawyer PR, et al. Cardiovascular effects of a meal: clinical implications. Clin Res 1982; *30*(1):7A.
36. Hill JO, DiGirolamo M, Heymsfield S. The thermic effect of food following ingested versus tube-delivered meals. Am J Physiol 1985; *248*:E370–E374.
37. Norryd C, Dencker H, Lunderquist A, et al. Superior mesenteric blood flow during digestion in man. Acta Chir Scand 1975; *141*:197–202.
38. Flatt JP. The biochemistry of energy expenditure. *In* Bray GA (ed). Recent Advances in Obesity Research. London, Newman, 1978: 211–228.
39. Hill JO, DiGirolamo M, Heymsfield S. A new method of measuring the thermic response to fuel. Am J Clin Nutr 1985; *42*:1290–1298.
40. Heymsfield SB, Hill JO, Evert M, et al. Energy expenditure during continuous intragastric infusion of dietary fuel: influence of formula infusion rate. Am J Clin Nutr 1987; *45*:526–533.
41. Galloway J, Stensby J, Heymsfield SB: Thermogenic response to IV hyperalimentation (HA). Clin Res 1979; *27*:226A.

42. West JB. Respiratory Physiology—The Essentials. Baltimore, Williams & Wilkins, 1974.

43. Gray BA, Rogers RM. Management of respiratory failure. *In* Baum GL, Wodinsky E (eds). Textbook of Pulmonary Diseases. 3rd ed. Boston, Little, Brown and Co, 1983.

44. Landsberg L, Young JB. Fasting, feeding and regulation of the sympathetic nervous system. N Engl J Med 1978; *298*:1295–1301.

45. Long CL, Schaffel N, Geiger W. Metabolic response to injury and illness: estimation of energy and protein needs from indirect calorimetry and nitrogen balance. JPEN 1979; *3*:452–456.

46. Askanazi J, Rosenbaum SH, Hyman AI, et al. Respiratory changes induced by the large glucose loads of total parenteral nutrition. JAMA 1980; *243*:1444–1447.

47. Askanazi J, Weissman C, Rosenbaum SH, et al. Nutrition and the respiratory system. Crit Care Med 1982; *10*:163–172.

48. Long CL. The energy and protein requirements of the critically ill patient. *In* Wright RA, Heymsfield SB (eds). Nutritional Assessment. Boston, Blackwell, 1984: 15–26.

49. Nutter DO. Exercise and the heart. *In* Hurst JW (ed). Update I: The Heart. New York, McGraw-Hill, 1979: 235–258.

50. Astrand P-O, Rodahl K. Textbook of Work Physiology. 2nd ed. New York, McGraw-Hill, 1977: 3.

51. Zahorska-Markiewicz B. Thermic effect of food and exercise in obesity. Eur J Appl Physiol 1980; *44*:231–235.

52. Waterlow JC. Classification and definition of protein-calorie malnutrition. Br Med J 1972; *3*:566–569.

53. Braunwald E. Pathophysiology of heart failure. *In* Braunwald WB (ed). Heart Disease: A Textbook of Cardiovascular Medicine. Philadelphia, WB Saunders, 1980: 453–471.

54. Schlant RC, Sonnenblick EH, Gorlin R. Normal physiology of the cardiovascular system. *In* Hurst JW (ed). The Heart. 5th ed. New York, McGraw-Hill, 1982: 75–114.

55. Guyton AC. Textbook of Medicine and Physiology. 6th ed. Philadelphia, WB Saunders, 1981: 52.

56. Heymsfield SB, Bethel R, Ansley JD, et al. Cardiac abnormalities in cachectic patients before and during nutritional repletion. Am Heart J 1978; *95*:584–594.

57. Gottdiener JS, Gross HA, Henry WL, et al. Effects of self-induced starvation on cardiac size and function in anorexia nervosa. Circulation 1978; *58*:425–433.

58. Nutter DO, Heymsfield SB, Murray TM, et al. The effect of chronic protein-calorie undernutrition in the rat on myocardial function and cardiac function. Circ Res 1979; *45*:144–152.

59. Abel RM, Grimes JB, Alonso D, et al. Adverse hemodynamic and ultrastructural changes in dogs' hearts subjected to protein-calorie malnutrition. Circulation 1977; *55*(Suppl 3).

60. Keys A. Circulation and cardiac function. *In* The Biology of Human Starvation. Vol I. Minneapolis, University of Minnesota Press, 1950: 607–634.

61. Ravussin E, Burnand B, Schutz Y, et al. Twenty-four hour energy expenditure and metabolic rate in obese, moderately obese, and control subjects. Am J Clin Nutr 1982; *35*:566–573.

62. Alexander JK, Dennis EW, Smith WG, et al. Blood volume, cardiac output and distribution of systemic blood flow in extreme obesity. Cardiovasc Res Cent Bull 1963; *1*:39–44.

63. DeGirolamo M, Esposito J. Adipose tissue, blood flow and cellularity in the growing rabbit. Am J Physiol 1975; *229*:107–112.

64. Messerli FH, Sundgaard-Riise K, Reisin ED, et al. Dimorphic cardiac adaptation to obesity and arterial hypertension. Ann Intern Med 1983; *99*:757–761.

65. Messerli FH, Sundgaard-Riise K, Reisin E, et al. Disparate cardiovascular effects of obesity and arterial hypertension. Am J Med 1983; *74*:808–812.

66. De Divitiis O, Fazio S, Petitto M, et al. Obesity and cardiac function. Circulation 1981; *64*:477–482.

67. Alexander JK, Pettigrove JR. Obesity and congestive heart failure. Geriatrics 1967; *22*(7):101–108.

68. Smith NL, Willius FA. Adiposity of the heart: a clinical and pathologic study of one hundred and thirty-six obese patients. Arch Intern Med 1933; *52*:911–931.

69. Alexander JK. The heart and obesity. *In* Hurst JW (ed). The Heart. 5th ed. New York, McGraw-Hill, 1982: 1584–1590.

70. Ford LE. Heart size. Circ Res 1976; *39*:297–303.

71. Grossman W, Jones C, McLaurin LP. Wall stress and patterns of hypertrophy in the human left ventricle. J Clin Invest 1975; *56*:56–64.

72. Schlant RC, Sonnenblick EH. Pathophysiology of heart failure. *In* Hurst JW (ed.) The Heart. 5th ed. New York, McGraw-Hill, 1982: 382–407.

73. Zak R. Cardiac hypertrophy and atrophy. *In* Opie L (ed). The Heart: Physiology, Metabolism, Pharmacology, Therapy. London, Grune & Stratton, 1984: 198–209.

74. Wehmann RE, Gregerman RI, Burns WH, et al. Suppression of thyrotropin in the low-thyroxine state of severe nonthyroidal illness. N Engl J Med 1985; *312*:546–552.

75. Curfman GD, O'Hara DS, Hopkins BE, et al. Suppression of myocardial protein degradation in the rat during fasting. Circ Res 1980; *46*:581–589.

76. Glass AR, Burman KD, Dahms WT, et al. Endocrine function in human obesity. Metabolism 1981; *30*(2):89–104.

77. Givers W. Synthesis and turnover of cardiac proteins. *In* Opie L (ed). The Heart: Physiology, Metabolism, Pharmacology, Therapy. London, Grune & Stratton, 1984: 30–39.

78. Sutton MGSJ, Plappert T, Grosby L, et al. Effects of reduced left ventricular mass on chamber architecture, load, and function: a study of anorexia nervosa. Circulation 1985; *72*:991–1000.

79. Roberts WC, Roberts JD. The floating heart or the heart too fat to sink: analysis of 55 necropsy patients. Am J Cardiol 1983; *52*:1286–1289.

80. Ravussin E, Burnand B, Schutz Y, et al. Energy expenditure before and during energy restriction in obese patients. Am J Clin Nutr 1985; *41*:753–759.

81. Vandewoude M, Vrints C, DeLeeuw I. Influence of intravenous hyperalimentation on cardiac dimensions and heart function. Clin Nutr 1982; *1*:193–199.

82. Alleyne GAO. Cardiac function in severely malnourished Jamaican children. Clin Sci 1966; *30*:553–562.

83. Smythe PM, Swanepoel A, Campbell JAH. The heart in kwashiorkor. Br Med J 1962; *7*:67–73.

84. Montgomery RD. Changes in the basal metabolic rate of the malnourished infant and their relation to body composition. J Clin Invest 1962; *41*:1653–1663.

85. Keys A, Henschel A, Taylor HL. The size and function of the human heart at rest in semi-starvation and in subsequent rehabilitation. Am J Physiol 1947; *50*:153–169.

86. Weinsier RL, Krumdieck PHCL. Death resulting from overzealous total parenteral nutrition: the refeeding syndrome revisited. Am J Clin Nutr 1980; *34*:393–399.

87. Isner JM, Roberts WC, Heymsfield SB, et al. Anorexia nervosa and sudden death. Ann Intern Med 1985; *102*:49–52.

88. Bray GA. Effect of caloric restriction on energy expenditure in obese patients. Lancet 1969; *2*:397–399.

89. Sweeney ME, Heymsfield SB, Heller T, et al. Cardiovascular and metabolic effects of short-term semi-starvation. Clin Res 1986; *34*:393A.

90. Van Itallie TB, Yang MU. Cardiac dysfunction in obese dieters: a potentially lethal complication of rapid, massive weight loss. Am J Clin Nutr 1984; *39*:695–702.

91. Sours HE, Fratalli VP, Brand CD, et al. Sudden death associated with very low calorie weight reduction regimens. Am J Clin Nutr 1981; *34*:453–461.

92. Kaltman AJ, Goldring RM. Role of circulatory congestion in the cardiorespiratory failure of obesity. Am J Med 1976; *60*:645–653.

93. Heymsfield SB, Smith JL, Redd S, et al. Nutrition support in cardiac failure. Surg Clin North Am 1981; *61*:636–653.

94. Pittman JG, Cohen P. The pathogenesis of cardiac cachexia. N Engl J Med 1964; *271*:403–409.

95. Pittman JG, Cohen P. The pathogenesis of cardiac cachexia (concluded). N Engl J Med 1964; *271*:453–460.

96. Blackburn GL, Gibbons GW, Bothe A, et al. Nutritional support in cardiac cachexia. J Thorac Cardiovasc Surg 1977; *73*:480–496.

97. Abel RM, Fischer JE, Buckley MJ, et al. Malnutrition in cardiac surgical patients. Arch Surg 1976; *111*:45–50.

98. Abel RM, Paul J. Failure of short-term nutritional convalescence to reverse the adverse hemodynamic effects of protein-calorie malnutrition in dogs. JPEN 1979; *3*:211–214.

99. Heymsfield B, Bleier J, Wenger N. Detection of protein-calorie undernutrition in advanced heart disease. Circulation (Suppl 3) 1977; *56*:102.

100. Wright RA, Heymsfield SB (eds). Nutritional assessment of the adult hospitalized patient. Boston, Blackwell Scientific, 1984.

101. Gibbons GW, Blackburn GL, Vitale J, et al. Pre- and post-operative hyperalimentation in the treatment of cardiac cachexia. J Surg Res 1976; *19*:439–444.

102. Hemysfield SB, Smith J, Hersh T. Home nasoenteric feeding for malabsorption and weight loss refractory to conventional therapy. Ann Intern Med 1983: *98*:168–170.

103. Heymsfield SB, Bethel R, Ansley JD, et al. Enteral hyper-alimentation: an alternative to central intravenous hyperalimentation. Ann Intern Med 1979; *90*:63–71.

104. Smith JL, Heymsfield SB. Enteral nutritional support: formula preparation from modular ingredients. JPEN 1983; *7*:280–288.

27

ANEMIAS

ALLAN J. ERSLEV

Nutritional anemia may very well be the most common malady in this world.[1] Starvation, malnutrition, and alcoholism are of course the somber causes of deficient intake of crucial hematinics, but of at least equal importance is the fact that growth, menstruation, and childbearing challenge the iron and folic acid content of even adequate diets. In order to understand and respond to the pathogenesis of these nutritional anemias, numerous animal and human studies have been carried out on the hematological effect of a deficiency of specific nutrients, vitamins, or trace minerals. However, when the results from these experimental studies are applied to the anemias observed in the field, it is soon realized that nutritional deficiencies rarely involve a single dietary component but usually are complex and multifactorial. Nevertheless, we have to be splitters rather than lumpers, and the description here of nutritional anemia will initially attempt to deal with the effect of the two major courses, iron and folic acid deficiency, one at a time.

Anemia is a hematological disorder characterized by too few red blood cells in circulating blood. Since its clinical manifestations are caused by reduced transport of oxygen from lungs to tissues, it is functionally better defined as a disorder with a reduced oxygen carrying capacity of blood or more conveniently with a reduced hemoglobin concentration. Under normal conditions the hemoglobin concentration is quite stable and maintained within a narrow range (14 to 17 g/dl for males and 12 to 15 g/dl for females). These ranges are set and maintained by a feedback control mechanism in which an oxygen sensor in the kidney responds to changes in the supply and demand for oxygen by regulating the production of a renal erythropoietic hormone, erythropoietin (Fig. 27–1). The proper functioning of this efficient but sluggish control depends on the presence of an intact kidney and a responsive bone marrow. Nutritional deficiencies rarely cause renal failure but unfortunately are the most common cause of bone marrow dysfunction.

CELLULAR KINETICS OF ERYTHROPOIESIS

The production of red blood cells under normal conditions is the prerogative of the bone marrow.

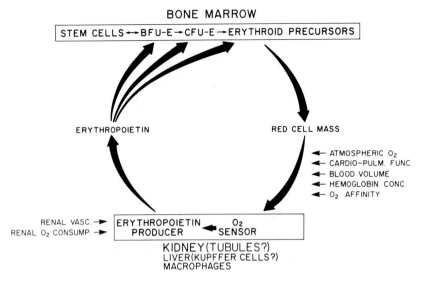

FIGURE 27–1. Feedback control of the red cell mass mediated in one limb by hemoglobin oxygen and in the other limb by erythropoietin. (From Erslev AJ, Gabuzda T. Pathophysiology of Blood. 3rd ed. Philadelphia, WB Saunders Company, 1985.)

Here a small number of pluripotential and self-perpetuating stem cells sustain compartments of unipotential progenitor cells (Fig. 27–2). These small mononuclear cells are morphologically similar to stem cells, but functionally they have become committed to single cell lines. Furthermore, they have lost the unlimited capacity for self-renewal characteristic of the stem cells. Consequently, their proliferation involves a certain degree of maturation and change, and unless finally differentiated to a precursor cell they die. How the stem cells are made to respond to the needs of the progenitor cell compartment is unknown, but it appears as if the stem cells are mainly dormant and are activated only when a depleted progenitor cell compartment needs replenishment.

The progenitor cells committed to the erythroid cell line proliferate extensively, and when cultured on a semisolid medium will display numerous subcolonies growing at a distance from the parent progenitor cell providing a burstlike pattern of growth (BFU-E) (Fig. 27–3). The initial proliferation of these bursts depends on the presence of certain non-specific burst-promoting factors generated by lymphocytes and mononuclear macrophages. Erythropoietin supplements the action of the burst-promoting factors and eventually becomes the primary growth factor for the CFU-E subcultures of the bursts (Fig. 27–4). However, in addition to its growth-promoting action it is a specific erythroid differentiating factor. When the maturation of the progenitor cells has made them ready for differentiation, erythropoietin will transform the CFU-E to the first of the precursor cells, a proerythroblast. The biochemical pathway of this blast transformation is unknown, but it cannot be carried out in the absence of erythropoietin. Subsequent proliferation and maturation are not dependent on the presence of erythropoietin, although it appears that it also has a certain growth-promoting effect on the early precursor cells.

The proliferation and maturation of the erythroid precursor cells are programmed to last 4 to 5 days but are affected by the presence or absence of certain nutritional components. Vitamin B_{12} and folic acid are necessary coenzymes for the synthesis of DNA,

HEMATOPOIESIS

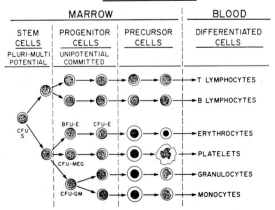

FIGURE 27–2. Outline of hematokinetics. CFU-S, colony-forming unit—spleen; CFU-GM, colony-forming unit—granulocytes, monocytes; CFU-MEG, colony-forming unit—megakaryocytes; BFU-E, burst-forming units—erythroid; CFU-E, colony-forming unit—erythroid. (From Erslev AJ, Gabuzda TG. Pathophysiology of Blood. 3rd ed. Philadelphia, WB Saunders Company, 1985.)

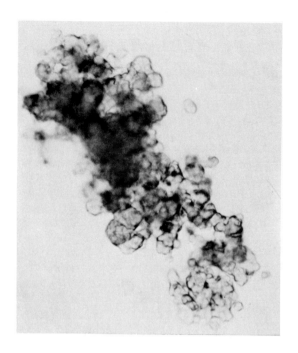

FIGURE 27–3. The appearance of a single burst-forming unit. In color it would be vividly red.

but their absence apparently does not cause a deletion of DNA synthesis but only abnormal synthesis. Certainly, patients with B_{12} and folic acid deficiency have normal or even increased proliferation of progenitor and precursor cells, resulting in a hyperplastic but ineffective erythropoiesis. Iron is needed for the synthesis of hemoglobin, and a deficiency results in the production of microcytic, hemoglobin-deficient red blood cells. However, there is also a decrease in the number of red cells produced, possibly owing to a lack of iron-containing enzymes necessary for normal cellular proliferation. In addition, other vitamins and trace metals may play a role in the formation of red cells and contribute to the fact that nutritional deficiencies are a major cause of red cell precursor failure and anemia.

The subsequent function and life span of mature red cells is only indirectly affected by nutritional deficiencies, since most structural defects are introduced during precursor cell development. However, changes in the lipid composition of plasma, caused by liver dysfunction, may affect the red cell membrane and impair red cell survival.

NUTRITIONAL DEFICIENCIES

Despite the abundance of iron in our environment and the presence of folic acid in most raw foods, the usual daily intake and absorption of these two hematinics are barely adequate to cover normal metabolic demands. Consequently, anemia may develop—if intake is reduced, true nutritional deficiency anemia; or if demands are increased, relative nutritional deficiency. True deficiency rarely occurs for other vitamins or minerals, despite claims by health food devotees, but relative deficiency is not unusual in patients whose metabolic demands are increased because of acquired or inborn errors of metabolism.

FIGURE 27–4. Kinetics of erythroid stem cells with hypothetical receptors for BPF (burst-promoting factor) and EPO (erythropoietin). (From Erslev AJ, Gabuzda T. Pathophysiology of Blood. 3rd ed. Philadelphia, WB Saunders Company, 1985.)

ERYTHROPOIESIS

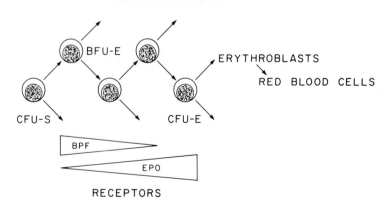

Iron

The average diet contains between 10 and 20 mg of iron of which 5 to 10 per cent or about 1 mg is absorbed. Although the daily need for iron in erythropoiesis and synthesis of various enzymes is 20 to 25 mg, most of this is obtained by recycling, and the 1 mg absorbed appears merely to balance losses in feces, sweat, and desquamated skin.[2] However, this is true only for males and postmenopausal women, while growing children and women in the reproductive age need about twice as much iron. It has actually been estimated that a relative nutritional iron deficiency exists in about 25 per cent of infants, 6 per cent of children, 15 per cent of menstruating women, and 30 per cent of pregnant women.[3,4] In contrast, absolute nutritional deficiencies are uncommon, even among alcoholics on an extremely inadequate diet, and one has to look for increased requirements for iron or excessive loss of iron in every patient who is found to be iron deficient.

The growth spurts of infancy, especially in low birth weight infants, and of adolescence are common times for iron deficiency to appear. The well-nourished infant fed on cow's milk is particularly susceptible because such a diet, although adequate in calories, is a poor source of iron. Fortunately, iron deficiency at birth is rare even if the mother is herself iron deficient. The onset of menstruation doubles the baseline physiologic requirement of 1 mg a day, and a young woman if anemic should probably be given a trial of supplemental iron before an exhaustive hematological search for an explanation is indicated. Pregnancy creates another increase in the daily requirement for iron, which is only initially offset by the cessation of menstruation (Fig. 27–5). The maternal red cell mass expands about 400 ml, corresponding to 400 mg of extra iron, and the fetus requires an additional 300 mg. At the time of birth there is again blood loss, and iron needed for lactation is about equal to what is lost in menstruation.

Surgical bypass of the duodenum, such as in the Billroth type II operation, may cause iron deficiency, since the duodenum is a major site of iron absorption. However, other intestinal malabsorptive conditions only rarely cause impaired absorption of iron. On the other hand, iron deficiency anemia is common after gastrectomy owing to lack of gastric acidity, which promotes absorption, and rapid gastrointestinal transit time, which may lead to oozing of blood.

In general, blood loss is the most important factor in the development of iron deficiency, both physiological as described above and pathological as exemplified by hookworm disease, which is estimated to involve almost half a billion of the world population. Gastrointestinal and uterine bleedings have to be considered first and ruled out in all patients with iron deficiency anemia. Aspirin and alcohol are common and often neglected causes of gastric blood loss. Urinary hematuria, hemoglobinuria, or hemosiderinuria should be ruled out, and one should never forget the existence of overenthusiastic blood donors.

IRON METABOLISM

Iron in food is present both as myoglobin iron in meat and as inorganic iron in plants, but normally only 5 to 10 per cent of the iron is absorbed. The absorption is promoted by gastric acidity and ascorbic acid, which reduces ferric iron to the more accessible ferrous iron. Several chelators in food may promote or hinder absorption, but impaired absorption is rarely a cause of iron deficiency. Actually the absorption, which takes place primarily in the duodenum and proximal jejunum, is finely tuned to admit enough iron to cover losses.[5] This feedback between the needs and the supplies of iron is still only vaguely understood. It has been proposed that there is an intraintestinal pool of transferrin which

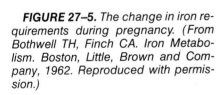

FIGURE 27–5. The change in iron requirements during pregnancy. (From Bothwell TH, Finch CA. Iron Metabolism. Boston, Little, Brown and Company, 1962. Reproduced with permission.)

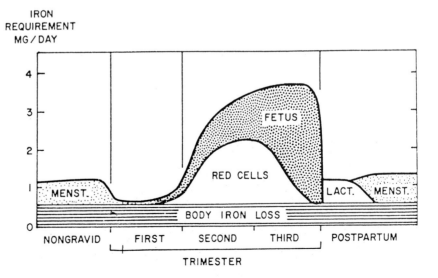

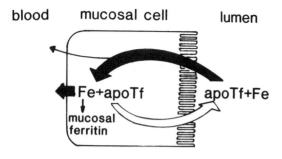

blood   mucosal cell   lumen

FIGURE 27–6. Model for the regulation of iron absorption. (From Huebers, HA, et al. Blood 1983; 61:289. Reproduced with permission.)

binds iron and promotes its entry into the mucosal cells. The size of this pool is in balance with the intracellular pool of transferrin, thereby promoting iron absorption when the pools of transferrin are high and decreasing it when they are low (Fig. 27–6). However, this hypothesis does not explain why the absorption is increased in response to increased erythropoietic activity even when transferrin levels are normal or low.

After absorption the iron is added to a pool of ferric iron bound to transferrin. Most of this pool is provided by reutilized hemoglobin iron from effete red cells. These cells are phagocytized by macrophages, and their iron is packed inside apoferritin protein shells to form molecules of ferritin, which may contain as many as 4000 atoms of iron each. The ferritin iron is either released into the circulation and bound to transferrin or compressed within lysosomes to amorphous aggregates of insoluble ma-

terial called hemosiderin. Hemosiderin granules are visible by light microscopy and provide poorly accessible iron storage. In a normal adult 500 to 1500 mg of iron is present as storage iron while 2500 mg of iron circulates as hemoglobin iron (1 ml of packed red cells contains about 1 mg of iron) (Fig. 27–7). The size of the body pool of storage iron is conveniently assessed by measurement of the concentration of serum ferritin. In normal males the serum ferritin is about 100 μg/ml (Fig. 27–8), but since serum ferritin is an acute phase protein this level is increased in infection, inflammation, or malignancy and may be unreliable as a measure of the stores. Under those conditions it is necessary to evaluate the amount of tissue iron present directly from iron stains of marrow particles.

The iron transported bound to transferrin constitutes only 4 to 5 mg, but it has a rapid turnover and provides the maturing erythroblasts in bone

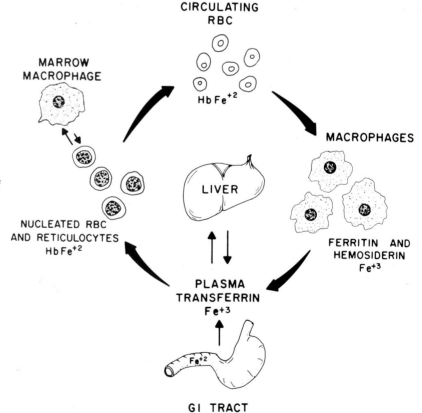

FIGURE 27–7. Metabolic pathways of iron. (From Erslev AJ, Gabuzda T. Pathophysiology of Blood. 3rd ed. Philadelphia, WB Saunders Company, 1985.)

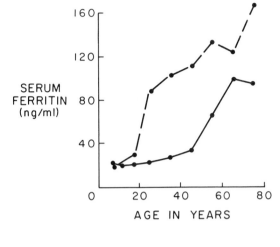

FIGURE 27–8. Normal serum ferritin values for men (interrupted lines) and women (solid lines) at different ages. (Adapted from Cook JD, Finch CA, Smith NJ. Blood 1976; 48:451.)

marrow with about 20 to 30 mg of iron a day for hemoglobin synthesis. The erythroblasts have receptors for the iron-transferrin complex, and this complex is pinocytosed into the cytoplasm of the erythroblasts and reticulocytes. Here the iron is split off and incorporated into heme, while the transferrin is regurgitated and reutilized as an iron carrier. Each transferrin molecule is able to ferry two atoms of iron, and it has been proposed that saturated, diferric transferrin will deliver its iron to erythroblasts more readily than will a monoferric transferrin molecule.[6] This may play a role in hindering the delivery of iron in iron deficiency anemia, in which the transferrin level is high and most of the molecules are monoferric, and enhance the delivery of iron in anemia of chronic disease, in which the transferrin level is low and more saturated.

IRON DEFICIENCY ANEMIA

The first change in development of iron deficiency is the loss of storage iron in the mononuclear macrophage system. A decrease in plasma ferritin concentration parallels this loss. After the stores of iron are used up the plasma iron concentration falls, at the same time stimulating an increase in the synthesis of transferrin and an increase in the absorption of iron from the intestine. The saturation of transferrin with iron falls from about 30 per cent to values often below 10 per cent. Erythrocyte protoporphyrin levels are increased secondary to the intracellular deficit of sufficient iron for heme synthesis. The measurements of these levels are being used increasingly for screening for iron deficiency. Anemia is the last change to be observed. At first only the hemoglobin concentration is decreased, and the number of red cells may actually be increased as a sign of increased erythropoietin production. However, as the anemia becomes more severe the absolute red cell count decreases, the cells become microcytic and hypochromic, with changes in size and shape (Fig. 27–9). The indices show a decrease in mean corpuscular volume (MCV), but using electronic counting equip-

ment the mean corpuscular hemoglobin concentration (MCHC) is rarely altered.

Iron deficiency per se may cause some characteristic signs and symptoms. The activities of certain iron-containing enzymes decrease, but this change may not be of pathophysiological significance. However, if iron deficiency is protracted, there may be changes in the curvature of the fingernails (spooning), the nails and hair become more brittle, and there may be glossitis and fissures around the edge of the mouth. Dysphagia with web formation in the upper esophagus is a rare complication of severe iron deficiency. There may be gastrointestinal blood losses, presumably owing to mucosal friability, and women may develop menorrhagia aggravating an already existent iron deficiency. The anemia itself is often well tolerated except when there is acute blood loss or cardiovascular limitations. The granulocytes do not seem to be affected. There may be an increase in the platelet count, especially in children; the reason for this increase is not clear.

Differential diagnosis between iron deficiency anemia and other causes of microcytosis is usually not difficult if one has laboratory facilities measuring serum iron, transferrin, and ferritin.[7] A low serum iron concentration is a hallmark of both iron deficiency anemia and the anemia of chronic disease, but serum transferrin concentration is elevated in iron deficiency and normal or low in anemia of chronic disease. On the other hand, serum ferritin is low in iron deficiency and normal or high in anemia of chronic disease. Thalassemia trait is a common cause of microcytosis but is characterized by a significant family history and normal iron studies.

MANAGEMENT

Iron compounds given by mouth are usually well absorbed but are often associated with some mild gastrointestinal symptoms; it is wise to begin slowly with one tablet a day (i.e., ferrous sulfate 300 mg) and work up to a total of three tablets a day. The response is usually gratifying after a few weeks of

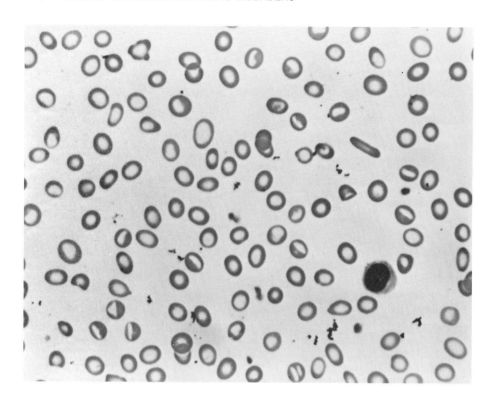

FIGURE 27–9. *Morphology of the red cells in serum iron deficiency anemia. (From Erslev AJ, Gabuzda T. Pathophysiology of Blood. 3rd ed. Philadelphia, WB Saunders Company, 1985.)*

treatment, with an increase in the hemoglobin concentration. However, the body stores may not be replenished until after several months of sustained medication. Prophylaxis against iron deficiency in menstruating or pregnant women does not require large doses of iron, and one tablet of ferrous sulfate a day should be adequate. If the patient does not respond to oral iron therapy, there may be two explanations—that the patient is not taking the medication, or that the blood is being lost as fast as it is being made. In either case parenteral iron can be used intramuscularly or intravenously. Iron given intravenously should be given slowly, preceded by a test dose; if tolerated, as in most individuals, it can be given at a rate of 1 to 2 g per session and the stores can be replenished rapidly.

Folic Acid

Folic acid and its derivatives are present in many different foods—leafy green vegetables, fruits, meats, eggs—and the minimal daily requirement of 50 μg should be met easily on even a marginal diet. However, much of the folic acid is not readily available, and the officially recommended daily intake is 400 μg, a more realistic figure.[8] When this is compared with the total body store of about 5000 μg, it can be seen that the body can easily be depleted of folic acid by sustained poor intake. Such depletion occurs far more easily than is the case for vitamin B_{12}, the body stores of which are about 1000 times as large as the officially recommended daily intake

of 5 μg. Nevertheless, folic acid is present in abundance, and one has to be on a severely limited diet in order not to meet the daily folic acid requirements.[9] Such limited diets, however, are not unusual; they are experienced, for example, by many elderly recluses who eat out of frying pans or live on tea and toast. Chronic alcoholics are also vulnerable because of limited intake of solid food and impaired hepatic metabolism of folic acid.[10,11] Furthermore, and probably of most importance, excessive cooking of vegetables, as is practiced in many countries, will destroy folic acid.[12]

These conditions will challenge the adequacy of folic acid intake, but will usually not alone cause an overt megaloblastic anemia. For this to happen the demand must also be increased, as is the case during growth and pregnancy.[13] It has actually been claimed that one third of all pregnant women in the world experience severe enough folic acid deficiency to develop megaloblastic anemia.[3] Fortunately, babies born of even severely depleted mothers rarely have folic acid deficiency. Conditions characterized by increased cellular proliferation such as hemolytic anemia,[14] exfoliative skin disease, thyrotoxicosis, and hyperalimentation also increase the demand for folic acid.[13] Malabsorption due to sprue or other intestinal disorders demands an increased intake of folic acid in order to prevent the development of megaloblastic anemia. In nontropical sprue or gluten-sensitive enteropathy folic acid deficiency is especially prominent, since the disease process primarily involves the upper reaches of the bowel, in which folic acid is absorbed.[15] Tropical sprue, on the other hand, involves the entire gut and causes impaired absorption of both folic acid and vitamin B_{12}.[16] Patients treated for seizure disorders with phenytoin derivatives may develop a folic acid–responsive megaloblastic anemia, but the pathogenesis is not clear. On the other hand, methotrexate-induced megaloblastosis appears to be due to impaired reduction of folic acid to its biologically active form tetrahydrofolic acid.

FOLIC ACID METABOLISM

Pteroylglutamic acid or folic acid is made up of pteroic acid (composed of pteridine with a para-aminobenzoic acid residue) and glutamic acid (Fig. 27–10). In food it exists as a polyglutamate, which must be broken down to a monoglutamate in the intestine to permit efficient absorption.[17] Following absorption the pteroyl moiety is reduced by the enzyme dihydrofolate reductase first to dehydrofolate and then to tetrahydrofolate. It is this reduction that is inhibited by minute concentrations of the chemotherapeutic compound methotrexate. Plasma folate exists almost entirely as an N^5-methyl tetrahydrofolate, but after cellular uptake the methyl group is removed and folic acid becomes biologically active as tetrahydrofolate. Its size and activity are increased by the addition of several glutamic acid residues, but the initial demethylation is the crucial process that renders it an important carrier and donor of one-carbon compounds such as formyl, methylene, hydroxymethyl, methenyl, formamine, and methyl. Since vitamin B_{12} is a coenzyme for demethylation and since vitamin B_{12} deficiency results in an increase in the concentration of inactive circulating methyl tetrahydrofolate, it has been suggested that B_{12} is the intracellular gate keeper for demethylation and activation of folic acid, the so-called methyl-trap hypothesis (Fig. 27–10).[18] The clinical interrelationship between folic acid and vitamin B_{12} is

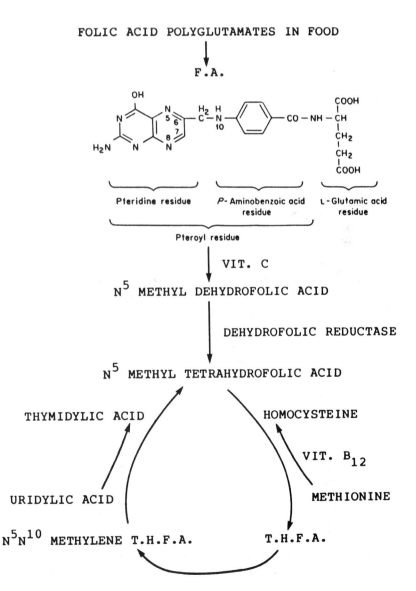

FIGURE 27–10. Outline of folic acid metabolism from food to the biologically active tetrahydrofolic acid (T.H.F.A.). This outline depicts the hypothesis of the methyl trap caused by vitamin B_{12} deficiency. It also shows one of the most important one-carbon transfers T.H.F.A. is involved in, the change from an RNA base, uridine, to a DNA base, thymidine.

unquestionable, but the trap hypothesis is still a hypothetical explanation for this relationship.[19]

The active intracellular tetrahydrofolates play a role in a number of metabolic reactions but are particularly important in the transformation of uridylate to thymidylate, or in other words in the synthesis of DNA and normal nuclear development (Fig. 27–10).

Although folic acid deficiency is not notable for its neurologic sequelae, rare inborn errors in the metabolism of folic acid have been associated with mental retardation. Consequently, the possibility that the common deficiency of folic acid during growth may be detrimental to normal mental development is a concern.[20]

FOLIC ACID DEFICIENCY ANEMIA

The signs and symptoms of folic acid deficiency primarily relate to the hemopoietic and gastrointestinal systems.[21] There is a moderate anemia, which is usually well tolerated in individuals with normal cardiac and pulmonary functions. Sclerae are often slightly icteric, the tongue is smooth and atrophic, and splenomegaly may be present. There may also be diarrhea or vague gastrointestinal complaints, even in patients without an underlying malabsorption disorder.

Laboratory examination discloses a macrocytic anemia with the presence of macro-ovalocytes on the blood smear (Fig. 27–11). Since folic acid deficiency involves the proliferation of all bone marrow precursor cells, there is also a reduction in the number of granulocytes and thrombocytes, but this is rarely severe enough to cause infections or hemorrhagic problems. The granulocytes display a characteristic multilobed appearance, and in a widely quoted study Herbert showed that the first laboratory evidence of folic acid deficiency was the appearance of multilobed granulocytes.[22] Distinctive morphologic changes are also present in the epithelial cells of the gastrointestinal tract, but the diagnosis rests on finding "megaloblastic" changes in bone marrow precursor cells. The bone marrow is extremely cellular with a preponderance of immature precursor cells. This is due to a partial maturation arrest as well as intramedullary destruction of maturing cells. All cell lines show evidence of impaired nuclear maturation, but these "megaloblastic" changes are most notable in the erythroid precursors. As these mature they display an arrest in nuclear development while cytoplasmic hemoglobinization proceeds undisturbed. This "nuclear-cytoplasmic dissociation" is a reflection of impaired DNA synthesis but intact RNA synthesis and results in the formation of large and short-lived macrocytes. The marrow granulocyte precursors also show distinctive changes, in particular, large horseshoe-shaped nuclear forms at the late stage of maturation (Fig. 27–11).

The diagnosis of folic acid deficiency anemia rests on the history, the bone marrow morphology, and measurements of the serum concentration of folic acid. Deficiency of vitamin B_{12} will cause almost identical changes in the bone marrow, but is rarely caused by poor nutrition. However, in questionable cases a serum concentration of folic acid of below 2.0 ng/ml indicates folic acid deficiency. Red cell folate concentration more accurately reflects tissue stores and is less than 135 ng/ml packed cells in deficient states. Despite these diagnostic aids, folic acid deficiency may be difficult to recognize in hospitalized patients partaking in a normal diet days before the diagnostic work-up is begun.

With treatment, the signs and symptoms promptly revert to normal within a few days. Megaloblastic changes and signs of premature red cell destruction such as elevated bilirubin and serum lactic dehydrogenase disappear. The reticulocyte count reaches a peak 7 to 10 days after onset of treatment, and the hemoglobin concentration slowly returns to normal. Concomitantly, diarrhea and other gastrointestinal symptoms improve even in patients with an unrelated malabsorptive disease. The usual therapeutic doses of folic acid are 1 to 5 mg daily. In patients with folic acid deficiency due to intoxication by amethopterin, which blocks the reduction of folic acid to tetrahydrofolic acid, folic acid treatment is of no use. In such patients the "rescue" is to use citrovorum factor, N^5-formyl tetrahydrofolic acid, which bypasses the block in reduction. Preventive treatment in patients with an increase in demand for folic acid, such as in growth or pregnancy, should be about 1 mg a day.

Other Nutrients

Combined folic acid and iron deficiency: As mentioned before, multiple deficiencies frequently occur in malnourished individuals.[23] This can lead to difficulties in the recognition of the cause of anemia, since the microcytosis of iron deficiency may cancel the macrocytosis of folic acid deficiency. In the bone marrow the folic acid–deficient megaloblastic features of red cell precursors may also be less characteristic and lead to diagnostic uncertainties. Fortunately, the megaloblastic features of granulocyte precursors are rarely altered by iron deficiency, and the presence of multilobed circulating granulocytes should always raise the suspicion of folic acid deficiency and thus demands a determination of the serum concentration of this vitamin.

Vitamin B_{12} deficiency is, as stated before, rarely caused by inadequate intake. The minimal daily requirement of 5 μg[8] is difficult not to meet even in a severely restricted diet, and only the strictest vegetarians should be suspected of having an absolute nutritional vitamin B_{12} deficiency. However, in patients with intestinal illnesses involving the distal ileum an absorption defect may lead to a relative

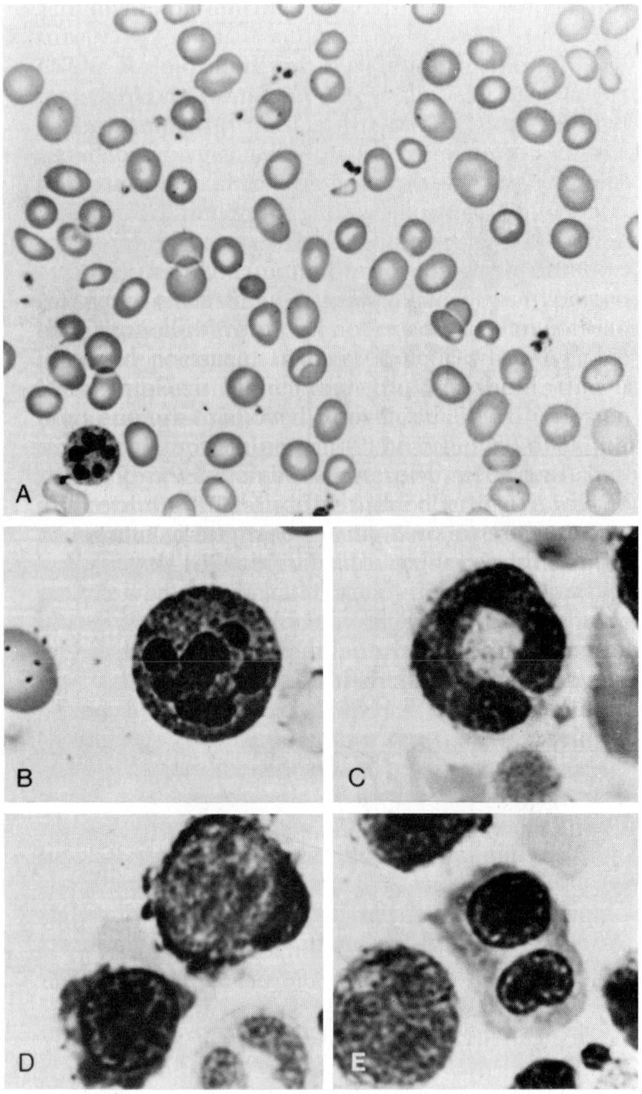

FIGURE 27–11. Morphologic manifestations of megaloblastic anemia. A, Blood film shows ovalomacrocytosis. B, Hypersegmented granulocyte. C, Large C-shaped band cell. D and E, Characteristic changes in marrow erythroid cells. (From Erslev AJ, Gabuzda T. Pathophysiology of Blood. 3rd ed. Philadelphia, WB Saunders Company, 1985.)

deficiency of vitamin B_{12}.[24] In patients with intestinal blind loops or with fish tapeworms, there is a competition for vitamin B_{12} between intestinal micro- or macroorganisms and the absorptive stretch of the ileum, occasionally causing a relative nutritional deficiency. The clinical manifestations of such a relative nutritional deficiency are almost identical with those of folic acid deficiency, and the differential diagnosis rests on determination of the serum concentration of vitamin B_{12}. Neurologic complications characteristic of the severe vitamin B_{12} deficiency found in patients with pernicious anemia due to lack of intrinsic factor should be looked for but are rarely observed in patients with a relative nutritional deficiency.

Nutritional pyridoxine or vitamin B_6 deficiency has not been demonstrated for certain to produce anemia. However, some patients with sideroblastic anemia may respond partially to the administration of pyridoxine without actually being pyridoxine deficient.[25] Deficiencies in other components of the vitamin B group such as *riboflavin* or *niacin* are also rarely if ever the cause of anemia.[26] However, a deficiency of vitamin A has been claimed to cause anemia frequently. This is especially the case for infants and for malnourished individuals in the developing countries, but it has not been recognized for certain in the United States. The manifestations are similar to those of iron deficiency anemia, with the production of microcytic and hypochromic red blood cells.

Vitamin C deficiency anemia is as rare as claims to the contrary are common. Although most patients with scurvy are anemic, the anemia rarely responds to vitamin C but rather to iron or folic acid. Nevertheless, vitamin C may have a supportive role in the reduction of folic acid to tetrahydrofolate and in the intestinal absorption of iron and should be added to the diet of patients with nutritional deficiencies of folic acid and iron.[26]

Vitamin E deficiency has been reported to cause a

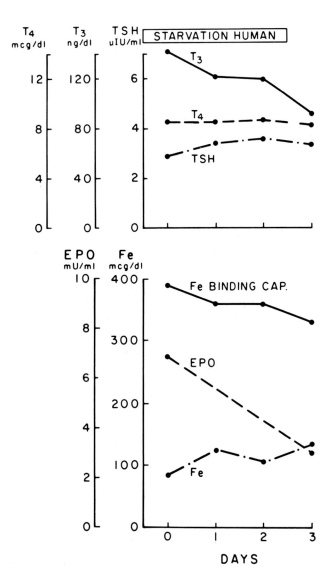

FIGURE 27–12. The effect of 4 days of absolute starvation in normal man on the serum levels of thyroid hormones, erythropoietin, iron, and transferrin.

hemolytic anemia in some premature babies, but otherwise has not been found to be responsible for overt anemia.

Copper deficiency has been reported to cause anemia in some infants and adults receiving parenteral alimentation. The anemia is hypochromic and microcytic and may be caused by an impaired iron metabolism induced by lack of copper.

In children severe protein deprivation (*kwashiorkor*) or protein and caloric deprivation (*marasmus*) cause anemia, but the pathogenesis is not clear. There is usually little change in the production of granulocytes and platelets, although the affected children have a decreased resistance to infection, but there is a striking erythroid hypoplasia of the bone marrow. There is also a reduction in the serum concentration of erythropoietin and in the levels of T_3 and T_4 (Fig. 27–12), and it appears that starvation will induce a hypothyroid state with reduced metabolic turnover and oxygen need.[27] Consequently, one aspect of the anemia is a physiologic adaptation to decreased metabolic activity. Another aspect is fluid imbalance with an increased plasma volume resulting in a dilution anemia. Finally, deficiencies in vitamins and essential amino acids may play a role, but such deficiencies often first become manifest during treatment with high-calorie diets.[26]

References

1. DeMaeyer E, Adiels-Tegman M. The prevalence of anemia in the world. World Health Stat Q 1985; *38*:302–316.
2. Erslev AJ, Gabuzda TG. Pathophysiology of Blood. 3rd ed. Philadelphia, WB Saunders, 1985: 87–97.
3. Herbert V. Anemias. *In* Paige DM (ed). Manual of Clinical Nutrition. Pleasantville, NY, Nutrition Publications, 1983: 35.1–35.24.
4. Cook JD, Lynch SR. The liabilities of iron deficiency. Blood 1986; *68*:803–809.
5. Charlton RW, Bothwell TH. Iron absorption. Ann Rev Med 1983; *34*:55–68.
6. Heubers HA, Finch CA. Transferrin: physiologic behavior and clinical implications. Blood 1984; *64*:763–767.

7. Cook JD. Clinical evaluation of iron deficiency. Semin Hematol 1982; *19*:6–18.
8. Food and Nutrition Board, National Research Council. Recommended Dietary Allowances. 9th ed. Washington, National Academy of Sciences, 1980.
9. Food and Nutrition Board, National Research Council. Folic Acid: Biochemistry and Physiology in Relation to the Human Nutrition Requirement. Washington, National Academy of Sciences, 1977.
10. Jandl JH, Lear AA. The metabolism of folic acid in cirrhosis. Ann Intern Med 1956; *45*:1027–1044.
11. Hillman RS, Steinberg SE. The effects of alcohol on folate metabolism. Ann Rev Med 1982; *33*:345–354.
12. O'Brien W. Acute military tropical sprue in Southeast Asia. Am J Clin Nutr 1968; *21*:1007–1012.
13. Colman N, Herbert V. Dietary assessment with special emphasis on prevention of folate deficiency. *In* Botez MI, Reynolds EH (eds). Folic Acid in Neurology, Psychiatry and Internal Medicine. New York, Raven Press, 1979: 63–74.
14. Jandl JH, Greenberg MS. Bone marrow failure due to relative nutritional deficiency in Cooley's hemolytic anemia. N Engl J Med 1959; *260*:461–468.
15. Jeffries GH, Weser E, Sleisenger MH. Malabsorption. Gastroenterology 1969; *56*:777–797.
16. Gardner FH. Tropical sprue. N Engl J Med 1958; *258*:791–835.
17. Beck WS. Metabolic aspects of vitamin B_{12} and folic acid. *In* Williams WJ, Beutler E, Erslev AJ, et al. (eds). Hematology. 3rd ed. New York, McGraw-Hill, 1983: 311–331.
18. Scott JM, Weir DG. The methyl folate trap. Lancet 1981; *2*:337–340.
19. Chanarin J, Deacon R, Lumb, et al. Cobalamin-folate interrelations: a critical review. Blood 1985; *66*:479–489.
20. Erbe RW. Inborn errors of folate metabolism. N Engl J Med 1975; *293*:753–757.
21. Erslev AJ, Gabuzda T. Pathophysiology of Blood. 3rd ed. Philadelphia; WB Saunders, 1985: 71–82.
22. Herbert V. Experimental nutritional folate deficiency in man. Trans Assoc Am Phys 1962; *75*:307–320.
23. Herbert V. Megaloblastic anemia with two nutrient deficiencies: two cases. Med Grand Rounds 1982; *1*:320–336.
24. Seethram B, Alpers DH. Absorption and transport of cobalamin (vitamin B_{12}). Ann Rev Nutr 1982; *2*:343–369.
25. Erslev AJ, Lear AA, Castle WB. Pyridoxine-responsive anemia. N Engl J Med 1960; *262*:1209–1214.
26. Oski FA. Anemia related to nutritional deficiencies other than vitamin B_{12} and folic acid. *In* Williams WJ, Beutler E, Erslev AJ, et al. (eds). Hematology. 3rd ed. New York, McGraw-Hill, 1983: 532–537.
27. Caro J, Silver R, Erslev AJ, et al. Erythropoietin production in fasted rats. Effect of thyroid hormones and glucose supplementation. J Lab Clin Med 1981; *98*:860–868.

28

RESPIRATORY DISEASES

JEFFREY ASKANAZI / SUSAN GOLDSTEIN
VLADIMIR KVETAN / JOHN M. KINNEY

Malnutrition in hospitalized patients is associated with functional deterioration, including reduced respiratory muscle strength and endurance[1-3] (associated with decreased diaphragmatic mass). Under these conditions a reduction of the ventilatory response to hypoxemia is observed.[4] In patients with chronic obstructive pulmonary disease (COPD) the development of malnutrition serves to exacerbate the already existing functional impairments. Unfortunately, weight loss is not only a serious development but also a common occurrence in chronic lung disease. As many as 40 per cent of patients diagnosed with COPD experience progressive weight loss, which is associated with a higher rate of mortality[5] in this subgroup. When weight loss develops in a patient with COPD, the average life expectancy is only 2.9 years.[6] In addition, these patients often become sedentary owing to shortness of breath upon exertion.

Chronic obstructive pulmonary disease is often categorized into two groups that characterizes the patient's disease state and general appearance. Emphysema patients are considered the "pink puffers" who have hyperinflated lungs and low body weight. Patients with chronic bronchitis are often termed "blue bloaters." The name refers to their tendency to be overweight and to retain carbon dioxide.[7] The former group tends to have lung deterioration that corresponds to the degree of nutritional depletion. In addition, the pink puffers can be further divided into those with normal levels of arterial CO_2 and CO_2 retainers. It appears that end-stage emphysema patients start to develop symptoms that are traditionally associated with chronic bronchitis, such as excessive mucosal secretions and CO_2 retention.

CLINICAL IMPACT AND ETIOLOGY OF WEIGHT LOSS

A number of investigators have observed an association between weight loss and clinical deterioration in patients with COPD. Sukumalchantra and

Williams[8] followed 44 COPD patients during a 5-year period and found that the maximal midexpiratory flow rate (MMF) and the lung diffusing capacity (D_{CO}) were reduced in the 12 patients who lost more than 10 per cent of their initial weight. In the 32 patients who had no weight loss, there was no change in the MMF; however, D_{CO} did drop significantly. Results of studies by Vandenbergh et al.[5] and Burrows[9] have shown that there is a progressive decline in body weight with advancing pulmonary disease. In addition, this progressive weight loss in COPD patients is associated with negative effects on lung function,[10] including an increase in mortality rates and an increased incidence of heart failure compared with those in COPD patients without weight loss.[1,11,12] Others have shown that weight loss in COPD patients is directly associated with the degree of obstruction to airflow and the severity of the disease.[1,11,13]

In malnourished patients without COPD, it has been shown that a severe reduction in body cell mass is associated with significantly lower respiratory muscle strength, specifically a lower peak inspiratory force ($P_I$max).[14] Contrary to popular belief these studies show there is reduced diaphragm weight, respiratory muscle strength, and endurance in malnourished patients without concomitant clinical signs of pulmonary disease.[2,3] In addition, an increased need for mechanical ventilator support has been observed in malnourished patients without COPD.[15,16] The respiratory muscles appear to be directly affected by undernutrition. This suggests that malnourished patients with COPD would face even greater demands.

It is apparent that weight loss does not occur in all patients with COPD. Openbrier et al.[17] investigated the nutritional status of two groups of COPD patients and found that nutritional depletion is more prevalent in patients with emphysema as compared with those with chronic bronchitis. Patients with emphysema are found to be somatically depleted of protein, and the degree of nutritional depletion is significantly correlated with the degree of lung dysfunction. Many investigators agree that the weight loss in patients with COPD is associated with a marasmic type of protein-calorie malnutrition[13,18] involving equal weight loss from all body compartments without a decline in serum albumin.

The cause of the weight loss in patients with COPD is poorly understood. A number of investigators have attributed this weight loss to a decrease in caloric intake.[1,19] More recently, however, investigators have suggested an additional cause of weight loss due to an increase in the total energy expenditure resulting from the underlying disease process. In malnourished patients with COPD, Hunter et al.[13] found that caloric intake was well above predicted energy needs, averaging 2535 kcal/day. Other studies, including our own, have supported the concept that weight loss is probably due to an increased resting energy expenditure.[20,21] We have demonstrated that energy expenditure was increased 15 per cent ($\pm$ 4 SE) prior to nutritional repletion and 27 per cent ($\pm$ 4 SE) during the nutritional repletion program. This is unlike the pattern we observe in malnourished surgical patients who are hypometabolic prior to nutritional repletion with an energy expenditure that equals predicted normal during a nutritional repletion program ($1.7 \times$ REE). The increase in resting energy expenditure may be due to an increased work of breathing. Since $\dot{V}_E$ was within normal limits in this group of patients, the increased work of breathing must have been due to a greater load per breath. It has been suggested that weight loss of COPD may be beneficial because metabolic demands are reduced and this leads to lower ventilatory requirements, alleviating the overworked respiratory muscles. Tirlapur and Afzal[22] have demonstrated that a low intake of calories and carbohydrate with concomitant weight loss decreases arterial P_{CO_2} and improves respiratory muscle strength in overweight hypercapnic patients with COPD. It is clear, however, that this is a different patient population with a less serious clinical picture. In normal-weight COPD patients such as in our patient population, weight loss appears to have negative consequences, such as deterioration in respiratory and skeletal muscle strength. Weight loss may be appropriate therapy for overweight patients to alleviate acute physiological abnormalities, but is inappropriate for COPD patients of normal body weight.

METABOLIC DEMAND AND VENTILATORY DRIVE

Nutritional intake not only influences lung function by altering body composition and improving defense mechanisms, but also influences respiratory function through alterations in metabolic demand and ventilatory drive. Increasing glucose intake is a stimulus to ventilation, primarily owing to increased CO_2 production. Carbohydrate is oxidized with a higher respiratory quotient than is lipid. Numerous researchers have reported a large rise in CO_2 production with the administration of hypertonic glucose,[23–25] which leads to respiratory distress in patients. This is especially true in patients with previously existing lung dysfunction. In malnourished unstressed patients, there is a marked rise in CO_2 production when intravenous solutions of glucose and amino acids are administered; the RQ may rise to 1.0 or above if lipogenesis occurs. In malnourished stressed patients, O_2 consumption as well as CO_2 production rises markedly with a more modest rise in the RQ. In either case the rise in CO_2 production will increase the level of ventilation required. Substitution of a fat emulsion for part of the glucose will decrease ventilatory demand.[26] Intravenous lipid infusions may decrease the diffusing capacity of O_2 across the alveoli;[27] however, this phenomenon has never been observed with an oral fat-based diet.

Recent studies have demonstrated that infusion of amino acids results in enhanced ventilatory response to a CO_2 stimulus.[28] Normal subjects receiving 5 per cent dextrose followed by intravenous infusion of amino acids demonstrated an enhanced sensitivity to CO_2 during the amino acid infusion. Increasing protein intake to 21 g of nitrogen per day with a fixed caloric intake to high levels further enhances the ventilatory response above that observed with a lower nitrogen intake (11 g/day). Increasing glucose intake alone in the absence of amino acids appears to have minimal effects on ventilatory sensitivity.[29] Since ventilatory drive may often be markedly increased in many patients with COPD,[30] further increases induced by nutritional support may be contraindicated. The COPD patients who received a high-carbohydrate diet in the present study had increased ventilation secondary to an increased CO_2 production similar to responses observed in patients without COPD. The effect of amino acid infusions to increase ventilatory drive and the effect of glucose infusions to increase CO_2 production suggest that both protein and glucose must be given in limited quantities. For this reason, a high-fat diet might be beneficial for the patient with severe dyspnea or the patient being weaned from mechanical ventilation. Recent studies by Takala et al.[31,32] demonstrate that the effect of amino acids on respiration is a function of the amino acid profile of the infusion. A solution enriched with the branched-chain amino acids has a greater effect on the minute ventilation–arterial Pa_{CO_2} regression than does an infusion of a commercial amino acid solution. The hypothesis presented by Takala et al. suggests that amino acids may serve to stimulate ventilation by alterations in neurotransmitter synthesis. Tryptophan is a precursor to serotonin and competes with the large neutral amino acids (including valine, leucine, and isoleucine) for brain uptake. Increases in valine, leucine, and isoleucine concentration in plasma could serve to reduce tryptophan uptake and hence serotonin production.[33] Since serotonin is regarded as a respiratory inhibitor, a reduction could serve to stimulate ventilation.[34]

RESPIRATORY AND SKELETAL MUSCLES

It has been demonstrated that respiratory muscle mass and function are compromised in both malnutrition and COPD. The diaphragm, being the principal muscle of respiration, is often used to exemplify the entire respiratory system. Malnutrition can result in deterioration in both peripheral[35] and respiratory muscle function[36] that exceeds the loss of muscle mass. In addition, malnourished patients undergoing nutritional repletion improve muscle function within 2 weeks, which is long before lean body mass is completely restored. This may indicate that the compromise in muscle function may be due, primarily, to low supply of short-term energy stores and/or biochemical adverse alterations of the remaining muscle cells. The changes of muscle function may be due to an increased intracellular calcium concentration found during hypocaloric dieting or a faulty Na-K ATPase cellular mechanism.[37]

Reports indicate that the diaphragm atrophies in malnourished patients[1,38] and may also atrophy in patients with COPD uncomplicated by malnutrition.[39] Thus, the combination of malnutrition and COPD may be particularly detrimental.[38] Arora and Rochester have shown that patients who are underweight have a reduced diaphragm muscle mass, area, and length independent of the disease state.[3] Diaphragm muscle area has been shown to be reduced in patients with COPD.[39] These same reports have suggested that there is a significant inverse correlation between diaphragmatic area and the extent of the pulmonary disease in patients with emphysema. However, others have shown that the dimensions of the diaphragm are within normal limits in patients with COPD whose body weight was normal at the time of death.[40] In a well-controlled study of elastase-induced emphysema in hamsters, remodeling of diaphragm structure occurred without any effect on mass.[40] Chronic increased respiratory workloads in rodents have also been shown to cause histochemical changes in muscle and an increased oxidative capacity of the diaphragm.[41] Patients with emphysema and weight loss have a reduction in diaphragm weight that exceeds the loss of body weight.[4] This is similar to the alterations in diaphragm weight observed in malnourished patients without lung disease. Sternocleidomastoid muscle thickness, assessed using anthropometric techniques, is reduced in patients with COPD who are of normal weight and even further reduced in COPD patients who have lost weight.[42] In summary, it would appear that COPD probably does not cause changes in diaphragm weight independent of changes in whole body weight but does appear to cause histological and biochemical adaptations in the diaphragm.

Studies have found that respiratory muscle strength is decreased with COPD.[43,44] In these studies respiratory muscle strength was measured using maximum static inspiratory and expiratory ($P_I$max, $P_E$max) pressures, and it was demonstrated that $P_I$max was uniformly reduced in patients as a function of the severity of the disease. In contrast, $P_E$max was not always reduced in chronic lung disease. This decrease in strength found in patients with COPD may be related to a general weakness of the respiratory muscles. Clark et al.[45] showed that there was a relation between increasing airway obstruction and decreasing amounts of ATP and phosphocreatine (PCr) in the intercostal muscles. Other investigators have observed decreased levels of ATP and PCr in intercostal and quadriceps muscles in patients with COPD in respiratory distress.[46] These low levels of ATP and PCr rose in response to nutritional therapy, and concurrently the patient's clinical condition improved.

A decrease in respiratory muscle endurance has also been demonstrated in COPD by measuring maximal voluntary ventilation (MVV).[47,48] In addition, malnutrition has negatve effects on MVV in patients without lung disease. Consequently, it would be expected that the effects of malnutrition and COPD in combination have a marked negative impact on MVV. In nutritionally depleted patients without COPD, a severe reduction in body cell mass appears to be associated with a reduction in inspiratory muscle strength.[14] In patients on mechanical ventilators it appears that nutritional status and supplementation have a major role in determining respiratory muscle strength and the overall clinical condition.[15]

NUTRITION AND THE PULMONARY PARENCHYMA

Numerous studies have reported varying degrees of apparent pulmonary dysfunction when intravenous fat emulsions (IVFE) are given. These changes have generally not been of sufficient magnitude to carry much clinical significance. The lung dysfunction observed has been attributed to an associated hyperlipemia. Recent studies, however, suggest that the associated impairment in lung function is due to alterations in pulmonary vascular tone (which results in ventilation/perfusion inequalities) caused by an IVFE-related increase in prostaglandin production. The polyunsaturated fatty acids in the IVFE serve as precursors to the prostaglandins. Owing to the varied effects of prostaglandins, infusion of IVFE may have profound physiological and pharmacological actions aside from the provision of lipid calories. These effects may in fact be beneficial to patients suffering from pulmonary disease. We have sug-

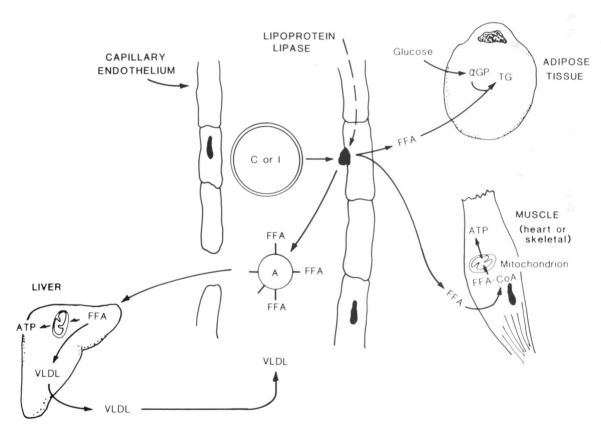

FIGURE 28–1. *Metabolic fat of chylomicrons or Intralipid particles. Chylomicrons (C) or Intralipid (I) particles interact with lipoprotein lipase, which is the rate-limiting enzyme responsible for Intralipid triglyceride degradation. The triglyceride is degraded into free fatty acids (FFA) and glycerol. (For clarity, glycerol is not shown.) In adipose tissue the FFA are reesterfied with α-glycerol-phosphate to triglyceride and stored. In muscle cells FFA is converted to its CoA ester and oxidized to yield ATP. A portion of the FFA released by lipoprotein lipase recirculates in the plasma bound to albumin (A). These FFA are readily taken up by liver, where they may be oxidized or converted to very low density lipoprotein (VLDL) and reenter the blood stream. (From Bryan H, Shennan A, Griffin E, et al. Intralipid—its rational use in parenteral nutrition of the newborn. Pediatrics 1976; 58:787. Reproduced with permission.)*

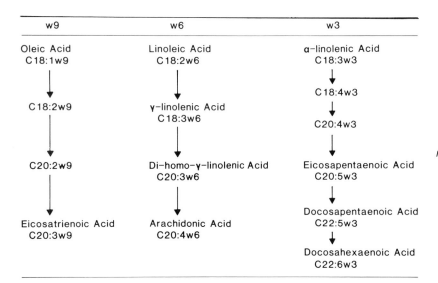

FIGURE 28–2. *The major polyunsaturated fatty acids.*

gested that long-term parenteral nutrition using lipid may result in a reduction in pulmonary inflammation.[49,50] It is our intent in this review to analyze the available data and put forth the hypothesis that lipid emulsions, when used appropriately, do not impair lung function but may actually be beneficial to the lung via alterations in prostaglandin synthesis and surfactant production.

PHYSIOLOGICAL EFFECTS OF IVFE ON THE LUNG

The effects of IVFE on lung function in humans have been studied in adult subjects with normal lungs and in both adult and pediatric patients with pre-existing lung injury. Greene et al.[51] first drew attention to the pulmonary effects of lipid by investigating the relationship between pulmonary diffusion and IVFE infusion. In 6 of 20 normal subjects they observed a transient increase in diffusion capacity following a single injection of IVFE. One subject showed a minor decrease in P_{O_2} after exercise. By preventing the increase in serum triglyceride level with heparin infusion, they could prevent the decrease in diffusion capacity. They therefore con-

TABLE 28–1. Characteristics and Components of IVFE's

	Intralipid	Liposyn
Fat source	Soybean oil	Safflower oil
Glycerin content	2.25%	2.5%
Particle size	0.5 μm	0.4 μm
Fatty acid composition		
Linoleic acid	54%	77%
Linolenic acid	8%	0.5%
Oleic acid	25%	13%
Palmitic acid	9%	7%
Osmolarity	280 mosm/L	300 mosm/L

From Hageman JR, Hunt CE. Clin Chest Med, 1986; 7:69. Reproduced with permission.

cluded that the hyperlipemia induced by the IVFE caused the decreased pulmonary diffusion capacity. In another study in normal subjects, Sundstrøm et al.[52] found that the pulmonary diffusion capacity for carbon monoxide (D_{CO}) and the alveolar-arterial difference in oxygen tension (AaD_{O_2}) decreased with lipid infusion. They found no change in pulmonary artery pressure. Talbott and Frayser[53] reported a decrease in arterial oxygen saturation (Sa_{O_2}) and a decrease in D_{CO} after IVFE infusion in 11 subjects. In a group of patients with atherosclerotic heart disease, Kuo et al.[54] also found a decrease in Sa_{O_2} when they infused IVFE.

There is indirect evidence that IVFE's may aggravate existing gas exchange abnormalities in acutely ill patients. This has been suggested by the observation that traumatic fat embolism following major fractures or acute pancreatitis can result in hypoxia and adult respiratory distress syndrome (ARDS) ("fat embolism syndrome").[55,56] Although the pathophysiology of the fat embolism syndrome is unclear, embolization of fat particles to the lungs and the release of vasoactive substances and platelets are thought to be important steps in the development of the syndrome.[57] Venus et al.[58] found that IVFE infusion in patients with disrupted alveolar capillary membrane (ARDS group) resulted in decreased oxygenation, increased intrapulmonary shunting, and increased mean pulmonary artery pressure. The changes were reversed once lipid infusion was discontinued.[51] They found no changes in these pulmonary variables in patients with intact alveolar capillary membrane (non-ARDS group). Van Deyk et al.,[59] however, found no changes in AaD_{O_2}, intrapulmonary shunting, or pulmonary artery pressure during infusion of IVFE in 16 patients with multiple injuries.

Pereira et al.[60] found that premature infants less than 1 week of age developed a decrease (in the 10 mm Hg range) in P_{O_2} levels during fat infusion.

They measured lung compliance, airway resistance, and functional residual capacity and did not find any changes in any of these measurements before or during IVFE infusion.

The decreased diffusion capability often reported after IVFE is a confusing measurement, because it does not allow one to distinguish between an increased thickness of the alveolar-capillary membrane, the red cell membranes, or the surface area available for gas exchange. The decreased diffusion capacity has been attributed to changes in alveolar capillary membrane due to deposition of fat particles in the reticuloendothelial system (RES)[60] and alteration in red cell membranes. Most often, however, a decreased diffusion capacity represents an increase in pulmonary shunt flow; this may be the cause of the alterations in oxygenation observed with the IVFE's.

One mechanism proposed for the pathogenesis of the respiratory dysfunction associated with IVFE infusion is the liberation of free fatty acids in the IVFE solution.

Previous studies have generally attributed the IVF-related alterations in lung function to increased TG levels.[51,52] However, more recent experimental studies in animals have not shown any relation between TG increases and lung function.[6] These studies have documented an increase in prostaglandin (PG) plasma levels during IVFE infusion; the PG alterations appear to cause the changes in lung function.[61] Inwood et al.[27] found no ventilatory changes in rabbits with normal lung function receiving IVFE. In rabbits with lung damage after pretreatment with oleic acid, they found an IVFE-related decrease in PaO_2 and increase in $AaPO_2$, both of which returned to baseline without TG normalization. Indomethacin prevented the changes in lung function despite the TG increase. McKeen et al.[62] found that IVFE caused pulmonary vasoconstriction, increased lung microvascular pressure, and arterial hypoxia in sheep. These effects were not changed by heparin-induced lipolysis clearing the plasma for TG, but were prevented and reversed by indomethacin. Gurtner et al.[63] reported that IVFE caused pulmonary vasoconstriction in the isolated perfused rabbit lung. This response to IVFE could be abolished by administration of indomethacin. In oleic acid damaged rabbit lungs, Hageman et al.[61] found an increased pulmonary production of vasodilatory PG's with an associated decrease in Po_2 in the lung injury group. Both the increased PG production and the decrease in Po_2 were blocked by indomethacin. These investigators found no correlation between lung function and hyperlipemia.

All these studies support the hypothesis that the IVFE-related changes in lung function are in fact PG-mediated. The effects can best be explained by changes in the distribution of intrapulmonary blood flow consequent to PG-mediated alterations in pulmonary vasomotor tone. The changes in blood flow lead to an increase in ventilation/perfusion ($\dot{V}_a/\dot{Q}$) inequalities, which can explain the PaO_2 and $P(A-a)O_2$ changes related to IVFE. In the lung-damaged groups, there was a lower baseline PaO_2 caused by secondary hypoxic vasconstriction; with vasodilators such as PGE_2 and PGI_2, the perfusion of poorly ventilated alveoli should increase. This in turn would increase the intrapulmonary right-to-left shunt and cause a further decrease in PaO_2. The same mechanism for hypoxia has been observed in other situations in which vasodilators have been given to patients with impaired lung function and $\dot{V}_a/\dot{Q}$ imbalance. In the normal lung groups with no baseline hypoxic vasoconstriction, the experimental studies showed no IVFE-associated PaO_2 decrease.

It is becoming increasingly evident that PG's play an integral role in regulating the functions of cells involved in immune and inflammatory reactions.[64]

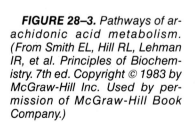

FIGURE 28–3. Pathways of arachidonic acid metabolism. (From Smith EL, Hill RL, Lehman IR, et al. Principles of Biochemistry. 7th ed. Copyright © 1983 by McGraw-Hill Inc. Used by permission of McGraw-Hill Book Company.)

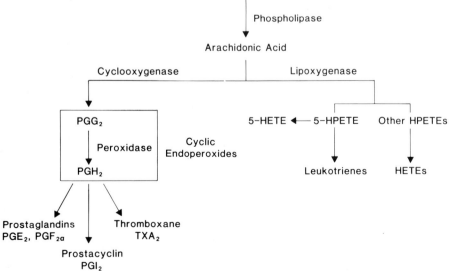

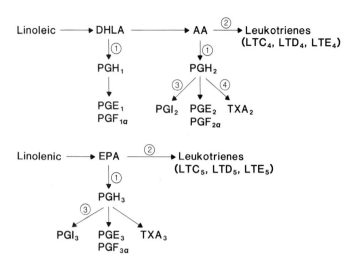

FIGURE 28–4. *The pathway of eicosanoid synthesis from polyunsaturated fatty acids. DHLA, di-homo-( )-linolenic acid; AA, arachidonic acid; EPA, eicosapentaenoic acid; TXA. thromboxane; 1, cyclo-oxygenase; 2, lipo-oxygenase; 3, prostacyclin synthetase; 4, thromboxane synthetase.*

Numerous in vivo and in vitro studies have established the suppressive effect of the E series of prostaglandins, prostacyclin, and some of the leukotrienes on various immunological and inflammatory responses. The thromboxanes and most of the leukotrienes are in general thought to have proinflammatory effects. Among the effects of the PGE's are inhibition of platelet aggregation, leukocyte chemotaxis, adherence and aggregation, phagocytosis, and vasculitis.

These studies suggest that the PG's or IVFE's may have a therapeutic potential as modulatory of immune and inflammatory responses. In our patients with cystic fibrosis, we have noticed a thinning of secretions, fewer pulmonary infections, and an overall clinical improvement after long-term TPN.[49,50] We have suggested that this may be due to an anti-inflammatory effect of the Intralipid mediated via PG synthesis, but further studies are needed to evaluate these findings properly. Long-term intravenous fat supplementation has been given to patients with CF in a number of circumstances. Some studies found that IVFE improved the fatty acid composition in plasma and the pulmonary function in children with CF, while others reported little or no improvement. It is not clear if the response of pulmonary inflammation is due to a correction of deficiency in fatty acids in CF or a pharmacological anti-inflammatory effect of the IVFE infusion. As outlined below, the variable responses may reflect different dose, rate, and duration of infusion. Promising effects have been reported with PGE₁ in adult respiratory distress syndrome (ARDS), but the drug is difficult to administer because of its systemic vasodilating properties. IVFE's may have similar effects, depending on the dose given. If so, it is possible that IVFE's would be more effective with fewer side effects, since PG's are local hormones and could be expected to function more effectively when local synthesis is stimulated as opposed to systemic infusion. Systemic infusion of prostaglandin results in low tissue levels with high blood levels. Infusion of fat results in high tissue levels of PG's with low systemic levels.

Effects of Dose, Rate, Duration, and Fatty Acid Content of IVFE Infusion

Infusion of IVFE and arachidonic acid has a mixed action on the pulmonary vascular bed. When IVFE is given as a bolus or rapid infusion, a vasoconstrictive response is reported; when IVFE is given as a slow infusion a vasodilating effect is seen. The reason for these results is unclear, but it has been suggested that an alteration in PG production is a factor since the vasomotor response is blocked by indomethacin. During a slow infusion it is likely that there is a net increase in vasodilating and anti-inflammatory PG's like PGE₂ and PGI₂. During a bolus or a rapid infusion, however, the excessive amount of substrate may overwhelm the enzymatic pathways for PGI₂ and PGE₂ metabolism, resulting in an increased production of potent vasoconstrictive PG's such as thromboxane TxA₂ (Fig. 28–6). In general, the anti-inflammatory PG's have a vasodilatory

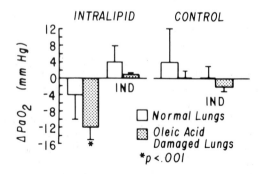

FIGURE 28–5. *Changes in PaO₂ occurring as a result of infusion over 1 hour of 4.0 ml/kg Intralipid. The only significant PaO₂ decrease occurred in the lung injury group. Bars: mean ± SEM. IND, indomethacin. (From Hageman JR, Hunt LE. Fat emulsions and lung function. Clin Chest Med 1986; 7:69. Reproduced with permission.)*

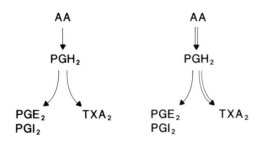

FIGURE 28–6. *Hypothetical explanation for the mixed response of infusion of arachidonic acid (AA). During a slow infusion* (left) *there may be a net increase in vasodilating (and anti-inflammatory) prostaglandins like PGE$_2$ and PGI$_2$. During a bolus or a rapid infusion* (right) *the excessive amount of AA may overwhelm the enzymes for PGE$_2$ and PGI$_2$ with a net increase of vasoconstrictive prostaglandins as thromboxane (TXA$_2$).*

effect on the pulmonary vascular bed in contrast to the vasoconstrictive effects of the proinflammatory thromboxanes. We have therefore suggested that the IVFE's exert an anti-inflammatory response when given as a slow infusion and may have a proinflammatory response when given as a bolus or rapid infusion. We have observed in cystic fibrosis patients that patients who receive IVFE report progressive thinning of secretions up to a point with increasing doses of Intralipid. Above a certain level of the rate of lipid infusion, however, the patients report that their secretions have gotten thicker; this may be due to the result of thromboxane production as linoleic acid saturates the PGE system.

Studies have shown that the amounts of PG's synthesized can be regulated by the level of precursor fatty acids as well as dose and rate of infusion of IVFE's. Since the PG synthesis is altered in this way by IVFE infusion, the fat emulsions may have significant pulmonary and nonpulmonary clinical effects related to known or postulated consequences of PG alterations. It may also be possible to use IVFE as a pharmacological agent to achieve PG-related anti-inflammatory, antiplatelet aggregation, changes in membrane function, and vasomotor tone responses. The simplistic notion that IVFE provides fat calories that either do or do not damage the lung should be rejected. Further studies are needed to delineate the complex and specific pathophysiological changes that occur and the precise role of IVFE in patients with lung disease.

References

1. Thurlbeck WM. Diaphragm and body weight in emphysema. Thorax 1978; *33*:483–487.
2. Arora NS, Rochester DF. Respiratory muscle strength and maximal voluntary ventilation in undernourished patients. Am Rev Respir Dis 1982; *126*:5–8.
3. Arora NS, Rochester DF. Effects of bodyweight and muscularity on human diaphragm muscle mass, thickness and area. J Appl Physiol 1982; *52*:64–70.
4. Baier H, Somani P. Ventilatory drive in normal man during semi-starvation. Chest 1984; *85*:222–225.
5. Vandenbergh E, Van de Woestijne KP, Gyselen A. Weight changes in the terminal stages of chronic obstructive pulmonary disease; relation to respiratory function and prognosis. Am Rev Respir Dis 1967; *95*:556–566.
6. Vandenbergh E, Van de Woestjne KP, Billiet L, et al. Evolution et propiostic de la bronchite chronique au stade de la retention de CO$_2$. Bull Physiopath Resp 1965; *1*:260.
7. Dornhorst AC. Respiratory insufficiency. Lancet 1955; *1*:1185.
8. Sukumalchantra Y, Williams MH. Serial studies of pulmonary function in patients with chronic obstructive pulmonary disease. Am J Med 1965; *39*:441–445.
9. Burrows BA, Nidon AH, Barclay WR, et al. Chronic obstructive lung disease: relationship of clinical and physiologic findings to the severity of airways obstruction. Am Rev Respir Dis 1964; *91*:665–678.
10. Driver AG, McAlevy MT, Smith JL. Nutritional assessment of patients with chronic obstructive pulmonary disease and acute respiratory failure. Chest 1982; *82*:568–571.
11. Renzetti AD, McClement DH, Litt BD: The Veterans Administration cooperative study of pulmonary function—mortality in relation to respiratory function in chronic obstructive pulmonary disease. Am J Med 1966; *41*:115–129.
12. Boushy SF, Adhikair PK, Sakamoto A, et al. Factors affecting prognosis in emphysema. Dis Chest 1964; *45*:402–411.
13. Hunter AMB, Carey MA, Larsh HW. The nutritional status of patients with chronic obstructive pulmonary disease. Am Rev Respir Dis 1981; *124*:376–381.
14. Kelly SM, Rosa A, Field S, et al. Inspiratory muscle strength and body composition in patients receiving total parenteral nutrition therapy. Am Rev Respir Dis 1984; *130*:33–37.
15. Bassili HR, Dietel M. Effect of nutritional support on weaning patients off mechanical ventilators. JPEN 1981; *5*:161–163.
16. Driver AG, LeBrun M. Iatrogenic malnutrition in patients receiving ventilatory support. JAMA 1980; *244*:2195–2196.
17. Openbrier DR, Irwin MM, Rogers RM, et al. Nutritional status and lung function in patients with emphysema and chronic bronchitis. Chest 1983; *88*:17–22.
18. Rogers RM, Dauber JH, Saunder MH, et al: Nutrition and COPD state-of-the-art minireview. Chest 1984; *85*:635–665.
19. Wilson NL, Wilson RHL, Farber SM. Nutrition in pulmonary emphysema. J Am Diet Assoc 1964; *45*:530—536.
20. Openbrier DR, Irwin MM, Dauber JH, et al. Factors affecting nutritional status and the impact of nutritional support in patients with emphysema. Chest 1984; *85*:675–695.
21. Heymsfield SP, Head A, Grossman G, et al. Mechanisms of cachexia in chronic obstructive pulmonary disease. (Abstract.) JPEN 1981; *5*:562.
22. Tirlapur V, Afzal M. Effect of low calorie intake on abnormal pulmonary physiology in patients with chronic hypercapnic respiratory failure. Am J Med 1984; *77*:987–994.
23. Askanazi J, Elwyn DH, Silverberg PA, et al. Respiratory distress secondary to a high carbohydrate load: a case report. Surgery 1980; *87*:596–598.
24. Covelli HD, Black JW, Olsen MV, et al. Respiratory failure precipitated by high carbohydrate loads. Ann Intern Med 1981; *95*:579–581.
25. Gieseke T, Gurushanthaiah G, Glauser FL. Effect of carbohydrates on carbon dioxide excretion in patients with airway disease. Chest 1977; *71*:55–58.
26. Askanazi J, Nordenstrom J, Rosenbaum SH, et al. Nutrition for the patient with respiratory failure: glucose vs fat. Anesthesiology 1981; *54*:373–377.
27. Inwood RF, Gora P, Hunt CE. Indomethacin inhibition of

Intralipid-induced lung dysfunction. Prostaglandins Med 1981; 6:503–514.

28. Askanazi J, Weissman C, Lasala P, et al. Effects of increasing protein intake on ventilatory drive. Anesthesiology 1984; 60:106–110.

29. Rodriguez J, Weissman C, Askanazi J, et al. Respiratory effects of glucose infusion. JPEN 1982; 5:573.

30. Milic-Emili J. Recent advances in clinical assessment of control of breathing. Lung 1982; 160:1–17.

31. Takala J, Askanazi J, Weissman C, et al. Changes in respiratory control induced by amino acid infusions. Crit Care Med, in press.

32. Takala J, Askanazi J, LaSala P, et al. Effects of branched chain enriched solutions of amino acids on respiratory control. In preparation.

33. Fernstrom JD, Larin F. Wurtman RJ. Correlation between brain tryptophan and plasma neutral amino acid levels following food consumption in rats. Life Sci 1973; 13:517.

34. Olson ED Jr, Dempsey JA, McCrimmon DR. Serotonin and the control of ventilation in awake rats. J Clin Invest 1979; 64:689.

35. Lopes J, Russell DM, Witwell J, et al. Skeletal muscle function in malnutrition. Am J Clin Nutr 1982; 36:602–610.

36. Fraser IM, Russell DM, Whittaker S, et al. Skeletal and diaphragmatic muscle function in malnourished COPD patients. (Abstract.) Am Rev Respir Dis 1984; 129:A269.

37. Russell DM, Walker PM, Leiter LA, et al. Metabolic and structural changes in skeletal muscle during hypocaloric dieting. Am J Clin Nutr 1984; 39:503–513.

38. Butler C. Diaphragmatic changes in emphysema. Am Rev Respir Dis 1976; 114:155–159.

39. Arora NS, Rochester DF. Effect of chronic obstructive pulmonary disease on diaphragm muscle dimensions. Am Rev Respir Dis 1982; 123:176.

40. Kelson SG, Wolanski T, Supinskli GS, et al. The effect of elastase-induced emphysema on diaphragmatic muscle structure in hamsters. Am Rev Respir Dis 1983; 129:330–334.

41. Keens TG, Chen V, Patel P, et al. Cellular adaptation of the ventilatory muscles to a chronic increased ventilatory load. J Appl Physiol 1978; 44:905–908.

42. Arora NS, Rochester DF. Effect of chronic airflow limitation (CAL) on sternocleidomastoid muscle thickness. Chest 1984; 85(Suppl):588.

43. Braun NMT, Rochester DF. Respiratory muscle strength in obstructive lung disease. Am Rev Respir Dis 1979; 117:91.

44. Rochester DF, Arora NS, Braun NMT, et al. The respiratory muscles in chronic obstructive lung disease. Bull Physiopathol Respir 1979; 15:951–975.

45. Clark TJH, Freedman S, Campbell EJM, et al. The ventilatory capacity of patients with chronic airway obstruction. Clin Sci 1969; 36:307–316.

46. Aldrich TK, Arora NS, Rochester DF. The influence of airway obstruction and respiratory muscle strength on maximal voluntary ventilation in lung disease. Am Rev Respir Dis 1982; 126:195–199.

47. Campbell JA, Hughes RL, Sahgal V, et al. Alterations in intercostal muscle morphology and biochemistry in patients with obstructive lung disease. Am Rev Respir Dis 1980; 122:679–686.

48. Gertz I, Hedenstierna G, Hellers G, et al. Muscle metabolism in patients with chronic obstructive lung disease and acute respiratory failure. Clin Sci Mol Med 1977; 52:395–403.

49. Askanazi J, Rothkopf M, Rosenbaum SH, et al. Treatment of cystic fibrosis with long term home parenteral nutrition. Nutr Int 1987; 3:277.

50. Skeie B, Askanazi J, Rothkopf M, et al. Long term parenteral nutrition and exercise tolerance in cystic fibrosis. Submitted, 1986.

51. Greene HL, Hazlett D, Demaree R. Relationship between Intralipid-induced hyperlipemia and pulmonary function. Am J Clin Nutr 1976; 29:127.

52. Sundstrøm G, Zauner CW, Mans A. Decrease in pulmonary diffusing capacity during lipid infusion in healthy men. J Appl Physiol 1973; 34:816.

53. Talbott GD, Frayser R. Hyperlipidaemia: a cause of decreased oxygen saturation. Nature 1963; 200:684.

54. Kuo PT, Whereat AF. Lipemia as a cause of arterial oxygen unsaturation, and the effect of its control in patients with atherosclerosis. Circulation 1957; 16:493.

55. Nixon JR, Brock-Utne JG. Free fatty acid and arterial oxygen changes following major injury: correlation between hypoxemia and increased free fatty acid levels. J Trauma 1978; 18:23.

56. Kimure T, Toung JK, Margolis S, et al. Respiratory failure in acute pancreatitis. A possible role for triglycerides. Ann Surg 1979; 189:509.

57. Peltier LF. Fat embolism—a current concept. Clin Orthop 1969; 66:241.

58. Venus B, Patel CB, Mathru M, et al. Pulmonary effects of lipid infusion in patients with acute respiratory failure. Crit Care Med 1984; 12:293.

59. Van Deyk K, Hempel V, Munch F, et al. Influence of parenteral fat administration on the pulmonary vascular system in man. Intensive Care Med 1983; 9:73.

60. Pereira GR, Fox WW, Stanley CA, et al. Decreased oxygenation and hyperlipemia during intravenous fat infusions in premature infants. Pediatrics 1980; 66:26.

61. Hageman JR, McCulloch K, Gora P, et al. Intralipid alterations in pulmonary prostaglandin metabolism and gas exchange. Crit Care Med 1983; 11:794.

62. McKeen CR, Brigham KL, Bowers RE, et al. Pulmonary vascular effects of fat emulsion infusion in ananesthetized sheep. J Clin Invest 1978; 61:1291.

63. Swan PK, Tibbals J, Duncan AW. Prostaglandin E$_1$ in primary pulmonary hypertension. Crit Care Med 1986; 14:72.

64. Vane JR: Prostaglandins as mediators of inflammation. In Samuelsen B (ed). Advances in Prostaglandin and Thromboxane Research. New York, Raven Press, 1976: 791–798.

29

RENAL DISEASES

ANDERS ALVESTRAND / JONAS BERGSTRÖM

There are several reasons why nutritional problems play a particularly important role in the treatment of patients with renal failure. First, impaired glomerular filtration results in decreased excretion of creatinine, urea, and several other nitrogenous, potentially toxic metabolites. Retention of such substances in the body fluids leads to the development of a toxic syndrome, uremia, which is associated with symptoms from the gastrointestinal tract and the central nervous system. The renal failure per se, the uremic intoxication, and also various endocrinological abnormalities secondary to the renal failure or uremia have metabolic effects that are of primary importance with respect to nutrition.

Second, the production of nitrogenous, potentially toxic metabolites depends directly on the intake of protein. Restriction of dietary protein therefore results in decreased accumulation of nitrogenous metabolites and elimination or alleviation of the uremic syndrome. For many years the conservative management of patients with advanced renal failure has been based on treatment with low-protein regimens. Such treatment requires that careful attention be paid to the nutritional status.

Finally, advanced renal failure is associated with disturbances in fluid and electrolyte balance that must be taken into consideration in the formulation of the nutritional management.

This chapter describes how various metabolic disturbances associated with impaired renal function and uremia may influence the nutritional status in patients with renal insufficiency and also discusses the nutritional management of patients with chronic and acute renal insufficiency.

COMPONENTS OF RENAL FAILURE THAT MAY REQUIRE MANAGEMENT

Disturbances in Fluid Balance and Electrolyte Metabolism: The Uremic State

Disturbances in water and electrolyte metabolism may be predominant in acute oliguric renal failure

531

and in the end stage of chronic renal disease, when tubular adaptability to the reduced glomerular filtration of water and electrolytes is insufficient to maintain homeostasis. An excessive intake of water may infrequently result in water intoxication with hypotonicity of the body fluids (low serum sodium), brain edema, twitching, convulsions, and coma due to osmotic water transport into the central nervous system.[1] Far more common is sodium retention with associated water retention, which may result in peripheral edema, pulmonary congestion, pleural effusion, ascites, congestive heart failure, and hypertension.

In chronic renal failure sodium homeostasis may be reasonably well preserved even when the glomerular filtration rate (GFR) is substantially reduced; this requires an adaptation of tubular reabsorption in the remaining nephrons to compensate for the reduction in glomerular filtration rate.[2] How this is achieved is far from clear, but it has been speculated that this adaptation involves the secretion of a natriuretic factor or hormone in response to accumulation of extracellular fluid.[3] Sodium reabsorption in the individual nephron of the diseased kidney is not only reduced, but may also vary over a much wider range than in the normal nephron in response to varying sodium intake.[4] However, owing to the loss of functioning nephron mass, the overall adaptability is reduced, which means that both sodium loading and low sodium intake are less well tolerated than in normal individuals. Although the majority of uremic patients tend to retain sodium and water, there is a subgroup of patients who tend to lose sodium and water on a normal sodium intake, and thus are at risk of developing extracellular dehydration with low blood pressure and further lowering of glomerular filtration rate. Such patients, who are frequently polyuric and may be markedly acidotic because of loss of bicarbonate by the kidneys, are important to identify since they constitute a subgroup from the therapeutic view. Likewise, some patients with acute renal failure may have a high urinary output of water and electrolytes in spite of severe reduction of the GFR.[5]

Another problem in uremia is metabolic acidosis due to inability of the remnant tubular mass to restore body buffers by regenerating bicarbonate and thus to eliminate an excess of hydrogen ions formed in the metabolism of the sulfur-containing amino acids of protein and of certain phosphate esters.[6] In patients with chronic renal failure acidosis generally does not occur until the GFR is reduced to about 25 ml/min or less. Bone carbonate participates as an extrarenal buffer, and acidosis is rarely severe even at filtration rates lower than 10 ml/min. In patients with interstitial nephritis, however, acidosis tends to occur earlier than in those with glomerulonephritis.[7] Also, in acute renal failure associated with markedly enhanced degradation of tissue protein and accelerated net acid retention, more severe acidosis may

develop. Metabolic acidosis leads to an increased rate of muscle protein breakdown and enhanced urea generation.[8,9] More severe metabolic acidosis stimulates compensatory hyperventilation and has an overall deleterious effect on several metabolic processes, particularly in the central nervous system. Furthermore, chronic acidosis may contribute to the metabolic bone disease of uremia by dissolving buffer salts from the skeleton.[10]

Hyperkalemia is another consequence of severely reduced renal function and may be especially marked in oliguric acute renal failure. A plasma potassium concentration above 7 mmol/L is life-threatening, since it may cause cardiac dysrhythmias and cardiac arrest due to ventricular fibrillation. Factors that promote hyperkalemia are enhanced cell catabolism and severe metabolic acidosis. Severe hyperkalemia is less commonly a problem in chronic renal failure, since tubular adaptation with increased secretion of potassium per nephron and enhanced fecal excretion of potassium to some extent compensate for reduction in nephron mass.[11] In contrast to the blunted effect of insulin in enhancing glucose uptake in uremia, the ability of insulin to increase potassium uptake by muscle is normal in patients with chronic renal failure.[12]

Impaired magnesium excretion by the kidneys may lead to hypermagnesemia, but only rarely to symptoms of magnesium intoxication except in patients with excessive magnesium intake, as from magnesium-containing antacids. Symptoms of magnesium intoxication are somnolence and ventricular arrhythmias.

All the aforementioned disturbances are at least to some extent amenable to treatment by conservative measures, including dietary manipulations.

Patients with acute or chronic end-stage renal failure may exhibit a number of toxic uremic symptoms even when water, electrolyte, and acid-base balance are apparently fully controlled.

The term uremia, which literally means urine in the body, is used to describe a condition that develops in severe renal failure and is characterized by disturbances in water and electrolyte metabolism, toxic symptoms caused by retained metabolites, and secondary endocrine disturbances.

Symptoms from the central nervous system (fatigue, somnolence, coma, cramps) and gastrointestinal tract (nausea, vomiting) predominate. Other typical symptoms and signs of uremia are anemia, bleeding tendency, itching, peripheral neuropathy, susceptibility to infection (impaired cellular immune response), and various metabolic disturbances such as glucose intolerance, lipid abnormalities, and abnormal metabolism of protein and amino acids.

The most obvious explanation provided for this diversity in symptomatology is that uremia is a generalized form of autointoxication by metabolites that are normally excreted by the kidneys.[13] There is strong evidence that at least some of these metabolites are products of protein metabolism, since increased protein intake may promote toxic symptoms, especially nausea and vomiting, whereas protein restriction alleviates these symptoms, generally in association with a decrease in blood urea concentration. This is not to say that urea per se is a major uremic toxin, but only that some important features of uremic toxicity are associated with accumulation of urea. Several other groups of compounds have been suggested to be uremic toxins, for example, phenols, aliphatic and aromatic amines, polyamines, indoles, and guanidines, some of them being derived from naturally occurring amino acids by the action of bacteria in the gut. Products of purine and pyridine metabolism, derived from breakdown of nucleic acids, have also been suggested to be uremic toxins, as have myoinositol and other polyols. So-called middle molecules, compounds that have larger molecular weights (350 to 2000 daltons) than the aforementioned small molecular compounds, also accumulate in the end stage of renal failure and are associated with toxic symptoms and in vitro toxicity in various bioassay systems.[14]

Disturbances in Amino Acids and Protein Metabolism

It is well recognized that patients with advanced renal failure have a tendency toward negative nitrogen balance and muscle wasting. This may be a consequence of poor food intake due to anorexia caused by uremic toxicity.

In chronic renal failure protein metabolism may also be affected by several factors, such as the uremic intoxication per se, hormonal derangements, and alterations in the metabolism of amino acids and other nutrients secondary to uremia or renal failure.

There is evidence that impaired protein synthesis as well as enhanced protein catabolism may contribute to diminution of lean body mass in uremia. Thus, protein synthesis in vitro is impaired in the presence of uremic plasma dialysate.[15] Increased protein synthesis is observed in the presence of postdialysis as compared with predialysis plasma dialysate, indicating that factors in uremia inhibit protein synthesis and that dialysis removes a great part of the inhibitor effect, which appears to be related to dialyzable molecules.

Increased muscle release of amino acids in experimental chronic uremia in rats[16,17] suggests that muscle protein catabolism is enhanced in uremia. However, direct measurements of amino acid balance across leg tissues in uremic patients demonstrated a general tendency toward decreased net amino acid release from leg tissues, suggesting that muscle catabolism is not increased in chronic uremia.[18,19] These results are in line with the observation of lower protein flux, i.e., a lower rate of breakdown and synthesis of protein in relation to protein intake

in nondialyzed uremic children than in normal children.[20] However, the possibility cannot be excluded that the decreased net release of amino acids and the low protein turnover observed in these studies reflect an adaptive response to depletion of muscle protein and intracellular amino acid pools, respectively.

Insulin is an anabolic hormone that enhances amino acid transport and stimulates protein synthesis. As discussed below, insulin-mediated glucose metabolism is severely impaired in uremic subjects. The primary site of this insulin resistance is the peripheral tissues, mainly muscle.[21] If the resistance to the action of insulin were also extended to amino acid metabolism, this might contribute to impaired muscle amino acid uptake and protein synthesis. Studies of the effect of insulin on amino acid and protein metabolism in uremic muscle have given controversial results. In rats with experimental acute or chronic renal failure, protein breakdown is poorly suppressed by insulin. Also, the ability of insulin to stimulate muscle protein synthesis is blunted.[16,22] In contrast, studies using the euglycemic clamp technique in combination with arterial and femoral venous catheterization and muscle biopsy showed that the effect of physiological hyperinsulinemia on plasma and muscle intracellular amino acid concentrations and leg amino acid exchange is similar in patients with chronic renal failure and control subjects.[18,23] These results suggest that insulin resistance in uremia does not extend to amino acid metabolism.

In renal failure muscle protein and amino acid metabolism may also be affected by increased secretion of parathyroid hormone. Both intact PTH and its N-terminal fragment have been shown to enhance muscle protein degradation and increase the release of alanine and glutamine.[24]

There are numerous reports of abnormal plasma amino acid concentrations in patients with chronic renal failure.[25,26] Among the consistent findings are high concentrations of several nonessential amino acids and low concentrations of essential amino acids, including the branched-chain amino acids valine, isoleucine, and leucine. The plasma concentration of tyrosine is low and the phenylalanine:tyrosine ratio is high. Many of the plasma amino acid abnormalities found in uremia are similar to those observed in protein malnutrition, and it has been suggested that they are in part attributable to dietary inadequacy. The largest pool of free amino acids, however, is not in the extracellular pool but in skeletal muscle. In untreated uremic patients a typical muscle intracellular amino acid pattern is observed with low concentration of valine but normal concentrations of leucine and isoleucine and low concentrations of threonine, lysine, and histidine. Intracellular levels of the methylated histidines are high.[27]

The mechanisms behind most of these amino acid abnormalities in uremia are not well understood. The low tyrosine concentration in uremia and the resulting high phenylalanine:tyrosine ratio, however, can be at least partly explained by impaired conversion of phenylalanine to tyrosine, which has been attributed to inhibition, by some uremic toxins, of phenylalanine hydroxylase activity.[28] Other, possibly hormonal, factors may also be involved in the altered metabolism of phenylalanine and tyrosine. The synthesis of histidine has been shown to be impaired to the extent that it becomes an essential amino acid in uremia.[29,30] It has also been found that histidine may be essential in health.[31]

The pathogenesis of the abnormal branched-chain amino acid patterns in muscle and plasma is not known. One can only speculate whether factors related to uremic intoxication per se or hormonal alterations contribute to the valine depletion and the abnormal distribution of isoleucine and leucine across the cell membrane.

Although the mechanism of most amino acid abnormalities is not known, determination of the amino acid pools in renal failure and uremia may have important clinical implications. Since there is evidence suggesting that protein synthesis rates are more closely related to intracellular as opposed to extracellular amino acid pools, measurement of intracellular amino acid levels may be of special interest.[32] Based on information on the intracellular pattern, amino acid supplements could be designed to specifically correct depleted amino acid pools or to compensate for metabolic changes caused by the renal failure or factors related to the uremic state. The dietary proportions of the individual essential amino acids become especially important in the nutrition of uremic patients, in whom accumulation of nitrogenous products is critical. For protein synthesis to proceed, each of the essential amino acids must be present simultaneously in the intracellular pool. If a given amino acid is present only in a limited amount, protein can be formed only as long as the supply of this limiting amino acid lasts. If one essential amino acid is missing from the pool, the remaining ones cannot be stored for later synthesis and will be catabolized for energy, thereby adding to the nitrogen load.

Recent studies in patients with near–end-stage renal failure have shown that some, but not all, intracellular amino acid abnormalities can be corrected by nutritional means, which take the specific amino acid abnormalities into consideration[27] (vide infra). Also, nitrogen balance studies have shown that normalization of intracellular amino acid pools may be associated with improved nitrogen utilization.[33]

Carbohydrate Intolerance

The existence of carbohydrate intolerance in patients with advanced chronic renal failure has been recognized for many years. Clinically this abnormality is characterized by normal or marginally increased fasting blood glucose levels and normal or moderately increased fasting insulin concentrations. Although this metabolic abnormality seldom causes any trouble in the clinical management of uremic patients, it may have important consequences with respect to protein and lipid metabolism and may be a major risk factor for the development of atherosclerosis.

Impaired beta cell response to glucose is observed in some uremic patients.[34] Results of recent studies show that secondary hyperparathyroidism in chronic renal failure is associated with impaired insulin secretion and also that parathyroidectomy results in improved glucose tolerance due to enhanced insulin secretion.[35,36] However, tissue insensitivity to the action of insulin, primarily in muscle, is the predominant factor contributing to the glucose intolerance in most patients with chronic renal failure.[21]

Little information is available concerning the mechanisms of the insulin resistance in uremia. Insulin binding to monocytes has been shown to be normal in uremic subjects,[37] suggesting that in chronic renal failure insulin resistance is caused by a postbinding intracellular defect in insulin action. The demonstration of improved carbohydrate tolerance after hemodialysis treatment[34,38] or protein restriction[39,40] suggests that some toxic metabolites may impair the insulin effect in uremia. A peptide in the middle molecular weight range that induces insulin resistance by an intracellular protein-dependent mechanism has recently been identified and partly characterized; this peptide seems to be specific for uremia.[41] Other studies, however, have failed to confirm that hemodialysis[42] or treatment with a low-protein diet[43] corrects the abnormal carbohydrate metabolism.

Increased circulating levels of glucagon have been implicated in the development of carbohydrate intolerance in uremia.[44,45] However, the demonstration in undialyzed uremic subjects of normal hepatic glucose production and the observation that hepatic glucose production is appropriately suppressed by insulin[18] indicate that gluconeogenesis is not enhanced in uremia and argue against a role for glucagon in the glucose intolerance of uremia.

The concentration of growth hormone, another diabetogenic hormone, is also frequently increased in renal failure,[46,47] but no correlation has been found between the presence of glucose intolerance or insulin resistance and growth hormone concentrations in individual patients with renal failure.

The abnormal carbohydrate metabolism may be responsible, in part, for the increased incidence of atherosclerotic complications in patients with renal failure. First, the hyperglycemia per se can lead to the production of abnormal circulating proteins such as glycosolated hemoglobin and may contribute to abnormalities in the structural proteins of capillary basement membranes in muscle and kidney tissue. Second, the insulin antagonism may result in hypertriglyceridemia and thereby add to the risk of accelerated atherogenesis. Insulin is one of the main regulators of lipoprotein lipase, the enzyme that regulates the removal of triglyceride from the circulation. If the insulin resistance also affects the activity of lipoprotein lipase, it may contribute to the impaired removal of triglycerides from plasma.

Hyperlipidemia and Atherosclerosis

Hypertriglyceridemia, mainly due to increase in very low density (VLDL) triglycerides and low density (LDL) triglycerides, is a common finding in uremia. Total cholesterol is generally normal, but the distribution is abnormal with a raised cholesterol:triglyceride ratio in VLDL and a lowered ratio in LDL. High density lipoprotein (HDL) cholesterol and triglycerides are low.[48] All these lipoprotein disturbances are considered to be potential risk factors for atherosclerosis. Several abnormalities in apolipoprotein composition of plasma lipoproteins have been identified in uremic patients.[49]

The most probable explanation for hypertriglyceridemia in uremia is a decreased removal of triglycerides due to reduced activity of plasma and tissue lipoprotein lipase and possibly also of hepatic lipoprotein lipase. An increased frequency of late pre-beta-lipoproteins in VLDL in uremia[50] further suggests that there is a delayed clearance of VLDL remnants. The activity of lecithin-cholesterol aryltransferase is also lowered in uremia, presumably owing to diminished synthesis. This enzyme is secreted by the liver into the blood, where it esterifies cholesterol on HDL and facilitates transfer of free triglycerides and cholesterol from VLDL and LDL to HDL; reduced activity may thus contribute to the decreased catabolism of lipoprotein in uremia. Increased production of VLDL triglycerides most likely also operates in chronic renal failure.[48]

Cardiovascular disease is a common cause of death in uremic patients on dialysis or after renal transplantation.[51] Based on autopsy findings it was suggested that prolonged hemodialysis may accelerate atherosclerosis.[52] However, there is no proof that dialysis per se affects progression of atherosclerosis in uremic patients. Rather, the high incidence of cardiovascular disease in hemodialysis patients is a consequence of events taking place before the patient is started on dialysis.[53–55] It is established that the lipid changes in uremia start early in the course of disease, which may mean many years of exposure to risk factors in the form of abnormal lipids before the patient reaches the end stage.[48] Whether this constitutes a real risk has not been established. Longstanding hypertension, however, is an established risk factor for atherosclerosis in renal failure.[56] Enhancement of the lipid abnormalities of uremia has been observed in patients treated with continuous ambulatory peritoneal dialysis (CAPD) and provided

with a continuous supply of glucose by the peritoneal route.[57,58] A direct correlation was observed between the amount of glucose instilled in the abdomen per day and the level of total and VLDL triglycerides.[58] Some of these patients also become obese. There is a suspicion that CAPD patients are especially at risk of developing accelerated atherosclerosis, but the observation time is still far too short to make a definite evaluation possible. There is a possibility that improved blood pressure control observed in CAPD patients counteracts such a tendency.

Disturbances in Calcium and Phosphorus Metabolism

The most obvious clinical evidence of the abnormal metabolism of calcium and phosphorus, which is universally present in renal failure, is hyperphosphatemia, hypocalcemia, and increased concentration in plasma of immunoreactive parathyroid hormone (PTH). Altered metabolism of vitamin D plays a central role in the development of these abnormalities, which in turn affect the metabolism of vitamin D.[59]

It is well recognized that the kidney is the major organ regulating the elimination of phosphorus and, thus, serum phosphorus concentration. Many investigators believe that retention of phosphate is the initiating factor for the development of secondary hyperparathyroidism.[60] Early in the course of renal failure retention of phosphorus results in transient periods of hyperphosphatemia and hypocalcemia, the latter stimulating secretion of PTH. The excess parathyroid hormone blocks the reabsorption of phosphorus and acts on bone to release calcium into the extracellular fluid. Normal plasma concentrations of calcium and phosphorus are thus restored, but at the price of an elevated circulating level of parathyroid hormone. As renal function deteriorates, increasingly high levels of parathyroid hormone are required to keep the plasma concentrations of calcium and phosphorus at normal levels. When the glomerular filtration rate is less than 25 to 30 ml/min and the renal excretion of phosphate cannot be increased further, manifest hyperphosphatemia and hypocalcemia develop; continued stimulus to increased secretion of PTH leads to enlargement of the parathyroid glands and aggravation of the hyperparathyroidism. However, this "trade-off hypothesis" has been challenged in that it has been proposed that dietary phosphate plays a role in the development of secondary hyperparathyroidism primarily through the inhibition of 1-hydroxylation of 25-hydroxyvitamin D_3.[61] 1,25-dihydroxyvitamin D_3 is synthesized in the kidney and is the most potent metabolite of vitamin D.[62] Impaired production and, hence, deficiency of this metabolite leads to inadequate intestinal absorption of calcium and negative calcium balance and also impairs the action of PTH on bone, which consequently results in hypocalcemia and hyperparathyroidism.

Secondary hyperparathyroidism together with deficiency of active vitamin D may lead to the development of renal osteodystrophy, a common, in some cases disabling, complication in patients with advanced renal failure.[63] Also, PTH impairs energy production, transfer, and utilization in both myocardium[64] and skeletal muscle,[65] and stimulates muscle protein breakdown.[24] Thus, both cardiovascular symptoms and the myopathy associated with uremia may be due partly to secondary hyperparathyroidism. Furthermore, PTH has been shown to exert deleterious effects on the hematopoietic and nervous systems as well.[66–68] As discussed above, excess of PTH may also suppress insulin secretion.[35,36] It has also been speculated that hyperparathyroidism can accelerate the progression of the renal failure by promoting calcium deposition in renal tissue.[69]

When discussing nutritional management in renal failure it is of particular importance to note that secondary hyperparathyroidism may be prevented or reversed by dietary means. It has been demonstrated that after experimental induction of renal failure in dogs by stepwise reduction of the renal parenchyma, hyperparathyroidism may be prevented if dietary phosphate is lowered in proportion to the reduction of renal function.[70] Considering the potentially serious consequences of secondary hyperparathyroidism, every effort should be made to prevent or minimize hypersecretion of parathyroid hormone in patients with renal failure.

Vitamins and Trace Elements

There is evidence that patients with uremia tend to develop deficiencies of certain water-soluble vitamins, because of either poor intake or altered metabolism. Low intake of vitamins may be due to loss of appetite, nausea and vomiting, and dietary restrictions. Low-protein diets always carry the risk of low intake of vitamins as well. In hemodialysis patients loss of water-soluble vitamins also occurs through the dialytic procedure. A few of the water-soluble vitamins appear to be especially critical. Thus, it has been shown that vitamin B_6 (pyridoxine) levels are low in uremic patients, both nondialyzed and dialyzed.[71] Ascorbic acid concentrations in blood are also decreased in a fraction of uremic patients maintained with dialysis.[72] Plasma levels of branched-chain amino acids are low in pyridoxine-deficient men with normal renal function.[73] Consequently, deficiency of pyridoxine may possibly be associated with the low concentrations of branched-chain amino acids in plasma and muscle in uremic patients. Folic acid deficiency with megaloblastic anemia has also been reported in hemodialysis patients,[74] although not confirmed by all investiga-

tors.[75,76] Hemodialysis patients may rarely have deficiency of vitamin B_{12}.[77]

With regard to the lipid-soluble vitamins the situation is partly different. Vitamin A is elevated in uremia,[78] as is serum retinol-binding protein. However, the high levels of vitamin A are not due solely to retention of retinol-binding protein (a protein which is normally catabolized in the kidney), since the vitamin A content of the liver in uremic patients is also considerably elevated.[79] Many characteristics of vitamin A intoxication, such as xerosis, pleuritis, and pigmentation, are also common in uremia. Vitamin A may enhance parathyroid hormone secretion and thus enhance renal osteodystrophy. There is also a possibility that hypervitaminosis A may contribute to the lipid changes in uremia. Vitamin D metabolism in uremia has been discussed earlier. There is no evidence that vitamin E and vitamin K requirements are changed in uremia.

Some trace elements may also become critical in uremia. The oral intake of iron may be low owing to loss of appetite, nausea and vomiting, and dietary restrictions. Although there is no evidence that iron absorption is impaired in renal failure, loss of iron can occur from the gastrointestinal tract because of occult bleeding,[80,81] especially if the patient takes medication with salicylate compounds. Unavoidable blood loss occurs in hemodialysis patients because small amounts of blood are sequestered in the dialyzer.[80] However, hemodialysis patients who require multiple blood transfusions may develop hemosiderosis with deposition of iron in liver and other organs.[82] Patients on chronic hemodialysis may develop proximal myopathy with muscle weakness owing to iron deposition in the skeletal muscle.[83] Iron status of uremic patients is best evaluated from serum ferritin levels, which correlate well with iron deposition in the bone marrow,[84] whereas serum iron and transferrin seem to have a poor diagnostic value in this respect.

Uremic patients have abnormal zinc metabolism and may be zinc deficient.[85] However, zinc content in muscle[86] and red cells[87,88] may even be increased in renal failure. Zinc deficiency has been held responsible for the persistence of gonadal dysfunction and impaired sexual function in uremic men despite adequate dialysis.[89] Zinc deficiency has also been held responsible for the impairment in taste and smell acuity. In patients on hemodialysis, supplementation with zinc was reported to improve taste perception and food intake.[90] However, other studies have not confirmed beneficial effects of zinc supplements on taste acuity and sexual function,[91,92] and no correlation was found between zinc concentrations in whole blood and plasma and taste and smell acuity.[88]

Critically low levels of other essential trace elements have not been established in blood or tissues of uremic patients. Thus, tissue selenium levels are normal.[93]

Overload with aluminum is known to be a major problem for dialysis patients.[94] The ability of the diseased kidneys to excrete aluminum is decreased in renal failure. The most important cause of aluminum loading is now probably the increased exposure to aluminum that results from the administration of phosphate-binding gel given to renal failure patients. Most of these preparations contain aluminum, some of which is absorbed. In most dialysis centers the elemental contaminants in water used for preparation of dialysate are now removed by reverse osmosis. However, any aluminum present in the dialysate may be transferred to the patient because of plasma binding of aluminum, which maintains a gradient from the dialysate to the patient.[95] Further accumulation of aluminum may result from the parenteral administration of nutritional solutions, which may contain aluminum.[96] Aluminum intoxication may cause encephalopathy and dementia[94] and is also responsible for uremic osteomalacic bone disease.[97] Furthermore, it has been suggested that aluminum intensifies anemia in uremic patients.[98]

SPECIFIC THERAPEUTIC APPROACHES

Water and Electrolyte Restrictions

Patients with renal failure may have reduced capacity to regulate water and sodium homeostasis. In patients who have a tendency to gain sodium and water (increasing weight, edema, congestive heart failure, hypertension), sodium restriction is indicated. However, it is usually not advisable to prescribe a sodium-free diet, since the ability to preserve sodium optimally may be blunted. Extreme sodium restriction also affects the palatability of the diet and is therefore intolerable for the majority of patients, especially if the diet is restricted with regard to protein as well.

Determination of the 24-hour output of sodium in the urine may be helpful in deciding how much sodium the patient tolerates. An amount of sodium equal to the output will maintain sodium balance. We usually recommend a prescribed limited dose of sodium chloride each day, generally 2 to 4 g as powder, provided in weighed doses. The salt can be used either in cooking or added to the food. If there is a tendency to sodium accumulation with these limited amounts of salt, a diuretic acting in the loop of Henle, preferably furosemide, is prescribed as required. The doses have to be increased with the severity of renal failure, some patients requiring 250 or 500 mg daily to maintain sodium homeostasis. One should beware of overtreatment, which leads to extracellular dehydration, postural hypotension, and further reduction of the glomerular filtration rate. Potassium depletion due to furosemide is only

rarely a problem in chronic renal disease, provided that the dosage of the diuretic is adequate in relation to the patient's tendency to retain salt.

When dietary sodium intake is restricted, water restriction is rarely required, since thirst diminishes and the patient adapts his or her intake of water in relation to the intake of salt. However, some patients have excessive thirst and accumulate water out of proportion to sodium and may thus develop hyponatremia. In such cases restriction of water intake to about 1.5 L per day or less may be indicated. Patients who have a tendency to lose sodium and water may develop extracellular dehydration and postural hypotension and may require extra sodium chloride, sometimes up to 10 to 12 g of salt or more. In such cases the extra sodium chloride may be given as tablets.

Because of the tendency to develop metabolic acidosis, most patients with advanced chronic renal failure require sodium bicarbonate. One should aim at keeping the standard bicarbonate concentration in plasma above 20 mmol/L, since (as discussed above) correction of acidosis, also of moderate degree, may suppress muscle protein degradation and urea formation.[8,9] This generally requires 2 to 4 g of sodium bicarbonate per day given orally as tablets. The dose is adjusted according to the patient's plasma bicarbonate level, some patients requiring much higher doses to be kept in acid-base balance. The administration of sodium bicarbonate also increases the body burden of sodium and may cause sodium retention. Again, this can be compensated for by treatment with diuretics (furosemide in advanced renal failure). The tendency to develop metabolic acidosis is also diminished by protein restriction, since the majority of the metabolically formed excess of hydrogen ions are generated when protein is catabolized. Oral phosphate binders (aluminum hydroxide) and calcium carbonate, which are given to uremic patients to control metabolic bone disease, also to some extent neutralize hydrogen ions and thus contribute to the control of acidosis.

Plasma potassium is usually normal or only moderately elevated in chronic renal failure, and specific treatment for hyperkalemia is rarely necessary. If hyperkalemia above 6.5 mmol/L persists in spite of adequate control of acid-base balance, it is recommended that the patient avoid food and drinks rich in potassium. If this does not help, potassium-binding anion exchange resins may be given by mouth on a chronic basis. Excessive supply of magnesium taken orally as magnesium-containing antacids should be avoided in renal failure, because of the risk of excessive hypermagnesemia and symptoms of magnesium intoxication.

At the end stage of chronic renal failure, when the patient is oliguric despite adequate fluid therapy and treatment with diuretics, the patient may require dialysis treatment and parenteral therapy with fluids, electrolytes, and nutrients, according to the principles used in acute renal failure.

Low-Protein Diets

In renal failure excessive intake of protein can enhance production of nitrogenous, potentially toxic waste products and increase uremic toxicity. Therefore, restriction of dietary protein has an obvious role in the management of patients with uremia, provided that good nutrition can be maintained. The basic concept of treatment with a low-protein diet is to provide a restricted amount of protein along with generous amounts of energy.

The minimum requirement of protein and the optimum proportions of amino acids in normal humans has been defined in carefully conducted nitrogen balance studies.[99,100] In order to achieve nitrogen balance in adults with normal renal function approximately 0.5 to 0.6 g of protein per kg body weight per day is required. Only 20 per cent of this has to be in the form of essential amino acids.[101] Nitrogen balance studies in uremic patients ingesting protein-restricted diets with a high content of high-quality protein (i.e., proteins rich in essential amino acids) have shown that 0.4 to 0.5 g of protein per kg of body weight per day is required to achieve nitrogen equilibrium.[102,103] Thus, the total protein requirement in uremic subjects is similar to that in normal subjects. The need for essential amino acids, however, appears to be greater in uremia.[104] In addition, the optimal proportions of essential amino acids are different in uremia.[27]

To keep the patient free from uremic symptoms, the protein intake must be gradually reduced as renal function deteriorates. It is, however, not settled when dietary protein should first be restricted in patients with chronic renal failure. As treatment with a low-protein diet is primarily a means to alleviate uremic toxicity, residual renal function is not the main guideline for reducing the protein intake. Although urea is probably only slightly toxic, the concentration of urea is correlated with accumulation of more toxic substances. In general, uremic symptoms appear when serum urea is as high as 25 to 30 mmol/L (BUN 80 to 100 mg/dl); this rarely occurs until the GFR is below 20 ml/min. Dietary protein, therefore, should be gradually reduced to maintain serum urea below approximately 30 mmol/L.

In patients with uremic symptoms such as general fatigue, nausea, and vomiting, restriction of dietary protein generally results in improvement of the general condition with alleviation of the uremic syndrome along with a decrease in the serum urea concentration. As emphasized by Walser,[105] the restriction of dietary protein results in a fall in serum urea that is proportionally greater than the reduction in protein intake. The nonurea component of

nitrogen excretion, 2.5 g/day (the nitrogen content of about 15 g of protein), is little affected. Thus, reduction of protein intake, for example from 80 to 40 g/day, will reduce net urea nitrogen production from 10.3 to 3.9 g/day. Serum creatinine, however, is not or only marginally affected. Initially only a moderate restriction of dietary protein to about 60 g/day (0.8 to 1 g/kg/day) may be necessary to eliminate uremic symptoms. When renal function deteriorates further, and the urea concentration increases, toxic symptoms reappear and further restriction of protein intake to about 40 g/day (0.5 to 0.6 g/kg/day) becomes necessary. Provided that a large proportion of the dietary protein is of high biological value, neutral nitrogen balance is maintained in patients whose uremia is not severe. It is doubtful, however, whether nitrogen equilibrium can be maintained in all patients with a diet providing 40 g of protein per day.[104]

In some cases, despite a relatively good general condition and a low serum urea level, the patient is observed to be slowly losing body weight. Muscle mass decreases and serum albumin and transferrin fall as signs of protein depletion. In all such cases the possibility that the actual daily protein intake does not amount to 40 g must be considered, careful evaluation of the dietary records should be performed, and the urea generation rate should be determined to assess protein intake (see below). When there is clinical evidence of negative nitrogen balance during treatment with the diet containing 40 g of protein, the balance can be improved if the diet is supplemented with 5 to 10 g of essential amino acids. It may even be wise to minimize the risk of wasting by supplementing the diet with a small amount of essential amino acids in all patients ingesting only 40 g of protein per day. The amino acid supplement is most conveniently given in tablets (see below).

Patients who experience marked uremic symptoms when on an unrestricted diet can, if the progression of the renal insufficiency is slow, manage for years on a diet providing 40 g of protein per day, and treatment by dialysis can be forestalled or postponed. As the renal function deteriorates further, urea accumulates and toxic symptoms develop in spite of the dietary restriction to 40 g of protein. The next step must then be to introduce a diet with more severe protein restriction.

In 1963 Giordano[106] showed that uremic patients on an extremely nitrogen-restricted diet (less than 3 g of protein per day) could be brought into positive nitrogen balance when given essential L-amino acids. It was initially thought that nitrogen sparing was mainly due to reutilization of urea (present in excessive amounts in uremia) for the synthesis of protein if dietary protein was restricted and adequate amounts of synthetic essential amino acids or protein of high biological value were provided. Hydrolysis of urea into ammonia by urease-producing bacteria takes place in the gut. When ammonia is taken up by the liver it can either be reconverted to urea or combined with carbohydrate to form nonessential amino acids, which can be incorporated into new protein. Later, however, it was shown that reincorporation of urea nitrogen into protein is small, amounting to no more than a few per cent.[107] The quantitatively small nutritional importance of urea recycling is further supported by the observation that nitrogen balance improved rather than worsened when urea degradation was suppressed by oral antibiotics.[108] An alternative explanation of why nitrogen balance is achieved and net production of urea decreases might be that metabolic adaptation may occur in response to a restriction in dietary protein content, resulting in more efficient reutilization of the amino acids liberated during protein breakdown.[109]

Giordano's concept of urea reutilization soon promoted clinical applications. Diets providing as little as 20 to 25 g of protein per day have been reported to maintain neutral nitrogen balance if almost all of the protein is of high biological value.[106,110] Several investigations, however, have shown that most patients are in negative nitrogen balance on diets providing this small an amount of protein.[103,111] Severe complications such as acidosis, hyperkalemia, hypophosphatemia, bleeding, and progressive peripheral neuropathy during long-term treatment with such regimens have been reported.[112–114] Another drawback with these diets is that very rigid restrictions of protein, which must be rich in essential amino acids and balanced with respect to human requirements, lead to monotonous and unpalatable diets and make it difficult for the patients to tolerate the regimen for prolonged periods.

AMINO ACID SUPPLEMENTATION

Another approach to nutrition with a protein-restricted diet in severe chronic uremia is to provide crystalline amino acid supplements of threonine, valine, isoleucine, leucine, methionine, phenylalanine, lysine, tryptophan, and histidine to a diet containing 15 to 20 g of unselected protein.[115] Since the demand for essential amino acids can be met by this supplement, there is no need to provide only dietary protein of high biological value. This makes it possible to compose diets that are much more palatable and variable and thus easier for the patients to accept. The supply of substantial amounts of nonessential amino acids with the diet may also involve a nutritional advantage. For protein synthesis to take place, nonessential as well as essential amino acids must be present. Although nonessential amino acids may be synthesized in the body from essential amino acids, urea, ammonia, and other nonessential amino acids, there are data indicating that nitrogen utilization is more efficient in uremia when both nonessential and essential amino acids are supplied.[116,117]

ENERGY REQUIREMENTS

The energy requirements for patients with advanced chronic renal failure are not settled. Results from studies using indirect calorimetry, however, suggest that basal energy expenditure is similar in undialyzed as well as dialyzed chronically uremic patients and normal subjects and that energy expenditure increases to the same extent in uremic as in normal subjects with exercise and after a test meal.[118] Adequate energy intake may become especially important in patients on low-protein diets with potentially marginal intake of essential amino acids. If the energy intake does not meet the requirements, some of the ingested protein will be used to meet energy demands and will then not be available for protein synthesis. In patients treated with a low-protein diet containing about 25 g of protein per day, Hyne et al.[119] observed a positive correlation between energy intake within the range of 35 to 55 kcal/kg and nitrogen balance. In this study, however, all patients were in varying degrees of negative nitrogen balance, indicating that the essential amino acid and/or protein requirements were not fulfilled. In patients treated with a 15 to 20 g protein diet and essential amino acid supplementation, positive nitrogen balance has been achieved with an energy intake of 25 to 50 kcal/kg.[104] Dietary energy requirements were studied by Kopple et al.[118] in nondialyzed chronic renal failure patients, who were fed diets providing 0.55 to 0.60 g of protein/kg/day and 0.45, 0.35, 0.25, or 0.15 kcal/kg/day. Nitrogen balance correlated directly with energy intake, whereas an inverse correlation was found between energy intake and urea generation. These results suggested that for clinically stable nondialyzed patients ingesting 0.55 to 0.60 g of protein/kg/day, a dietary energy intake of approximately 35 kcal/kg/day is most likely to maintain neutral or positive nitrogen balance and reduce net urea generation. Based on available information it can, thus, be concluded that a daily intake of at least 35 kcal/kg should meet the energy requirements in adult men and women doing light physical work, provided that the requirements of dietary proteins and essential amino acids are met, but a larger amount of energy should probably be recommended to subjects performing heavier work.

However, in patients with advanced renal failure dietary energy intake tends to be lower than normal. Although taste recognition, especially for sweet and bitter, is impaired in uremia,[120] many patients develop aversion to sweet products and may have difficulties in obtaining sufficient amounts of energy. A substantial part of the energy needs can, however, be provided in the form of electrolyte- and protein-free starch products. Caloreen, a mixture of glucose polymers prepared from corn starch, can be added to a variety of foods without perceptible increase in sweetness.[121] It is rapidly converted to glucose, but, with an osmolality in solution of only one fifth of that of glucose, Caloreen is less likely than glucose to cause diarrhea. Additional energy can also be administered in pasta made from protein-free flour (Aprotene).

20 GRAM PROTEIN DIET

About 15 years ago a nutritional regimen was worked out that, in both the short term and the long term, has been successful with respect to nutritional maintenance and patient acceptance.[115] The basis for this nutritional regimen is a diet with a content of unselected protein of about 18 to 20 g/day, which is supplemented with essential amino acids. A high energy intake is encouraged, preferably at least 35 kcal/kg/day. About 50 per cent of the energy is derived from carbohydrates and 50 per cent from fat. A substantial part of the energy must come from low-electrolyte, low-protein sources.

Essential amino acids (10 to 15 g/day) are most conveniently supplied in tablets. (The optimal composition of essential amino acid supplements is discussed below.)

This dietary regimen is primarily intended for patients with chronic uremia who cannot be maintained free from toxic symptoms or in whom serum urea increases to above 30 to 35 mmol/L (BUN 80 to 100 mg/dl) while they are on a 40 g protein diet.

A prerequisite of a successful outcome of treatment with the supplemented diet is in general that the patients can be detoxified before the amino acid preparation is supplied. This can be attained by an initial treatment period (1 to 2 weeks) with the low-protein diet alone. When reduction of serum urea and alleviation of the uremic syndrome have been obtained, amino acids are supplied. If possible, detoxification by performing dialysis once or twice is preferred, since the period on the unsupplemented low-protein diet, during which the nitrogen balance is negative, will then be shortened. Essential amino acids can usually be instituted when serum urea concentration has decreased to 25 to 30 mmol/L. Supplementation of the diet with essential amino acids results in positive nitrogen balance, and a further reduction of the serum urea concentration is often observed.

It is important that water, electrolyte, and acid-base balances be well controlled. Patients are allowed a liberal salt intake, a prerequisite of success with the dietary therapy. The low-protein diet should be made salt-poor with a sodium content of less than 10 to 15 mmol/day. Individual salt intake can then be more easily controlled. Patients are usually advised to season the food with 2 to 3 g of table salt per day, and, if necessary, additional sodium is given in tablets. Sodium bicarbonate (in tablets) should be given in sufficient amounts to keep the plasma bicarbonate concentration within the normal range. To allow the liberal salt intake it is often necessary to prescribe a diuretic acting in the ascending limb of Henle's loop (see above).

The success of the conservative dietary treatment with amino acid supplementation is dependent on whether the patient adheres to the prescribed diet. It is recommended that the patient be admitted to the ward when the low-protein diet is instituted. The effect of the treatment can then be closely supervised, and the patient then also gets the opportunity to learn what the nutritional regimen involves. Dietary education of the patient and adaptation of the diet to the individual taste of the patient call for expertise, and the value of assistance by a skilled, interested, and imaginative dietician in these tasks cannot be exaggerated.

Many studies of the efficacy and acceptability of a dietary regimen of 15 to 25 g of unselected protein with essential amino acid supplementation have been performed in nondialyzed chronic renal failure patients.[122] In most of these studies the diet has been supplemented with amino acid preparations containing threonine, valine, isoleucine, leucine, methionine, phenylalanine, lysine, and tryptophan in the proportions recommended by Rose[99] for normal humans, and also containing histidine. Generally 14 to 20 g/day of amino acids have been given.

Switching from free protein intake or moderately reduced protein intake to more markedly reduced protein intake supplemented with essential amino acids leads to a decrease in serum or blood urea and a reduction in the urea:creatinine ratio. Normal values are frequently obtained in patients with low serum albumin, but initially normal values remain unchanged. Increases in transferrin, C3 and other complement factors, prealbumin, and cholinesterase are observed during therapy with the dietary regimen. All these findings support the conclusion that essential amino acids are beneficial as a supplement to low-protein diets in nondialyzed patients with chronic renal failure. However, restricted intake of unselected protein supplemented with essential amino acids appears to offer little advantage over a selective diet that provides 40 g of protein of high biological value, except that the unselected supplemented diet is preferred and patient compliance is better.[123]

Nitrogen balance studies performed after a short period of treatment with essential amino acids, generally after an initial adaptation period on a protein-restricted diet only, showed positive or neutral nitrogen balance in most patients.

Only a few nitrogen balance studies have included patients treated with a low-protein diet and essential amino acids over longer periods of time (more than 3 months). In such studies, in adult patients receiving essential amino acids in the proportions recommended by Rose for normal humans and histidine, the mean nitrogen balance was found to be negative.[115,124,125] Long-term treatment with this regimen did not normalize abnormalities in intracellular amino acid concentrations typically observed in uremia.[27] Positive nitrogen balance and reversion toward normal intracellular amino acid levels, however, were observed after long-term treatment with an 18 to 20 g protein diet supplemented with a modified amino acid preparation with changed proportions between the branched-chain amino acids (valine > leucine > isoleucine).[27,33] The modified formula also contained threonine in higher proportion and tyrosine.[23,27] These results support the suggestion that protein metabolism and nitrogen utilization may be improved by normalization of the intracellular amino acid pattern.

SUPPLEMENTATION WITH NITROGEN-FREE ANALOGUES

As an attempt to further reduce the necessary accumulation of waste nitrogen, Schloerb[126] and Richards et al.[127] first suggested that nitrogen-free analogues of essential amino acids might replace the amino acids in the nutrition of the uremic patient. The rationale for replacement of essential amino acids by their nitrogen-free analogues was, as Rose first suggested, that the carbon skeleton and not the amino acid itself is the indispensable part of the essential amino acid, and that essential keto acids are transaminated by nonessential amino acids, producing the corresponding essential amino acids and nonessential keto acids. In other words, essential amino acids may be provided without simultaneously increasing the amount of nitrogen that must be excreted. It has been shown in animal experiments that all essential amino acids except lysine and threonine may be synthesized in the body.[128] It has also been demonstrated that the alpha-keto analogues can substitute for all essential amino acids except lysine and threonine in both healthy and uremic subjects.[129,130] Mitch and Walser[131,132] demonstrated that uremic subjects can utilize the hydroxy analogues of methionine and phenylalanine as substitutes for the corresponding amino acids. The hydroxy analogues are oxidized to the respective keto analogues by dehydrogenases present in various tissues and then transaminated to the corresponding essential amino acids.

There are, at least theoretically, several reasons why it might be advantageous to supplement a low-protein diet with a keto acid preparation instead of essential amino acids. Some results suggest that keto acids may improve nitrogen utilization and decrease urea generation more than can be accounted for by transamination.[133] It has been suggested that leucine and its keto analogue alpha-keto-isocaproate (KICA) might spare nitrogen by affecting regulatory mechanisms for protein synthesis and degradation.[134]

Leucine, apparently alone among the physiological amino acids, stimulates protein synthesis and decreases protein degeneration in both skeletal and heart muscle.[135,136] The stimulatory effect of leucine appears to be restricted to the amino acid itself, whereas KICA, or one of its degradation products,

has the ability to suppress protein breakdown. However, these results were obtained in in vitro studies, and it is not clear whether leucine and KICA have similar protein-sparing effects in vivo.

Supplementation of a low-protein diet with a keto acid preparation could be advantageous in patients with near-end-stage renal failure. In these patients nitrogen supply must be more restricted than is possible with a low-protein diet plus supplementary essential amino acids, in order to obviate excessive accumulation of nonprotein nitrogen and thus prevent or alleviate uremic symptoms. Another potential advantage might be that supplementation of a less protein-restricted diet with a keto acid preparation could result in the same total nitrogen supply and the same nitrogen-sparing effect as that obtained with a more protein-restricted diet and essential amino acid supplementation. Clinical results, however, indicate that keto analogue supplementation has no substantial nutritional benefit in uremic patients who ingest a 40 g protein diet, probably because the degradation of the keto analogues is enhanced when dietary protein intake is increased.[137,137a] Also, keto acid supplementation can generally be instituted immediately when the patient is switched to the low-protein diet, so that no detoxification is required as is often necessary when essential amino acids are given. Positive nitrogen balance has been obtained within 3 to 10 days after reduction of dietary protein intake to about 20 g/day and supplementation of the diet with nitrogen-free analogues.[133,138] Side effects, on the other hand, seem to be more frequent with keto acid supplementation than when essential amino acids are given. In commercially available preparations the analogues have been provided as calcium salts, and gastrointestinal intolerance may be caused by the high calcium content of the preparation. Hypercalcemia and hypophosphatemia have been observed in a significant fraction of patients on long-term therapy but have rarely been severe or symptomatic.[139] Mild hypophosphatemia and hypercalcemia may even be beneficial, by suppressing parathyroid hormone production.[140] The fall in plasma inorganic phosphate has been suggested to be due to improved build-up of cellular tissue, induced by keto acid supplementation. However, since the effect seems to persist over long periods of time,[124,125] hypophosphatemia could conceivably be due to reduced intestinal absorption of phosphate, because of increased intestinal binding of phosphate to the calcium administered with the keto acids.

Clinically, preparations containing nitrogen-free analogues of valine, isoleucine, leucine, methionine, and phenylalanine plus the essential amino acids threonine, lysine, histidine, and tryptophan as such have been used as supplements to diets providing 15 to 25 g of unselected protein in uremic patients. The clinical results of such therapy have been comparable to those obtained with amino acid–

supplemented diets, with alleviation of the uremic syndrome and maintenance of nitrogen balance.[141]

Several studies, reviewed by Kampf et al.,[123] have shown that nitrogen balance after short-term treatment (less than 2 months) may become positive or neutral when a low-protein diet is combined with a keto acid/amino acid preparation. The composition of the analogue preparations used in most of these studies has been based on requirements of the essential amino acids of normal subjects, but the relative amounts of the branched-chain keto acids have been increased to compensate for the relatively higher degree of degradation of these analogues by the liver. After long-term treatment (longer than 3 months) with this regimen the average nitrogen balance was negative, and derangements in plasma and intracellular amino acid patterns similar to those in patients treated with a low-protein diet and essential amino acids (in the proportions recommended by Rose) were observed, suggesting imbalanced amino acid supply.[142]

The optimal composition of essential amino acid analogue preparations is highly dependent on the degree of conversion of the analogues to their corresponding essential amino acids. Halliday et al.[143] gave ^{13}C-labeled alpha-keto analogues of valine and phenylalanine orally or intravenously to three healthy subjects and four uremic individuals who served as their own controls. Levels of $^{13}CO_2$ in expired air and of ^{13}C-labeled keto acids in urine were determined, and plasma and, in some cases, intramuscular concentrations of total and ^{13}C-labeled free valine and phenylalanine were measured. The degree of conversion of these two alpha-keto acids into essential amino acids was on the order of 25 to 50 per cent, regardless of route of administration or subjects' health. Epstein et al.[144] measured decarboxylation of ^{14}C-alpha-ketoisovaleric acid by determining $^{14}CO_2$ in expired air in normal subjects and two uremic patients on low-protein diets supplemented with EAA and KIVA in place of valine. Carboxylation was calculated to be 22 to 32 per cent; thus 68 to 78 per cent might have been available for protein synthesis at this very low protein intake. Apart from these two studies there have been no direct measurements of the degree of conversion of branched-chain keto acids or other essential keto acids in uremic patients. However, using tracer techniques in animal experiments, Tungsanga et al. recently showed that the nutritional efficiency of ketoisocaproic acid as a substitute for leucine was higher in uremic rats than in control rats.[145]

Several formulations with modified contents of essential amino acids and analogues have been tested as supplements to a diet containing 20 to 25 g of mixed-quality protein in patients with advanced chronic renal failure.[146] These supplements have been designed to minimize or reverse the amino acid abnormalities rather than to meet the normal requirements for the essential amino acids. To avoid the side effects (gastrointestinal distress and clinically significant hypercalcemia) that some patients experience when analogues are given as calcium salts, the analogues have been given as mixed salts between branched-chain keto analogues and the basic amino acids (ornithine, lysine, and histidine). Encouraging long-term results with respect to nutritional effects and tolerability were reported for one of these formulations, which was designed to have the same proportions of the branched-chain amino acids as the modified essential amino acid formula discussed above. The mixture contained very little methionine, and phenylalanine and tryptophan were not included in any form.[147]

In spite of the above-mentioned drawbacks of providing the keto acids as calcium salts, the rationale for giving the branched-chain amino acid analogues as salts of basic amino acids, at all, is not clear. The basic amino acids contain two nitrogen atoms, and the nitrogen intake is thus doubled when a branched-chain amino acid is substituted for by its keto analogue given as the salt of a basic amino acid. As discussed above, there is no firm evidence that supplementation with the keto analogues of the branched-chain acids involves any advantage other than reduction of nitrogen intake.

Guidelines for Judging Efficacy of Treatment with Low-Protein Diets

In patients with severe renal insufficiency and especially those who are treated with low-protein regimens, the resistance to even light complications may be impaired. A slight further reduction of the renal function may lead to markedly increased uremic intoxication. Also, nitrogen balance may become negative and uremic symptoms may reappear in association with a trivial respiratory infection. These patients should therefore be regularly assessed by a physician.

A deterioration of the patient's general condition with a rise in serum urea may be due to a further impairment of renal function, which then should be reflected by a rise in serum creatinine. A rise in serum urea and reappearance of uremic symptoms without a concomitant increase in serum creatinine suggests that nitrogen metabolism is affected by some extrarenal factor. The influence of such factors should also be suspected if treatment fails initially. Factors that increase protein catabolism and lead to a rise in serum urea include inadequate energy intake, infection and fever, potassium deficiency, cardiac insufficiency, severe acidosis, and corticosteroid therapy. In many cases the treatment can be continued with improved results if the cause of the accelerated rate of protein catabolism can be corrected.

A prerequisite for a successful outcome of treatment with a low-protein regimen in patients with renal failure is that the patient adhere to the prescribed diet. If the protein intake is higher than recommended, the uremic intoxication will not be alleviated and the patient's symptoms will persist. On the other hand, too low a protein intake involves the risk of protein malnutrition.

The degree of adherence to a prescribed protein intake can be assessed by the serum urea:creatinine ratio, as discussed by Kopple and Coburn.[148] The serum urea concentration is affected by renal function, protein intake, and the rate of protein breakdown, whereas the serum creatinine level depends primarily on renal function. Hence, by calculating the serum urea:creatinine ratio, the influences on the serum urea level of renal function on the one hand and of protein intake and protein breakdown on the other can be evaluated separately. In a metabolic steady state the serum urea:creatinine ratio does not change and can be used to assess protein intake. The relation between the serum urea:creatinine ratio and protein intake, however, may be influenced by urine flow, as urea clearance may fall disproportionately to creatinine clearance when urine flow is low, and also by muscle mass. Therefore, the serum urea:creatinine ratio is of value primarily for the continuous assessment of protein intake in the individual patient.

A better method to estimate the protein intake quantitatively is to determine the protein catabolic rate (PCR). Urea is the predominant product of protein catabolism, and PCR can, in the metabolic steady state, be calculated from the following equation:[149]

$$PCR = \frac{(0.028 \times UAR) + (0.031 \times BW)}{0.154}$$

where UAR is the urea appearance rate (or net urea production), which is the sum of the total amount of urea excreted in the urine and the change of total body urea per 24 hours (moles/24 hours). The non-urea nitrogen excretion is calculated as $0.031 \times$ body weight (kg).

If serum urea is constant, urea appearance is equal to urinary urea excretion. If serum urea is not constant, the change in total body urea can be approximated from the equation:

$$body\ urea = serum\ urea \times 0.6 \times BW$$

Under conditions of metabolic balance PCR will equal protein intake. In patients with constant body weight PCR may thus give a good quantitative estimate of the amount of protein ingested.

During treatment with a protein-restricted diet the nutritional status of the patient must be periodically monitored. As discussed below, it is also important to detect and evaluate malnutrition in dialysis patients. Unfortunately there is no single method for nutritional evaluation that is applicable and sensitive to all situations. Body weight gives only an estimate of tissue weight even if the patient has not developed clinical edema, and is of limited value in the nutritional evaluation of dialysis patients, in whom body water may fluctuate considerably. By measuring mid upper arm circumference and triceps skinfold thickness (TSF) the arm muscle circumference (AMC) may be calculated as follows:

$$AMC\ (cm) = mid\ upper\ arm\ circumference\ (cm)\\ - 0.314 \times TSF\ (mm)$$

AMC, which gives an evaluation of the somatic protein compartment, is highly interrelated with other nutritional variables[150] and is, therefore, of special value in the assessment of protein energy malnutrition. Grip strength, which can be measured in seconds by use of a hand-grip dynamometer, also appears to be a sensitive indicator of the nutritional status.[151]

In addition, the concentrations of certain serum proteins such as albumin and transferrin can be used to evaluate the visceral protein compartment. It should be emphasized that acute nutritional changes are not reflected by changes of the above anthropometric parameters or serum albumin and transferrin, which are of value primarily for the continuous assessment of the nutritional status in patients during prolonged therapy with protein restriction or dialysis.

Prealbumin and retinol-binding protein are among the most sensitive indicators of nutrition[152] when renal function is normal. In chronic renal failure the concentrations of these low molecular weight proteins are increased, probably because of decreased catabolism and excretion. Nevertheless, results of studies of nutritional assessment of hemodialysis patients suggest that prealbumin and retinol-binding protein, which have short turnover time, may reflect more acute changes in the availability of nutrient supply, if they are determined repeatedly in individual patients.[150] Young et al. reported that in nonfasting hemodialysis patients the plasma concentration of valine was the single nutritional parameter that showed the highest degree of correlation with other nutritional parameters.[150] However, this observation was not confirmed in patients studied in the fasting state.[153]

As discussed above, reliable information on acute changes in the nutritional status in renal failure patients may not be obtained by assessments of anthropometric parameters or determination of plasma proteins. Direct measurements on skeletal muscle, representing the largest cellular mass and nitrogen store in the body, may therefore be of special value in patients with renal insufficiency. Muscle DNA content is considered a reliable reference standard in normal and undernourished adults.[154] Starvation and refeeding are accompanied by rapid changes in muscle RNA content.[155] The ratio of noncollagen, alkali-soluble protein to DNA is considered as an estimate of the cytoplasmic volume of a single cell, and the RNA:DNA ratio is an index of the capacity of the cell to synthesize proteins. Thus, determination of nucleic acid and protein content in muscle tissue obtained by needle aspiration may be a valuable tool for nutritional assessment at a cellular level and can be used to monitor the response to nutritional therapy in individual patients.[156]

Outcome of Treatment with Low-Protein Diets

It has been suggested that patients who have been treated for prolonged periods with protein-restricted diets may not well withstand the multiple stresses of hemodialysis and transplantation.[157] In particular, it has been claimed that atherosclerosis develops at an accelerated rate in patients treated with protein restriction prior to hemodialysis treatment as compared with patients starting early on dialysis.[158] There is, however, little evidence in support of these misgivings. In a group of 68 patients who were treated for a mean of 215 days (30 to 840 days) with a diet containing 15 to 20 g of protein per day supplemented with essential amino acids or keto analogues beyond the time when they could not be supported by moderate protein reduction (40 g of protein per day), results concerning mortality and life expectancy were at least as good as for patients on dialysis.[159] These findings do not support the contention that prolonged dietary treatment accelerates atherosclerosis. The diet in this study was not modified to provide increased amounts of polyunsaturated fat or reduction in disaccharides. Attman and Gustafson,[160] who studied the influence of treatment with a similar low-protein regimen, could not find any deterioration in total lipids and lipoproteins over an average period of 9½ months in spite of continuous reduction in renal function over the observation period. Moreover, patients treated with this type of low-protein regimen showed no change in body cell mass and energy stores as estimated by body weight and determination of total body water and total body potassium.[161] Finally, no clinical evidence of malnutrition, serum protein depletion, or progressive neuropathy has been found in patients treated with 18 to 25 g of protein per day supplemented with essential amino acids.[162] All of these results indicate that patients with far advanced renal failure can safely be treated for prolonged periods with low-protein regimens such as those described above and that dialysis treatment thereby can be forestalled. Nevertheless, it is of utmost importance that patients treated with protein restriction be carefully supervised (see above) and that dialysis treatment and intensified nutritional therapy be instituted if signs of malnutrition appear.

Treatment of Calcium-Phosphorus Abnormalities

Treatment aimed at preventing the development of secondary hyperparathyroidism should be instituted early in the course of renal failure. When GFR is higher than 25 to 30 ml/min, normal plasma levels of calcium and phosphate are generally observed. The phosphate concentration, however, is kept within the normal range only because the circulating level of PTH is elevated. Therefore, treatment of hyperphosphatemia should preferably be initiated before hyperphosphatemia is clinically evident. Such treatment includes dietary phosphate restriction and oral administration of phosphate-binding aluminum hydroxide gels to increase fecal phosphate excretion. As discussed above, such treatment may, however, involve the risk of aluminum intoxication. Initially a marked phosphate restriction may be accomplished by excluding milk from the diet. As renal function worsens, the amount of phosphate being excreted becomes very low. It is then necessary to eliminate all foods high in phosphorus, especially dairy products, to prevent retention of phosphate.

Treatment of hyperphosphatemia is facilitated by protein restriction. The daily supply of phosphate with a normal diet is 1.0 to 1.8 g or more, whereas a 40 g protein diet provides about 0.6 to 0.9 g of phosphate and a 20 g unselected protein diet about 0.4 to 0.6 g of phosphate per day. If a substantial part of the energy intake is supplied as electrolyte-free oligosaccharides and only selected proteins of vegetable origin are included in the diet, the phosphate may be reduced further. Such diets, however, are not well tolerated.

As discussed above, calcium balance is often negative in patients with renal failure due to deficiency of 1,25-dihydroxyvitamin D_3 and impaired intestinal calcium absorption. Moreover, dietary calcium intake is often low in uremic patients. Thus, a 40 g protein diet contains 400 to 500 mg and a 20 g protein diet only 200 to 300 mg of calcium.

Dietary supplements of calcium are therefore indicated in patients with a restricted protein intake and also in hemodialysis patients, in whom intake of dairy products is often restricted to reduce the phosphate load. Positive calcium balance may be obtained in uremic patients when the intake of calcium exceeds 1200 to 1500 mg/day.[62] Thus, it seems reasonable to recommend a calcium supplement that provides about 1000 mg/day of elemental calcium. Calcium supplements, however, should not be given before serum phosphorus is corrected by phosphate restriction and phosphate-binding antacids.

If normalization of serum calcium cannot be obtained by oral calcium supplementation, treatment with vitamin D is required. 1,25-dihydroxyvitamin D_3, which is the most potent metabolite of vitamin D with respect to calcium absorption, is now commercially available. Initially, a daily dose of 0.25 to

0.5 μg is given, which is slowly increased until normocalcemia is achieved. The dose must be carefully monitored to avoid hypercalcemia, which may lead to further impairment of renal function. Hypercalcemia also involves the risk of soft tissue calcification, especially if serum phosphorus is high, and treatment with vitamin D must not be initiated until serum phosphorus can be safely controlled.

Lipid-Lowering Regimens

In view of the fact that we do not know exactly the importance of the lipid changes in uremia, although they may be atherogenic, it is still of interest that dietary manipulation can change the lipid patterns. Decreasing dietary carbohydrate intake to 20 to 35 per cent of total calories ingested leads to a significant fall in postprandial insulin response, VLDL secretion, and plasma triglyceride concentration.[163,164] The consumption of a diet rich in polyunsaturated fatty acids has been shown to normalize increased serum triglycerides and to increase lowered HDL cholesterol, suggesting that the diet may be effective for prevention of atherosclerosis.[165] In patients with CAPD lipid abnormalities, restriction of oral carbohydrate intake to 240 to 250 g/day and minimum use of high-glucose dialysate appears to prevent further increase in serum triglycerides.[57]

Perhaps of equal value is increased exercise. Goldberg et al.[166] reported on hemodialysis patients who showed significant improvement in oxygen consumption and exercise tolerance within 4 to 7 months of exercise training. The plasma triglycerides decreased and the HDL increased. This was a carefully controlled study, that is not applicable to all patients, but it clearly indicates that greater use may be made of sensible exercise. Other ways of manipulating blood lipids in uremia are by giving lipid-lowering drugs. Clofibrate should be used only after careful consideration of the risk, and the doses should be reduced in uremic patients. In this connection, it is of interest that the plasma level of L-carnitine decreases profoundly while patients are undergoing hemodialysis.[167] Carnitine has been administered orally or intravenously to dialysis patients in varying doses and has been found to have a lowering effect on triglycerides and free fatty acids, whereas cholesterol is not changed. Therapy also resulted in elevation of both plasma and muscle concentrations of L-carnitine. Giving DL-carnitine may induce a myasthenia-like syndrome in patients on long-term hemodialysis,[168] an effect that can be prevented by treatment with L-carnitine. The clinical value of L-carnitine therapy has yet to be finally evaluated.

Treatment of Vitamin and Trace Element Abnormalities

As discussed above, plasma levels of vitamin B$_6$ (pyridoxine) are low in uremic patients. A pyridoxine supplement of 5 to 10 mg/day is therefore recommended, since pyridoxal phosphate is a coenzyme for transamination reactions. Such supplementation may be of special importance in patients on low-protein diets.

Although deficiency of folic acid and vitamin C is not consistently found in dialyzed or conservatively treated uremic patients, supplementation with 1 mg/day of folic acid and 100 mg/day of vitamin C is usually recommended.[169]

Supplementation of vitamin D is discussed in the preceding section. Since accumulation of vitamin A may be deleterious in uremia, polyvitamin preparations containing vitamin A should be avoided.

Iron deficiency due to inadequate dietary intake, intestinal blood loss, and, in dialysis patients, sequestration in the dialyzer may sometimes become clinically important and contribute to the anemia of renal failure. However, iron supplementation should not be be given routinely to all patients because iron overload may be present, in which case the serum ferritin concentration is high. To patients with low serum ferritin, oral supplementation with iron should be given. Ferrosulfate, 0.3 g three times daily half an hour after meals, has been recommended for such patients.[169] If the patient cannot be nourished orally or cannot tolerate oral iron therapy, parenteral iron administration is indicated. Whether supplementary zinc administration is needed remains controversial, and no definite recommendations can be made. Oral zinc, for example 50 mg of elemental zinc per day as zinc acetate, may be tried in male dialysis patients with gonadal dysfunction and in patients complaining of impaired taste perception.[170]

Nutritional Therapy in Hemodialysis Patients

Several recent reports have documented that protein-energy malnutrition is frequently present in patients treated with maintenance hemodialysis therapy.[150,153,171,172] It is generally accepted that suboptimal nutritional status is associated with increased morbidity and may contribute to poor rehabilitation and poor quality of life. Immune alterations strikingly similar to those observed in malnutrition have been documented in hemodialysis patients,[173] suggesting that protein-energy malnutrition may be a risk factor for infection and septicemia in such patients.

In 120 hemodialysis patients, Acchiardo et al.[174] found that a subgroup with a mean protein intake of 0.63 g/kg/day had a mortality of 14 per cent per year while groups of patients with higher intakes, 0.93, 1.02, and 1.29 g/kg/day, had a mortality of only 4, 3, and 0 per cent, respectively. The number of hospitalizations per year was also much higher in the patients with the lowest intake of protein. The authors concluded that protein malnutrition is the main factor in morbidity and mortality of hemodialysis patients. This conclusion is supported by the results of other studies as well.[153,175]

PROTEIN REQUIREMENT

It has long been recognized that dietary requirements of protein are higher during intermittent dialysis than in normal subjects and nondialyzed uremic patients.[176] However, there is no consensus about the amount of dietary protein that is necessary to maintain nitrogen balance in patients on intermittent hemodialysis. Subjects with normal renal function have a minimum daily protein requirement of about 0.5 g/kg/day.[99,100] Results of nitrogen balance studies in patients on twice a week maintenance dialysis suggested that approximately 0.75 g/kg/day of high biological value protein is necessary to maintain nitrogen equilibrium[177] or a slightly positive nitrogen balance.[178]

According to more recent long-term studies, this amount of protein may not be adequate. Signs of malnutrition have been observed in substantial fractions of apparently well-rehabilitated patients on maintenance hemodialysis, who had a daily protein intake of about 1 g/kg/day.[179,180]

In contrast, nondialyzed uremic patients may be in nitrogen balance on 0.5 to 0.6 g/kg/day of high-quality protein[111] or less if the diet is supplemented with essential amino acids[33] or their keto analogues.[138,147] Hence, the increased protein requirements of hemodialysis patients cannot be attributed to uremia, but must be a consequence of the hemodialysis treatment.

There is now evidence that the hemodialysis procedure per se is a strong catabolic stimulus. Borah et al.[181] studied nitrogen balance during intermittent hemodialysis therapy on high (1.4 g/kg) and low (0.5 g/kg) protein intake. They found that during ingestion of the low-protein diet the nitrogen balance was markedly negative on dialysis days and also slightly negative on nondialysis days, resulting in a negative cumulative balance for the study period. During ingestion of the high-protein diet nitrogen balance was still negative on dialysis days but positive on nondialysis days, and the cumulative balance for the study period was zero.

Ward, Farrell, et al. studied the effect of hemodialysis on protein catabolism by comparing urea appearance rate during dialysis and in the interdialytic period.[182,183] The rate was about 30 per cent higher during dialysis than off dialysis, which confirmed that the dialytic procedure is a catabolic stimulus. This figure may be an underestimation if the catabolic effects of dialysis extend beyond the period of dialysis into the interdialytic period. Furthermore, calculating protein degradation from urea appearance does not take into account losses of free amino acids from the extra- and intracellular amino acid pools, which may have to be replaced by degradation of protein.

During hemodialysis average losses of free amino acids in the dialysis fluid have been reported to be 5 to 8 g per dialysis,[184-188] of which about one third are essential amino acids. In addition 4 to 5 g of peptide-bound amino acids are lost per dialysis;[184,186] thus, the total losses of amino acids are about 10 to 13 g per dialysis.[184,187,188] In fasting patients losses of amino acids were smaller with than without glucose in the dialysate,[184] but in nonfasting patients addition of glucose to the dialysate could not reduce the free amino acid loss during routine hemodialysis.[185] Obviously, the losses of free and bound amino acids during dialysis are insufficient to account completely for the increased protein requirements in hemodialysis patients compared with nonuremic individuals and nondialyzed uremic patients. Hence, one has to conclude that additional factors, not related to the dialytic removal of amino acids (and glucose), are involved.

Results of recent studies indicate that accelerated protein breakdown associated with hemodialysis may be caused by interaction between blood and artificial membranes in a dialyzer. The release of amino acids from leg tissues (representing mainly muscle) was measured in healthy subjects before and after sham dialysis (i.e., in vivo passage of blood through a cuprophane dialyzer but with no circulating dialysate). The results indicate that the net release of amino acids increased by about 100 per cent 5 to 6 hours after the start of sham dialysis. This response was prevented by indomethacin, suggesting that the enhanced protein catabolism is mediated by prostaglandins.[189]

NUTRITIONAL SUPPLEMENTATION IN HEMODIALYSIS PATIENTS

If dietary protein and energy are inadequate to compensate for the catabolic factors associated with hemodialysis, the nutritional status will be impaired, and wasting will develop in the long run. Indeed, marginal or insufficient dietary intake of nutrients is common in hemodialysis patients.[153] Altered taste acuity, possibly caused by zinc deficiency, or restrictions of salt and fluid may make the diet unpalatable and may lead to inadequate food intake. Additional causes of anorexia include heavy medication, including oral phosphate binders, and also depression.

Nutritional assessment and determination of optimal nutrition are thus of primary importance in the treatment of patients on maintenance hemodialysis. Although wasting may be obvious in advanced cases, patients with milder degrees of malnutrition may be more difficult to identify. Several excellent papers dealing with nutritional evaluation in patients on dialysis have recently been published.[150,190,191] Some of the more commonly used methods for assessing nutritional status in uremia have been discussed earlier in this chapter.

Attempts have been made to compensate for the amino acid losses and increased protein requirements in regular hemodialysis patients by supplementation with essential amino acids orally[192–196] or intravenously.[172,190,197] The clinical biochemical results of such supplementation have been presented in a recent review.[122] On the basis of measurement of visceral proteins as well as plasma amino acids, some authors conclude that the effect of essential amino acid supplementation is questionable, at least in hemodialysis patients with a relatively high protein intake.[190,195,198]

Decreased intracellular levels of valine were observed in hemodialysis patients with an estimated protein intake of about 1 g/kg/day, suggesting that the intake of valine was inadequate and that the diet should be supplemented.[142]

Whereas it is debatable whether amino acid supplementation has any beneficial effects in well-nourished patients on a diet containing 1 g of protein/kg/day or more, oral or intravenous supplementation of essential amino acids between or during dialysis treatments is clearly indicated in patients with dietary intake less than this or in those who are septic or otherwise hypercatabolic. In patients with marginally low dietary protein intake, 5 to 10 g of essential amino acids may be administered orally in tablets. If this mode of administration is not feasible, amino acids can be infused during the dialysis procedure. It is then probably valuable to administer nonessential as well as essential amino acids. If nonessential amino acids are not supplied, synthesis from essential amino acids must make up for the nonessential amino acids lost into the dialysate. Furthermore, synthesis of dispensable amino acids may be impaired in uremia. The nutritional value of providing a general (nonessential plus essential amino acid) mixture is suggested by studies by Piraino et al.[172] Superior results with respect to weight gain and normalization of plasma amino acid concentrations were observed in catabolic chronic hemodialysis patients when essential and nonessential amino acids were infused during each dialysis for 5 months as compared with supplementation with only essential amino acids.

Energy requirements for patients on maintenance hemodialysis have not been well defined. Probably the minimum daily intake for the adult patient should exceed 35 kcal/kg/day. In many patients this requirement is not fulfilled,[153] and they should therefore be encouraged to supplement the diet with high-energy compounds, such as Caloreen. As in the case of amino acids, energy can also be administered during the dialysis procedure. However, when the dialysate glucose concentration is 200 to 450 mg/dl, only a rather small amount of glucose (25 to 50 g) is taken up during a hemodialysis treatment of 4 to 5 hours. Addition of glucose (200 mg/dl) to the dialysate prevents the hypoglycemia observed during glucose-free dialysis. As discussed above, it is not settled whether this amount of glucose may also lower dialysis-induced protein catabolism. From a practical point of view, dialysate glucose has been observed to be associated with less postdialysis fatigue and reduced fluid removal problems.[156] On the other hand, addition of glucose to the dialysis fluid involves an increased risk of pyrogenic reactions secondary to bacterial growth, and in most centers glucose dialysate is not used routinely.

In patients with inadequate dietary intake, protein and energy may alternatively be supplied in nutritional solutions that the patient may drink with meals. Patients with anorexia, however, often prefer to slowly sip small volumes hour by hour and may in this way ingest substantial amounts of protein and energy each day. In patients who cannot comply with such regimens, nutritional support can be given by feeding some of these solutions enterally via some of the thin, fine polyvinyl chloride feeding tubes that are now available. These tubes, which can be left in site for several weeks without complications, do not cause great discomfort and allow the patient to ingest food in a normal manner. If, by any of these means, the intake of protein and energy may be increased and the nutritional status improved, the anorexia can often be alleviated or eliminated.

An easy way of providing protein and energy to patients who cannot meet the requirements by oral intake is to infuse amino acids together with glucose and fat during the hemodialysis treatments. The amino acids and energy should preferably be infused throughout the hemodialysis procedure. Wolfson et al.[187] have recently shown that the net loss of amino acids into the dialysate does not exceed about 10 per cent of the amount infused. Approximately 40 g of amino acids can be administered together with glucose and fat, providing approximately 800 kcal, in a volume of 800 ml. Owing to the high blood flow, hypertonic (50 per cent) glucose solutions can be infused into the venous line without causing damage to the peripheral vessels. If nutrients are administered throughout the hemodialysis procedure, the infused amino acids and glucose may replace losses during the dialysis and thereby reduce catabolism. The risk of fluid overload may also be lowered if water can be removed by ultrafiltration as it is infused. However, little is known about the utilization of amino acids infused during HD. One may speculate whether factors that promote the HD-associated increase in net protein breakdown may influence protein synthesis as well as protein catabolism. Continuous infusion may therefore be preferred before infusion during the HD procedures only, although this makes the use of a central venous catheter necessary.

Protein supplementation by i.v. infusion of amino acids is expensive and, in spite of the foregoing potential advantages, it therefore seems reasonable to restrict parenteral infusion of amino acids to patients in whom supplementation by the oral route or by means of infusion through a nasogastric feeding tube is not possible. Parenteral nutrition is often necessary in HD patients with septicemia or other infectious illnesses and also in association with surgery. In such clinical settings the protein catabolic rate can be markedly raised and can amount to 100 to 150 g/day or more, in which case the principles of the nutritional management situation do not differ from those applied in the treatment of hypercatabolic patients with acute renal failure (see below).

Nutritional Management in Acute Renal Failure

Despite recent advances in dialysis treatment, the mortality rate in acute renal failure remains as high as prior to the dialysis era. Acute tubular necrosis occurring with trauma or following complications to surgery or septicemia is associated with a mortality rate of 40 to 80 per cent.[199] This persistently high mortality is probably a reflection of the fact that an increased number of severely injured or critically ill patients now get improved intensive care and survive long enough for acute renal failure to become clinically evident. In contrast, mortality in patients with acute tubular necrosis secondary to dehydration or following administration of nephrotoxins is markedly lower, ranging from 10 to 30 per cent.[199]

Extreme catabolism is most probably a major contributing factor to the persistently high mortality in patients with acute renal failure after trauma or surgery. The protein catabolic rate may amount to 150 to 200 g of protein per 24 hours.[200] Because of underlying disease, many patients have an impaired nutritional status prior to the renal damage. Since many patients are not able to eat, overt malnutrition and wasting often ensue or are worsened. Malnutrition is associated with impaired wound healing and immunocompetence, and infections are common in the course of acute renal insufficiency. Indeed, sepsis is the most frequent cause of death in acute renal failure.[201] It has also been suggested that malnutrition may adversely affect the healing of the renal injury and thus the rate of recovery from renal failure.[202] Therefore, nutritional management probably is of major importance for the outcome of patients with acute renal insufficiency.

The optimal nutritional therapy in patients with acute renal failure is, however, difficult to define. The nutritional requirements depend on the clinical setting and can certainly differ considerably between patients with different degrees of renal failure and catabolism. Moreover, the evaluation of various nutritional regimens is very difficult in the clinical situation because of the great number of variables involved in patients with acute renal failure.

The goals of nutritional management in patients with acute renal failure should be to improve and maintain an optimal nutritional status without inducing uremic symptoms or disturbing fluid and electrolyte balance. Indeed, this is a formidable task; in patients undergoing severe catabolic stress, energy and protein requirements may be markedly increased. In addition, acute renal failure is commonly associated with oliguria or anuria, which necessitates careful supervision of fluid and electrolyte balances and makes parenteral nutrition more difficult.

Before the advent of dialysis, protein restriction was employed as a mean to alleviate the uremic toxicity, and 100 to 200 g/day of carbohydrate was supplied to reduce protein catabolism. Kleinknecht et al.,[201] however, showed that overall mortality could be significantly reduced in patients with acute renal failure of various etiologies who underwent early and frequent dialysis. By dialysis potentially toxic products of tissue breakdown, which may impair or inhibit protein synthesis or cause other metabolic disturbances, are eliminated and improved conditions of utilization of administered nutrients are created. Dialysis also enables elimination of excess fluid by ultrafiltration. Complete parenteral nutrition using a crystalline full-profile (essential and nonessential) amino acid solution with glucose and a lipid emulsion (Intralipid) was employed by Lee et al.[203]

PROTEIN SUPPLY IN ACUTE RENAL FAILURE

Even since hemodialysis has been generally available the emphasis in the nutritional management of patients with acute renal failure has been based on protein restriction. Applying the principles of the Giordano-Giovanetti diet, Abel et al.[204] treated patients with acute renal failure parenterally with 11.5 g of essential amino acids and hypertonic glucose. Such therapy was reported to retard the rate of rise of blood urea nitrogen and to decrease the need for or frequency of dialysis in acute renal failure. The observation of decreased concentrations of serum phosphate and potassium was suggested to imply increased protein synthesis and incorporation of these substances into intracellular structures.

In a controlled, prospective study Abel et al.[205] found that patients who received parenteral nutrition with 13.5 g of essential amino acids and hypertonic glucose had an increased rate of survival from an episode of renal failure as compared with patients who received only hypertonic glucose. There was no difference in overall hospital survival between the two patient groups. The authors concluded that the amino acid therapy resulted in decreased mortality. They also suggested that treatment with essential amino acids increased the rate of recovery of renal function. Such effects have not been observed by other investigators. Animal studies on the effect of amino acids in acute renal failure have given divergent results. In a study of rat kidney slices, infusion of amino acids was observed to enhance renal cellular membrane regeneration after mercuric chloride–induced acute renal failure.[202] In contrast, in rats with myohemoglobinuric or mercury-induced acute renal failure, infusion of various doses of amino acids was not consistently associated with abbreviated course or improved survival.[206]

Several authors have reported on parenteral nutrition in groups of patients with acute renal failure.[207,208] In general, parenteral administration of 13 to 20 g of essential amino acids and 1500 to 2000 kcal/day has resulted in a decline in the rise of serum urea, potassium, and phosphorus, whereas nitrogen balance, when studied, has been negative.

The rationale for supplying small quantities of only essential amino acids to patients with acute uremia was that urea could be reutilized for the synthesis of nonessential amino acids. As discussed above, however, it has been shown that reincorporation of urea nitrogen into protein is small and of minor nutritional importance.[107] Less than 100 per cent of free amino acids from muscle protein breakdown can be reutilized for protein synthesis. In the hypercatabolic state an inadequate supply of protein involves the risk of amino acid deprivation. As synthesis of nonessential amino acids, which are as necessary for protein synthesis as the essential amino acids, may be required in uremia,[209,210] it has been suggested that nonessential as well as essential amino acids should be provided in acute renal failure.

However, in a retrospective study Freund et al.[211] reported that patients who receive essential and nonessential amino acids (total about 23 g/day) had a horrendous mortality of 91 per cent as opposed to a 75 per cent survival rate for patients treated with 14 g of essential amino acids only.

In a later prospective and controlled study Feinstein et al.[200] compared the effect of parenteral nutrition with glucose alone, glucose with 21 g/day essential amino acids, or glucose with 21 g/day essential amino acids and 21 g/day nonessential amino acids in acutely uremic patients. No differences in recovery of renal function or survival between the treatment groups were observed. Nitrogen balance was negative in all treatment groups and was associated with low plasma concentrations of several essential amino acids, similar to changes observed in malnutrition. These data suggest that larger quantities of amino acids and possibly energy are required for the enhanced rate of anabolism that is needed to counterbalance the accelerated catabolism. Inadequate protein synthesis also entails the risk of impaired wound healing and infection, which, apart from being risk factors in themselves, may further enhance protein breakdown.

As discussed in the previous section, positive or neutral nitrogen balance can be obtained in patients with advanced, stable chronic renal failure ingesting a low-protein diet that provides 15 to 25 g of unselected protein, if the diet is supplemented with 7.5 to 10 g of essential amino acids or a preparation containing essential amino acids and nitrogen-free analogues. It is difficult to conceive, however, that

the principles of nutrition applied in the treatment of patients with stable chronic renal failure are valid in the management of patients with acute renal failure, in whom protein catabolism is often highly accelerated.

It should be emphasized that the catabolic rate varies to a great extent between individual patients. The most accelerated catabolism is observed in patients with acute renal failure following burns or multiple trauma and in septicemia, whereas in patients with acute renal failure of "medical" etiologies, such as nephrotoxic injuries from drugs or contrast media, the protein catabolic rate can be normal or only slightly increased. It seems reasonable to believe that the requirements for protein depend on the degree of catabolism and that the supply of protein, therefore, should be individualized.

As discussed earlier, net protein degradation can be estimated based on the appearance of urea nitrogen. A simplified way of estimating the degree of protein breakdown has been suggested by Lee,[212] who, employing the rate of rise of blood urea, defined patients with acute renal failure as normocatabolic (daily blood urea rise 4 to 8 mmol/L, 30 to 60 g protein breakdown/day), moderately catabolic (daily blood urea rise 8 to 12 mmol/L, 60 to 85 g protein breakdown/day), or hypercatabolic (daily blood urea rise >12 mmol/L, >85 g protein breakdown/day). Irrespective of the method used to evaluate protein degradation, such grouping, which of course always will be arbitrary, may be of use in the discussion of nutritional support of patients with acute renal failure.

In patients with a normal rate of catabolism, treatment with a protein-restricted diet (15 to 20 g of protein/day) supplemented with 8 to 12 g of essential amino acids (including histidine) may be used to prevent uremic symptoms and to avoid dialysis treatment or to reduce the frequency of dialysis.

Oliguria, however, makes such a nutritional regimen difficult or impossible. Fluid balance must be carefully supervised in every patient with acute renal failure. To avoid overhydration, the daily fluid administration must not exceed the losses. In a 70-kg subject insensible losses amount to 700 to 800 ml/day, whereas about 200 ml of water is produced metabolically. Thus, the basic need of fluid amounts to about 500 to 600 ml/day. For fluid equilibrium to be maintained, this volume plus the urinary volume should be supplied each day. To these basic losses should also be added any fluid lost from the gastrointestinal tract by nasogastric tubes, fistulas, and stool. Patients with abnormal losses from the gastrointestinal tract and also patients with excessive evaporation, such as from burns, with all probability have enhanced catabolism, however, and should not be subjected to protein restriction.

In hypercatabolic patients larger amounts of protein must be supplied to prevent or diminish negative nitrogen balance. Dialysis should then be instituted and should be applied as frequently as necessary to enable adequate nutritional support. In general dialysis treatment is required three or four times weekly, but daily dialysis may be necessary. If gastrointestinal function is normal, oral nutrition should be preferred. In patients without gastrointestinal dysfunction but in whom oral nutritional intake is not sufficient, the food may be supplemented with nutritional solutions given through a fine nasogastric tube. When gastrointestinal function is impaired, however, total parenteral nutrition must be instituted. Supply of protein or amino acids by a nasogastric tube or parenterally should be initiated as soon as it is evident that the patient cannot meet the nutritional demands by the oral route. Such nutrition, however, should not be started until the uremic state is controlled by adequate dialysis. The optimal composition of the amino acid solutions still needs to be investigated. It is not established whether the preparation should be limited to essential amino acids only or should include nonessential amino acids as well. The only well-controlled study addressing this issue[200] does not answer the question, partly because the total amount of amino acids administered was probably inadequate. As discussed above, there are several suggestions that nonessential amino acids may limit nitrogen utilization in acute renal failure, and consequently we believe that both essential and nonessential amino acids, tentatively in equal amounts, should be administered.

ENERGY SUPPLY IN ACUTE RENAL FAILURE

It is generally believed that the increased energy requirement in severe postsurgical and septic states is equally high or goes up even further when acute renal failure supervenes. In only a few studies, however, has energy expenditure been measured in patients with acute renal failure. In one study of 29 mechanically ventilated patients with acute renal failure associated with multiple trauma or postsurgical complications, resting energy expenditure (as determined through the measurement of oxgyen consumption) was found to be elevated by 20 to 50 per cent above normal.[213] Forsberg et al.[214] measured energy expenditure by continuous indirect calorimetry in nine mechanically ventilated patients with postsurgical sepsis and acute renal failure. Energy expenditure was on average 126 per cent of estimated basal metabolic rate. Of particular note is that the mean energy expenditure in these acute renal failure patients was 18 per cent lower than that in eight matched patients with postoperative sepsis requiring mechanical ventilation but without impaired renal function. Consequently, these results do not support the assumption that energy requirements are higher in patients with acute renal failure than in comparable patients with normal renal function.

The energy requirements, like those for protein, are markedly different among individual patients.

There is no direct quantitative correlation between energy metabolism and protein metabolism. Knowledge of the breakdown of protein, which can be estimated fairly well by the determination of urea generation, does not provide any reliable information on energy requirements. Ideally, energy requirements should therefore be estimated through the measurement of energy expenditure by indirect calorimetry. To avoid negative energy balance the supply of energy should probably exceed energy expenditure by 15 to 20 per cent. When the energy expenditure cannot be measured by indirect calorimetry, the energy requirement should be estimated to be similar to that in patients in the same clinical setting but with normal renal function. In most cases the energy requirements probably amount to about 30 kcal/kg/day and only seldom exceed 35 kcal/kg/day, and they are most likely lower than previously thought.[215–217]

The energy requirements should be covered by both glucose and fat. It is necessary to supply certain amounts of carbohydrates to prevent the production of ketones. The basal requirements in an adult subject are at least 100 g or 20 per cent of the energy. Hypertonic glucose (50 per cent) should be infused slowly into a central vein.

Hypermetabolism and hypercatabolism in patients with trauma and septicemia are associated with impaired glucose metabolism. Administration of excessive amounts of glucose in such patients may increase the metabolic stress and lead to enhanced release of catecholamines, accelerated metabolism with increased oxygen consumption, and increased production of carbon dioxide, which in patients with impaired respiratory function may cause respiratory insufficiency.[215] Moreover, impaired glucose metabolism, mainly caused by peripheral resistance to insulin, is almost universally present in uremia. Insulin (1 IU/3 to 5 g of glucose) should therefore be given to promote cellular glucose uptake. Besides its effect on blood glucose, insulin stimulates the transfer of amino acid across the cell membrane and stimulates protein synthesis, and might therefore be of particular importance in the treatment of malnourished patients. Blood glucose should be monitored regularly. The use of fat emulsions (Intralipid 20 per cent) is advantageous, inasmuch as a high amount of energy can be supplied in a small volume (2000 kcal/L). An additional advantage is the simultaneous supply of essential fatty acids. Also of practical importance is that fat emulsions, owing to low osmolality, may be infused in peripheral low flow veins. There are no indications that the intravenous infusion of fat interferes with the dialysance of artificial kidney membranes.[203]

In both chronic[218,219] and acute renal failure,[220] however, the rate of fat elimination is slower than normal. Based on available information on triglyceride clearance in chronically uremic subjects and in metabolically stable patients with acute renal failure, a fat intake of 1 g/kg/day appears to be a safe dosage level.[220] According to our own experience infusions of 500 ml of 20 per cent Intralipid per day are well tolerated. In other acute conditions, such as the postoperative state, trauma, and sepsis, accelerated rates of fat elimination have been reported.[221,222] Thus, it is conceivable that in certain cases such factors may influence the rate of fat clearance. When parenteral fat is infused in patients with renal failure for prolonged periods, adequate fat elimination should be ensured by measurements of plasma triglyceride concentration. A simple method to avoid significant hyperlipidemia would be to control serum before fat is infused and postpone the administration should serum be lipemic.

HEMODIALYSIS AND CONTINUOUS ARTERIOVENOUS HEMOFILTRATION IN ACUTE RENAL FAILURE

As discussed above, dialysis treatment should be instituted early when acute renal failure is associated with accelerated catabolism. Employing modern dialysis and ultrafiltration techniques, daily or near daily hemodialysis treatments may permit the supply of 70 to 80 g of protein, 3000 kcal, and 3000 ml of fluid per day. Hemodialysis should probably be preferred to peritoneal dialysis, since the latter involves substantially greater losses of amino acids and proteins and is also associated with an increased risk of respiratory complications in this category of patients.

Critically ill patients with multiple organ failure are often hemodynamically unstable and may not tolerate effective hemodialysis treatment. Especially in this group of patients, but also in other acute renal failure patients, continuous arteriovenous hemofiltration (CAVH) may be the most appropriate method of treatment.[223–225]

In CAVH, using large-bore catheters inserted into the femoral artery and vein and the patient's own blood pressure, arterial blood is circulated through a hemofilter. Systemic blood pressure provides the driving force to achieve sufficient blood flow across the filter for ultrafiltration. Ultrafiltrate, composed of plasma water and non–protein-bound small- and middle-weight solutes, passes through the membrane of the filter and is drained to a collection bag. The filtration rate amounts to 8 to 15 L/day. The urea concentration rate in the ultrafiltrate is almost identical to that in arterial blood, and the total daily urea removal is the ultrafiltrate concentration of urea times the ultrafiltrate volume. In moderately catabolic patients the convective transport of solutes may be sufficient to inhibit excessive accumulation of urea and other uremic substances. In hypercatabolic patients, however, CAVH may have to be supported by intermittent hemodialysis to relieve the uremic intoxication. The filtered volume is replaced by a saline solution that is modified to replace all the plasma water constituents except urea, creatinine,

and other unwanted uremic solutes. One of the major advantages to the use of CAVH in acute renal failure is that a part of the fluid volume removed by filtration may be replaced by infusion of nutritive solutions. Since large volumes are filtered daily, practically unlimited volumes may be infused and large amounts of glucose, amino acids, and fat can thus be administered through continuous infusion.

It is evident that the metabolic derangements associated with acute renal failure are far from fully elucidated. Also, as discussed above, the guidelines for nutritional management are not always based on scientifically well-founded data. Thus, problems such as how much protein and energy should be supplied in hypercatabolic patients with acute renal failure and whether only essential amino acids or a more complete mixture of amino acids should be administered call for prospective studies. Acute renal failure is often only one component in a complicated clinical setting in traumatized or septic patients with multiple organ failure. In such cases the mortality rate is influenced by several factors other than nutrition, and mortality is probably not the best indicator of the efficacy of treatment. The nitrogen and energy balance and other nutritional parameters should therefore be studied in individual patients during randomized periods with different nutrition as well as in large groups of patients in similar clinical settings.

INFLUENCE OF DIETARY MANAGEMENT ON THE PROGRESSION OF CHRONIC RENAL FAILURE

It is a general experience that once renal failure has advanced to a certain point, further deterioration is almost inevitable even if the underlying cause is removed and complicating factors such as hypertension and urinary infection are controlled. Mitch et al.[226] have reported that in most cases of chronic renal insufficiency, the reciprocal of serum creatinine declines linearly with time (i.e., the rate of deterioration is constant) and that this linear decrease is observed even as renal failure becomes nearly terminal. This observation makes it possible to estimate the effect of therapy on progression in individual patients.

Until lately the aims of nutritional management in chronic renal failure have been to optimize the nutritional status of the patient and/or to alleviate uremic toxicity. Recently, however, several experimental and clinical studies have shown that the course of renal failure may be affected by dietary changes. Thus, it has been demonstrated[227] that phosphate restriction can prevent the development of interstitial nephropathy in subtotally nephrectomized rats, presumably because deposition of calcium phosphate in the tissues is prevented. It has also been shown that the progression may be retarded in patients treated with a phosphate-restricted diet,[228] and it has been suggested that improved control of serum phosphate and reduction of the calcium × phosphate product might be involved in the retardation of renal failure.[69] Likewise, the progression of renal failure has been slowed in patients treated with protein restriction[229–231] supplemented with essential amino acids or keto acid preparations. The effect of restriction of phosphorus and protein, respectively, has not been separated clearly, since dietary restriction of phosphorus entails restriction of protein and vice versa. The lack of effect of treatment with a low-phosphate diet on the progression of renal failure in some patients[232] and also our own observations that retardation of renal insufficiency in patients treated with a low-protein diet and essential amino acids is not consistently associated with improvement in calcium and phosphorus metabolism,[231] suggest that preservation of renal function may be mediated by restriction of dietary protein per se.

Hostetter et al.[233] have speculated that the final common outcome of chronic renal disease depends on some critical loss of renal mass. Compensatory hyperperfusion of remnant glomeruli might result in sclerotic destruction. This suggestion is supported by the observation that in partially nephrectomized rats severe restriction of dietary protein intake can partly prevent glomerular hyperfiltration and reduce the structural abnormalities in remnant glomeruli. This effect is apparently not dependent on improved phosphate control, since in this study the phosphate content of the low-protein diet was similar to that of the control diet. It should be emphasized that the effect of protein restriction on glomerular hyperfiltration in remnant nephrons was found in rats with experimental renal failure and that there is lack of evidence that the same mechanism is operating in human renal disease. It cannot be excluded, however, that the hyperfiltration hypothesis may also be relevant to patients with chronic renal failure of various etiologies. Available clinical data from different groups,[230,231] although anecdotal or not well controlled, strongly suggest that progression of end-stage renal failure in humans may be retarded or halted by treatment with a low-protein diet supplemented with essential amino acids or keto acids. Since acute enhancement of glomerular filtration occurs after a protein meal,[234,235] it is conceivable that hyperfiltration and further destruction of the renal parenchyma may be avoided or delayed by the protein restriction. This may have important clinical implications in the future, especially if it can be shown that this principle of treatment is operative in early renal failure as well. Recently it has also been suggested that the abnormalities in lipid metabolism that arise in the nephrotic syndrome and in chronic renal failure may themselves lead to further renal damage.[236] Prospective randomized studies are required to confirm the present findings and to evaluate by which mechanisms protein restriction and lipid abnormalities affect progression of renal failure.

References

1. Arieff AI, Guisado R. Effects on the central nervous system of hypernatremic and hyponatremic states. Kidney Int 1976; 10:104–116.
2. Bricker NS. On the pathogenesis of the uremic state. An exposition of the "trade-off hypothesis." N Engl J Med 1972; 286:1093–1099.
3. De Wardener HE, Clarkson EM. The natriuretic hormone: recent developments. Clin Sci 1982; 63:415–420.
4. Bricker NS, Fine LG, Kaplan M, et al. "Magnification phenomenon" in chronic renal disease. N Engl J Med 1978; 299:1287–1293.
5. Bradley SD, Anderson RJ. Nonoliguric acute renal failure. Am J Kidney Dis 1985; 6:71–80.
6. Relman AS. The acidosis of renal disease. Am J Med 1968; 44:706–713.
7. Gonic HC, Kleeman CR, Rubini ME, et al. Functional impairment in chronic renal disease. Nephron, 1969; 6:28–49.
8. May RC, Kelly RA, Mitch WE. Mechanisms for defects in muscle protein metabolism in rats with chronic uremia. Influence of metabolic acidosis. J Clin Invest 1987; 79:1099–1103.
9. Papadoyannikis NJ, Stefanidis CJ, McGeown M. The effect of the correction of metabolic acidosis on nitrogen and potassium balance of patients with chronic renal failure. Am J Clin Nutr 1984; 40:623–627.
10. Lemann J Jr, Litzow JR, Lennon EJ. The effects of chronic acid loads in normal man. Further evidence of the participation of bone mineral in the defense against chronic metabolic acidosis. J Clin Invest 1966; 45:1608–1614.
11. van Ypersele de Strihou C. Potassium homeostasis in renal failure. Kidney Int 1977; 11:491–504.
12. Alvestrand A, Smith D, Wahren J, et al. Insulin-mediated potassium uptake by splanchnic and leg tissues in uremic and healthy subjects. Am J Physiol 1984; 246:E174–E180.
13. Bergström J, Fürst P: Uraemic toxins. In Drukker W, Parsons FM, Maher JF (eds). Replacement of Renal Function by Dialysis. The Hague, Martinus Nijhoff's Publishers, 1983: 354–390.
14. Middle Molecules in Uremia and Other Diseases: Analytical Techniques, Metabolic Toxicity and Clinical Aspects. Proceedings of the Symposium on Present Status and Future Orientation of Middle Molecules in Uremia and Other Diseases, Avignon, France, 1980. Artif Organs 1981; 4:Suppl 4.
15. Delaporte C, Gros F, Anagnostopoulos T. Inhibitory effects of plasma dialysate on protein synthesis in vitro: influence of dialysis and transplantation. Am J Clin Nutr 1980; 33:1407–1410.
16. Garber AJ. Skeletal muscle protein and amino acid metabolism in experimental chronic uremia in the rat. J Clin Invest 1978; 62:623–632.
17. Harter HR, Karl IE, Klahr S, et al. Effects of reduced renal mass and dietary protein intake on amino acid release and glucose uptake by rat muscle in vitro. J Clin Invest 1979; 64:513–523.
18. DeFronzo RA, Smith D, Alvestrand A. Insulin action in uremia. Kidney Int 1983; 24(Suppl 16):102–104.
19. Deferrare G, Garibotto G, Robaudo C, et al. Leg metabolism of amino acids and ammonia in patients with chronic renal failure. Clin Sci 1985; 69:143–151.
20. Conley SB, Rose GM, Robson AM, et al. Effects of dietary intake and hemodialysis on protein turnover in uremic children. Kidney Int 1980; 17:837–846.
21. DeFronzo RA, Alvestrand A, Smith D, et al. Insulin resistance in uremia. J Clin Invest 1981; 67:563–568.

22. Mitch WE. Amino acid release by the hindquarter and urea appearance in acute uremia. Am J Physiol 1981; *241*:415–419.

23. Alvestrand A. Amino acid metabolism in patients with chronic renal failure. Clin Nutr 1985; *4*(Suppl):14–23.

24. Garber AJ. Effects of parathyroid hormone on skeletal muscle protein and amino acid metabolism. J Clin Invest 1983; *71*:1806–1821.

25. Gulyassy PF, Aviram A, Peters JH. Evaluation of amino acid and protein requirements in chronic uremia. Arch Intern Med 1970; *126*:855–859.

26. Young GA, Parsons FM. Plasma amino acid imbalance in patients with chronic renal failure on intermittent dialysis. Clin Chim Acta 1970; *27*:491–496.

27. Alvestrand A, Bergström J, Fürst P. Plasma and muscle free amino acids in uremia: influence of nutrition with amino acids. Clin Nephrol 1982; *18*:297–305.

28. Young GA, Parsons FM. Impairment of phenylalanine hydroxylation in chronic renal insufficiency. Clin Sci Mol Med 1973; *48*:89–97.

29. Bergström J, Fürst P, Josephson B, et al. Improvement of nitrogen balance in a uremic patient by the addition of histidine to essential amino acid solutions given intravenously. Life Sci 1970; *9*(Part II):787–794.

30. Fürst P. ¹⁵N studies in severe renal failure. II. Evidence for the essentiality of histidine. Scand J Clin Lab Invest 1972; *30*:307–312.

31. Kopple JD, Swendseid ME. Evidence that histidine is an essential amino acid in normal and chronically uremic man. J Clin Invest 1975; *55*:881–891.

32. Li JB, Fulks RM, Goldberg AL. Evidence that the intracellular pool of tyrosine serves as a precursor for protein synthesis in muscle. J Biol Chem 1973; *248*:7272–7275.

33. Alvestrand A, Ahlberg M, Bergström J, et al. Clinical results of long-term treatment with low protein diet and a new amino acid preparation in chronic uremic patients. Clin Nephrol 1983; *19*:67–73.

34. DeFronzo RA, Tobin JD, Rowe JW, et al. Glucose intolerance in uremia. Quantification of pancreatic beta cell sensitivity to glucose and tissue sensitivity to insulin. J Clin Invest 1978; *62*:425–435.

35. Akmal M, Massry SG, Goldstein DA, et al. Role of parathyroid hormone in the glucose intolerance of chronic renal failure. J Clin Invest 1985; *75*:1037–1044.

36. Mak RHK, Bettinelli A, Turner C, et al. The influence of hyperparathyroidism on glucose metabolism in uremia. J Clin Endocrinol Metab 1985; *60*:229–233.

37. Smith D, DeFronzo RA. Insulin resistance in uremia mediated by postbinding defects. Kidney Int 1982; *22*:54–62.

38. Hampers CL, Soeldner JS, Doak PB, et al. Effect of chronic renal failure and hemodialysis on carbohydrate metabolism. J Clin Invest 1966; *45*:1719–1731.

39. Snyder D, Pulido LB, Kagan A. Dietary reversal of the carbohydrate intolerance in uremia. Proc Eur Dial Transplant Assoc 1968; *5*:205–213.

40. Mak RH, Turner C, Thompson T, et al. The effect of a low protein diet with amino/keto acid supplements on glucose metabolism in children with uremia. J Clin Endocrinol Metab 1986: *63*:985–989.

41. McCaleb ML, Izzo MS, Lockwood DH. Characterization and partial purification of a factor from uremic human serum that induces insulin resistance. J Clin Invest 1985; *75*:391–396.

42. Swenson RS, Weisinger J, Reaven GM. Evidence that hemodialysis does not improve the glucose tolerance of patients with chronic renal failure. Metabolism 1974; *23*:929–936.

43. Attman PO, Gustavsson A. Lipid and carbohydrate metabolism in uremia. Influence of treatment with protein-reduced diet and essential amino-acids. Nutr Metabol 1980; *24*:261–266.

44. Bilbrey GL, Faloona GR, White MG, et al. Hyperglucagonemia of renal failure. J Clin Invest 1974; *53*:841–847.

45. Sherwin RS, Bastl C, Finkelstein FO, et al. Influence of uremia and hemodialysis on the turnover and metabolic effects of glucagon. J Clin Invest 1976; *57*:722–731.

46. Wright AD, Lowry C, Fraser TR, et al. Serum growth hormone and glucose tolerance in renal failure. Lancet 1968; *2*:798–801.

47. Samaan N, Freeman RM. Growth hormone levels in severe renal failure. Metabolism 1970; *19*:102–113.

48. Norbeck HE, Carlson LA. The uremic dyslipoproteinemia: its characteristics and relations to clinical factors. Acta Med Scand 1981; *289*:489–504.

49. Attman PO. Dietary treatment in uremia. Renal function, protein and lipid metabolism. Thesis. Näringsforskning 1979; *23*:40–59.

50. Norbeck HE, Carlson LA. Increased frequency of late prebeta lipoproteins (LP beta) in isolated serum very low density lipoproteins in uraemia. Eur J Clin Invest 1980; *10*:423–426.

51. Brunner FP, Brynger H, Chantler C, et al. Combined Report on Regular Dialysis and Transplantation in Europe IX, 1978. Proc Eur Dial Transplant Assoc 1979: *16*:3–82.

52. Lindner A, Charraa B, Sherrard DJ, et al. Accelerated atherosclerosis in prolonged maintenance hemodialysis. N Engl J Med 1974; *290*:697–701.

53. Burke JF, Francos GC, Moore LL, et al. Accelerated atherosclerosis in chronic-dialysis patients—another look. Nephron 1978; *21*:181–185.

54. Rostand SG, Gretes JC, Kirk KA, et al. Ischemic heart disease in patients with uremia undergoing maintenance hemodialysis. Kidney Int 1979; *16*:600–611.

55. Nicholls AJ, Catto GRD, Edward N, et al. Accelerated atherosclerosis in long-term dialysis and renal transplant patients: fact or fiction? Lancet 1980; *1*:276–278.

56. Vincenti F, Amend WJ, Abele J, et al. The role of hypertension in hemodialysis-associated atherosclerosis. Am J Med 1980; *68*:363–369.

57. Turgan C, Feehally J, Bennett S, et al. Accelerated hypertriglyceridemia in patients on continuous ambulatory peritoneal dialysis—a preventable abnormality. Int J Artif Organs 1981; *4*:158–160.

58. Lindholm B, Karlander SG, Norbeck HE, et al. Glucose and lipid metabolism in peritoneal dialysis. *In* La Greca G, Biasioli S, Ronco C (eds). Proc 1st Int Course on Peritoneal Dialysis. Milan, Wichtig Editore, 1982: 217–231.

59. David DS. Mineral and bone homeostasis in renal failure. *In* David DS (ed). Calcium Metabolism in Renal Failure and Nephrolithiasis. New York, John Wiley & Sons, 1977: 1–76.

60. Slatopolsky E, Rutherford WE, Hruska K, et al. How important is phosphate in the pathogenesis of renal osteodystrophy? Arch Intern Med 1978; *138*:848–852.

61. Llach F, Massry SG. On the mechanism of secondary hyperparathyroidism in moderate renal failure. J Clin Endocrinol Metab 1985; *61*:601–606.

62. DeLuca HF. The kidney as an endocrine organ involved in calcium homeostasis. Kidney Int 1973; *4*:80–88.

63. Parfitt AM. Clinical and radiographic manifestations of renal osteodystrophy. *In* David DS (ed). Calcium Metabolism in Renal Failure and Nephrolithiasis. New York, John Wiley & Sons, 1977: 145–196.

64. Baczynski R, Massry SG, Kohan R, et al. Effect of parathyroid hormone on myocardial energy metabolism in the rat. Kidney Int 1985; *27*:718–725.

65. Baczynski R, Massry SG, Kohan R, et al. Effect of parathyroid hormone on energy metabolism of skeletal muscle. Kidney Int 1985; *28*:722–727.

66. Massry SG. Pathogenesis of the anemia of uremia: role of secondary hyperparathyroidism. Kidney Int 1983; *24*(Suppl 16):204–207.

67. Argov Z, Melamed E, Katz S. Hyperparathyroidism presenting with unusual neurological features. Eur Neurol 1971; *24*:449–461.

68. Avram MM, Iancu M, Morrow D, et al. Uremic syndrome

in man: new evidence for parathormone as a multisystem neurotoxin. Clin Nephrol 1979; *11*:59–62.

69. Walser M. Does dietary therapy have a role in the predialysis patient? Am J Clin Nutr 1980; *33*:1629–1637.

70. Slatopolsky E, Bricker NS. The role of phosphorus restriction in the prevention of secondary hyperparathyroidism in chronic renal disease. Kidney Int 1973; *4*:141–145.

71. Kopple JD, Mercurio K, Blumenkrantz MJ, et al. Daily requirement for pyrodoxine supplements in chronic renal failure. Kidney Int 1981; *19*:694–704.

72. Sullivan JF, Eisenstein AB. Ascorbic acid depletion during hemodialysis. JAMA 1972; *220*:1697–1699.

73. Park YK, Linswiler H. Effect of vitamin B_6 depletion in adult man on the plasma concentration and the urinary excretion of free amino acids. J Nutr 1971; *101*:185–192.

74. Kopple JD, Swendseid ME. Vitamin nutrition in patients undergoing maintenance hemodialysis. Kidney Int 1975; 7(Suppl 2):S79–84.

75. Milman N. Serum vitamin B_{12} and erythrocyte folate in chronic uraemia and after renal transplantation. Scand J Haematol 1980; *25*:151–157.

76. Hemmelöff Andersen KE. Folic acid status of patients with chronic renal failure maintained by dialysis. Clin Nephrol 1977; *8*:510–513.

77. Bastow MD, Woods HF, Walls J. Persistent anemia associated with reduced serum vitamin B_{12} levels in patients undergoing regular hemodialysis therapy. Clin Nephrol 1979; *11*:133–135.

78. Werb R. Vitamin A toxicity in hemodialysis patients. Int J Artif Organs 1979; *2*:178–180.

79. Yatzidis H, Digenis P, Fountas P. Hypervitaminosis A accompanying advanced chronic renal failure. Br Med J 1975; *3*:352–353.

80. Linton AL, Clark WF, Driedger AA, et al. Correctable factors contributing to the anemia of dialysis patients. Nephron 1977; *19*:95–98.

81. Rosenblatt SG, Drake S, Fadem S, et al. Gastrointestinal blood loss in patients with chronic renal failure. Am J Kidney Dis 1982; *1*:232–236.

82. Schafer AI, Cheron RG, Dluhy R, et al. Clinical consequences of acquired transfusional iron overload in adults. N Engl J Med 1981; *304*:319–324.

83. Bregman H, Gelfand MC, Winchester JF, et al. Iron-overload–associated myopathy in patients on maintenance haemodialysis: a histocompatibility-linked disorder. Lancet 1980; *2*:882–885.

84. Milman N, Christensen TE, Strandberg-Pedersen N, et al. Serum ferritin and bone marrow iron in non-dialysis, peritoneal dialysis and hemodialysis patients with chronic renal failure. Acta Med Scand 1980; *207*:201–205.

85. Mahajan SK, Prasad AS, Rahbani P, et al. Zinc metabolism in uremia. J Lab Clin Med 1979; *94*:693–698.

86. Rudolph H, Alfrey AC, Smythe WR. Muscle and serum trace element profile in uremia. Trans Am Soc Artif Int Organs 1973; *19*:456–465.

87. Cornelis R, Mees L, Ringoir S, et al. Serum and red blood cell Zn, Se, Cs and Rb in dialysis patients. Min Elec Metab 1979; *2*:88–93.

88. Vreman HJ, Venter C, Leegwater J, et al. Taste, smell and zinc metabolism in patients with chronic renal failure. Nephron 1980; *26*:163–170.

89. Antoniou LD, Sudhaker T, Shalhoub RJ, et al. Reversal of uremic impotence by zinc. Lancet 1977; *2*:895–898.

90. Atkin-Thor E, Goddard BW, Onion J. Hypogeusia and zinc depletion in chronic dialysis patients. Am J Clin Nutr 1978; *31*:1948–1951.

91. Zetin M, Stone RA. Effects of zinc in chronic hemodialysis. Clin Nephrol 1980; *13*:20–25.

92. Brook AC, Johnston DG, Ward MK, et al. Absence of a therapeutic effect of zinc in the sexual dysfunction of hemodialysed patients. Lancet 1980; *2*:618–619.

93. Smythe WR, Alfrey AC, Craswell PW, et al. Trace element abnormalities in chronic uremia. Ann Intern Med 1982; *96*:302–310.

94. Alfrey AC, LeGendre GR, Kaehny WD. The dialysis encephalopathy syndrome—possible aluminum intoxication. N Engl J Med 1976; *294*:184–188.

95. Kaehny WD, Alfrey AC, Holman RE, et al. Aluminum transfer during hemodialysis. Kidney Int 1977; *12*:361–365.

96. Targoff CM, Coburn ME, Ament WJ, et al. Bone disease with total parenteral nutrition, a new syndrome. *In* Norman AW, Schaefer K, Herrath D (eds). Vitamin D: Basic Research and Its Clinical Application. Hawthorne, NY, De Gruyter, 1979: 1171–1172.

97. Platts MM, Goode GC, Hislop JS. Composition of the domestic water supply and the incidence of fractures and encephalopathy in patients on home dialysis. Br Med J 1977; *2*:657–660.

98. Short AI, Winney RJ, Robson JS. Reversible microcytic hypochromic anemia in dialysis patients due to aluminum intoxication. Proc Eur Dial Transplant Assoc 1980; *17*:226–233.

99. Rose WC. The amino acid requirements of adult man. Nutr Abstr Rev 1957; *27*:631–647.

100. Hegsted DM. Variation in requirements of nutrients—amino acids. Fed Proc 1963; *22*:1424–1430.

101. Munroe HN. Amino acid requirements and metabolism. *In* Wilkinson AW (ed). Parenteral Nutrition. London, Churchill Livingstone, 1972: 33.

102. Herdon RF, Freeman S, Cleveland AS. Protein requirements in chronic insufficient patients. A study of the nitrogen minimum. J Lab Clin Med 1958; *52*:235.

103. Ford J, Phillips ME, Toye FE, et al. Nitrogen balance in patients with chronic renal failure on diets containing varying quantities of protein. Br Med J 1969; *1*:735–740.

104. Fürst P, Ahlberg M, Alvestrand A, et al. Principles of essential amino acid therapy in uremia. Am J Clin Nutr 1978; *31*:1744–1755.

105. Walser M. Nutritional management of chronic renal failure. Am J Kidney Dis 1982; *1*:261–275.

106. Giordano C. Use of exogenous and endogenous urea for protein synthesis in normal and uremic subjects. J Lab Clin Med 1963; *62*:231–246.

107. Varcoe R, Halliday D, Carson ER, et al. Efficiency of utilization of urea nitrogen for albumin synthesis by chronically uraemic and normal man. Clin Sci Mol Med 1975; *48*:379–390.

108. Mitch WE, Walser M. Effect of oral neomycin and kanamycin in chronic uremic patients. II. Nitrogen balance. Kidney Int 1977; *11*:123–128.

109. Young VR. Some metabolic and nutritional considerations of dietary protein restriction. *In* Mitch WE (ed). The Progressive Nature of Renal Disease. New York, Churchill Livingstone, 1986: 263–283.

110. Giovannetti S, Maggiore Q. A low-nitrogen diet with proteins of high biological value for severe chronic uraemia. Lancet 1964; *1*:1000–1003.

111. Kopple JD, Coburn JW. Metabolic studies of low protein diets in uremia. I. Nitrogen and potassium. Medicine 1973; *52*:583–595.

112. Berlyne GM, Shaw AB. Giordano-Giovannetti diet in terminal renal failure. Lancet 1965; *2*:7.

113. Kopple JD, Sorensen MK, Coburn JW, et al. Controlled comparison of 20-g and 40-g protein diets in the treatment of chronic uremia. Am J Clin Nutr 1968; *21*:553–564.

114. Lange K, Lonergan ET, Semar M, et al. Transketolase inhibition as a mechanism in uremic neuropathy. *In* Kluthe R, Berlyne G, Burton B (eds). Uremia. Stuttgart, Georg Thieme Verlag, 1972: 24–32.

115. Bergström J, Fürst P, Noree LO. Treatment of chronic uremic patients with protein-poor diet and oral supply of essential amino acids. I. Nitrogen balance studies. Clin Nephrol 1975; *3*:187–194.

116. Rogers QR, Chen DM, Harper AE. The importance of dispensable amino acids for maximal growth in the rat. Proc Soc Exp Biol Med 1970; *134*:517–522.

117. Pennisi AJ, Wang M, Kopple JD. Effects of low nitrogen

diets in uremic and control rats. Fed Proc 1976; 35:257–260.

118. Kopple JD, Monteon FJ, Shaib JK. Effect of energy intake on nitrogen metabolism in nondialysed patients with chronic renal failure. Kidney Int 1986; 29:734–742.

119. Hyne BEB, Fowell E, Lee HA. The effect of caloric intake on nitrogen balance in chronic renal failure. Clin Sci 1972; 43:679–688.

120. Burge JC, Park HS, Whitlock CP, et al. Taste acuity in patients undergoing long-term hemodialysis. Kidney Int 1979; 15:49–53.

121. Berlyne GM, Booth EM, Brewis RAL, et al. A soluble glucose polymer for use in renal failure and caloric deprivation states. Lancet 1969; 1:689–692.

122. Bergström J, Alvestrand A. Therapy with branched chain amino acids in chronic uremia. In Adibi SA, Fekl W, Langenbeck U, et al. (eds). Branched Chain Amino and Keto Acids in Health and Disease. Basel, S Karger, 1984: 391–422.

123. Kampf D, Fischer HC, Kessel M. Efficacy of an unselected protein diet (25 g) with minor oral supply of essential amino acids and keto analogues compared with selective protein diet (40 g) in chronic renal failure. Am J Clin 1980; 33:1673–1677.

124. Fröhling P, Schmicker R, Vetter K, et al. Conservative treatment with keto acid and amino acid supplement low-protein diets in chronic renal failure. Am J Clin Nutr 1980; 33:1667–1672.

125. Vetter K, Fröhling P, Kaschube I, et al. Therapie der chronischen Niereninsuffizienz mit Ketosteril im Rahmen der sogenannten "Schwedendiät." Wissenschaftliche Informationen 1980; 13:419–451.

126. Schloerb PR. Essential amino acid administration in uremia. Am J Med Sci 1966; 252:650–659.

127. Richards P, Metcalfe-Gibson A, Ward E, et al. Utilisation of ammonia nitrogen for protein synthesis in man, and the effect of protein restriction and uremia. Lancet 1967; 2:7521–7523.

128. Walser M, Lund P, Ruderman NB, et al. Synthesis of essential amino acids from their alpha-keto analogues by perfused rat liver and muscle. J Clin Invest 1973; 52:2865–2877.

129. Richards P, Brown CL, Houghton BJ, et al. Synthesis of phenylalanine and valine by healthy and uremic men. Lancet 1971; 2:128–134.

130. Rudman D. Capacity of human subjects to utilize keto analogues of valine and phenylalanine. J Clin Invest 1971; 50:90–96.

131. Mitch WE, Walser M. Nitrogen balance in uremic subjects receiving the hydroxy-analogue of methionine and branched-chain ketoacids as substitutes for the respective amino acids. Clin Nephrol 1977; 8:341–344.

132. Mitch WE, Walser M. Utilization of calcium L-phenyllactate as a substitute for phenylalanine by uremic subjects. Metabolism 1977; 26:1041–1046.

133. Walser M. Ketoacids in the treatment of uremia. Clin Nephrol 1975; 3:180–186.

134. Mitch WE, Walser M, Sapir DG. A comparison of nitrogen-sparing by leucine and its keto-analogue in fasting subjects. Clin Res 1979; 27:373.

135. Buse MG, Reid SS. Leucine: a possible regulator of protein turnover in muscle. J Clin Invest 1975; 56:1250–1261.

136. Chua B, Siehl DL, Morgan HE. Effect of leucine and metabolites of branched-chain amino acids on protein turnover in heart. J Biol Chem 1979; 254:8358–8362.

137. Hecking E. Supplementation with essential amino acids or alpha keto analogues in patients on long-term hemodialysis. Int J Artif Organs 1980; 3:127–137.

137a.Kang CW, Tungsanga K, Walser M. Effect of the level of dietary protein utilization of alpha-ketoisocaproate for protein synthesis in man. Am J Clin Nutr 1986; 43:504–509.

138. Bergström J, Ahlberg M, Alvestrand A, et al. Metabolic studies with keto acids in uremia. Am J Clin Nutr 1978; 31:1761–1766.

139. Mitch WE, Gelman B, Walser M. Hypercalcemia and hypophosphatemia in uremic patients receiving essential amino acids or N-free analogues. Kidney Int 1977; 12:530.

140. Barsotti G, Morelli E, Guiducci A, et al. Reversal of hyperparathyroidism in severe uremics following very low-protein and low-phosphorus diet. Nephron 1982; 30:310–313.

141. Mitch WE, Collier VU, Walser M. Treatment of chronic renal failure with branched-chain keto acids plus other essential amino acids or their nitrogen-free analogues. In Walser M, Williamson JR (eds). Metabolism and Clinical Implications of Branched-Chain Amino and Keto Acids. New York, Elsevier/North Holland, 1981: 587–592.

142. Alvestrand A, Fürst P, Bergström J. Intracellular amino acids in uremia. Kidney Int 1983; 24(Suppl 16):S9–16.

143. Halliday D, Madigan M, Chalmers RA, et al. The degree of conversion of alpha-keto acids to valine and phenylalanine in health and uremia. Q J Med 1981; 50:53–62.

144. Epstein CM, Chawla RK, Wadsworth A, et al. Decarboxylation of alpha-ketoisovaleric acid after oral administration in man. Am J Clin Nutr 1980; 33:1968–1974.

145. Tungsanga K, Kang CW, Walser M. Utilization of alpha-ketoisocaproate for protein synthesis in chronically uremic rats. Kidney Int 1986; 30:891–894.

146. Walser M, Mitch WE, Abras E. Supplements containing amino acids and keto acids in the treatment of chronic uremia. Kidney Int 1983; 24(Suppl 16):285–289.

147. Mitch WE, Abras E, Walser M. Long-term effects of a new keto acid–amino acid supplement in patients with chronic renal failure. N Engl J Med 1984; 311:48–53.

148. Kopple JD, Coburn JW. Evaluation of chronic uremia. Importance of serum urea nitrogen, serum creatinine and their ratio. JAMA 1974; 227:41–44.

149. Maroni BJ, Steinman TI, Mitch WE. A method for estimating nitrogen intake of patients with chronic renal failure. Kidney Int 1985; 27:58–65.

150. Young GA, Swanepoel CR, Croft MR, et al. Anthropometry and plasma valine, amino acids, and proteins in the nutritional assessment of hemodialysis patients. Kidney Int 1982; 21:492–499.

151. Klidjian AM, Archer TJ, Foster KJ, et al. Detection of dangerous malnutrition. JPEN 1982; 6:119–121.

152. Ingenbleek Y, van den Schrieck HG, de Nayer P, et al. Albumin, transferrin and the thyroxine-binding prealbumin/retinol-binding protein (TBPA-RBP) complex in assessment of malnutrition. Clin Chim Acta 1975; 63:61–67.

153. Wolfson M, Strong CJ, Minturn D, et al. Nutritional status and lymphocyte function in maintenance hemodialysis patients. Am J Clin Nutr 1984; 37:547–555.

154. Gordon EE, Kowalsky K, Fritts M. Muscle proteins and DNA in rat quadriceps during growth. Am J Physiol 1966; 210:1033–1040.

155. Millward DJ, Waterlow JC. Effect of nutrition on protein turnover in skeletal muscle. Fed Proc 1978; 37:2283–2290.

156. Guarnieri G, Toigo G, Situlin R, et al. Muscle biopsy studies in chronically uremic patients: evidence for malnutrition. Kidney Int 1983; 24(Suppl 16):187–193.

157. Ritz E, Mehls O, Gilli G, et al. Protein restriction in the conservative management of uremia. Am J Clin Nutr 1978; 31:1703–1711.

158. Bonomini V, Feletti C, Scolari MP, et al. Atherosclerosis in uremia: a longitudinal study. Am J Clin Nutr 1980; 33:1493–1500.

159. Alvestrand A, Ahlberg M, Fürst P, et al. Clinical experience with amino acid and keto acid diets. Am J Clin Nutr 1980; 33:1654–1659.

160. Attman PO, Gustafson A. Lipid and carbohydrate metabolism in uremia. Eur J Clin Invest 1979; 9:285–292.

161. Attman PO, Ewald J, Isaksson B. Body composition during long-term treatment of uremia with amino acid supple-

mented low protein diet. Am J Clin Nutr 1980; 33:801–810.

162. Bergström J, Lindblom U, Noree LO. Preservation of peripheral nerve function in severe uremia during treatment with low protein high calorie diet and surplus of essential amino acids. Acta Neurol Scand 1975; 51:99–109.

163. Sanfelippo ML, Swenson RS, Reaven GM. Response of plasma triglycerides to dietary change in patients on hemodialysis. Kidney Int 1978; 14:180–186.

164. Cattran DC, Steiner G, Fenton SSA, et al. Dialysis hyperlipidemia: response to dietary manipulations. Clin Nephrol 1980; 13:177–182.

165. Tsukamoto Y, Okubo M, Yoneda T, et al. Effects of a polyunsaturated fatty acid-rich diet on serum lipids in patients with chronic renal failure. Nephron 1982; 31:236–241.

166. Goldberg AP, Hagberg JM, Delmez JA, et al. Exercise training improves abnormal lipid and carbohydrate metabolism in hemodialysis patients. Trans Am Soc Artif Intern Organs 1979; 25:431–437.

167. De Felice SL, Klein MI. Carnitine and hemodialysis—a minireview. Curr Ther Res 1980; 28:195–198.

168. Bazzato G, Mezzina C, Ciman M, et al. Myasthenia-like syndrome associated with carnitine in patients on long-term hemodialysis. Lancet 1979: 1:1041–1042.

169. Kopple JD. Nutritional therapy in kidney failure. Nutr Rev 1981; 39:193–206.

170. Mahajan SK, Abbasi AA, Prasad AS, et al. Effect of oral zinc therapy on gonadal function in hemodialysis patients. Ann Intern Med 1982; 97:357–361.

171. Thunberg BJ, Swamy A, Cestero RVM. Cross-sectional and longitudinal nutritional measurements in maintenance hemodialysis patients. Am J Clin Nutr 1981; 34:2005–2012.

172. Piraino AJ, Firpo JJ, Powers DV. Prolonged hyperalimentation in catabolic chronic dialysis therapy patients. JPEN 1981; 5:463–477.

173. Mattern WD, Hak LJ, Lamanna RW, et al. Malnutrition, altered immune function, and the risk of infection in maintenance hemodialysis patients. Am J Kidney Dis 1982; 1:206–218.

174. Acchiardo SR, Moore LW, Latour PA. Malnutrition as the main factor in morbidity and mortality of hemodialysis patients. Kidney Int 1983; 24(Suppl 16):199–203.

175. Degoulet P, Legrain M, Reach I, et al. Mortality risk factors in patients treated by chronic hemodialysis. Nephron 1982; 31:103–110.

176. Comty CA. Long-term dietary management of dialysis patients. J Am Diet Assoc 1968; 54:439–444.

177. Ginn HE, Frost A, Lacy WW. Nitrogen balance in hemodialysis patients. Am J Clin Nutr 1968; 21:385–393.

178. Kopple JD, Shinaberger JH, Coburn JW, et al. Optimal dietary protein treatment during chronic hemodialysis. Trans Am Soc Artif Organs 1969; 15:302–308.

179. Schaeffer G, Heinze V, Jontofsohn R, et al. Amino acid and protein intake in RDT patients. A nutritional and biochemical analysis. Clin Nephrol 1975; 3:228–233.

180. Kluthe R, Lüttgen FM, Capetianu T, et al. Protein requirements in maintenance hemodialysis. Am J Clin Nutr 1978; 31:1812–1820.

181. Borah MF, Schoenfeld PY, Gotch FA, et al. Nitrogen balance during intermittent dialysis therapy of uremia. Kidney Int 1978; 14:491–500.

182. Ward RA, Shirlow MJ, Hayes JM, et al. Protein catabolism during hemodialysis. Am J Clin Nutr 1979; 32:2443–2449.

183. Farrell PC, Hone PW. Dialysis-induced catabolism. Am J Clin Nutr 1980; 33:1417–1422.

184. Kopple JD, Swendseid ME, Shinaberger JH, et al. The free and bound amino acids removed by hemodialysis. Trans Am Soc Artif Organs 1973; 19:309–313.

185. Ono K, Sasaki T, Waki Y. Glucose in the dialyzate does not reduce the free amino acid loss during routine hemodi-

alysis of non-fasting patients. Clin Nephrol 1984; 21:106–109.

186. Hecking E, Distler A, Dörr R, et al. Aminosäurenverlust im Dialysat: Beweis für die Notwendigkeit der parenteralen oder oralen Substitution von Aminosäurengemischen bei Dialysepatienten? Akt Ernährungsmed 1977; 1:15–20.

187. Wolfson M, Jones MR, Kopple JD. Amino acid losses during hemodialysis with infusion of amino acids and glucose. Kidney Int 1982; 21:500–506.

188. Tepper T, van der Hem GK, Klip HG, et al. Loss of amino acids during hemodialysis: effect of oral essential amino acid supplementation. Nephron 1981; 29:25–29.

189. Bergström J, Alvestrand A, Gutierrez A. Acute and chronic metabolic effects of hemodialysis. In Smeby LC, Jørstad S, Widerøe T-E (eds). Immune and Metabolic Aspects of Therapeutic Blood Purification Systems. Basel, Karger, 1986: 254–273.

190. Guarnieri G, Faccini L, Lipartiti T, et al. Simple methods for nutritional assessment in hemodialyzed patients. Am J Clin Nutr 1980; 33:1598–1607.

191. Blumenkrantz MJ, Kopple JD, Gutman RA, et al. Methods for assessing nutritional status of patients with renal failure. Am J Clin Nutr 1980; 33:1567–1585.

192. Llach F, Franklin SS, Maxwell MH. Dietary management of patients in chronic renal failure. Nephron 1975; 14:401–412.

193. Phillips ME, Havard J, Howard JP. Oral essential amino acid supplementation in patients on maintenance hemodialysis. Clin Nephrol 1978; 9:241–248.

194. Ganda OP, Aoki TT, Soeldner JS, et al. Hormone-fuel concentrations in anephric subjects. J Clin Invest 1976; 57:1403–1411.

195. Hecking E, Köhler J, Zobel R, et al. Treatment with essential amino acids in patients on chronic hemodialysis: a double blind cross-over study. Am J Clin Nutr 1978; 31:1821–1826.

196. Acchiardo S, Moore L, Cockrell S. Effect of essential amino acids (EAA) on chronic hemodialysis (CHD) patients (PTS). Trans Am Soc Artif Organs 1982; 28:608–613.

197. Hiedland A, Kult J. Long-term effect of essential amino acids supplementation in patients on regular dialysis treatment. Clin Nephrol 1975; 3:234–239.

198. Ulm A, Neuhäuser M, Leber HW. Influence of essential amino acids and keto acids on protein metabolism and anemia of patients on intermittent hemodialysis. Am J Clin Nutr 1978; 31:1827–1830.

199. Anderson RJ, Schrier RW. Clinical spectrum of oliguric and nonoliguric acute renal failure. In Brenner BM, Stein JH (eds). Contemporary Issues in Nephrology: Acute Renal Failure. New York, Churchill Livingstone Inc, 1980; 6:1–16.

200. Feinstein EI, Blumenkrantz MJ, Healy M, et al. Clinical and metabolic responses to parenteral nutrition in acute renal failure. Medicine 1981; 60:124–137.

201. Kleinknecht D, Jungers P, Chanard J, et al. Uremic and nonuremic complications in acute renal failure: evaluation of early and frequent dialysis on prognosis. Kidney Int 1972; 1:190–196.

202. Toback FG, Havener LJ, Dodd RC, et al. Phospholipid metabolism during renal regeneration after acute tubular necrosis. Am J Physiol 1977; 232:216–222.

203. Lee HA, Sharpstone P, Ames AC. Parenteral nutrition in renal failure. Postgrad Med J 1967; 43:81–91.

204. Abel RM, Abbott WM, Fischer JE. Acute renal failure: treatment without dialysis by total parenteral nutrition. Arch Surg 1971; 103:513–514.

205. Abel RM, Beck CH, Abbott WM, et al. Improved survival from acute renal failure after treatment with intravenous essential L-amino acids and glucose. N Engl J Med 1973; 288:695–699.

206. Oken DE, Sprinkel FM, Kirschbaum BB, et al. Amino acid therapy in the treatment of experimental acute renal failure in the rat. Kidney Int 1980; 17:14–23.

207. Blumenkrantz MJ, Kopple JD, Koffler A, et al. Total par-

enteral nutrition in the management of acute renal failure. Am J Clin Nutr 1978; *31*:1831–1840.

208. Blackburn GL, Etter G, Mackenzie T. Criteria for choosing amino acid therapy in acute renal failure. Am J Clin Nutr 1978; *31*:1841–1853.

209. Berlyne GM, Bazzard FJ, Booth EM, et al. The dietary treatment of acute renal failure. Q J Med 1967; *36*:59–83.

210. Richards P. Nutritional potential of nitrogen recycling in man. Am J Clin Nutr 1972; *25*:615–625.

211. Freund H, Atamian S, Fischer JE. Comparative study of parenteral nutrition in renal failure using essential and nonessential amino acid containing solutions. Surg Gynecol Obstet 1980; *151*:652–656.

212. Lee HA. The nutritional management of renal diseases. *In* Dickerson WT, Lee HA (eds). Nutrition in the Clinical Management of Disease. London, Edward Arnold, 1978: 210–235.

213. Mault JR, Bartlett RH, Dechert RE, et al. Starvation: a major contribution to mortality in acute renal failure? Trans Am Soc Artif Organs 1983; *29*:390–395.

214. Forsberg E, Carlsson M, Thörne A, et al. Energy expenditure in long-term critically ill patients with acute renal failure. Fourth Congress on Nutrition and Metabolism in Renal Disease, Williamsburg, VA, October 10–13, 1985.

215. Askanazi J, Carpentier YA, Elwyn H. Influence of total parenteral nutrition on fuel utilization in injury and sepsis. Ann Surg 1980; *191*:40–46.

216. Long CL, Schaeffel N, Geiger JW, et al. Metabolic response to injury and illness. Estimation of energy and protein needs from indirect calorimetry and nitrogen balance. JPEN 1979; *3*:452–456.

217. Macfie J, Holmfield JHM, King RFGJ, et al. Effect of the energy source on changes in energy expenditure and respiratory quotient during total parenteral nutrition. JPEN 1983; *7*:1–5.

218. Chan MK, Varghese Z, Persaud JW, et al. Fat clearance before and after heparin in chronic renal failure—haemodialysis reduces postheparin fractional clearance rate of Intralipid. Clin Chim Acta 1980; *108*:95–111.

219. Russel GI, Davies TG, Walls J. Evaluation of the intravenous fat tolerance test in chronic renal disease. Clin Nephrol 1980; *13*:282–286.

220. Druml W, Widhalm K, Laggner A, et al. Fat elimination in acute renal failure. Clin Nutr 1982; *1*:109–115.

221. Hallberg D. Elimination of exogenous lipids from the blood stream. Acta Physiol Scand 1965; *65*(Suppl 254):1–23.

222. Robin AP, Nordenström J, Askanazi J, et al. Plasma clearance of fat emulsions in trauma and sepsis: use of a three-stage lipid clearance test. JPEN 1980; *4*:505–510.

223. Kramer P, Kanfhold G, Gröne HJ, et al. Management of anuric intensive-care patients with arteriovenous hemofiltration. Int J Artif Organs 1980; *3*:225–230.

224. Kramer P, Böhler J, Kehr A, et al. Intensive care patients of continuous arteriovenous hemofiltration. Trans Am Soc Artif Organs 1982; *28*:28–32.

225. Golper TA. Continuous arteriovenous hemofiltration in acute renal failure. Am J Kidney Dis 1985; *6*:373–376.

226. Mitch WE, Walser M, Buffington GA, et al. A simple method of estimating progression of chronic renal failure. Lancet 1976; *2*:1326–1328.

227. Ibels LS, Alfrey AC, Hant L, et al. Preservation of function in experimental renal disease by dietary restriction of phosphate. N Engl J Med 1978; *298*:122–126.

228. Maschio G, Oldrizzi L, Tesitore N, et al. Effects of dietary protein and phosphorus restriction on the progression of early renal failure. Kidney Int 1982; *22*:371–376.

229. Kluthe R, Oeschlen D, Quirin H, et al. Six years experience with a special low-protein diet. *In* Kluthe R, Berlyne G, Burton B (eds). Uremia, International Conference on Pathogenesis and Therapy. Stuttgart, Georg Thieme Verlag, 1971: 50.

230. Barsotti G, Guiducci A, Ciardella F, et al. Effects on renal function of a low-nitrogen diet supplemented with essential amino acids and ketoanalogues and of hemodialysis and free protein supply in patients with chronic renal failure. Nephron 1981; *27*:113–117.

231. Alvestrand A, Ahlberg M, Bergström J. Retardation of the progression of renal insufficiency in patients treated with low-protein diet. Kidney Int 1983; *24*(Suppl 16):S268–272.

232. Barrientos A, Arteaga J, Rodicio JL, et al. Role of control of phosphate in the progression of chronic renal failure. Min Electr Metab 1982; *7*:127–133.

233. Hostetter TH, Rennke HG, Brenner BM. Compensatory renal hemodynamic injury: a final common pathway of residual nephron destruction. Am J Kidney Dis 1982; *1*:310–314.

234. Pullman TN, Alvings AS, Dern RJ, et al. The influence of dietary protein intake on specific renal function in normal men. J Lab Clin Med 1954; *44*:320–332.

235. Bergström J, Ahlberg M, Alvestrand A. Influence of protein intake on renal hemodynamics and plasma hormone concentrations in normal subjects. Acta Med Scand 1985; *217*:189–196.

236. Moorhead JF, Chan MK, El-Nahas M. Lipid nephrotoxicity in chronic progressive glomerular and tubulo-interstitial disease. Lancet 1982; *2*:1309–1311.

30

THE RENAL TRANSPLANT PATIENT

CHARLES T. VAN BUREN / BARRY D. KAHAN

Physicians who treat patients with renal insufficiency have commonly used nutritional manipulation to influence the metabolic consequences of kidney failure. Much of the focus has been upon limitation of protein intake, since azotemia and elevation in serum creatinine were noted to be expected perturbations associated with renal failure. In an era prior to widespread use of hemodialysis to maintain patients with end-stage renal disease, Giordano[1] and Giovannetti[2] reported that the use of very low quantities of high-biological-value protein led to decreased azotemia and even to positive nitrogen balance in patients with chronic renal failure.

Although specific dietary regimens have been a mainstay for the management of patients with chronic renal disease, little attention has been given to dietary prescription once the patient has undergone successful renal transplantation. The questions that would appear to be relevant to nutritional management of renal transplant patients include: What are the fundamental aberrations in lipid, carbohydrate, or protein metabolism associated with chronic renal failure? What is the relevance of preoperative nutritional status to immune responsiveness to an allograft after transplantation? What is the influence of immunosuppressive drugs upon metabolism of nutrients? Can specific nutritional regimens favorably influence the outcome of the recipient of an allograft?

METABOLIC CHANGES IN CHRONIC RENAL FAILURE

Although the metabolic changes affected by severe renal impairment are widespread, the biochemical derangements most directly associated with kidney failure are azotemia and elevation in serum creatinine. Although the precise nature of uremic toxins remains to be defined, blood urea nitrogen (BUN) remains a focus of clinical attention. Administration of an exogenous urea load in normal individuals fails to lead to clinical signs and symptoms of uremia.[3] However, if the BUN is increased to 150 mg/dl for more than a week by adding urea to the dialysis bath of patients undergoing otherwise standard hemodialysis, the patients develop uremic symptoms.[4] Current evidence suggests that urea is not directly responsible for these changes, but rather accumulation of ammonia and other toxic urea metabolites. Nevertheless, urea serves as a useful indicator of dialysis efficacy. The National Dialysis Study reported that dialysis regimens that persistently maintained BUN below 80 mg/dl were associated with fewer uremic complications than were less rigorous regimens.[5]

Creatinine, the other nitrogenous waste commonly used to measure level of renal function, is a dehydration product of the creatine and creatine phosphate stores of striated, smooth, and cardiac muscle. Each day 1.7 per cent of the total creatine pool is converted to creatinine.[6] Thus the amount of creatinine produced daily is related to the body muscle mass. The total excretion of creatinine also may be affected by dietary intake. Baked meat may add up to 3.2 mg of creatinine per gram of ingested cooked meat daily.[7] Thus diet and body habitus will determine the total creatinine load that must be cleared. With progressive loss of renal function, creatinine clearance decreases, with resultant increased serum creatinine levels.

Because creatinine is primarily filtered by the kidney, with only a small portion of the excreted load secreted by the proximal tubule, serum creatinine levels have been used as an approximation of glomerular filtration rate. Thus a doubling of serum creatinine reflects a loss of 50 per cent of remaining renal function.[8] Once the patient has approached end-stage renal disease requiring dialysis support (creatinine clearance <10 to 15 ml/min), serum creatinine levels become less clinically useful, since the steady-state serum creatinine will reflect muscle mass far more than residual renal function or efficacy of dialysis.

Because of impaired excretion of BUN and creatinine in patients with renal disease, many of the traditional studies used to determine protein requirements are limited in this population. Nitrogen balance studies are complicated because the urea nitrogen normally excreted in the urine instead is removed in the dialysis bath or accumulates in the body fluids as freely miscible urea. To adapt to these alterations in paths of nitrogen loss, nitrogen balance studies are used in renal falure patients to calculate the urea nitrogen appearance rate. This value is calculated by the following formula:[9]

$$UNA = U_u + \Delta$$
UNA = Urea nitrogen appearance
U_u = Urinary urea nitrogen (grams)
Δ = Change in body urea nitrogen
Δ = $(BUN_{END} - BUN_{INITIAL}) (0.60\ BW) + (BW_{END} - BW_{INITIAL}) (BUN_{FINAL})$

This method for calculating urea production presumes that the urea generated either is excreted in the urine or accumulates in the urea pool, that is, the total body water. This formula should be used during an interdialytic study period, since an ongoing dialysis treatment would require measurement of the urea nitrogen loss in the dialysate. Once the urea nitrogen appearance is calculated, nitrogen balance may be calculated from the following formula:

$$Balance\ N = Intake\ N - UNA - 2.5\ g/day$$

with 2.5 g/day representing the amount of non-urea nitrogen loss on a daily basis.[10]

Early investigations of nitrogen utilization in renal disease focused upon use of essential amino acid–enriched low-protein regimens. This was based upon the observation that rats fed essential amino acids and ^{15}N-labeled urea as a nitrogen source had a much greater incorporation of the radioactive isotope into body protein than animals fed the isotopically labeled urea while maintained on a mixture of essential and nonessential amino acids.[11] The authors reasoned that ammonia released in the gut by bacterial hydrolysis of urea could be used to manufacture nonessential amino acids for protein synthesis. Thus, urea was not an end product of protein catabolism, but could be recycled for tissue anabolism.

Giordano, in 1963, described the first clinical application of this laboratory observation.[1] At the time of the study hemodialysis, though long used for management of acute renal failure, had been used successfully for the management of chronic renal failure for less than 5 years. Indications for chronic dialysis included electrolyte abnormalities, fluid overload, or azotemia associated with uremic symptoms. The other putative toxins of uremia and the complications of inadequate dialysis, such as uremic neuropathy and pericarditis, were not well recognized. In this historical context Giordano sought to limit nitrogen intake to essential amino acids to decrease azotemia, hence the need for dialysis. He documented positive nitrogen balance and weight gain in 7 of 8 uremic patients maintained on a high-carbohydrate 15 g protein equivalent diet. Accompanying these clinical signs of improved nutrition was a decrease in blood urea while serum creatinine remained stable. The need for the essential amino acids was demonstrated by an increase in azotemia and onset of negative nitrogen balance when the carbohydrate in the diet was given alone. These observations were confirmed by Giovannetti in a series of chronic renal failure patients placed on a high-carbohydrate, low-protein diet.[2]

The Giordano-Giovannetti diet, which consisted of concentrated carbohydrate and limited amounts of protein high in essential amino acid content, became a mainstay for the management of chronic renal failure patients for the next several years. Unfortunately, the bland, monotonous character of the diet led to poor patient compliance. Patients who were spared dialysis therapy on this regimen often developed bleeding disorders, neuropathy, and hypophosphatemia. Moreover, in the group of chronically malnourished patients these authors studied, even a diet with inadequate amounts of protein could result in positive nitrogen balance. Without other criteria being used to test whether patients' long-term nutrition was improved, the hypothesis that a prolonged state of protein anabolism resulted remained unproved.

In 1968, Kaye described a young woman with renal failure who had been managed on a low protein intake.[12] The patient presented with ascites, hypertension, peripheral edema, and the appearance of general malnutrition. Assessment by anthropometric measurement was consistent with this diagnosis, while isotopic studies revealed a significant increase in total body water. Daily dialysis and provision of 2 to 3 g/kg/day of protein in the diet resulted in slight weight gain, dramatic loss of body water, resolution of hypertension, and restoration of body cell mass. This description of the problems of protein restriction in the chronic dialysis patient had followed observations of Giordano and others that maintaining nitrogen balance in these patients while on 20 to 30 g protein diets was difficult.[13] During that decade the efficiency of hemodialysis had improved, enabling many physicians to prescribe more liberal protein intake without requiring more lengthy dialysis.

Studies of the specific metabolic abnormalities in chronic renal failure have provided a more precise definition of the nutritional requirements of uremic patients. Such investigations have at times been confounded by the difficulty of accurately determining nitrogen equilibrium in patients with end-stage kidney disease, especially if the patient is being dialyzed. Bergstrom reconfirmed that positive nitrogen balance could be established in nondialyzed chronic renal failure patients fed an oral nonprotein diet supplemented by intravenous infusion of eight essential amino acids.[14] This positive nitrogen balance could be improved by adding histidine to the amino acid infusion. Others have since confirmed the requirement for histidine in renal failure.

Another metabolic alteration induced by the uremic state is reflected in the low plasma concentration of tyrosine found in renal failure patients.[15] This abnormality persists even when dietary supplements of phenylalanine, the amino acid precursor of tyrosine, are provided. Both decreased synthesis of tyrosine by the enzyme phenylalanine hydroxylase and more rapid degradation of tyrosine by induction of tyrosine aminotransferase are documented metabolic consequences of uremia.[16, 17]

Disturbances of other plasma amino acid patterns reflect altered utilization in chronic renal failure. Many dialysis patients have a decreased ratio of essential to total plasma amino acid concentrations (E/T ratio). Venous levels of the three branched-chain amino acids, valine, leucine, and isoleucine, are depressed in uremic individuals.[15] These abnormalities, while frequently found in the patients with renal failure, are similar to amino acid patterns associated with malnutrition. To further complicate matters, depression of plasma amino acid concentrations may not reflect intracellular stores. Indeed, analysis of muscle biopsy specimens reveals normal or supranormal intracellular levels of isoleucine and leucine while simultaneously obtained venous amino acid levels are depressed.[18] Thus, attempts to base definition of nutritional status on peripheral amino acid levels in chronic renal failure are not well founded.

Better understanding of these changes in amino acid metabolism has led to the use of alternative methods of dietary management of patients with renal failure. Following the successful control of azotemia by essential amino acid diets in patients with chronic renal failure, Richards et al.[19] suggested that alpha-keto analogues of the essential amino acids similarly could maintain positive nitrogen balance. The mechanism for this anabolic effect is unclear. Early speculation centered upon increased urea clearance rates in the gut due to higher blood levels of urea; ammonia derived from this source could then be used for synthesis of nonessential amino acids. Walser demonstrated, however, that urea clearance does not increase proportionally to serum urea levels.[20] Furthermore, the theory that essential amino acids or their alpha-keto analogues promoted synthesis of nonessential amino acids from urea nitrogen has not been validated. In fact, on such diets no more than 6 per cent of ^{15}N-labeled urea could be found incorporated in albumin, discounting promotion of urea recycling as the means by which essential amino acids have their salutary effect.[21] Walser has documented that alpha-keto analogues of the essential amino acids maintain positive nitrogen balance in uremic patients.[22] Furthermore, this positive balance continues even after the infusion of keto analogues has been discontinued. Mild infections may reverse such gains, and such restricted diets suffer from limitations similar to those of essential amino acid regimens. At present alpha-keto analogues of amino acids are not a practical means of maintaining protein anabolism in renal failure patients.

Uremia also influences carbohydrate metabolism. Hyperglycemia is a common biochemical feature of the uremic state, and patients with chronic renal failure have abnormally elevated serum glucose levels following an intravenous or oral glucose load.[23] Paradoxically, plasma insulin levels are elevated and decrease at a slower rate following a glucose load than they do in a normal response.[24] This may in part be explained by the presence of elevated levels of proinsulin, an inactive precursor of insulin that is indistinguishable from the active hormone by standard radioimmunoassay.[25] The prolonged elevation of plasma insulin may also be due to a decrease in the catabolism of this protein. Plasma glucagon levels are elevated in renal failure, and may lead to a diminished hypoglycemic effect of exogenously administered insulin.[24] Finally, hyperkalemia, acidosis, and other metabolic derangements may combine to result in a state of relative insulin resistance and baseline hyperglycemia.

The abnormalities observed in insulin and glucagon metabolism in renal failure patients may in part account for observed changes in lipid metabolism. Patients with chronic renal failure manifest hypertriglyceridemia, primarily due to an increase in very low density lipoproproteins (pre beta band, VLDL).[26] This increase is due in large part to a decrease in triglyceride clearance.[27] Following an oral fat load, peak postprandial triglyceride levels are higher and decrease more slowly in chronic renal failure patients than in nonuremic patients with hyperlipemia.[28] The decreased clearance of lipids is also observed following infusion of Intralipid, a commercially available fat emulsion.[29] Lipoprotein lipase and hepatic lipase activity are decreased in patients with renal failure, suggesting a possible mechanism for the observed decrease in triglyceride clearance.[30] These changes, in turn, may be secondary to the observed hyperinsulinemia previously described in patients with renal disease.

Therapy for this hypertriglyceridemia is directed toward decreasing the proportion of carbohydrate-derived calories in the diet. A 20 per cent reduction in the carbohydrate content of the diet resulted in a significant decrease in plasma triglyceride levels in a study of patients with chronic renal failure.[31] In a study similar to reported studies of nonuremic patients, raising the proportion of polyunsaturated fats in the diet resulted in lower plasma triglycerides in patients with chronic renal failure.[32] Finally, in both experimental and clinical studies increased exercise enhanced insulin sensitivity, increased peak oxygen consumption, and decreased serum triglyceride levels in subjects with chronic renal failure.[33]

Abnormalities in amino acid, lipid, and carbohydrate metabolism in renal failure affect the protein requirements of chronic renal failure (CRF) patients. Although initial studies suggested that nondialyzed CRF patients required less dietary protein to remain in nitrogen equilibrium than did normal adults, most evidence suggests that CRF patients require 0.5 to 0.6 g/kg/day of protein, a substantial portion of which must be high in essential amino acids.[34] This is similar to the requirement of 0.56 g/kg/day of protein established as a minimum daily adult requirement by the WHO.[35] Dialysis adversely affects this equilibrium, increasing the rate of protein catabolism.[10] In addition, dialysis results in loss of 0.5 to 2.0 g of amino acids per hour of dialysis time.[36] Blood drawn for routine laboratory tests or bleeding associated with coil rupture or clotting represents yet another drain upon protein stores of dialysis patients.

Peritoneal dialysis, which has undergone a renaissance in the form of chronic peritoneal dialysis (continuous ambulatory peritoneal dialysis, CAPD), is a much more stressful method of dialysis for the body's protein synthetic reserves. From 10 to 22 g of protein may be lost per day of CAPD.[37] This loss increases even further in the face of the inflammatory response of peritonitis. Finally, patients with renal disease may have further sources of protein loss in the form of proteinuria due to glomerulonephritis or accelerated protein catabolism resulting from corticosteroid treatment of glomerulonephritis or lupus erythematosus. These demands to replace increased losses and inefficient protein metabolism, superimposed upon individuals who are anorectic or nauseated by the systemic manifestations of renal disease, are a major reason why the minimum protein requirements for hemodialysis patients are 1 g/kg/day, and for CAPD patients range up to 1.4 g/kg/day of dietary protein.

PREOPERATIVE NUTRITIONAL STATUS

Heidland et al. have studied supplementation of high-protein diets with essential amino acids provided enterally or parenterally.[38] While these studies have demonstrated improved serum protein levels and positive nitrogen balance in patients given 10 to 15 g of essential amino acids as a supplement to 1 mg/kg/day maintenance protein intake, other investigators have not demonstrated a benefit of such therapy.[39] Problems arise in comparing results, since authors often fail to define the nutritional status of patients prior to the initiation of a study or to use as basal diets regimens that contain an inadequate amount of protein. Furthermore, as revealed in a prospective study of patients being evaluated as potential renal transplant recipients, criteria used for the assessment of malnutrition in other patient populations are not necessarily applicable to patients with renal failure.

At The University of Texas Medical School at Houston, 170 consecutive patients were evaluated over an 18-month period as potential candidates for renal transplants by the Organ Transplantation Division. While these patients were being evaluated medically they had dietary histories taken specifically checking for recent weight loss, had standard anthropometric determinations performed, and had as part of their biochemical assessment studies of BUN, serum creatinine, transferrin, C3, C4, albumin, IgG, IgA, IgM, and complete blood count with differential. In addition, all patients were tested for cutaneous response to five microbial antigens, whole blood spontaneous blastogenesis (an index of leukocyte metabolic activity), peripheral blood total and active T cell count, and panel mixed lymphocyte blastogenic response (a measure of the patient's response to alloantigen). These last four tests have correlated well with the immune response of patients to a renal allograft. Patients who are relatively hyporesponsive as assessed by immune response testing will have fewer rejection episodes and a better chance of maintaining allograft function.[40]

The results of this prospective screening were provocative.[41] Malnutrition was defined by a 10 per cent or greater weight loss, a subnormal dry body weight, and a triceps skinfold thickness that was less than 80 per cent of normal. No correlation was observed between nutritional status as defined by these criteria and serum urea nitrogen, creatinine, C3, C4, immunoglobulin, or transferrin levels. A significant correlation was found between serum albumin and nutritional status, as has been previously described. No correlation was found between nutritional status and the four important predictors of immune response to a renal allograft: anergy, low active T cell numbers, low panel mixed lymphocyte culture (MLC) response, and low spontaneous blastogenesis. Thus the association between immune function and nutritional status described by others is not found in patients with chronic renal failure. Any study that purports to examine the effect of dietary manipulation on nutrition in CRF must define objective criteria of malnutrition that are useful for the population to be studied.

This caveat is of prime importance in the treatment of patients with acute renal failure (ARF). These patients are especially at risk for the development of malnutrition, since they face the accelerated protein catabolism associated with stress states and acute illnesses. The treatment options, however, are limited by the volume of calorie-containing fluid that may be provided to these patients, who often have other organ system disease. Congestive failure and hepatic decompensation may compromise an otherwise vigorous nutritional support program. Gastrointestinal motility disturbances commonly present lead to total parenteral support of these critically ill patients.

The first application of the principles enunciated by Giovannetti and Giordano in the clinical setting of acute renal failure was by Wilmore and Dudrick in 1969.[42] Central venous infusion of a hypertonic dextrose–essential amino acid mixture was used to nourish a 42-year-old patient with acute renal failure secondary to sepsis. On this regimen the man recovered renal function while healing a duodenal fistula. Dudrick et al. extended this experience in a series of ten patients with either acute or chronic renal failure.[43] Several of the patients recovered from bouts of acute tubular necrosis on this regimen, and all patients demonstrated metabolic and clinical improvement.

The use of this intravenous formula was studied in an animal model of ARF.[44] Bilaterally nephrectomized beagle puppies were placed in four treatment groups. The animals received one of the following nutritional supports: chow diet; intravenous infusion of 70 per cent dextrose; or 70 per cent dextrose and essential amino acids. The D_{70}-EAA infusion was the only regimen that delayed the development of azotemia in this animal model of ARF. This study emphasized that the potential benefit of this hypertonic dextrose–essential amino acid solution was to delay the need for hemodialysis in the setting of ARF.

In a prospective clinical study, Abel, Fischer, et al. compared a central infusion of 50 per cent dextrose with an infusion of 50 per cent dextrose and essential amino acids (D_{50}-EAA) as a means of nutritional support for patients in ARF.[45] There was no decreased dialytic interval in the group receiving D_{50}-EAA as compared with the control group. Hospital survival was not significantly altered. However, patients recovered renal function faster on the D_{50}-EAA regimen and thus required less dialysis. Moreover, there was a significantly decreased mortality in that group of ARF patients requiring dialysis who received D_{50}-EAA as compared with the group that received D_{50}. This is the first, and to date the only, study to demonstrate a benefit of hypertonic dextrose–essential amino acid solutions in patients requiring dialysis for acute renal failure.

Other investigators have failed to confirm these results. EAA–hypertonic glucose infusions have been demonstrated to be no different from hypertonic dextrose alone in reversing the morbidity and mortality of ARF.[46] Some investigators have found nonessential amino acid regimens equally effective as EAA regimens in treating patients with ARF,[47] while Freund et al. have demonstrated increased mortality in ARF patents administered EAA–nonessential amino acid–hypertonic dextrose formula compared with those receiving hypertonic dextrose alone.[48] Thus there is no consensus as to the most effective parenteral nutrition regimen to use in patients with renal failure.

Much of the debate regarding this question of what nutritional regimen is most effective in patients with ARF must then be based upon knowledge of the pathophysiology of renal failure. Unlike at the time of the original studies described by Abel and Fischer, hemodialysis is no longer regarded as a therapy to be cautiously applied in the setting of ARF. Indeed, studies suggest that frequent and aggressive hemodialysis reduces the morbidity and mortality of this condition.[49] Given the normal increase in protein catabolism associated with hemodialysis or CAPD, there is little rationale for limiting protein intake to 2.5 per cent EAA alone, as advocated in the original Abel-Fischer regimen. Any regimen must provide between 1 and 1.4 g/kg/day of amino acids or protein to attempt to maintain nitrogen equilibrium. Given the previously described abnormalities in lipid clearance, such a regimen should also include glucose and exogenous insulin as required to provide nonnitrogen calories.

This reasoning has led to the use of a modified renal failure formula at our institution (Table 30–1). This regimen has been used successfully in over 30 patients with renal failure or renal dysfunction. Twenty-four of these patients were treated following renal transplantation for periods from 1 week to 6 months. Catheter-related sepsis has not been a problem despite the immunosuppressed condition of these patients. Moreover, in seven of these patients improved renal allograft function was noted following the institution of total parenteral nutrition. Patients either maintained dry body weight or gained body cell mass while receiving this infusion. Because of the fluid load necessary to deliver adequate calories, cooperation with involved nephrologists using ultrafiltration and aggressive dialysis is a necessary part of the total nutritional management.

IMMUNOSUPPRESSION AND POSTOPERATIVE NUTRITION

Little attention has been directed toward the appropriate nutritional regimen to be used post transplantation. Most patients who have received renal allografts are currently maintained upon a regimen of corticosteroids and another nonspecific immunosuppressant to combat rejection of the allograft. Azathioprine, a midazole derivative of 6-mercaptopurine, has served as a mainstay of immunosuppression since its first clinical use in 1962.[50] Generally, 50 to 90 per cent of patients who receive a renal allograft will experience a rejection episode.[51,52] These rejection episodes are commonly treated with corticosteroid therapy. Regimens for maintenance immunosuppression and antirejection therapy used at the University of Texas at Houston are listed in Table 30–2.

Corticosteroid therapy has been associated with well-described metabolic consequences. Pharmacologic doses of steroids induce hyperglycemia and hypertriglyceridemia and increase gluconeogenesis.[53,54] Much of the increase in nitrogen catabolism observed with steroids is due to mobilization of amino acids from muscle stores. 3-Methylhistidine, a marker of muscle metabolism, increases dramatically in rats administered corticosteroids.[55] In addi-

TABLE 30–1. Parenteral Nutrition Formula for Renal Failure Patients

600 ml	D_{70}
200 ml	5% essential amino acids
200 ml	8.5% Freamine III

$MgSO_4$, Ca gluconate, NaCl, $KHPO)_4$
KCl (as needed)
Insulin, albumin (as needed)
5 ml MVI (daily)

TABLE 30–2. Regimen for Immunosuppressive Agents Used at the University of Texas Medical School at Houston

	Immunosuppressive Therapy	
	Prednisone	*Cyclosporine*
Day 1	120 mg/day (oral)	6 mg/kg/day (IV)
Day 2	100 mg/day (oral)	6 mg/kg/day (IV)
Day 3	80 mg/day (oral)	14 mg/kg/day (oral)
Day 4	60 mg/day (oral)	14 mg/kg/day
Day 5	45 mg/day (oral)	14 mg/kg/day
Day 6	40 mg/day (oral)	14 mg/kg/day
Day 7	30 mg/day (oral)	14 mg/kg/day

Week 2

12 mg/kg/day

Rejection Therapy
IV Methylprednisolone

Day 1	1500 mg/day
Day 2	200 mg/day
Day 3	160 mg/day
Day 4	120 mg/day
Day 5	100 mg/day
Day 6	80 mg/day
Day 7	60 mg/day
Day 8	45 mg/day
Day 9	40 mg/day
Day 10	30 mg/day

tion, sodium and fluid retention, hypokalemia, and hypertension are all recognized consequences of steroid therapy.

To combat these observed catabolic responses associated with high-dose corticosteroids, several investigators have attempted to increase protein intake following transplantation. Cogan et al. examined a high-calorie (33 kcal/kg/day), high-protein (1.3 g/kg/day) post-transplantation diet versus a low-calorie (20 kcal/kg/day), low-protein (0.73 g/kg/day) regimen.[56] High urea nitrogen production rates were demonstrated in both groups, with no difference noted in urea generation based upon the diet provided. In contrast, nitrogen balance studies demonstrated nitrogen equilibrium in patients on the high-protein diet, compared with persistent negative nitrogen balance in those on the low-protein hypocaloric diet. Although the authors demonstrated that negative nitrogen balance was not a necessary consequence of corticosteroid therapy, the limitation of nitrogen balance as the only index of protein catabolism in patients with rapidly changing renal function is an inherent problem with the study. More importantly, the use of protein and calorie intakes that are inadequate to meet the needs of patients with renal failure raises questions regarding the validity of the observations in the "control group." Other observers have suggested that negative nitrogen balance is a phenomenon observed in transplantation even with more ideal protein diets.[57]

Whittier et al. addressed the benefit of high-nitrogen, low-carbohydrate diets in 12 post-transplant patients.[58] Patients were randomly assigned to control or experimental groups. Control patients received 30 kcal/kg/day and approximately 1 g/kg/day of protein and 3 g/kg/day of carbohydrate; patients in the experimental group received an isocaloric regimen averaging 2 g/kg/day of protein and 1g/kg/day of carbohydrate. Experimental patients demonstrated a significant improvement in nitrogen balance compared with control patients, and in addition were "less cushingoid" in appearance. These data appear to confirm Cogan's observation that markedly increasing dietary protein can largely prevent the catabolic effect of corticosteroids.

Although these studies suggest that dietary intervention can alter the metabolic response to high-dose corticosteroids, the influence of diet upon the immune response itself has been largely neglected. Most of the observations have focused upon deficiency states. Thus, protein malnutrition, zinc deficiency, and various vitamin deficiencies have all been demonstrated to lead to depressed cellular immunity.[59–61] No clinically defensible experiment could induce these deficiency states in immunosuppressed transplant patients. Early investigations at the University of Texas Medical School at Houston demonstrated that restriction of dietary nucleotides alone could decrease the immune response. Rejection of a subcutaneously transplanted alloreactive tumor in a mouse could be delayed in animals maintained upon a casein diet that was isocaloric and isonitrogenous with standard chow. This diet did not increase the efficacy of azathioprine.[62]

Further studies demonstrated that patients fed a nucleotide-free diet (NFD) had significantly less cardiac allograft rejection, graft-versus-host disease, in vivo and in vitro mixed lymphocyte proliferative responsiveness, and sensitization to PPD as compared with control groups fed standard chow or NFD + 0.25 per cent RNA.[63–65] The response appeared to be primarily directed against the T lymphocyte. Responses to lipopolysaccharide, a T cell independent antigen, were unaltered.[63] Although initially these findings contradicted the dogma that pyrimidines and purines are bases which are not required by the body because of de novo synthesis of these compounds, Cohen et al. had observed that G_1 phase thymocytes and G_1 phase peripheral T lymphocytes do not have de novo purine synthetic activity.[66] B cells require exogenous nucleotides for optimal antibody production.[67] Proliferative responses of lymphoid cells appear to require provision of exogenous nucleotides.[68] Thus, the concept that a body compartment such as the T lymphocyte stores might require exogenous purine or pyrimidine bases during immune stimulation is supported by other experimental observations.

These observations also appeared to contradict the studies that have demonstrated improved immune function in patients maintained on parenteral nutrition, which represents a form of nucleotide-free regimen.[69] Most of these observations have compared immune function in malnourished patients and in those supported by total parenteral nutrition (TPN).[70] The experimental studies have suggested that NFD does not abrogate the immune response, but instead delays maturation of a primary cellular immune response. Thus these observations do not conflict with the studies demonstrating improved skin test reactivity, a secondary immune event, in patients on TPN.

The important question remaining was whether the NFD improved the efficacy of standard immunosuppression. The mainstay of clinical immunosuppressive therapy has changed with the advent of cyclosporine. This novel endecapeptide has been demonstrated to profoundly suppress cellular immune responses to lectins or alloantigens.[71, 72] Clinical use of cyclosporine has demonstrated improved allograft survival, decreased incidence of rejection and infection after transplantation, and decreased need for corticosteroid therapy.[73, 74] Many European centers have sought to use cyclosporine alone, without steroids, in transplant patients.[75] Calne has reported that 30 per cent of his cyclosporine-treated allograft recipients never require corticosteroid therapy.[76] Thus in the current cyclosporine era the influence of diet upon corticosteroid side effects may be far less relevant.

To test the effect of diet upon cyclosporine therapy, mice receiving an H_2-incompatible cardiac allograft were maintained upon NFD, NFD + RNA, or chow and randomized to receive a 4-day course of cyclosporine (14 mg/kg/day) or olive oil vehicle by gavage feeding. This short course of cyclosporine alone failed to prolong allograft survival. NFD did significantly improve allograft survival and when combined with cyclosporine therapy proved synergistic in effect in further prolonging allograft survival.[77] Thus, NFD can augment the efficacy of cyclosporine therapy. The action of the diet appears to be directed primarily against helper T lymphocytes.[78] Following immunostimulation, NFD-fed mice demonstrate lower numbers of Lyt-1+ lymphocytes, a murine marker of the helper T lymphocyte. Similarly, production of interleukin 2, a lymphokine produced by activated T cells, is decreased in mice deprived of dietary nucleotides.[78] These changes are similar to those observed following cyclosporine therapy, and may explain why the NFD has proved so useful to increasing the effect of cyclosporine.

Because of these experimental observations, all patients at the University of Texas Medical School at Houston are maintained upon a nucleotide-free diet (Table 30–3) in addition to cyclosporine and prednisone therapy. Although the effect of this diet has yet to be documented clinically, the incidence of allograft rejection (35 per cent) and allograft survival (83 per cent) reported with this regimen has remained competitive with the best reports in the literature.[79] The future of dietary manipulation to in-

TABLE 30–3. Nucleotide-Free Diet

Foods Eliminated from the Nucleotide-Free Diet:

All meat, fish, poultry, soups and
sauces derived from:

Peas	Asparagus
Beans	Cauliflower
Lentils	English peas
Spinach	Celery
Mushrooms	Wheat germ
Radishes	Bran

**Major Sources of Protein on the
Nucleotide-Free Diet:**

Eggs
Cheese
Milk products

fluence immune responsiveness and response to corticosteroids will remain uncertain until the mechanisms underlying the observed phenomena are elucidated.

Thus, profound changes in body metabolism occur with the onset of renal failure. The hormonal milieu, the requirements for protein, and the metabolism of various substrates change in patients with poor renal function. Assessment of nutritional status and monitoring of the utilization of dietary constituents must be altered to allow for problems encountered in studying patients with renal failure. Increased protein requirements and decreased utilization of lipid and glucose are several of the important changes observed with the onset of renal failure. Prescribing nutritional therapy before or after transplant must allow for these differences. Finally, the impact of diet upon post-transplant catabolic responses and upon immune response appears to be an exciting area for future exploration.

References

1. Giordano C. Use of exogenous and endogenous urea for protein synthesis in normal and uremic subjects. J Lab Clin Med 1963; 62:231–246.
2. Giovannetti S, Maggiore Q. A low nitrogen diet with protein of high biological value for severe chronic uremia. Lancet 1964; 1:1000–1003.
3. Javid M. Urea—new use of an old agent. Surg Clin North Am 1958; 38:907–928.
4. Johnson WJ, Hagge WH, Wagoner RD, et al. Effects of urea loading in patients with far advanced renal failure. Mayo Clin Proc 1972; 47:21–29.
5. Lowrie EG, Laird NM, Parker TF, et al. The effect of hemodialysis prescription on patient morbidity: report from the National Cooperative Dialysis Study. N Engl J Med 1981; 305:1176–1181.
6. Crim MC, Callaway DH, Margen S. Creatine metabolism in men: creatine pool size and turnover in relationship to creatine intake. J Nutr 1976; 106:471–481.
7. Camara AA, Arn KD, Reimer A, et al. The twenty-four hour endogenous creatinine clearance as a clinical measure of the functional status of the kidneys. J Lab Clin Med 1951; 37:743–763.
8. Kassirer JP. Clinical evaluation of kidney function—glomerular function. N Engl J Med 1971; 285:385–389.
9. Kopple JD. Nutritional therapy in kidney failure. Nutr Rev 1981; 39(5):193–206.
10. Borah MF, Schoenfeld PY, Gotch FA, et al. Mitogen balance during intermittent dialysis therapy of uremia. Kidney Int 1978; 14:491–500.
11. Rose WC, Dekker EE. Urea as a source of nitrogen for the biosynthesis of amino acids. J Biol Chem 1956; 233:107–121.
12. Kaye M, Comty C. Nutritional repletion during dialysis. Am J Clin Nutr 1968; 21:583–589.
13. Giordano C, Esposito R, DePascale C, et al. Dietary treatment in renal failure. In Proceedings at Third International Congress of Nephrology. Vol. 3. Washington, 1966. Basel, S. Karger, 1967: 214–225.
14. Bergstrom J, Furst P, Josephson B, et al. Improvement of nitrogen balance in a uremic patient by the addition of histidine to essential amino acid solutions given intravenously. Life Sci 1970; (II) 91:787–794.
15. Furst P, Ahlberg M, Alvestrand A, et al. Principles of essential amino acid therapy in uremia. Am J Clin Nutr 1978; 31:1744–1755.
16. Swendseid ME, Wang M, Vyhmeister I, et al. Amino acid metabolism in the chronically uremic rat. Clin Nephrol 1975; 3:240–246.
17. Sapico V, Shea L, Litwack G. Translocation of inducible tyrosine amino-transferase to the mitochondrial fraction. J Biol Chem 1974; 249:2122–2129.
18. DeFronza RA, Felig P. Amino acid metabolism in uremia. Am J Clin Nutr 1980; 33:1378–1386.
19. Richards P, Metcalfe-Gibson A, Ward EE, et al. Utilization of ammonia nitrogen for protein synthesis in man, and the effect of protein restriction and uremia. Lancet 1967; 2:845–849.
20. Walser M. Urea metabolism in chronic renal failure. J Clin Invest 1974; 53:1385–1392.
21. Varcoe R, Halliday D, Carson ER, et al. Efficiency of utilization of urea nitrogen for albumin synthesis by chronically uremic and normal man. Clin Sci Mol Med 1975; 48:379–390.
22. Walser M, Coulter W, Dighe S, et al. The effect of keto-analogues of essential amino acids in severe chronic uremia. J Clin Invest 1973; 52:678–690.
23. Swenson RS, Weisinger J, Reaven GM. Evidence that hemodialysis does not improve the glucose tolerance of patients with chronic renal failure. Metabolism 1974; 23:929–936.
24. Feldman HA, Singer I. Endocrinology and metabolism in uremia and dialysis: a clinical review. Medicine 1974; 54:345–376.
25. Mako M, Block M, Starr J, et al. Proinsulin in chronic renal and hepatic failure. Clin Res 1973; 21:631.
26. Reaven GM, Swenson RS, Sanfelippo ML. Uremic hypertriglyceridemia. Am J Clin Nutr 1980; 33:1476–1484.
27. Sanfelippo ML, Swenson RS, Reaven GM. Reduction of plasma triglycerides by diet in subjects with chronic renal failure. Kidney Int 1977; 11:54–59.
28. Chan MK, Varghese Z, Moorhead JR. Lipid abnormalities in uremia, dialysis and transplantation. Kidney Int 1981; 19:625–637.
29. Norbeck HE: Serum lipoproteins in chronic renal failure. Acta Med Scand 1981; 649:1–49.
30. Goldberg AP, Appelbaum-Bowden OM, Bierman EL, et al.: Increase in lipoprotein lipase during clofibrate treatment on hypertriglyceridemia in patients on hemodialysis. N Engl J Med 1979; 301:1073–1076.
31. Sanfelippo ML, Swenson RS, Reaven GM: Response of plasma triglycerides to dietary changes in patients on hemodialysis. Kidney Int 1978; 14:180–190.
32. Gokal R, Mann JI, Oliver DO, et al. Dietary treatment of hyperlipidemia in chronic hemodialysis patients. Am J Clin Nutr 1978; 31:1915–1918.
33. Zabetakis PH, Gleim GW, Pasternak FL, et al. Long duration submaximal exercise conditioning on hemodialysis patients. Clin Nephrol 1982; 18:17–22.

34. Kopple JF, Swendseid M. Evidence that histidine is an essential amino acid in normal and chronically uremic man. J Clin Invest 1975; 55:881–891.

35. Energy and protein requirements. Report of a joint FAO/WHO Ad Hoc Expert Committee. WHO Tech Rep Ser 522, 1973.

36. Bilbrey GL, Faloona GR, White MG, et al. Hyperglucagonemia of renal failure. J Clin Invest 1974; 53:841–847.

37. Moncrief JW, Popovich RP, Nolph KD, et al. Clinical experience with continuous ambulatory peritoneal dialysis. Am Soc Artif Intern Organs 1979; 2:114–118.

38. Heidland A, Kult J. Long term effects of essential amino acid supplementation in patients on regular dialysis treatment. Clin Nephrol 1975; 3:234–239.

39. Ulm A, Neuhaser M, Leber HW. Influence of essential amino acids and keto acids on protein metabolism and anemia of patients on intermittent hemodialysis. Am J Clin Nutr 1978; 31:1827–1830.

40. Kerman RH, Floyd M, Van Buren CT, et al. Prediction of allograft survival based on pretransplant nonspecific immunocompetence. Transplant Proc 1981; 13:1533–1535.

41. Van Buren CT, Kerman RH, Van Buren D, et al. Correlation of immune responsiveness with nutritional indices in chronic renal failure patients. JPEN 1979; 3:524.

42. Wilmore D, Dudrick SJ. Treatment of acute renal failure with intravenous essential L-amino acids. Arch Surg 1969; 99:669–673.

43. Dudrick SJ, Steiger E, Long JM. Renal failure in surgical patients: treatment with intravenous essential acids and hypertonic glucose. Surgery 1970; 68:180–186.

44. Van Buren CT, Dudrick SJ, Dworkin AB, et al. Effects of intravenous essential L-amino acids and hypertonic dextrose on anephric beagles. Surg Forum 1972; 23:83–84.

45. Abel RM, Beck CH, Abbott WM, et al. Improved survival from acute renal failure after treatment with intravenous essential L-amino acids and glucose. N Engl J Med 1973; 288:695–699.

46. Feinstein EI, Blumenkrantz MJ, Healy M, et al. Clinical and metabolic responses to parenteral nutrition in acute renal failure: a controlled double blind study. Medicine 1981; 60:124–137.

47. Sofio C, Nicora R. High caloric essential amino acid parenteral therapy in acute renal failure. Acta Chir Scand (Suppl) 1976; 466:98–99.

48. Freund H, Atamian S, Fischer JE. Comparative study of parenteral nutrition in renal failure using essential and nonessential amino acid containing solutions. Surg Gynecol Obstet 1980; 151:652–656.

49. Kleinknecht D, Jungers D, Chanard J, et al. Uremic and nonuremic complications in acute renal failure: evaluation of early and frequent dialysis on prognosis. Kidney Int 1972; 1:190–196.

50. Calne RY, Alexandre GPJ, Murray JE. A study of the effects of drugs in prolonging survival of homologous renal transplants in dogs. Ann NY Acad Sci 1962; 99:743–761.

51. Kerman RH, Floyd M, Van Buren CT, et al. Improved allograft survival of strong immune responder–high risk recipients with adjuvant antithymocyte globulin therapy. Transplantation 1980; 30:450–454.

52. Sutherland DER, Fryd DS, Strand MH, et al. Results of the Minnesota randomized prospective trial of cyclosporine versus azathioprine-antilymphocyte globulin for immunosuppression in renal allograft recipients. Am J Kidney Dis 1985; 5:318–327.

53. Baxter JD, Tyrrell JB. The adrenal cortex. In Felig P, Baxter JD, Broadus AE, et al. (eds). Endocrinology and Metabolism. New York, McGraw-Hill, 1981: 415–417.

54. Illingworth DR, Connor WE. Disorders of lipid metabolism. In Felig P, Baxter JD, Broadus AE, et al. (eds). Endocrinology and Metabolism. New York, McGraw-Hill, 1981: 925–926.

55. Tomas FM, Monro HM, Young VR. Effect of glucocorticoid administration on the rate of muscle protein breakdown in vivo in rats as measured by urinary excretion of NT-methylhistidine. Biochem J 1979; 178:139–146.

56. Cogan MG, Sargent JA, Yarbrough SG, et al.: Prevention of prednisone induced negative nitrogen balance. Ann Intern Med 1981; 95:158–161.

57. Steinmuller DR, Richards C, Novick A, et al. Protein catabolic rate post transplant. Dial Transplant 1983; 12:504–507.

58. Whittier FC, Evans DH, Dutton S, et al. Nutrition in renal transplantation. Am J Kidney Dis 1985; 6:405–411.

59. Chandra RK. Immunocompetence in undernutrition. J Pediatr 1972; 81:1194–1200.

60. Golden MH, Golden BE, Jackson AA. Effect of zinc on thymus of recently malnourished children. Lancet 1977; 2:1057–1059.

61. Alexander JW, Stinnett JD. Changes in immunologic function. In Fischer JE (ed). Surgical Nutrition. Toronto, Little, Brown, 1983: 541–542.

62. Van Buren D, Rudolph F, Kahan BD, et al. The effect of a purine-free diet on EL4 tumor growth in the allogeneic host. JPEN 1980; 4:590.

63. Van Buren CT, Kulkarni A, Schandle VB, et al. The influence of dietary nucleotides on cell mediated immunity. Transplantation 1983; 36:350–352.

64. Kulkarni SS, Bhateley DC, Zander AP, et al. Functional impairment of T-lymphocytes in mouse radiation chimeras by a nucleotide free diet. Exp Hematol 1984; 12:694–699.

65. Van Buren CT, Kulkarni AD, Rudolph FB. Nucleotide deprivation retards delayed cutaneous hypersensitivity (DCH). JPEN 1985; 9:117.

66. Cohen A, Barankiewicz J, Lederman HM, et al. Purine metabolism in human T lymphocytes: role of purine nucleoside cycle. Can J Biochem Cell Biol 1984; 62:577–583.

67. Seegmiller JE, Watanabe T, Schreier MH. The effect of adenosine on lymphoid cell proliferation and antibody formation. In Purine and Pyrimidine Metabolism (Ciba Foundation Symposium). Amsterdam, Elsevier, May, 1977.

68. Nishida Y, Okudaira K, Tanimoto K, et al. The differences in purine metabolism between T and B lymphocytes. Exp Hematol 1980; 8:593–598.

69. Copeland EM, Daly JM, Dudrick SJ. Nutrition as an adjunct to cancer treatment in the adult. Cancer Res 1977; 37:2451–2457.

70. Law DK, Dudrick SJ, Abdou NI. Immunocompetence of patients with protein-calorie malnutrition. The effects of nutritional repletion. Ann Intern Med 1973; 79:545–550.

71. Borel JF, Feurer C, Gubler HU, et al. Biological effects of cyclosporin A: a new antilymphocytic agent. Agents Actions 1976; 6:468–475.

72. Borel JF, Feuer C, Magnee C, et al. Effects of new antilymphocytic peptide cyclosporin A in animals. Immunology 1977; 32:1017–1025.

73. Najarian JS, Ferguson RM, Sutherland DER, et al. A prospective trial of the efficacy of cyclosporine in renal transplantation at the University of Minnesota. Transplant Proc 1983; 15:438–441.

74. Kahan BD, Van Buren CT, Flechner SM, et al. Cyclosporine immunosuppression mitigates immunologic risk factors in renal allotransplantation. Transplant Proc 1983; 15:2469–2478.

75. European Multicentre Trial Group: Cyclosporine in cadaveric renal transplantation: one year followup of a multicentre trial. Lancet 1983; 2:986–989.

76. Merion RM, White DJG, Thiru S, et al. Cyclosporine: five years' experience in cadaveric renal transplantation. N Engl J Med 1984; 310:148–154.

77. Van Buren CT, Kulkarni AD, Rudolph FB. Synergistic effect of a nucleotide free diet and cyclosporine on allograft survival. Transplant Proc 1983; 15:2967–2968.

78. Van Buren CT, Kulkarni AD, Fanslow WC, et al. Dietary nucleotides: a requirement for helper/inducer T lymphocytes. Transplantation 1985; 40:694–697.

79. Kahan BD, Wideman CA, Flechner SM, et al. Impact of cyclosporine on renal transplant practice at the University of Texas Medical School at Houston. Am J Kidney Dis 1985; 5:288–295.

31

NEOPLASTIC DISEASES

JOHN M. DALY / ARLEEN K. THOM

The link between malnutrition and cancer has been well established. Anorexia resulting from malignant disease is commonly implicated in the development of malnutrition with decreased nutrient intake and weight loss. In the absence of adequate exogenous nutrients, the body utilizes endogenous fuel reserves to satisfy the ongoing requirements of both host and tumor for energy and protein. In patients with tumors obstructing portions of the alimentary tract, the presence of the malignant growth is sufficient to reduce nutrient ingestion. In other patients, clinical malnutrition develops out of proportion to decreases in good intake, and is thought to arise from interference by the tumor in the host's energy utilization and substrate metabolism. It has also been suggested that tumors deplete nutrient reserves by selectively utilizing substances intended for normal tissue metabolism. Compounding the effects of the tumor on nutrient availability to the host are the nutritionally depleting effects of oncological therapies administered singly or sequentially. The site of the tumor or the extent of the operative resection may limit ingestion and absorption of nutrients via the gastrointestinal tract. Radiation therapy may produce stomatitis, enteritis, and malabsorption, whereas chemotherapy often induces anorexia, nausea, vomiting, diarrhea, and mucosal ulcerations. Thus, the cancer itself and aggressive therapy to eradicate it often produce a variety of symptoms that lead to weight loss and nutritional depletion. For example, DeWys et al.[1] noted substantial weight loss in 40 per cent of patients with breast cancer and in 80 per cent of patients with carcinoma of the pancreas and stomach. Using standard methods of nutritional assessment, Nixon et al. documented substantial losses of adipose tissue and visceral and skeletal muscle in a series of hospitalized cancer patients.[2]

The term "cancer cachexia" describes a group of symptoms and signs—inanition, anorexia, weakness, tissue wasting, and organ dysfunction—characteristic of the malignant process. Cachexia, nearly ubiquitous in patients with advanced metastatic malignant disease, also occurs in patients with localized disease. Its relationship to tumor burden, disease stage, and cell type is inconsistent, and no single theory satisfactorily explains the cachectic state. A variety of etiological factors can occur simultaneously or sequentially to produce cachexia (Fig. 31–1).

Several physiological derangements have been cited as possible explanations for the anorexia that attends malignant disease. Abnormalities in taste sensation, such as an increased threshold for sweetness and a reduced threshold for sour and salty flavors, have been demonstrated. Deficiencies of zinc and other trace minerals also contribute to alterations in taste sensation. Patients with hepatic metastases attended by some degree of hepatic insufficiency may develop anorexia and nausea as a result of difficulty in clearing lactate produced by anaerobic tumor metabolism of glucose. It has been suggested that undefined substances released by certain tumors on the feeding center in the hypothalamus reduce oral intake. Studies to elucidate the specific metabolic processes that affect nutrient intake in cancer patients have noted changes in serum norepinephrine[3] and plasma free tryptophan concentrations.[4] Results of parabiosis experiments performed by Lucke et al.[5] indicate the existence of a transferable humoral factor that produces abnormalities characteristic of the tumor-bearing state in the non–tumor-bearing rat. Theologides[6] proposed that tumor peptides acting through neuroendocrine cells and neuroreceptors alter metabolic pathways. Odell and Watson[7] showed that most cancer patients have increased plasma levels of substances that cross-react immunologically with a wide variety of hormones. Nakahara[8] described a "toxohormone" capable of mimicking abnormalities seen in cancer cachexia. Krause et al.[4] postulated that abnormalities in central nervous system serotonin metabolism may be responsible for the anorexia associated with cancer.

The local effects of the tumor are more readily explained than the systemic effects, particularly when the tumor arises from or impinges on the alimentary canal. Patients with cancer of the oral cavity, pharynx, and proximal esophagus have diminished intake because of odynophagia or dysphagia due to partial or complete obstruction. Esophagitis may develop in association with the malignant obstruction, or ulceration may occur. Patients with gastric cancers often have reduced gastric capacity with partial gastric outlet obstruction and suffer frequent bouts of nausea and vomiting. Intestinal malignancies may result in partial intestinal obstruction or blind-loop syndrome and inferfere with nutrient absorption. Intestinal fistulas may occur owing to the malignancy or after radiotherapy. Pancreatic carcinomas frequently lead to exocrine enzyme deficiencies, bile salt unavailability, and malabsorption syndromes.

ABNORMALITIES OF ENERGY REQUIREMENTS

The extent of malnutrition associated with cancer is often greater than that which can be explained solely on the basis of diminished intake. This observation has led several investigators to evaluate derangements of nutrient metabolism associated with the tumor-bearing state. Malignant disease also appears to affect resting metabolic rate and therefore energy requirements (Fig. 31–2). Using indirect calorimetry, Bozzetti et al. measured resting metabolic expenditure in 65 cancer patients and found it to be elevated in 60 per cent of these patients.[9] Elevated resting metabolic rates were noted despite weight loss and evidence of malnutrition in these patients. There was, in fact, a strong correlation between the increase in resting metabolic expenditure and the extent of weight loss in these patients. Warnold et

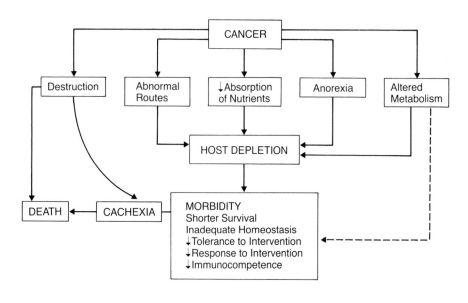

FIGURE 31–1. *Mechanisms by which cancer disturbs host homeostasis, leading to cachexia and death.*

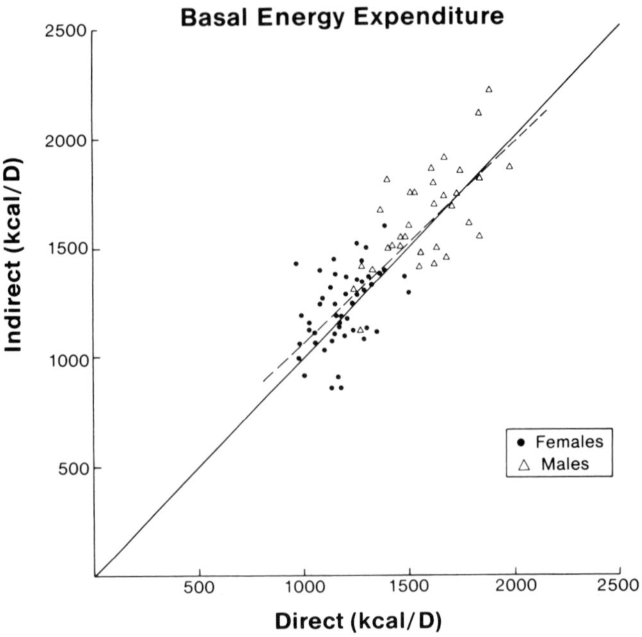

Basal Energy Expenditure

FIGURE 31–2. Comparison of basal heat release measured by direct calorimetry in 74 healthy subjects. (From Daly JM, Heymsfield SB, Head CA, et al. Am J Clin Nutr 1985; 42:1170–1174. © Am J Clin Nutr, American Society for Clinical Nutrition. Reproduced with permission.)

al. found that total energy expenditures and resting metabolic rates of cancer patients were significantly greater than those of controls.[10] Mean basal energy expenditure (BEE) was increased in a group of patients with small cell lung carcinoma studied by Shike et al.[11] Patients who responded to chemotherapy showed a significant decrease in mean BEE, while nonresponders exhibited no change in this variable. The findings obtained in these various studies of energy expenditure imply that cancer induces a hypermetabolic state that contributes to nutrient depletion. Results of other studies, however, fail to support this conclusion. In a review article, Young found that increased resting metabolism is not a consistent finding among cancer patients.[12] Nevertheless, it is apparent that the cancer patient's adaptation to starvation is abnormal.

Fuerer et al. noted that the Harris-Benedict equation accurately predicts energy expenditure in 80 per cent of healthy controls and 60 per cent of stable hospitalized patients when compared with resting energy expenditure actually measured by indirect calorimetry.[13] However, when 200 hospitalized cancer patients were evaluated, most patients fell out of the predicted range of energy expenditure, with 33 per cent being hypometabolic, 26 per cent hypermetabolic, and 41 per cent normometabolic (Fig. 31–3). The only parameter that correlated with abnormal metabolic rate was the duration of disease, with the hypermetabolic patients having a significantly longer duration of disease compared with normometabolic patients (33 vs. 13 months).[14] When a more uniform population of malnourished cancer patients, 173 patients with gastrointestinal cancers,

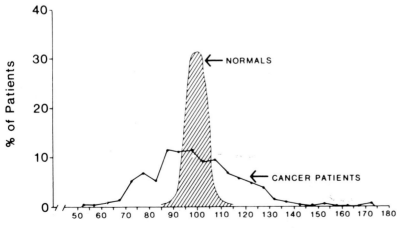

FIGURE 31–3. Distribution of measured resting energy expenditure in "normals" and in 200 cancer patients. (From Knox LS, Crosby LO, Feurer ID, et al. Ann Surg 1983; 197:152–162. Reproduced with permission.)

was studied, 36 per cent were hypometabolic, 22 per cent were hypermetabolic, and 42 per cent were normometabolic, with the degree of weight loss and tumor burden similar between groups. Within this population, Dempsey et al. noted that the primary tumor site was important.[15] Patients with pancreatic and hepatobiliary tumors were more frequently hypometabolic while patients with stomach cancer were more frequently hypermetabolic. These studies indicate the range of energy requirements that exists in cancer patients experiencing similar degrees of weight loss. These measurements, however, are all static single measurements and do not fully describe the dynamic, long-term situation.

ABNORMALITIES IN SUBSTRATE METABOLISM

In addition to abnormalities in energy measurements, a multitude of laboratory and clinical studies have noted metabolic derangements in tumor-bearing hosts[16] (Table 31–1).

Carbohydrates

Several tumor models in mice, rats, and rabbits have been evaluated using radiolabeled amino acids to determine their effect on serum glucose levels and rates of gluconeogenesis. Tumors uniformly produce decreased glucose tolerance and varying degrees of hypoglycemia. Animals with the most severe hypoglycemia were those that failed to increase the rate of gluconeogenesis in response to tumor growth.[17] Weight-losing, malnourished cancer pa-

tients have been found to have an increased rate of conversion of alanine to glucose, a decreased ability to oxidize exogenous glucose, and an increased rate of lactate production.[18] Studies using radiolabeled pyruvate to evaluate Cori cycle activity showed particularly high glucose recycling in 6 of 8 cancer patients. When ^{14}C-alanine and ^{14}C-glucose infusions were performed in seven patients with esophageal cancer and in seven non–cancer patients, this metabolic change was reconfirmed, but found to be reversible by infusion of TPN.[19]

Increased turnover rates of glucose and glycerol were found in 11 cancer patients based on infusions of ^{3}H-glucose and ^{14}C-glucose. This increase in glucose turnover may be related to the inappropriately high energy consumption seen in patients with cancer cachexia. Lundholm et al. concluded that high glucose turnover may account for over 40 per cent of the increased oxygen consumption seen in cancer cachexia.[20] Burt et al. evaluated peripheral tissue metabolism in 6 patients with esophageal cancer and 6 control patients by sampling arterial and deep venous blood from the forearm. Cancer patients had an increased uptake of glucose and an increased release of lactic acid compared with controls. They also had an increased release of amino acids from muscle with abnormal plasma aminograms distinct from well-nourished, non–cancer patients and patients with simple starvation. Decreased serum insulin and increased serum glucagon levels were also demonstrated.[21] Eight cancer patients and 7 control patients were evaluated with glucose flux determinations and indirect calorimetry in the basal and refed states. Cancer patients had a markedly increased rate of glucose recycling, with an elevated glucose flux that remained despite refeeding. Although the cancer patients did not demonstrate inhibition of endogenous production of glucose with refeeding, they had a similar improvement in nitrogen balance as the control patients. The increase in glucose flux accounted for 41 per cent of daily glucose intake, and would account for an 0.8 to 0.9 kg weight loss over 30 days.[22]

Fats

The presence of tumor-induced cachexia may occur in association with elevated serum triglyceride levels as well as decreased serum glucose and insulin concentrations. Hollander et al. found that tumor-bearing mice gained significantly less weight and had less body lipid with a small, slowly growing human melanoma than with a large, rapidly growing murine sarcoma.[23] Devereux et al. postulated that there is a tumor-associated lipid-mobilizing factor acting in the development of cancer cachexia.[24]

Whole-body lipolysis in patients can be estimated by measurements of glycerol turnover. Eden et al. studied cancer patients with and without weight loss

TABLE 31–1. Metabolic Comparison of Starved and Tumor-Bearing Humans

Parameter	Starved	Tumor-Bearing
Similar Responses		
Glucose tolerance	D	D
Whole-body glucose recycling	I	I
Gluconeogenesis from alanine	I	I
Total plasma amino acids	D	D
Different Responses		
Basal metabolic rate	D	I
Blood glucose	D	NC
Blood lactate	NC	I
Serum insulin	D	NC
Plasma glucagon	I	NC
Urinary nitrogen excretion	D	NC
Whole-body glucose turnover	D	I
Whole-body protein turnover	D	NC
Whole-body protein synthesis	D	NC
Whole-body protein catabolism	I	NC
O_2 consumption	D	NC
CO_2 production	D	NC
Respiratory quotient (RQ)	D	NC

D, significant decrease; I, significant increase; NC, no significant change.

Adapted from Brennan MF. N Engl J Med 1981; *305*:375–382.

and compared them with non–cancer patients with and without weight loss. Cancer patients with weight loss had elevated fasting plasma glycerol levels and glycerol turnover rates. Concomitantly, glycerol oxidation was 25 to 30 per cent of glycerol turnover in these patients, whereas in lean normal subjects after a short fast it is 60 per cent of glycerol turnover. In this study, the rate of glycerol turnover was related to the serum insulin level.[25]

Protein

Evaluation of tumor effects on protein metabolism has been performed in both animals and patients. Tyrosine flux was studied in the NEDH/C rat implanted with the RNC-254 fibrosarcoma. Pair-fed as well as ad lib–fed non–tumor-bearing animals were used as controls. Overall weight gain was similar in the tumor-bearing and non–tumor-bearing pair-fed animals, but the tumor grew proportionally more than the host, resulting in less gain in host weight. Significant increases in liver weight, whole-body tyrosine flux, and tyrosine incorporation into protein were noted when tumor weight reached 10 per cent of total body weight. In this advanced stage of tumor growth there was a significant increase in protein turnover without changes in amino acid oxidation or net whole-body protein catabolism. This metabolic response is different from injury and infection, where increases in protein turnover are associated with increased amino acid oxidation and increased net protein catabolism.[26]

In a study by Oram-Smith et al., tumor-bearing rats were given one of four intravenous feedings: (1) full TPN (D25W + 2.5 per cent AA); (2) amino acids only (2.5 per cent AA); (3) low calorie, no protein (D2.5W); and (4) only calories without protein (D25W). Animals with tumors had increased hepatic protein synthesis when on the low-protein or low-calorie diets, with no change in liver protein synthesis noted in tumor-bearing, fully nourished animals. Tumor protein synthesis was decreased only in the animals that received the no-protein, low-calorie diet.[27] Therefore, malnourished tumor-bearing animals demonstrated an increase in hepatic protein synthesis, possibly in response to a hormonal or chemical factor released by the tumor. These results have been substantiated by in vitro studies done on freshly isolated rat hepatocytes.[28]

Using isolated rat hepatocytes from tumor-bearing rats and non–tumor-bearing, pair-fed controls, the production of secretory and nonsecretory proteins has also been studied. An enhanced rate of protein synthesis was noted in the hepatocytes from the tumor-bearing animals which was proportional to the tumor burden, reaching statistical significance when the tumor was 5 per cent of the total body weight.[28] This increase in protein synthetic activity

due to the presence of malignancy exacts a high metabolic cost, estimated at 2.0 kcal/g, and may account for much of the increased energy expenditure and elevated metabolic rate seen in some cancer patients.

Lundholm et al. obtained biopsies of rectus abdominis muscle in 43 cancer patients and 55 matched control patients who were undergoing operation. They documented increased activity of several enzymes of muscle protein degradation and decreased activity of several enzymes of muscle protein synthesis in the cancer patients.[29] In particular, the activities of cathepsin-D and glucuronidase were increased and the activities of hexokinase, phosphofructokinase, lactate dehydrogenase, and cytochrome c oxidase were decreased. These investigators noted a decrease in incorporation of glucose into glycogen in the cancer patients. In the skeletal muscle, the activity of cathepsin-D correlated with the rate of protein degradation only in the cancer patients. These metabolic changes were reported to be unrelated to the degree of prior weight loss and current nutritional status, indicating that metabolic abnormalities may precede cancer cachexia.

Waterhouse noted that immunoglobulin production was maintained in cachectic tumor patients with normal or elevated serum IgG, IgM, and IgA levels and elevated or normal immunoglobulin synthetic and disappearance rates.[18]

Evaluation of body composition in cancer patients has been accurately performed using gamma neutron activation to measure total body nitrogen, a whole-body counter to measure total body potassium, and tritiated water to measure total body water. Twenty-nine male and 22 female cancer patients were evaluated as well as 10 normal patients of each sex. Patients were grouped into categories of tumor type—hematological, lung, gastrointestinal, and head and neck. Patients with solid tumors had a 5 to 25 per cent weight loss, but patients with hematologic malignancies had minimal weight loss. Cohn et al. found that patients with solid tumors had marked reduction in skeletal muscle tissue with conservation of visceral proteins. Loss of total body potassium was accounted for by the loss of skeletal muscle, although TBK was not a good predictor of total body nitrogen. The highest percentage of body fat that was lost was 50 per cent.[30]

Whole-body protein turnover was studied by Heber et al. in 12 patients with non–oat-cell lung cancer and the results compared with 6 age-matched, healthy controls.[31] Patients were studied under metabolic ward conditions and underwent ^{14}C-lysine infusion for protein turnover determination and ^{3}H-glucose infusion for assessment of glucose production. Urinary 3-methylhistidine and urinary cortisone were also measured. The data are summarized below:

	Control	Cancer
Protein turnover (g/kg/day)	2.12 ± 0.38	3.15 ± 0.51
Glucose production (mg/kg/min)	2.18 ± 0.06	2.84 ± 0.16
3-Methylhistidine (μmol/g Cr/day)	71 ± 8	106 ± 11
Urinary cortisone (mg/day)	47 ± 8	69 ± 9

Increased protein turnover rate correlated inversely with the percent ideal body weight, probably as a result of malnutrition in the cancer patients. Tumor protein turnover could not entirely account for the increased whole body protein turnover. Thus, Heber et al. questioned whether these abnormalities are localized to the region of the tumor or are more systemic in nature.[31]

Burt et al. studied protein turnover employing the ^{15}N-glycine tracer technique.[32] Patients with localized carcinoma of the distal esophagus were randomized to receive enteral or parenteral feeding. Patients were evaluated at the initiation of the study and after 2 weeks of feeding. Patients had similar baseline rates of whole-body protein turnover, synthesis, and catabolism which were greater than in normal fasting volunteers.[33] Feeding by jejunostomy reversed negative nitrogen balance and resulted in an increase in whole-body protein turnover. Similarly, TPN increased protein turnover and synthesis and decreased protein catabolism.[34]

These investigators found an optimal increase in serum insulin that resulted in maximal whole-body protein synthesis, which then exceeded that of catabolism. Thus, refeeding with increased protein turnover, synthesis, and catabolism appears to be related to the increase in endogenous insulin levels.

Endocrine Abnormalities

Insulin plays a key role in energy metabolism. An abnormality of insulin production is frequently found in cancer patients, with more extreme changes in cancer patients with weight loss and cachexia. Eden et al. demonstrated that changes in serum insulin concentration affect the rate of glycerol turnover.[25] When malnourished non–cancer patients are refed with an enteral diet they demonstrate an increase in serum insulin levels. This insulin response has been shown to be blunted in cancer patients.[22] Adrenal catecholamine production may be abnormal in cancer patients. In a study of glycerol turnover, urinary excretion of vanillylmandelic acid was higher in weight-losing cancer patients, although there was no significant difference in serum catecholamine levels.[25]

Thyroid hormone levels have been found to be decreased in some cancer patients, despite a normal or elevated basal metabolic rate. A decreased serum T_3 concentration was found to correlate with the degree of malnutrition, irrespective of the presence of cancer.[35] Administration of growth hormone may improve utilization of nutrients.[36]

Host immunological function is frequently depressed in cancer patients owing to histological type, stage of disease, age, radiation therapy, and malnutrition. In animal studies, in which factors can be controlled, delayed cutaneous hypersensitivity has been assessed. Tumor-bearing animals rendered PPD-negative by a protein-free diet became PPD-positive when fed with TPN or allowed to eat a regular diet. Although animals fed the regular diet continued to lose weight (−17 g vs. +14 g for TPN), many regained the ability to mount a positive PPD.[37]

Immune function was evaluated in dogs who underwent 21 days of protein-calorie malnutrition followed by refeeding with TPN. With malnutrition there was a decrease in serum levels of IgG, C3, and peripheral lymphocyte counts. Dionigi noted a decrease in lymphocyte blastogenesis to PHA and a decrease in neutrophil chemotaxis. TPN was able to restore humoral immunity, although the dogs retained measurable deficiencies of the cellular immune system. The serum IgG, IgM, C3, and neutrophil chemotaxis returned to normal or supranormal levels, but there was no improvement in lymphocyte count or T cell function assay.[38]

Additional metabolic changes associated with weight loss in cancer patients include changes in body composition, such as increased extracellular fluid and total body sodium and decreased intracellular fluid and total body potassium. This extracellular fluid expansion may obscure underlying nutritional deficits. Cohn et al. found that in patients who lost weight, total body potassium was diminished out of proportion to total body nitrogen.[30] On the basis of this finding, it appeared that the endogenous nutrient losses in these patients were primarily from the skeletal muscle component, since muscle accounts for only 45 per cent of total body nitrogen but 80 per cent of total body potassium. Significant losses of total body fat were also apparent among patients in this series. More studies using these direct methods of whole body analysis are needed to elucidate further the changes in body composition that occur in cancer patients.

Two conclusions can be drawn regarding the frequency of weight loss and malnutrition in cancer patients: (1) nutrient intake is decreased as a result of multiple factors; and (2) the tumor-bearing state alters the expected metabolic response to starvation with inhibition of the expected normal conservation of endogenous nutrient stores. The normal adaptation to starvation involves an overall reduction in total caloric expenditure for preservation of the visceral proteins essential to sustaining important body functions; to attain this end, there is increased reliance on fat rather than protein for energy production. In the cancer patient, not only is there remodeling of protein, but there is also continual catabolism of amino acids for glucose production and a failure to utilize available and more efficient oxidative pathways. The added stress of the tumor-bearing state accelerates erosion of both fat and lean body mass.

CONSEQUENCES OF MALNUTRITION

The sequelae of nutritional depletion in the cancer patient are severe. In a review of 500 autopsy reports for cancer patients, Warren found that cancer cachexia accounted for at least 22 per cent of cancer deaths.[39] He noted that this estimate was probably conservative, since cachexia was implicated as an ancillary contributor to the deaths of many other cancer patients. The protein-calorie deprivation that results from the cachectic state leads not only to obvious weight loss but also to compromise of the visceral and somatic protein compartments vital to enzymatic, structural, and mechanical function. Impairment of immunocompetence and increased susceptibility to infection frequently result. The effect on immune function is often exacerbated by debilitating courses of chemotherapy and radiation therapy. Moreover, poor wound healing, wound dehiscence, prolonged ileus, extended hospitalization, and increased morbidity and mortality following various surgical procedures have all been linked to poor nutritional status in cancer patients. Extensive nutrient depletion may also alter the course of necessary antineoplastic therapy, precluding the administration of proper drug and irradiation doses by diminishing the patient's toxicity threshold.

NUTRITIONAL ASSESSMENT

In surgical patients, malnutrition is associated with delayed wound healing, decreased resistance to infection, and other potential complications. Implementation of perioperative nutritional intervention results in reversal of markers associated with malnutrition, such as improvement in short half-life serum protein levels and reversal of skin test anergy. In turn, improvement in these markers by perioperative nutritional intervention is associated with reduced postoperative morbidity and mortality. Assessment of operative risk, therefore, requires qualitative and quantitatve methods of nutritional assessment. Nutritional assessment techniques correlate physiological and body compositional aberrations with useful clinical markers that are associated with malnutrition. Standard methods for assessing nutritional status include a history and physical examination, anthropometric measurements, laboratory determinations, and measurement of immune competence.

Nutritional assessment should be undertaken in all patients under consideration for nutritional support and should be used as a guideline to quantitate the degree of malnutrition.

History and Physical Examination

Nutritional deficits may be generalized or may involve only specific nutrients. Certain clinical entities are associated with generalized nutritional deficiencies. For example, alcoholism is associated with protein-calorie malnutrition, as well as deficits of various vitamins and minerals including niacin and zinc. Specific operative procedures may be implicated in individual vitamin and mineral deficiencies. Ileal resection or diversion may result in steatorrhea with deficiencies in fat-soluble vitamins and magnesium.

A complete dietary history may also give clues to underlying deficiencies, including a history of recent weight loss or the use of fad diets. The medical history should evaluate prior operations that may have resulted in nutritional deficits, such as folate deficiency as a result of a prior gastrectomy. Additionally, a history of chronic illness such as pancreatic insufficiency may indicate deficiencies of the fat-soluble vitamins. The social history may help explain underlying deficiencies by revealing poverty, alcoholism, and fad diets, which have all been implicated in malnutrition. Finally, a careful systems review should uncover symptoms associated with anorexia and weight loss. Nausea and vomiting, diarrhea, melena, abdominal pain, dysphagia, peripheral edema, and fever are often present in disease states that are associated with protein-calorie malnutrition.

A careful physical examination should identify which patients are malnourished. Overall patient appearance should be noted. Although most patients will not be obviously emaciated, pallor, edema, skin lesions, and muscle wasting are clinical indications of malnutrition. The integument often provides specific and general signs of nutritional deficiency states. Loss of hair is associated with protein deficiency. Loss of subcutaneous fat may be associated with calorie depletion. Iron deficiency may be the cause of spoon-shaped nails. Niacin deficiency (pellagra) may result in a symmetrical, hyperpigmented skin rash over body parts exposed to sunlight.

The oral cavity is commonly affected in malnutrition. The absence of teeth or the presence of caries may have contributed to the underlying deficiency. Glossitis is associated with vitamin B deficiency, and swollen, bleeding gums are associated with vitamin C deficiency.

Muscle wasting is the most recognizable sign of protein-calorie malnutrition, and it may be associated with peripheral edema. All muscle groups may be affected, although signs may be more obvious in the hypothenar muscles of the hand and the muscles of facial expression.

Anthropometric Measurements

Anthropometry is the science that deals with the measurement of the size, weight, and proportions of the human body. Body proportions or composition may be analytical methods to determine total body nitrogen, potassium, and water. For the most part, however, these methods are not clinically useful. More simplified methods of determining body composition have been used, and standardized anthropometric measurements have been compared with direct body composition analyses. These are helpful in determining nutritional status, particularly in groups rather than in individuals, and in serial determinations within a single patient.

The body may be divided into six compartments: fat, skin and skeleton, extracellular mass, plasma protein, viscera, and somatic protein mass (Fig. 31–4). Assessment of the various compartments is useful in quantifying the type and degree of deficits present. Assessing compartment losses is important not only for determining nutrient needs but also because each compartment serves various functions, which may be affected by individual deficits.

SOMATIC PROTEIN MASS

Anthropometric measurements of somatic protein mass (skeletal muscle) are body weight and mid upper arm muscle circumference.

Body weight should be measured upon hospital admission in all surgical patients and can be compared to ideal body weight, derived from the Metropolitan Life Insurance tables. However, a comparison of actual body weight to ideal body weight may have little clinical applicability owing to the wide range of weights for any given frame size. In addition, obesity is prevalent in our society, so that actual weight may be similar to ideal weight even though substantial recent weight loss may have occurred. More useful is the comparison of body weight to known recent weight. Insufficient caloric intake re-

sults in increased utilization of endogenous fat and protein stores for caloric needs, which results in weight loss. Extracellular sodium and water may be retained in protein-depleted patients, causing an underestimation of malnutrition when determined by body weight. However, loss of weight over a prolonged period (weeks) is usually specific for decreased energy intake in relation to energy needs.

The mid upper arm circumference is a simple anthropometric estimate of skeletal muscle mass. The mid upper arm is defined as the midpoint between the olecranon and the acromial process. The circumference of the arm muscle at this point calculated using the triceps skinfold thickness is compared with results in standard tables. Less than 60 per cent of standard is considered abnormal.

BODY FAT MASS

Depletion of body fat is an indicator of inadequate caloric intake relative to energy needs. Body fat is determined anthropometrically by measurement of skinfold thickness. This method is justified because subcutaneous fat accounts for approximately 50 per cent of total body fat. Various sites can be used for measurement of skinfold thickness, including thigh, calf, biceps, suprailiac, and chin. The summation of measurements taken at three or four different sites (Durnin's equation) may also be utilized. However, the most common method for assessing subcutaneous fat has been the use of triceps and subscapular skinfolds. Apart from the ease of measurements, the use of triceps and subscapular skinfolds tend to be more accurate than other skinfolds in edematous patients.

Laboratory Determinations

Estimation of somatic and visceral protein mass can be obtained by laboratory tests. Depletion of somatic mass can be determined by measurement of

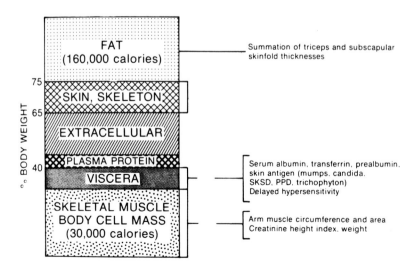

FIGURE 31–4. Normal adult body composition as relative percentages of body weight. Measurements for fat, viscera, and skeletal muscle body cell mass are listed.

24-hour urinary creatinine excretion in the presence of normal renal function. Creatinine is the breakdown product of creatine, a liver-synthesized energy molecule that is stored in skeletal muscle. By measurement of the 24-hour urinary creatinine excretion in the absence of renal impairment, one can indirectly assess skeletal muscle mass. Known 24-hour urinary creatinine levels for normal adults of similar sex and height can be compared with actual patient measurements. The ratio of the patient's 24-hour urinary creatinine excretion to normal values, expressed as a percentage, is called the creatinine-height index (CHI). A CHI of 100 per cent indicates normal lean body mass. Depletion of lean body mass should result in a CHI of less than 80 per cent. Nevertheless, this methodology suffers from the use of "ideal" values found in tables and from the difficulties encountered in obtaining an accurate 24-hour urine collection.

Visceral protein mass is estimated by measurement of plasma transport protein concentrations. The ideal measurable plasma protein should have a short half-life (high rate of synthesis and catabolism) with few factors altering catabolism. Current laboratory methods measure plasma levels of albumin, transferrin, prealbumin, and retinol-binding protein.

Serum albumin is not an ideal transport protein for estimation of visceral protein mass. Its metabolic half-life is approximately 20 days. Albumin is present to a great extent in the extravascular space, which affects its rate of catabolism. Albumin can be mobilized from this pool into the vascular space. Additionally, hydrational changes may affect serum concentrations. Thus, serum concentrations may not adequately assess visceral protein mass, particularly in the acute setting. Nevertheless, depressed serum albumin concentrations are associated with chronic visceral protein mass depletion when plasma levels fall below 3.0 g/100 ml.

Plasma transferrin concentration is a better estimate of visceral protein mass because it has a metabolic half-life of 8 days and has a smaller total body pool. Nevertheless, hepatic transferrin synthesis rates may be affected by different nutrient deficiencies including iron deficiency, which can mask underlying protein depletion.

Finally, short half-life proteins, such as prealbumin and retinol-binding protein, have been used for estimation of visceral protein mass. Prealbumin is involved in the transport of thyroid hormone. It has a metabolic half-life of 2 days. However, it is rapidly depressed in patients with traumatic injuries or sepsis who are not malnourished. Retinol-binding protein has a metabolic half-life of 12 hours. This serum protein is considered unreliable in patients with renal failure because it is cleared by the kidneys. Additionally, it is sensitive to other factors, including stress, which has limited its clinical use.

Immunocompetence

Anergy to skin-test antigens has been shown to be a predictor of septic complications. Although delayed cutaneous hypersensitivity is usually considered a test specifically for cell-mediated immunity, both cell-mediated and humoral immune responses are interrelated. Specifically, subsets of T lymphocytes, T helper and T suppressor cells, interact with B cells, allowing and controlling the ability of B cells to produce antibodies. Therefore, depression of T cell function as measured by anergy to skin-test antigens helps assess the ability of the patient to mount an immune response to injury and infection. Various skin test antigens used include mumps virus, tuberculin, and *Candida* sp. A positive response has a diameter of induration greater than 5 mm. A patient is considered anergic if induration fails to form to all skin-test antigens, although a graded system of immune responsiveness may be used.

The immune system may be depressed by patient age, trauma, inhalational anesthetic agents, drugs, malignancy, and oncological therapy, as well as malnutrition. Reversal of skin test anergy in malnourished patients has been demonstrated following nutritional repletion. This supports the belief that nutritional intervention is useful in immune-suppressed patients. Nevertheless, because of the complexity of the immune system, as well as the ability of various factors to alter the immune response, delayed hypersensitivity skin testing should be considered as complementary to other means of assessing nutritional status.

Accuracy of Nutritional Assessment

There is no complete agreement on the accuracy and usefulness of the various techniques used to determine nutritional status. This is due to the lack of one specific, accurate test to which the other techniques of nutritional assessment may be compared. The prognostic nutritional index (PNI) is an attempt to correlate various methods of nutritional assessment with the occurrence of postoperative morbidity and mortality through stepwise regression analyses.[40]

$$PNI\ (\%) = 158 - 16.6\ (ALB) - 0.78\ (TSF) - 0.20\ (TFN) - 5.8\ (DH)$$

where PNI is an estimate of the risk of a complication occurring in an individual patient, ALB is the serum albumin concentration (g/100 ml), TSF is the triceps skinfold thickness (mm), TFN is the serum transferrin concentration (mg/100 ml), and DH is delayed cutaneous hypersensitivity reactivity to any of three recall antigens (0, nonreactive; 1, 5 mm induration, 2, >5 mm induration). In a prospective study, the PNI was accurate in predicting which surgical patients were at a high risk for postoperative morbidity and mortality.[41] Application of perioperative nutritional support to patients considered to be at high risk significantly reduced postoperative morbidity and mortality.[42]

The history and findings from physical examination by trained observers have been prospectively compared with anthropometric data, laboratory data, delayed cutaneous hypersensitivity, and highly sophisticated direct body composition analysis as a method of nutritional assessment. Two clinicians trained in nutritional assessment techniques independently examined 59 patients and categorized them into one of three groups, those who were normal, those with mild malnutrition, and those with severe malnutrition. The two examiners agreed on the classification in 48 of the 59 patients (81 per cent). Furthermore, the clinical evaluation of nutritional status was then compared with the objective measurements. There was a significant correlation in all tests with the clinical status except for total lymphocyte count. The clinical status was also able to separate the patients into groups with significantly different mean values for six of the nine objective measurements. Finally, these investigators demonstrated that the morbidity of these patients correlated with the clinical nutritional status.[43] However, it should also be noted that objective evaluation of nutritional status also correlates with clinical outcome and allows a means of quantitating nutritional status changes with nutrient supplementation. These evaluations, however, should be considered as adjuncts to and not replacements for a thorough medical history-taking and a complete physical examination.

ENTERAL NUTRITION

Utilization of an intact gastrointestinal tract for nutritional support should be the initial step in alimentation. The use of large-bore tubes with bolus "home-style" feeding was used in past years but was not well accepted owing to significant patient discomfort that develops with prolonged use of this technique. Recent technical advances, however, have improved the quality of the equipment, the method of delivery, and the spectrum of available nutrient formulas.

Malnourished cancer patients with an intact gastrointestinal tract should initially be given enteral nutritional support. The specific disease processes affecting oral nutrition are diverse. In general, cancer patients who are unable to eat, unwilling to eat, unable to eat enough, or unwilling to eat enough should be considered for enteral nutritional support.

Patients with upper gastrointestinal or oral malignancies commonly develop problems resulting in an inability to eat. Many patients develop difficulty in chewing or swallowing because of their underlying disease process. Additionally, radiation therapy or chemotherapy treatment for various malignancies may result in stomatitis, mucositis, or nausea, which may affect oral intake. Finally, some patients may have a functional intestinal tract but may be unable to eat owing to proximal intestinal atrophy, obstruction, or fistula.

Cancer patients who require enteral nutritional supplementation may be supported through various routes of administration. These routes are oral, nasoenteric, and enteric (gastrostomy or jejunostomy). The selection of the route of administration should be based on the underlying indication for nutritional support. In general, cancer patients with only moderately insufficient oral intake may be given oral supplementation with aggressive dietary counseling. Patients with more severe deficiencies or higher nutrient needs commonly require tube feedings.

Use of silicone rubber or polyurethane small-bore feeding tubes has significantly reduced patient discomfort caused by older, large-bore, inflexible nasogastric tubes. Longer catheters with mercury-weighted ends may be used for nasoduodenal feedings. For patients who require long-term enteral support, surgically placed gastrostomy or jejunostomy catheters are more permanent routes for feedings. These feeding enterostomies have become a routine part of complicated surgical procedures by some surgeons for intestinal decompression and better nutritional support.

Gastric feedings are advantageous in some patients. Osmolality of the feeding formula is rarely a consideration with gastric feedings, because of the ability of the stomach to dilute hyperosmolar solutions. Additionally, bolus feedings may be utilized, reducing patient care time. However, gastric outlet obstruction, obtundation, and laryngeal incompetence are considered contraindications to gastric feeding because of the high incidence of aspiration.

Jejunal feedings require continuous pump infusions. Diarrhea is more commonly encountered with jejunal than with gastric feedings owing to the delivery of hyperosmolar feedings into the small intestine. The presence of hyperosmolar solutions in the intestine results in diffusion of water into the intestinal lumen. In order to reduce the incidence of diarrhea, jejunal feedings should be started with dilute solutions, with the concentration of feedings increased only after the patient is tolerating adequate volumes. If diarrhea persists, antiperistaltic agents may be added to the feeding formula or the delivery rate may be decreased.

Dietary Formulations

Currently available dietary formulations may be divided among blenderized formulas, nutritionally complete commercial formulas, chemically defined formulas, and modular formulas.

Blenderized tube feedings may be composed of any food that can be blenderized. These may be prepared at home or may be commercial preparations. Caloric distribution of these formulas should parallel a normal diet. Blenderized formulas are indicated most often for cancer patients with feeding gastrostomies who are unable to eat by mouth.

Nutritionally complete commercial formulas vary in protein, carbohydrate, and fat composition. Several are flavored and are considered suitable for oral supplementation. Several formulas utilize sucrose or glucose as carbohydrate sources and are suitable for lactose-deficient patients. Commercial formulas are convenient, sterile, and low in cost and are the most frequently used diets given to patients requiring tube feedings.

Chemically defined formulas are commonly called elemental diets. The nutrients are provided in a predigested and readily absorbed form. These diets are not often used in oral feedings, since the presence of amino acids in the formula markedly reduces its palatability. They are useful for patients with digestive disturbances, such as those with radiation enteritis or pancreatic insufficiency. However, they are more expensive than nutritionally complete commercial formulas and are hyperosmolar, which may cause cramping and diarrhea.

Modular formulations include special formulas used for specific nutrient needs or because of organ dysfunction. Single-nutrient formulas are used to modify other enteral formulas, tailoring them for specific needs. Patients with renal or hepatic failure may require specialized modular formulas that take into account underlying fluid and amino acid abnormalities.

Complications

Complications of enteral nutrition may be considered mechanical, gastrointestinal, or metabolic. Mechanical problems relate to the placement and care of tubes used for feedings. In general, placement of the tubes should be followed by radiological verification of proper intraluminal placement. Intraoperative placement of a jejunostomy can be verified by the instillation of saline into the catheter while compressing the jejunum immediately distal to the catheter. Placement of small-bore nasogastric tubes should always be verified radiologically prior to initiation of feedings, particularly in obtunded patients or patients with poor cough reflex. The presence of peritoneal irritative symptoms in patients being fed through a jejunostomy warrants further evaluation to ensure that dislodgement of the catheter has not resulted in the intraperitoneal delivery of feedings. Attachment of the stomach or small bowel to the anterior abdominal wall reduces the chance of accidental intraperitoneal catheter dislodgement.

Gastrointestinal side effects of enteral feedings are common. These inlude abdominal distention, diarrhea, and vomiting. Gastric feedings usually are better tolerated by bolus infusion. However, the presence of 200 ml or more residual volume may indicate gastric atony or distal obstruction. Feedings should be stopped in patients with this much residual volume. Proper monitoring of residual volume reduces the incidence of vomiting. Patients being fed intragastrically should be started on small amounts of full-strength formulas, with gradually increasing volumes as tolerated.

Patients are more likely to develop diarrhea when being fed through a jejunostomy than when other delivery routes are used. The presence of the hyperosmolar feeding in the proximal small intestine results in a passive diffusion of water into the lumen to render the intraluminal contents isotonic. If the infusion rate is too rapid for a given osmolality, diarrhea occurs. Therefore, patients with jejunostomies should be able to tolerate a sufficient volume of the infusate before the concentration is increased. If diarrhea occurs, either an antiperistaltic agent should be added to the infusate or else its rate of delivery decreased until symptoms abate. Finally, each patient should be matched to a defined formula. This would reduce the incidence of gastrointestinal side effects in patients with lactose intolerance caused by infusion of a lactose-based carbohydrate source. Additionally, patients not demonstrating a specific need for elemental diets could be fed by other nutritionally balanced commercial formulas, which may be less hyperosmolar and less expensive.

Metabolic complications can occur with enteral feedings. Glucose intolerance can result from the relative infusion of too much glucose. Patients on tube feedings, particularly those with constant infusions, should be monitored serially for blood and urine glucose levels. Diabetic patients may require exogenous insulin or a lower rate of nutrient delivery.

Hypertonic dehydration can result from the intraluminal loss of free water. Free water can be given to reduce the chance of this occurring. Infusion rates can also be reduced if the problem develops.

Tube feedings may be contraindicated in situations of severe gastrointestinal dysfunction, upper gastrointestinal bleeding, intractable vomiting, and diarrhea. Nasogastric feedings are contraindicated in obtunded patients.

PARENTERAL NUTRITION

The ability to provide complete intravenous feedings to patients in a clinically practical manner has been appreciated since the late 1960's. The application of total parenteral nutrition (TPN), as an adjunct or as primary therapy, to a variety of clinical situations has resulted in its general acceptance as a safe, clinically useful tool. Although relatively few major advances in the delivery techniques of TPN have been made since 1968, widespread application of TPN has resulted in a greater understanding of underlying physiological principles. In turn, this has allowed a standardization of methodology with a resultant decrease in complications associated with TPN.

Indications

The initial application of TPN was to provide supportive care in critically ill patients with severe nutritional deficiencies. More recent studies have demonstrated its usefulness not only in patients who were nutritionally depleted but also in those who required only maintenance of their nutritional state. The ability to improve clinical outcome through the judicious application of TPN has been demonstrated in several disease states. It has been difficult to demonstrate improved clinical outcome in patients with cancer undergoing chemotherapy by the addition of TPN, although cellular immunity and nutritional status may be improved. One difficulty in conducting these clinical trials in a randomized prospective fashion is the ethical dilemma of not feeding patients who are severely malnourished. Patients less severely depleted have a lower mortality with end points that are harder to measure. Therefore, the evidence for improved clinical outcome in these situations may continue to be indirect.

TPN should be initiated in cancer patients who are malnourished or, as a result of their medical care, are unable to maintain their current nutritional state and who cannot maintain an adequate enteral intake or do not have a functional gastrointestinal tract. TPN should be continued in patients whose clinical condition is improved by the application of this therapy.

Complications

Potential complications of TPN may be divided into technical, infectious, and metabolic complications.

Although subclavian vein catheterization is a widely used technique, it is not free of potential complications. These complications can be minimized by rigid adherence to the previously described techniques. If the catheter is placed by those who have done few catheterizations, adequate supervision can further reduce the incidence of complication. Arterial puncture during catheterization is indicated by the filling of the syringe with bright red blood. The needle should be withdrawn and firm pressure applied for several minutes. Pneumothorax is the most common potential technical complication. This may be suggested if air is aspirated into the syringe during insertion. The needle should be withdrawn and the patients observed for signs of respiratory distress. A chest radiograph should be obtained to rule out pneumothorax and to check the catheter position after all insertions. TPN should not be initiated until the chest roentgenogram is reviewed. This will reduce the incidence of hydrothorax. Catheter embolism is an iatrogenic complication that may occur when the catheter is withdrawn through the needle used for insertion, either for repositioning of the catheter or after a failed venipuncture. Joint withdrawal of the catheter and needle should eliminate this complication.[44]

Infectious complications associated with TPN are potentially serious. Contamination may occur owing to faulty techniques of catheter insertion or maintenance, infusion of contaminated solutions, or use of the subclavian catheter for other purposes such as infusion of medications. Cancer patients receiving TPN are predisposed to infectious complications because of the nature of the underlying disease, their nutritional state, and interference with host defense mechanisms as a result of treatment.

Management of cancer patients who become febrile while receiving TPN requires a methodical approach because of the potential seriousness of catheter sepsis. A diligent examination and fever work-up should be instituted to rule out other potential sources of the fever. Failure to demonstrate another cause requires removal of the nutrient solution and tubing. Cultures of the solutions, peripheral blood, and central venous blood should be taken. Positive cultures, cardiovascular instability, or persistent fever require replacement of the indwelling catheter. To avoid complications associated with catheter reinsertion, the catheter may be changed over a guide wire. The tip of the removed catheter should be cultured and broad-spectrum antibiotics initiated if blood cultures continue to remain positive.

Infusions of hypercaloric solutions may result in glucose intolerance. A normal adult can utilize 0.5 g of glucose per kilogram per hour. For a 70-kg man, this extrapolates to utilization of 3500 kcal/day.

The ability of patients to metabolize large glucose loads is directly related to their ability to mount an insulin response to the infused glucose. Studies conducted on the insulin response in nondiabetic patients receiving TPN have demonstrated several points:

1. Abrupt initiation of hypercaloric feedings results in insulin levels four to six times basal levels by 6 hours.

2. Continued infusion is associated with lowering of both the insulin and glucose levels.

3. The glucose tolerance test was normal during TPN, which demonstrates the ability of the normal pancreas to increase insulin production if faced with increasing glucose load.

4. Cessation of TPN does not usually result in rebound hypoglycemia.

Diabetic patients cannot mount an insulin response or have an inadequate hormonal response.

To avoid osmotic diuresis, TPN is maintained at a rate that results in blood glucose levels below 225 mg/dl and urinary glucose levels below 2 g/dl. Patients with diabetes mellitus or persistent glycosuria will require exogenous administration of crystalline insulin, which may be added to the nutrient solution in dosages up to 60 units per 1000 kcal to achieve a reduction in blood glucose concentration.

EFFECTS OF NUTRITIONAL SUPPLEMENTATION AND DEPRIVATION

Although the relationship between cancer, dietary intake, and the nutritional status of the patient is complex, there are three aspects to consider when evaluating the impact of nutritional support in the tumor-bearing host. The first is the effect on the host. This is measured in improvements in weight, protein levels, energy stores, organ and muscle function, and immune status, and can be evaluated in clinical and animal studies. The second is the effect on the tumor, measured by changing rates of tumor growth. This is best studied in animal models with well-characterized tumors. In these systems changes in rates of tumor growth may be more easily measured, and attributed to the dietary manipulation, as can the tumor incidence. The third is the effect on the response to and tolerance of antineoplastic therapy, which may be altered by changes in dietary therapy.

Host Nutritional Status and Substrate Metabolism

The rationale for providing increased amounts of amino acids in cancer patients is based on the finding that a tumor-associated stimulation of host liver gluconeogenesis from lactate and amino acid precursors occurs which provides much of the glucose metabolized by human and animal neoplasms. Malnourished cancer patients have twice the glucose turnover and four times the Cori cycle activity of similarly malnourished non–cancer patients. In 1975, Steiger et al. analyzed body weight, liver weight, and serum albumin levels in adenocarcinoma-bearing rats after 10 days of parenteral nutrition.[45] Tumor-bearing animals given parenteral amino acids alone, hypercaloric glucose alone, or hypocaloric glucose exhibited nitrogen wasting with markedly negative nitrogen balances.

In 1977, Oram-Smith et al. measured nitrogen balance in this same experimental system and demonstrated nitrogen equilibrium in animals receiving TPN.[27] In 1980 Buzby et al. demonstrated significant host weight gain and positive nitrogen balance over a 4-day period in animals given adequate amino acids and calories. Fat-based TPN was slightly more effective than carbohydrate-based TPN in promoting weight gain in this study.[46]

Daly et al.[37] and Ota et al.[47] demonstrated that increased body weight of hepatoma-bearing Buffalo rats occurred with either oral or parenteral nutrition. Provision of an isocaloric protein-free diet resulted in continued weight loss. Daly et al. subsequently demonstrated that oral protein repletion of malnourished Sprague-Dawley rats with Walker-256 carcinosarcoma accelerated both tumor and host growth within 48 hours.[48] In animals with small tumor burdens (less than 5 per cent of carcass weight), oral nutritional repletion resulted in a return to normal of serum albumin concentration, liver and muscle protein content, and carcass weight within 6 days of initiating nutritional repletion (Figs. 31–5 and 31–6). In malnourished animals with large tumors (greater than 25 per cent of carcass weight), serum albumin concentration returned to normal, but liver and muscle protein content and carcass weight remained significantly lower after oral repletion com-

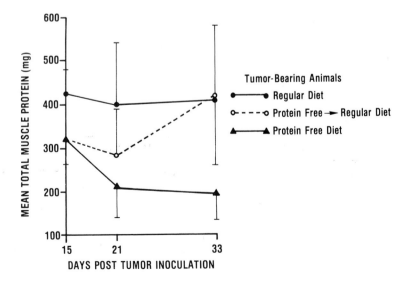

FIGURE 31–5. Nutritional repletion of tumor-bearing rats resulted in an increase in total muscle protein with a return to the levels in rats fed regular diets by day 33. (Adapted from Daly JM, Copeland EM, Dudrick SJ, et al. J Surg Res 1980; 28:507–518.)

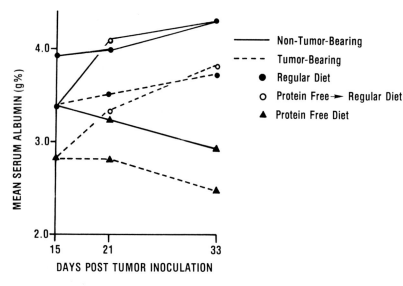

FIGURE 31–6. Nutritional repletion of tumor-bearing and non–tumor-bearing rats resulted in a rapid increase in mean serum albumin concentration to the levels in rats fed regular diets by day 21. (From Daly JM, Copeland EM, Dudrick SJ, et al. J Surg Res 1980; 28:507–518. Reproduced with permission.)

pared with those measurements in well-nourished tumor-bearing animals.

In 1977, Cameron et al. demonstrated that TPN could prevent weight loss characteristically seen in hepatoma-bearing rats given ad libitum oral feeding.[49] However, no significant change in duration of survival was observed in animals receiving TPN and, in fact, tumor growth was stimulated out of proportion to increases in host weight gain. In 1983, Popp et al. found similar results in sarcoma-bearing Fischer-344 rats given TPN (Fig. 31–7).[50] Although carcass weight increased with TPN administration, mean tumor weight increased to a greater extent than lean carcass weight with increased levels of substrate infusion.

Immunocompetence

Both humoral and cellular immunity are depressed in animals with severe protein restriction. Law et al. in 1974 demonstrated decreased titers of antibodies, decreased number of IGM-producing cells, decreased in vitro lymphocyte response to mitogens, and decreased delayed hypersensitivity in Sprague-Dawley rats after 6 weeks of protein-free nutrition.[51] Protein repletion 48 hours before antigen stimulation was necessary for full expression of the immune response.

In 1978, Daly et al. demonstrated that only 30 per cent of Buffalo rats bearing Morris hepatoma demonstrated a positive delayed hypersensitivity response to intradermal PPD after 2 weeks on an oral protein-free diet.[37] Protein repletion with 7 days of TPN or oral ad libitum feeding restored PPD-immunocompetence to 91 and 78 per cent of animals, respectively. Only 17 per cent of animals remaining on protein-free diets for the 7-day period demonstrated PPD skin test reactivity. Body weight significantly increased in animals receiving protein repletion; continued loss of weight occurred in animals given the protein-free diet. Thus, restoration of immunocompetence and body weight was observed in malnourished tumor-bearing animals receiving adequate protein and calories.

FIGURE 31–7. Tumor weight changes during intravenous nutritional support ranging from 33 to 167 per cent of normal rat caloric intake. AAD. oral amino acid diet. (From Popp MB, Wagner SC, Brito OJ. Host and tumor responses to increasing levels of intravenous nutritional support. Surgery 1983; 94:300–308. Reproduced with permission.)

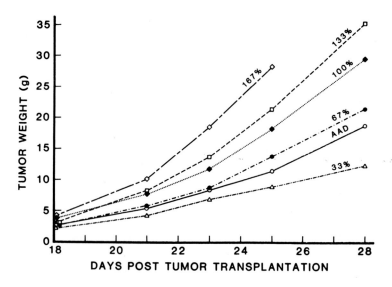

A prospective randomized controlled study that was done to evaluate the role of preoperative TPN on postoperative morbidity and mortality in gastrointestinal cancer patients also evaluated several immunologic parameters. The TPN treated patients developed significant increases in prealbumin, retinol-binding protein, transferrin, C4, C3A, IgA, IgM, and IgG preoperatively. They also had statistically fewer major complications (19/59 vs. 11/66) and less mortality (11/59 vs. 3/66) than the control patients.[52]

Tumorigenesis, Tumor Growth, and Nutritional Support

Numerous studies have shown that protein-calorie deprivation results in a reduced incidence of spontaneous tumorigenesis and a decreased rate of establishment of transplanted tumors. Tannenbaum and Silverstone in 1953 reported that protein and calorie restriction significantly inhibited spontaneous tumorigenesis in many tumor systems in the mouse and rat.[53] Refeeding significantly stimulated both spontaneous tumorigenesis and tumor development in transplantable tumor models. In 1950 Green et al. documented delayed establishment of transplanted Walker-256 carcinosarcoma in protein-depleted rats.[54] In 1971 Ross et al. demonstrated a reduced incidence of spontaneous benign and malignant tumors with underfeeding in rats.[55] In this study, a pattern of tumorigenesis was established early in life and remained stable with subsequent nutritional changes.

Carcinogen-induced tumors are also influenced by provision of nutrients. White in 1961 reported that protein-calorie deprivation significantly reduced the incidence of numerous carcinogen-induced malignancies in rats and mice.[56] In 1973, Moore et al. confirmed this finding in DMBA-induced breast tumors in Sprague-Dawley rats.[57] Thus, protein-calorie deprivation in animal/tumor systems is associated with a decreased incidence of spontaneous and carcinogen-induced tumors and inhibition of tumor establishment with transplantable tumors.

Once tumor establishment occurs, subsequent tumor growth is significantly influenced by nutrition. Tumor volume, tumor weight, cellular mitotic activity, synthesis of DNA, RNA, and protein, and cell cycle changes have been used as parameters of tumor growth. Several investigators have documented accelerated tumor growth in rat and mouse models with ad libitum oral feeding of protein and carbohydrate diets. In 1978, Daly et al. demonstrated significant stimulation of the Walker-256 carcinosarcoma in Sprague-Dawley rats within 48 hours of initiating oral nutritional repletion in previously malnourished animals.[37] A similar rate of increase in tumor volume was demonstrated in the Morris hepatoma of orally repleted Buffalo rats. Stimula-

tion of tumor growth was not selective, however, as evidenced by a constant ratio of tumor weight to host weight in nutritionally depleted and repleted animals. Starvation, combined reduction of protein and calories, and oral feeding of protein-free diets have resulted in decreased tumor growth in several tumor systems including the Walker-256 carcinosarcoma, mammary adenocarcinoma, and rat sarcoma.

Accelerated tumor growth has been noted with provision of parenteral nutrition. In 1975, Steiger et al. demonstrated increased growth of the AC-33 mammary adenocarcinoma in Lewis/Wistar rats with TPN.[45] Parenteral amino acids with or without hypertonic dextrose were responsible for tumor stimulation in this system. Although no change in the ratio of tumor weight to body weight was observed, stimulation of tumor protein synthesis and a significant increase in the percentage of tumor cells synthesizing DNA occurred with the provision of TPN. In 1976, Cameron and Pavlat demonstrated increased growth and a higher index of mitotic activity in the Morris hepatoma of Buffalo rats receiving intravenous nutrition.[58] In 1981, Cameron observed increased ^{3}H-thymidine uptake in tumor cells of animals receiving total parenteral nutrition (TPN).[59] In their study preferential growth of the Morris hepatoma occurred with parenteral nutrition as evidenced by a significant increase in the ratio of tumor weight to host body weight. In 1983, Popp et al. reported similar results in methylcholanthrene-induced sarcomas in Fischer-344 rats.[50] Tumor growth occurred to a greater extent than growth of the host lean body mass with excessive TPN administration. A direct correlation was observed between tumor weight and the rate of nutrient substrate infusion in this study.

Isolated studies have reported no significant stimulation of tumor growth with parenteral nutrition. In 1982, Kishi concluded that 7 days of TPN did not accelerate growth of the Walker-256 carcinosarcoma in Wistar rats.[60] However, a greater than twofold increase in tumor weight occurred in animals receiving TPN compared with animals given D5W in their study. Although a level of statistical significance (p <0.05) was not achieved, a small number of animals were studied and a definite trend toward increased tumor growth occurred in animals given TPN. In 1985, King et al. studied changes in tumor weight, protein content, and ^{3}H-thymidine uptake in comparison with oral feeding.[61] However, protein intake was 25 per cent greater in animals receiving oral diets. Relative to fasting animals and groups of rats receiving oral nutrition, TPN with glucose and TPN with fat resulted in a significant increase in tumor weight. Thus, the majority of experimental evidence demonstrates that nutritional repletion of malnourished rats and excessive nutrient administration stimulates growth of animal tumors.

In an attempt to retard tumor growth selectively, several investigators have induced specific dietary deficiencies in tumor-bearing animals. In 1959 Munro and Clark measured the RNA content in hepatoma and host liver in rats fed a 25 per cent protein diet compared with animals fed an isocaloric, protein-free diet.[62] Although no change occurred in RNA content of tumor tissue, a decrease in RNA content of host liver was observed in rats ingesting the protein-free diet. In 1977, Ota et al. measured protein content and found similar results in Buffalo rats with Morris hepatomas.[47] In animals given protein-free diets, tumor protein content remained unchanged while liver protein content decreased. In 1980, Daly et al. similarly demonstrated no change in protein content of Walker-256 carcinosarcoma in Sprague-Dawley rats given protein-free diets.[63] The tumor was able to effectively incorporate protein at the expense of host tissue during periods of dietary protein restriction. In 1977, Reilly et al. demonstrated decreased growth of MCA-induced sarcomas in rats during starvation;[64] however, DNA specific activity increased in the tumor and decreased in host liver. These studies confirmed the concept of the tumor as a "nitrogen trap" and documented that tumors are successful competitors with host tissues for nutrient substrates during periods of limited dietary supply.

Deficiencies of selective amino acids have resulted in continued tumor growth and host nutritional depletion. Studies performed in rats, mice, and hamsters with essential amino acid deprivation demonstrates minimal tumor inhibition. In fact, accelerated tumor growth has been observed with moderate leucine restriction in adenocarcinoma-bearing mice and with exclusive administration of branched-chain amino acids in AC-33 adenocarcinoma of rats.

Two studies have documented selective tumor inhibition with diets deficient in specific amino acids. In 1973 Jose and Good fed tumor-bearing mice casein-restricted diets to reduce plasma levels of cysteine, methionine, and tryptophan.[65] A reduction in the ratio of tumor weight to host body weight occurred and was associated with a reduction in serum blocking antibody. The authors hypothesized that tumor inhibition in mice given casein-restricted diets occurred by decreasing titers of serum blocking antibody without altering cell-mediated immunity. In 1971, Theuer demonstrated preferential reduction in the growth rate of BW20232 adenocarcinoma of C57BL mice fed diets deficient in phenylalanine, valine, or isoleucine.[66] A proportional reduction in tumor and host weight occurred using oral diets deficient in tryptophan, threonine, leucine, or methionine.

Selective starvation of tumor cells with maintenance of normal host cells has been attempted by inducing specific deficiencies of micronutrients, including vitamins, trace metals, and electrolytes. In a rat model, folate deficiency impaired growth of the Walker-256 carcinosarcoma but did not alter growth of the Murphy-Strum lymphosarcoma.[67] Regardless of its effects on tumor growth, prolonged folate deprivation causes significant toxicity. Pantothenic acid deficiency caused fibrosarcoma growth retardation in rats; however, host growth was impaired to a similar degree.[68] Decreased riboflavin availability has been induced by administering riboflavin analogues such as lyxoflavin and galactoflavin. Tumor regression occurred after administration of these riboflavin analogues; however, host effects were not documented.[69]

Pyridoxine-deficient diets and pyridoxine inhibitors have independently been shown to cause tumor regression in several rat and mouse models. Vitamin A and its derivatives are effective inhibitors of chemical carcinogenesis in multiple epithelial systems including mammary gland and urinary bladder. Animals fed diets deficient in retinoids (vitamin A and its natural and synthetic analogues) develop an increased number of malignancies following exposure to chemical carcinogens.[70] The effect of vitamin C on cancer development is controversial, but several studies indicate that vitamin C decreases the incidence of squamous cell carcinoma in mice exposed to ultraviolet radiation.[71] Vitamin K antagonists or dietary deficiency of vitamin K significantly reduced the number of spontaneous metastases in mice with Lewis lung carcinoma.[72]

Trace metal deficiencies, particularly of zinc and magnesium, influence tumor growth under experimental conditions. DeWys and Pories in 1972 demonstrated significant reduction of tumor establishment in zinc-deficient animals transplanted with either Walker-256 sarcoma or Lewis lung carcinoma.[73] The duration of survival of zinc-deficient animals was significantly greater than the length of survival in pair-fed control animals. Zinc-deficient animals with L1210 leukemia similarly demonstrated increased duration of survival compared with control animals. The toxicity of prolonged zinc deficiency, however, precludes dietary deprivation of this trace metal for extended periods. Young and Parsons reported 40 per cent reduction in growth of the Yoshida hepatoma and Walker sarcoma in magnesium-deficient rats.[74] Similar results were observed by Mills et al. in 1983 in transplanted mammary adenocarcinoma in rats.[75]

Potassium deficiency has been shown to effectively inhibit tumor growth in tumor-bearing animals. Isolated potassium deficiency decreased growth of the Yoshida hepatoma and Walker-256 carcinosarcoma in rats by 30 to 60 per cent. With combined deficiencies of potassium and magnesium, tumor growth was reduced by 45 to 85 per cent. Ryan et al. demonstrated similar growth inhibition of ascitic tumor cells in vivo with potassium depletion.[76]

Surgery and Nutritional Support

Many cancer patients are malnourished, with the reported incidence of greater than 10 per cent weight loss varying from 10 to 50 per cent.[1, 77, 78] These patients are at increased risk of postoperative complications and mortality. Several prospective randomized trials have been undertaken to evaluate the role of TPN in abrogating this in the preoperative cancer patient. Interpretation of these studies is hindered by the small number of patients evaluated, and the amount and duration of TPN. A review by Brennan[79] lists 10 such clinical trials, with only the series by Muller et al. involving more than 100 patients.[52, 80]

The first study to show a statistical decrease in operative complications was by Heatley et al.,[81] where the incidence of wound infections was decreased from 11 of 36 in controls to 3 of 39 in preoperative TPN-treated patients.

Muller et al. randomized cancer patients to three treatment groups. Approximately 60 per cent of patients had some degree of malnutrition. Sixty-six patients received 10 days of preoperative TPN consisting of 1.5 g of amino acid/kg and 45 kcal/kg body weight/day given as 11 g glucose/kg. Fifty-nine control patients received a 2400-kcal regular diet. A third group of 46 patients received TPN with one half of their nonprotein calories given in the form of a lipid emulsion. The TPN significantly (p <0.05) reduced the incidence of complications (19/59 vs. 11/66) and mortality (11/59 vs. 3/66).[52]

The arm of the study involving TPN with lipid was prematurely terminated owing to higher complication (17/46) and mortality (10/46) rates in these patients, although these are similar to the control group. The investigators suggested that the high fat content led to decreased macrophage and granulocytic function.

When they looked at specific subgroups of patients, they found the greatest reduction in complication risk to occur in patients with carcinoma of the upper gastrointestinal tract.

A nonrandomized study that evaluated perioperative TPN in patients undergoing resections for esophageal carcinoma showed improved survival and decreased postoperative complications with TPN (Fig. 31–8).[82]

Chemotherapy and Nutritional Support

Few well-controlled animal studies have been performed to objectively determine the influence of nutritional status on host toxicity from chemotherapy. Steiger et al. administered 5-fluorouracil to Lewis-Wistar rats receiving either TPN or parenteral 5 per cent dextrose.[45] In animals receiving TPN, positive nitrogen balance and significant weight gain occurred despite chemotherapy administration. In 5-fluorouracil–treated animals given 5 per cent dextrose, nitrogen balance was negative and weight loss occurred. However, TPN did not prevent the myelosuppressive activity of the 5-fluorouracil, as both

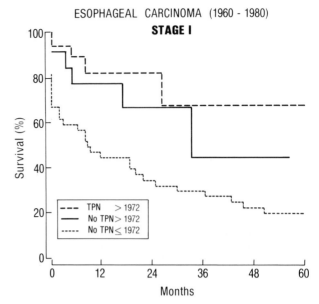

FIGURE 31–8. Five-year survival curves for patients with Stage I esophageal cancer show a significant improvement in survival with total parenteral nutrition over concurrent patients not receiving TPN and over patients treated from 1960 to 1972. (Adapted from Daly JM, Massar E, Giacco G, et al. Ann Surg 1982; 196:203–208.)

groups of animals demonstrated an identical degree of peripheral leukopenia. In 1975, Souchen et al. demonstrated a lower incidence of gastrointestinal toxicity to 5-fluorouracil and a twofold increase in mean survival rate in animals receiving TPN compared with rats receiving an oral diet.[83]

In 1982, Torosian et al. demonstrated a significant reduction in methotrexate toxicity with improved nutritional status in Lewis-Wistar rats with AC-33 adenocarcinoma.[84] Clinical signs of toxicity including hair loss, lethargy, diarrhea, and leukopenia were reduced in well-nourished animals compared with protein-depleted animals. At high doses of methotrexate (20 mg/kg), 100 per cent mortality occurred in malnourished animals versus no mortality in the well-nourished group. In 1984, Mihranian et al. documented decreased plasma clearance and increased serum levels of methotrexate in malnourished animals, accounting for increased drug toxicity.[85] Grossie et al. suggest that increased methotrexate toxicity in malnourished rats was related to reduced liver and bone marrow levels of dihydrofolate reductase, the major enzyme inhibited by methotrexate.[86]

Tumor Response to Chemotherapy

Although stimulation of tumor growth by nutrient administration has been generally regarded as detrimental to the host, laboratory studies have demonstrated that these changes in tumor metabolism may be exploited to therapeutic advantage. In 1981,

Daly et al. reported improved tumor response to chemotherapy in rats provided with continuous parenteral or intrajejunal feeding.[87] It was postulated that continuous substrate administration stimulated tumor cell proliferation and significantly improved tumor response to chemotherapy. Reynolds et al. demonstrated similar results with oral nutritional repletion of Sprague-Dawley rats with Walker-256 carcinosarcoma treated with methotrexate.[88] In 1983, Torosian et al. demonstrated improved tumor response to chemotherapy in AC-33–bearing Lewis-Wistar rats receiving 48 hours of parenteral nutrition.[89] After only 2 hours of TPN, a significant increase in the percentage of S-phase tumor cells, or DNA-synthesizing cells, was demonstrated. Improved antineoplastic activity was observed with cycle-specific agents (methotrexate, Adriamycin) but not with cycle-nonspecific chemotherapy (Cytoxan). This phenomenon occurred independent of host nutritional status and was primarily due to the amino acid moiety in TPN. Selective potentiation of tumor cytotoxicity appeared to occur, as no increase in host toxicity was demonstrated.

Several randomized and nonrandomized clinical trials have been conducted to evaluate TPN as an adjunct to chemotherapy.[90] These studies have demonstrated an improvement in host nutritional status with nutritional support but no improvement in treatment outcome (Table 31–2).

Nixon et al. evaluated the effect of TPN on toxicity of chemotherapy, response to therapy, and overall survival in patients with metastatic large bowel cancer.[101] They stratified 50 patients as to degree of weight loss (0 to 6 per cent, 6 to 12 per cent, 12 to 24 per cent), and randomized patients to receive TPN or their usual oral diets. Patients had metastatic cancer to multiple sites with a slightly higher incidence of liver metastasis in the TPN group. Because of the small number of patients, they were unable to evaluate the effect of TPN on clinical complications or response to chemotherapy. They found no difference in survival between TPN and control patients with 12 to 24 per cent weight loss. There was a trend toward decreased survival with TPN in patients with less weight loss, and in the stratum of 0 to 6 per cent weight loss, the TPN patients had a statistically significant shorter lifespan (66 vs. 398 days, $p = 0.02$), although this group contained only 18 patients.

Forty-two patients with advanced diffuse lymphoma were randomized to receive TPN or oral feeding during aggressive chemotherapy. No impact was noted on overall survival or response to chemotherapy. Nitrogen balance was not monitored, but based on measurements of serum proteins, triceps skinfold thickness, and arm circumference, the patients appeared to maintain their nutritional status with oral intake alone. The major morbidity noted from the TPN was an 11 per cent incidence of symptomatic subclavian vein thrombosis.[97]

A randomized, prospective study of 30 patients with Stage III testicular cancer comparing TPN with D5W infusion during administration of chemotherapy showed no difference in patient morbidity or response rates. There was a measurable improvement in weight loss during the chemotherapy in the patients treated with TPN.

These studies are by no means conclusive, but they do suggest that: (1) cancer patients tolerate TPN with an acceptable complication rate; (2) TPN does not appear to stimulate human tumor growth in humans; (3) nutritional morbidity in cancer patients undergoing chemotherapy is a consequence of progression of the disease and aggressive therapy; and (4) TPN does not improve tumor response to therapy.

Radiotherapy and Nutritional Support

As an intensive form of local antineoplastic therapy, toxic effects of radiotherapy are localized to the tissue adjacent to the tumor bed.

Radiotherapy perhaps has the greatest impact on host nutrition when used to treat head and neck malignancies. Here the side effects of radiotherapy

TABLE 31–2. Effect of TPN As an Adjunct to Chemotherapy

Investigators	Tumor	Response Difference	Randomized	Malnourished
Copeland et al.[91]	Mixed	+	No	Yes
Souchon et al.[83]	Colon	+	No	Yes
Lanzotti et al.[92]	Lung: non–oat-cell	+	No	Yes
Issell et al.[93]	Lung: non–oat-cell	+	Yes	Yes
Jordan et al.[94]	Lung: non–oat-cell	+/−	No	No
Valdivieso et al.[95]	Lung: oat-cell	+/−	Yes	Yes/no
Clamon et al.[96]	Lung: oat-cell	−	Yes	No
Popp et al.[97]	Lymphoma	−	Yes	No
Levine et al.[98]	Lymphoma	−	Yes	No
Shamberger et al.[99]	Sarcoma	−	Yes	No
Samuels et al.[100]	Testicular	−	Yes	No
Nixon et al.[101]	Colon	−	Yes	Yes

+, difference in response to TPN vs. CTRL; −, no difference in response.
Adapted from Copeland EM. JPEN 1986; 10:337–342.

affect both the patient's ability to eat and his or her subjective enjoyment of eating by reducing taste and smell. The side effects are worse in the first months after treatment, with xerostomia, mucositis, taste changes, and sialitis developing in a dose-related fashion. Changes in taste may be particularly unpleasant to the patient, with the greatest loss of bitter and acid tastes. These changes may take from a few months to a year to return to normal.

A review of 122 patients with squamous cell carcinomas of the oral cavity, oropharynx, and hypopharynx evaluated the degree of weight loss during radiotherapy. The average weight loss was 8.2 lb, with over 90 per cent of patients losing weight.[102] No attention was given to nutritional support in these patients. In a prospective randomized trial evaluating tube versus oral feeding, head and neck cancer patients were able to adjust their tube feedings to meet their nutritional requirements during treatment with radiation therapy.[78] Those patients who had irradiation to the oral cavity had significantly less weight loss during therapy with tube feedings than with oral feedings alone (0.7 vs. 7.8 per cent).

Radiation to the thorax as well as the head and neck may lead to esophagitis, with the potential for fistula or stricture formation.

Radiation to the upper abdomen may reduce gastric acidity or lead to gastritis and ulcer formation. Patients with these side effects may have nausea, vomiting, or diarrhea. Radiation enteritis may develop throughout the small or large bowel resulting in dilated, thickened bowel with decreased absorptive capacity. Deficiencies in fat,[103] protein,[104] glucose, and electrolyte absorption have also been reported.

SUMMARY

Cancer patients may develop anorexia and diminished nutrient intake as a result of their disease. Specific derangements in substrate metabolism and energy utilization have been demonstrated in cancer patients and animal tumor models. These patients had measurable changes in body composition, with erosion of body protein and fat stores followed by significant weight loss. Further studies are currently under way to elucidate changes in the hormonal milieu, neurotransmitter release, or specific polypeptide production that may also occur in cancer patients. These systemic alterations vary with the type of tumor, the extent of the tumor burden, and the duration of disease.

Clinically, cancer patients are frequently malnourished at the time of diagnosis, or develop progressive malnutrition during the course of their disease. This cancer-related malnutrition has a negative prognostic value, and may interfere with administration of maximal antitumor therapy.

The use of nutritional support in the cancer patient, whether by the enteral or parenteral route, can improve the nutritional status of the cancer patient, and may increase the tolerance for surgery, chemotherapy, or radiotherapy. Perioperatve nutritional support may impact on survival, with the greatest improvement apparent in patients with gastrointestinal malignancies. Nutritional support may also decrease the risk of complications in patients who would otherwise be at increased risk secondary to malnutrition.

Our current body of knowledge of protein, fat, and carbohydrate metabolism in the cancer patient, and of the impact of nutritional support, is rapidly expanding. Future research directed at applying this information by manipulating substrate supply and utilization may lead to significant benefits for the cancer patient.

References

1. DeWys WD, Begg C, Lavin PT, et al. Prognostic effect of weight loss prior to chemotherapy in cancer patients. Am J Med 1980; 60:491–497.
2. Nixon DW, Heymsfield SB, Cohen AE, et al. Protein calorie undernutrition in hospitalized cancer patients. Am J Med 1980; 68:683–690.
3. Nichols MB, Maickel RP, Yim CKW. Brain catecholamine alterations accompanying development of anorexia in rats bearing the Walker-256 carcinoma. Life Sci 1985; 36:2223–2231.
4. Krause R, Humphrey C, Meyenfeldt M, et al. A central mechanism for anorexia in cancer: a hypothesis. Cancer Treat Rep 1981; 65(Suppl 5):15–21.
5. Lucke B, Berwick M, Zeckwer I. Liver catalase activity in parabiotic rats with one partner tumor bearing. J Natl Cancer Inst 1952; 13:681–686.
6. Theologides A. Cancer cachexia. Cancer 1979; 43:2004–2012.
7. Odell WD, Watson AR. Hormones from tumors: are they ubiquitous? Am J Med 1980; 68:317–318.
8. Nakahara W. A chemical basis for tumor host relations. J Natl Cancer Inst 1960; 24:77–86.
9. Bozzetti F, Pagnoni AM, DelVecchio M. Excessive caloric expenditure as a cause of malnutrition in patients with cancer. Surg Gynecol Obstet 1980; 150:229–234.
10. Warnold I, Lundholm K. Schersten T. Energy balance and body composition in cancer patents. Cancer Res 1978; 38:1801–1807.
11. Shike M, Russel DM, Detsky AS, et al. Changes in body composition in patients with small cell lung cancer. The effect of total parenteral nutrition as an adjunct to chemotherapy. Ann Intern Med 1984; 101:303–309.
12. Young VR: Energy metabolism and requirements in the cancer patient. Cancer Res 1977; 37:2336–2347.
13. Feurer ID, Crosby CO, Mullen JL. Measured and predicted resting energy expenditure in clinically stable patients. Clin Nutr 1984; 3:27–34.
14. Knox LS, Crosby LO, Feurer ID, et al. Energy expenditure in malnourished cancer patients. Ann Surg 1983; 197:152–162.
15. Dempsey DT, Mullen JL. Macronutrient requirements in the malnourished cancer patient. Cancer 1985; 55:290–294.
16. Brennan MF. Total parenteral nutrition in the cancer patient. N Engl J Med 1981; 305:375–382.
17. Shapot VS, Blinov VA. Blood glucose levels and gluconeo-

genesis in animals bearing transplantable tumors. Cancer Res 1974; *34*:1827–1832.

18. Waterhouse C. How tumors affect host metabolism. Ann NY Acad Sci 1974; *230*:86–93.

19. Waterhouse C, Jeanpretre N, Keilson J. Gluconeogenesis from alanine in patients with progressive malignant disease. Cancer Res 1979; *39*:1968–1972.

20. Lundholm K, Edstrom S, Karlberg I, et al. Glucose turnover, gluconeogenesis from glycerol, and estimation of net glucose cycling in cancer patients. Cancer 1982; *50*:1142–1150.

21. Burt ME, Aoki TT, Gorschboth LM, et al. Peripheral tissue metabolism in cancer-bearing man. Ann Surg 1983; *198*:635–691.

22. Eden E, Edstrom S, Bennegard K, et al. Glucose flux in relation to energy expenditure in malnourished patients with and without cancer during periods of fasting and feeding. Cancer Res 1984; *44*:1718–1724.

23. Hollander DM, Ebert EC, Roberts AI, et al. Effects of tumor type and burden on carcass lipid depletion in mice. Surgery 1986; *100*:292–297.

24. Devereux DF, Redgrave TG, Lod MF, et al. Tumor-associated metabolism in the rat is a unique physiologic entity. J Surg Res 1985; *38*:149–153.

25. Eden E, Edstrom S, Bennegard K, et al. Glycerol dynamics in weight-losing cancer patients. Surgery 1985; *97*:176–184.

26. Kawamura I, Moldawer LL, Keenan RA, et al. Altered amino acid kinetics in rats with progressive tumor growth. Cancer Res 1982; *42*:824–829.

27. Oram-Smith JC, Stein TP, Wallace HW, et al. Intravenous nutrition and tumor host protein metabolism. J Surg Res 1977; *22*:499–503.

28. Warren RS, Jeevanandam M, Brennan MF. Protein synthesis in the tumor-influenced hepatocyte. Surgery 1985; *98*:275–282.

29. Lundholm K, Bylund AC, Holm J, et al. Skeletal muscle metabolism in patients with malignant tumor. Eur J Cancer 1976; *12*:465–473.

30. Cohn SH, Gartenhaus W, Sawitsky A, et al. Compartmental body composition of cancer patients by measurement of total body nitrogen, potassium, and water. Metabolism 1981; *30*:222–229.

31. Heber D, Chlebowski RT, Ishibashi DE, et al. Abnormalities in glucose and protein metabolism in noncachectic lung cancer patents. Cancer Res 1982; *42*:4815–4850.

32. Burt ME, Stein TP, Brennan MF. A controlled randomized trial evaluating the effects of enteral and parenteral nutrition on protein metabolism in cancer-bearing man. J Surg Res 1983; *34*:303–314.

33. Jeevanandam M, Lowry SF, Horowitz AD, et al. Influence of increasing dietary intake on whole body protein kinetics in normal man. Clin Nutr 1986; *5*:41–48.

34. Burt ME, Stein TP, Schwade JG, et al. Whole body protein metabolism in cancer-bearing patients. Cancer 1984; *53*:1246–1254.

35. Persson H, Bennegard K, Lundberg P, et al. Thyroid hormones in conditions of chronic malnutrition. Ann Surg 1985; *201*:45–52.

36. Manson JM, Wilmore DW. Positive nitrogen balance with human growth hormone and hypocaloric intravenous feeding. Surgery 1986; *100*:188–196.

37. Daly JM, Copeland EM, Dudrick SJ. Effects of intravenous nutrition on tumor growth and host immunocompetence in malnourished animals. Surgery 1978; *84*:655–658.

38. Dionigi R, Zonta A, Dominioni L, et al. The effects of total parenteral nutrition on immunodepression due to malnutrition. Ann Surg 1977; *185*:467–474.

39. Warren S. The intermediate cause of death in cancer. Am J Med Sci 1932; *184*:610–615.

40. Mullen JL, Buzby GP, Waldman TG, et al. Prediction of operative morbidity and mortality by preoperative nutritional assessment. Surg Forum 1979; *30*:80–82.

41. Buzby GP, Mullen JL, Matthews DC, et al. Prognostic nutritional index in gastrointestinal surgery. Am J Surg 1980; *139*:160–166.

42. Mullen JL, Buzby GP, Matthews, DC, et al. Reduction of operative morbidity and mortality by combined preoperative and postoperative nutritional support. Ann Surg 1980; *192*:604–613.

43. Baker JP, Detsky AS, Wesson DE, et al. Nutritional assessment: a comparison of clinical judgement and objective measures. N Engl J Med 1982; *306*:969–972.

44. Daly JM, Long JM. Intravenous hyperalimentation: techniques and potential complications. Surg Clin North Am 1981; *61*:583–592.

45. Steiger E, Oram-Smith J, Miller E, et al. Effects of nutrition on prevalence of neoplasms in the rat. J Natl Cancer Inst 1971; *51*:1095–1113.

46. Buzby GP, Mullen JL, Stein TP, et al. Host-tumor interaction and nutrient supply. Cancer 1980; *45*:2940–2948.

47. Ota DM, Copeland EM, Strobel HW, et al. The effect of protein nutrition on host and tumor metabolism. J Surg Res 1977; *22*:181–188.

48. Daly JM, Copeland EM, Dudrick SJ, et al. Nutritional repletion of malnourished tumor-bearing and nontumor-bearing rats: effects on body weight, liver, muscle, and tumor. J Surg Res 1980; *28*:507–518.

49. Cameron, IL, Ackley WJ, Rogers W. Responses of hepatoma-bearing rats to total parenteral hyperalimentation and to ad libitum feeding. J Surg Res 1977; *23*:189–195.

50. Popp MB, Wagner SC, Brito OJ. Host and tumor responses to increasing levels of intravenous nutritional support. Surgery 1983; *94*:300–308.

51. Law DK, Dudrick SJ, Abdou NI. The effect of dietary protein depletion on immunocompetence; the importance of nutritional repletion prior to immunologic induction. Ann Surg 1974; *179*:168–173.

52. Muller JM, Dienst C, Brenner U, et al. Preoperative parenteral feeding in patients with gastrointestinal carcinoma. Lancet 1982; *1*:68–71.

53. Tannenbaum A, Silverstone H. Nutrition in relation to cancer. Adv Cancer Res 1953; *1*:451–501.

54. Green JW, Benditt EO, Humphreys EM. The effect of protein depletion on the host response to transplantable rat tumor Walker 256. Cancer Res 1950; *10*:769–774.

55. Ross MH, Bras G. Lasting influence of early caloric restriction on prevalence of neoplasm in the rat. J Natl Cancer Inst 1971; *51*:1095–1113.

56. White FR. The relationship between underfeeding and tumor formation, transplantation, and growth in rats and mice. Cancer Res 1961; *21*:281–290.

57. Moore C, Tittle PW. Muscle activity, body fat, and induced rat mammary tumors. Surgery 1973; *73*:329–332.

58. Cameron IL, Pavlat WA. Stimulation of growth of a transplantable hepatoma in rats by parenteral nutrition. J Natl Cancer Inst 1976; *56*:597–601.

59. Cameron IL. Effect of total parenteral nutrition on tumor-host responses in rats. Can Treat Rep 1981; *65*(Suppl):93–99.

60. Kishi T, Iwasawa Y, Hiroshi I, et al. Nutritional responses of tumor-bearing rats to oral or intravenous feeding. JPEN 1982; *6*:295–300.

61. King WWK, Boelhouwer RU, Kingsworth AN, et al. Total parenteral nutrition with and without fat as substrate for growth of rats and transplanted hepatocarcinoma. JPEN 1985; *9*:422–427.

62. Munro HN, Clark CM. The influence of dietary protein on the metabolism of ribonucleic acid in rat hepatoma. Br J Cancer 1959; *13*:324–335.

63. Daly JM, Copeland EM, Dudrick SJ, et al. Nutritional repletion of malnourished tumor-bearing and nontumor-bearing rats; effects on body weight, liver, muscle and tumor. J Surg Res 1980; *28*:507–518.

64. Reilly JJ, Goodgame JT, Jones DC, et al. DNA synthesis in rat sarcoma and liver. The effect of starvation. J Surg Res 1977; *22*:281–286.

65. Jose DG, Good RA. Quantitative effects of nutritional es-

sential amino acid deficiency on immune responses to tumors in mice. J Exp Med 1973; *137*:1–9.

66. Theuer RC. Effect of essential amino acid restriction on the growth of female C57BL mice and their implanted BW10232 adenocarcinomas. J Nutr 1971; *101*:223–232.

67. Demetrakopoulos GE, Brennan MF: Tumoricidal potential of nutritional manipulations. Cancer Res 1982; *42*(Suppl):756s–765s.

68. Montanez G, Murphy AE, Dunn M. Influence of pantothenic acid deficiency on the viability and growth of rat fibrosarcoma. Cancer Res 1951; *11*:834–838.

69. Stoerk MC, Emerson CA. Complete regression of lymphosarcoma implants following temporary induction of riboflavin deficiency in mice. Proc Soc Exp Biol Med 1949; *70*:703–707.

70. Rogers AE, Herndon BJ, Buoberne PM. Induction by dimethylhydrazine of intestinal carcinoma in normal rats and rats fed high and low levels of vitamin A. Cancer Res 1978; *33*:1003–1009.

71. Dunham WB, Zuckerkandl E, Reynolds R, et al. Effects of intake of L-ascorbic acid on the incidence of dermal neoplasms induced in mice by ultraviolet light. Proc Natl Acad Sci USA 1982; *79*:7532–7536.

72. Hilgard P. Experimental vitamin K deficiency and spontaneous metastases. Br J Cancer 1977; *35*:891–892.

73. DeWys W, Pories W. Inhibition of a spectrum of animal tumors by dietary zinc deficiency. J Natl Cancer Inst 1972; *48*:375–381.

74. Young GA, Parsons FM. The effects of dietary deficiencies of magnesium and potassium on the growth and chemistry of transplanted tumors and host tissues in the rat. Eur J Cancer 1977; *13*:103–113.

75. Mills BJ, Higgins PJ, Broghamer WL, et al. Magnesium depletion inhibits growth of established tumors. Fed Proc 1983; *42*:1312.

76. Ryan MP, Smyth H, Hingerty D. Effect of magnesium and potassium deficiencies on composition and cell growth in ascites tumor cells in vivo. Life Sci 1969; *8*:485–489.

77. Daly JM, Dudrick SJ, Copeland EM. Evaluation of nutritional indices as prognostic indicators in the cancer patient. Cancer 1979; *43*:925–931.

78. Belghiti J, Longonnet F, Bourstyn E, et al. Surgical implications of malnutrition and immunodeficiency in patients with carcinoma of the esophagus. Br J Surg 1983; *70*:339–341.

79. Brennan MF. Malnutrition in patients with gastrointestinal malignancy. Significance and management. Dig Dis Sci 1986; *31*:775–905.

80. Muller JM, Keller HW, Brenner U, et al. Indications and effects of preoperative parenteral nutrition. World J Surg 1986; *10*:53–63.

81. Heatley RV, Williams RHP, Lewis MH. Pre-operative intravenous feeding—a controlled trial. Postgrad Med J 1979; *55*:541–545.

82. Daly JM, Massar E, Giacco G, et al. Parenteral nutrition in esophageal cancer patients. Ann Surg 1982; *196*:203–208.

83. Souchon EA, Copeland EM, Watson P et al. Intravenous hyperalimentation as an adjunct to cancer chemotherapy with 5-fluorouracil. J Surg Res 1975; *18*:451–454.

84. Torosian MH, Buzby GP, Presti ME, et al. Reduction of methotrexate toxicity with improved nutritional status. Surg Forum 1982; *33*:109–112.

85. Mihranian MH, Wang YM, Daly JM. Effects of nutritional depletion and repletion on plasma methotrexate pharmacokinetics. Cancer 1984; *54*:2268–2271.

86. Grossie VB, Ho DHW, Loo TL. Effect of malnutrition on methotrexate toxicity and tissue levels of dihydrofolate reductase in the rat. Cancer Treat Rep 1982; *66*:85–89.

87. Daly JM, Reynolds HM, Copeland EM, et al. Effects of enteral and parenteral nutrition on tumor response to chemotherapy in experimental animals. J Surg Oncol 1981; *16*:79–96.

88. Reynolds HM, Daly JM, Rowland BJ, et al. Effects of nutritional repletion on host and tumor response to chemotherapy. Cancer 1980; *45*:3069–3074.

89. Torosian MH, Mullen JL, Miller EE, et al. Adjuvant, pulse total parenteral nutrition and tumor response to cycle-specific and cycle non-specific chemotherapy. Surgery 1983; *94*:291–299.

90. Copeland EM. Intravenous hyperalimentation and cancer. A historical perspective. JPEN 1986; *10*:337–342.

91. Copeland EM, MacFadyen BV Jr, Lanzotti VJ, et al. Intravenous hyperalimentation as an adjunct to cancer chemotherapy. Am J Surg 1975; *129*:167–173.

92. Lanzotti VJ, Copeland EM, George SL, et al. Cancer chemotherapeutic response and intravenous hyperalimentation. Cancer Chemother Rep 1975; *59*:437–439.

93. Issell BV, Valdivieso M, Zaren HA, et al. Protection against chemotherapy toxicity by IV hyperalimentation. Cancer Treat Rep 1978; *62*:1139–1143.

94. Jordan WM, Valdivieso M, Franman C, et al. Treatment of advanced adenocarcinoma of the lung with floraflur, dosorubicin, cyclophosphamide and cisplatin (FACP) with intensive hyperalimentation. Cancer Treat Rep 1981; *65*:197–206.

95. Valdivieso M, Bodey GP, Benjamin RS. Role of hyperalimentation as an adjunct to intensive chemotherapy for small cell bronchogenic carcinoma. Cancer Treat Rep 1981; *65*:145–151.

96. Clamon GH, Feld R, Evans WK, et al. Effect of adjuvant central IV hyperalimentation in survival and response to treatment of patients with small cell lung cancer: a randomized trial. Cancer Treat Rep 1981; *69*:167–177.

97. Popp MB, Fisher RI, Wresley R, et al. A prospective randomized study of adjuvant parenteral nutrition in the treatment of advanced diffuse lymphoma: influence on survival. Surgery 1981; *90*:195–203.

98. Levine AS, Brennan MF, Ramo A. Controlled clinical trials of nutritional intervention as an adjunct to chemotherapy, with a comment on nutrition and drug resistance. Cancer Res 1982; *42*:744–781.

99. Shamberger RC, Brennan MF, Goodgame JT, et al. A prospective, randomized study of adjuvant parenteral nutrition in the treatment of sarcomas: results of metabolic and survival studies. Surgery 1984; *96*:1–11.

100. Samuels ML, Selig DE, Ogden S, et al. IV hyperalimentation and chemotherapy for stage III testicular cancer: a randomized study. Cancer Treat Rep 1981; *65*:615–627.

101. Nixon DW, Moffitt S, Lawson DH, et al: Total parenteral nutrition as an adjunct to chemotherapy of metastatic colorectal cancer. Cancer Treat Rep 1981; *65*(Suppl 5):121–128.

102. Donaldson SS: Nutritional consequences of radiotherapy. Cancer Res 1977; *37*:2407–2413.

103. Reeves RJ, Sanders AP, Isley JK, et al. Fat absorption studies and small bowel X-ray studies in patients undergoing Co^{60} teletherapy and as radium application. Am J Roentgenol 1965; *94*:848–851.

104. Goodner CJ, Moore TE, Bowers JZ, et al. Effects of acute whole body X-irradiation on the absorption and distribution of Na^{22} and H^{3}OH from the gastrointestinal tract of the fasted rat. Am J Physiol 1955; *183*:475–478.

32

FOOD ALLERGY

RANJIT K. CHANDRA / SHAKUNTLA PURI

Adverse reactions to foods as the cause of both acute and chronic symptoms have been recognized for centuries. An immediate problem arising soon after the ingestion of an unusual food item, for example the development of facial swelling after eating oysters, is readily and often correctly attributable to food hypersensitivity. The link between chronic symptoms and food allergy is more difficult to establish, particularly if the involved dietary element is eaten frequently. Nevertheless, several recent studies using acceptable critical criteria of diagnosis have documented the role of food hypersensitivity in the genesis of a variety of chronic or recurrent clinical problems in at least a proportion of patients with such disorders as migraine, inflammatory bowel disease, and irritable bowel syndrome.

FOOD ALLERGY AND FOOD INTOLERANCE

It is important to make a clear distinction between *food allergy* or hypersensitivity, in which one or more immunological reactions can be demonstrated, and *food intolerance,* which denotes adverse reactions to dietary elements but without documentation of an underlying immunological process.[1,2] The concept that immunological reactions underlie allergy dates back to Von Pirquet. We know that there are at least four types of basic immunological reactions that mediate physiological and pathological response to both external and internal noxious agents.[3] These involve the participation of immunoglobulins of several major isotypes and of sensitized lymphocytes. The antigen-antibody-lymphocyte reactions result in the release of chemical mediators with vasoactive and other properties, ultimately producing the diverse range of symptoms and signs characteristic of allergic disorders,[4] such as angioedema, urticaria and other skin rashes, wheezing, and rhinitis. The true incidence of food allergy is difficult to estimate because of the differences among groups of patients investigated, the criteria for diagnosis, the bias on the part of the investigator, and the frequent difficulty of differentiating immunological from non-immunological causes of adverse symptoms attributable to foods.[5,6] The occurrence of allergy to cow's milk protein has been variably reported in 0.3 to 7.5 per cent of all infants; a conservative reasonable estimate of its incidence among randomly selected infants would be 1 per cent. The prevalence of allergy to other foods is even more difficult to estimate precisely.

Food intolerance, on the other hand, may be a more frequent phenomenon. It includes all non-immunological abnormal reactions to foods, with such diverse causes as psychological aversion, enzyme deficiencies (for example, lactose intolerance), and reactions to preservatives (for example, tartrazine) and nonavoidable food additives (for example, tetracyclines and penicillin in meat and dairy products). In some instances, psychological aversion to certain foods may be so strong as to produce marked physical symptoms and it may become very difficult to distinguish it from true intolerance with a defined biochemical process.[2] A list of some examples of nonimmunological causes of food intolerance is given in Table 32–1. Enzyme deficiencies can result in profound intolerance to certain carbohydrates and amino acids, the common examples being galactosemia and phenylketonuria. Shellfish contain toxins that produce swelling and numbness of lips, mouth, face, and limbs as well as nausea, vomiting, and debilitating, life-threatening neurological signs. A heat-stable neurotoxin with curare-like activity has been isolated from shellfish and is responsible for such severe symptoms. Aflatoxin in peanuts, cyanide in fruit pits, and pressor amines in bananas may be the cause of clinical problems. Chance contaminants or deliberately added substances, for example, pesticides, tetracyclines, penicillin, dyes, tartrazine, or nitrites, can be the source of a variety of nonimmunological adverse reactions to food.

In some instances, although the causal association of food ingestion and clinical manifestations can be established on the basis of history and temporal events, the pathogenetic mechanisms may not be clear and thus a label of either food allergy or food intolerance cannot be assigned with certainty. Repeated observations and the use of a wide variety of investigative tools may ultimately reveal the nature of the pathogenetic mechanisms involved.

In this chapter, the main focus is on food allergy and the terms "allergy" and "hypersensitivity" are used interchangeably.

TABLE 32–1. *Foods Commonly Causing Allergic Reactions*

Milk	Nut
Egg	Chocolate
Wheat	Orange
Fish	Tomato
Peanut	Soy

PHYSIOLOGY

There is a popular notion that the mucosal surface of the gastrointestinal tract is impermeable to antigens. There are increasing data, however, to support the theory that macromolecules do cross this barrier in variable amounts that may have limited nutritional significance but are sufficient to induce an immune response. This transport of antigenic molecules is more extensive in premature and newborn infants.[7] However, normal adults also show development of antibodies after a physiological load of an antigen; for example, after a large meal one can detect small amounts of antigen in the circulation.

Antigen Absorption

Food antigens undergo proteolytic hydrolysis in the small intestine. A small variable amount of this escapes digestion and runs the risk of becoming absorbed as intact macromolecules. When a sufficient number of these molecules come in contact with intestinal microvilli, they are taken into the cell by the process of pinocytosis. Once inside the cell, they form phagosomes into which are released intracellular lysosomal enzymes, which further tend to degrade the proteins. It has been suggested that specific receptors for certain proteins may facilitate the uptake of antigens and their transportation intracellularly. Small quantities of food antigens escape this breakdown to enter the intercellular spaces and subsequently the lymphatics and blood stream. It is now known that membrane or M ("microfold") cells interposed between columnar epithelial cells play an important role in antigen uptake.[8] These cells are devoid of microvilli and have very little glycocalyx; these features facilitate uptake of macromolecules. Moreover, lymphocytes and macrophages are in intimate contact with such cells and take up the released antigen. This is the first step for sensitization.

Factors Controlling Antigen Transport

Both immunological and nonimmunological host defense factors are involved in the control of antigen transport through the gut.

Nonimmunological mechanisms include:

1. Intestinal proteolytic breakdown of macromolecules so that the ingested protein loses its antigenicity.

2. Intestinal flora. Through competitive inhibition normal intestinal flora prevent the growth of potential pathogenic organisms and thus infectious damage to the intestinal mucosal barrier. The interruption of the mucosal barrier and the immature epithelium that replaces it during the recovery phase of infection are important factors in increased intestinal absorption of antigens following acute gastroenteritis.

3. Intestinal secretions. Mucus covering the epithelial surface of the gut prevents attachment of the antigen to the cell surface.

4. Gastric activity. The combined digestive effect of gastric acid and pepsin helps in the initiation of degradation of macromolecules and prevents the growth of pathogenic bacteria.

5. Intestinal motility allows mechanical clearance of pathogenic organisms and also causes decreased adherence of antigenic substances to intestinal surfaces.

6. Liver as host defense. The reticuloendothelial system of the liver acts as the second line of defense against biologically active substances that have traversed the small intestinal wall and have gained entrance into the portal circulation.

Immunological mechanisms, both local and systemic responses, help in antigenic exclusion. Lymphoid tissue in the Peyer's patches of the gastrointestinal tract contain IgA precursor cells.[9] Intestinal contents including antigenic macromolecules gain access to these lymphoid cells through specialized epithelial cells, called M cells, referred to above. M cells by virtue of few microvilli, poorly developed glycocalyx, and absence of lysosomal organelles are specially adapted for intact antigen transport. Antigen processing occurs in the lymphoid cells that mature into early B cells destined to become plasma cells for antibody formation. T helper cells present in the Peyer's patches help in this B cell maturation. This may be one of the reasons why patients with T cell defects (ataxia-telangiectasia, for example) have an associated IgA deficiency.

IgA-bearing lymphoblasts migrate to mesenteric lymph nodes for further maturation and then via the thoracic duct enter the blood circulation, from which they ultimately home into the lamina propria of the small intestine, epithelium, and other mucosal surfaces. Homing of plasma cells to these surfaces is regulated by the presence of antigen, the secretory component of IgA, and other unknown factors. Maternal transplacental antibody and the secretory IgA antibody, acquired from milk produced by the enteromammary immune system, influence neonatal processing of enteric antigen and may have an impact on the development of systemic and local immune responses later in life. Antibodies synthesized in the lamina propria are transported on to the intestinal surface after coupling with the secretory component in the epithelial cells. On the surface the secretory antibody is retained in the mucous coat, forming an "antiseptic point." By blocking the binding sites of antigens on the bacterial cell wall, these antibodies interfere with adhesion of these substances to epithelial surfaces, preventing their absorption and entry into systemic circulation.

Immunological Mechanisms

The exact immunological mechanisms have not been well documented for every type of clinical reaction due to food allergy. However, both humoral and cell-mediated immune components are involved in the pathogenesis. Immune reactions to foods may involve one or more of the four classic types of hypersensitive reactions described by Gell and Coombs.[10]

Type I Reaction. Also known as immediate hypersensitivity, this type of reaction follows antigen combination with reaginic or homocytotropic antibody on the surface of mast cells or basophils. This combination results in a sequential activation of intracellular metabolic events culminating in the release of vasoactive amines, such as histamine and slow-reacting substance.[11] The clinical manifestations include abdominal pain, cramps, vomiting, diarrhea, rhinitis, asthma, urticaria, and systemic anaphylaxis.

IgE is the principal reaginic antibody in man. Homocytotropic IgG_4 antibodies, however, may also play a role in rare instances.

Type II Reaction. Also known as cytotoxic hypersensitivity response, this reaction involves the interaction of complement-fixing antibodies to antigens which are an integral part of, or are fixed to, the surface of various cells. The reaction results in cell wall damage. Milk-induced thrombocytopenia may be caused by this type of reaction.

Type III Reaction. Also known as the Arthus response or immune complex disease, this reaction results when circulating immune complexes of food antigen and the specific antibody are deposited in tissues, often blood vessels, and initiate complement activation. Small immune complexes produced in antigen excess fix complement poorly and cannot be cleared from the circulation by the reticuloendothelial system. The symptoms, which consist of gastrointestinal, renal, pulmonary, or joint manifestations, appear within a few hours to a few days and last for days or weeks.

Type IV Reaction. Also known as delayed hypersensitivity, this reaction involves an interaction between antigen and sensitized T lymphocytes. Lymphocyte proliferation occurs, and a variety of soluble mediators collectively called lymphokines are released. It is possible that some gastrointestinal symptoms and signs of food allergy and chronic pulmonary disease are manifestations of this type of reaction. Development of skin lesions following hypersensitization with poison ivy and other contactants is an example of cell-mediated immune response.

DETERMINANTS OF FOOD HYPERSENSITIVITY

Antigens

Food proteins ingested by an individual, because of their foreign nature, can induce an immune response if absorbed intact through the gastrointestinal tract. During infancy, the child receives cow's milk proteins in formula feeds or very small amounts of cow's milk or other proteins secreted in breast milk.[12–14] Cow's milk contains three times more protein than human breast milk. Animal studies have shown that some milk formulas are more sensitizing than others and that raw cow's milk is very sensitizing. Heat treatment of milk reduces the antigenicity of the proteins. Pasteurization also helps in reducing antigen reaction. It modifies casein so that less tough curd is formed in the stomach.

Beta-lactoglobulin is one of the major proteins in cow's milk whey proteins, but is absent from human breast milk.[15] It is not surprising that approximately 85 per cent of cow's milk allergies are due to beta-lactoglobulin.

Most studies have reported no consistent association between a particular food and a particular symptom. However, some workers have linked specific manifestations to particular foods. For example, skin manifestation such as eczema and urticaria have been linked to egg protein, abdominal pain to fish, and oral mucosal reactions to peanuts.

Host

A breach in immune or nonimmune mechanisms controlling macromolecular entry results in antigen absorption in excessive amounts, thus sensitizing the individual. Several factors are involved in this sensitization.

Genetics. Offspring of parents with allergies have a higher risk of developing atopy.[16] Prospective clinical studies have documented a greater risk of subsequent allergic disorders in offspring of allergic patients (about 70 per cent incidence with bilateral and 58 per cent incidence with unilateral parental history). A genetic regulation of IgE production has been suggested. There is a significant correlation between serum IgE levels of parents and their children. Approximately 77 per cent of offspring from a biparental atopic background, 43 per cent with one atopic parent, and 17 per cent with no history of parental allergy had high IgE levels. It has been suggested that parental IgE measurements can have predictive value in terms of IgE levels and subsequent development of allergy in their offspring.

The clear association between HLA type and the development of allergy has not been documented so far. However, study of families with allergies and population studies have provided some evidence for this linkage.

Alterations in Bowel Permeability. The intestinal epithelial surface of newborn premature infants is more permeable to ingested food antigens than that of older infants and adults.[7] This has been attributed to the immaturity of epithelial cells, which have been shown to have greater power to engulf antigen mol-

ecules. Conditions causing mucosal damage also result in enhanced antigen absorption either through the damaged epithelium or through immature cells replacing the damaged tissue. This has been shown to occur during the recovery phase of acute gastroenteritis, with alcohol ingestion, and with the use of hyperosmolar elemental feeds. Severe malnutrition through decreased epithelial cell turnover can also result in enhanced pinocytosis of macromolecules; moreover, secretory IgA is also low in undernourished patients.[17,18]

Alterations in Immune Response. Early exposure to massive amounts of antigen during the neonatal period causes T cell suppression of immune responses, leading to immune tolerance. On the other hand, deficiency of cellular immunity may permit antigen uptake. This may explain the presence of milk antibodies in patients with T cell dysfunction like Wiskott-Aldrich syndrome, systemic lupus erythematosus, and IgA deficiency. The other well-known association is the frequent occurrence of an opsonic function defect and of C2 deficiency in patients with food allergy.

Alterations in Secretory IgA. Secretory IgA by blocking the attachment sites of antigenic molecules prevents their adherence to mucosal epithelium. Breast milk provides this antibody to the neonate, whose system is immature. This may explain in part the protective role of breast feeding in development of atopy in infants with positive family history of high cord blood IgE levels.[19–21] Several studies have demonstrated the presence of circulating immune complexes containing food antigens in patients with IgA deficiency.

Alterations in Local IgE Response. It has been suggested that children with food allergies are high IgE responders, both at the local intestinal level and at the systemic level. For example, patients with hemorrhagic proctitis have an excess of IgE-producing cells in the rectum, and they show intolerance to milk. IgE response through mast cell degranulation causes local anaphylaxis with mucosal injury. This may result in increased antigen absorption, thus setting a stage for nonreaginic sensitization.

CLINICAL MANIFESTATIONS

Food allergy is manifested clinically by a wide range of symptoms and signs from abdominal pain to generalized anaphylaxis (Fig. 32–1, Table 32–2). This diverse nature of presentation is influenced by factors such as the age of the patient, the amount and quality of food antigens ingested, and the type and extent of associated medical problems.[2,22]

Infants. Cow's milk allergy usually starts around the age of 2 months or within 2 or 3 weeks of introduction of cow's milk in the infant's diet. It is often manifested as recurrent vomiting or diarrhea. The infant may develop eczema either as the only

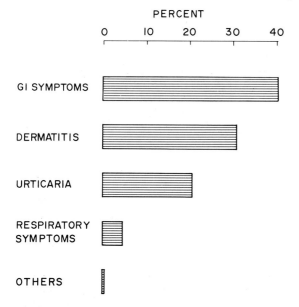

FIGURE 32–1. Prevalence of symptoms in patients with proven food allergy.

symptom or in association with a bowel disturbance. Recent observations suggest that cow's milk protein allergy may underlie ulcerative colitis in at least one half of patients presenting during infancy. Associated features related to the respiratory tract and skin such as rhinorrhea, asthma or urticaria may be present. There seems to be a distinction between cow's milk allergy in breast-fed and formula-fed babies. Breast-fed infants, being exposed to smaller amounts of antigen, are more sensitized and tend to have severe reactions that may last for several years. In formula-fed babies, on the other hand, allergy is triggered by large amounts of antigen which, with time, can cause immune tolerance. Anaphylactic reactions are not a common feature of cow's milk allergy in infants. Prick tests are not always positive. This type of allergy subsides spontaneously; therefore, a gradual return to cow's milk feeding should be tried after several months.

Older Children. Symptoms may occur because of allergy to milk or other food antigens (Table 32–3). The disorder usually presents as gradual onset of abdominal pain after a meal which may take the form of recurrent colic, stomach ache or vague abdominal pain. Children may develop iron deficiency anemia from chronic intestinal blood loss or growth retardation from malabsorption or protein-losing enteropathy. Recurrent asthma or other respiratory symptoms and eczema may occasionally be the presenting features. Nonspecific symptoms include irritability, temper tantrums, fatigue, and headache. Although the evidence is still conflicting, there are reports suggesting that food hypersensitivity plays a role in inflammatory bowel disease and celiac disease. Patients with ulcerative colitis have several atopic manifestations, and increased IgG and IgM antibodies to milk in the circulation have been observed in patients with ulcerative colitis. Secondary development of food allergy is well known in patients with gluten-sensitive enteropathy.

Introduction of an appropriate hypoallergenic diet causes remission of symptoms within hours to days.[23] They may, however, persist up to 2 weeks. The natural course of allergy in children is often complete remission in 7 to 10 years. They may, however, continue to show positive skin tests or develop other allergies, for example, hay fever.

Adults. In adult life, nonimmunological causes of food intolerance are much more common. The presenting manifestations of food allergy in this age group may be classic allergic symptoms as in childhood—gastrointestinal disorders, urticaria, asthma, or anaphylaxis. However, other presentations are not uncommon. These may include hemorrhagic proctitis from cow's milk intolerance. Patients with arthritis may show exacerbation of symptoms on exposure to milk, and this is associated with positive skin tests to milk and the presence of milk-specific IgG antibodies in circulation. Other foods may also be involved. Hyperactivity, tension-fatigue syndrome, migraine headaches, exacerbation of steroid-sensitive nephrotic syndrome, and thrombocytopenia are some of the other manifestations of food allergy occasionally reported in the literature.

TABLE 32–2. Symptoms and Signs of Food Allergy

Gastrointestinal	Respiratory	Cutaneous
Vomiting	Rhinorrhea	Dermatitis
Abdominal pain	Postnasal discharge	Eczema
Abdominal distention	Sneezing	Urticaria
Diarrhea	Cough	Angioedema
Malabsorption	Recurrent croup	
Occult bleeding	Bronchospasm	
Protein-losing enteropathy	Serous otitis media	
Hematological	**Neurological**	**Miscellaneous**
Anemia	Irritability	Sudden infant death syndrome
Eosinophilia	Restlessness	Enuresis
Thrombocytopenia	Hyperactivity	
	Fatigue	
	Migraine	

TABLE 32–3. *Examples of Nonimmunological Adverse Reactions to Foods*

Clinical Features	Predisposing Factor	Offending Substance
Diarrhea, abdominal cramps	Lactose deficiency	Lactose in milk
Vomiting, neurologic problems	—	Saxitoxin in shellfish
Vomiting, diarrhea, neurologic symptoms	—	Botulinal toxin derived from *Clostridium botulinum*
Diarrhea, pain, fever, dizziness, weakness	—	*Salmonella* or *Staphylococcus* poisoning
Vomiting, pain, salivation, diarrhea, sweating, blurred vision	—	Mushroom poisoning
Headache, fever, depression, weakness	—	Solanine alkaloid in potato skins
Hemolytic anemia	Glucose- 6-phosphate dehydrogenase deficiency	Fava beans, drugs
Paroxysmal atrial tachycardia	—	Caffeine
Bronchospasm	—	Metabisulfite in wine and salads
Urticaria	—	Benzoates and food dyes
Headache	—	Wine, cocoa, cheese, monosodium glutamate (MSG)

From Chandra RK. Food Intolerance. New York, Elsevier, 1984: 104. Reproduced with permission.

DIAGNOSIS

Evaluation of patients with suspected food allergy is a diagnostic challenge. Translating subjective symptoms into objective evidence of food intolerance and proving an immunological basis for such symptoms is a formidable task for the physician investigating such an individual. Patients with nonspecific symptoms, mental ill health, an obsessional neurosis for certain foods and ideas biased by previously given scientific or unscientific advice create even further problems in diagnosis.

Food Exclusion and Challenge

At the present time this method remains the mainstay of clinical diagnosis. Properly performed, it helps in providing valuable information about the patient's tolerance to foods.[24] Following a careful detailed history, the patient is provided with a food diary in which he records the diet on one side and symptoms on the other. The object is to correlate any offending food with symptoms, and this helps in planning an exclusion and challenge diet. If there is any evidence of specific food intolerance, the patient is started on an elimination diet removing the suspected food. Otherwise, an empirical elimination diet that omits several common food allergens is used.[25]

If symptoms disappear on an elimination diet, the next phase of evaluation is done. In this a challenge test, which can be performed under two circumstances, is done. If the patient is symptom-free on a diet but the specific allergen is not known, the omitted foods are introduced in stages until a satisfactory maintenance diet is achieved or until symptoms recur. When there is a suspicion about a single food, the challenge test is carried out using a double-blind placebo control technique in order to obtain objectivity.

Food challenge tests are not without the risk of side effects. They should therefore be performed under supervision, usually in a hospital setting, and the patient must be informed of the potential danger. A single positive reaction to a double-blind food challenge, such as diarrhea, vomiting, hives, or asthma, should be taken as an evidence of reaction to the particular food. In the case of subjective symptoms, however, it is important to substantiate a number of positive test responses to a suspected food along with totally negative placebo test results.

Many foods contain a variety of intentional and unintentional food additives. Many of these, even in trace quantities, can produce untoward effects as a result of allergy, intolerance, or idiosyncrasy. For example, tartrazine, because of its cross-reaction with aspirin, can precipitate asthma in aspirin-sensitive individuals. When a food additive like this is suspected as a cause of an untoward reaction, a "fresh food diet"—a challenge test with commonly used substances given in capsule form—can be tried to see if a remission of symptoms results.

Skin Testing

Skin testing is the most widely used diagnostic procedure in the evaluation of food allergy.[26] Water-soluble extracts of foods are applied to the back of the forearm and the underlying skin is pricked or scratched. Intradermal skin testing is no longer used for food antigens. The concentration of extract used is 1:10 or 1:20 w/v. Skin mast cells of sensitized patients have antigen-specific IgE on their surface. Interaction of this IgE with the applied antigen triggers a response that results in mast cell degranulation and development of a local wheal and flare reaction in 10 to 15 minutes. Unfortunately, both false-positive and false-negative responses to food extracts are frequent. These may be attributed to factors like antigen preparation, skin conditions, immunological mechanisms underlying the symptoms, interpretation of response, and the technique used.

RAST

The radioallergosorbent test (RAST) is the in vitro demonstration of IgE against the specific food antigen.[27] In this test, the patient's serum is incubated with paper discs to which the food antigen is attached. Antigen-specific IgE present in the patient's serum attaches to the antigen. The nonspecific IgE is washed away, and the Ag-IgE complex is again incubated with radiolabeled anti-IgE. Measurement of the radioactive anti-IgE attached to the patient's IgE that is directed to the antigen on the paper disc gives quantitative assessment of antigen-specific IgE. Clinically, RAST is used when skin testing might produce severe reactions like anaphylaxis, in patients with generalized eczema or dermatographism. However, RAST has some disadvantages and requires expensive equipment and reagents.

Precipitating and Hemagglutinating Antibodies

Precipitating antibodies of IgG and IgM classes can be detected in patients with food allergy by the technique of double immunodiffusion in agar. The sensitivity of the test can be increased by using Plexiglas reservoirs and a thin layer of agar to facilitate antibody diffusion. This is a relatively simple test but requires experience in its performance and interpretation. It is most helpful in milk-induced chronic pulmonary disease or Heiner syndrome. Positive results are, however, also seen in celiac disease, cystic fibrosis, IgE deficiency, Down syndrome, and Wiskott-Aldrich syndrome, in patients convalescing from acute gastroenteritis, and also in healthy individuals, especially young infants. Therefore, any condition that allows abnormal transport of food antigen can result in high titers of specific antibodies in the serum. Thus this test cannot be assumed to be of value in making a positive diagnosis, but high titers of antibodies do afford a clue concerning the possibility of an accompanying disorder.

Complement Activation

Nonreaginic immunological mechanisms of food allergy involve the activation of the complement system. A fasting pre-test blood sample is obtained and the patient is challenged with the suspected food allergen (e.g., cow's milk, egg) in a physiological amount. A second blood sample is drawn 90 minutes later. Immunoelectrophoresis is done, using monospecific antiserum to C3. Complement activation is indicated by the presence of C3 split products in the post-challenge test. However, this test is positive in less than 5 per cent of all patients with food allergy.

Other Tests

The diagnostic tests remaining to be described are not of much practical help. They either employ complicated techniques or are invasive, and their diagnostic value is questionable.

Eosinophilia. Eosinophilia (count > 400 eosinophils/mm^3) may be present in about one fourth to one half of patients with cow's milk allergy. Increased eosinophils may also be found locally, as in nasal smear, gastric contents, stools, or mucosal biopsy specimens.

Serum Immunoglobulins. Selective IgA deficiency and other dysgammaglobulinemias are associated with a high prevalence of food allergy.

Circulating Immune Complexes. Circulating antigen–IgG antibody complexes in low titer are seen frequently in healthy infants in response to small amounts of antigen transport across the intestinal mucosa. However, IgE immune complexes if present can be of pathogenetic importance. These are detected by Raji cell radioimmunoassay or C1q binding.

Lymphocyte Proliferation and Lymphokine Release. Lymphocytes, when activated, produce a variety of lymphokines, including leukocyte migration inhibition factor (LIF). The validity of this test has been investigated extensively for the diagnosis of food intolerance. Significantly positive tests in challenge-proven milk-tolerant patients as compared with controls have been reported, with reversal of the test toward normal in children who had become tolerant to milk. This test requires considerable manual skill and experience. However, once this is achieved, the results are reproducible.

Leukocyte Histamine Release. Peripheral blood leukocytes are mixed with the suspected allergen and the amount of histamine released in excess of that from control leukocytes not exposed to the allergen is estimated. The test is often false positive and therefore lacks specificity.

Plasma Histamine. Elevated levels of plasma histamine have been observed in a small proportion of allergic subjects challenged with oral or subcutaneous food provocation.

Intestinal Permeability. It has been suggested that increased intestinal permeability is an important predisposing factor in the development of food allergy. This has been shown recently in patients with eczema and other manifestations of food allergy (Fig. 32–2).

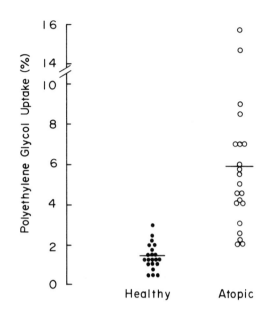

FIGURE 32–2. *Absorption of polyethylene glycol in healthy subjects and in those with food allergy.*

Coproantibodies. Because of a high rate of false-positive results, the presence of fecal antibodies is of little diagnostic value.

Intestinal Biopsy. Small bowel biopsy has been recommended by some gastroenterologists for the diagnosis of food allergy. The changes induced by food allergens are nonspecific and are therefore not pathognomonic of food hypersensitivity. Moreover, food challenge may produce only an extraintestinal manifestation in the presence of normal mucosa. Immunofluorescence studies for the presence of plasma cells and immune complexes may provide useful information.

DIFFERENTIAL DIAGNOSIS

Food allergy, as discussed under clinical manifestations, has multisystemic presentations. The conditions to be considered in the differential diagnosis, therefore, depend on the clinical presentation in a given patient.[2]

Lactase Deficiency. An important alternate diagnosis to cow's milk allergy is lactose malabsorption. This may be difficult to distinguish clinically, especially at the initial presentation, as cow's milk protein allergy and lactose intolerance may coexist. Mucosal damage produced by cow's milk allergy may produce secondary lactase deficiency and consequently lactose intolerance. The diagnosis of lactase deficiency can be verified by a lactose tolerance test or a hydrogen breath test.

Celiac Disease. Celiac disease is an important consideration in the differential diagnosis of food allergy. The two conditions sometimes coexist. Transient cow's milk hypersensitivity in patients with celiac disease is documented. Transient gluten intolerance accompanying cow's milk allergy has also been described. Infants with celiac disease are symptom-free before the introduction of solids in their diet. Malabsorption starts when gluten (wheat, barley, or rye) is introduced into the diet. The diagnosis depends upon the characteristic changes in the intestinal biopsy. These changes may, however, sometimes be indistinguishable from the nonspecific histological changes of food allergy. Improvement of these changes on a gluten-free diet may be helpful. There are reports of high diagnostic reliability of the fluorescent immunosorbent test for gliadin antibody.

Cystic Fibrosis. Cystic fibrosis may present as malabsorption and/or pulmonary system involvement. The digestive and pulmonary systems are also the most common end organs of food allergy. In cystic fibrosis, malabsorption, which affects all dietary components, can be corrected by supplementation with pancreatic enzymes. The diagnosis is established by the finding of an elevated level of sweat chloride.

Gastroenteritis. Cow's milk intolerance may follow transiently on an acute episode of gastroenteritis. However, after regeneration of the mucosa, which may take several weeks, tolerance to cow's milk is established gradually. The history of intolerance to cow's milk after an episode of diarrhea, with no such intolerance symptom before that, and the use of stool cultures and other laboratory tests usually help in establishing a diagnosis.

Galactosemia. Galactosemia is a disorder of galactose metabolism due to congenital deficiency of galactose-1-phosphatase, uridyl transferase, or galactokinase. It manifests itself in early infancy as vomiting, diarrhea, failure to thrive, jaundice, and cataracts. The diagnosis is established by demonstrating low levels of the enzyme in red blood cells.

Immunodeficiencies. Children with immunodeficiencies, such as selective IgA deficiency or B or T cell defects, may present with persistent diarrhea, failure to thrive, frequent respiratory tract infection, and skin rashes. Immunological screening studies should, therefore, be done in such patients. These conditions also may include food allergy as part of their clinical picture.

Intestinal Parasitic Infestation. Gastrointestinal manifestations from parasitic infestations like *Giardia lamblia* or *Strongyloides stercoralis* may be important in the differential diagnosis in low socioeconomic and poor hygienic conditions. Stools should be analyzed for ova and parasites if the diagnostic possibility of infestation is entertained.

Rhinitis. Chronic rhinitis alone or in association with other features is the most common respiratory tract manifestation of food allergy in young children. However, hypersensitivity to inhalants is seen more often as a cause of allergic rhinitis, especially in older children and adults. A history of seasonal symptoms and positive skin tests and RAST for inhalants favor this type of allergy. Vasomotor rhinitis, eosinophilic nonallergic rhinitis, and upper respiratory tract infections are the other conditions that should be ruled out.

Pulmonary Disease. In a child presenting with wheezing, a number of conditions other than bronchial asthma need to be considered. These include bronchiolitis, anomalies of the trachea or bronchi, vascular rings, foreign body, bronchopulmonary aspergillosis, recurrent aspiration (e.g., from achalasia), heart failure, and mediastinal masses. Foods can be an important etiological factor in idiopathic pulmonary hemosiderosis.

Respiratory disease due to food ingestion is mediated largely by non-IgE mechanisms, although mixed responses are also seen. These patients often have precipitating antibodies or high levels of IgG_4 antibody specific to cow's milk protein.

Skin Disorders. Dermatological manifestations are the most frequent symptoms of food allergy and include dermatitis, eczema, urticaria, and angioedema. Skin lesions from other causes should be included in the differential diagnosis of these lesions. Seborrheic dermatitis is a condition characterized by scaly erythematous lesions appearing on the scalp and may extend to involve the face and other parts of the body. Acrodermatitis enteropathica, a disease due to an inherited defect of zinc absorption, presents in early infancy as eczematous and vesiculobullous lesions, diarrhea, failure to thrive, hair loss, and increased susceptibility to infections. Serum zinc levels are low and the skin lesions respond to zinc supplementation. Drugs, viral infections, candidiasis, and insect bites are some of the other causes of skin rashes.

MANAGEMENT

Prevention of Sensitization. During the newborn period, the immune mechanisms are immature and the intestinal mucosa has increased permeability. There is, therefore, the greatest risk of antigen absorption and consequent sensitization at this stage. Following an episode of acute gastroenteritis, there is increased mucosal permeability.[7] The importance of breast feeding during these periods cannot be overemphasized. It has been recommended that infants should be exclusively breast-fed for at least 4 months. Breast milk contains secretory IgA and immunoreactive cells, which provide both local and systemic mechanisms of antigen handling and exclusion, consequently preventing sensitization.[28] Another mechanism by which breast feeding protects against sensitization is by changing the intestinal flora. Intestinal flora of artificially fed babies are gram negative with a predominance of *Escherichia coli*, whereas breast-fed babies have predominantly gram-positive bifidobacteria. *E. coli* antitoxin

(formed in response to this colonization) acts as a powerful adjuvant, and even small amounts of antigen absorbed through the gut result in IgE antibody formation. Exclusive breast feeding reduces the prevalence of atopic disease, such as eczema. This is particularly important in high-risk infants of parents with allergic disorders.[19–21]

If a mother cannot breast feed, the infant should be given a nutritionally adequate elemental hydrolysate-based or soya-based infant formula. Weaning should be started at 4 months of age with cereals, preferably rice cereal; addition of meats, vegetables, and fruits should then be considered. Foods derived from cow's milk and eggs are to be avoided, particularly if these are the foods to which the parents are allergic. Partial breast feeding should be continued for many months.

Elimination of Allergens from the Diet. Avoidance of food to which the patient is sensitized is most important to alleviate the clinical manifestations of food allergy. However, this approach is not always practical or as simple as it sounds. A single foodstuff that has a clear-cut allergenic effect and is taken only occasionally is simple to eliminate from the diet. However, with multiple allergens from commonly used foods and with nonspecific symptoms, particularly of the non–IgE-mediated type, the therapeutic success of elimination diets is reduced. Under these circumstances a correct and detailed history, knowledge of foodstuffs containing the allergen, an understanding attitude, and the cooperation of the patient and his or her family are essential. The essential part of this approach is to provide a well-balanced diet with sufficient protein content. An example of an oligoallergenic diet is given in Table 32–4.

Prevention of Allergen Absorption and Mast Cell Degranulation. Breast milk, by virtue of its humoral and cellular elements such as antibodies, leukocytes,

---

TABLE 32–4. An Example of an Oligoantigenic Diet

One cereal, e.g., rice (including rice flour)
One meat, e.g., lamb or mutton—2 servings per day (including sheep's liver, sheep's liver, etc.)
One vegetable, e.g., cabbage, cauliflower and Brussels sprouts
One fruit, e.g., apple (including purée. uncolored apple juice and apple jelly)
Milk-free margarine, e.g., Tomar Kosher
Boiled goats' milk (1 pint/day)
One oil, e.g., sunflower
Sugar, golden syrup, sago, tapioca, salt, water, tea, coffee
Comprehensive vitamin and mineral supplements (including trace elements) may be needed—selected brands should be coloring and preservative free.

Imaginative cooking can produce a varied and attractive diet from a limited range of foods such as this, but the help of a dietitian is essential to ensure such a diet is nutritionally adequate and acceptable. It is maintained for only 3–4 weeks, after which other foods are reintroduced one after the other. If it is unsuccessful, another oligoantigenic diet, including none of the foods in the first one, should be instituted.

From Soothill JF, Hayward AR, Woud CBS (eds). Paediatric Immunology. London, Blackwell, 1983: 264. Reproduced with permission.

and antibacterial and antiviral factors, protects against penetration of intestinal mucosa by potential food allergens. The role of oral sodium cromoglycate is controversial in this respect. Sodium cromoglycate blocks the degranulation of local mast cells in the intestinal mucosa. Consequently this prevents an increase of intestinal permeability, which, if it occurred, would lead to enhanced absorption of macromolecules and formation of immune complexes.

Hyposensitization. The studies conducted so far regarding the use of hyposensitization in order to acquire immunological tolerance have not provided sufficiently good clinical results. Its role, therefore, has not been as clearly established in food allergy as it is for respiratory allergy. Increasing doses of properly diluted food allergen are used over a period of 4 to 5 months. The beneficial results of oral hyposensitization reported in some studies, particularly in cow's milk allergy, have been debated; they may be attributable to a spontaneous development of tolerance and change in sensitivity, which occurs frequently with age in cow's milk allergy.

Symptomatic Treatment. Symptomatic treatment may be used before the diagnosis of food allergy has been made and the offending allergen has been identified. It is also useful in cases in which the preventive measures described above have failed to control the symptoms. The nature of the treatment used depends on the type and severity of symptoms and their frequency and duration.

References

1. Chandra RK (ed). Food Allergy. St. John's, Newfoundland, Nutrition Research Education Foundation, 1987.
2. Chandra RK (ed). Food Intolerance. New York, Elsevier, 1984.
3. Heiner DC (ed). Food allergy. Clin Rev Allergy 1984; 2:1–94.
4. May CD, Bock SA. A modern clinical approach to food hypersensitivity. Allergy 1978; 33:166–188.
5. Nelson HS. The atopic diseases. Ann Allergy 1985; 55:441–447.
6. Krause RM. Epidemiology of allergic disease. J Allergy Clin Immunol 1986; 78:953–958.
7. Walker WA. Antigen handling by the gut. Arch Dis Child 1978; 53:527–533.
8. Owens RL, Jones AL. Epithelial cell specialization within human Peyer's patches. Gastroenterology 1974; 66:189–199.
9. Cornes JS. Number, size and distribution of Peyer's patches in the human small intestine. Gut 1965; 6:225–232.
10. Gell PGH, Coombs RRA (eds). Clinical Aspects of Immunology. Oxford, Blackwell, 1975: 453.
11. Metcalfe DD. Chemical mediators of allergic reactions. *In* Chandra RK (ed). Food Allergy. St. John's, Newfoundland, Nutrition Research Education Foundation, 1987: 117–136.
12. Donally HH. The question of elimination of foreign protein (egg protein and cow milk) in woman's milk. J Immunol 1930; 19:15–40.
13. Stuart CA. Passage of cow milk protein in breast milk. Clin Allergy 1984; 14:533–535.
14. Van Asperen PP, Kemp AS, Mellis CM. Immediate hypersensitivity reactions on the first known exposure to the food. Arch Dis Child 1983; 58:253–256.
15. Bjorksten B. Prediction and prevention of allergy in childhood. *In* Chandra RK (ed). Food Allergy. St. John's, Newfoundland, Nutrition Research Education Foundation, 1987: 343–359.
16. Marsh DG, Bias WB. The genetics of atopic allergy. Immunogenetics 1978; 6:248–259.
17. Chandra RK. Reduced secretory antibody response to live attenuated measles and poliovirus vaccines in malnourished children. Br Med J 1975; 2:583–585.
18. Srisinha S, Suskind RM, Edelman R. Secretory and serum IgA in children with protein-energy malnutrition. Pediatrics 1975; 55:166–173.
19. Chandra RK, Puri S, Cheema PS. Predictive value of cord blood IgE in the development of atopic disease and role of breast feeding in its prevention. Clin Allergy 1985; 15:517–522.
20. Businco L, Marchetti F, Pelligrini G. Prevention of atopic disease in "at risk newborns" by prolonged breast feeding. Clin Allergy 1983; 51:296–304.
21. Saarinen IM. Prophylaxis for atopic disease. Clin Rev Allergy 1984; 2:151–167.
22. Bock SA. Food sensitivity. Am J Dis Child 1980; 134:973–982.
23. Collins-Williams CC. Allergy to foods other than cow's milk. *In* Chandra RK (ed). Food Intolerance. New York, Elsevier, 1984.
24. Mathew DJ, Taylor B, Normal AP, et al. Prevention of eczema. Lancet 1977; 1:321–324.
25. Taylor S. Elimination diets. *In* Chandra RK (ed). Food Allergy. St. John's, Newfoundland, Nutrition Research Education Foundation, 1987.
26. Bock SA. Proper use of skin tests with food extracts in diagnosis of hypersensitivity to foods in children. J Allergy 1977; 7:375–383.
27. Aas K, Johansson SGO. The radioallergosorbent test in the in vitro diagnosis of multiple reaginic allergy. J Allergy 1971; 48:134–142.
28. Chandra RK. Immunological aspects of human milk. Nutr Rev 1978; 36:265–272.

33

IMMUNITY AND INFECTION

RANJIT K. CHANDRA

The concept that diet influences resistance to disease has been recognized for centuries. It is only recently, however, that the immunological mechanisms underlying nutrition-infection interactions have been delineated. It is also known that several individual nutrients play an important role in the regulation of immunity. The subject has been the focus of much recent work and has been summarized in several recent reviews and monographs.[1-10]

It is established that immune deficiency states increase susceptibility to infection. Malnourished subjects are also at risk of severe life-threatening infection. Thus it is logical to infer that nutritional deficiency may result in immune deficiency and a higher incidence and severity of infectious illness. Indeed several epidemiological surveys have confirmed this,[11] and recent work suggests that malnutrition is the commonest cause of secondary immune deficiency.[3]

The most prominent and consistent change in the immunocompetence of malnourished subjects occurs in cell-mediated immunity. Other mechanisms of host resistance that may show significant alterations in nutritional imbalance are the complement system, phagocyte function, mucosal antibody response, and antibody affinity.[12] The interpretation of work in this area must be undertaken cautiously. Animal data cannot always be extrapolated to the human situation; a case in point is the demonstration in mice of *enhanced* cell-mediated immunity in the presence of protein deficiency. Certainly, in kwashiorkor and other syndromes of protein deficiency in man, cell-mediated immunity is always *decreased*. Human malnutrition is usually a composite of multiple nutritional deficiencies set against a background of multiple infections. On the other hand, experimental animals are housed in hygienic environments and fed well-defined diets deficient in a single nutrient. These are some possible reasons for differences in the results of studies in laboratory animals and man. The age of the subject tested, dose of antigen employed, the use of adjuvants, and the presence of control serum in in vitro tests are other important determinants of the immune responses elicited in malnutrition.

Another issue of great practical significance is the threshold of immunodeficiency that is relevant for increased risk of disease. We know that the complement C3 level must be reduced to less than 30 per cent of control before it can decrease opsonic function. Thus it is important to define the extent of immunity dysfunction that is important clinically.

In this chapter, the epidemiological and clinical observations pertaining to nutrition-infection interactions are reviewed, the phenomenology of lymphoid tissue changes and immunity dysfunction is described, and examples are provided of the practical significance of these observations.

CLINICAL AND EPIDEMIOLOGICAL OBSERVATIONS

The results of surveys of malnourished populations in developing countries have suggested that infections are more severe and of longer duration among those with reduced weight for height. The data on increased incidence of infections are less convincing. Field surveys in Asia and the Americas have confirmed the intimate association of nutritional deficiencies, growth failure, and infectious illness,[11] particularly diarrheal disease.[13] In a prospective study in Mexican children followed weekly from birth to 5 years of age, moderate malnutrition correlated significantly with the duration and severity of episodes of infectious disease and to a lesser extent with the incidence of diarrheal disease in the age period 8 to 18 months. The majority of hospitalized children with severe forms of malnutrition have an associated infection at the time of admission; this is more often observed in kwashiorkor than in marasmus. A Pan American Health Organization survey of childhood mortality patterns in the Americas showed that 57 per cent of children under 5 years of age who died had signs of intrauterine and/or postnatal nutritional growth retardation as either the primary or an associated cause of death. These data are critically reviewed elsewhere.[6, 33]

Many infectious diseases run a more severe course in nutritionally deprived children. For example, measles is known to produce fatal giant-cell pneumonia in children with kwashiorkor. It is interesting that there is an unexplained geographical difference in measles-associated morbidity and mortality—the frightening severity of measles in West African infants with kwashiorkor has not been observed in undernourished children in Asia and other regions.[14,15] Herpes virus infection is often generalized and fatal in kwashiorkor; adrenal, hepatic, and cerebral hemorrhages are seen at autopsy and there is a conspicuous lack of inflammatory response. Septicemia due to gram-negative microorganisms and respiratory infections caused by *Pneumocystis carinii* frequently complicate moderate to severe protein-energy malnutrition.

Undernourished populations usually have a heavier load of parasites. This is not to say that nutritional deficiency necessarily leads to heavy parasite infestation—the reverse is probably often true. However, in laboratory animals experimental protein deficiency generally facilitates protozoal and helminthic infection. The variable effects of nutrition on disease produced by various pathogens is shown in Table 33–1.

TABLE 33–1. Infectious Diseases Influenced by Nutritional Status

	Influence		
	Definite	*Variable*	*Slight*
Bacterial	Tuberculosis Bacterial diarrhea Cholera Leprosy Pertussis Respiratory infections	Diphtheria *Staphylococcus* *Streptococcus*	Typhoid Plague Tetanus Bacterial toxins
Viral	Measles Rotavirus diarrhea Respiratory infections Herpes	Influenza	Small pox Yellow fever ARBO encephalitis Poliomyelitis
Parasitic	*Pneumocystis carinii* Intestinal parasites Trypanosomiasis Leishmaniasis Schistosomiasis	Giardiasis Filariasis	Malaria
Fungal	Candidosis Aspergillosis	Mold toxins	
Other		Syphilis Typhus	

ARBO, arthropod-borne virus.

MORPHOLOGICAL AND MICROBIOLOGICAL CHANGES

The thymus is smaller and lighter in children who die of malnutrition compared with the findings in well-nourished controls. Histopathologically, there is ill-defined demarcation between the cortex and medulla. There are fewer than normal lymphoid cells, and Hassall corpuscles are crowded, dilated, degenerate, and occasionally even calcified. There is cellular depletion of thymus-dependent areas in the spleen and lymph nodes. In the intestine, lymphoid aggregates are small, and the numbers of intraepithelial lymphocytes and of submucosal plasma cells are reduced (Table 33–2). Clinically, the effects of malnutrition on lymphoid organs are reflected in the small size of the tonsils.

The pattern of microorganisms isolated from malnourished subjects (Table 33–3) reflects the findings in primary immunodeficiency states.

IMMUNOLOGICAL FINDINGS

The mechanisms of host resistance are outlined in Table 33–4. It is important to emphasize that these processes act in concert rather than in isolation.[16] Thus the deficiency of one facet of immunity is often compensated for by normal responses in other aspects of host resistance.

Cell-Mediated Immunity

Impaired cell-mediated immunity in moderate to severe undernutrition has been extensively reported.[17–23] Several types of evidence have been collected: cutaneous delayed hypersensitivity to a battery of ubiquitous recall antigens or after deliberate sensitization with a chemical agent; the proportion and number of circulating T lymphocytes; lymphocyte DNA synthesis induced by mitogens and antigens; production of soluble mediators of immunological reactivity in response to mitogens and antigens; mixed lymphocyte response; and rejection of skin homografts.

The profound structural changes in the thymus and other lymphoid organs of severely malnourished patients may be expected to result in both nu-

TABLE 33–2. *Number of Plasma Cells (Mean ± S.D.) in the Jejunal Mucosa, by Immunoglobulin Class**

	IgA	IgM	IgG
Malnourished persons	52 ± 15 (57 ± 16)	31 ± 10 (33 ± 11)	9 ± 3 (10 ± 3)
Well-nourished persons	91 ± 17 (80 ± 15)	19 ± 5 (18 ± 4)	4 ± 2 (4 ± 2)

*No. of cells per tissue segment of 6 μm × 500 μm. Figures in parentheses are percentages of all plasma cells.

TABLE 33–3. *Organisms Often Isolated from Patients with Immune Deficiencies*

Group	Pathogens
Bacteria	*Staphylococcus*
	Streptococcus
	Pneumococcus
	Pseudomonas
	Serratia
	Aerobacter
	Klebsiella
	Mycobacterium
Fungi	*Candida*
	Aspergillus
	Nocardia
	Histoplasma
Viruses	Herpes
	Measles
	Varicella
	Cytomegalic inclusion
	Hepatitis
	Epstein-Barr
	Vaccinia
Parasites	*Pneumocystis carinii*
	Giardia lamblia

merical and functional alterations in T lymphocytes. The proportion and number of rosette-forming T cells in the peripheral blood is reduced[24–27] (Fig. 33–1). There is a proportionate increase in "null" cells which do not bear the conventional surface markers of mature T and B lymphocytes. These null cells contain large amounts of terminal deoxynucleotidyl transferase activity[28] and in the presence of thymosin can convert to rosetting cells in vitro.[29] This would suggest that the majority of null cells are incompletely differentiated T lymphocytes. Faulty maturation is probably the result of reduced thymic hormone activity.[30]

The availability of monoclonal antibodies specific for various subsets of lymphocytes and the techniques of cell sorting and immunofluorescence microscopy have permitted investigation of changes in the number and function of T cell subpopulations. Malnourished patients have a pronounced reduction in the proportion of T4 helper cells (Fig. 33–2) and a moderately reduced proportion of T8 cytotoxic

TABLE 33–4. *Host Defenses*

Specific Immunological Responses
Immunoglobulins and antibodies
  Serum
  Secretory
Cell-mediated immunity
  T lymphocytes (e.g., helper, suppressor, cytotoxic)
  Killer cells

Nonspecific Factors of Resistance
Skin and mucous membranes
Mucus
Visceral and ciliary movements
Phagocytes
Complement system
Opsonic function
Iron-binding proteins (transferrin, lactoferrin)
Interferon
Lysozyme
Febrile

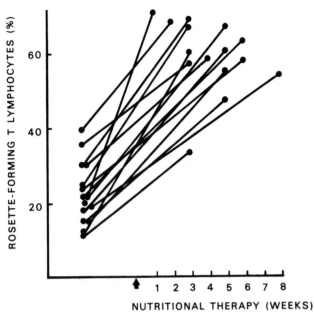

FIGURE 33–1. *Rosette-forming T lymphocytes are reduced in protein-energy malnutrition and increase rapidly back to within the normal range on nutritional supplementation.*

suppressor cells; proportions return to normal when the patients recover.[31,32] These findings suggest a reduction in either the number of such cells or the density of antigen molecules on cell surfaces. Changes may also occur in lymphocyte migration. Undernourished animals show reduced homing of labeled lymph node cells.[33]

Skin reactions of the delayed hypersensitivity type are usually impaired in kwashiorkor and marasmus.[17–25] Failure of both afferent and efferent limbs of the immune response may be involved. Lymphocyte stimulation response to mitogens is reduced, which is largely explainable by a reduction of responding T cells. Furthermore, sera of malnourished individuals contain certain inhibitory factors. These include α_2-macroglobulin, IgE, acute phase

reactant glycoproteins, bacterial products and α_1-fetoprotein.

These alterations in T cell number and function are easily reversed by providing nutritional supplements to undernourished individuals (Fig. 33–1). The restoration of the immune response is very quick, and it has been suggested that immunocompetence can be employed as a sensitive, albeit nonspecific, index of nutritional status. The one group of individuals who do not show a dramatic recovery on nutritional supplements are small-for-gestational-age, low-birth-weight infants. Such children may continue to have reduced number of T cells and impaired in vitro proliferation responses for many months and even years after birth.[34] The intergenerational effect of malnutrition on immune response has been clearly documented in laboratory animals.[36] The clinical significance of these observations requires follow-up of such infants.

Malnutrition is a composite of deficiencies of many nutrients. It has been shown that many dietary factors, including iron, selenium, zinc, folate, vitamin A, pyridoxine, and lipids influence cell-mediated immunity. Moreover, even subclinical deficiencies of some nutrients may alter T cell function.

Humoral Immunity

Immunoglobulins and antibodies provide an effective defense against many microorganisms, promote phagocytosis, and prevent the attachment of pathogens to epithelial cells. In malnutrition, the number of B cells is normal. There is polyclonal hyperimmunoglobulinemia. This is mainly the result of repeated bacterial and parasitic infections. Also, reduced suppressor cell activity may contribute to this. Rarely, a young marasmic infant, without gross infection, may have low levels of serum IgG and other immunoglobulins. Serum IgE is moderately elevated, more so in those with parasites. The metabolic turnover of IgG is increased in those with infection and reduced in infants without infection. Antibody responses in malnourished individuals and animals have been extensively studied and are reviewed elsewhere. In general, antibody response is normal, particularly if the dose of the antigen is appropriate, adequate numbers of boosters are given, and an adjuvant is employed. Antibody affinity is decreased.[37] T cell–dependent antigens may elicit a lower response in malnourished individuals compared with well-nourished ones. Antibody response in infected malnourished subjects is decreased (Fig. 33–3).

Mucosal surfaces are protected by a number of nonspecific factors as well as secretory IgA (sIgA). The latter is decreased in the saliva and nasopharyngeal secretions of malnourished patients.[38,39] The specific sIgA antibody response to viral vaccines, for example, polio virus and measles, is decreased.[38]

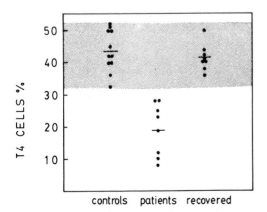

FIGURE 33–2. *Helper T4 cells are decreased in number in protein-energy malnutrition and revert back to normal proportion after nutritional recovery.*

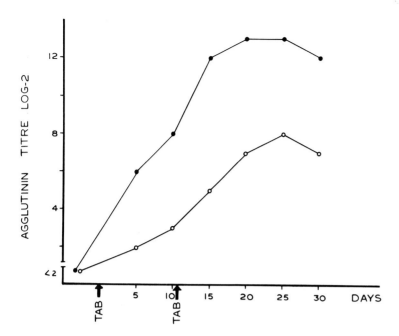

FIGURE 33–3. Serum antibody response to TAB (typhoid, paratyphoid A and B) vaccine in malnourished children with (○) and without (●) infection.

These changes in mucosal immune barrier may result in a higher incidence of septicemia and intestinal colonization, and in suboptimal protection after immunization.

In malnourished individuals phagocytosis is normal but intracellular bacterial killing is reduced.[40,41] The importance of using a discriminatory ratio of bacteria to phagocytes has been stressed recently.

Opsonic activity is related to the concentration of plasma employed in in vitro techniques. At a concentration of 5 per cent or higher, the ability of the serum to opsonize particles is comparable for both well-nourished and undernourished individuals; however, at greater dilutions the serum of malnourished children has a lower opsonic activity.[2]

The complement system contributes to the opsonic function of plasma. In malnutrition, the levels of C3, Factor B, and many other complement components are decreased.[2,42,43] The reduction in C3 is more marked in those with associated infection (Fig. 33–4). Reduced C3 levels are the result of decreased synthesis as well as increased utilization.[42]

Changes in lysozyme, interferon, and interleukin 1 and 2 production have been noted recently. These alterations in host immunity may also contribute to increased severity of infections in malnutrition.

Isolated deficiencies of single nutrients in man are rare; data from studies in laboratory animals suggest that cell-mediated immunity and antibody responses to T cell–dependent antigens is decreased in deficiencies of zinc, iron, copper, vitamins A, B_6, and E, and folic acid. Information on other nutrients is less consistent. The data on the effects of single nutrients on immunity have been recently reviewed.[5,44–46]

PRACTICAL SIGNIFICANCE

There is much of clinical importance in recent observations in the area of nutrition and immunity.

First, immunological tests can be used as functional indices of nutritional assessment.[12] Second, preoperative anergy may signify an enhanced risk of postoperative complications (Table 33–5). Those who show negative response to a battery of recall antigens have a fivefold increase in infection and mortality. The predictive value of this observation has been reviewed elsewhere[47] and is summarized in Table 33–6. Third, the correction of nutritional deficiency in the elderly may be expected to improve their immune responses.[48] Fourth, antibody response to conventional vaccination procedures may be condi-

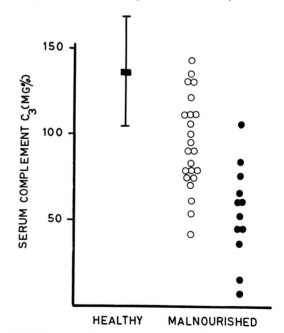

FIGURE 33–4. Serum complement levels in malnourished children with (●) and without (○) infection. The mean and 2 SD limits for well-nourished healthy children are shown as a bar.

TABLE 33–5. *Reliability of Preoperative Anergy (Absence of Delayed Cutaneous Hypersensitivity) in Predicting Postoperative Malnutrition–Associated Complications*

Outcome	Sensitivity (%)	Specificity (%)	Positive Predictive Value (%)	Negative Predictive Value (%)
Sepsis	61 (50–80)	74 (62–90)	28 (14–39)	92 (84–97)
Mortality	49 (37–60)	74 (60–88)	25 (21–29)	91 (90–92)

Data are shown as mean (and range) of values obtained from several studies, largely based on adults undergoing major surgery for a variety of primary diagnoses

TABLE 33–6. *Nutritional Status and Skin Reactivity as Predictors of Postoperative Sepsis and Mortality in Adults Undergoing Major Surgery*

	Number of Patients	Number with Sepsis (%)*	Number of Deaths (%)
Nutritional status:†			
Malnourished	51	12 (23.5)	2 (3.9)
Well nourished	160	9 (5.6)	1 (0.6)
Skin reactivity:‡			
Anergic	59	14 (23.7)	2 (3.4)
Reactive	152	7 (4.6)	1 (0.6)

*Postoperative wound infection, positive blood culture, pneumonia.

†Based on clinical, anthropometric (weight for height < 80%), and biochemical (albumin < 3.0 g/dl) data.

‡To one or more of: *Candida, Trichophyton,* streptokinase-streptodornase, tetanus toxoid, tuberculin.

tioned by nutritional status.[38,49] Fifth, one must caution against the excessive intake of certain trace elements. This practice may also compromise immunocompetence, as observed recently in the case of zinc.[50] Finally, nutrition may be a significant contributing factor to the development of such ill-understood entities as cancer[1] and acquired immune deficiency syndrome[51] and the occurrence of complications such as opportunistic infections.

References

1. Chandra RK, Newberne PM. Nutrition, Immunity and Infection, Mechanisms of Interactions. New York, Plenum, 1977.
2. Chandra RK. Immunology of Nutritional Disorders. London, Edward Arnold, 1980.
3. Chandra RK. Immunodeficiency in undernutrition and overnutrition. Nutr Rev 1981; 39:225–231.
4. Good RA. Nutrition and immunity. J Clin Immunol 1981; 1:3–9.
5. Beisel WR. Single nutrients and immunity. Am J Clin Nutr 1982; 35:417–418.
6. Chandra RK. Nutrition, immunity and infection: present knowledge and future directions. Lancet 1983; 1:688–691.
7. Gurr MI. The role of lipids in the regulation of the immune system. Prog Lipid Res 1983; 22:257–287.
8. Keusch GT, Wilson CS, Waksal SD. Nutrition, host defenses, and the lymphoid system. In Gallin JI, Fauci AS (eds). Advances in Host Defense Mechanisms. Vol. 2. New York, Raven Press, 1983: 275–359.
9. Dowd PS, Heatley RV. The influence of undernutrition on immunity. Clin Sci 1984; 66:241–248.
10. Johnston PV. Dietary fat, eicosanoids, and immunity. Adv Lipid Res 1985; 21:103–141.
11. Scrimshaw NS, Taylor CE, Gordon JE. Interactions of nutrition and infection. WHO Monograph Series, 57, 1968.
12. Chandra RK. Immunocompetence as a functional index of nutritional status. Br Med Bull 1981; 37:89–94.
13. Tomkins A. Nutritional status and severity of diarrhoea among pre-school children in rural Nigeria. Lancet 1981; 1:860–862.
14. Sinha DP. Measles and malnutrition in a West Bengal village. Trop Geogr Med 1977; 19:125–134.
15. Smedman L, Lindeberg A, Jeppsson O, et al. Nutritional status and measles: a community study in Guinea-Bissau. Ann Trop Pediat 1983; 3:169–176.
16. Chandra RK. Primary and Secondary Immunodeficiency Disorders. Edinburgh, Churchill Livingstone, 1983.
17. Harland PS. Tuberculin reactions in malnourished children. Lancet 1965; 2:719–721.
18. Smythe PM, Brereton-Stiles GG, Grace HJ, et al. Thymolymphatic deficiency and depression of cell-mediated immunity in protein-calorie malnutrition. Lancet 1971; 2:939–943.
19. Chandra RK. Immunocompetence in undernutrition. J Pediatr 1972; 81:1194–1200.
20. Neumann CG, Lawlor GJ Jr, Stiehm ER, et al. Immunologic responses in malnourished children. Am J Clin Nutr 1975; 28:89–104.
21. Ziegler HD, Ziegler PB. Depression of tuberculin reaction in mild and moderate protein-calorie malnourished children following BCG vaccination. Johns Hopkins Med J 1975; 137:59–64.
22. Kielmann AA, Uberoi IS, Chandra RK, et al. The effect of nutritional status on immune capacity and immune responses in preschool children in a rural community in India. Bull WHO 1976; 54:477–483.
23. Sinha DP, Bang FB. Protein and calorie malnutrition, cell-mediated immunity, and B.C.G. vaccination in children from rural West Bengal. Lancet 1976; 2:531–534.
24. Chandra RK. Rosette-forming T lymphocytes and cell-mediated immunity in malnutrition. Br Med J 1974; 3:608–609.
25. Ferguson AC, Lawlor GJ Jr, Neumann CG, et al. Decreased rosette-forming lymphocytes in malnutrition and intra-uterine growth retardation. J Pediatr 1974; 85:717–723.
26. Bang BG, Mahalanabis D, Mukherjee KL, et al. T and B lymphocyte rosetting in undernourished children. Proc Soc Exp Biol Med 1975; 149:199–202.
27. Puri V, Misra PK, Saxena KC, et al. Immune status in malnutrition. Indian J Pediatr 1980; 17:127–132.
28. Chandra RK. T and B lymphocyte subpopulations and leukocyte terminal deoxynucleotidyl-transferase in energy-protein malnutrition. Acta Paediatr Scan 1979; 68:841–845.
29. Jackson TM, Zaman SN. Effect of thymopoietin on rosette formation in vitro in malnutrition. Clin Exp Immunol 1980; 39:717–721.
30. Chandra RK. Serum thymic hormone activity in protein-energy malnutrition. Clin Exp Immunol 1979; 38:228–230.
31. Chandra RK, Gupta S, Singh H. Inducer and suppressor T cell sets in protein-energy malnutrition. Analysis by monoclonal antibodies. Nutr Res 1982; 2:21–26.
32. Chandra RK. Numerical and functional deficiency in T helper cells in protein energy malnutrition. Clin Exp Immunol 1983; 51:126–132.
33. Chandra RK. The nutrition-immunity-infection nexus: The enumeration and functional assessment of lymphocyte subsets in nutritional deficiency. Nutr Res 1983; 3:605–615.
34. Chandra RK. Fetal malnutrition and postnatal immunocompetence. Am J Dis Child 1975; 129:450–454.
35. Moscatelli P, Bricarelli FD, Piccinini A, et al. Defective im-

munocompetence in foetal undernutrition. Helv Paediatr Acta 1976; *31*:241–247.

36. Chandra RK. Antibody formation in first and second generation offspring of nutritionally deprived rats. Science 1975; *190*:289.

37. Chandra RK, Chandra S, Gupta S. Antibody affinity and immune complexes after immunization with tetanus toxoid in protein-energy malnutrition. Am J Clin Nutr 1984; *40*:131–134.

38. Chandra RK. Reduced secretory antibody response to live attenuated measles and poliovirus vaccines in malnourished children. Br Med J 1975; *2*:583–585.

39. Watson RR, Reyes MA, McMurray DN. Influence of malnutrition on the concentration of IgA, lysozyme, amylase and aminopeptidase in children's tears. Proc Soc Exp Biol Med 1978; *157*:215–219.

40. Seth V, Chandra RK. Opsonic activity, phagocytosis and bactericidal capacity of polymorphs in undernutrition. Arch Dis Child 1972; *47*:282–284.

41. Schopfer K, Douglas SD. Neutrophil function in children with kwashiorkor. J Lab Clin Med 1976; *88*:450–461.

42. Chandra RK. Serum complement and immunoconglutinin in malnutrition. Arch Dis Child, 1975; *50*:225–229.

43. Haller L, Zubler RH, Lambert PH. Plasma levels of complement components and complement haemolytic activity in protein-energy malnutrition. Clin Exp Immunol 1978; *34*:248–252.

44. Chandra RK, Dayton DH. Trace element regulation of immunity and infection. Nutr Res 1982; *2*:721–733.

45. Chandra RK. Trace elements and immune response. Immuno Today 1983; *4*:322–325.

46. Vyas D, Chandra RK. Functional consequences of iron deficiency. *In* Stekel A (ed). Iron Deficiency. New York, Raven Press, 1973.

47. Puri S, Chandra RK. Nutritional regulation of host resistance and predictive value of immunologic tests in assessment of outcome. Pediatr Clin N Am 1985; *32*:499–516.

48. Chandra RK, Joshi P, Au B, et al. Nutrition and immunocompetence of the elderly: effect of short-term nutritional supplementation on cell-mediated immunity and lymphocyte subsets. Nutr Res 1982; *2*:223–232.

49. Chandra RK, Puri S. Nutritional support improves antibody response to influenza virus vaccine in the elderly. Br Med J 1985; *291*:705–706.

50. Chandra RK. Excessive intake of zinc impairs immune responses. JAMA 1984; *4*:322–325.

51. Jain VK, Chandra RK. Does nutritional deficiency predispose to acquired immune deficiency syndrome? Nutr Res 1984; *4*:537–543.

34

METABOLIC RESPONSE TO INFECTION

WILLIAM R. BEISEL

Infectious diseases are the most common kinds of illness to afflict mankind; on a global basis they account for more deaths each year than any other form of disease. Even the normally healthy person will experience multiple episodes of individual infection throughout a lifetime. Because of the natural defense mechanisms of the body and, on occasion, the added assistance of antimicrobial therapy, the normally healthy person will usually be able to control most kinds of infecting microorganisms and recover fully from infectious illnesses after only a brief period of incapacitation.

Having a multiplicity of innate resistance mechanisms and the capacity to develop specific immunity against previously experienced antigens, normal persons are able to prevent or eliminate an invasion by microorganism species that are typically present in the usual body flora and surrounding environment, and to do so without experiencing overt disease. The human host is hardly ever free of small localized inflammatory lesions on the skin and mucous membrane surfaces, but these seldom lead to a generalized illness. However, microorganisms with high degrees of virulence, or those which penetrate anatomical barriers in unusually large numbers, can overcome the initial resistance mechanisms of the normal person to initiate an acute infectious process, with or without clinical disease. These infections are usually followed by a full recovery, but they may become subacute or chronic, or if sufficiently severe, they may overwhelm host defenses and progress to a fatal outcome.

Any process that serves to eliminate or weaken one or more of the normal host resistance mechanisms will increase the opportunity for an invading infectious microorganism to produce clinical disease.[1] Congenital deficiencies involving a nonspecific (or generalized) host defensive mechanism or an immune system component, traumatic processes that penetrate normal anatomical barriers and allow mi-

---

The views of the author do not purport to reflect the positions of the Department of the Army or the Department of Defense.

croorganisms to enter the tissues, the presence of foreign bodies, or the development of diverse disease processes or malignancies can all increase the opportunities for an infectious microorganism to produce disease.[1,2]

On a worldwide basis, the malnutrition associated with poverty and famine is a highly important cause of depressed host resistance, and this can lead, in turn, to life-threatening serious infections. Furthermore, severe disease processes such as malignancy, trauma, cardiac decompensation, and pulmonary, hepatic, or renal dysfunction can each lead to a malnourished state that weakens host resistance mechanisms and predisposes the patient to an invasion by microorganisms. Such superimposed infections are often caused by opportunistic organisms that lack the virulence factors necessary to produce disease in a healthy person.

Host nutrition and infectious illnesses are therefore closely interrelated. These interrelationships can best be understood by learning how an infectious process affects the nutritional status of the host, and, conversely, how an altered nutritional state can influence host resistance or susceptibility to an infection.

CONCEPTS OF INFECTION-INDUCED EFFECTS ON NUTRITION

Acute febrile illnesses typically stimulate a broad and complex, but highly predictable, array of metabolic and physiological responses.[3,4] These predictable responses are considered to be "generalized" or "nonspecific" because they are similar and consistent despite the nature of the infectious agent or inflammatory response that causes them.[5] These generalized acute-phase responses appear to be purposeful, in that they are initiated by endogenous control mechanisms. These responses apparently serve to enhance all nonspecific and antigen-specific defensive mechanisms that help to eliminate invading microorganisms and repair residual damage.[1,2] The metabolic and physiological responses to a generalized infection induce nutritional losses from body stores. These losses generally reflect the severity and duration of an illness.[3,4] Losses of body nutrients are also influenced by the age, sex, and previous nutritional status of the patient, and by the presence of any underlying medical or surgical problems. Infection-induced nutritional losses are influenced by a complex array of biochemical, metabolic, and endocrine responses and by the release of endogenous mediators from certain specialized body cells.[6,7] These responses are related to the progression and regression of the infectious process itself.[3] The sequential patterns of these metabolic and physiological responses develop and then regress in a relatively orderly and predictable manner. Infections that become localized cause additional forms of nutrient loss.

Metabolic and physiological reactions during a generalized acute-phase response to an infectious illness are closely coordinated.[1,6] The acute-phase response is characterized by the generation of fever and hypermetabolism, the production of leukocytic and inflammatory actions, and the secretion of hormones and endogenous mediators. Also, skeletal muscle protein undergoes rapid catabolism in order that amino acids already present within the body can be redistributed and used to manufacture additional glucose and a variety of unique proteins. Other changes in the metabolism of nitrogen, carbohydrates, lipids, minerals, and vitamins are included in the generalized acute-phase response to infection.

Localized infections can also result in metabolic and nutritional derangements that may be superimposed on the responses due to the generalized forms of infection. However, the consequences of a localized infection, such as diarrhea, may cause the nutritional losses to exceed (in both speed and magnitude) the losses of a generalized infection that does not produce diarrhea.

Nutritional losses incurred during an infectious illness cannot be sustained indefinitely. When the supplies of readily mobilized nutritional substrates such as the amino acids become exhausted, the resultant deficiencies can seriously weaken the ability of the body to defend itself against a subsequent or intercurrent infection, or to repair infection-induced damages in various organs and tissues.[2-4] Thus, there is a tendency for the sequence of infection and malnutrition to develop into a synergistic cycle, with each new infection causing more profound nutritional losses. Such a vicious cycle, or downhill spiral, is seen most often in the young children of underdeveloped nations, but it is also a common consequence of serious medical or surgical illnesses or trauma. Unless nutritional support is provided as an integral part of therapy for patients with severe disease with septic complications, life-threatening nutritional deficits can occur, even in the most modern of medical treatment centers.

Generalized infectious illnesses are thus typified by a concomitant acceleration of both anabolic and catabolic phenomena.[3] During the hypermetabolic state that characterizes febrile infections, glycogen stores, fat depots, newly synthesized glucose, and skeletal muscle protein are utilized or consumed in excess amounts through physiologically controlled, apparently purposeful molecular mechanisms.[8] This process has colorfully been termed "septic autocannibalism."[9] These catabolic mechanisms serve to generate endogenous nutrient substrates from stores already present within the body. This process is used to provide metabolic energy and substrate molecules which help activate and sustain a variety of host defensive mechanisms used to control or terminate the infection. Although these complex anabolic and catabolic responses occur in generalized infections of all varieties, and although these responses appear to have ultimate benefit for host survival, the catabolic phenomena are not without their nutritional costs.[4]

All host defensive systems are dependent upon anabolic phenomena that lead to the production of new protein molecules.[1] Creation of many varieties of highly specialized proteins would thus appear to be one of the major purposes of the generalized acute-phase metabolic response during an infectious process.[10] New proteins must be synthesized during the creation of additional phagocytic cells, fibroblasts, clones of specialized lymphocytes, and antigen-specific plasma cells needed for the production of immunoglobulins. Hepatic cells must produce various "acute-phase" proteins for secretion into plasma, as well as additional enzymes and metallothioneins for their own intracellular use. Protein and peptide hormones are synthesized by endocrine glands.[11] Lymphokines, monokines, lysozyme, and interferons are also produced by various body cells in direct support of host defensive mechanisms.[12] The body seems willing to sacrifice components of its nonessential tissues in order to achieve these objectives. However, if these endogenous supplies of free amino acids and other nutrients become exhausted and cannot be resupplied, the continued presence of an infectious process may then lead to widespread functional failure of many intracellular processes, and, ultimately, to the failure of multiple organs and to death of the host.[9]

CONCEPTS OF NUTRITIONAL EFFECTS ON HOST RESISTANCE

The nutritional status of a patient before, during, and after an infectious illness can influence the adequacy of general host resistance mechanisms as well as immune system competence.[1,2,13] The immune system provides the body with a capacity to respond to specific foreign antigens. The immune system is enormously complex and highly integrated, with regulatory checks and balances that control each response. The immune system, with all its components, is rapidly responsive, continually vigilant, and highly precise in its ability to recognize and detect foreign antigens. Intercellular mechanisms serve to amplify the immunological response to foreign antigens, and to provide a superb capacity for "memory," by quickly responding to previously encountered antigens.

Generalized nonimmunological aspects of host defense are composed of native, natural or antigen-nonspecific resistance mechanisms. Like the immune system, these nonspecific mechanisms have cellular, humoral, and secretory components. These defenses are considered nonspecific because they respond similarly to a wide variety of different diseases and inflammatory or traumatic processes.[1] Lymphoid tissues of the immune system, macrophages, and other nonspecific host defensive cells have an ability to influence each other. These cells accomplish this communication by the production and release of various enzymes, biologically active molecules, and endogenous mediators. They also produce substances that can react directly or indirectly, and in a synergistic manner, to reduce or prevent the growth of invading microorganisms.[10,12]

Infectious or parasitic organisms initiate bidirectional interactions with the defensive mechanisms of the host, both immunological and nonspecific. The influences of nutritional status on these defensive mechanisms and on microorganisms survival are also complex.[1] In most bacterial diseases, serious malnutrition is detrimental to survival.[1] Some viral diseases, however, may not progress as rapidly or become as severe in a person who is severely malnourished. This curious phenomenon results from the necessity of viruses to utilize the molecular mechanisms of host cells in order to replicate. Viral growth may thus be reduced if the host is suffering from nutrient deprivations that impair cellular metabolic processes.[2]

METABOLIC RESPONSES DURING ACUTE UNCOMPLICATED INFECTIONS

When pathogenic microorganisms penetrate body defenses to begin an infectious process, the first interactions are with individual body cells. These initial interactions are dependent in large measure upon the species of invading organisms and the kinds of body cells that respond to the invaders.[1] Microorganisms that usually replicate in extracellular locations are handled by cells with phagocytic capabilities, such as neutrophils, blood monocytes, and tissue macrophages. On the other hand, viruses and obligate intracellular bacteria or parasites must enter some specific type of host cell (such as a hepatocyte, lymphocyte, or nerve cell) to begin their multiplication.

Metabolic changes begin to occur almost immediately in a host cell that interacts with an invading organism. This interaction can involve a burst of cellular respiration when phagocytosis is initiated, the consumption of nutrients by obligate intracellular bacteria and parasites, or in cells invaded by a virus, the takeover and control of molecular pathways within host cells by enzymes released by the virus. A phagocytic event is generally followed by phagosome formation, an activation of cationic proteins, proteases, hydrolases, lysozyme, and myeloperoxidases, and ultimately by the generation of superoxide, singlet oxygen, and other reactive oxygen radicals.[3]

During the initial phases of an infection, the incubation period, metabolic responses are largely confined to the cells that are interacting with the invading organisms. Detectable changes in body-wide metabolic processes are initially quite subtle.

However, with the appearance of generalized symptoms and fever, widespread changes in body metabolism begin to appear.[1] These changes are easily measured and, in combination, they constitute the metabolic acute-phase responses to a generalized acute uncomplicated infection. These generalized changes are initiated by endogenous cellular products released in direct response to the invading microorganism, to toxic substances produced or released by some varieties of pathogenic microorganisms, or to biologically active substances released from cells that participate in an inflammatory reaction.[6,7,10,12,14] Once an infectious process has induced a generalized symptomatic illness, metabolic responses are remarkably consistent in their characteristic patterns of multiple organ participation and in their sequential evolution.[3,4]

Stereotypical Patterns of Generalized Response

Generalized infectious illnesses of all varieties lead to a highly predictable series of biochemical, metabolic, and hormonal responses.[3,5] In combination with fever and anorexia, these responses lead to both the hypermetabolism and hypercatabolism that cause losses of somatic cell protein and a depletion of body nutrient stores. Negative balances with losses of nitrogen and other intracellular constituents, and a decrease in body weight, typify the expected consequences of the generalized increase in metabolic activity during fever.[3,15]

Although nutritional depletion must be recognized as the most prominent consequence of an acute infectious illness, the sequential array of changes in body metabolism actually represents an admixture of both anabolic and catabolic components.[3] Each 1° C of fever causes basal oxygen consumption of the body to increase by about 13 per cent.[15] The resultant increase in cellular energy needs and expenditures occurs at the same time that food intake is diminished by anorexia. In the face of a diminished intake of nutrients, cellular energy needs are supplied chiefly by substrates derived from sources already contained within body tissues.[15] Free amino acids, mobilized through catabolic processes in skeletal muscle and somatic proteins, are used as an important source of the extra energy needed during fever.[8,15]

Redistribution of certain trace elements accompanies the acute febrile illness and is a part of the stereotypical response to infection.[6,16] Iron and zinc are both redistributed through mechanisms that lead to their storage in the liver and other tissue.[3] Copper, on the other hand, increases in plasma because of an increased hepatic synthesis of ceruloplasmin, one of the acute-phase protein reactants.[3,10]

The generalized host metabolic responses may be modified by a number of factors. These include the severity and duration of an infection or its possible progression to subacute or chronic phases, the age and sex of the patient, the presence of genetic resistance factors or partial immunity, coexisting disease or trauma, and the pre-existing nutritional status of the host. Upon this generalized array of expected stereotypical metabolic changes may be superimposed some additional metabolic consequences of the infections that become localized within certain anatomical sites or organ systems.[2,3]

The number of discrete metabolic responses during infectious illnesses is large and complex. Accordingly, responses discussed in the following paragraphs will be grouped into major categories of change, and will include those of protein, carbohydrate, and fat metabolism as well as changes in vitamin, electrolyte, mineral, and trace element metabolism.

Changes in Protein, Amino Acid, and Nitrogen Metabolism

Body proteins are both synthesized and catabolized at an accelerated rate during acute febrile infections, but the varieties of proteins selected for synthesis are considerably different from those of the normal state.[10]

Protein Catabolism. The accelerated catabolism of skeletal muscle protein during febrile infection is stimulated by endogenously produced mediators that activate the proteolytic enzymes of muscle cells.[17–20] These mediators are now grouped under the name interleukin 1.[12] Although proteolysis in skeletal muscle can be quite extensive during severe illness, this process appears to be of ultimate value for host survival.[4] Skeletal muscle protein typically contains a metabolically dynamic, nutritionally balanced, labile "bank" of amino acids. With severe trauma, infection, or widespread inflammatory states, the labile sources of amino acids in skeletal muscle protein can be mobilized quickly for use in meeting the high-priority defensive needs of the host. Accelerated proteolysis in skeletal muscle releases free amino acids for the synthesis elsewhere of new proteins and for the generation of metabolic energy.[21,22] Proteolysis may also be accelerated in cardiac muscle.[20]

Extracellular proteins can also be utilized, or consumed in excess, as they participate in defensive functions. The acute-phase reactants, fibronectin, fibrin, and other coagulation system proteins, and components of the complement and kinin systems are catabolized in greater amounts.[10,20–28]

Amino Acid Metabolism. Branched-chain amino acids released during proteolysis can be metabolized within the muscle cells as immediate sources of energy.[22] The direct cellular oxidation of branched-chain amino acids also serves to generate amino nitrogen groups, which can subsequently be joined to pyruvate or other carbon sources via the action of aminotransferase enzymes. This molecular mechanism leads to the de novo synthesis of alanine and glutamine within muscle cells.[22] As a result, the intracellular amino acid composition of muscle is markedly altered during sepsis.[29] Further, the free amino acids that emerge from muscle tissue during early infection-induced catabolism do not coincide exactly with the amino acid composition of normal skeletal muscle protein. Owing to the sequential metabolic destruction of branched-chain amino acids (leucine, valine, and isoleucine) and the synthesis of alanine and glutamine in muscle cells, the percentage of free amino acids entering the plasma is relatively low in branched-chain group members but is increased in both alanine and glutamine.[22]

Because of the accelerated release of amino acids derived from skeletal muscle protein, plasma concentrations might be expected to increase. On the other hand, the anorexia-induced decline in dietary proteins and amino acids during infection, along with a diminished intestinal capacity to absorb nutrients, would tend to diminish free amino acid concentrations in plasma. Another phenomenon that influences these concentrations is the accelerated uptake of free amino acids by cells of the liver and other tissues for their use in protein synthesis or gluconeogenesis. The same endogenous interleukin 1 mediator that stimulates the accelerated proteolysis in skeletal muscle also stimulates the accelerated uptake of free amino acids by the liver.[6,7] As a result, the ultimate concentration of each free amino acid in plasma, during each stage of the infectious process, is dependent upon the divergent forces that control the rates of input or removal from the plasma pool. In overwhelming sepsis, plasma free amino acid patterns become severely deranged.[30,31]

Amino acids contribute an important substrate for the accelerated gluconeogenesis that takes place in the liver during acute infection.[22] During this accelerated gluconeogenesis, the nitrogenous component of alanine contributes an important substrate for an accelerated hepatic synthesis of urea.[8] Amino nitrogen, generated during transamination reactions associated with the increased utilization of amino acids for gluconeogenesis, is metabolized to produce urea. This process accounts for almost all of the infection-related increase in urea excretion.[8]

Most of the amino acids released into plasma during muscle proteolysis can be utilized either for the synthesis of new proteins or for energy production. However, only some of the tryptophan and phenylalanine released from muscle can be employed in the production of new proteins and, as a result, these two amino acids generally accumulate in excess in the plasma.[21] However, to compensate for this, the body accelerates the metabolic pathways that are normally used to degrade these two potentially toxic amino acids.

Some tryptophan can be utilized for the production of serotonin via a metabolic pathway controlled by phenylalanine hydroxylase, and some is metabolized to indoleacetic acid by the action of tryptophan-2-monooxygenase. The largest portion of excess tryptophan, however, is metabolized via the kynurenin pathway, which is controlled by the rate-limiting enzyme tryptophan oxygenase.[21] Induction of this hepatic enzyme is stimulated during infection but its induction requires the permissive presence of cortisol. Tryptophan entering the kynurenin pathway is converted into kynurenin and/or other metabolic products. These kynurenin metabolites are then excreted via the urine as diazo reactants.[21]

Phenylalanine can normally be converted to tyrosine by the action of phenylalanine hydrolase, but during infection the phenylalanine:tyrosine ratio in plasma generally increases. During severe sepsis increases may also occur in the plasma values of sulfur-containing amino acids, including taurine, cystine, and methionine. Similarly, a rise in the plasma concentration of free proline is to be expected during severe sepsis. The increase in plasma proline shows close correlation with a sepsis-induced accumulation of lactate and a decline in peripheral resistance and oxygen consumption.[32] Therefore, proline can serve as an excellent indicator of disease severity. Increased concentrations of proline in sepsis may be attributable to impaired hepatocyte capabilities and a reduced ability of Krebs cycle enzymes to function.[32]

Certain amino acids become methylated after they have first been incorporated into a body protein. When one of these proteins molecules is degraded, the methylated amino acids cannot generally be reused for the synthesis of new proteins or for other purposes, and therefore the free methylated amino acids are typically excreted into the urine without further change.[3] Histidine, lysine, and arginine can all be methylated in this manner. Measurements of the excretion of 3-methylhistidine can be used to obtain indirect information about the rates of catabolic degradation of proteins that contain it. Although the source of 3-methylhistidine appears to be limited to the contractile proteins, actin and myosin, increased 3-methylhistidine secretion in the urine generally parallels the losses in total body nitrogen and the overall catabolism of skeletal muscle protein.[3] Based on similar concepts, the post-transcriptional hydroxylation of proline produces hydroxyproline in collagen. An increase in plasma or urinary hydroxyproline is thus indirectly indicative of an excessive rate of degradation of connective tissue protein.[3]

Protein Synthesis. Protein synthesis is essential for maintaining all body defense mechanisms. Proteins are needed for the creation of new cells that participate in killing the invading organisms, for the function of immune defenses, or for the repair of structural damage. Specific new (or additional) body proteins must be also manufactured for metabolic uses within cells that contribute to host defense, or for secretion by cells into extracellular body fluids. In infection as in health, each protein to be synthesized requires the activation of a cell nucleus genome, the transcription of its messenger RNA, the production of RNA-containing ribosomes, and the assembly of free intracellular amino acids into the nascent protein chain.[33,34] In some instances sugars, lipid components, or trace elements must be added, and sometimes a precursor protein molecule may be formed that must subsequently be cleaved to a smaller size for functional activity to occur.

Protein synthesis is required for the production and function of phagocytic neutrophils, monocytes and macrophages, and various subsets of lymphocytes. Fibroblasts must also be formed to assist in repair of damaged tissues. Cells must produce the proteins required for maintenance of their intracellular organelles, endoplasmic reticulum, and exterior cell wall structures and receptors. Protein hormones and various hormone-like proteinaceous substances such as the lymphokines, monokines, and interleukins must also be synthesized during acute infections.

Hepatic cells must synthesize numerous enzymes and certain unique intracellular proteins such as metallothionein, hemosiderin, and ferritin.[3,16,21,35] A large variety of proteins must be produced during infection for secretion or release into the plasma.[10] These include the several different types of immunoglobulin, antimicrobial factors such as interferon, lysozyme, transferrin, and lactoferrin, components of the coagulation, complement, and kinin systems, fibronectin, and a variety of acute-phase reactant serum glycoproteins. These acute-phase proteins include alpha-1-acid glycoprotein, haptoglobin, ceruloplasmin, fibrinogen, various components of the complement system, and C-reactive protein.[10] Although neither the molecular nor physiological functions of some of these individual acute-phase reactant proteins is known with certainty, as a group they appear to increase the ability of the body to remove infectious microorganisms from the circulation, to enhance immune responsiveness, and to block the effects of any harmful proteases or free hemoglobin that might gain access to the plasma.

The anabolic activity that creates these various proteins needed for host defense is overshadowed clinically by the more prominent wasting effects of illness.

Nitrogen Balance. Body balances of nitrogen become negative soon after the onset of fever in most acute infections. Negative nitrogen balances are largely due to catabolic processes and the use of amino acids for energy production during the hypermetabolic period.[3,4] Negative balances can be ascribed only in small part to anorexia and the reduction in dietary nitrogen intake during infection. This rapid loss of body nitrogen during infection contrasts with a tendency for nitrogen losses to be minimized during simple starvation. Urea is a predominant component in the loss of urinary nitrogen, but urinary losses of ammonia and other nitrogen-containing components such as creatinine, uric acid, alpha amino nitrogen, and diazo reactants are also increased.[8] During acute febrile illness, 20 g or more of nitrogen may be lost per day.[4]

Changes in Carbohydrate Metabolism

The production of glucose is accelerated in patients with sepsis or other forms of febrile infection.[3,8,15] The increased glucose production during surgical sepsis is so great that it may not be slowed by infusions of 5 per cent dextrose.[36] This stimulation of gluconeogenesis is brought about by a combination of several hormones acting in concert, and also by the increased availability within the liver of the substrates necessary for enhanced gluconeogenesis.[11] Although manufacture of some glucose can also occur in the kidneys, little is known about the magnitude of renal gluconeogenesis in the infected host.

Although hyperglycemia and increased rates of gluconeogenesis typify the onset of a febrile infection, the capability of the body to sustain high glucose production cannot always be continued.[37,38] If the infectious process causes hepatocellular necrosis, or a functional failure of metabolic processes within hepatic cells, glucose production can also be diminished. Endotoxin or other microbial products may interfere with the ability of the liver to synthesize phosphoenolpyruvate carboxykinase,[39] a cortisol-induced enzyme that is necessary for the production of glucose from three-carbon compounds.

Hypoglycemia can also result from an insufficient supply of new substrate. This may occur in infants or aged individuals who lack a sizeable pool of "labile" nitrogen in their skeletal muscles, or hypoglycemia can be a problem in severe or protracted sepsis after the "labile" pool of endogenous body amino acids has become exhausted.[8]

Hormonal and Substrate Influences. Glucagon and the catecholamines stimulate the accelerated production and release of glucose by their ability to activate hepatic adenylate cyclase. Catecholamine effects, however, are generally not prominent unless cardiovascular hypotension intervenes.[40] During most acute infections, the production of adrenal glucocorticoid steroids and growth hormone is also increased. These hormonal stimuli for glycolysis and gluconeogenesis occur in the face of modest increases in rates of secretion and plasma concentrations of insulin. This infection-stimulated secretion of insulin, at a time when dietary intake is reduced by anorexia, is a unique phenomenon, inasmuch as insulin secretion typically declines to its lowest possible physiological values during periods of starvation.[11]

The hormonal settings that stimulate gluconeogenesis are assisted by the presence within the liver of all of the usual substrates for hepatic production of glucose.[8] These include lactate, pyruvate, glycerol, alanine, and the other gluconeogenic amino acids. The increased availability of certain of these substrates can be accounted for by the increased output of alanine from skeletal muscle, and of lactate produced by heightened metabolism of body tissues. The shunting of three-carbon compounds to the liver as lactate, pyruvate, and glycerol, and then back to the tissues as six-carbon glucose may be considered a "futile cycle," but this process does yield cellular energy substrates and permits the production of heat, as needed during fever.[3] Similarly, the synthesis of alanine in muscle, and its degradation in the liver to produce both glucose and urea, is an energy-inefficient mechanism, but it also serves to generate carbohydrate fuel during periods of fever.[8]

Glucose Tolerance. Early in the course of febrile infections, glucose tolerance tests become abnormal. Baseline glucose concentrations also tend to be somewhat increased. The rise of blood glucose following a glucose meal or a glucose infusion reaches higher than normal values, and the subsequent decline is slower.[3] The content of the glucose pool of the body may increase two to three times above normal in septic patients. The turnover and oxidation rates for glucose may also double, as may the rates of conversion of alanine to glucose.[36] Because these infection-induced increases in blood glucose values occur in the face of somewhat higher than normal plasma insulin values, some degree of cellular insulin resistance seems likely. This could be due to alterations in the number, or affinity, or insulin receptors on body cell surfaces, but information regarding this possibility has yet to be clarified.[11]

Changes in Fat Metabolism

Although body lipid metabolism does not exhibit changes as dramatic as those of protein or carbohydrate, endogenous fat stores of the body continue to provide a major source of necessary calories during acute infectious diseases.[41,42] Like stores of other nutrients, these lipid depots can also become depleted if an illness progresses to a prolonged chronic state. Because of sustained or high plasma insulin values, the release of free fatty acids from triglyceride stores may be partially inhibited during acute infections, although this action may be overcome by a high catecholamine output during sepsis.[41] On the other hand, the production of fatty acids and triglycerides by the liver is enhanced. In fact, if exogenous carbohydrate is administered in amounts too large to permit their concomitant oxidation by a febrile patient, the excess carbohydrate will be used for lipogenesis, as in periods of health. In some bacterial infections, especially gram-negative ones, accumulation of triglycerides in plasma may become large enough to cause the plasma to take on a characteristic milky appearance, as is typical of some hyperlipidemias.[42]

The algebraic summation of the input and removal rates for each type of plasma lipid will determine its individual concentrations. Infectious illnesses result in a wide range of plasma lipid values, with some reports describing declining lipid concentrations, while other evidence points to an increase of some lipids in plasma.[42] This diversity is especially true for cholesterol concentrations, which may increase, decrease, or remain constant; in fact, biphasic changes can occur during the course of a single infection.

The free fatty acids of plasma tend to decrease.[43] This is due, in part, to a decline in the plasma albumin that serves as their major transport protein. Free fatty acid values may also decline because of increased rates of uptake and utilization by the liver, and/or decreased release from triglyceride stores. On the other hand, twofold to threefold increases in rates of glycerol turnover in septic patients would suggest an increased release of free fatty acids from stored triglycerides. This may occur with no increase in plasma glycerol,[41] which can be used rapidly for gluconeogenesis. Additionally, the uptake and utilization of free fatty acids by skeletal muscle and the myocardium may be diminished in gram-negative sepsis or endotoxemia.[22]

During infection, the hepatic synthesis of new fatty acids from the two-carbon units of acetate appears to be accelerated. At the same time, the liver may accelerate its uptake of free fatty acids from the plasma.[42] Triglycerides, as well as their lipoprotein carriers, are also produced at an accelerated rate by the liver.[42] The lipoproteins serve to transport triglycerides and other lipid moieties into the plasma. Typically, however, the liver accumulates an excess of triglycerides during periods of infection, and these triglycerides may coalesce to form numerous lipid droplets in the hepatocytes, thus creating a histological appearance of fatty metamorphosis of liver.

Short- and medium-chain fatty acids are readily transported into hepatic cell mitochondria during infection, but the transport of longer-chain fatty acids into the mitochondria may be impaired. However, carnitine, which contributes to the mitochondrial uptake of fatty acids, does not appear to be in short supply. The degradation of fatty acids to two-carbon units within the mitochondria appears to proceed normally, but the subsequent synthesis of ketone bodies may be inhibited, at least in part.[43] Although some ketogenesis may continue, the overall amounts of ketone bodies that are formed by the mitochondria during infection appear to be much lower than the amounts typically produced by patients with degrees and durations of starvation similar to those seen in infected patients.[22,43] The heightened secretion of insulin during infection has been postulated as the cause for both the accelerated synthesis of fatty acids by the liver and the apparent inhibition of ketone body production.[43]

Although hypertriglyceridemia can be explained, in part, by the increased hepatic production of triglycerides and lipoproteins, there may be some slowing of triglyceride uptake by peripheral fat cells during infection. This is due to a decrease in the activity of peripheral, heparin-sensitive lipases that assist in the clearance of triglycerides from plasma.[44]

Changes in Vitamin Metabolism

Relatively little is known about alterations in vitamin metabolism during infectious illness, although it is the general consensus that vitamins are utilized in greater amounts than normal, and that body vitamin stores become depleted.[3] Acute infections have been followed, in some instances, by the onset of classic vitamin A deficiency states or by beriberi, pellagra, or scurvy.[45] Such complications of infection generally are seen only in persons whose antecedent nutritional state was poor. Blood concentrations of vitamin A, vitamin C, and pyridoxine may decline during acute bacterial and viral illnesses, malaria, and chronic tuberculosis.[3] Depressed vitamin concentrations have also been found to occur in the blood and tissues of laboratory animals with experimental infections. Riboflavin excretion generally increases in urine in parallel with losses of body nitrogen.[3]

There can be no doubt that an adequate availability of vitamins is necessary to permit the full maintenance of functionally adequate host defenses.[13] The adrenal cortex normally contains large amounts of vitamin C, and these stores become depleted during active steroidogenesis.[11] Neutrophils also contain large amounts of vitamin C, and these stores are also depleted during phagocytosis. The group B vitamins, vitamin C, and folic acid all contribute to the adequacy of phagocytic activity by host cells.[1,13] A number of vitamins, including vitamin A, riboflavin, nicotinamide, pyridoxine, vitamin B_{12}, vitamin E, and folate all appear to contribute to the immune functions of B and T lymphocytes, as well as to macrophage activities.[13] The antioxidant activity of vitamin E may help to protect cellular lysosomes, as reported in leprosy.[1] Parasitic infestations of the gut, especially those involving tapeworms, may divert intestinal vitamins to the parasites and thereby reduce the amounts absorbed for use by the host.[1,3]

Some antimicrobial drugs can influence vitamin metabolism. Pyridoxine depletion has been noted in patients receiving isoniazid. On the other hand, patients with tuberculosis may become overly sensitive to vitamin D and may then develop hypercalcemia.[3]

Changes in Electrolyte Metabolism and Acid-Base Balance

Fluid and electrolyte balance metabolism problems can have a profound effect on the outcome of infectious illnesses. The body tends to retain an excess of both extracellular salt and water unless severe or protracted vomiting and diarrhea are component parts of the infection and cause undue losses of intestinal and gastric fluids.[3]

Overhydration. In typical infections, an increased secretion of aldosterone causes salt to be retained by the kidneys.[11] An excess of body water may also be retained. In some diseases, such as Rocky Mountain spotted fever, the hemorrhagic fevers, and infections that localize within the cranial vault, an exaggerated secretion of antidiuretic hormone from the posterior pituitary gland may occur in a physiologically inappropriate manner.[11] Overproduction of antidiuretic hormone causes body water to be retained in excess, thereby initiating a dilutional hyponatremia with the possibility of a life-threatening fluid overload.

Dehydration. On the other hand, protracted diarrhea causes isoosmotic losses of intestinal electrolytes and fluids. In high-volume diarrheas such as occur in Asiatic cholera or *Escherichia coli* enterotoxemia, the principal losses of intestinal electrolytes involve sodium, potassium, and bicarbonate.[46] With lower-volume diarrheic losses of body fluids, or with chronic diarrheas, the loss of body potassium is greater than that of sodium, and only little bicarbonate is lost. Conversely, with vomiting, there is a loss of gastric hydrochloric acid. These isoosmotic losses via the gut can result in a serious depletion of extracellular water, with concomitant hemoconcentration and acid-base imbalances.[3]

Alterations in pH. Complications of various infectious diseases can produce every known type of derangement in acid-base balance. The onset of fever is accompanied by accelerated respiration. This tachypnea causes an exaggerated loss of carbon dioxide.[3] The respiratory alkalosis that ensues is typically seen during all early febrile infections and it persists for varying periods of time. The initial alkalosis may then be replaced by other variants of acid-base imbalance as various metabolic and physiological responses to illness begin to evolve. If the exchange of pulmonary gases is blocked because of congestion or consolidation of alveolar spaces, as in pneumonia or other pulmonary infections, retention of carbon dioxide can then lead to respiratory acidosis.[3] Similarly, if respiratory muscle function becomes impaired by paralysis in diseases such as poliomyelitis, tetanus, or botulism, respiratory acidosis will also emerge.

As an infectious process proceeds, acid metabolites tend to accumulate. These can swing the acid-base equilibrium in the direction of metabolic acidosis. With high fevers or septic shock, the production and accumulation of lactic acid are markedly increased. With severe sepsis, an increased shunting of pulmonary circulation blood will further reduce arterial blood oxygenation.[47,48] The metabolic acidosis due to any of these causes can seriously affect body cellular functions if an infection is severe and protracted.

The development of metabolic alkalosis is seen only rarely in an infectious disease, but it can occur during severe persistent diarrheas that deplete the body of potassium.[46]

Changes in Mineral and Trace Element Metabolism

With the onset of symptomatic infectious illnesses, a number of changes occur in mineral and trace element metabolism. Sizable losses of all principal intracellular elements occur. Such losses tend to be proportional to the concomitant losses of body nitrogen. Magnesium, potassium, and phosphorus losses are of this variety, as are losses of sulfur and zinc. The loss of intracellular elements can be demonstrated in vitro by subjecting tissue culture cells to a chlamydial infection.[49] If the infectious illness is associated with muscle paralysis, muscle tissue losses are still greater, and a concomitant disuse atrophy of bone will cause additional losses of the principal bone minerals, calcium and phosphorus.

Unusual, but transient, changes in phosphorus excretion are associated with respiratory alkalosis. During periods of heat-induced tachypnea, inorganic phosphates may virtually disappear for a time from urine and sweat. Despite this transient retention, major losses of phosphorus eventually occur during febrile infections along with concomitant losses in other minerals. Losses of intracellular potassium also parallel those of nitrogen in generalized infections.[3] Should diarrhea occur as a component of the illness, fecal losses of potassium and magnesium are increased disproportionately.

Although major changes in calcium balance have not been associated with infectious illnesses, other than those producing muscular paralysis, changes in calcium metabolism are undoubtedly of importance at the cellular level.[3] Because of the actions of calmodulin within cells, rates of flux of calcium across cellular membranes may be altered during acute infection. This phenomenon helps to modulate the actions of many hormones and perhaps of some of the endogenous mediators.

Three of the trace elements show unique changes in their concentration in plasma during infections and other inflammatory states. These changes are due principally to a redistribution of these elements within the body. This redistribution is initiated by the actions of the endogenous mediator interleukin 1, which stimulates the hepatic accumulation of iron and zinc and also leads to the hepatic secretion of copper as a component of ceruloplasmin.[6,7]

Within several hours after the release of interleukin 1 by monocytes and macrophages that are activated by phagocytosis or other stimuli, the liver begins to accumulate both iron and zinc. Although zinc cannot normally be stored in large amounts within the liver, interleukin 1 stimulates the hepatic synthesis of intracellular metallothioneins.[35] These unique proteins bind zinc and retain it within hepatocytes during the course of acute infections.[50] On the other hand, iron is sequestered through its incorporation into hemosiderin and ferritin in various tissue storage sites.[6,7,16] The zinc and iron tend to remain in their sequestered sites throughout the duration of an active infectious process, and because of this, the availability of iron and zinc is reduced for physiological release or utilization in other sites. A diminished intestinal absorption of iron also contributes to the hypoferremia of infection.[16]

The same mediator that stimulates the liver to sequester iron and zinc, interleukin 1, also causes the liver to synthesize and release large quantities of the acute-phase reactant proteins, one of which is ceruloplasmin.[10] The rise in serum copper is somewhat slower than the decline in plasma iron and zinc, and copper concentrations remain elevated for a somewhat longer period after an infection has been cured. The return of plasma copper to normal baseline values is dependent upon the rather long half-disappearance time of ceruloplasmin.

CONTROL MECHANISMS FOR THE METABOLIC RESPONSES

Virtually all normal metabolic pathways and intracellular molecular control mechanisms become involved in one or more ways in helping the body to survive an invasion by infectious microorganisms. The normal physiological control mechanisms used for adjusting cellular metabolic functions continue to retain their importance in regulating many of the metabolic alterations during infectious processes. But in addition to these usual physiological controls (that include both neuronal and hormonal components), the body possesses a normally inactive, ancillary, hormone-like control mechanism that can be brought rapidly into play whenever it is needed. This mechanism serves to initiate the generalized acute-phase metabolic responses to any acute infectious, traumatic, or pathological process that includes, as a component, a prominent inflammatory reaction. This standby control mechanism begins to function whenever blood monocytes or tissue macrophages are activated.[7,10,12,14] This will occur if these cells engage in phagocytosis or are stimulated by any of a variety of immunological or chemical substances. With activation, these phagocytic cells rapidly synthesize and release endogenous mediator proteins. When released into the circulation, these hormone-like mediators stimulate generalized defensive responses throughout the body. Such responses should be viewed as physiological reactions rather than as pathological events. These mediator-induced responses include the development of fever, the appearance of leukocytosis, the production of acute-phase reactants by the liver, the acceleration of skeletal muscle proteolysis, the increased flux of free amino acids into and out of the plasma pool, the redistribution of certain trace elements, the release of certain hormones, the generation of energy-yielding substrates, and, also, the activation of cells of the immunological system.[7,10,12,14] Anorexia is another prominent component of the generalized host response, but the initiating mechanism remains unidentified.

In addition to the controls exerted by neurological stimuli, hormones, and hormone-like endogenous mediators, a number of physiological events produce secondary influences on host metabolism. Fever has an important influence on all body cells by stimulating increased basal metabolic activity and oxygen consumption.[15] The inflammatory process in localized areas causes initial physiological changes and metabolic alterations in local cells. These local events can progress in severity to cause single or disseminated areas of acute pathology and necrosis, or the inflammatory process can evolve into a more chronic granulomatous reaction.

Role of the Endogenous Mediators

Endogenous mediators are released from phagocytic cells following: (1) the onset of a localized inflammatory response, (2) an infection by microorganisms that do not invade body cells, or (3) the death of host cells caused by microorganisms that replicate in intracellular locations. Localized phagocytic cells, mast cells and other tissue cells, and the circulating leukocytes and platelets all give off biologically active substances, either as secreted products or as cellular enzymes or other constituents liberated at the time of cell necrosis. Most of these endogenous substances are locally active, but some exert their effects only after escaping from the localized area. When macrophages and monocytes become activated, they produce the highly important endogenous mediator interleukin 1, which has widespread functions throughout the body in stimulating or triggering various generalized acute-phase defensive measures.[6,7,10,12,14]

The mechanism for releasing interleukin 1 represents a nonspecific type of host response, in that many different kinds of stimuli can lead to activation of the system that causes the cellular production and release of this hormone-like substance.[12] Interleukin 1 is believed to be a small protein that circulates in the form of monomers, dimers, or trimers. A unifying concept[12] postulates that interleukin 1 may act in a manner roughly parallel to the known actions of several hormones and of some toxins that stimulate a series of distinct and successive events after attachment to cellular membrane receptors. A number of hormones have been shown to exert their initial action by binding to cell surfaces and stimulating the activity of cell membrane adenylate cyclase. When activated, this enzyme generates intracellular cAMP. The cAMP acts as a second, intracellular messenger that directly triggers some unique function of the stimulated cell. The cellular effect produced by the hormone depends on the biological role of the particular cell stimulated, triggered by its molecular response to cAMP. The analogous proposed action of interleukin 1 also involves an initial binding to the cell surface, followed by the activation of cell membrane phospholipase A2. This action of interleukin 1 is similar to that of calcium ionophores, which cause an increase in calcium uptake by the cell, thereby activating effects in various types of cells identical to those of interleukin 1.[12] Following calcium uptake and the activation of phospholipase A2, there occurs a hydrolysis of phospholipids contained in the surface membrane of the cell, and the intracellular release of arachidonic acid. Arachidonic acid is analogous to cAMP in this unifying concept in that it stimulates subsequent steps of cellular activity. Again, the subsequent steps are dependent upon the responsive molecular mechanisms characteristic of the cell itself. Cells that possess an active cyclooxygenase pathway convert arachidonic acid into one of the prostaglandins, and thereby account for certain aspects of the biological activity of interleukin 1. On the other hand, cells that convert arachidonic acid to one of the leukotrienes initiate other actions known to be stimulated by interleukin 1.[12]

The cells possessing cyclooxygenase pathways include neurones, fibroblasts, and skeletal muscle contractile cells; in these cells, the actions of interleukin 1 can be blocked by certain drugs, such as aspirin or ibuprofen, that can inhibit the cyclooxygenase pathway.[12] In the temperature regulating center of the brain, the release of prostaglandin leads in turn to neuronal stimuli that produce fever. In skeletal muscle cells, prostaglandins lead to the activation of cellular proteases that cause the degradation of skeletal muscle protein. In fibroblasts, the release of prostaglandin activates collagenases that contribute to the destruction of collagen in various arthritic diseases.[12]

Conceptually, the leukotrienes could have the responsibility to serve as intracellular messengers for cellular actions of interleukin 1 that are not inhibited by the cyclooxygenase blockers. Effects of interleukin 1 not blocked by these drugs include the initiation of leukocyte production, the release of pancreatic islet hormones, and the numerous metabolic changes occurring in hepatocytes, including the accelerated uptake of amino acids, zinc, and iron and the triggering of the mechanisms for producing proteins included in the acute-phase reactant group.[12]

Interleukin 1 is now used as a single common name for several previously described substances, including lymphocyte activating factor, endogenous pyrogen, leukocytic endogenous mediator, and leukocytosis promoting (or inducing) factor.[12] It is not known if all these endogenous mediators exist as a single molecular species, or if they actually represent a family of closely related molecules. The exact structure is not known for any of the substances currently termed interleukin 1. However, it may be concluded that interleukin 1 is the key mediator of the generalized nonspecific acute-phase host response to microbial invasion or other inflammatory processes, that interleukin 1 acts in a hormone-like manner during infection and inflammation, and that the biological activities of interleukin 1 account for numerous aspects of the acute-phase reaction.[7,10,12,14]

Actions of interleukin 1 demonstrated in vitro support this concept. Stimulation of hepatocytes in culture leads to a production of fibrinogen,[51] in vivo actions on bone marrow colony cells cause an increase in their proliferation,[52] actions on skeletal muscle induce proteolysis,[17,18] effects on articular fibroblasts stimulate the release of collagenase,[53] and actions on the isolated pancreas result in the induction of insulin secretion.[54] Accordingly, secondary mediation of interleukin 1 activities by the central nervous system or other hormones need not be postulated. Some stimulating effects of interleukin 1, however, require the permissive presence of glucocorticoids.[55] These hormones must be present to allow hepatocytes to induce the production and secretion of acute-phase reactants that are not produced by the liver during normal health.[55]

It is generally believed that the major actions of interleukin 1 are beneficial for host defenses. This mediator has been shown to appear in the plasma of patients shortly before the onset of symptomatic infectious illnesses and to persist throughout the course of illness.[56] The production of fever increases body metabolic rates, and the production of insulin leads to glucose utilization. The heightened uptake of amino acid by the liver, when combined with the accelerated proteolysis of skeletal muscle, makes possible the gluconeogenic activities of the liver as well as the ability of hepatocytes to synthesize various enzymes, metallothioneins, and the acute-phase reactant proteins.[3,7,10,15]

The action of interleukin 1 on the lymphoid systems is a stimulatory one.[12] Interleukin 1 does not cause lymphocytes to proliferate, but rather it directly enhances the overall activity of B lymphocytes to express surface markers and to produce immunoglobulins.[12] It also stimulates certain T lymphocyte subsets to produce interleukin 2, which in turn stimulates proliferatve activity. Working in concert, interleukin 1 and interleukin 2 thus act as an amplifying mechanism, enabling the immune system to respond more quickly and more positively to the presence of new foreign antigens.

On the other hand, not all of the actions of the interleukin 1 mediators may be helpful to the host. By stimulating the production of collagenases by articular fibroblasts, interleukin 1 may actually contribute to damage within joint spaces during arthritic processes.[12,54] Excessively high fevers can also be dangerous to the host, triggering convulsive seizures and other harmful effects.[15]

Role of Hormones

A number of hormones play a role in the metabolic responses to infection, although the hormonal effects in some instances are of limited duration and magnitude. As a rule, host resistance is optimal when endocrine functions are normal. Too much or too little of certain hormones tends to be detrimental.[11]

Adrenal Hormones. An increased secretion of adrenal glucocorticoid hormones begins with, or shortly before, the onset of fever during most symptomatic infections.[11] However, the maximal increase in the daily rates of cortisol production during early illness generally achieves values only two to five times normal. During early illness, plasma cortisol loses its circadian periodicity and tends to maintain concentrations near, or slightly above, the plasma concentrations normally reached during peak morning hours. The increase in glucocorticoid secretion is accompanied by smaller increases in the output of adrenal ketosteroids and pregnanetriol. These ACTH-mediated adrenocortical responses do not persist beyond the onset of recovery. In fact, if an infection becomes subacute or chronic, the production and urinary excretion of adrenal corticosteroids and ketosteroids generally falls below normal.[11]

If an infectious illness progresses to an agonal stage or is complicated by the onset of septic shock, a functional failure of hepatic enzyme systems may lead to an inability of the liver to metabolize free cortisol to its water-soluble metabolites. Plasma cortisol concentrations may then increase markedly. On the other hand, if a hemorrhagic diathesis leads to adrenal gland infarction, glucocorticoid production may cease.[11]

As fever progresses, aldosterone secretion begins to increase gradually.[11] The aldosterone increase does not coincide in timing with the more rapid increases of plasma cortisol. Following cessation of fever, aldosterone secretion typically abates rather gradually, in contrast to the sharp decrease usually seen with cortisol secretion. The heightened production of aldosterone contributes to a renal retention of salt and water during acute infectious diseases. Loss of tissue constituents or body weight during an infection may be masked somewhat by a retention of extracellular fluids. In critically ill patients with septic shock, plasma aldosterone values may fall despite the fact that renin concentrations are increased.[57]

A tendency for excessive body water to accumulate during severe infections has also been attributed to an inappropriate secretion of antidiuretic hormone. Because of fluid retention during fever, the early convalescent period is often characterized by a diuresis of excess fluids.

Glucoregulatory Hormones. The glucoregulatory hormones are also intimately involved in host responses during febrile illnesses.[8,11,43] Fasting plasma concentrations of insulin, glucagon, cortisol, catecholamines, and growth hormone all tend to be increased, and the hepatic production and release of glucose is accelerated as a consequence. The increases in plasma glucagon are considerably greater than those of insulin, so that the molar ratio of insulin to glucagon tends to decrease.[43] Insulin effectiveness in peripheral tissues also seems to be impaired during febrile illness,[11,30] suggesting that some factor in the sick patient is able to alter the cellular uptake or manner of response to elevated plasma concentrations of insulin.

The production of catecholamines may increase slightly during, and even before, the onset of symptoms in mild infections.[58,59] However, catecholamine values are markedly increased during severe infections, especially those accompanied by hypotension.[31] The tissue of patients with bacterial sepsis may not respond to the catecholamines in a fully normal manner. In any event, the net response to the effects of glucoregulatory hormones during early infection is to increase the production of glucose and the release of glucose from glycogen stores. In the event of substrate depletion or hepatocellular dysfunction, gluconeogenesis cannot be sustained and hypoglycemia may occur.

Thyroid Hormones. Thyroid hormone responses do not appear to play a major role in influencing host metabolism during infection. Although thyroid hormone concentrations in plasma tend to decline during early stages of illness, the thyroid gland seems to respond quite slowly.[11,60] This combination of events cause a biphasic sequence of thyroid hormone concentrations in plasma. Early in infection, an accelerated disappearance of plasma T_4 and T_3 is typical. These changes are accompanied by reciprocal increases in reverse T_3.[60] Such phenomena are due primarily to cellular effects occurring outside the thyroid gland, although the binding avidity of plasma proteins for various thyroid hormones may be altered as well. These plasma changes are indicative of an increased utilization and deiodination, plus an altered metabolism of thyroid hormones by the liver, blood leukocytes, and other peripheral tissues.[11] This decline in plasma concentrations of the thyroid hormones is not met, as would normally be expected, by an outpouring of hormones from the thyroid gland. Rather, a sluggish response by the pituitary-thyroid axis seems to allow for a depression

in major thyroid hormone values during the early stages of infection. However, later during recovery, the thyroid gland output of its hormones tends to rebound, and hormonal values in plasma may actually overshoot their normal concentrations for a time.[11,60]

Role of Pathophysiological Events

Fever. Fever is probably the most easily recognized clinical and physiological component of the generalized acute-phase host response during early infection. Fever alters host metabolic functions by increasing the rates of intracellular metabolism in proportion to the amount of increase in body temperature.[3,15] Metabolic processes within cells are generally accelerated, and the consumption of oxygen is also stimulated. Fever may help to amplify and accelerate some of the other metabolic effects of interleukin 1.[12] There is evidence that the ability of lymphocytes to function and to secrete immunoglobulins is enhanced at the higher body temperatures achieved during the clinical fevers seen with most infectious illnesses.

Anorexia. Anorexia also plays a role in influencing host metabolic activities by decreasing the intake of dietary nutrients.[3] This decrease in availability of new, exogenous substrates, at a time when fever is causing body tissues to speed up their metabolism, forces the utilization of substrates that are already present in endogenous tissue stores and depots of the body. Because of fever, the metabolic responses to a diminished dietary intake due to infection-induced anorexia are considerably different from those seen when the diminution of dietary intake is due to simple starvation.[3]

With simple starvation, body-wide adaptive metabolic responses quickly become operative. These responses are directed toward a maximal conservation of the body stores of nitrogen. Thus, during simple starvation, body energy metabolism is rapidly transformed to an almost totally fat-dependent economy. Free fatty acids and ketones are produced in excess, and these rapidly become the major fuels used to supply cellular needs. Cells of the central nervous system rapidly induce new enzymes that allow the brain to utilize ketone bodies instead of glucose as a major source of energy. Both the production and use of glucose are then minimized, along with the need to use amino acids as substrates for energy production. These adaptations serve to conserve body nitrogen stores and to reduce the output of urinary nitrogen to minimal values, approximately 2 to 3 g in the starving adult who is otherwise normal.[61] These starvation-induced mechanisms for nitrogen conservation are not initiated during the anorexia of acute infectious illnesses. Rather, body nitrogen stores are actively mobilized and consumed, both as an important direct energy source and as the additional substrates needed to produce glucose for meeting the added caloric needs induced by the presence of fever.[3] At the same time, body ketone production is minimized rather than increased.[43] As a result of infection-induced metabolic responses, negative balances of nitrogen are magnified despite the presence of anorexia, rather than being reduced as in simple starvation.

Inflammation. The development of a localized inflammatory response is attended by the usual symptoms of heat, redness, swelling, and pain. These symptoms are each related to metabolic and physiological events that take place in the localized region.[62] The initial cellular injury liberates biologically active substances that stimulate local vasodilatation, capillary wall "stickiness," and an ingress of leukocytes, which amplify the local responses. The release of locally active substances includes proteolytic enzymes liberated from the lysosomal contents of degraded phagocytes, histamine from mast cells, and serotonin from blood platelets. Fibrinogen deposition in and around zones of inflammation helps to limit the area of cellular damage. Fibrin deposition also helps to minimize the escape of proteolytic enzymes from the zone of inflammation. Eventually, the fibrin strands contribute to the healing process.[3]

As described in earlier paragraphs, the inflammatory process serves to activate local monocytes and macrophages, causing them to release interleukin 1 and other monokines.

Septic Shock. The hypotensive shock that accompanies some infections, especially gram-negative ones, causes additional changes in body metabolism. These changes are due to the slowing and stagnation of blood flow, to red cell pooling, and ultimately to a diminished delivery of oxygen to peripheral vascular beds.[31,37,47,48,63–65] The resultant pathological conditions are accompanied by an exaggerated production of lactic acid and other acidic metabolic wastes. Under these circumstances, individual cells of various organs and tissues cannot maintain their normal metabolic capacity to perform biochemical and physiological functions. With the metabolic failure of individual cells, functional failure of single or multiple organs will follow. All of these phenomena represent pathological changes that are superimposed upon, but are not a part of, the generalized early metabolic and physiological responses to an infectious illness.

Localized Infections. The localization of an infectious process within a single organ system can also disrupt the function of individual cells and the organ itself. The metabolic consequences differ from, but may be superimposed upon, the generalized acute-phase metabolic responses to an infectious process. Hepatitis viruses or other viruses with hepatic trophism can directly affect the function of individual liver cells and lead to death of hepatocytes. Such a viral localization can seriously impair hepatic function for varying periods of time. Since the liver plays a highly important role in support of the generalized acute-phase metabolic responses to infection, loss of hepatic functions can have serious consequences.[37] The most important of these involve the inability to produce and secrete bile acids, to manufacture glucose, and to degrade or metabolize potentially toxic substances. Dangerous hypoglycemia is of possible clinical importance in severe hepatitis. Failure to metabolize free amino acids in a normal manner may be expected to lead to hepatic encephalopathy, as manifested by characteristic neuromuscular contractions and eventually by coma. During the course of acute viral hepatitis, generally in the second week, the sequestration of iron within the liver can no longer be maintained, and hyperferremia can result.[3] Disturbances in the binding of zinc to its plasma carrier molecules (proteins and certain amino acids) have also been described during acute viral hepatitis.[3]

Similarly, acute nephritis can lead to physiological disruptions of kidney function and to the changes in body metabolism typically associated with renal failure and uremia. As previously mentioned, severe pulmonary consolidation or respiratory muscle paralysis can lead to an impaired exchange of respiratory gases, anoxia, and derangements in acid-base metabolism. Myocarditis or pericarditis can produce cardiovascular system dysfunction. In addition, infections that become localized within the cranial vault can often stimulate an inappropriate secretion of antidiuretic hormone, followed by an abnormal accumulation of total body water and the possibility of a fluid overload in the cardiovascular system.[3,11]

NUTRITIONAL CONSEQUENCES OF ACUTE INFECTIOUS ILLNESS

All symptomatic acute infectious illnesses generate biochemical and metabolic responses that influence the nutritional status of the host. The major nutritional consequences are the result of a depletion of body nitrogen and the loss of elements that are normally found in intracellular locations.[3] Losses of bony minerals and extracellular electrolytes can also occur under circumstances described in previous paragraphs. In addition, most generalized infections cause some loss of vitamin stores, although infection-induced vitamin depletion seldom becomes clinically overt in patients seen in the "developed" nations.

The magnitude of these individual nutrient losses is dependent on several factors, including the severity of illness, the magnitude of fever, and the duration of illness.[3] These factors, in turn, may hinge upon the pre-illness presence of any cellular or humoral immunity that can provide some degree of protection from the invading microorganism. Nutritional losses will also be influenced by the antecedent nutritional status of the patient at the time the infectious process begins. Chronic severe infections, such as tuberculosis, can markedly deplete the body of its nutritional stores and lead to a dangerous state of cachexia. On the other hand, parasitic infestations that establish a chronic symbiotic relationship with the host may have little apparent effect on nutritional status.

Depletion of Stored Body Nutrients

A depletion of the nutrients stored in body tissues does not generally begin during an infectious process until after the onset of symptoms and fever. Metabolic changes within single cells during the period of an incubating illness are generally too subtle to cause a measurable nutritional depletion, although biochemical values in plasma or tissues may be influenced.[3]

Nitrogen Losses. With the onset of fever, the combination of anorexia and the enhanced production of glucose from amino acid substrates leads to the hepatic synthesis of urea.[8] Urinary losses of urea plus those of other nitrogenous compounds such as creatinine, uric acid, alpha-amino nitrogen, and the diazo reactants, in combination with varying degrees of anorexia, produce sizeable losses of body nitrogen.[3] Additional nitrogen can be lost directly through sweat or exudates, or via a loss of blood, if hemorrhage is a part of the infectious process. Sources of amino acids that constitute the so-called "labile nitrogen" pool within the body are located chiefly in skeletal muscle and other somatic tissues. Since these pools are finite and of relatively limited size (even in a normal healthy adult), they can become severely depleted by a week-long period of illness.[3,9] Rates of nitrogen loss are usually greatest during the first few days of fever. Thereafter, the daily losses of body nitrogen begin to taper off gradually even though fever persists.[3,4] After a febrile period of 2 to 3 weeks, continued losses of nitrogen become almost negligible, and the body re-establishes a new equilibrium in nitrogen balance despite the fact that the infectious process is still active. This new equilibrium, however, is generally re-established only when the body is markedly cachectic.[3,4]

Loss of Intracellular Nutrients. Body stores of the intracellular elements tend to be lost in relative proportion to the rates of nitrogen loss and to the normal ratio of nitrogen to each element present in skeletal muscle tissue. Elements generally lost in proportion to the losses of nitrogen include magnesium, potassium, phosphorus, zinc, and sulfur.[3] Phosphorus losses, however, may be initially minimized by the disappearance of inorganic phosphates from the urine and sweat during the period when respiratory alkalosis and hyperventilation are taking place. On the other hand, losses of phosphate may be increased if there is body immobilization (through paralysis or other factors of illness) sufficient to produce a disuse atrophy of bone. In such instances, excess bone mineral components such as calcium and phosphorus will be lost proportionately.[3] No evidence is available concerning a total-body depletion of other trace elements during infection.

Under normal conditions of health, carbohydrate stores of glycogen in tissues are quite small, but they can be used to supplement ongoing gluconeogenesis as may be required to meet cellular needs for carbohydrate fuels.[8] An infection places special demands on body systems for generating carbohydrate fuels, but these demands can generally be met as long as cellular gluconeogenic mechanisms remain functional and an adequate supply of gluconeogenic substrates can be supplied.[15] In severe or protracted infections, especially those associated with sepsis caused by endotoxin-containing bacteria or those associated with hepatocellular dysfunction, hypoglycemia and a depletion of cellular glycogen stores may be expected.[37,64] Little is known about how body cells provide (or fail to provide) carbohydrate components for the glycoproteins produced during periods of infection.

Body lipid stores are rarely depleted during the initial phases of an acute infectious illness. However, if the illness becomes subacute or chronic, fat stores will gradually be utilized to supply metabolizable free fatty acid substrates, and eventually body fat depots will become depleted.

Adequate data are not available to demonstrate chronic or measurable losses of most body vitamins. In contrast, an increase in urinary riboflavin may occur in parallel with the increased loss of body nitrogen.[3] Any depletion of body stores of other vitamins must be estimated by a lowered concentration in body fluids or cells, or, more rarely, by the specific appearance during illness of a clinically evident avitaminosis.

Conservation and Replacement of Nutrients. The depletion of body nutrients during even a mild, self-limited, short-term infection may take weeks to be restored following clinical recovery from the illness.[3,4] The depletion of nutrient stores is generally most marked shortly after the acute illness has been cured. Stores of lost body nutrients begin to be replaced during convalescence, but they are replenished only gradually. Although the nutritional losses incurred during a brief mild infection are of no great clinical importance, the same cannot be said regarding febrile infections that are severe or protracted. Careful attention to the state of body nutrition during the course of subacute and chronic infections can reduce or even prevent some of the expected depletions.[66] The maintenance during illness of an adequate intake of caloric sources derived from carbohydrate and lipid nutrients can help to minimize ongoing losses of other body nutrients, especially those involving nitrogenous compounds. If an adequate caloric intake can be maintained, the intake of high-quality protein or a balanced amino acid mixture need not be appreciably higher than normal in order to maintain nitrogen balance.[66] However, administration of nutrient mixtures that are high in their content of branched-chain amino acids seems to provide some positive benefit in helping to prevent the depletion of body nitrogen stores during serious infections.[66]

Therapeutic attempts to maintain an adequate intake of essential nutrients and energy sources take on greater importance in acute infectious illnesses of marked severity and long duration. The normally healthy, well-nourished individual who develops an easily treated or short-lived infectious illness will not suffer an appreciable depletion of body nutrients stores. Such brief illnesses do not require unusual efforts to maintain nutrient intakes during their acute course. Following clinical recovery, the body will be able to reaccumulate, over a period of time, all nutrients that were lost.[3] However, if an illness persists, or if a series of complications or secondary infections develop, the total loss of nutrients will become sizable unless prevented by appropriate nutritional therapy. If nutritional support is neglected in such instances, serious depletions of body nitrogen and stores of other essential nutrients can be anticipated.

Sequestration or Redistribution of Body Nutrients

The sequestration or redistribution of certain nutrients during infection appears to be a purposeful, physiologically controlled mechanism for assisting in body defenses against invading microorganisms.

Iron. The most prominent example of such a nutrient redistribution is the sequestration of iron within tissue stores of hemosiderin and ferritin during infectious or inflammatory states. Concomitantly, plasma iron concentrations decline, sometimes to almost nondetectable values, especially in pyogenic bacterial infections. The decline in plasma iron and the accumulation of iron in body stores begins within hours after the onset of fever or symptomatic illness. This phenomenon appears to be mediated by an action of interleukin 1. Iron sequestration then persists until the infectious disease is cured.[16]

If an infectious disease continues into a chronic state, the sequestered iron remains unavailable for use in red blood cell production. This physiological retention of iron in storage sites can lead to the so-called anemia of infection. This form of anemia resembles iron deficiency anemia, in that the red blood cells are hypochromic and microcytic and the plasma iron values are low.[16] However, in infection adequate or higher than normal amounts of iron can be demonstrated in reticuloendothelial storage sites within the liver, spleen, and bone marrow. Further, total iron binding values in plasma tend to be reduced in infections, whereas plasma ferritin values are high.

The depressed iron binding capacity and high ferritin values of infection are the reverse of changes seen in simple iron deficiency anemia.[16]

It is not certain if plasma transport proteins such as transferrin or lactoferrin play a mechanistic role in helping iron to enter storage depots during infection.[67] It is also controversial whether the accumulation of hepatic iron is caused by an accelerated uptake of iron by the liver, or a diminished release of iron from the liver. In any event, the normal flux of iron between plasma and tissue stores is altered so as to allow iron to accumulate within body storage sites. Iron is not normally lost from the body in excess quantities during most infectious diseases, unless there is overt bleeding or other losses of whole blood.[16]

The sequestration of iron appears to be an important factor in reducing the ability of iron-requiring bacteria to proliferate within body tissues. When iron enters tissue depots during infection, the plasma carrier proteins for iron (i.e., transferrin and lactoferrin) become less saturated.[16] Because the affinity constant of these proteins for binding the iron in plasma is greater than the iron binding affinity of any bacterial siderophore, the unsaturated transferrin and lactoferrin molecules provide an important mechanism for withholding free iron from its potential availability to bacterial invaders.[16] Many bacteria cannot proliferate if they lack sufficient iron, and they secrete iron-binding siderophores in an attempt to acquire iron from surrounding environments. In this regard, the release of lactoferrin by neutrophils in localized inflammatory lesions provides an additional mechanism for ensuring that extracellular iron is bound to a host protein and that its availability is thereby denied for bacterial growth. Concentrations of iron in the proper range are also necessary for some bacteria to produce toxic substances. Because of this, the reduced availability of iron can also serve to protect the body by diminishing bacterial toxin production.

In patients with severe protein malnutrition and a depletion of body nitrogen stores, a reduced ability to synthesize iron-binding plasma proteins can reduce the effectiveness of these proteins as direct antimicrobial factors. In some clinical situations, it has proved dangerous to administer therapeutic iron in large amounts to patients who are severely depleted of body protein and who have reduced concentrations of transferrin in their plasma.[68] If plasma free iron-binding proteins are diminished, they can easily be saturated by any iron given as nutritional therapy, and iron can thus be made available to bacterial invaders. Severely malnourished patients may harbor dangerous pathogens (such as bacteria causing tuberculosis or brucellosis, or malarial parasites) without manifesting symptomatic illness; if iron is given before protein malnutrition is corrected, these infections may flare up in a dramatic and dangerous manner.[16]

Zinc. Zinc is another element sequestered in the liver by the action of a purposeful physiological mechanism induced by infection.[3,7,35] Presumably the sequestration of zinc is also beneficial for host resistance, but evidence for this is less than adequate. Like iron, zinc accumulates within the liver in response to stimulation by interleukin 1.[7] The accumulation of zinc in storage forms requires an initial de novo synthesis of metallothionein by the hepatocytes.[35] The sequestration phenomenon proceeds, however, with surprising speed, and zinc concentrations in plasma begin to decline within a few hours after the onset of symptoms or fever.[35,50] Because the binding of zinc to alpha-2-macroglobulin in plasma is quite strong, the concentrations of total plasma zinc do not fall proportionately to values as low as those of iron. In fact, reductions of plasma zinc during acute infections rarely fall to below 50 per cent of normal.[3,7]

Copper. Another example of the physiological redistribution of body minerals is the hepatic production and secretion of greater than normal quantities of ceruloplasmin and the copper it contains.[3,10] Ceruloplasmin is one of the acute-phase reactant proteins induced by interleukin 1, and is produced by the liver. The increase in plasma copper during infection is somewhat more gradual than the rapid declines in iron and zinc, and because of the relatively long half-life of ceruloplasmin in plasma, copper concentrations decline gradually over a period of time after an acute infection has been cured.[3,10]

Pathological Redistributions. In some diseases associated with a dysfunction of cellular metabolic processes, excess quantities of sodium accumulate within body cells. Intracellular sodium cannot be returned in a normal manner to the extracellular fluids, apparently because the functional capacity is impaired in the sodium-pumping mechanisms of external cellular membranes. Accumulation of sodium within cells should be regarded as an example of a pathological redistribution of a body element rather than a purposeful physiological mechanism destined to help with host survival.[3]

Since the liver plays a prominent role in the sequestration and redistribution of trace elements during infection, it is not surprising that these processes may be disrupted during diseases such as hepatitis that cause functional failure in molecular mechanisms of hepatocytes. During the second week of acute hepatitis, plasma iron can become abnormally elevated, apparently because the liver fails to retain its stores of iron.[3,16] During hepatitis, there are also unexplained changes in the ability of plasma proteins components to bind zinc as macroligands, and excess amounts of zinc–amino acid microligands may be lost via the urine.[3]

Functional Effects of Malnutrition on Host Defensive Mechanisms

Loss of body nutrients and the depletion of nutrient pools generally results in a diminished capacity of host resistance mechanisms to function normally.[1,13,69,70] The depletion of body proteins and amino acid stores reduces the ability of the body to synthesize new proteins. All body defensive mechanisms are ultimately dependent on an ongoing synthesis of new proteins, but various aspects of host defense are affected to different degrees by protein deficiency.[1,13,70] Protein deficiency, especially if combined with a deficiency in energy-yielding substrates, can reduce the ability of the body to maintain the structural integrity of the anatomical barriers that normally prevent the entry of microorganisms into body tissues. Protein deficiencies also contribute to a diminished ability of mucosal and dermal surfaces to produce important secretions that normally contain antimicrobial factors, such as lysozyme, secretory IgA, or the gastric acidity required to inactivate certain bacteria.[1,70] More important, protein malnutrition causes an atrophy of body lymphoid tissues such as the thymus, the tonsils, the lymph nodes, and lymphoid follicles throughout the body.[1,13] The greatest atrophy occurs in areas normally occupied by T lymphocytes, but, in contrast, B lymphocyte and plasma cell areas are generally preserved.[1,13] These histological changes are in keeping with clinical observations that cell-mediated immune functions are more severely depressed in protein malnutrition than is humoral immunity.[70]

Deficiencies of vitamins are known to reduce the functional capacity of some of the immune system responses.[13,69] This problem is most important with deficiencies of vitamins that are necessary for the replication of cellular DNA.[13] Lack of vitamins that influence nucleic acid metabolism (i.e., vitamins B_{12}, B_6, and A and folic acid) can reduce the ability of T lymphocytes to function normally. This impairs the ability of the body to maintain an adequate cell-mediated immunity.

Deficiencies of vitamin C are especially important because they impair the functional ability of neutrophils to migrate when stimulated by chemotactic substances.[13,69] In clinical terms, severe vitamin C deficiency states are accompanied by an inability of the body to develop an inflammatory reaction.

A lack of vitamin A is important because it reduces the competence of both B and T cells of the immune system and because it interferes with the integrity of body surface structures.[13,69]

A lack of the essential fatty acids impairs the ability of body cells to maintain the normal composition of their extracellular membranes. This deficiency can have a deleterious effect on cellular functions important in host defenses, especially those of lymphocyte populations.[13,69]

Deficiencies of trace elements can have important consequences in terms of host defense. A lack of iron is especially important because many of the mechanisms required by neutrophils to kill ingested organisms are dependent on iron-containing myeloperoxidases.[13,69] Iron deficiency also leads to impaired function of B and T cells.

Zinc deficiency has important effects both on immune system competence and on the structural integrity of dermal and mucosal membranes. A lack of zinc can lead to anatomical disruptions of mucosal and epithelial barriers that normally prevent the invasion of pathogenic microorganisms. Zinc is an essential element required for synthesis of cellular nucleic acids, and therefore zinc deficiency is especially deleterious to the T cells of the lymphoid system, which are necessary for maintaining cell-mediated immunity.[13,69] Deficiencies of copper, magnesium, and selenium can also cause depressed immunocompetence.

Convalescent Period Nutrition

The early convalescent period, immediately after a successful cure of an infectious disease, is a nutritionally highly important but often neglected period in the longitudinal course of an illness.[3] The immediate convalescent period represents a time when the nutritional stores of the body are quantitatively most depleted. Although the typical patient no longer has symptoms of illness and has regained a feeling of well-being, residual nutritional deficiencies at that time make the body quite susceptible to another superimposed infectious disease.

Early convalescence is also a time of unique nutritional opportunity.[3] Any potential danger that might result from the forced feeding of a patient during acute symptomatic illness is no longer a threat. The anorexia of illness is generally replaced during the early convalescent period by the return of a normal appetite, or even by some degree of hyperphagia. This latter phenomena is most commonly seen in children. If highly nutritious foods are fed during this period of increased appetite, children may quickly be able to re-establish their normal nutritional pools, regain their normal rate of growth, or even achieve a catch-up in growth that corrects any infection-induced growth lags.[3] A similar period of increased appetite may also occur in adult patients who have recovered from an infection. From a nutritional point of view, the early convalescent period thus represents a "window of opportunity" that can be utilized to gain a relatively rapid repletion of the key nutrients that are lost during infection.[3] These nutrients can be resupplied during convalescence without the potential danger of complicating the recovery process or upsetting normal host defense mechanisms. However, unless nutrients are supplied in greater than normal amounts following an illness, the reaccumulation of body nutrient stores may take a protracted period, varying from weeks to months, depending upon the extent of infection-induced depletions.

The nutritional repletion of a person who has been seriously or chronically ill with infection and has endured severe nutritional depletion is especially important. Nutritional repletion will help to prevent reinfections that could initiate a downhill cycle or spiral of infection, worsening malnutrition, and repeated reinfections.

The immunodeficiency syndrome produced by malnutrition can generally be reversed with relative ease, and in a short time, if good nutritional support is provided.[2] There is evidence that some functional components of the complex immune system will recover their competence faster than other components during periods of nutritional rehabilitation. Thus, for short periods of time, refeeding may produce less-than-balanced functional interrelationships among various components of the immune system. However, the dangers of a long-continued, nutritionally induced immunodeficiency state are certainly greater than any potential problems that may arise from transient immune system imbalances during periods of nutritional rehabilitation.

One problem of potential clinical concern during nutritional rehabilitation, as described earlier, is that of iron overload in a protein-depleted patient.[68] Optimal treatment strategy should ensure that protein deficiencies are corrected and that plasma transferrin concentrations are re-established before the initiation of parenteral or oral iron therapy.[16] Latent infections should be treated concurrently if they can be recognized, and any re-emerging infection should be considered as an important threat.

Transitions of Infections from Acute to Subacute, Chronic, or Terminal Stages

Relatively complete data are available to define the typical pattern of metabolic and nutritional responses to an acute mild infectious disease.[3] Relatively good data are also available concerning the presence of changes in nutritional status and body composition in patients with chronic infectious illnesses and in patients with infectious complications of terminal medical and surgical diseases or malignant states.[9] However, very little is known about the metabolic, hormonal, and nutritional transitions that take place when an acute infection begins to evolve into a subacute or chronic stage, or when an acute infection becomes superimposed upon another severe disease process.

Attempts have been made to categorize and define such transitions using systematic measurements of a variety of hormonal and biochemical laboratory tests, plus physiological measurements of cardiovascular and respiratory functions.[48] Useful categories to define the immediate clinical status of a patient are based upon the concept that the initial, generalized acute-phase metabolic responses associated with acute sepsis, trauma, or both in combination are physiologically induced and controlled. These generalized responses cause the classification of a patient to change from a normal "R," or reference, state to an abnormal but physiologically regulated "A" state that represents a typical compensated stress response to sepsis or trauma.[48,65] If the acute infectious process is cured, these generalized "A" state responses abate.

Little is known about the progression of events or the control mechanisms that characterize a transition of a generalized infection to a subacute or chronic disease. However, such a transition is generally associated with a continuing low-grade or intermittent fever, a further gradual wasting of body stores of somatic proteins and fat, the development of an anemia, a diminishing of output of adrenal steroids, and a gradual transformation of body composition to that of a wasted, cachectic state.[2–4] This wasting process is accompanied, as a rule, by the development of immunological dysfunction and anergy, with defects in cell-mediated immunity being most profound.[13] Chronically infected individuals may lose their delayed dermal hypersensitivity responsiveness to all of the common antigens to which they had previously been sensitized. The nutritionally wasted, chronically infected individual has a markedly diminished ability to respond to secondary, superimposed infections by generating a fever or an appropriate leukocytosis.[1–4] Such patients may be unable to generate an inflammatory response or a granulomatous reaction in response to localized microorganisms or foreign antigens.

The occurrence of a protracted septic process creates difficult problems in a traumatized patient or in someone with a coexisting medical or surgical illness or malignancy.[9,29–32,37,47,48,64,65] If the nutritional status of the patient cannot be restored in the continued presence of these complex illnesses, physiologically controlled defensive mechanisms and cellular functions are likely to become incompetent. The abilities of modern medical and surgical techniques to prolong the lives of seriously ill patients and the introduction of drugs with antimetabolic or anti-immunological functions have combined to increase the incidence of patients who develop serious malnutrition. Thus, secondary infections with opportunistic organisms are all-too-common problems in our most modern medical centers.

With protracted sepsis and malnutrition, the earlier metabolic, hormonal, and immunological responses are again altered, marking a transition of a patient from the abnormal but physiologically controlled "A" state to a clearly pathological condition defined as the "B," "C," or "D" state.[48] The "B" state predominantly represents a progression of illness in which there is a failure of the hyperdynamic cardiovascular response to supply peripheral cellular needs. This failure is manifested by narrowed arteriovenous oxygen differences indicative of reduced oxygen extraction in tissues and by severe metabolic acidosis.[48] In the "C" state, marked septic

hypotensive shock, despite increased cardiac output, is complicated by respiratory insufficiency.[47,48,65] Physiological derangements in the respiratory distress syndrome are associated with an inadequate oxygenation of the blood, pulmonary circulation shunting, and retention of carbon dioxide in the "C" state. The "D" state is characterized by a transition of illness to include primary myocardial failure rather than peripheral vascular system dysfunction.

In addition to these pulmonary or cardiovascular complications of severe sepsis and injury, the lack of key nutrients (including oxygen) soon leads to the ultimate functional breakdown of vital intracellular mechanisms. Functional breakdown of biochemical and molecular systems of body cells can become widespread. When many vital organs or tissues are affected, multiple organ system failure ensues.[63,64] The medical and surgical approaches to managing complex problems of this sort are covered in other chapters of this book.

SUMMARY

The development of acute generalized infectious illnesses and serious inflammatory reactions is accompanied by the occurrence of a large number of interrelated host defensive measures. These constitute the generalized acute-phase response to infection, inflammatory states, or complex trauma. These responses include the development of fever and hypermetabolism, the production of a leukocytic response, the accelerated proteolysis of skeletal muscle, the generation of free amino acids from body somatic protein catabolism, the production of a number of hormones, the synthesis by the liver of acute-phase reactant proteins and of various intracellular enzymes, the acceleration within the liver of gluconeogenesis and lipogenesis with a relative suppression of ketogenesis, the redistribution and/or sequestration of various trace elements, and, importantly, the stimulation of immune system activity. These components of the acute-phase generalized, nonspecific metabolic response to acute infection are triggered by the release from activated monocytes and tissue macrophages of endogenous mediators which are currently grouped under the term interleukin 1.

The metabolic, hormonal, and physiological components of the generalized response to infectious diseases are quite uniform from one infection to another. The generalized acute-phase responses appear to have special survival value by stimulating a large variety of nonspecific host defenses as well as by activating the immune system. This latter phenomenon increases the functional capacity of lymphocytes to develop cellular and humoral immunity against specific antigens contained within the invading microorganism.

The magnitude of these generalized responses is

governed by the severity and duration of illness. However, these generalized acute-phase responses are not without their costs to the body, for they result in a wasting of muscle mass, an increased consumption of body nutrients (especially the amino acids), and absolute losses from the body of nitrogen and elements normally present inside body cells. The nutritional costs of infection are influenced importantly by the height and duration of fever, and to a lesser degree by the presence of anorexia. Infection-induced depletions of body nutrients serve to weaken host resistance.

Infections that become localized in single organ systems cause additional changes in host metabolism and nutritional losses that are superimposed upon the generalized metabolic responses described in preceding paragraphs. The complications of some infections can result in major derangements of acid-base balance and of salt and water metabolism. If acute infections are not cured rapidly, they may progress to subacute or chronic illnesses accompanied by a severe depletion of body nutrients and an eventual failure of host defensive mechanisms. Severe progressive infections can also lead to functional derangements in the respiratory and cardiovascular systems, hypotensive shock, tissue anoxia, and cardiac failure. The accompanying inability of individual body cells to maintain normal functions can also give rise to multi-organ failure and death.

References

1. Beisel WR. Nutrition, infection, specific immune responses, and nonspecific host defenses: a complex interaction. *In* Watson RR (ed). Nutrition, Disease Resistance, and Immune Function. New York, Marcel Dekker, 1984: 3–34.
2. Beisel WR. Effects of infection on nutritional status and immunity. Fed Proc 1980; 39:3105–3108.
3. Beisel WR. Metabolic effects of infection. *In* Chandra RK (ed). Progress in Food and Nutrition Science. New York, Pergamon Press, 1984.
4. Beisel WR. Magnitude of the host nutritional responses to infection. Am J Clin Nutr 1977; 30:1236–1247.
5. Wiles JB, Cerra FB, Siegel JH, et al. The systemic septic response: does the organism matter? Crit Care Med 1980; 8:55–60.
6. Beisel WR. Mediators of fever and muscle proteolysis. N Engl J Med 1983; 308:586–588.
7. Beisel WR, Sobocinski PZ: Endogenous mediators of fever-related metabolic and hormonal responses. *In* Lipton JM (ed). Fever. New York, Raven Press, 1980: 39–48.
8. Beisel WR, Wannemacher RW Jr. Gluconeogenesis, ureagenesis, and ketogenesis during sepsis. JPEN 1980; 4:277–285.
9. Cerra FB, Siegel JH, Coleman B, et al. Septic autocannibalism. A failure of exogenous nutritional support. Ann Surg 1980; 192:570–580.
10. Powanda MC, Beisel WR. Hypothesis: leukocyte endogenous mediator/endogenous pyrogen/lymphocyte-activating factor modulates the development of nonspecific and specific immunity and affects nutritional status. Am J Clin Nutr 1982; 35:762–768.
11. Beisel WR. Alterations in hormone production and utilization during infection. *In* Powanda MC, Canonico PG (eds). Infection. The Physiologic and Metabolic Responses of the Host. Amsterdam; Elsevier/North-Holland Biomedical Press, 1981: 147–172.
12. Dinarello CA. Interleukin-1. Rev Infect Dis 1984; 6:51–95.
13. Levy JA. II. Nutrition and the immune system. *In* Stites DP, Stobo JD, Fudenberg HH, et al. (eds). Basic and Clinical Immunology. 4th ed. Los Altos, CA, Lange Medical Publications, 1982: 297–305.
14. Borstein DL. Leukocyte pyrogen: a major mediator of the acute phase reaction. Ann NY Acad Sci 1982; 389:323–337.
15. Beisel WR, Wannemacher RW Jr, Neufeld HA. Relation of fever to energy expenditure. *In* Kinney JM (ed). Assessment of Energy Metabolism in Health and Disease. Columbus, OH, Ross Laboratories, 1980: 144–150.
16. Beisel WR. Iron nutrition: immunity and infection. Res Staff Phy 1981; 37–42.
17. Clowes GHA Jr, George BC, Villee CA Jr, et al. Muscle proteolysis induced by a circulating peptide in patients with sepsis or trauma. N Engl J Med 1983; 308:545–552.
18. Baracos V, Rodemann HP, Dinarello CA, et al. Stimulation of muscle protein degradation and prostaglandin E_2 release by leukocytic pyrogen (interleukin-1). A mechanism for the increased degradation of muscle proteins during fever. N Engl J Med 1983; 308:553–558.
19. Astrom E, Friman G, Pilstrom L. Human skeletal muscle in bacterial infection: enzyme activities and their relationship to age. Scand J Infect Dis 1977; 9:193–195.
20. Ilback N-G. Striated Muscle in Infection. Uppsala, Sweden, University of Uppsala, 1983; Thesis. 686:1–49.
21. Powanda MC, Dinterman RE, Wannemacher RW Jr, et al. Tryptophan metabolism in relation to amino acid alterations during typhoid fever. Acta Vitaminol Enzymol (Milano) 1975; 29:164–168.
22. O'Donnell TF Jr, Clowes GHA Jr, Blackburn GL, et al. Proteolysis associated with a deficit of peripheral energy fuel substrates in septic man. Surgery 1976; 80:192–200.
23. Mosher DF. Changes in plasma cold-insoluble globulin concentration during experimental Rocky Mountain spotted fever infection in rhesus monkeys. Thromb Res 1976; 9:37–45.
24. Fearon DT, Ruddy S, Schur PH, et al. Activation of the properdin pathway of complement in patients with gram-negative bacteremia. N Engl J Med 1975; 292:937–940.
25. Fine D, Mosher D, Yamada T, et al. Coagulation and complement studies in Rocky Mountain spotted fever. Arch Intern Med 1978; 138:735–738.
26. Wing DA, Yamada T, Hawley HB, et al. Model for disseminated intravascular coagulation: bacterial sepsis in rhesus monkeys. J Lab Clin Med 1978; 92:239–251.
27. Mason JW, Kleeberg U, Dolan P, et al. Plasma kallikrein and Hageman factor in gram-negative bacteremia. Ann Intern Med 1970; 73:545–551.
28. Satterwhite TK, Hawiger J, Burklow SL, et al. Degradation products of fibrinogen and fibrin in bacteremia due to gram-negative rods. J Infect Dis 1973; 127:437–441.
29. Askanazi J, Carpentier YA, Michelsen CB, et al. Muscle and plasma amino acids following injury. Influence of intercurrent infection. Ann Surg 1980; 192:78–85.
30. Freund HR, Ryan JA Jr, Fischer JE. Amino acid derangements in patients with sepsis: treatment with branched chain amino acid rich infusions. Ann Surg 1978; 188:423–430.
31. Marchuk JB, Finley RJ, Groves AC, et al. Catabolic hormones and substrate patterns in septic patients. J Surg Res 1977; 23:177–182.
32. Cerra FB, Caprioli J, Siegel JH, et al. Proline metabolism in sepsis, cirrhosis and general surgery. Ann Surg 1979; 190:577–586.
33. Little JS. Synthesis, transport, and secretion of plasma proteins by the livers of control and *Streptococcus pneumoniae*–infected rats. Infect Immun 1978; 22:585–596.
34. Thompson WL, Wannemacher RW Jr. Effects of infection and endotoxin on rat hepatic RNA production and distribution. Am J Physiol 1980; 238:G303–G311.

35. Sobocinski PZ, Canterbury WJ Jr, Mapes CA, et al. Involvement of hepatic metallothioneins in hypozincemia associated with bacterial infection. Am J Physiol 1978; *234*:E399–E406.

36. Long CL, Kinney JM, Geiger JS. Nonsuppressibility of gluconeogenesis by glucose in septic patients. Metabolism 1976; *25*:193–201.

37. Cerra FB, Siegel JH, Border JR, et al. The hepatic failure of sepsis: cellular versus substrate. Surgery 1979; *86*:409–422

38. Nolan JP. The role of endotoxin in liver injury. Gastroenterology 1975; *69*:1346–1356.

39. McCallum RE, Seale TW, Stith RD. Influence of endotoxin treatment on dexamethasone induction of hepatic phosphoenolpyruvate carboxykinase. Infect Immun 1983; *39*:213–219.

40. Wilmore DW, Long JM, Mason AD Jr, et al. Mediator of the hypermetabolic response to thermal injury. Ann Surg 1974; *180*:653–699.

41. Carpentier YA, Askanazi J, Elwyn DH, et al. Effects of hypercaloric glucose infusion on lipid metabolism in injury and sepsis. J Trauma 1979; *19*:649–654.

42. Beisel WR, Fiser RH Jr. Lipid metabolism during infectious illness. Am J Clin Nutr 1970; *23*:1069–1079.

43. Neufeld HA, Pace JG, Kaminski MV, et al. A probable endocrine basis for the depression of ketone bodies during infectious or inflammatory state in rats. Endocrinology 1980; *107*:596–601.

44. Kaufmann RL, Matson CF, Rowberg AH, et al. Defective lipid disposal mechanisms during bacterial infection in rhesus monkeys. Metabolism 1976; *25*:615–624.

45. Scrimshaw NS, Taylor CE, Gordon JE. Interactions of nutrition and infection. WHO Monograph Series 1968; *57*:148–166.

46. Watten RH, Morgan FM, Songkhla YN, et al. Water and electrolyte studies in cholera. J Clin Invest 1959; *38*:1879–1889.

47. Clowes GHA Jr, Hirsch E, Williams L, et al. Septic lung and shock lung in man. Ann Surg 1975; *181*:681–692.

48. Siegel JH, Giovannini I, Coleman B. Ventilation:perfusion maldistribution secondary to the hyperdynamic cardiovascular state as the major cause of increased pulmonary shunting in human sepsis. J Trauma 1979; *19*:432–460.

49. Chang GT, Moulder JW. Loss of inorganic ions from host cells infected with *Chlamydia psittaci*. Infect Immun 1978; *19*:827–832.

50. Cousins RJ. Relationship of metallothionein synthesis and degradation to intracellular zinc metabolism. Dev Toxicol Environ Sci 1982; *9*:251–262.

51. Rupp RG, Fuller GM. The effects of leucocytic and serum factors on fibrinogen biosynthesis in cultured hepatocytes. Exp Cell Res 1979; *118*:23–30.

52. Schlick E, Hartung K, Piccoli M, et al. The capacity of biological response modifiers (BRM) to induce the secretion of colony stimulating factor(s) by murine macrophages and human monocytes. Fed Proc 1983; *42*:1221.

53. Mizel SB, Dayer J-M, Krane SM, et al. Stimulation of rheumatoid synovial cell collagenase and prostaglandin production by partially purified lymphoyte-activating factor (interleukin-1). Proc Natl Acad Sci USA 1981; *78*:2474–2477.

54. Filkins JP, Yelich MR. Mechanism of hyperinsulinemia after reticuloendothelial system phagocytosis. Am J Physiol 1982; *242*:E115–E120.

55. Thompson WL, Abeles FB, Beall FA, et al. Influence of the adrenal glucocorticoids on the stimulation of synthesis of hepatic ribonucleic acid and plasma acute-phase globulins by leucocytic endogenous mediator. Biochem J 1976; *156*:25–32.

56. Wannemacher RW Jr, Pekarek RS, Klainer AS, et al. Detection of a leukocytic endogenous mediator-like mediator of serum amino acid and zinc depression during infectious illnesses. Infect Immun 1975; *11*:873–885.

57. Zipser RD, Davenport MW, Martin KL, et al. Hyperreninemic hypoaldosteronism in the critically ill: a new entity. J Clin Endocrinol Metab 1981; *53*:867–873.

58. Gruchow HW. Catecholamine activity and infectious disease episodes. J Human Stress 1979; *5*:11–17.

59. Buescher EL, Belfer ML, Artenstein MS, et al. A prospective study of corticosteroid and catecholamine levels in relation to viral respiratory illness. J Human Stress 1979; *5*:18–28.

60. Wartofsky L. The response of the thyroid gland and thyroid hormone metabolism to infectious disease. Horm Res 1974; *5*:112–128.

61. Cahill GF Jr. Starvation in man. Clin Endocrinol Metab 1976; *5*:397–415.

62. Lewis T. Inflammation as a disease mechanism. *In* Sweifach BJ, Grant L, McCluskey RT (eds). The Inflammatory Process III. 2nd ed. New York, Academic Press, 1974: 515–518.

63. Bell RC, Coalson JJ, Smith JD, et al. Multiple organ system failure and infection in adult respiratory distress syndrome. Ann Intern Med 1983; *99*:293–298.

64. Border JR, Chenier R, McMenamy RH, et al. Multiple systems organ failure: muscle fuel deficit with visceral protein malnutrition. Surg Clin North Am 1976; *56*:1147–1167.

65. Siegel JH, Cerra FB, Coleman B, et al. Physiological and metabolic correlations in human sepsis. Surgery 1979; *86*:163–193.

66. Wannemacher RW Jr, Kaminski MV Jr, Neufeld HA. Protein-sparing therapy during pneumococcal infection in rhesus monkeys. JPEN 1978; *2*:507–518.

67. Van Snick JL, Masson PL, Heremans JF. The involvement of lactoferrin in the hyposideremia of acute inflammation. J Exp Med 1974; *140*:1068–1084.

68. Murray MJ, Murray AB. Starvation suppression and refeeding activation of infection. An ecological necessity? Lancet 1977; *1*:123–125.

69. Beisel WR. Single nutrients and immunity. Am J Clin Nutr 1982; *35*:415–468.

70. Chandra RK, Newberne PM. Nutrition, Immunity, and Infection. New York, Plenum Press, 1977: 1–246.

35

NUTRITIONAL MANAGEMENT OF THE INFECTED PATIENT

J. WESLEY ALEXANDER

Nutrition-infection interactions have had a major influence on human development since the beginning of recorded history.[1] Before the 18th century, the world population remained relatively stable because large numbers of people died from epidemics, which included diarrheal diseases, measles, smallpox, typhus, malaria, typhoid fever, and plague. While the nature of these infectious diseases was not understood until less than 100 years ago, it was clear that overcrowding, poverty, hunger, and famine with its associated undernutrition set the stage for rampant epidemics that caused the death of as much as 80 to 90 per cent of a regional population such as a city or province.[1,2] It is difficult to know which was more important in the natural decline of death from infection and rise in the world population, but improved hygiene, socioeconomic improvements, and better food supplies all played important roles.[3,4]

Even in modern times, the relative impacts of these various factors are not easily separated, but it is a fact that undernutrition predisposes to a variety of infectious diseases. As an example, Chandra[5] reports that the mortality among young children in rural India is inversely proportional to their weight. In children with weight for height less than 60 per cent of normal, the mortality rate was 18 per cent compared with 7 per cent when the children were 61 to 70 per cent of the weight for height and only 1 per cent when their weight was greater than 80 per cent of normal. Infectious diseases in malnourished individuals in industrialized societies as well as underdeveloped countries are associated with more frequent and severe complications than in persons who are not malnourished.[6,7] Malnutrition increases susceptibility to bacterial, parasitic, and fungal infections more than viral or plasmodial infections.[5,6,8] Viral infections and malaria may, in fact, be more frequent and more severe in well-fed individuals than in the malnourished. Excessive quantities of vitamins in the diet may also decrease resistance to certain viral infections,[9] and iron may increase the mortality in some bacterial infections.[10] Thus, nutrition may have both good and bad effects during infection. The complexities of the interaction of nutrition and infection will be examined in this chapter.

INFECTION IN MALNOURISHED SUBJECTS

Although a relationship between malnutrition and infectious disease has been recognized for over a century, there are still many considerations that are far from clear. Numerous animal studies have shown altered resistance to infection associated with malnutrition (Table 35–1). In general, undernutrition may provide some protection against certain viruses and some intracellular pathogens, but malnutrition, especially protein deficiency, usually predisposes to infections by a wide variety of microbes, especially extracellular bacterial and fungal pathogens.

Much of our understanding of nutrition-infection interrelationships in man has come from investigations of malnutrition in underdeveloped countries. Diarrhea and respiratory infections are the principal causes of death in the world today.[18,19] Shann et al.[19] reported that of the 15 million children under the age of 5 who die each year, 96 per cent are in the Third World and about one third die from pneumonia. Some infections may be devastating in undernourished individuals. As an example, the death rates from measles in children from poor rural and urban areas exceeds those of the affluent societies by 200- to 400-fold, with case fatality rates ranging from 20 to 40 per cent. Santos et al.[7] point out that nutritional deficiency is an associated cause in 47 per cent of deaths from all causes in children under the age of 5 in a study of 13 Latin American cities. When an infectious disease was the cause of death, 61 per cent of the patients had associated malnutrition contributing to the death. Black et al.[20] and Guerrant et al.[21] emphasize that diarrhea occurs commonly because of malnutrition but also aggravates the malnourished state, leading to weight loss, stunted growth, and increased susceptibility to a variety of infections. The potential role of local mucosal immunities is implicated in these infections.

It is also clear that malnutrition is a common occurrence in hospitalized patients in developed countries and that preceding malnutrition leads to an increased incidence of infectious complications. As examples, Jensen et al.[22] showed that 54 per cent of malnourished patients developed postoperative complications, compared with only 11 per cent of well-nourished patients. Meguid,[23] in a study of patients undergoing major abdominal surgery for cancer, reported that 33 per cent of well-nourished patients had one or more complications, whereas 65 per cent of malnourished patients had complications (p<0.001) and more than twice as many of the malnourished patients died. Pine et al.,[24] in a discriminate analysis of determinants of organ malfunction or death in patients with intra-abdominal sepsis, demonstrated that malnutrition was a major contributing factor. Malnutrition was also found to be an important factor in the development of surgical infections by Dionigi et al.[25]

Various protocols have been designed to determine how nutritional assessment of the patient can be useful in predicting outcome. In general, the anthropometric tests have been shown to be ineffective

TABLE 35–1. Effect of Malnutrition on Infection

Type of Malnutrition	Increased Resistance to:	Decreased Resistance to:
Acute starvation	*Listeria monocytogenes* Some virus infection	*Salmonella* and other bacterial infections
Acute protein		*Listeria* *Streptococcus pneumoniae* *Staphylococcus aureus* *Candida* Influenza *Salmonella* Mycobacteria *Pneumocystis*
Chronic protein-energy	Malaria	*Pseudomonas* Most extracellular bacteria, including *Escherichia coli* Most intracellular bacteria
Vitamin A		*Salmonella*, many other bacteria, viruses, and protozoa
Vitamin C	Malaria	Most bacterial infection
Thiamine	Many viruses	Poliomyelitis, many bacteria
Pantothenic acid	Myelitis virus, protozoal infection	Many bacteria
Folic acid and vitamin B_{12}	Lymphocytic choriomeningitis	*Shigella*

This table represents only a partial review to exemplify some of the problems related to interpretation of nutrition-infection interactions. See references 9 and 11 to 17 for further information.

predictors for individual patients. The most useful schemes have come from cluster analysis[26] and prognostic nutritional indices[27-29] which take into account several factors such as serum albumin, serum transferrin, triceps skinfold, and delayed hypersensitivity response. In certain studies, simple markers such as serum transferrin have been found to be useful predictors of complication rates.[30-32] Delayed type hypersensitivity skin testing has been found to be a significant predictor of both mortality and septic complications by Meakins et al.[33-35] but unfortunately there are numerous other variables, such as the presence of sepsis itself, that will alter the results of this test. It is obvious from all of the reported studies that malnutrition causes significant reduction in both specific and nonspecific immunological resistance of individual subjects to the development of infection. Testing of immune competence provides some degree of prediction of the susceptibility of individual patients to the development of infections, but it is more useful for population studies than for the individual patient. This is not surprising since there are numerous variables of nutrition that may influence immune competence to a specific infection in different ways.

IMMUNOLOGICAL CONSEQUENCES OF UNDERNUTRITION

Malnutrition can affect every segment of the immune system. Table 35-2 lists immunological perturbations that have been reported following both general and specific nutritional depletion. These changes are discussed in more detail in Chapter 33, and comprehensive reviews of the effects of single nutrient effects in immunological function have been presented elsewhere.[36,37]

What is important is that these immunodeficiencies can be corrected by vigorous nutritional support,[38,39] sometimes within a very short period of time.[40] Ahlstedt et al.[41] showed that the increased susceptibility to infections by *E. coli* by malnourished mice could be restored to normal by refeeding for

only 1 day. However, specific variables of immunological resistance to infection may take much longer to correct, up to 2 weeks.[42]

In a retrospective study, Mullen et al.[27] found that preoperative total parenteral nutrition in patients who were found to be at high risk, as determined by a calculated prognostic nutritional index, reduced postoperative complications 2.5-fold and major postoperative sepsis reduced sixfold. These studies strongly suggest that resistance to most types of infection, especially those caused by extracellular bacterial pathogens, is markedly improved by nutritional restoration of malnourished subjects.

THE EFFECTS OF SEPSIS ON NUTRITIONAL STATUS

The nutritional consequences of infection are very important to the host and in planning dietary treatment protocols.[6-8] In general, infection causes anorexia with decreased food intake resulting in decreased availability of substrate for synthesis (Table 35-3). Fever and a hypermetabolic state cause increased requirements overall, and altered metabolism may contribute to changes in the needs for certain nutrients such as vitamin C or arginine. There may be increased losses associated with increased ureagenesis or from either wounds or the intestinal tract.

In children with marasmus, infection commonly precipitates kwashiorkor, and similar rapid deterioration of nutritional status can be seen in hospitalized patients in highly developed nations. During infection there is a sequestration of iron and zinc, which may have a protective mechanism,[10] but iron levels may fall drastically.

Nonspecific effects of infection on the immune system include activation of the complement cascade with consumption of complement components. There is subsequently a rise in most complement components, especially C3, which may rise to more than twice normal values.[44] Sakamoto et al.[45] have shown that levels of C1, 4, 2, and 3 were all increased

TABLE 35-2. Effect of Malnutrition on Immune Function

Type of Malnutrition or Deficiency	T Cell Function	DST	B Cell Function	Macrophage Function	Neutrophil Function	Complement
Chronic protein-energy	↓↓	↓↓	↓ to variable	↓	↓	↓ esp C2, C3
Protein	N or ↓	↓	↓ to variable	↓↓	↓	↓ esp C2, C3
Lipid	↓		↓		↓	
Zinc	↓↓	↓↓	N	variable	↓	
Iron	↓	↓	N	↓	↓	
Pyridoxine (vitamin B₆)	↓	↓	↓	↓	↓	
Pantothenic acid	↓	↓	↓↓			
Folate and vitamin B₁₂	↓	↓	variable		↓ (?)	↓ C3
Vitamin C	variable	↓	N		variable	
Vitamin A	↓	↓	↓			
Thiamine	↓		↓			

DST, delayed type hypersensitivity skin test. N, normal. No entry indicates insufficient or conflicting data.

TABLE 35–3. Nutritional Consequences of Infection

Decreased food intake
Increased requirements
Increased losses from wounds, intestinal tract,
  or urinary tract
Altered metabolism

by the presence of infection in both normally fed and protein-malnourished animals, although levels of all these complement components as well as CH_{50} were markedly depressed by protein malnutrition. Complement activation characteristically causes a sudden drop in the number of circulating neutrophils, followed shortly by an increase in their numbers. There is activation of neutrophils associated with their binding to complement fragments, particularly C5a, with an associated altered function. The increased production of neutrophils in itself causes an increased nutritional demand. Anergy usually develops during infection and may be a combination of both altered immune response and malnutrition. Soon after bacterial challenge, there may be a reduction in circulating immunoglobulins followed shortly by an increased synthesis. Infection causes increased ureagenesis with increased nitrogen losses from the urinary tract as well as the intestine. The stress reaction is associated with an increase in the catabolic hormones, namely adrenocortical steroids (such as cortisol), glucagon, and catecholamines. This, in concert with the production of interleukin 1, which is generated by the activation of mononuclear phagocytes by complement degradation products, is associated with a catabolic response and breakdown of proteins, particularly in the skeletal muscle. Protein requirements generally go up during infection. Since the nutritional requirements cannot be met from exogenous sources, there is increased utilization of endogenous fuels. Glycogen stores are rapidly depleted, and the available energy therefore comes largely from protein degradation through gluconeogenesis. Energy requirements are met by mobilization of lipids from adipose tissues and protein from skeletal muscle. Selective shunting of available amino acid supply into the synthesis of acute-phase proteins, some of which may have a survival advantage, may make protein deficiencies more acute. Characteristically, there is decreased synthesis of transferrin and albumin, which characteristically fall to very low levels with acute infection. In the already malnourished individual these consequences may be particularly disastrous.

Perhaps of equal importance, liver function may be seriously compromised during infection.[46] While such liver abnormalities can be caused by malnutrition itself, they are more likely to result from endotoxin effects and/or complement activation. The important observation, however, is that with abnormal function of the liver, this central organ may be unable to process nutrients in an orderly fashion to keep pace with the protein synthesis needed for optimal nonspecific resistance to infection.

NUTRITION IN THE HYPERMETABOLIC BURNED SUBJECT

Patients with sepsis and patients with severe thermal injury have some similarities related to nutritional requirements, although there are obvious differences. Both are hypermetabolic, have complement activation, and are often acutely malnourished. Since more is known about nutrition in burn injury, this will be discussed in some detail. With the advent of topical therapy some 20 years ago, many patients with large burns lived for a longer period of time, only to succumb ultimately from sepsis. It was noted that weight loss was a substantial problem following major thermal injury of 40 per cent or more of the body surface area, and weight losses of 20 to 30 per cent of preburn weight were not uncommon. With the realization that malnutrition probably played a significant role in outcome following burn injury, wholesale nutritional supplementation began to be used in 1969 and 1970. In an analysis of the causes of burn deaths at our institution for a 5-year period before aggressive nutritional supplementation was instituted compared with the 5-year period immediately afterward, it was apparent that there was an abrupt 80 per cent reduction in deaths from septicemia and burn wound sepsis that occurred at the end of 1970.[47] Even so, infectious complications continued to be the major cause of death in patients with greater than 50 per cent injury who survived the initial period of hospitalization.

Because of persistently low levels of serum albumin and serum transferrin in patients with large burns and because of the similarities of immune defects following burn injury and those documented following protein-energy and pure protein deprivation in experimental animals, a study was instituted to determine whether simple protein supplementation would be of benefit following severe burn injury.[48] Patients were randomly assigned to receive either a diet of normal composition with 15 per cent of calories provided as proteins or a diet that was supplemented with milk whey protein to provide 22 per cent of calories as proteins. Forty-four per cent of the patients in the control group died as a result of infection, compared with none in the high-protein group ($p < 0.03$). In patients receiving the high-protein diet (but actually fewer calories) there were significantly fewer infections, fewer days that the patients required treatment with antibiotics, and higher levels of serum protein and protein components such as albumin and transferrin, as well as evidence of better support of all immunological functions tested. Thus, it was clear that protein supplementation had a beneficial effect on outcome in humans with large burns.

Because of the problems of rigid control of the diet in human subjects, an animal model was developed that involved placement of a gastrostomy into guinea pigs, exiting the tube in the intrascapular area so that they could continuously be fed a liquid diet by pump-controlled infusions while being unrestrained in their cages. At least a week after the gastrostomy placement, the animals were burned with a standardized burn of 30 per cent of the total body surface area (TBSA). Dietary support using infusions of a highly defined diet, the content of which could be regulated at will, was then begun. Measurements during all of these studies have included daily weight, nitrogen balance, estimation of diarrhea (if any), and terminal measurements of albumin; transferrin; liver and gut weight, fat, and protein contents; muscle weight and protein content; and central carcass weight after evisceration and skinning of the animals.

Initial studies showed that guinea pigs with 30 per cent full-thickness burns developed a progressive hypermetabolic response as measured by indirect calorimetry, increasing oxygen consumption to 50 per cent above baseline by the end of 2 weeks postburn, representing an average expenditure of 175 kcal/kg/day.[49] Different caloric intakes (100, 150, 175, or 200 kcal/kg/day) did not alter the hypermetabolic response, but there was insufficient nutritional support when less than 175 kcal/kg/day was given.

In one set of experiments, seven defined combinations of caloric and protein intake were studied for 14 days in 97 guinea pigs bearing a 30 per cent full-thickness burn.[50] With a caloric intake of 175 kcal/kg/day, equaling the measured energy expenditure, the animals receiving 10 per cent of calories as protein had a significantly greater postburn weight loss (p < 0.05) and muscle mass depletion (p < 0.05), and significantly lower muscle nitrogen concentration (p < 0.05), serum albumin level (p < 0.01), and liver nitrogen content (p < 0.01). With the same caloric intake but with 20 or 30 per cent of calories as protein, the weight loss and the muscle wasting were reduced, but not abolished, and the serum albumin level and liver nitrogen content were normalized. With diets containing 200 kcal/kg/day, the muscle tissue was unaltered when animals were given 20 per cent of calories as protein. They had a lower weight loss and a higher serum albumin level (p < 0.01), but also greater fatty infiltration of the liver (p < 0.01). At both levels of caloric intake, the nitrogen balance correlated significantly with the level of nitrogen intake but did not correlate with the changes of body weight. All things considered, the best metabolic and nutritional results were obtained with diets that provided a caloric intake that paralleled the measured energy expenditure and contained 20 to 30 per cent of calories as protein.

Early full feeding (within 2 hours of burn) compared with adaptation over 3 days not only eliminated mortality and weight loss but maintained gut mucosal integrity to a much better degree.[51] Amazingly, feeding the diet at full concentration within 2 hours of injury reduced the hypermetabolic response by 80 per cent. The mechanism whereby immediate enteral feeding after burn injury reduced postburn hypermetabolism and catabolism was studied in 57 burned guinea pigs (30 per cent TBSA) divided into three groups: A (n = 19), given 175 kcal/kg/day beginning 2 hours after burn; B (n = 20), given 175 kcal/kg/day with an initial 72-hour adaptation period; C (n = 18), given 200 kcal/kg/day with the same adaptation period as B. Resting metabolic expenditure (RME) on PBD 13 was lowest in group A (109 per cent of preburn level) compared with group B (144 per cent, p < 0.001) and group C (137 per cent, p < 0.01). On PBD 1, group A had the greatest jejunal mucosal weight and thickness (p < 0.001), and mucosal weight had negative correlations with plasma cortisol (r = 0.829, p < 0.001) and glucagon (r = 0.888, p < 0.001). Two weeks after burn, urinary vanillylmandelic acid (VMA) excretion and plasma cortisol and glucagon were lowest in group A (p < 0.05 to p < 0.01). These hormones also significantly correlated with RME (p < 0.01). These findings suggest that immediate postburn enteral feeding can prevent hypermetabolism via preservation of gut mucosal integrity and prevention of excessive secretion of catabolic hormones.

Experiments were designed to investigate the effect of exogenous lipid as an energy source and determine the optimal carbohydrate:lipid ratio. Forty-five guinea pigs with catheter gastrostomy received a 30 per cent TBSA full-thickness flame burn.[52] After burn they were given intragastric tube feedings using five diets at different dietary lipid compositions: 0, 5, 15, 30, and 50 per cent of nonprotein calories. Total calories administered (175 kcal/kg/day), protein content and composition (20 per cent of total calories), total volume, and vitamin and mineral content were constant in all animals. At postburn day (PBD) 14, body weight, carcass weight and muscle weight were the greatest in 0 per cent and 5 per cent lipid groups, and the least in 30 per cent and 50 per cent lipid groups. Serum transfusion was highest in the 5 per cent and 15 per cent lipid groups, and lowest in the 30 per cent and 50 per cent groups. Total nitrogen content in muscle and cumulative nitrogen balance were best in the 15 per cent lipid group. This indicated that dietary lipid levels between 5 and 15 per cent of the nonprotein calories are optimal for nutritional support after burn injury and higher levels should not be given.

Increased synthesis of prostaglandins has been implicated in mediation of the metabolic and immune response after burn. The prostaglandin precursor linoleic acid also participates in the regulation of the immune response. The effect of linoleic acid or oleic acid as the sole source of lipid in the diet and the effect of indomethacin treatment on the metabolism and survival following burn injury were studied.[52a]

Eighteen female burned guinea pigs (30 per cent TBSA) with previously placed catheter gastrostomies were divided into three groups. Groups A, B, and C received 10 per cent of total calories as linoleic acid, oleic acid, or Microlipid (linoleic 73.7 per cent, oleic 15.0 per cent), respectively. Indomethacin (2 mg/kg/day) was administered to group C animals through gastrostomy tubes from 2 days before burn until PBD 14. After an initial 3-day adaptation period, all animal groups received continuous isocaloric (175 kcal/kg/day, 70 per cent of total calories as polycose, and 20 per cent as whey protein) intragastric tube feedings until PBD 14. In these experiments, the whey protein was not supplemented with arginine. Postburn 24-hour urine volume was significantly highest in the group C (A = 65 ± 11, B = 48 ± 15, C = 108 ± 6 ml/kg/day; $p < 0.02$). Resting metabolic expenditure (RME) on PBD 3 was lowest in group C (114 per cent of preburn level) compared with group A (125 per cent, $p < 0.10$) and group B (129 per cent, $p < 0.02$). Mean survival time after burn in group A (9.3 ± 1.0 days) was shortest compared with group B (12.6 ± 1.0 days, $p < 0.04$) and group C (13.2 ± 1.2 days, $p < 0.05$). Dinitrofluorobenzene (DNFB)-dependent ear swelling in animals of group C on PBD 13 showed a 73 per cent increase (average ear swelling increase in guinea pigs with 30 per cent TBSA burns and normal diets was 26 per cent). This study suggested that dietary linoleic acid may adversely influence immunocompetence after burn and that indomethacin may delay the hypermetabolic response and improve immune defense after burn.

Recently, branched-chain amino acid (BCAA) enriched diets have become commercially available and widely used in stressed patients. Nevertheless, there is very little information about the effect of this kind of nutritional support in severely burned individuals. Seventy-one burned guinea pigs (30 per cent TBSA) with previously placed catheter gastrostomies were divided into six groups. Groups I, II, and III received 10, 20, and 30 per cent of total calories as whey protein, respectively. The other three groups received BCAA supplementation to increase BCAA to 50 per cent of total amino acids compared with 21.5 per cent BCAA content in whey protein. Group IV received the same amount of nitrogen as group I, group V the same as group II, and group VI the same as group III. After an initial 3-day adaptation period, all animals in all groups received continuous isocaloric (175 kcal/kg/day) intragastric tube feeding until PBD 14. No BCAA group showed evidence of any beneficial effect in various nutritional parameters when compared with the corresponding whey protein group with isonitrogenous intake. Furthermore, the data indicated that when nitrogen intake is too low or very high, BCAA supplementation has an adverse effect.[53]

A study was done to compare effectiveness of the immediate postburn parenteral (IV) versus enteral (IG) feedings. Twenty-eight guinea pigs bearing 30 per cent BSA burn were divided into two groups. The IG group was fed continuously by gastrostomy tube and the IV group was fed by central venous catheter. Both groups had dual (both) catheters. Each group received 175 kcal/kg/day with the same nutrients beginning 2 hours after burn. Body weight (BW) in the IV group decreased much faster than that in the IG group until PBD 8 (per cent of initial BW on PBD 2: IG = $95.0 \pm 1.7\%$, IV = $89.7 \pm 1.2\%$, $p < 0.05$; on PBD 8: IG = $91.6 \pm 1.8\%$, IV = $84.1 \pm 1.6\%$, $p < 0.02$). Plasma cortisol on PBD 1 was higher in the IV group than in the IG group (123.6 ± 23.4 vs. 61.7 ± 9.0 μg/dl, $p < 0.02$), and on PBD 14 a similar trend was found (163.3 ± 33.3 vs. 72.6 ± 6.2 μg/dl). The IG group had significantly heavier jejunal mucosal weight than the IV group on PBD 1 and 14. Mucosal weight had negative correlation with cortisol on PBD 1 ($r = 0.729$, $p < 0.01$). This study suggested that immediate postburn enteral nutrition provides better nutritional support and preserves gut mucosal integrity better than parenteral nutrition. However, this highly defined diet did not prevent hypermetabolism.

Another study was done to compare the effects of intact protein versus free amino acids as the sole source of nitrogen. Twenty-one guinea pigs (400 g) were given a 30 per cent BSA, full-thickness burn and then divided into two groups. Both groups were fed isocaloric diets (175 kcal/kg/day) by continuous gastric infusion. One group (n = 12) received a diet containing whey protein (WP) while the other group (n = 9) received an otherwise identical diet containing free amino acids in a whey protein pattern (AA). After 14 days, the animals were sacrificed. WP was found to maintain body weight better than AA (95 vs. 89 per cent, $p < 0.02$). The cumulative nitrogen balance was better in the WP group ($+1184 \pm 194$ vs. -242 ± 94 mg, $p < 0.001$). WP animals showed statistically significant benefits in the following parameters: liver (L), gut mucosa (GM), and gastrocnemius (G) weights, and in serum albumin (Alb), transferrin (Tf) and C3 levels.

	WP	**AA**
L (g)	19.7 ± 1.2	15.7 ± 1.0
GM (g/10 cm)	0.53 ± 0.04	0.28 ± 0.04
G (g)	1.12 ± 0.03	1.02 ± 0.04
Alb (g/dl)	3.0 ± 0.1	1.9 ± 0.1
Tf (% nl)	150 ± 9	94 ± 14
C3 (% nl)	150 ± 8	110 ± 10

It can only be concluded that intact protein is superior to free amino acids for the nutritional support of the burned guinea pigs.

All of these studies have given indication that the nutritional needs in seriously burned subjects are markedly different from normal individuals and different from what is currently being given to patients in most burn units (Table 35–4). The similarities

**TABLE 35–4. Summary of Nutritional Needs in Seriously Burned Subjects
(50% TBSA) Based Upon Clinical and Animal Studies**

	For Burned Subject	For Normal Subject
Increased caloric load	2800–3000 kcal/m²/day	1500 kcal/m²/day
Increased protein (high quality)	22% of calories	15% of calories
Arginine supplementation	2% of calories	—
Decreased fat intake	10% of calories	40% of calories

BCAA supplementation offers no nutritional advantage and may be harmful.
Increased vitamins (2 to 5 times RDA) and minerals are recommended.
Intact protein is better than amino acid solution containing the same amino acid distribution.
Feeding by the enteral route provides better nutritional support than the intravenous route.
Feeding by the enteral route immediately after burn injury prevents hypermetabolism (in animals).

between burned patients and septic patients suggest that septic patients may also be getting inappropriate nutritional support.

ALTERATION OF FUEL UTILIZATION DURING SEPSIS

Sepsis is associated with increased levels of cortisol, glucagon, and catecholamines. Bessey et al.[54] have recently shown that infusion of these hormones causes some but not all of the features of hypermetabolism. Major features associated with sepsis are increased metabolic rate and oxygen consumption, accelerated net protein breakdown, negative nitrogen balance, and alteration of carbohydrate metabolism. The extent of these changes relates to both the extent of injury or infection and the magnitude of the catabolic hormone response, and they are associated with elevated blood glucose concentrations, increased endogenous glucose production, altered insulin levels, and profound insulin resistance.[54]

Nanni et al.[55] have suggested that septic patients become more dependent than nonseptic patients on lipid fuels for oxidative metabolism. In patients receiving total parenteral nutrition, Stoner et al.[56] showed that fat oxidation continued despite infusion of excess glucose. Dahn et al.[57] have done studies in nonseptic hypermetabolic patients requiring parenteral nutrition and in seriously ill septic subjects, noting an elevation of triglyceride during lipid infusions that was higher in the septic patients. The rate of lipid clearance appeared identical in both septic and nonseptic patients, and hepatic ketogenic capacity did not appear to be impaired in septic patients. Wannemacher et al.[58] also showed that lipid calories were effectively used for protein sparing during pneumococcal infections in rhesus monkeys. The protein-sparing effect of lipid emulsions was not related to its glycerin content.[59] Askanazi et al.[60] have shown in man that endogenous fat is preferentially used during sepsis as a fuel and energy source and that administration of a large glucose load did not totally suppress net fat oxidation. Instead, there was an increase in the $\dot{V}O_2$, continued oxidation of fat, and an apparent increase in the conversion of glucose to glycogen.

Milewski et al.[61] studied intracellular free amino acids in undernourished patients with or without sepsis. They found that associated with sepsis, there was significant reduction in muscle glutamine, lysine, tyrosine, valine, leucine, isoleucine, phenylalanine, and methionine, suggesting an increased catabolic rate. In another interesting investigation, Kingsland et al.[62] studied the metabolism of glutamate in patients during sepsis compared with that in healthy controls. Increased urinary excretion of aspartate was observed in control patients following glutamate administration, but in the septic patients there was increased excretion of glutamine. Deamination predominated over transamination during the metabolism of glutamate, although the half-life of glutamate was the same in the control and septic patients. This study showed that the mechanisms of individual amino acid metabolism were much different in septic than in control patients. Metabolism in the liver might be particularly disordered, as evidenced by the studies of Caruana et al.,[63] who showed that hepatocellular necrosis of the liver is characteristic of sepsis; this suggests that many of the metabolic changes and utilization of amino acids in septic patients may be related to liver function per se.

NUTRITION DURING SEPSIS

Several specific problems related to nutrition-infection interaction that occur in septic individuals make generalized recommendations for nutritional support quite difficult. These include the following considerations:

1. Susceptibility to infection is organism-dependent and may involve different resistance mechanisms.

2. The effects of infection on host defense and nutritional status are also somewhat organism-dependent.

3. Good nutritional status may increase susceptibility to certain infections, especially those of viral origin.

4. Nutrition during infection may benefit the infecting organism more than the patient.

5. The severity of infection and the severity of the associated or predisposing malnutrition are con-

founding factors that markedly influence potential therapeutic approaches via nutrition.

6. There may be an effect of alterations in intestinal flora on both immunity of the host and nutritional response.

That acute starvation may improve resistance to infection has been shown by several animal studies (see Table 35–1). However, in such studies, the animals were not previously hypermetabolic. Using mice, Murray and Murray[15] showed that when animals were infected with *Listeria monocytogenes*, mortality was actually increased and survival time shortened in animals force-fed to normal energy intakes. Infected animals allowed ad libitum feeding with only 50 per cent of the intake of controls had better survival than animals that had normal energy intakes using identical diets. In a somewhat different type of study, Petersen et al.[64,65] showed that normal rats challenged with an *E. coli* hemoglobin adjuvant peritonitis had 66 per cent survival, compared with 15 per cent survival for protein-depleted animals. When the protein-depleted animals were refed with regular diets, they had 60 per cent survival, but when they were repleted with intravenous hyperalimentation, the mortality was no better than in protein-depleted controls. Thus, the route of the administration of nutrients may have an effect on outcome just as it does following burn injury.

Obesity or hyperlipidemia may have an effect on the resistance to viral and bacterial infections.[17,37] Marginally malnourished dogs have higher resistance to clinical disease caused by distemper virus than do normal or obese dogs. Hypercholesterolemic diets suppress the resistance to *Listeria monocytogenes*. This may be in part because high intakes of the polyunsaturated fatty acids are immunosuppressive, inhibiting a number of lymphocytic functions such as mitogen stimulation.[66] Linoleic acid is particularly effective in reducing immune responses. Cleary and Pickering[67] showed in vitro that commercial fat emulsion acts as a particulate stimulus to activate and exhaust metabolic pathways of neutrophils. In addition, the fat emulsion increases the numbers and availability of Fc receptors on the neutrophils. Lipid emulsion may impair reticuloendothelial system function as well as granulocyte migration and bactericidal capacity. In addition, when used for parenteral nutrition, it may impair bacterial clearance and enhance bacterial virulence in mice.[68] Weinberg[10] has clearly demonstrated that increased amounts of iron in the diet may increase the susceptibility to bacterial infection.

RECOMMENDATIONS

The uncomfortable implication of the above review is that not very much solid information is known about the optimal composition of dietary formulas for support of nutrition in patients who have on-going sepsis. Only highly controlled but empirical experiments in well-designed animal studies will answer some of the many important questions related to optimal nutritional support during sepsis and provide models for testing in humans.

It is anticipated that intense high-calorie feedings may have an adverse effect on many infections and that basal maintenance or even hypocaloric diets may be more beneficial.

It is likely that a higher proportion of the dietary intake during sepsis should be provided by high-quality protein and that supplementation with certain amino acids, such as arginine or the branched-chain amino acids, especially leucine, may be beneficial.

With the clear evidence that fat is harmful in many instances during sepsis even though lipids may be used preferentially as a fuel, the proportion of the diet providing lipid calories should probably be reduced (perhaps to about 10 to 15 per cent of total calories).

Since free amino acids (compared with intact protein) have an adverse effect following burn injury, it is reasonable that these should be avoided in enteral diets whenever possible in favor of intact protein with a high biological value.

Since enteral nutrition is clearly superior to intravenous nutrition in burn injury, the gut should be used whenever possible in the septic patient. This might have an additional beneficial effect by providing increased support of liver function and perhaps by decreasing the endotoxin load from the gut.[69] Also, intravenous feedings may not be as effective as enteral feedings because of an inability to provide an optimal amino acid mix intravenously.

It is apparent that excessive amounts of iron (and possibly zinc) should not be administered during acute infection since their nutritional properties may benefit the infecting organism more than the patient.[10,26,37] While vitamin deficiencies may clearly increase susceptibility to infection, it is not known whether vitamin excesses may preferentially benefit the organism during ongoing, extracellular bacterial infections.[36,37]

Definitive recommendations regarding nutritional support of the septic patient are obviously very tenuous. An intense amount of investigation is needed to settle the many unanswered questions and provide guidance for management of a difficult and continuing problem of major clinical importance.

Acknowledgment

Portions of the studies described herein were supported by USPHS Grant AI 12936 and the Shriners of North America.

References

1. McNeill WH. Plagues & People. Garden City, Anchor, 1977.
2. Alexander JW, Stinnett JD. Changes in immunologic function. *In* Fischer JE (ed). Surgical Nutrition. Boston, Little, Brown, 1983: 535–549.
3. Bollett AJ. The rise and fall of disease. Am J Med 1981; 70:12–16.
4. Scrimshaw NS, Taylor CE, Gordon JE. Interactions of nutrition and infection. WHO Monograph Series, 1968: 57.
5. Chandra RK. Nutrition, immunity, and infection: present knowledge and future directions. Lancet 1983; 1:688–691.
6. Shizgal HM. Nutrition and immune function. Surg Ann 1981; 13:15–29.
7. Santos JI, Arredondo JL, Vitale JJ. Nutrition, infection and immunity. Pediatr Ann 1983; 12:182–194.
8. Neumann CG, Jelliffe DB, Jelliffe EFP. Interaction of nutrition and infection. A factor important to African development. Clin Pediatr 1978; 17:807–812.
9. Lee CM, Aboko-Cole GF. The interaction of nutrition and infection: a succinct review. J Natl Med Assoc 1979; 8:765–777.
10. Weinberg ED. Iron and susceptibility to infectious disease. Science 1974; 184:952.
11. Petro TM, Chien G, Watson RR. Alteration of cell-mediated immunity to *Listeria monocytogenes* in protein-malnourished mice treated with thymosin fraction V. Infect Immun 1982; 37:601–608.
12. Wing EJ, Barczynski LK, Boehmer SM. Effect of acute nutritional deprivation on immune function in mice I. Macrophages. Immunology 1983; 48:543–550.
13. Sobrado J, Maiz A, Kawamura I, et al. Effect of dietary protein depletion on nonspecific immune responses and survival in the guinea pig. Am J Clin Nutr 1983; 37:795–801.
14. Wing EJ. Effect of acute nutritional deprivation of host defenses against *Listeria monocytogenes*—macrophage function. *In* Eisenstein TK, Actor P, Friedman H (eds). Host Defenses to Intracellular Pathogens. New York, Plenum, 1983: 245–250.
15. Murray MJ, Murray AB. Anorexia of infection as a mechanism of host defense. Am J Clin Nutr 1979; 32:593–596.
16. Jakab GJ, Warr GA, Astry CL. Alterations of pulmonary defense mechanisms by protein depletion diet. Infect Immun 1981; 34:610–622.
17. Watson RR, Petro TM. Resistance to bacterial and parasitic infections in the nutritionally compromised host. CRC Crit Rev Microbiol 1984; 10:297–315.
18. Walsh JD, Warren KS. Selective primary health care: an interim strategy for disease control in developing countries. N Engl J Med 1979; 301:967–974.
19. Chann F, Gratten M, Germer S, Hazlett D, et al. Aetiology of pneumonia in children in Goroka Hospital, Papua New Guinea. Lancet 1984; 2:537–541.
20. Black RE, Brown KH, Becker S. Malnutrition is a determining factor in diarrheal duration, but not incidence, among young children in a longitudinal study in rural Bangladesh. Am J Clin Nutr 1984; 37:87–94.
21. Guerrant RL, Kirchhoff LV, Shields DS, et al. Prospective study of diarrheal illnesses in northeastern Brazil: patterns of disease, nutritional impact, etiologies, and risk factors. J Infect Dis 1983; 148:986–997.
22. Jensen S, Møller-Peterson, Madsen P. Prognostisk ernaeringsindeks.Sammenhaeng mellem den praeoperatve ernaeringstilstand og det postoperative forløb. Ugeskr Laeger 1983; 145:1531–1533.
23. Meguid MM, Debonis D, Meguid V, et al. Nutritional support in cancer. Lancet 1983; 2:230–231.
24. Pine RW, Wertz MJ, Lennard ES, et al. Determinants of organ malfunction or death in patients with intra-abdominal sepsis. A discriminant analysis. Arch Surg 1983; 118:242–249.
25. Dionigi P, Dionigi R, Nazari S, et al. Nutritional and immunological evaluations in cancer patients. Relationship to surgical infections. JPEN 1980; 4:351–356.
26. Nazari S, Dionigi R, Comodi I, et al. Preoperative prediction and quantification of septic risk caused by malnutrition. Arch Surg 1982; 117:266–274.
27. Mullen JL, Buzby GP, Matthews DC, et al. Reduction of operative morbidity and mortality by combined preoperative and postoperative nutritional support. Ann Surg 1980; 192:604–613.
28. Dempsy DT, Buzby GP, Mullen JL. Nutritional assessment in the seriously ill patient. J Am Coll Nutr 1983; 2:15–23.
29. Morath MA, Miller SF, Finley RK, et al. Clinical value of the prognostic nutritional index in burn patients. J Burn Care Rehab 1984; 5:294–299.
30. Casey J, Flinn WR, Yao JST, et al. Correlation of immune and nutritional status with wound complications in patients undergoing vascular operations. Surgery 1983; 93:822–827.
31. Zagoren AJ, Burday M, Sonn RL, et al. Predicting postoperative complications by determinations of serum albumin, total lymphocyte count, and total neutrophil count. J Am Osteopath Assoc 1983; 82:768–773, 1983.
32. Ogle CK, Alexander JW, MacMillan BG. The relationship of bacterium to levels of transferrin, albumin and total serum protein in burned patients. Burns 1981; 8:32–38.
33. Meakins JL, Pietsch JB, Bubenick O, et al. Delayed hypersensitivity: indication of acquired failure of host defenses in sepsis and trauma. Ann Surg 1977; 186:241–250.
34. Christou NV, McLean APH, Meakins JL. Host defense in blunt trauma: interrelationships of kinetics of anergy and depressed neutrophil function, nutritional status, and sepsis. J Trauma 1980; 20:833–841.
35. Ing AFM, Meakins JL, McLean APH, et al. Determinants of susceptibility to sepsis and mortality: malnutrition vs anergy. J Surg Res 1982; 32:249–255.
36. Beisel WR, Edelman R, Nauss K, et al. Single-nutrient effects on immunologic functions. Report of a workshop sponsored by the Department of Food and Nutrition and its Nutrition Advisory Group of the American Medical Association. JAMA 1981; 245:53–58.
37. Beisel WR. Single Nutrients and Immunity. Bethesda, MD, American Society for Clinical Nutrition, 1982: 417.
38. Dowd PS, Heatley RV. The influence of undernutrition on immunity. Clin Sci 1984; 66:241–248.
39. Rhoads JE. The impact of nutrition on infection. Surg Clin North Am 1980; 60:41–47.
40. Law DK, Dudrick SJ, Abdou NI. The effect of dietary protein depletion on immunocompetence: the influence of nutritional repletion prior to immunologic induction. Ann Surg 1974; 179:168.
41. Ahlstedt S. Experimental *Escherichia coli* 06 infection in mice. III. Effects of malnutrition, immunization and nutritional restoration. Acta Path Microbiol Scand [C] 1981; 89:15–22.
42. Dionigi R, Zonta D, Diminioni L, et al. The effects of total parenteral nutrition on immunodepression due to malnutrition. Ann Surg 1977; 185:467.
43. Barbul A, Sisto DA, Wasserkrug HL, et al. Nitrogen sparing and immune mechanisms of arginine: differential dose-dependent responses during post injury hyperalimentation. Curr Surg 1983; 408:114–116.
44. Alexander JW. Changes in the immune system after injury and injury related sepsis. *In* Wesdorp IC, Soeters PB (eds). Clinical Nutrition '81. Edinburgh, Churchill-Livingstone, 1982: 301–304.
45. Sakamoto M, Ishu S, Nishioka K. Level of complement activity and components C1, C4, C2, and C3 in complement response to bacterial challenge in malnourished rats. Infect Immun 1981; 32:553–556.
46. Royle GT, Kettlewell MGW. Liver function tests in surgical infection and malnutrition. Ann Surg 1981; 192:192–194.
47. Alexander JW, MacMillan BG. Hospital infections in burns. *In* Bennett JV, Brachman P (eds). Nosocomial Infections. Boston, Little, Brown, 1979: 335–353.
48. Alexander JW, MacMillan BG, Stinnett JD, et al. Beneficial

effects of aggressive protein feeding in severely burned children. Ann Surg 1980; *192*:505–517.

49. Dominioni L, Stinnett JD, Fang C-H, et al. Gastrostomy feeding in normal and hypermetabolic burned guinea pigs: a model for the study of enteral diets. J Burn Care Rehab 1984; *5*:100–105.

50. Dominioni L, Trocki O, Fang C-H, et al. Enteral feeding in burn hypermetabolism: nutritional and metabolic effects of different levels of calorie and protein intake. JPEN 1985; *9*:269–279.

51. Mochizuki H, Trocki O, Dominioni L, et al. Mechanism of prevention of postburn hypermetabolism and catabolism by early enteral feeding. Ann Surg 1984; *200*:297–310.

52. Mochizuki H, Trocki O, Dominioni L, et al. Optimal lipid content for enteral diets following thermal injury. JPEN 1984; *8*:638–646.

52a. Alexander JW, Saito H, Trocki O, et al. The importance of lipid type in the diet after injury. Ann Surg 1986; *204*:1–8.

53. Mochizuki H, Trocki O, Dominioni L, et al. Effect of a diet rich in branched chain amino acids on severely burned guinea pigs. J. Trauma 1986; *26*:1077–1085.

54. Bessey PQ, Watters JM, Aoki TT, et al. Combined hormonal infusion simulates the metabolic response to injury. Ann Surg 1984; *200*:264–281.

55. Nanni G, Siegel JH, Coleman B, et al. Increased lipid fuel dependence in the critically ill septic patient. J Trauma 1984; *24*:14–30.

56. Stoner HB, Little RA, Frayn KN, et al. The effect of sepsis on the oxidation of carbohydrate and fat. Br J Surg 1983; *70*:32–35.

57. Dahn MS, Kirkpatrick JR, Blasier R. Alterations in the metabolism of exogenous lipid associated with sepsis. JPEN 1984; *8*:169–173.

58. Wannemacher RW Jr, Kaminski MV Jr, Neufeld HA, et al. Protein-sparing therapy during pneumococcal infection in rhesus monkeys. JPEN 1978; *2*:507–518.

59. Wannemacher RW Jr, Kaminski MV Jr, Dinterman RE, et al. Use of lipid calories during pneumococcal sepsis in the rhesus monkey. JPEN 1982; *6*:100–105.

60. Askanazi J, Carpentier YA, Elwyn DH, et al. Influence of total parenteral nutrition on fuel utilization in injury and sepsis. Ann Surg 1980; *191*:40–46.

61. Milewski PJ, Threlfall CJ, Heath DF. Intracellular free amino acids in undernourished patients with or without sepsis. Clin Sci 1982; *62*:83–91.

62. Kingsland PA, Kingsnorth A, Royle GT, et al. Glutamate metabolism in malnutrition and sepsis in man. Br J Surg 1981; *68*:234–237.

63. Caruana JA Jr, Montes M, Camara DS, et al. Functional and histopathologic changes in the liver during sepsis. Surg Gynecol Obstet 1982; *154*:653–656.

64. Petersen SR, Kudsk KA, Carpenter G, et al. Malnutrition and immunocompetence: increased mortality following an infectious challenge during hyperalimentation. J Trauma 1981; *21*:528–533.

65. Kudsk KA, Carpenter G, Petersen S, et al. Effect of enteral and parenteral feeding in malnourished rats with *E. coli*–hemoglobin adjuvant peritonitis. J Surg Res 1981; *31*:105–110.

66. Weyman C, Belin J, Smith AD, et al. Linoleic acid as an immunosuppressive agent. Lancet 1975; *2*:33.

67. Cleary TG, Pickering LK. Mechanisms of intralipid effect on polymorphonuclear leukocytes. J Clin Lab Immunol 1983; *11*:21–26.

68. Fischer GW, Hunter KW, Wilson SR. Diminished bacterial defences with intralipid. Lancet 1980; *2*:819–820.

69. Deitch EA, Maejima K, Berg R. Effect of oral antibiotics and bacterial overgrowth on the translocation of the GI tract microflora in burned rats. J Trauma 1985; *25*:385–392.

36

WOUND HEALING

WILLIAM H. GOODSON III / THOMAS K. HUNT

Wound nutrition is in fact whole-body nutrition. Wound tissue can locally absorb an amino acid and incorporate that substrate into new structural protein, but this is an uncommon mechanism and has been demonstrated more as a laboratory curiosity than in the actual course of wound nutrition.[1] In a clinical sense nutrition for wound healing is a complex system of local and remote energy and substrate use.

Local nutritional needs are obvious. Amino acids and sugar are needed as substrate for collagen and proteoglycan synthesis; fibroblasts need glucose or another energy source to synthesize messenger RNA and DNA for replication and to form the high-energy bonds required for amino acid transfer and protein synthesis; energy is needed for migration of fibroblasts and epithelial and endothelial cells.

In addition to energy consumption in the wound, there are many cells and proteins that are synthesized elsewhere and transported in a ready-to-use form to the wound (Table 36–1). Bone marrow produces platelets, polymorphonuclear leukocytes, and monocytes. The liver synthesizes fibronectin, complement, and glucose in situations of stress or fasting All of these are transported to the wound via the blood. This transport, along with transport of oxygen for energy metabolism, collagen synthesis, and host defense mechanisms, requires muscular strength for respiration and maintenance of cardiac output. Thus, proper wound healing depends upon a complex system of energy transportation, delivery, and use.

EVENTS OF NORMAL HEALING

Injury, either accidental or surgical, destroys tissue and presents a series of problems that must be solved before tissue integrity can be restored. Mesodermal cells move in to fill the gap in injured tissue. These cells, beginning with the inflammatory cells, arrange themselves in a characteristic pattern of inflammatory cells, fibroblasts, and new vessels which has been called the "wound module." These

TABLE 36–1. Elements of Wound Healing and Site Where Nutrition Is Used for Synthesis

Element	Role	Site of Nutrition Use for Synthesis
Cellular		
Platelet	Hemostasis Growth factors	Bone marrow
Polymorphonuclear leukocyte	Phagocytosis Bacterial killing	Bone marrow
Macrophage	Wound autodebridement Growth factors	Bone marrow
Fibroblast	Synthesize collagen matrix Wound contraction	Wound
Endothelium	Neovascularization	Blood vessels in or near wound
Structural		
Thrombin and other coagulation factors	Hemostasis Interact with other cells	Liver
Fibronectin	Collagen–cell interaction	Liver
Collagen	Wound strength	Wound
Proteoglycans	In wound matrix, exact role undefined	Wound
Nutritional		
Glucose	Energy for wound cells Substrate for proteoglycans	Diet, liver (glycogen, gluconeogenesis, lactate recycling)
Vitamins	Necessary cofactors	Diet (stored in liver)
Amino acids	Structure of wound matrix Cell synthesis	Muscles (protein breakdown), liver (transamination), diet
Trace minerals	Enzyme cofactors	Diet (stored in bone [calcium] and liver)

cells fill the space of the wound and synthesize the repair matrix. They make only one product, though a complex one, the collagen matrix or scar tissue. The wound module, like any other specialized tissue, has its own nutritional needs and its own physiological features.

After injury the first problem is hemostasis, which requires the cascade of coagulation factors and the specific action of platelets, which are synthesized in the liver and bone marrow, respectively. Hemostasis has a very high priority in the body economy, and therefore coagulation precursors are not usually depleted except in extreme states of malnutrition. They provide specific elements that are assumed to be vital for satisfactory wound healing, but the elements themselves are synthesized in areas remote from the wound. As platelets provide hemostasis they also release a growth factor called platelet-derived growth factor (PDGF), which is the first of several wound factors that are important for healing.[2,3] PDGF, like similar factors from macrophages (see below), stimulates the growth of new blood vessels, without which a wound cannot heal.

Even under the best of circumstances there is inevitably some contamination of a wound with bacteria. The wound is a warm, moist environment, and in the absence of a specific compensatory response even small numbers of bacteria would rapidly grow and multiply. Fortunately, with adequate circulation there is usually rapid delivery of polymorphonuclear leukocytes, which by nonspecific killing mechanisms are able to eliminate small numbers of bacteria quickly. These cells also are synthesized in the bone marrow and are brought to the wound by the circulation. Polymorphonuclear leukocytes have the additional need for molecular oxygen. This molecular oxygen is used for intracellular killing of bacteria and is provided by the circulation. If polymorphonuclear leukocytes are placed in a hypoxic environment such as hypoperfused tissue their oxygen-dependent, nonspecific bacterial killing mechanisms are less effective and infection is more likely and more severe.[4]

Normal leukocytes consume some glucose at rest and increase their glucose consumption approximately eightfold to tenfold when phagocytosing bacteria.[5] This explains how the need for glucose increases sharply when infection occurs. Leukocytes from patients with chronic severe malnutrition are capable of only about half the increase in glucose use during phagocytosis.

Even in a small, clean, incised wound millions of cells die. They die of physical disruption, of desiccation on exposure to air, and of chemical injury on exposure to "antiseptic" or nonphysiologic solutions. This disruption extends beneath the wound's surface even after sharp debridement or creation of a clean wound. These fragments of dead cells and desiccated tissue must be debrided. A process of autodebridement (self-cleaning) of a wound is accomplished primarily by tissue macrophages (the tissue phase of previously circulating monocytes) which also derive ultimately from bone marrow.

In addition to debriding wounds, macrophages release separate factors that stimulate angiogenesis and fibroplasia. Experiments on the role of macrophages have demonstrated the following:

1. If macrophages are eliminated from an animal, healing will be impaired.

2. Preparations of macrophages in cornea or wound attract blood vessels to grow toward them.

3. Media in which macrophages are grown stimulate endothelial and fibroblast growth.

No other wound cell shows this range of capabilities. In a teleological sense their pivotal importance seems to be the best of evolutionary economy: this cell is similar to the most primitive cells used by invertebrates to "plug" holes in their integument.

The macrophage may also be the central cell in the body's recognition of injury. Tissue hypoxia in a wound has long been suspected to be a major stimulus to the growth of the wound module.[6] The central area of a wound is invariably hypoxic (see discussion of wound metabolism, below), and products of anaerobic metabolism such as lactate stimulate cell growth in wounds. Studies with rabbit ear chambers show that the wound module grows toward the central, hypoxic zone, but if the hypoxia in the central area of the wound is corrected to atmospheric oxygen tension the growth of the wound is retarded or even stopped.[7] In culture macrophages make more angiogenesis factor when lactate is added to the media or if the culture is made hypoxic and then accumulates lactate. It seems likely that, in addition to their role in debriding wounds, macrophages also function to translate a specific stimulus—hypoxia or wound lactate—into specific growth factors, which in turn promote growth of new blood vessels and fibroblasts.

After release of growth factors by platelets and macrophages the major growth and consumption of energy shifts to the wound, where replication of fibroblasts, synthesis of collagen in the extracellular matrix by the fibroblasts, and the growth and development of new blood vessels in the area of the wound become major energy users. Blood vessels need the support provided by collagen, and collagen is provided by fibroblasts, which in turn need oxygen and nutrition from the blood. This creates interdependent growth.

Fibroblasts originate in the wound itself and are presumably stimulated to grow there by platelet- and macrophage-derived growth factors acting in concert with insulin and somatomedin. Fibroblasts replicate best in moderate hypoxia and multiply in experimental wounds near functioning vessels in which the oxygen tension is 35 to 40 mm Hg. Their ultimate source is still debated. Some postulate a fibrocyte lying in wait for injury or other need. Other investigators assume that fibroblasts are specialized

or dedifferentiated smooth muscle cells that arise largely from the adventitia of blood vessels. Whichever cell is the source, it is clear that fibroblasts multiply in the area of wounds. If a wound is irradiated sufficiently there is no growth of fibroblasts and no wound healing. Fibroblasts have specific nutritional requirements for oxygen, structural substrate, nutritional substrate, trace minerals, and vitamins. Using these substrates they synthesize two major categories of products necessary for wound healing, collagens and proteoglycans.

The amino acid hydroxyproline constitutes about 15 per cent of collagen and is rarely found elsewhere. For this reason hydroxyproline is often used as a marker for the collagen content of various tissues. It cannot be incorporated directly into new collagen molecules, however. Instead, as the collagen molecule is synthesized on the ribosomes of the fibroblast, proline is incorporated into its structure. These proline residues and some of the lysine residues are hydroxylated, once the basic molecule has been synthesized, by an essential intraribosomal step that requires the presence of iron, ascorbic acid, alpha-ketoglutarate, and molecular oxygen. As a practical point, only lack of ascorbic acid and lack of oxygen are potential clinical problems, except in infants, whose healing probably can also be retarded by iron deficiency. Newly synthesized and hydroxylated collagen is then assembled into a triple helix. The cross-linked organization of this triple helix requires the presence of hydroxyproline and hydroxylysine. Because only the unhydroxylated form of the amino acids can be used to synthesize collagen, the deficiency of any of the cofactors for proline hydroxylation to hydroxyproline, particularly oxygen, can limit the formation of collagen.

Collagen synthesis is achieved in several stages during the growth of the wound module. First, fibroblasts replicate in a region of moderate hypoxia and lactate concentration. Here they receive the signal to prepare for collagen synthesis. As a result of this environment the ribosomal network and enzymes are prepared for collagen synthesis and some collagen synthesis begins. However, collagen cannot be synthesized rapidly in low oxygen tensions. When growth of the wound module (specifically, the new vessels) around the fibroblast is complete, the module acquires an oxygen supply and collagen is synthesized rapidly. Although there is a moderate gradient of glucose into even large dead spaces, the supply of glucose for wound metabolism is usually adequate if blood glucose is sufficient.

The hydroxylation of proline to hydroxyproline in the formation of collagen requires molecular oxygen. This process cannot borrow oxygen from other molecules. Extensive laboratory studies have shown that collagen formation by fibroblasts depends on oxygen. Collagen is only slowly synthesized below a pericellular PO_2 of 20 mm Hg. Maximum collagen synthesis is reached at levels of about 100 to 120 mm Hg. Accumulation of collagen in experimental wounds is decreased in animals breathing 12 per cent oxygen (equivalent to an altitude of about 12,000 ft) and is moderately increased in those breathing 40 per cent oxygen. The central wound PO_2 is below 20 mm Hg in animals kept in 12 per cent oxygen. In human subjects the average oxygen tension in the center of a wound reaches 35 to 45 mm Hg between the third and seventh days after operation. This range can be described as "adequate," but certainly does not allow maximum collagen formation. Administration of oxygen by face mask at this time can raise tissue oxygen and collagen deposition. This suggests a paradox. Low PO_2 stimulates fibroplasia and angiogenesis and starts collagen synthesis, but higher PO_2 makes more collagen. The fact is, however, that modest increases of wound edge PO_2 do not materially affect the central hypoxia.

The oxygen content of the central part of a human wound depends on four major factors: the oxygen tension in the blood circulating to the area of the wound; the rate of blood flow through the capillaries near the wound; the distance from the central portion of the wound to the nearest capillary; and the oxygen consumption by cells between the nearest blood vessel and the central portion of the wound.[8] Oxygen is a convenient marker, since it is readily measured in tissue, but it also reflects the delivery of nutrition to a wound; therefore, local tissue PO_2 is a convenient index of blood perfusion.

If hypoxia is present because of decreased blood flow, one can assume that other substrate materials are also deficient because of decreased perfusion. Like delivery of oxygen, delivery of substrate to a wound is determined by the circulation of blood in the area of the wound, the content of substrates in the blood, the distance from the nearest blood supply to the wound, and the competitive consumption of substrate by other cells in the wound area.

It is important to remember that collagen not only is formed in a wound, but is remodeled as well. Beginning almost as soon as a wound is created, there is a breakdown of pre-existing collagen. Usually more collagen is synthesized than destroyed, and therefore the wound gains tensile strength. However, these processes can proceed independently; specifically, collagen lysis can continue in the absence of synthesis. If lysis predominates, wounds lose strength. This occurs in scurvy, or vitamin C deficiency: collagen synthesis ceases, lysis continues, and old wounds reopen.

ENERGY NEEDS OF WOUNDS

In the simplest sense collagen synthesis is the desired result of normal healing. Collagen is a protein and as such requires approximately 1 kilocalorie for the formation of each gram. A volume of granulation tissue a fraction of a millimeter thick and 3 cm square weighs approximately 500 mg and contains at least 10 mg of collagen. Collagen constitutes only a portion of granulation tissue. In addition to collagen it has proteoglycans, millions of new cells, new blood vessels, and serum proteins, all elements that require synthesis. The energy needs of small wounds are minor relative to the overall energy economy of the body, but a large wound such as a burn or peritonitis can rapidly become the dominant factor in body nutrition.

Wounds accumulate lactate, a product of incomplete oxidation of glucose. Lactate may indicate inefficient extraction of energy from available nutrition because of the relative hypoxia found in damaged tissue and/or tissue under repair.[9] When oxidized to water and carbon dioxide a mole of glucose yields three times as many moles of ATP or calories of energy as when oxidized only to lactate. This inefficiency is the metabolic price of having cells function in the wound at the leading edge of the available nutrition where there is limited perfusion, high competition between cells for oxygen, and insufficient oxygen for complete energy extraction. In addition, some wound cells (i.e., macrophages) apparently "choose" to oxidize glucose only to lactate since even in a well-oxygenated culture they still make lactate. (Some researchers have studied wounds created by injection of inflammatory agents into muscle. The metabolism in these wounds is less anaerobic, probably reflecting the more efficient baseline circulation of muscle compared with that of uninjured subcutaneous tissue.[10])

Lactate formed in a wound is carried away by the circulation to the liver, where it is recycled to glucose by the Cori cycle. This requires energy, further reducing the useful energy extracted for each mole of glucose, but normal liver has excellent perfusion and if uninjured is able to assume this role of chemical supplier and recycler of carbon fragments just as it does for anaerobically metabolizing muscle. It is sufficiently important to conserve the limited oxygen in a wound that the body is willing to "pay double" for the energy it receives from glucose—it receives less energy in the wound than would be available with more oxygen and it spends more energy to recycle the partially used glucose fragments (lactate) to make new glucose. The liver also provides serum factors, complement and fibronectin, in addition to its role in early wound healing. Synthesis of these proteins requires adequate nutrition, and, along with other serum proteins such as albumin and transferrin, they are depressed in chronically malnourished patients.

Whole-body metabolic needs are always increased by injury, trauma or burn, but there is a much greater energy need if sepsis is superimposed on the injury. Infected wounds consume complement and other nonspecific proteins used to resist and opsonize bacteria. Combined with the nutrition needed to synthesize and operate polymorphonuclear leukocytes (the burst of glucose use during phagocytosis) these requirements can equal or exceed the local use of energy in the wound for the simple processes of collagen formation and remodeling. Much of the energy for these needs is consumed outside the wound, but it is still part of the energy economy of satisfactory healing.

In a situation of stress, body protein mass becomes a source of substrate for healing, and the amount of protein available relates to survival. Some is used as individual amino acids, but again the liver has a major role as the supplier that converts the protein mass into glucose. Sustained synthesis, particularly during sepsis, is energy-expensive. Body potassium stores reflect this whole-body cell mass of protein. Persons who have depleted protein stores, as shown by depleted total body potassium, have more complications following surgery, longer recovery, higher mortality, and, specifically, more wound problems.[11]

Bone marrow supplies platelets, polymorphonuclear leukocytes, and monocytes. If there is major injury or if infection is added to a wound, there is a substantial and continuing need for these cells. This taxes the ability of the bone marrow to replicate, and in severe chronic stress the bone marrow can be depleted.

ROLE OF THE CIRCULATION IN NUTRITION SUPPLY TO THE WOUND

Adequate wound nutrition requires wound circulation to deliver substrate and the presynthesized materials, such as inflammatory cells. Adequate or increased circulation allows oxygen delivery for better substrate use and resistance to infection and also supplies glucose for energy requirements and amino acids for protein synthesis.

Various factors can cause a decrease in wound perfusion. Most important of these is decreased vascular volume.[8] Hypovolemia caused by inadequate fluid resuscitation, blood loss, diuretics, or hemodialysis will decrease vascular volume and therefore decrease subcutaneous blood flow by reflex vasoconstriction. Adequate circulation requires good filling pressures, and if cardiac output is depressed by either primary cardiac injury or sepsis there will be decreased circulation of the peripheral tissue. Nicotine inhaled in cigarette smoking causes vasoconstriction. This again restricts circulation of the subcutaneous tissue and limits wound nutrition.

Conspicuously absent from the list of factors limiting wound circulation is anemia. It has been shown clinically that anemia down to a packed cell volume of approximately 20 does not restrict wound circulation[12] and experimentally does not decrease tensile strength or collagen contents of wounds.[13,14] Low hematocrit levels are associated with a decreased "reserve" for oxygen delivery during exercise, but are not usually rate-limiting to supply of nutrition or oxygen for wound healing purposes.

SPECIFIC NUTRITIONAL NEEDS FOR WOUNDS

Various experiments have shown needs for specific substances and trace materials in wound healing. Diets deficient in arginine or histidine lead to poor healing. Specific amino acids such as methionine or lysine have been shown by some authors to partially restore healing in seriously protein-depleted animals when given as single agents. As a practical point, however, attempts to restore adequate healing by giving single amino acids are not of clinical use, and there are few required nutrients that commonly become depleted in wounds in the absence of obvious total-body protein-calorie malnutrition.

Vitamin A, stored in large quantities in the liver, is required for an adequate inflammatory response in wound healing. Not only is it necessary for normal inflammatory response, but in the presence of steroids, which usually suppress inflammation, vitamin A can restore the inflammatory response.[15–19] This has been demonstrated experimentally and clinically. Excess vitamin A, however, can lead to an excessive inflammatory response and can be harmful in and of itself. For this reason supplemental vitamin A is usually given only in a dose of about 20,000 to 25,000 U for 10 days. This dose usually saturates the liver. Vitamin A is the most commonly deficient vitamin.

The B vitamins are unlikely to be depleted in the absence of general malnutrition, but they do have an important role. Thiamine (vitamin B_1) is necessary for lysyl oxidase (which is necessary for condensation of hydroxlysine molecules to make lysine-lysine links, which in turn give collagen much of its strength). Thiamine deficiency causes a decrease in total collagen, especially type III. It is thought that this occurs because of the need for thiamine for normal cell energy metabolism.[20] Pantothenic acid (vitamin B_5) deficiency is associated with decreased wound strength and decrease in number of fibroblasts on histological section, probably because of an effect of cell replication.[21]

Vitamin C is required for the hydroxylation of proline during the formation of collagen and is therefore a necessary wound nutrient. As discussed, in the absence of vitamin C collagen lysis can continue despite interruption of collagen synthesis. Therefore, wounds that were previously sound may be weakened by continued lysis of collagen. This can lead to reopening of old wounds, which is one of the classic symptoms of scurvy.

Vitamin D does not have a direct, local role in wound healing, but it is needed for calcium hemostasis. Calcium ion is a necessary cofactor for normal coagulation and many enzyme systems. Under usual circumstances liver stores of vitamin D in conjunction with bone reserves of calcium will meet all needs. Major exceptions occur in patients with malabsorption syndromes, in which vitamin D is not absorbed, and patients with fractures, who may need up to 800 IU a day of vitamin D, which is two times the usually recommended dose.[22]

Vitamin E has achieved an unusual role in the mind of the lay public as being beneficial for healing. There have only been a few laboratory tests of this vitamin and they have shown the opposite—vitamin E retards healing[23] and fibrosis.[24] Both of the authors of this chapter have encountered patients whose healing seemed retarded by doses of vitamin E over 1000 IU per day. Of course, some vitamin E is necessary for normal fat metabolism, but daily doses probably should not exceed 100 IU unless there is another specific need for the vitamin.

Vitamin K, like vitamin D, has no direct role in the wound, but it does have a role in coagulation, which is a prerequisite of healing. Clinically, vitamin K deficiency is most often encountered in newborns, patients with malabsorption, and those taking coumadin-type anticoagulants.

Zinc is a necessary cofactor for collagen formation. It is lost in the urine during stress and weight loss and tends to be clinically depleted in patients with chronic malnutrition, chronic metabolic stress, or chronic diarrhea. Zinc is thought to be needed for nucleic acid synthesis in cell replication and mRNA formation and directly for protein synthesis. Zinc normally accumulates in wounds during healing. Healing is deficient when zinc is deficient; supplemental zinc, given as 220-mg zinc sulfate tablets, can correct this deficiency.[25–28] Serum zinc levels are depressed by chronic steroid administration. Therefore it is usually given with vitamin A to treat or prevent steroid-retarded healing.

Several other minerals are needed for normal healing. Magnesium, which is often depleted by chronic diarrhea or intestinal fistulas, is a necessary cofactor for enzymes in protein synthesis and as such is needed for normal healing. Copper is needed for erythrocyte formation and as a cofactor for the enzyme lysyl oxidase. If lysyl oxidase is deficient, collagen will not gain normal strength by cross-linking. Body needs for other trace minerals—manganese, molybdenum, cobalt, chromium, selenium—are known, but specific roles for them in wound healing have not been defined.

HORMONE REQUIREMENTS TO ALLOW UTILIZATION OF NUTRITION

In addition to specific nutritional requirements for wounds, there must be an adequate hormone environment to allow the utilization of substrate by wounds. The most common deficiency in this regard occurs in diabetes mellitus. It appears that the initiation of cell growth and collagen synthesis requires insulin, but once these processes are under way the presence of insulin may not be required for the continuation of synthesis. For Type I or juvenile-onset diabetics absence of insulin restricts the ability of fibroblasts and other cells to use glucose for cell replication and synthetic needs. Experimentally, it is most important in the early phases of healing.[29] Animals given adequate amounts of insulin for the first several days of a healing experiment heal normally even if insulin is withdrawn during the later phases. Similarly, when insulin antibodies are used to retard healing, the effect is like that of malnutrition.[30] Adult-onset or Type II diabetes does not usually represent a limitation of the ability to use glucose in the wound. Instead, the problems with wound healing in subjects with Type II diabetes seem as much related to the presence of adipose tissue, with its relative hypoperfusion, as to an actual failure to use glucose. Insulin is required for cell replication in almost all cell culture systems.

THE EFFECT OF MALNUTRITION ON WOUND HEALING

Starvation sufficient to produce weight loss of approximately 20 per cent delays the gain of tensile strength of experimental wounds in animals.[31–33] Feeding methionine or lysine alone sometimes restores healing disproportionately in these animals, so a deficiency of methionine and cysteine or lysine is thought to be particularly important in the mechanism of retarded healing in malnutrition, although these results are not universally accepted.[34–37] Specific deficiencies of arginine and histidine have been associated with poor healing.[38–41]

The estimate that a 20 per cent loss of body weight can be tolerated before wound healing is retarded assumes the absence of sepsis. With sepsis, a large portion of energy is diverted into white cell replication, containment of the infection by phagocytosis and lysosomal killing of bacteria, and the increased thermogenesis of fever; therefore preoperative loss of body mass is less well tolerated. Nutrition can be restored preoperatively either parenterally or orally. There are some experimental data to suggest that at least the tolerance of bacterial insult is greater with oral rather than with parenteral feeding. However, this has not been thoroughly substantiated in clinical experience. It is clear that parenteral nutrition is superior to no preoperative nutrition in severely malnourished patients.

Systematic experimental studies are few in human subjects. Using a technique they have validated carefully in animal studies, Flint, Haydock, et al.[42,43] have demonstrated decreased collagen accumulation in a small, standardized subcutaneous wound in patients who were moderately to severely malnourished.

Their preliminary studies indicate that the length of time required for restoration of healing may be shorter than is presently assumed. They have found evidence of improved healing with a period of parenteral nutrition that averaged about 11 days.[44] It may be that nutrition sufficient to restore liver protein synthesis and bone marrow function, without measurable repletion of body protein stores, is adequate for wound healing, assuming that this nutrition is sustained during the healing process. In other clinical studies Casey et al.[45] and Dickhaut et al.[46] have shown that wound complications and failure of an amputation to heal primarily, respectively, are more common in patients with preoperative depression of serum albumin, but they have not evaluated preoperative restoration of nutrition. Bozzetti et al.[47] evaluated an unrandomized group of patients receiving parenteral nutrition after proctectomy and found a trend toward higher hydroxyproline content in biopsies of granulation tissue than is usual in patients not receiving parenteral nutrition after a similar operation.

SUMMARY

Wound nutrition, like any massive building organization, uses a combination of in-situ and remote synthesis. Elements of coagulation, infection control, and wound autodebridement are synthesized at sites remote from the wound. Structural elements—proteoglycans, collagen—are synthesized in situ. The cells that produce structural elements and the systems to nourish these cells (new blood vessels) also grow locally in the wound. Careful attention to the substrate, vitamin, trace mineral, and energy requirements both in situ and remote from the wound is needed to promote maximum possible healing.

References

1. Niinikoski J, Kivisaari J, Viljanto J. Local hyperalimentation of experimental granulation tissue. Acta Chir Scand 1977; 143:201–206.
2. Knighton DR, Thakral KK, Hunt TK. Platelet-derived angiogenesis: an initiator of the healing sequence. Surg Forum 1980; 31:226–228.
3. Knighton DR, Hunt TK, Thakral KK, et al. Role of platelets and fibrin in the healing sequence. Ann Surg 1982; 196:379–388.
4. Knighton DR, Halliday B, Hunt TK. Oxygen as an antibiotic: the effect of inspired oxygen. Arch Surg 1984; 119:199–204.
5. Selvaraj RJ, Bhat KS. Metabolic and bactericidal activities of leukocytes in protein-calorie malnutrition. Am J Clin Nutr 1972; 25:166–174.
6. Hunt TK, Connolly WB, Aronson SB, et al. Anaerobic metabolism and wound healing: an hypothesis for the initiation and cessation of collagen synthesis in wounds. Am J Surg 1978; 135:328–332.
7. Knighton DR, Silver IA, Hunt TK. Regulation of wound-healing angiogenesis—effect of oxygen gradients and inspired oxygen concentration. Surgery 1981; 90:262–270.
8. Chang N, Goodson WH III, Gottrup F, et al. Direct measurement of wound and tissue oxygen tension in postoperative patients. Ann Surg 1983; 197:470–478.
9. Wilmore DW, Aulick LH, Mason AD, et al. Influence of the burn wound on local and systemic response to injury. Ann Surg 1977; 186:444–458.
10. Caldwell M, Shearer J, Morris A, et al. Evidence for aerobic glycolysis in lambda-carrageenan-wounded skeletal muscle. J Surg Res 1984; 37:63–68.
11. Walesby RK, Goode AW, Bentall HH. Nutritional status of patients undergoing valve replacement by open heart surgery. Lancet 1978; 1:76–77.
12. Jensen JA, Goodson WH III, Vasconez L, et al. Wound healing in anemia: a case report. West J Med 1986; 144:465–467.
13. Macon WL, Pories WJ. The effect of iron deficiency anemia on wound healing. Surgery 1971; 69:792–796.
14. Chvapil M, Hurych J, Ehrlichova E. The effect of iron deficiency on the synthesis of collagenous and noncollagenous proteins in wound granulation tissue and in the heart of rats. Exp Med Surg 1968; 26:52–60.
15. Hunt TK, Ehrlich HP, Garcia JA, et al. Effect of vitamin A on reversing the inhibitory effect of cortisone on healing of open wounds in animals and man. Ann Surg 1969; 170:633–641.
16. Bark S, Rettura G, Goldman D, et al. Effect of supplemental vitamin A on the healing of colon anastomosis. J Surg Res 1984; 36:470–474.
17. Herrmann JB, Woodward SC. An experimental study of wound healing accelerators. Am Surg 1972; 38:26–34.
18. Lee KH, Fu C-C, Spencer MR, et al. Mechanism of action of retinyl compounds on wound healing. III: Effect of retinoic acid on homologs on granulation formation. J Pharm Sci 1973; 62:895–899.
19. Salmela K, Ahonen J. The effect of methylprednisolone and vitamin A on wound healing. I. Acta Chir Scand 1981; 147:307–312.
20. Alvarez OM, Gilbreath RL. Thiamine influence on collagen during the granulation of skin wounds. J Surg Res 1982; 32:24–31.
21. Grenier JF, Aprahamian M, Genot C, et al. Pantothenic acid (vitamin B$_5$) efficiency on wound healing. Acta Vitaminol Enzymol 1982; 4:81–85.
22. Hey H, Lund B, Sorensen OH, et al. Delayed fracture healing following jejunoileal bypass surgery for obesity. Calcif Tissue Int 1982; 34:13–15.
23. Ehrlich HP, Tarver H, Hunt TK. Inhibitory effects of vitamin E on collagen synthesis and wound repair. Ann Surg 1972; 175:235–240.
24. Kagoma P, Burger SN, Seifter E, et al. The effect of vitamin E on experimentally induced peritoneal adhesions in mice. Arch Surg 1985; 120:949–951.
25. Sandstead HH, Henriksen LK, Greger JL, et al. Zinc nutriture in the elderly in relation to taste acuity, immune response and wound healing. Am J Clin Nutr 1982; 36:1046–1059.
26. Henzel JH, DeWeese MS, Lichti EL. Zinc concentrations within healing wounds. Arch Surg 1970; 100:349–357.
27. Pories WJ, Henzel JH, Rob CG, et al. Acceleration of wound healing in man with zinc sulphate given by mouth. Lancet 1967; 1:121–124.
28. Barcia PJ. Lack of acceleration of healing with zinc sulfate. Ann Surg 1970; 172:1048–1050.
29. Goodson WH III, Hunt TK. Wound healing in well-controlled diabetic men. Surg Forum 1984; 35:614–616.
30. Weringer EJ, Kelso JM, Tamai IY, et al. The effect of antisera to insulin, 2-deoxyglucose-induced hyperglycemia and starvation on wound healing in normal mice. Diabetes 1981; 30:407–410.
31. Irvin TT. Effects of malnutrition and hyperalimentation on wound healing. Surg Gynecol Obstet 1978; 146:33–37.
32. Ward MWN, Danzi M, Lewin MR, et al. The effects of subclinical malnutrition and refeeding on the healing of ex-

perimental colonic anastomoses. Br J Surg 1982; 69:308–310.

33. Daly JM, Vars HM, Dudrick SJ. Effects of protein depletion on strength of colonic anastomoses. Surg Gynecol Obstet 1972; *134*:15–21.

34. Csoka-Nemeth M. Uptake of ^{35}S-methionine and ^{35}S-chondroitin sulphate by the carrageenan granuloma in rats of different ages. Gerontologia 1966; *12*:217–225.

35. Irvin TT. The effect of methionine on colonic wound healing in malnourished rats. Br J Surg 1976; *63*:237–240.

36. Rosenberg BF, Caldwell FT. Effect of a single amino acid supplementation upon the rate of wound contraction and wound morphology in protein-depleted rats. Surg Gynecol Obstet 1965; *121*:1021–1027.

37. Stare FJ (ed). Wound healing in rabbits with a lysine deficiency. Nutr Reviews 1967; *25*:125–127.

38. Fitzpatrick DW, Fisher H. Histamine synthesis, imidazole dipeptides, and wound healing. Surgery 1982; *91*:430–434.

39. Fitzpatrick DW, Fisher H. Carnosine, histidine and wound healing. Surgery 1982; *91*:56–60.

40. Barbul A, Rettura G, Levenson SM, et al. Wound healing and thymotropic effects of arginine: a pituitary mechanism of action. Am J Clin Nutr 1983; *37*:786–794.

41. Seifter E, Rettura G, Barbul A, et al. Arginine: an essential amino acid for injured rats. Surgery 1978; *84*:224–230.

42. Flint MH, Haydock DA, Hyde KF, et al. The efficacy of subcutaneous Gore-Tex implants in monitoring wound healing response in experimental protein deficiency. Connective Tissue Res, in press.

43. Haydock DA, Hill GL. Impaired wound healing in surgical patients with varying degrees of malnutrition. JPEN 1986; *10*:550–554.

44. Haydock DA, Hill GL. Improved wound healing in surgical patients receiving intravenous nutrition. Br J Surg 1987; *74*:320.

45. Casey J, Flinn WR, Yao JST, et al. Correlation of immune and nutritional status with wound complications in patients undergoing vascular operations. Surgery 1983; *93*:822–827.

46. Dickhaut SC, DeLee JC, Page CR. Nutritional status: importance in predicting wound-healing after amputation. J Bone Joint Surg 1984; *66A*:71–75.

47. Bozzetti F, Terno G, Longoni C. Parenteral hyperalimentation and wound healing. Surg Gynecol Obstet 1975; *141*:712–714.

37

THE PERIOPERATIVE PATIENT

GRAHAM L. HILL

Starvation and weight loss are almost universal accompaniments of surgical illness. The surgical pathology, anorexia, fear, starvation necessitated by investigations, and the operative procedure itself all lead to malnutrition of a greater or lesser extent. Often this is taken as an accepted part of the experience in hospital and little may be done to either assess or improve the nutritional status of undernourished patients who require surgery. Techniques are now available to provide total nutritional requirements; nevertheless these may be expensive, require more time in hospital, and are not without danger. It is also difficult to quantify cost effectiveness of nutritional therapy in surgical patients.

In this chapter current research and its practical applications will be fully discussed, but it will become clear that much more needs to be done. There is a real need to define more clearly those circumstances in which patients will require perioperative nutrition and to carry out careful controlled studies in selected patients.

INDICATIONS FOR NUTRITIONAL THERAPY PRIOR TO MAJOR SURGERY

Around 50 years ago a Cleveland surgeon, Hiram Studley,[1] looked carefully at a number of factors he felt might contribute to the high mortality after gastrectomy for peptic ulcer disease. Carefully controlling for the age of the patient, the operating surgeon, and the type and length of the procedure, he found a striking correlation between the magnitude of preoperative weight loss and postoperative mortality. Close study of his paper shows that the cause of most of the deaths that occurred was respiratory infection and this was frequently complicated by wound dehiscence. Modern surgery with prophylactic antibiotics, better anesthetic and fluid balance techniques, improved suture materials, and vigorous physiotherapy has inbuilt safeguards to minimize the types of complications that occurred in Studley's patients. Hence the relationship between the preoperative nutritional state and the outcome of surgery is much less clear nowadays. Nevertheless, a number of recent prospective studies have shown that severely malnourished subjects are still at increased risk of developing complications after major surgery.[2–11] In this section, available information on the abnormal biology of undernourished surgical patients will be reviewed and studies on the effect of short-term nutritional repletion will be described. Practical clinical guidelines for the treatment of preoperative patients requiring nutritional therapy will then be set down.

Biology of Malnourished Surgical Patients Awaiting Major Surgery

CLINICAL CATEGORIES

A common denominator of all surgical illness is the oxidation of fat and erosion of the body protein mass. In patients who are not retaining water, this results in weight loss. Surgical patients who have lost a lot of weight fall into two broad categories. Firstly there is *marasmus*, which results from an overall deficit in food intake; the patient is consequently emaciated owing to wasting of body stores of fat and skeletal muscle. The effects are most apparent where these tissues normally give the figure its rounded appearance, hence the patient appears to be composed of skin and bone (Fig. 37–1). Secondly there is *kwashiorkor* (visceral attrition), which is much less common in surgical patients, and intermediate forms of mild degree are not infrequent. Here, subcutaneous fat is generally well preserved but muscle wasting is prominent, being associated with low plasma albumin and low levels of other transport proteins. Nutritional edema can occur but is not common in adult surgical patients (Fig. 37–2).

BODY COMPOSITION

In Chapter 4 it was shown that total body weight loss is accompanied by an equivalent proportion of weight being lost from most of the organs of the body. With severe weight loss body composition studies have shown that cellular protein, particularly that of skeletal muscle, is wasted. It is currently believed that the structural proteins (tendon, bone, etc.) are not wasted in most malnourished patients. As the body loses weight extracellular fluid accumulates but there is considerable loss of intracellular fluid that occurs pari passu with the loss of cellular protein.[12] Thus a malnourished patient who is losing weight may be said to have a shrinking body cell mass surrounded by a growing "sea" of extracellular fluid (Fig. 37–3).

METABOLIC CHANGES

As wasting occurs resting metabolic expenditure falls. The proportional reduction in metabolic expenditure is greater than the proportional reduction in weight. There is conservation of body nitrogen, an increased utilization of body fat, and an adaptation of the brain to use ketones as fuel. There are also profound alterations in muscle metabolism with reduction in key enzymes of glucose utilization, suggesting impairment of glucose utilization particularly under conditions of stress.[13]

ABNORMALITIES OF BODY FUNCTION IN MALNOURISHED PATIENTS

Psychologically, the intellect remains clear but there is a personality change, with inability to concentrate,

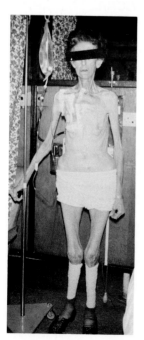

FIGURE 37–1. Adult marasmus. The effects of wasting on both fat and muscle are most apparent where these tissues give the figure its rounded appearance.

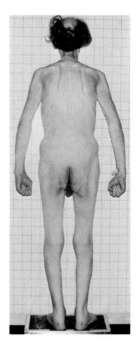

FIGURE 37–2. *Adult kwashiorkor. This patient has lost 30 per cent of his body weight and his plasma albumin is 26 g/L. There is a mild ankle edema. Subcutaneous fat is relatively well preserved.*

irritability, and apathy. Along with the wasting of *skeletal muscle* there is a selective atrophy of the Type II muscle fibers with a consequent increase in muscle fatigability.[13,14] *Respiratory function* may be profoundly affected. Malnourished patients have a reduced capacity to sustain adequate levels of ventilation from effects on both the central nervous system and respiratory muscles. Neural ventilatory drive is impaired and inspiratory and expiratory muscular weakness is demonstrable.[15] The function of the *cardiovascular system* is also impaired in malnourished patients, with bradycardia, low systolic and diastolic blood pressure, low venous pressure, reduced cardiac output, and reduced heart size.[16] The *gastrointestinal tract* is also affected. Achlorhydria and diarrhea are frequent. There is a reduction in organ size, villous atrophy, and brush border enzyme deficiencies.[17] *Hepatic function* is also impaired.[18] The *endocrine system* is not uniformly affected. Growth hormone is decreased, but thyrotrophic and adrenotrophic hormones are unaffected, as are corticosteroids. Gonadal atrophy leads to loss of libido and amenorrhea in the female.

Hepatic secretory proteins are all reduced in patients suffering from protein-energy malnutrition. Since total hepatic protein is reduced during fasting, it is to be expected that the plasma concentration of albumin, prealbumin, transferrin, retinol-binding protein, and other proteins secreted by the liver would be low. The rate of decline in the plasma levels of these proteins due to reduced synthesis is proportional to their half-life. Albumin, which has a very long half-life, does not fall rapidly in the plasma as the result of deficient nutrient intake, whereas

Components of Fat Free Body of 95 Adult Surgical Patients

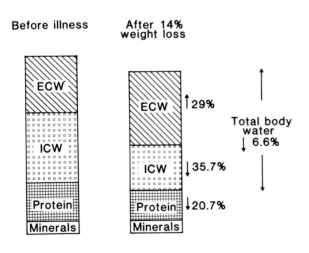

Before illness

After 14% weight loss

ECW ↑29%

ICW ↓35.7%

Protein ↓20.7%

Minerals

Total body water ↓6.6%

FIGURE 37–3. *The average change in composition of the fat-free body mass in 95 surgical patients with a significant weight loss. Note the marked redistribution of body water.*

levels of prealbumin, transferrin, and retinol-binding protein fall rapidly because their half-lives are considerably shorter. Low levels of plasma proteins in patients presenting for major surgery[19,20] are correlated with many other indices of malnutrition (Fig. 37–4). Since plasma albumin may act as an amino acid donor at the site of injury, and may be an important transporter of sulfur-containing amino acids, zinc, and fatty acids (all of which are important in wound healing), it is not difficult to understand that low levels of plasma albumin may have profound effects on wound healing. Likewise, transferrin may protect against wound infection by reducing the availability of iron to invasive organisms, and when plasma levels of transferrin are low in patients presenting for major surgery there appears to be an increased number of postoperative septic complications.[7]

It has not been easy to show a close association between *wound healing* and malnutrition in adult surgical subjects. There is ample evidence that protein deficiency is associated with impaired wound healing in animals, and there are data showing that hypoalbuminemia is associated with impaired healing in incised forearm wounds in adult patients.[21] Very recently, using a new method to study the wound healing response, it has been shown that early protein-energy malnutrition is associated with an impaired response that is similar to that seen in patients with severe weight loss.[22] Thus it appears that malnourished patients have slow healing, although scar formation is thought to be normal.[23]

Immune function has been carefully studied in malnourished children and has recently been the subject of intense investigation in adult surgical subjects.[24] Protein-calorie malnutrition is commonly associated with an acquired immune deficiency. Of the two recognized extreme variants of protein-energy malnutrition, kwashiorkor is characterized by an impairment in protein synthesis manifested by depression in serum albumin levels and relatively severe immune deficiency. In marasmus the serum albumin levels are better maintained and the immune function appears to be less severely affected.[25] Generally speaking, the in vivo skin tests show defective immune function in marasmus but the in vitro tests do not. In kwashiorkor in vitro function may also be normal.

THE PROFOUND EFFECT OF SEPSIS ON THE BIOLOGY OF SURGICAL MALNUTRITION

The important metabolic differences between the patient who is septic and starving and the one who is starving but free of sepsis are discussed in Chapter 34. Generally speaking, the metabolic effects of sepsis on the surgical patient are profound. Loss of cellular protein and gain in extracellular fluid are more marked, plasma proteins fall rapidly, and immune function is usually impaired. Although firm scientific data are lacking, it is assumed that many of the adverse functional effects of malnutrition that have just been outlined are more marked when the patient is septic. Of great clinical importance is the fact that septic patients do not respond adequately to nutritional therapy; it is necessary for the surgeon to control the infection first before effective nutritional repletion can be undertaken.[26,27]

Effects of Short-Term Nutritional Repletion

Clinical experience confirms that many patients with severe malnutrition look and feel better, begin to respond to their infective process, and start to heal their wounds within a week or two of beginning nutritional therapy. Underweight subjects who are not clinically septic seem to respond best, whereas

	Wt.L	Wt.	Fat	A.M.C	Alb	Tra	Pre	R.B.P	Lip	Hae
Weight Loss										* –·49
Weight			*** ·79	*** ·89			* ·48		** ·54	
Fat				** ·54					* ·43	
A.M.C.							* ·44		* ·46	* ·47
Albumin						** ·54	** ·53	** ·61		** ·55
Transferrin							*** ·66	*** ·68		
Prealbumin								*** ·86		* ·48
R.B.P.									* ·46	*** ·65
ß Lipoprotein										
Haemoglobin										

*p< 0·05;   **p< 0·01;   ***p< 0·001.

FIGURE 37–4. Low levels of plasma proteins are correlated with many other indices of malnutrition. Matrix of partial correlation coefficients controlling for age and height in 24 adult surgical patients, for anthropometric measurements, plasma proteins, and hemoglobin. A.M.C., arm muscle circumference; R.B.P., retinol-binding protein. (From Young GA, Hill GL. Am J Clin Nutr 1981; 34:166–172. © Am J Clin Nutr, American Society for Clinical Nutrition. Reproduced with permission.)

septic patients often appear to obtain little benefit. *Body composition studies* have demonstrated that nutritional therapy results in a rapid accumulation of fat and glycogen and a slow accumulation of protein.[26,28] Later, cellular protein and intracellular fluid accumulate and extracellular fluid shrinks; as a consequence total body water remains much the same. These effects are observed over a period of weeks and months, rather than the 10 or 14 days that are required or available to the clinician who is prescribing preoperative nutritional therapy before embarking on a major surgical procedure. Nevertheless, there are some potentially useful effects of short-term intravenous nutrition which have recently been demonstrated in the clinical setting. With adequate energy intake *metabolic expenditure* rises, liver and muscle *glycogen* are restored, and body *fat* is laid down.[27] There is a partial restoration of Type II *muscle* fibers, which may be associated with increased muscular endurance.[13,14] Available evidence suggests that some malnourished patients will have improved *ventilatory function* with short-term nutritional repletion,[15] although many questions concerning respiratory function remain unanswered. Similarly, there are some data that encourage the belief that intravenous nutrition improves *cardiac function* in malnourished patients.[29] *Gastrointestinal function* responds more effectively to enteral than to parenteral nutrition,[17] and the response is fairly rapid. *Hepatic secretory proteins* respond rapidly to effective nutritional replenishment. Although plasma albumin shows little effect in the short term, plasma transferrin and prealbumin return to normal levels in 1 or 2 weeks provided the patient is in positive nitrogen balance. It does not appear to be possible to restore plasma protein levels to normal in patients who are clinically septic.[30] The effect of short-term nutritional repletion on *wound healing* has only recently been studied. It appears that the wound healing response returns to normal in some patients after a week or two of intravenous nutrition; this is seen particularly in patients who are in positive nitrogen balance.[31] In patients who are very malnourished and in whom there is no evidence of sepsis *immune competence*, as assessed by delayed hypersensitivity skin testing, may be restored in about 2 to 5 weeks.[25]

In conclusion, it may be said that there are experimental data that appear to show improvement in a number of organ functions over a period of approximately 1 to 2 weeks in patients who are being fed intravenously. In other words there are some scientific data to support the conclusion that preoperative nutrition given to "at risk" patients may be beneficial. In subjects in whom continuing sepsis is a problem, available evidence suggests that if positive nitrogen balance cannot be achieved and low levels of plasma proteins cannot be restored to normal, then there seems to be little favorable effect on organ function.[32] Although much more work will be required before these conclusions can be verified,

they form the basic platform on which a number of the recommendations on preoperative nutrition in this book are based.

Identification of Subjects at Risk

It is claimed that indices of nutritional state can identify subsets of patients at high risk of postoperative complications and that these indices are useful tools for the selection of candidates for preoperative nutritional support.[2-4] Profound weight loss,[1] some anthropometric indices,[5,6] tests of muscle function,[6] measurements of plasma proteins—including albumin,[5,33] transferrin,[7] and prealbumin,[34] and combinations of these[3] (which are usually called prognostic nutritional indices)—have all been used as indicators of risk of postoperative nutrition-associated complications. They are said by those who use them to indicate the need for nutritional repletion prior to the operation itself. A comparison of these indicators of risk was recently made (Table 37–1). Measurements of weight loss and a variety of anthropometric indices are not clear indications of risk, but it can be seen that measurements of grip strength and low levels of plasma proteins are to some extent indicators of risk of postoperative complications. The various prognostic indices, which are largely determined by plasma protein levels, have little more to offer. Thus the indices of hepatic and muscle function are more helpful in identifying patients at risk of nutrition-associated complications. This is perhaps not unexpected if the risks themselves are considered. Morbidity and mortality in surgical patients usually derive from the failure of an essential body system rather than from exhaustion of energy or protein stores. For the survival of a patient the function of these body systems is probably more important than the absolute amount of protein or energy they contain. It seems reasonable therefore to conclude that patients particularly at risk should be able to be picked out by thorough physical examination and nutritional assessment, the findings of which are then related to abnormalities in specific organ systems. In the study outlined in Table 37–1 it was found that a thorough clinical examination which assessed major organ function proved to be as effective as any other indicator in identifying subjects at risk.[34] For clinical purposes then, a fairly adequate assessment of malnutrition and its associated risks can be obtained from a good history of dietary intake and energy output and a careful physical examination to assess the effects of protein depletion on each of the main organ systems. Plasma albumin should also be measured. *As a general guideline, body weight loss 15 to 20 per cent below well weight accompanied by clinical evidence of muscle weakness (respiratory and limb) and impaired physical endurance should alert the clinician to the possibility of increased risk of nutrition-associated complications. If the*

TABLE 37–1. *Comparison of Nutritional Indices As Indicators of Surgical Risk*

	Indicator	Cutoff*	Sensitivity %	Specificity %	Positive Predictive Value %	Negative Predictive Value %	Overall Predictive Value %	Statistical Data† X^2	p
Age	Age	>73 yrs	30	83	29	84	74	3.5	NS
Anthropometry	WL	>16%	31	84	30	85	75	4.4	<0.05
	BMI	<3rd%	30	75	22	83	67	0.5	NS
	TSF	<3rd%	21	80	19	84	70	0	NS
	MAMC	<3rd%	26	83	25	87	73	1.1	NS
Indices of function	GS (males)	<64 kPa	40	87	38	88	79	4.3	<0.05
	GS (females)	<47 kPa	30	83	21	89	76	0.3	NS
	Albumin	<35 g/L	33	82	29	85	73	4.2	<0.05
	Transferrin	<174 mg/dl	41	86	40	87	78	14.2	<0.001
	Prealbumin	<12 mg/dl	43	87	43	87	79	18.9	<0.001
Prognostic indices	Philadelphia	>45	35	83	32	85	75	6.5	<0.05
	Boston	>−0.7	30	84	30	84	74	3.8	<0.05
	Leeds	<−1.0	46	85	40	87	78	18.0	<0.001
Clinical judgment	Surgeon's assessment	>98 mm	32	83	27	86	75	2.0	NS
	Thorough clinical assessment	>60%	41	85	32	89	78	6.3	<0.025

*Each indicator was set such that 17 to 20% of patients were in high-risk group.
†Complication rates in high-risk versus low-risk groups.
WL, weight loss; BMI, body mass index; TSF, triceps skinfold; MAMC, midarm circumference; GS, grip strength; kPa, kilopascals; NS, not significant.
Data from Pettigrew and Hill. Br J Surg 1986; 73:47–51. Note that in this retrospective study of 218 patients undergoing major abdominal surgery, grip strength, plasma proteins, and a thorough examination all pointed out a group of patients at increased risk.

plasma albumin level is less than 32 g/L it is likely that sepsis is present or has been in the recent past, and that postoperative septic complications and impaired wound healing are a likely possibility.

Effects of Nutritional Therapy on the Outcome of Surgery

There have been a number of prospective studies in which patients undergoing major gastrointestinal surgery have been given courses of intravenous nutrition in an attempt to reduce the postoperative complication rate. Williams and colleagues[35] allocated 74 patients with a preoperative diagnosis of esophageal or stomach cancer into one of two groups. Both patient groups received oral multivitamin supplementation and were presented with a diet containing approximately 15 g of nitrogen and 3000 kcal. In addition, the treated group received between 2 and 3 L of a standard intravenous nutrient solution for a period of 7 to 10 days preoperatively. In the postoperative period all patients who had undergone an esophageal anastomosis were fed parenterally from the second postoperative day, and this was continued until an adequate oral intake was possible. For the remainder, assessment was made within the first 48 hours following surgery as to whether or not a satisfactory oral intake was likely by the third day. If this was thought to be unlikely, parenteral nutrition was resumed or commenced at that time. The two groups were closely matched in terms of their age, sex, and pathology. Following

surgery the hospital stay was the same in both groups, and there was a similar mortality and a similar anastomotic leakage rate; the only statistically significant difference was an increased number of wound infections in the control group. Close analysis of their data showed that the effect of preoperative parenteral nutrition significantly reduced the incidence of postoperative wound infection, but this benefit was most marked in those patients in whom plasma albumin was less than 30 to 35 g/L prior to the onset of the intravenous nutrition. The authors concluded that the clinical benefit would seem to be principally confined to these patients.

Another prospective study was done by Müller and colleagues in Cologne.[36] They studied the effect of 10 days of preoperative nutrition in all their patients undergoing surgery for gastrointestinal cancer whether malnourished or not. It is important to understand that in this study prophylactic antibiotics (which are associated with a marked reduction in the incidence of postoperative infection and are as a consequence used routinely in most gastrointestinal units around the world) were not used. For this reason the results are not typical of what might be expected in a normal clinical practice. Nevertheless, there was decreased sepsis and decreased mortality in those patients who were treated with preoperative intravenous nutrition (Fig. 37–5).

Another smaller prospective study was conducted by Holter and Fischer.[37] Patients with gastrointestinal cancer who had lost more than 10 lb over the 2- or 3-month period immediately prior to admission were randomly assigned either to receive parenteral

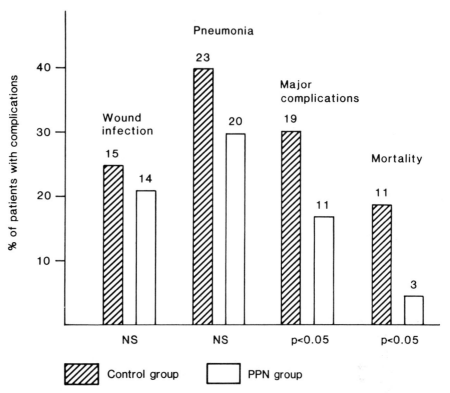

FIGURE 37–5. *Comparative clinical trial of preoperative total parenteral nutrition (PPN) in patients with gastrointestinal cancer. (Redrawn from Müller JM, Brenner U, Dienst C, et al. Lancet 1982; 1:68–71, with permission.)*

nutrition or not. Total parenteral nutrition was commenced 72 hours prior to surgery and was continued for a 10-day period postoperatively, or until 1500 kcal were taken by mouth. Thirty patients who had lost greater than 10 lb were randomly selected to receive intravenous nutrition and 26 patients who had lost greater than 10 lb were randomly selected not to receive parenteral nutrition. There was no statistical difference in the postoperative complication rate in either group. The study is taken as evidence that 3 days of preoperative parenteral nutrition is insufficient to influence the postoperative course.

Mullen[38] in Philadelphia studied retrospectively 145 patients who had been assessed by his nutritional support service. The course of preoperative nutrition had been selected arbitrarily by a variety of operating surgeons and in this way the study cannot be regarded as a prospective randomized trial; nevertheless, there are some lessons to be learned from it. Fifty patients received at least 7 days of effective and adequate intravenous nutrition and 95 patients received no preoperative nutritional support. The two study groups were similar in terms of age, sex, distribution, nutritional status on admission, and underlying disease process. In Figure 37–6, which is a summary of his findings, it can be seen that those patients who received intravenous nutrition for 7 days or longer had a markedly reduced incidence of complications.

These studies, taken together with the information already outlined that suggests that in some pa-

tients a short course of nutritional repletion is beneficial, make it seem reasonable to conclude that 1 to 2 weeks of preoperative intravenous nutrition should be considered for many malnourished patients prior to embarking on major surgery. If all malnourished patients were treated in this way, only about 10 per cent of those patients presenting for routine elective surgery would require treatment.[10] In reality the proportion is probably less than 5 per cent.

General Guidelines for the Practicing Surgeon

Although very sophisticated decision trees have been suggested for selecting patients for preoperative nutrition,[39] in clinical practice the process can be made more straightforward (Fig. 37–7). There are three factors that must be considered when a patient is presented as a possible candidate for preoperative nutritional support: his or her *nutritional state with its associated functional impairment*, the magnitude of the *projected operative procedure*, and the anticipated *response to the nutritional therapy*. The use of the schema shown in Figure 37–7 is best illustrated by three clinical examples.

Case 1. A male patient aged 65 years with 25 per cent weight loss presented with clinical evidence of wasting, associated muscular weakness and breathlessness on walking at a normal pace. His plasma

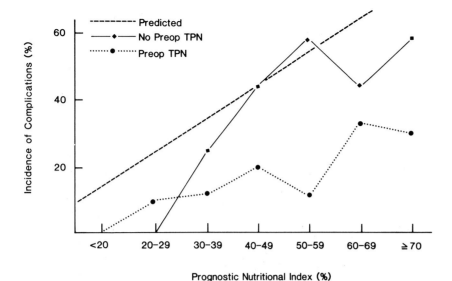

FIGURE 37–6. Incidence of complications versus prognostic nutritional index (PNI). In patients who received preoperative total parenteral nutrition (TPN) and in patients who received no preoperative TPN, the incidence of complications increases with increasing PNI. In patients who received no preoperative TPN the incidence of complications approaches that predicted by the prognostic nutritional index. The effect of preoperative TPN is to shift the curve downward and to the right. (Redrawn from Mullen JL. Surg Clin North Am 1981; 61:465–487).

albumin was normal. He complained of dysphagia secondary to adenocarcinoma of the gastric cardia and required a total gastrectomy—a procedure associated with a high complication rate. Referring to Figure 37–7, it is clear that since he was malnourished with clinical evidence of functional impairment and the planned operative procedure was to be a large one with a significant morbidity, he should be considered for preoperative nutritional repletion. He was wasted but there was no clinical evidence of sepsis. It could therefore be anticipated that he would respond effectively to a 2-week course of intravenous nutrition and could readily be put into positive nitrogen balance. Thus a 2-week course of preoperative intravenous nutrition (35 kcal/kg/day and 300 mg N/kg/day) was prescribed.[27] Intravenous nutrition was continued for a 2-week period postoperatively. No postoperative complications were encountered.

Case 2. A male patient aged 57 years presented with a vesicocolic fistula secondary to colonic diver-

ticular disease. He had 18 per cent weight loss and clinical evidence of fat and protein depletion. He was afebrile but felt weak and depressed. His plasma albumin was 28 g/L. It was clear that he was malnourished with consequent functional impairment and therefore at high risk from postoperative septic complications. The planned operative procedure was to be a large one with a 10 to 15 per cent morbidity. Since he was not septic at the time it could be anticipated that he could be put into positive nitrogen balance by appropriate intravenous nutrition. He was encouraged to ambulate and received a 2-week course of intravenous nutrition before surgery (Fig. 37–7). The left colon and upper rectum together with the fistula were resected, and the patient resumed eating on the fourth postoperative day and suffered no postoperative complications.

Case 3. A female patient had undergone a total colectomy for chronic ulcerative colitis 5 weeks before. She developed a high-output enterocutaneous fistula 7 days after surgery and had been severely ill

Decision Tree For Preoperative Nutrition

FIGURE 37–7. Simplified decision tree for selecting patients for preoperative nutritional therapy.

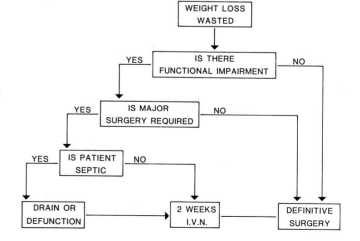

since with a swinging fever, partial wound dehiscence, and impaired renal function. Weight loss was not recorded, but physical examination revealed ample fat stores, although the muscle bellies of biceps and triceps felt soft and wasted. She had generalized edema. She was listless and confined to bed. Plasma albumin was 22 g/L. It was clear that she was malnourished and required nutritional repletion. The definitive operative procedure required to correct the fistula would be relaparotomy, total dissection of the intestine, excision of the fistula, and reanastomosis—a formidable procedure with a significant morbidity.[40] The associated sepsis indicated that intravenous nutrition would not have a significant effect on body composition or organ function. Thus, a limited laparotomy was performed before nutritional therapy was started, the abdomen was drained of pus and feces, and a loop jejunostomy was performed above the fistula to divert the fecal stream. A definitive fistula operation was not done (Fig. 37–7). A day later, as soon as the patient was stable, intravenous feeding was commenced. The patient, now free of sepsis, rapidly improved. Definitive fistula closure was undertaken 6 weeks later when the patient was in a sound nutritional state. The period of 6 weeks rather than 2 weeks was chosen on technical (not nutritional) grounds.[40] Intravenous nutrition was continued for 2 weeks postoperatively. About this time the patient began to eat, and 1 week later she was discharged, well, from the hospital.

The Problem Patient

Sometimes it is not at all clear if the patient will respond to nutritional therapy for sepsis until after intravenous nutrition has been commenced. On some occasions the septic focus can be quite difficult to find, and ultrasound, computerized axial tomography (CAT), or isotopic scans using autogenous neutrophils labeled with indium-111 are required before it can be anatomically located and drainage performed. Nevertheless, nutritional therapy will not be effective until the sepsis is controlled, and every effort must be made to do this. Where the sepsis is extensive or when the site of abscess is not certain, a full laparotomy should be undertaken with a thorough exploration of the peritoneal cavity. It is important for the surgeon to understand that definitive surgery should not be undertaken at this stage. It is wise to confine the procedure to location and drainage of sepsis and to defunctionalization if that seems appropriate. Once the sepsis is controlled the patient will respond to nutritional therapy, and a definitive procedure can be conducted in due course.

INDICATIONS FOR NUTRITIONAL THERAPY AFTER MAJOR SURGERY

Normal Response to Surgery and Postoperative Fatigue

After surgery a combination of starvation and increased catabolism occurs, resulting in a loss of body fat and protein. The extent of this loss depends upon the nutritional state of the patient prior to surgery, the extent of the operation itself, and the presence or absence of postoperative complications, particularly septic complications. The composition of such tissue loss has been analyzed for very major surgery, and an average loss of 4 kg in patients undergoing rectal incision is made up of 1 kg of protein, 1.3 kg of fat, and 1.8 kg of water.[28] The effects of such a loss are difficult to measure because of the widespread influences on physiological and psychomotor performances. However, for most patients undergoing surgery it appears to be unimportant,[41] although postoperative tiredness persists for months after major surgery or injury, long after the nutritional, endocrine, and metabolic changes associated with it have subsided. Little is known about the syndrome because of the difficulty of defining and measuring physical fitness, but it may well be related to the preoperative nutritional state just as much as to the extent of postoperative metabolic effects.[42] Studies involving chronic semistarvation, physical immobilization, and short-term sedation all demonstrate diminished intellectual and psychomotor performances.[43] These factors in varying degree are present in preoperative patients, so that the postoperative fatigue syndrome is, in part at least, a continuation of the preoperative decline in psychological function. It is not known if postoperative nutritional therapy sufficient to prevent tissue loss would prevent postoperative fatigue.

Malnutrition in the Postoperative Period

Postoperative malnutrition does exist and a number of studies have documented that it is more common than previously thought.[44] In clinical practice postoperative malnutrition occurs in three broad groups of patients. In some patients *pre-existing malnutrition* is untreated prior to surgery and hence persists after surgery. Postoperative malnutrition occurs in some patients directly *as a result of the surgical procedure itself.* But the most severe form of postoperative malnutrition occurs in those patients who have developed a *complication* of the surgical procedure.

PRE-EXISTING MALNUTRITION AS A CAUSE OF POSTOPERATIVE MALNUTRITION

When malnourished patients are subjected to a major surgical procedure in which further oxidation of both fat and protein occurs, protein-energy malnutrition may develop to a marked degree. Very wasted patients may show surprisingly little response to surgical trauma and, provided eating is resumed promptly, little weight may be lost. However, there is little margin for error (Fig. 37–8), and it is important to remember that after most major gastrointestinal surgery only 50 per cent of normal oral intake is taken over the first two postoperative weeks.[45] Thus, a patient who presents for a major procedure having already lost 20 to 30 lb may lose a further 10 lb as a result of the operation before normal oral intake is restored. It may take months before this weight is regained and normal body function restored.[43]

POSTOPERATIVE MALNUTRITION OCCURRING AS A RESULT OF THE SURGICAL PROCEDURE

After a particularly difficult anastomosis in the esophagus, stomach, duodenum, small bowel, pancreas, or biliary tract it is not uncommon for the surgeon to forbid normal food intake until all risk of anastomotic breakdown has passed, usually about the tenth or twelfth postoperative day. Since adequate voluntary food intake will not be achieved for another 2 weeks or so,[45] all but those patients who are normally nourished will suffer an overall weight loss of more than 20 lb unless some form of enteral or parenteral feeding is instituted (see Chapter 4).

Patients who have undergone massive bowel resection for Crohn's disease, tumor, or infarction are unable to consume orally an adequate intake until compensatory bowel adaption has occurred. Most adult subjects have about 6 meters of small intestine, and unless 70 to 80 per cent of this has been resected there is unlikely to be a major nutritional or metabolic problem.[46] Patients with less bowel than this will have diarrhea in the first postoperative weeks, which will be made considerably worse by attempts at oral feeding. Intravenous nutrition is required until the daily output of stool is less than 1.5 liters. Without such treatment profound protein-energy malnutrition will result. Some patients with lesser resections also develop diarrhea in the period immediately after oral intake has commenced, and steps must be taken to ensure that malnutrition does not develop as a consequence.

POSTOPERATIVE COMPLICATIONS AS A CAUSE OF MALNUTRITION

Whenever a major complication develops in the postoperative period there is a high chance that protein-energy malnutrition will occur as a direct consequence. Protein-energy deficit develops simply because oral intake is delayed, but if sepsis is present energy output is raised as well. A good example of this is the patient with an intra-abdominal abscess presenting during the second postoperative week. The patient is nauseated, his or her metabolic expenditure is raised, and there is a paralytic ileus. The lack of energy intake, together with the increased energy output, results in a large energy deficit which will continue until the abscess is drained and the patient resumes eating. Even then, it will be another 10 or 12 days before normal voluntary food intake will be resumed, and during that time only 50 per cent of the required energy will be consumed.[45] Although there are some patients with huge fat and protein stores who may be able to cope with such a nutritional assault, many others will require nutritional support when such complications develop. The patient who develops a high-output small bowel fistula will have a much greater problem. Not only must oral intake cease but the accompanying sepsis results in raised energy expenditure. Thus, the energy deficit will continue until the fistula

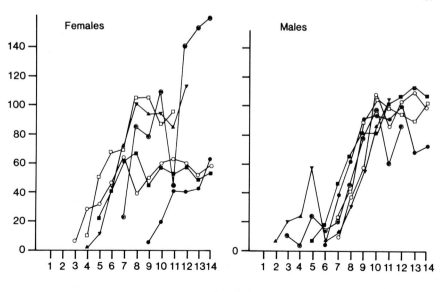

FIGURE 37–8. Daily postoperative voluntary food intake (energy) expressed on the vertical axis as a percentage of the food intake at home prior to surgery. (From Hackett AF, Yeung CK, Hill GL. Br J Surg 1979; 66:416. Reproduced with permission).

Days postop.

closes, either spontaneously or directly by surgery. Such a patient will require nutritional support for at least 6 weeks, and the surgeon should institute intravenous nutrition soon after the establishment of the fistula when sepsis is controlled to avoid the otherwise inevitable protein-energy malnutrition.

Prevention of Protein-Energy Malnutrition after Surgery

At the present time three methods are used clinically in an attempt to prevent protein energy malnutrition after surgery: *fine needle catheter jejunostomy* feeding, intravenous *isotonic amino acids*, and *intravenous hyperalimentation* all have their advocates, have been shown to limit protein loss after surgery, and are thought to have some clinical benefits.

FINE NEEDLE CATHETER JEJUNOSTOMY

Although some surgeons recommend the use of a dual tube for short-term feeding and decompression, the technique is not widely used. More often, when it is anticipated that enteric feeding will be required in the postoperative period, fine needle catheter jejunostomy is recommended. As a general rule the technique of jejunostomy feeding should be reserved for patients in whom the surgeon knows that voluntary food intake will be delayed, and in these circumstances it is of real value. Surprisingly, an extra 2000 kcal/day or so provided in this way does not impair voluntary food intake.[47] The details of catheter insertion and administration of the diet are described fully elsewhere.[48]

PROTEIN-SPARING THERAPY WITH ISOTONIC AMINO ACID SOLUTIONS

Infusion of dextrose free amino acid solutions has been proposed as a method with fewer technical and metabolic problems than intravenous hyperalimentation for sparing body protein in patients after major surgery. The concept is to promote low glucose and low insulin levels in plasma, allowing mobilization of endogenous fat stores, and satisfy energy deficit by ketogenesis.[49] There is no doubt that this treatment has a protein-sparing effect under very controlled conditions, but when it was used in patients undergoing very major surgery (in whom it was most needed) no clinical benefit could be found. In fact, studies of plasma proteins and plasma amino acids suggest that this treatment is not nearly as effective as a full course of intravenous nutrition, and for this reason we do not recommend its use.[50]

PREVENTION OF POSTOPERATIVE MALNUTRITION WITH INTRAVENOUS HYPERALIMENTATION

A number of workers have shown that protein and fat loss can be prevented by the administration of intravenous hyperalimentation in the postoperative period. It has been much harder, however, to demonstrate any positive clinical benefit to patients in whom postoperative complications have not occurred. In one prospective controlled study hospital convalescence and the healing time of large perineal wounds was shorter and accepted nutritional markers were favorably affected, much more so than when amino acids without an energy source were used.[50] The effectiveness of hyperalimentation in preventing malnutrition from occurring when postoperative complications have developed is an accepted clinical fact, and the improved survival of

TABLE 37–2. Energy and Nitrogen Requirements in General Surgical Patients

Nutritional and Metabolic Category	Energy (kcal/kg⁻¹/day⁻¹)	Nitrogen (mg/kg⁻¹/day⁻¹)	Remarks
Normally nourished: preoperative	40	250	Glucose calories above this level are not oxidized. Patients will be in energy and nitrogen balance.
Normally nourished: postoperative	40	300	Energy requirements do not increase significantly but increased nitrogen loss occurs due to decrease in protein synthesis.
Depleted: no stress	40	300	Aim is to replenish body fat stores and lean body mass. Energy needs are low with nutritional depletion and moderate gains in fat and protein will occur.
Depleted and stressed	45	350	Energy stores and protein compartment are depleted but energy requirements and protein loss are high. Need to match losses and provide extra nitrogen for repletion. Part of calorie load should be given as fat. (We suggest a 50:50 glucose-fat mix.)
Normally nourished and stressed	50	400	This group has the highest requirements for energy and nitrogen although the aim is to prevent loss, not to replete. Since glucose is not utilized sufficiently to provide adequate energy intake some of the energy is provided as fat (50:50 glucose-fat mix for ease of administration).

From Hill GL, Church JM. Br J Surg 1984; *71*:1–9. Reproduced with permission.

patients who develop postoperative enterocutaneous fistulas is an overwhelming testimony of this.[40]

Treatment of Postoperative Malnutrition

Though dietary supplements can treat patients with marginal postoperative malnutrition,[51] replacement with both protein and energy is essential to treat established malnutrition. Whenever the intestine can be used for either continuous orogastric feeding or enteral feeding, it is preferable to use these routes for they are safer and there is evidence to show that they can be just as effective as intravenous nutrition.[52] In many instances when major complications are present, intravenous nutrition has to be used because the intestine is unable to cope. The energy and protein intake and the provision of these in correct proportions in these circumstances is set out in Table 37-2. Further details are discussed elsewhere in this book and in the literature.[27]

References

1. Studley HO. Percentage of weight loss. A basic indicator of surgical risk in patients with chronic peptic ulcer. JAMA 1936; *106*:458–460.
2. Buzby GP, Mullen JL, Matthews DC, et al. Prognostic nutritional index in gastrointestinal surgery. Am J Surg 1980; *139*:160–167.
3. Mullen JL, Buzby GP, Matthew DC, et al. Reduction of operative morbidity and mortality by combined preoperative and postoperative nutritional support. Ann Surg 1980; *192*:604–613.
4. Rainey-MacDonald CG, Holliday RL, Wells GA, et al. Validity of a two-variable nutritional index for use in selecting candidates for nutritional support. JPEN 1983; *7*:15–20.
5. Hickman DM, Miller RA, Rombeau JL, et al. Serum albumin and body weight as predictors of postoperative course in colorectal cancer. JPEN 1980; *4*:314–316.
6. Klidjian AM, Foster KJ, Kammerling RM, et al. Relation of anthropometric and dynamometric variables to serious postoperative complications. Br Med J 1980; *281*:899–901.
7. Kaminski MV, Fitzgerald MJ, Murphy RJ, et al. Correlation of mortality with serum transferrin and anergy. JPEN 1977; *1*:27.
8. Irvin TT, Hunt TK. Effect of malnutrition on colonic healing. Ann Surg 1974; *180*:765–772.
9. Cruse PJE, Foord R. A five-year prospective study of 23,649 surgical wounds. Arch Surg 1973; *107*:206–210.
10. Warnold I, Lundholm K. Clinical significance of preoperative nutritional status in 215 non cancer patients. Ann Surg 1984; *199*:299–305.
11. Marshman R, Fisher MM, Coupland GAE. Nutritional status and postoperative complications in an Australian hospital. Aust NZ J Surg 1980; *50*:516–519.
12. Beddoe AH, Streat SJ, Hill GL. The hydration of the fat-free body in protein depleted patients. Am J Physiol 1986; *249*:E227–233.
13. Church JM, Choong SY, Hill GL. Abnormalities of muscle metabolism and histology in malnourished patients awaiting surgery: effects of a course of intravenous nutrition. Br J Surg 1984; *71*:563–569.
14. Russell DM, Jeejeebhoy KN. The assessment of the functional consequences of malnutrition. Nutritional Abstracts and Reviews, Clinical Nutrition Series A 1983; *53*:863–877.
15. Rochester DF, Esau SA. Malnutrition and the respiratory system. Chest 1984; *85*:411–415.
16. Abel RM, Grimes JB, Alonso D, et al. Adverse hemodynamic and ultrastructural changes in dog hearts subjected to protein-calorie malnutrition. Am Heart J 1979; *97*:733–744.
17. Betzhold J, Howard L. Enteral nutrition and gastrointestinal disease. *In* Rombeau JL, Caldwell MD (eds). Enteral and Tube Feeding. Philadelphia, WB Saunders, 1984: 338–361.
18. Grant JP. Clinical impact of protein malnutrition on organ mass and function. *In* Blackburn GL, Grant JP, Young VR (eds). Amino Acids—Metabolism and Medical Applications. Boston, PSG Wright, 1983: 353–354.
19. Young GA, Hill GL. Assessment of protein-calorie malnutrition in surgical patients from plasma proteins and anthropometric measurements. Am J Clin Nutr 1978; *31*:429–435.
20. Young GA, Hill GL. Evaluation of protein-energy malnutrition in surgical patients from plasma valine and other amino acids, proteins and anthropometric measurements. Am J Clin Nutr 1981; *34*:166–172.
21. Lindstedt E, Sandblom P. Wound healing in man: tensile strength of healing wounds in some patient groups. Ann Surg 1975; *181*:842–846.
22. Haydock DA, Hill GL. Improved wound healing response in surgical patients receiving intravenous nutrition. Br J Surg, 1987; *74*:320–323.
23. Temple WJ, Voitk AJ, Snelling FT, et al. Effect of nutrition, diet and suture material on long term wound healing. Ann Surg 1975; *182*:93–97.
24. Superina R, Meakins JL. Delayed hypersensitivity, anergy and the surgical patient. J Surg Res 1984; *37*:151–174.
25. Bistrian BR, Sherman M, Blackburn GL, et al. Cellular immunity in adult marasmus. Arch Intern Med 1977; *137*:1408–1411.
26. Streat SJ, Beddoe AH, Hill GL. Aggressive nutritional support does not prevent protein loss despite fat gain in septic intensive care patients. J Trauma 1987; *27*:262–266.
27. Hill GL, Church JM. Energy and protein requirements of general surgical patients requiring intravenous nutrition. Br J Surg 1984; *71*:1–9.
28. Hill GL, McCarthy ID, Collins JP, et al. A new method for the rapid measurement of body composition in critically ill surgical patients. Br J Surg 1978; *65*:732–735.
29. Abel RM, Fischer JE, Buckley MJ, et al. Malnutrition in cardiac patients: results of a prospective randomised evaluation of early postoperative total parenteral nutrition (TPN). Acta Chir Scand 1976; *466*:77.
30. Church JM, Hill GL. Assessing the efficacy of intravenous nutrition in general surgical patients—dynamic nutritional assessment using plasma proteins. JPEN 1987; *11*:135–139.
31. Haydock DA, Flint MH, Hill GL. Effects of intravenous nutrition on wound healing. Aust NZ J Surg 1984; *54*:169–170.
32. Hill GL, Church JM, Macfie J. Unpublished data.
33. Brown R, Bancewicz J, Hamid J, et al. Failure of delayed hypersensitivity skin testing to predict postoperative sepsis and mortality. Br Med J 1982; *284*:851–853.
34. Pettigrew RA, Hill GL. Indications of surgical risk and clinical judgement. Br J Surg 1986; *73*:47–51.
35. Williams RHP, Heatley RV, Lewis MH, et al. Preoperative parenteral nutrition in patients with stomach cancer. *In* Baxter DH, Jackson GM (eds). Clinical Parenteral Nutrition. Chester, England, Geistlich Education, 1977: 52–59.
36. Müller JM, Brenner U, Dienst C, et al. Preoperative parenteral feeding in patients with gastrointestinal carcinoma. Lancet 1982; *1*:68–71.
37. Holter AR, Fischer JE. The effects of perioperative hyperalimentation on complications in patients with carcinoma and weight loss. J Surg Res 1977; *23*:31–34.
38. Mullen JL. Consequences of malnutrition in the surgical patient. Surg Clin North Am 1981; *61*:465–487.
39. Detsky AS, Mendelson RA, Baker JP, et al. The choice to

treat all, some or no patients undergoing gastrointestinal surgery with nutritional support: a decision analysis approach. JPEN 1984; 8:245–253.

40. Hill GL. Operative strategy in the treatment of enterocutaneous fistulas. World J Surg 1983; 7:495–501.

41. Christensen T, Kehlet H. Postoperative fatigue and changes in nutritional status. Br J Surg 1984; 71:473–476.

42. Postoperative fatigue. Lancet 1979; 1:84–85.

43. Keys A, Brozek J, Henshel A, et al. The Biology of Human Starvation. Minneapolis, University of Minnesota Press, 1950.

44. Hill GL, Blackett RL, Pickford I, et al. Malnutrition in surgical patients—an unrecognised problem. Lancet 1977; 1:689–692.

45. Hackett AF, Yeung CK, Hill GL. Eating patterns in patients recovering from major surgery—a study of voluntary food intake and energy balance. Br J Surg 1979; 66:415–518.

46. Bambach CP, Hill GL. Long term nutritional effects of extensive resection of the small intestine. Aust NZ J Surg 1982; 52:500–506.

47. Yeung CK, Young GA, Hackett AF, et al. Fine needle catheter jejunostomy—an assessment of a new method of nutritional support after major gastrointestinal surgery. Br J Surg 1979; 66:727–732.

48. Rombeau JL, Caldwell MD. Enteral and Tube Feeding. Philadelphia, WB Saunders, 1984.

49. Blackburn GL, Flatt JP, Clowes GHA, et al. Peripheral intravenous feeding with isotonic amino acid solutions. Am J Surg 1973; 125:447–454.

50. Young GA, Hill GL. A controlled study of protein sparing therapy after excision of the rectum. Ann Surg 1980; 192:183–191.

51. Isaksson B, Edlund Y, Gelin LE, et al. The value of protein enriched diet in patients with peptic ulcer. Acta Chir Scand 1959; 118:418–427.

52. Yeung CK, Smith RC, Hill GL. Effect of an elemental diet on body composition: a comparison with intravenous nutrition. Gastroenterology 1979; 77:652–657.

38

THE INTENSIVE CARE PATIENT

JOHN M. KINNEY / PETER FURST / DAVID H. ELWYN
YVON A. CARPENTIER

The development of total parenteral nutrition and the associated use of chemically formulated diets for the acutely ill patient, particularly the type of patient found in modern intensive care units, has developed since World War II in many ways parallel to the development of intensive care units themselves.

Various changes in medical care during the 1940's and 1950's led to the modern intensive care unit. During World War II the United States Army hospitals concentrated recently injured combat casualties into "shock wards" where special supplies and staff could manage resuscitation more efficiently. During the 1950's bioengineers were developing equipment for mechanical ventilation after the initial success of the iron lung in ventilating patients who were victims of poliomyelitis or other forms of neurological disease associated with respiratory failure. This approach was given tremendous emphasis by the very severe polio epidemics that occurred in the 1950's, particularly in Scandinavia. Efforts to provide mechanical ventilation for the victims of this disease were thought by many to have stimulated the early grouping of patients requiring acute ventilatory assistance into respiratory intensive care units. During the early 1960's it became apparent that continuous monitoring of the electrocardiogram could provide an early warning system of dangerous arrhythmias in patients at risk because of cardiac disease. Therefore, units were designed that would group patients of this type where the concern was not so much for intensive care as for intensive monitoring. These factors all followed the contribution of specialized postoperative nursing care to the development of modern neurosurgery, particularly intracranial operations for brain tumors. This specialized nursing care preceded the generalized acceptance of the importance of postanesthesia recovery rooms for general surgical patients, which came about during the 1950's. The rapid growth of open-heart surgery during the 1960's was also felt to have depended greatly upon specialized grouping of postoperative cardiac patients into units able to provide intensive monitoring along with specialized ventilatory and circulatory care. In the 1970's most hospitals caring for adult medical and surgical patients were expected to have a general intensive care unit and perhaps specialized units for cardiac monitoring and for respiratory care. This specialization in intensive care has been followed by specialized units set aside for trauma care, burn care, renal failure, and so forth.

Modern hospital nutrition has had a somewhat similar development to modern intensive care units. In the 1930's isotonic saline solutions and glucose solutions were available for intravenous administration but not as widely used as later because of the incidence of pyrogenic reactions. In 1940 Elman introduced the concept of providing a source of amino acids by infusing protein hydrolysates intravenously. It was then recognized that the negative nitrogen balance that characterized many hospitalized patients could not be dealt with simply by providing adequate amounts of intravenous nitrogen unless appropriate calories were provided. Hypertonic solutions of glucose that were sufficient to provide the necessary calories could not be given by a peripheral vein. Therefore, extensive work was undertaken to develop an intravenous fat preparation; however, the early preparations were associated with many undesirable effects. By 1960, Wretlind had developed an intravenous fat emulsion with an extremely low incidence of undesirable reactions. This led to the introduction of balanced intravenous nutrition including fat, carbohydrate, and protein for patients who required periods of intravenous nutrition at a time when their intestinal function was not available. Such nutrition could sometimes be given by peripheral vein, thus avoiding the problems of hypertonic glucose solutions when given by peripheral vein. At about the same time in the United States the concept of introducing an intravenous catheter for monitoring of central venous pressure became an acceptable procedure in clinical management. Dudrick and Rhoads were studying intravenous nutrition at a time when the only commercial fat preparation available in the United States was withdrawn from the market. They then introduced the concept of feeding patients on the basis of a hypertonic glucose solution mixed with amino acids, vitamins, and minerals and given through a central vein. This "hyperalimentation" developed wide popularity in the United States during the 1970's when a commercial fat preparation was not available in this country. Since 1975, when commercial fat became available, its use has been guided by two schools of thought. One group provides one to two units of intravenous fat per week in order to prevent an essential fatty acid deficiency, while others administer a significant proportion of calories as fat each day, feeling that a balanced intravenous intake probably has certain advantages over giving only glucose as a source of nonprotein calories.

The past decade has seen the growth of specialization in intravenous nutrition just as in intensive care units. Various solutions, particularly of different amino acid compositions, have been developed with the intent of providing specific treatment for particular clinical conditions. It is increasingly clear that the response of any patient to nutritional support, whether enteral or parenteral, depends upon the underlying metabolic state. How intense is the catabolic stimulus? How long has the catabolic stimulus existed and how much weight loss and tissue depletion has occurred? Is the depleted patient still facing the catabolic drive of residual infection or is the patient now in an anabolic state as would occur after prolonged partial starvation? The following sections emphasize metabolic changes as background for considering the response to nutritional support.

ENERGY METABOLISM

JOHN M. KINNEY / PETER FURST

Physicians have long recognized that the rate of weight loss with acute illness or injury seemed to be correlated with the severity of the clinical problem. While day-to-day changes in body weight are strongly influenced by changes in body water, there is a general correlation between the rate of sustained weight loss and the cumulative loss of nitrogen. During the decade after World War I, it was suggested by certain surgeons that the severe weight loss after major injury was the result of the injury causing large increases in resting energy expenditure (REE). This idea was extended to suggest that perhaps the REE could become greater than the energy supplied by fat mobilization from adipose tissue. If this situation occurred, then tissues would turn to body protein as a source of nonspecific fuel with an associated increase in nitrogen excretion. This idea of extremely high levels of REE after major injury led to a sense of resignation on the part of many surgeons when faced with severe weight loss because no means of high-calorie nutritional support was available. Lack of interest in attempting to treat this weight loss was also compounded by the idea that the catabolic breakdown of body tissue, after injury, was triggered by hormones from the adrenal cortex and that this response was an obligatory part of the metabolic response to injury.

During the 1960's, Kinney and co-workers[1] undertook the study of the REE in various types of surgical disease and injury. There was considerable surprise to learn that major surgical operations were followed by distinct increases in nitrogen excretion, while increases in the REE ranged only as high as 10 per cent, with some patients having no change in REE. Convalescence from multiple injury, particularly if fractures of the extremities or pelvis were involved, was associated with increases of REE of 10 to 25 per cent that lasted for 2 to 3 weeks while there was an increase in nitrogen excretion. The presence of fever from bacteremia was found to increase the REE approximately 7 per cent for each degree F (13 per cent for each degree C) above normal body temperature as demonstrated by DuBois. And, thus, the common range of increase of REE was 20 to 30 per cent for most surgical infections. However, if the infection involved an extensive inflammatory response, such as acute peritonitis or empyema, the REE might be increased by 30 to 50 per cent. Extensive third-degree burns were commonly treated in the 1960's with the burn surfaces left open to the ambient air with some antibacterial agent applied to the surface. The rooms for such patients were often not heated above normal room temperature so that the radiative, as well as the evaporative, cooling in such patients was very high. The REE of these patients was found to be between 40 and 100 per cent above normal. Preliminary studies were interpreted to indicate that this increased heat loss was driving the resting hypermetabolism.[2] Chapter 39 presents evidence for an opposing point of view, which is that the primary cause of the hypermetabolism is the increased heat production of internal organs responding to the burn injury and that the increased heat loss is largely secondary. The management of patients with extensive thermal injuries has made considerable progress these past 20 years. Resuscitation is usually prompt, pulmonary injury is recognized and treated, excision of the burn surface is started soon after the injury, and closed dressings, which prevent evaporative cooling, have often replaced the former method of open treatment. Under these conditions, the burn patient usually has an REE that is only 20 to 40 per cent above normal.

Individuals who have undergone prolonged partial starvation, without an acute catabolic stimulus such as infection, will show a curvilinear decrease in REE.[3] Therefore, the REE of a cross-section of hospitalized patients will range from approximately − 30 per cent to +40 per cent of the normal value. The REE of each individual represents the balance between increases due to catabolic influences and decreases due to tissue depletion.

An increase in resting energy expenditure raises many important questions regarding the various mechanisms that contribute to the increase in REE and whether the increase is of particular importance to convalescence, or whether pharmacological agents will allow future physicians to abolish this hypermetabolism without penalizing the objectives that hypermetabolism is intended to accomplish during convalescence. Hypermetabolism at the cell level involves the production and utilization of ATP for various forms of metabolic work. Prominent among these forms is the energy used for ion transport, protein synthesis, osmotic work, nerve transmission, and "futile cycles." Futile cycles were originally considered in relation to the glycolytic pathway, but analogous forms of futile cycles have been seen to occur in the triglyceride turnover of adipocytes, and perhaps in the rapid turnover of proteins in certain highly active cells. Muscle tissue appears to be the major component of extensive weight loss, and muscle protein breakdown is the largest contributor to the nitrogen excretion after injury. Therefore, the energy compounds that can be measured in needle biopsies of human skeletal muscle (Table 38–1) are of particular interest to follow during the convalescence of patients after various forms of disease and injury.

Muscle Energy Metabolism

It is conceivable that certain metabolic functions such as energy generation and transmembrane transport may be impaired in the catabolic state. Our approach to this problem has been to study the intracellular energy metabolism directly by analyzing muscle tissue obtained by percutaneous needle biposy[4-6] from patients suffering from malnutrition or hypermetabolism. Indeed, muscle tissue is considered to be relatively resistant to metabolic insult when compared with the brain, liver, or kidney. Therefore, any observed changes in muscle tissue can be expected to correlate with more severe abnormalities in other organs.

In severe malnutrition profound changes were observed in cellular energy metabolism in muscle tissue in 12 depleted patients.[7] Compared with normal values,[8] the contents of ATP and PCr were markedly decreased and that of ADP reduced to a lesser degree, whereas the level of AMP was found to be elevated (Fig. 38–1). The content of muscle glycogen was considerably decreased and muscle free glucose concentration revealed a fourfold elevation compared with the normal mean values (Fig. 38–2). There was no sign of anaerobic metabolism due to hypoxia in the muscle tissue as shown by a normal lactate level (Fig. 38–2). All patients received intensive nutritional therapy for 30 days; 1 week with TPN, followed by treatment with an elementary synthetic diet. Of the 12 patients, 4 died within 1 week, whereas the remaining 8 patients recovered and the muscle biopsy could be repeated after 30 days of nutritional treatment. The initial severely abnormal pattern was fully normalized as a result of the successful nutritional therapy.

TABLE 38–1. Potential Energy Reserves of the Muscle Cells

	Dry Weight (μmol/g)	Available Energy (μmol P/g Dry Weight)
ATP	24.6	9.8 (40%)
Phosphorylcreatine	76.8	61.4 (80%)
Glycogen	365 glucosyl units	1,060 (anaerobic)
		14,200 (aerobic)
Triglyceride	48.6	24,520

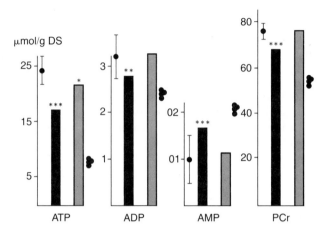

FIGURE 38–1. *The content of energy-rich phosphates in muscle tissue acquired from severely malnourished patients before (solid bar) and after (stippled bar) intensive nutritional therapy (n = 8), compared with range of normal values[8] indicated as mean ± SD on left side of each graph. Four patients died within the first week of treatment; muscle phosphate values for these patients are indicated by dots on right side of each graph. Significant differences from normal values are indicated: ***p < 0.001; **p < 0.01; *p < 0.05.*

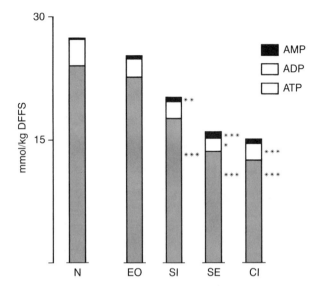

FIGURE 38–3. *Effect of injury and sepsis on the levels of muscle adenine nucleotides compared with normal values[8] (N). EO, elective operations;[11,12] SI, severe injury;[9,10] SE, sepsis;[9,10] CI, critical illness.[20] Significant decreases from normal values are indicated: ***p < 0.001; **p < 0.01; *p < 0.05.*

Severe trauma and sepsis are associated with a decreased content of energy-rich phosphates in muscle[9,10] (Fig. 38–3). The changes in high-energy phosphate in muscle were found to be parallel to alterations seen in liver.[8] Interestingly, in severe trauma or sepsis the decrease in ATP and total adenine nucleotides (TAN) persisted 30 days after injury.[9] In these conditions the major intracellular cations potassium and magnesium were also significantly decreased[11,12] and, surprisingly, the intracellular concentrations of these ions remained low in late convalescence.[12] Although the etiology of the observed changes in muscle composition is not yet clarified, it is possible that energy metabolism in muscle tissue could be related to these findings. Nevertheless, the fact that ATP and TAN remain low even in late convalescence might suggest that the skeletal muscle cells remain metabolically deranged to the extent that a normal intracellular potassium or magnesium content cannot be maintained. Further studies are urgently warranted to evaluate whether the described changes in cellular energy metabolism affect membrane transport and the sodium pump system.

Surgical trauma does not seem to be associated with appreciable changes in high-energy phosphates (Fig. 38–3) when the patients are adequately nourished with amino acids, carbohydrates, and fat.[13,14] In contrast, patients receiving amino acids alone demonstrate a decrease in ATP, ADP, and PCr.[13] These results suggest that small amounts of glucose are important for maintenance of cellular energy levels. It is tempting to speculate that if small amounts of glucose will prevent a decline in energy-rich phos-

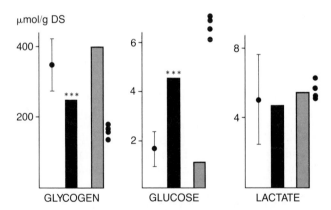

FIGURE 38–2. *The content of glycogen, free glucose, and lactate in muscle tissue acquired from severely malnourished patients before (solid bar) and after (stippled bar) intensive nutritional treatment (n = 8), compared with range of normal values[8] indicated as mean ± SD. Four patients died within first week of treatment; glycogen, glucose, and lactate values for these patients are indicated by dots on right side of each graph. Significant differences from normal values are indicated: ***p < 0.001.*

phates following surgical injury, greater amounts may prove useful in preventing decreases in energy level during major trauma and sepsis.

Low Energy Charge—A Cellular Expression of the Catabolic State

It might be evident that the normal balance between the utilization and production of adenine and adenine nucleotides is disturbed in catabolic situations. Obviously ATP resynthesis under pathological conditions, as in severe catabolism or in malnutrition-malabsorption, is dependent on the rate of energy expenditure in the muscle cells. The active carbohydrate stores in muscle and liver are very limited, and consequently, at least during chronic prolonged catabolism, the decreased adenine pool probably is a result of adaptive changes in the enzymatic system responsible for ATP resynthesis. Another possibility is that the decrease is limited to the same specific pool, for example, the sarcoplasmic or mitochondrial pool. It remains, thus, to be determined whether the diminished adenine pool is a result of a decreased capacity to resynthesize ATP or is secondary to other cell changes, such as a lower mitochondrial number due to long-term immobilization and subsequent adaptation, as might be the case in patients suffering from rheumatoid arthritis.[15]

In discussing the regulation of glycolysis and respiration, the relative concentrations of ADP and ATP in the cell are the most important controlling elements. When ATP is utilized in many biosynthetic reactions it undergoes pyrophosphate cleavage to yield AMP, whereas in muscular contraction ADP is the primary product of ATP utilization. At any given moment, a living cell contains not only ATP and ADP, but also AMP.[16] Atkinson and Walton[17] proposed the energy charge concept for the adenylate pool. The energy charge of the ATP-ADP-AMP system can easily be calculated for any given set of concentrations of ATP, ADP, and AMP by the equation:

$$\text{Energy charge} = \frac{1}{2} \times \frac{\text{ADP} + 2\,\text{ATP}}{\text{AMP} + \text{ADP} + \text{ATP}}$$

Because many regulatory enzymes in both catabolic and anabolic pathways are responsive to AMP, ADP, or ATP as modulators, Atkinson has suggested that the regulation of pathways that produce and utilize high-energy phosphate bonds is a function of the energy charge of the ATP-ADP-AMP system, which runs optimally in a steady state and strongly resists any deviations from it. Several enzymes that catalyze reactions in glycolysis or the citric acid cycle are either inhibited by ATP or stimulated by AMP. These enzyme reactions are, thus, activated at a low energy charge in the adenylate pool. Other reactions utilizing ATP for biosynthesis or production of storage compounds will be enhanced at high energy charge, but inhibited at a low one.[16,17]

In patients with hypercatabolism liver failure, respiratory failure,[19] untreated malnutrition or malabsorption,[7] or critical illness,[20] we found a low energy charge potential (Table 38–2). This would mean a decreased capacity for biosynthetic reactions and for production of energy storage compounds. Such a situation is often referred to as a catabolic state, and it has repeatedly been noted that the aforementioned situations are associated with excessive tissue breakdown and wasting. It is thus conceivable that the low energy charge seen during chronic or acute illness is the cellular expression of the "catabolic state."

Sick Cell Syndrome—Irreversible Cellular Damage?

There were patients who did not survive despite both nutritional and clinical treatment. As illustrated in Figures 38–1 and 38–2, in the four patients in whom aggressive nutritional therapy failed, more profound deviations from the normal range were apparent than in the patients in whom the therapy resulted in a recovery from their severe condition. Thus, compared with the normal values, the reductions of ATP and glycogen were considerable, corresponding to 70 and 65 per cent, respectively, whereas the content of AMP increased 100 per cent and measurement of free glucose revealed an eightfold elevation.

This latter abnormality is of special interest when one considers that free glucose is present in only minute quantities in normal muscle. A passive accumulation of this solute indicates an impairment of enzymatic, synthetic, and transport processes. The increase of free glucose is apparently correlated to the decrease in energy charge (ATP). Thus, cellular viability might ultimately be dependent upon the rate of intracellular energy expenditure and be limited at low levels of available free energy.

Nevertheless, by employing suitable therapeutic means the distorted pattern of energy-rich compounds can be normalized and the energy charge potential restored simultaneously with patient survival. This is emphasized in Figure 38–4, which shows that the energy charge potential, although considerably decreased, could be re-established in the normal range by aggressive nutritional therapy. On the other hand, the four patients who did not survive despite intensive treatment revealed extremely low energy charge potentials far outside of the range of levels shown by the recovered patients. The main inquiry, thus, would be whether the extent of hypercatabolism in these situations exceeded the limit at which the cellular damage can be considered irreversible. It is reasonable to assume that in these fatal cases the patients were no longer responsive to the applied therapeutic efforts. Consequently, the question may also be raised whether a markedly de-

TABLE 38–2. *Energy Charge Potentials in Various Conditions*

Condition (No. Patients)	Energy Charge Potential	Reference
Normal (80)	0.939 ± 0.00014	8
Malnutrition		
Before nutritional therapy (10)	0.916 ± 0.0095***	7
After nutritional therapy (6)	0.930 ± 0.0214	
Malabsorption (10)	0.921 ± 0.0082	7
Critically ill patients		
Acute (12)	0.928 ± 0.0094**	7,20
Chronic (15)	0.913 ± 0.0301**	7,20
Liver failure (12)	0.927 ± 0.0081***	18
Respiratory failure (10)	0.928 ± 0.0093**	19
Severe trauma (8)	0.920 ± 0.0125***	9,10
Sepsis (6)	0.912 ± 0.0293***	9,10
Surgical trauma		
Hip replacement (12)	0.942 ± 0.0099	13
Colon resection (22)	0.936 ± 0.0028	14
Rheumatoid arthritis (25)	0.931 ± 0.0019	15

**p < 0.01; ***p < 0.001.

creased energy charge potential is to be interpreted as a sign of irreversibility.

One can assume that the coupling of oxidation and phosphorylation in the mitochondria is seriously disturbed in catabolic conditions. The extent to which mitochondrial coupling can be reduced and still recover must be the scope of future studies. Another important question to be addressed is whether prolonged surgical hypermetabolism in the absence of shock may be associated with a decreased coupling efficiency, producing a situation in which the patient has increased demands for oxidative substrate, gas exchange, and heat while producing relatively less ATP for tissue and organ work. Future studies of catabolic patients, aimed at elucidating which steps in energy exchange have undergone primary changes, will be needed to guide rational clinical and nutritional therapy.

PROTEIN METABOLISM

DAVID H. ELWYN

Starvation, malnutrition, injury, and sepsis all have effects on nitrogen metabolism that must be considered with respect to the ICU patient. Superimposed on these are effects of diseases of the kidney, liver, or intestinal tract, which have been considered more specifically in other chapters. Loss of lean body mass (LBM), or more specifically body cell mass (BCM), can result in impaired host defense and increased morbidity and mortality with surgery. Starvation, malnutrition, injury, and sepsis each have characteristic effects on the rate of weight loss, the composition of weight loss, and the response to nutrients provided to prevent or minimize losses or to restore lost tissue.

Rates of Nitrogen Losses

Since the work of Cuthbertson, increased urinary excretion of nitrogen has been a hallmark of physical injury.[21] In severe cases this may reach 35 g N per day,[22] the equivalent of more than 1 kg of lean body mass. Since both N excretion and N balance are affected by dietary intake, quantitative comparisons of N balance in different pathophysiologic states must be made under similar dietary conditions. Takala and Klossner[23] have suggested that comparisons of N balance, made while patients are receiving infusion of 5 per cent dextrose as the sole nutrient, provide a useful index of the severity of trauma. In this condition, negative N balance is eight times greater in patients with severe burns, and six times greater with severe injury than in normal subjects (Table 38–3). Nitrogen balance in postoperative patients

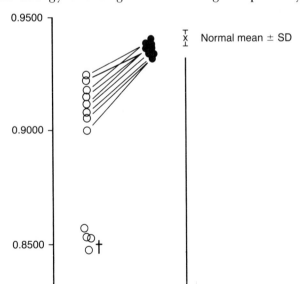

FIGURE 38–4. *Energy charge potential in muscle tissue before (○) and after (●) 30 days of intensive nutritional therapy, compared with the normal value (mean ± SD). Four patients died within the first week of treatment (open circles at bottom). The main inquiry: whether the extent of catabolism in these patients exceeded the limit at which the cellular damage can be considered irreversible.*

TABLE 38–3. Nitrogen Balance during 5 Per Cent Dextrose Infusion

Pathophysiologic State	Nitrogen Balance (mean ± SD)	
	mg/kg/day	*g/70 kg/day*
Severe burns	−380 ± 70	−27 ± 5
Severe injury	−260 ± 90	−18 ± 6
Postradical bladder cystectomy	−172 ± 47	−12 ± 1.3
Sepsis	−163 ± 84	−11.4 ± 5.9
Post total hip replacement	−96 ± 25	−6.7 ± 1.8
Malnourished	−90 ± 20	−6.3 ± 1.4
Normal subjects	−45 ± 3	−3.2 ± .2
Normal subjects after a 10–14 day fast	−30 ± 1	−2.1 ± .1

Data from Elwyn DH.

lies in between the normal value and that of accidental injury and depends on the severity of operation, being more negative after cystectomy than after total hip replacement. The nitrogen balance of septic patients is comparable to those after radical cystectomy. Normal subjects who were fasted prior to infusion of 5 per cent dextrose had a 50 per cent reduction in N excretion (Table 38–3). Malnourished patients who were not septic and were remote from injury or surgery nevertheless had rates of N excretion twice those of normal subjects, and three times those of normal subjects with prior fasting.

Composition of Weight Losses

Weight loss during starvation consists almost exclusively of body cell mass and fat[25] (Fig. 38–5). There are no significant changes in extracellular

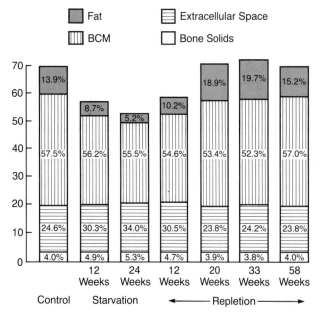

FIGURE 38–5. *Calculated tissue composition of weight loss and weight gain associated with partial starvation. Calculations are made from data in the study reported by Keys and co-workers.[25]*

fluid, blood volume, or bone solids, although as the body shrinks the relative proportions of these compartments increase, to the point that pitting edema is observed in prolonged starvation.[26] Proportional losses of water and N are for the most part quite constant and in the ratio found in BCM of approximately 25:1 (4:1 for water:protein ratio). In the first 2 to 3 days there may be transiently greater excretion of water associated with losses of extracellular fluid and sodium on the one hand[7] and with glycogen and potassium on the other.[8] Although N is distributed about 60:40 between BCM and extracellular structures (in bone, tendons, connective tissue, etc.), losses of N in starvation or fasting are almost entirely from the BCM. Therefore changes in N content under these conditions represent changes in BCM and more specifically the protein content of BCM, which represents its metabolically active component.

The ratio of fat to BCM during weight loss will depend on the dietary content of energy and N as well as the pathophysiological state of the subject.[9] Otherwise normal adult subjects who gain or lose weight on diets close to energy requirements gain or lose mainly adipose tissue. However, deposition or loss of fat requires increase or decrease in the size of supporting tissues such as muscle or blood vessels. Under these conditions the composition of tissue loss is approximately 0.5 g BCM to 1 g of fat. The energy content of BCM is approximately 0.8 kcal/g mainly due to protein, while that of fat is 9.5 kcal/kg. In terms of energy stored or utilized the contribution of protein and fat are in the proportion of 0.4:9.5; that is, protein accounts for only 4 per cent of the energy content of weight loss or gain on diets close to energy requirements. During fasting the ratio of BCM to fat losses is 2.6:1, which in caloric terms is 2.1/9.5, with protein supplying 18 per cent of the energy content. The composition of weight loss in elective surgery is very similar to that during fasting; in one study[27] ratios of BCM to fat ranged from 1.7:1 for women to 2.6:1 for men. In severe accidental injury the ratio of BCM to fat is even higher,[27] 4.4:1, corresponding to a caloric ratio of 3.5:9.5, with protein accounting for 29 per cent of energy content.

These studies of postoperative and injured patients were performed before widespread use of parenteral nutrition, and these patients were provided with infusions of 5 per cent dextrose and the amounts of orally ingested food considered appropriate on clinical grounds. Had they been fasted completely, rates of weight loss and the ratios of BCM to fat would have been higher; had they received parenteral or enteral supplements these rates would have been lower. The degree of physical activity is also important since exercise will have a marked effect on rates of fat loss, but little effect on rates of protein loss.

The ratio of BCM to fat losses is important on two counts; as observed previously[27] it demonstrates that (1) even under the most catabolic conditions, fat is the major source of endogenous energy, and that protein can, at most, supply 30 per cent of energy requirements; and (2) estimates of the composition of weight loss can provide goals for nutritional therapy, since it will usually be desirable to restore fat and BCM in the proportions that were lost.

Although starvation has little or no effect on the absolute amount of extracellular fluid (ECF), both injury and sepsis cause increases in ECF. In the short term, repletion therapy may improve morbidity more in relation to its role in reducing excess ECF than because of its effect on N balance and restoration of BCM.[30]

Tissue Sites of Weight and Nitrogen Losses

After 12 and 24 weeks of starvation with energy intakes only 50 per cent of initial requirements, there were marked losses in body cell mass and fat but no change in extracellular fluid (ECF), blood volume, or bone solids.[30] Thus N losses occur almost entirely from BCM and there is very little extracellular loss.

All cellular tissues lose weight during starvation except brain, and for most tissues the losses are roughly proportional to losses in body weight (Table 38–4). In fasting rats, early losses are most dramatic for the liver and gastrointestinal tract, which may lose 60 per cent of their weight in 3 to 4 days;[31] muscle losses are proportionally much smaller, and since rats can survive only 7 to 8 days of fasting, muscle loss is not as extensive as in humans. In liver and muscle there is increased hydration and fatty infiltration, so that weight losses underestimate the extent of protein losses.[32] Humans tolerate fasting for much longer periods than rats because body fat stores are much greater in comparison to daily energy expenditure. As a result, in long-term fasting or starvation muscle losses may be proportionally greater than for any other organ or tissue. Since muscle is larger than all other organs combined, at any stage of nutritional depletion or repletion, the biggest source or sink for protein is skeletal muscle. Whether or not humans demonstrate the rapid losses of liver and gastrointestinal tract seen in rats remains to be determined.

Losses of organ function accompany these losses

TABLE 38–4. Weight Loss of Emaciated Bodies at Autopsy

	Causes of Death		
	Chronic Infection	Cachexia	Tumor
Body weight	44	39	38
Heart	31	35	33
Liver	28	42	33
Kidney	16	36	28
Brain	3	5	3

Figures show percentage of weight lost from each site.
Adapted from Grant JP. *In* Blackburn GL, et al. Amino Acids: Metabolism and Medical Application. Littleton, MA, Wright PSG, 1983: 347–358.

in weight and protein, and all organs are affected. It was formerly thought that critical organs such as the heart and respiratory system were protected from malnutrition. It is now apparent that this is not so, and that in malnutrition serious functional decrements can occur in both systems.[32,33] During malnutrition itself the demands on the pulmonary and circulatory systems are reduced and may not strain their residual capacities. However, the increase in metabolic rate associated with sudden refeeding can cause congestive heart failure and even death.[25] The increased CO_2 production associated with refeeding, particularly of carbohydrate, can precipitate pulmonary distress and prevent weaning from respirators.[34] Thus it is important to start refeeding programs slowly with severely malnourished patients.

The gastrointestinal tract suffers atrophy of both mucosa and smooth muscle, resulting in decreased motility and malabsorption as well as diarrhea, flatulence, and increased incidence of peptic ulcers. With extreme wasting the gut becomes "paper thin."[32] As with the heart, sudden refeeding may be dangerous. Both liver and kidney show functional effects of starvation.[32] Even brain function is affected by malnutrition,[25] even though losses of brain protein are minimal. Anecdotal accounts indicate that malnutrition may lead to comatose states that can be reversed by intravenous nutrition.[35]

Malnutrition also reduces immunocompetence, primarily through reduced production of acute-phase reactants and of white blood cells. The detailed effects of malnutrition on the immune system are treated elsewhere in this volume.

Repletion of protein is fastest for rapidly turning over plasma proteins and for the immune system, which responds to refeeding within days to weeks. Skeletal muscle function will also show some improvement within a few weeks;[36] however, full recovery in terms of both protein content and function, after severe malnourishment, takes many months or even years to achieve.[25]

Response to Nutrients

Nitrogen balance is a complex function of protein, carbohydrate, and fat intake, always assuming an adequate supply of all other nutrients. The magnitude of the effect of changing any one of these will depend on the amounts of all three in the diet. The effect of increasing only carbohydrate is illustrated for surgical patients in Figure 38–6. At low caloric intakes there is an increase in N balance of 7.5 mg for each kcal of carbohydrate; at about 50 per cent of energy requirements this changes abruptly to 2.5 mg N/kcal. Quantitatively similar effects occur in normal subjects. The large N sparing effect of carbohydrate at low energy intakes is not shared by fat. This is related to the amount of glucose, 100 to 150 g or 375 to 500 kcal, required daily by the brain. On

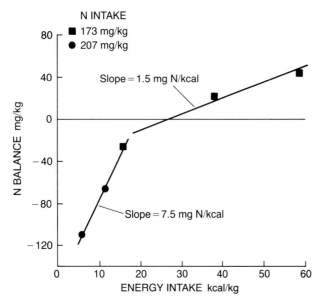

FIGURE 38–6. *Nitrogen balance at various levels of calorie intake in postoperative (■) and depleted (●) patients. (From Elwyn DH. Nutritional requirements of adult surgical patients. Crit Care Med 1980; 8:9–20.© Williams & Wilkins Company, Baltimore. Reproduced with permission.)*

carbohydrate-free diets over 160 g protein, or 26 g N, is required to synthesize this glucose, and if this amount of protein is not provided in the diet it must be provided from endogenous sources.[37] Fat can provide only one tenth of its weight as glucose; therefore dietary fat cannot replace dietary glucose or protein as a source of glucose for the brain. Above 150 g/day the N sparing effect of glucose is much smaller (Fig. 38–6), and this smaller effect of glucose is shared by fat.

In the normal adult, increasing protein intake above minimum requirements causes only transient increases in so called "labile protein;" at steady state, positive N balance cannot be achieved at any level of N intake if the subject is at zero energy balance. By contrast, nutritionally depleted adult patients can achieve markedly positive N balance at zero energy balance,[38] as shown in Figure 38–7, which relates N intake and energy balance to N balance and fat balance. This demonstrates: (1) that increasing either N intake or energy intake will increase N balance; (2) that the composition of tissue restored (BCM:fat) that results from increasing N intake is very different from that achieved by increasing energy intake; thus an N intake of 290 mg/kg and an energy balance of +11 kcal/kg will restore 2 g/kg of BCM to 1 g/kg of fat, while N intake of 150 mg/kg and energy balance of +20 kcal/kg restores 1 g/kg BCM to 2 g/kg of fat; (3) that markedly positive N balance can be achieved at zero or even negative energy balances, and that, since the effect of energy intake on N balance is small, large errors in estimating energy requirement will have little effect on N balance; and (4) that N requirements, to achieve zero N balance at zero en-

ergy balance, are much higher for hospitalized malnourished adult patients, 120 mg/kg, than for normal subjects, 70 mg/kg.

Not shown in Figure 38–7 is the large variability of N balance in this population. The SD is about 20 mg N/kg/day so that in using Figure 38–7 for an individual it should be kept in mind that 95 per cent of the population will fall within ± 40 mg N/kg of the value shown. The calorie to N ratio required for repletion of malnourished patients will depend on the tissue composition desired. To restore tissue with BCM:fat ratios in the range of 4:1 to 2:1 requires calorie:N ratios close to 100:1; a calorie:N ratio of 300 will restore tissue with a composition of 0.5 part BCM to 1 of fat.

Injured or septic patients have larger N requirements than normal subjects or malnourished patients (Table 38–3). If they are not significantly malnourished they will not achieve positive N balances except at very high energy intakes, since, as they have not lost significant amounts of body cell mass, there is little or nothing to restore. After elective operation of moderate severity there are obligatory losses of 15 to 20 g N in the first 3 to 4 days which cannot be prevented by providing more than adequate amounts of energy and N by either enteral or parenteral routes.[39] After 4 days, however, all patients had returned to zero N balance. With severely stressed patients the obligatory N losses are much greater and even with high nutrient intakes may per-

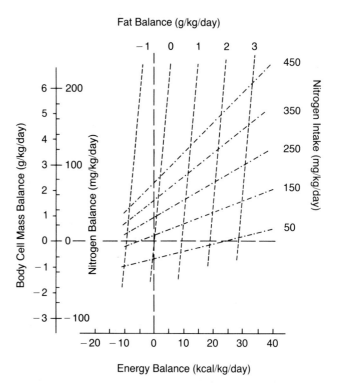

FIGURE 38–7. *Relations between nitrogen or lean body mass balance, fat balance, energy balance, and nitrogen intake. (Adapted from Shaw SN, et al. Am J Clin Nutr 1983; 37:930–940.)*

sist for a week or more. This is illustrated for severely burned or injured patients given energy at 45 to 50 kcal/kg/day and N intakes ranging from 0 to 300 mg/kg/day (Fig. 38–8). Nitrogen balance improved with increasing N intake up to 200 mg/kg but showed no change above this, even though the patients were in negative N balance of −3.5 g/day, or approximately −50 mg/kg/day. While N balance might be improved by greatly increasing energy intake, the amounts given already exceeded requirements, and further increases would markedly raise energy expenditure and deposit excessive amounts of fat. For most severely burned or injured patients this uncorrectable hypercatabolic state is transient, lasting for days to weeks. Losses of 3 to 4 g N/day, roughly 100 g/day of BCM, can be readily restored after the patient improves. For patients with chronic sepsis or multiple organ failure, who may already be malnourished, inability to maintain, much less restore, BCM is more of a problem and may significantly add to morbidity and mortality. It has not yet been demonstrated that there is any optimal nutritional therapy that can significantly improve the prognosis of such patients.

Amino Acid Composition

Nitrogen balance is dependent not only on the total amount of protein in the diet, but also on the amino acid composition. The crystalline amino acid solutions available for parenteral nutrition all have similar compositions with respect to nonessentials. A particular problem is that the low solubility of the semi-essential amino acids, tyrosine and cystine, severely limits how much can be given. Glutamine, because of its chemical instability, cannot be used in intravenous mixtures. Despite these problems, and differences between solutions, there is little evidence as yet to indicate that one or another of the commercial preparations is better or worse with respect to N balance in adult patients.

There is some evidence to show that protein hydrolysates are not as good as crystalline amino acid solutions.[41,42] This appears to be due to the inability of sick patients, in contrast to normal subjects, to effectively utilize the small peptides that make up a substantial fraction of protein hydrolysates.[43]

Considerable efforts have been made to explore the potential clinical benefits of solutions enriched with branched-chain amino acids (BCAA). The major use has been in hepatic encephalopathy, in which they have been shown to return the abnormal plasma amino acid pattern, very high concentrations of methionine and aromatic amino acids, toward normal[44] and to reduce morbidity and mortality.[45] Others have found little or no improvement in morbidity,[46] and there remains some controversy. Under some conditions enriched BCAA solutions have also been shown to improve N balance in both injured rats and patients. However, other studies have failed to show any improvement in N balance even with severely catabolic patients.[23] It seems that evidence is as yet insufficient to adopt enriched BCAA mixtures as a therapeutic agent for improving N balance in injury and sepsis.

Enteral versus Parenteral Feeding

Maintenance of gut morphology and function requires enterally administered nutrients.[47] With parenteral nutrition there is a decrease in both quantity and function of the intestinal mucosa. With respect to whole body N balance, there is some disagreement as to whether the two routes of administration are equivalent.[48] A number of studies indicate that, where equivalent intakes can be achieved, nitrogen balance is equally good with either enteral or parenteral nutrition. However, other studies showed that enteral feeding gave significantly less negative values than parenteral feeding, 10 to 20 g N over the first 3 to 4 days after moderate surgery. However, this is probably not sufficient reason of itself to choose enteral over parenteral nutrition. Even if there is no important difference between the two with respect to N balance, the enteral approach seems preferable (1) because of its effects on intestinal mucosa, (2) because it is cheaper, and (3) because it obviates the need for a central catheter. However, enteral nutrition is contraindicated in cases in which intestinal absorption is inadequate, there is danger of aspiration, or diarrhea is excessive.

Rates of Protein Synthesis and Degradation

Unidirectional rates of protein synthesis and degradation in humans have recently been reviewed.[21] Methods used include: (1) whole-body turnover studies in which isotopic amino acids are given by bolus or constant infusion, and the specific activity of precursor and degradation products (CO_2, urea,

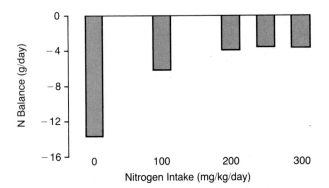

FIGURE 38–8. Effect of nitrogen intake on nitrogen balance in patients with severe injury or burn. (Data from Larsson J, et al. Clin Nutr [Special Suppl] 1984; 4:0.4.)

ammonia) are determined as a function of time in blood, urine, and breath; (2) measurement of synthesis rates in muscle and blood by sampling protein from these tissues in studies similar to whole body studies; and (3) measurement of 3-methylhistidine excretion in urine, or arteriovenous difference of 3-methylhistidine, as a measure of the unidirectional rate of muscle protein breakdown. Urinary 3-methylhistidine excretion must be interpreted with caution, since under some conditions gut may be a major contributor. These methods rely on many assumptions, which have not all been verified. The results are of interest in order to better understand the processes by which diet and disease effect changes in N balance and related gains or losses in body cell mass. However, as yet, the findings in this area add little of clinical significance to what can be determined by traditional methods of measuring N balance and indirect calorimetry. Starvation or malnutrition appears to decrease turnover, whereas feeding large amounts, particularly of protein, increases protein turnover. However, it should be kept in mind that there is an increase in both synthesis and degradation, and therefore increasing protein intake will not necessarily increase net synthesis. As noted earlier, after a certain point, increasing protein intake has no further effect on N balance in normal or hypercatabolic patients who are in energy balance. The effects of severe injury or sepsis are to increase whole-body protein turnover and to greatly increase degradation of muscle protein.

Neuroendocrine Mediation of the Hypercatabolic Response

It seems likely that the hypercatabolism and hypermetabolism of injury are adaptive responses, improving survival at a time when the organism has increased nutrient requirements but cannot obtain food. Some have speculated that the characteristic increase in breakdown of muscle protein is mainly to provide energy. However, as shown earlier, even under the most severe catabolic conditions, protein supplies only 30 per cent of energy requirements, the rest being supplied by fat, which provides 70 per cent or more. Furthermore, fat mobilization is increased with injury to a greater extent than fat oxidation.[49-51] It seems more reasonable to associate the increased protein breakdown with glucose requirements of both the brain and the wound. In the absence of nutrient intake only a small fraction of this glucose requirement can be met from fat, and most must be obtained from protein. In normal subjects, fasting lowers plasma glucose; there is a marked increase in production of ketones, which can spare 50 per cent or more of brain glucose requirements. As a result, there is a marked decrease in muscle protein breakdown. Injured or septic patients during fasting are both hyperglycemic and hyperinsulinemic; this

suppresses ketone formation and therefore brain glucose requirements, and the amounts of muscle protein breakdown are much higher in injured or septic patients than in normal subjects. The hyperglycemia makes it possible to supply the very large amounts of glucose needed by the wound,[52] which is glycolyzed but not oxidized. Despite the hyperglycemia, which in normal subjects would suppress fat oxidation, most of the energy expended by the body as a whole and by tissues other than brain and the wound is obtained from fat in subjects who are fasting or given 5 per cent dextrose.[51] Even with high glucose intakes, gluconeogenesis and fat oxidation remain at much higher levels than are seen in normal subjects.[51]

These metabolic changes appear to be mediated by increases in sympathetic activity and production of cortisol and glucagon; they can be simulated in normal subjects by simultaneous infusion of cortisol, glucagon, and epinephrine at rates to produce plasma concentrations seen in injury or sepsis. The ability of sepsis or injury to effect these neuroendocrine changes is mediated by two pathways. One involves the afferent nervous system; the other involves one or a family of peptide hormones, variously known as endogenous pyrogen, leukocyte endogenous mediator, cachectin, and interleukin 1.[53]

CARBOHYDRATE AND FAT METABOLISM

YVON A. CARPENTIER

Metabolic Response to Injury

The response to injury is essentially conditioned by hormonal and humoral mediators. Hormones seem to play a major role in the metabolic response, while humoral mediators—released by white blood cells—could be mainly involved in the inflammatory response. The metabolic response consists of two different phases, described as early as 1932 by Sir David Cuthbertson:[54]

1. The initial ebb phase of variable duration, characterized by low cardiac flow and tissue perfusion, during which substrate utilization and most cell functions are depressed in most tissues of the body.

2. The subsequent flow phase, characterized by high cardiac outflow and increased energy expenditure and nitrogen excretion. During this hypermetabolic phase, insulin release is high but most of its metabolic effects are counteracted by the elevated levels of catecholamines, glucagon, and cortisol. This hormonal imbalance leads to an increased mobilization of amino acids and free fatty acids (FFA) from peripheral muscles and adipose tissue stores. A portion of these released substrates is used for energy

production, either directly, as glucose, or after being remodeled in the liver, as triglycerides. Another portion of amino acids participate in the synthesis of proteins in the liver (where production of acute-phase reactants is markedly stimulated by humoral mediators) as well as in the immune system and for the healing of damaged tissues.

Although this hypermetabolic phase comprises both catabolic and anabolic processes, the net result is a significant loss of both protein and fat. This also leads to a modification of body composition characterized by a reduction in both protein and fat compartments, while extracellular, and to a lesser extent intracellular, water compartments are relatively enlarged.

The extent of the changes occurring during both these phases is directly related to the severity of the injury or the septic condition. It should be pointed out that minor surgical trauma—such as many elective operations—does not increase energy expenditure but significantly affects fat and protein metabolism. It should also be emphasized that the metabolic response to injury or sepsis is influenced by the pre-injury nutritional status of the patients: the limited response exhibited by severely depleted patients is accompanied by a higher incidence of morbidity and mortality.[55]

During the ebb phase, priority has to be given to the resuscitation; the role of nutritional support is very limited until adequate tissue perfusion has been restored. By contrast, the lack of nutritional support during the hypermetabolic flow phase results in a fast and severe nutritional depletion.

Kinetic measurements of glucose and FFA metabolism as well as data obtained by indirect calorimetry have shown that:

1. The relationship between plasma substrate concentration and turnover found in normal subjects does not apply to hypermetabolic patients. The elevation in plasma concentration is much less marked than the increase in turnover rate and therefore significantly underestimates the extent of the alteration.[56,57]

2. Oxidative metabolism is turned toward preferential utilization of fat substrate in the hypermetabolic phases.[58]

Complementary information is derived from a recent study on septic dogs;[59] simultaneous measurements of both FFA and very-low-density-lipoprotein triglyceride (VLDL-TG) turnover and oxidation rates have provided evidence that, while fat oxidation is essentially derived from circulating FFA in normal animals, plasma triglycerides significantly participate in energy production during sepsis. In this condition, hepatic recycling of plasma FFA leads to an augmented production of VLDL-TG concomitant with increased rates of removal and oxidation. These data are in agreement with measurements of increased plasma clearance and oxidation rates of exogenous (intravenous) fat emulsions in hypermetabolic patients.[60]

Differences in Energy Metabolism between Acutely Ill and Depleted Patients

Chronic partial starvation and post-injury hypermetabolism are both associated with an increased participation of fat in energy metabolism. Although some degree of nutritional depletion can be present in hypermetabolic critically ill patients and interfere with their metabolic response, it is appropriate to analyze some features specific to each condition:

1. Total energy expenditure and nitrogen output are increased in hypermetabolic patients but decreased in prolonged fasting.

2. Plasma concentrations of insulin and glucose, as well as the rate of hepatic glucose production, are increased in hypermetabolic patients but decreased in prolonged fasting.

3. Although plasma glycerol and FFA concentration are similarly elevated in both conditions, the turnover rate of these substrates is much higher in hypermetabolic patients.

4. Plasma clearance and oxidation rates of exogenous triglycerides are higher in hypermetabolic than in depleted patients.

These differences in substrate kinetics and hormonal milieu suggest that the high level of fat utilization observed in both conditions would be conditioned by different factors; it would be mainly due to the limited amount of carbohydrate available for energy production in prolonged fasting, while peripheral resistance toward glucose utilization would play a preponderant role during the hypermetabolic phase. This opinion is supported by the different metabolic response to massive IV glucose administration observed in both types of patients.

Influence of TPN on Features of the Metabolic Response

The administration of fat-free TPN (largely exceeding the energy expenditure and consisting of glucose and amino acids, with a lipid intake limited to the provision of essential fatty acids) induces different effects in depleted and hypermetabolic patients.[61] In depleted patients, such a large glucose load has no significant effect on oxygen consumption but induces a marked elevation in CO_2 production. The respiratory quotient (RQ) values increase above 1.0, indicating that, in terms of net oxidation, all the calories are then provided and that the excess glucose is converted into fat; new fat synthesis exceeds endogenous fat oxidation, and thus fat balance is positive. In hypermetabolic patients, a proportionately similar glucose load induces a significant increase in oxygen consumption together with a marked elevation in CO_2 production. The resulting RQ values remain below 1.0, indicating a persistent net oxidation of lipids. The negative fat balance can result either from a limitation of glucose oxidation or from a marked stimulation of fat oxidation. In addition, this indicates that a significant proportion of nonoxidized glucose cannot be converted into fat and is disposed of and stored in other carbohydrate forms, such as glycogen. This impairment in the utilization of large glucose loads by critically ill patients is accompanied by a further increase in the already elevated urinary excretion of catecholamines, which suggests that excessive glucose intake could act as an additional stress.[62]

In both depleted and hypermetabolic patients, the higher CO_2 production in response to massive glucose load induces a marked increase in minute ventilation; this response can precipitate pulmonary decompensation in patients with impaired or limited ventilatory function. In such conditions, switching from a fat-free to a fat-containing TPN—while keeping similar calorie intake—quickly results in decreases in both CO_2 production and minute ventilation. These changes, directly related to the composition of calorie intake, can markedly improve the clinical condition of nonventilated patients; they have allowed patients to be weaned off artificial ventilation after receiving ventilatory support during fat-free TPN. Besides reducing insulin requirements and the risks associated with hyperglycemia, fat-containing TPN has also been demonstrated to induce a lower incidence of liver dysfunction than fat-free TPN; this is likely related to a lesser accumulation of newly synthesized triglycerides and stored glycogen in the liver.

The demonstration of a faster plasma clearance and higher oxidation rate of exogenous lipids in hypermetabolic patients and the clinical benefits previously mentioned have led to recommendations for an increased proportion of fat in the calorie intake of critically ill patients. Many patients have been infused with fat emulsions for prolonged periods without presenting any detectable clinical complications. However, some reports on possible side effects of IV fat emulsions need to be carefully considered:

1. In vitro addition of Intralipid to the plasma of critically ill patients results in most cases in the agglutination of the fat particles.[63,64] This phenomenon, commonly called creaming, is positively correlated to the concentration of acute phase proteins—namely, C-reactive protein—and negatively to albumin levels. This observation has not been documented in vivo, and the clearance of exogenous fat has been found to be normal in patients whose plasma was inducing agglutination of fat particles. However, if this phenomenon was taking place, even to a minor extent, in the circulating plasma, these agglutinated compounds would be a rather poor substrate for lipoprotein in lipase and

could therefore follow abnormal pathways and be removed in the reticuloendothelial system.

2. Impaired functions of PMN leukocytes, monocytes and macrophages, directly related to the increase in plasma triglyceride concentration, have been observed in subjects infused with fat emulsions;[65,66] these alterations have been explained by the phagocytosis of exogenous particles.[67] However, controversial results have been reported by authors who found, in similar conditions, a stimulation of some monocyte and macrophage functions.[68,69] These conflicting results suggest that some changes in cell functions are more likely to be related to changes in membrane composition. Significant exchanges of both phospholipids and free cholesterol have been observed between exogenous lipid particles and circulating cell membranes.[70,71]

Although the relevance of these findings to clinical practice is still unclear, they suggest a need for more caution in fat administration to critically ill patients. Not only the total daily lipid intake but also the rate of infusion and the phospholipid:triglyceride ratio of fat emulsions should be carefully considered in order to avoid massive loads of various lipid components in the plasma. Obviously, transient accumulation of lipids cannot be detected by visual recognition of lactescence on plasma triglyceride determination in samples drawn 4 to 6 hours after fat infusion. Plasma concentration of triglycerides, phospholipid, and cholesterol should also be monitored during fat infusion in order to adjust the lipid intake and rate of infusion according to the individual's tolerance of each component. This recommendation appears to be even more important when one considers that exogenous lipids do not simply disappear from the plasma after having accomplished their role as energy suppliers, but are very active as artificial lipoproteins during their short intravascular life.

Influence of Exogenous Fat Emulsions on Lipoprotein Metabolism

Despite their differences in composition with endogenous chylomicrons, exogenous particles exchange various lipid and protein components with the other lipoproteins.

In vitro[72] and in vivo[73] studies have demonstrated a very high affinity of exogenous lipids for C-2, C-3 and E apoproteins, which play a crucial role in the catabolism of chylomicrons. The transfer of these apoproteins from HDL to artificial particles is related to the lipid load and reproduces in exogenous particles a pattern very close to that of intravascular circulating chylomicrons.

In vitro and in vivo studies have also shown that, similarly to endogenous TG-rich VLDL and chylomicrons, exogenous particles can donate triglycerides to cholesterol-rich LDL and HDL and, in a reciprocal manner, accept esterified cholesterol transferred from LDL and HDL.[74,75] These exchanges are dependent upon the concentration and types of triglycerides in the emulsion.[76] Besides these exchanges of neutral lipids and apoproteins, transfer of exogenous phospholipids to endogenous lipoproteins has also been demonstrated. These interactions can significantly modify the composition of both exogenous particles and endogenous lipoproteins. Since exogenous particles are progressively enriched with esterified cholesterol while being depleted of triglycerides, it becomes essential to determine the removal site of these "exogenous remnants." It will be particularly interesting to find out whether or not the absence of apoprotein B on these "exogenous remnants" affects the affinity of receptors specific to endogenous lipoprotein remnants. It should also be quite relevant to determine whether the modifications observed in the composition of endogenous lipoproteins will change their metabolic pathways and affect cholesterol metabolism, especially when long-term repeated fat infusions have to be considered.

Amount of Carbohydrate versus Amount of Fat in Daily Intake

The optimal amount of energy intake to be given to critically ill patients should theoretically result in obtaining a zero energy balance without inducing any worrisome complications.

Besides the specific needs of some tissues for glucose and the essential role of some unsaturated fatty acids for the synthesis of cell membranes and various prostaglandins, the calorie requirements of most tissues of the body can, from a theoretical point of view, be entirely covered either with carbohydrate or with fat.

However, the metabolic utilization of either energy substrate, being subject to considerable individual variability and influenced by the type and the severity of the illness or injury, cannot be precisely predicted for a given patient. Administering either substrate in excess of the maximal oxidation rate would result in the accumulation of nonutilized compounds and possibly induce severe side effects. These risks can be reduced by combining both types of substrates in TPN calorie intake and ideally, by monitoring their metabolic utilization. General recommendations cannot be made concerning the precise amount of carbohydrate and exogenous fat to be included in the TPN regimen of critically ill patients. From a practical viewpoint, nutritional support could be started with fat representing 30 to 50 per cent of total calorie intake and the regimen subsequently adjusted by taking into account metabolic utilization of each substrate as well as the development of complications.

Results of studies currently in progress could in the future offer the possibility of improving the utilization of fat as energy substrate by adding L-carnitine or using alternative substrates such as medium-chain triglycerides, but no convincing data are presently available.

References

Energy Metabolism

1. Kinney JM. The application of indirect calorimetry to clinical studies. *In* Kinney JM, Munro HN, Buskirk E (eds). Assessment of Energy Metabolism in Health and Disease. Proceedings of an International Symposium, Prouts Neck, ME, 1978. Columbus, OH, Ross Laboratories, 1980:42.
2. Kinney JM, Caldwell FT Jr. Fever: etiology, physiologic and metabolic effects, and management in surgical patients. *In* Sabiston DC (ed): Davis-Christopher Textbook of Surgery. 12th ed. Philadelphia, WB Saunders, 1981: 178.
3. Keys A, Brozek J, Henschel A, Mickelsen O, Taylor HL. The Biology of Human Starvation. Vol. 1. Minneapolis, University of Minnesota Press, 1950: Chapter 17.
4. Bergstrom J. Muscle electrolytes in man. Scand J Clin Lab Invest 1962; *14*(Suppl 68):1–110.
5. Edwards RHT, Maunder C, Lewis PD, et al. Percutaneous needle biopsy in the diagnosis of muscle diseases. Lancet 1973; 2:1070.
6. Bergstrom J. Percutaneous needle biopsy of skeletal muscle in physiological and clinical research. Scand J Clin Lab Invest 1975; *35*:609.
7. Furst P. Intermediary energy metabolism for catabolic state with special regard to muscle tissue. *In* Wilkinson AW, Cuthberston DP (eds). Metabolism and the Response to Injury. London, Pitman Medical, 1976: 94–112.
8. Harris RC, Hultman E, Nordesjo L. Glycogen, glycolytic intermediates and high-energy phosphates determined in biopsy samples of musculus quadriceps femoris of man at rest. Methods and variance of values. Scand J Clin Lab Invest 1974; *33*:109.
9. Liaw KY, Askanazi J, Michelsen CB, et al. Effect of injury and sepsis on high-energy phosphates in muscle and red cells. J Trauma 1980; *20*:755.
10. Liaw KY. Effect of injury, sepsis and parenteral nutrition on high-energy phosphates in human liver and muscle. JPEN 1985; *9*:28.
11. Bergstrom J, Furst P, Chao L, et al. Changes of muscle water and electrolytes with severity of trauma. Acta Chir Scand (Suppl) 1979; *494*:139.
12. Bergstrom J, Furst P, Larsson J, et al. Influence of injury on muscle water and electrolytes. Effect of severe injury, burns and sepsis. Acta Chir Scand, in press.
13. Liaw KY, Askanazi J, Michelsen CB, et al. Effect of postoperative nutrition on muscle high energy phosphates. Ann Surg 1982; *195*:12.
14. Vinnars E, Holmstrom B, Schildt B, et al. Metabolic effects of four intravenous nutritional regimes in patients undergoing elective surgery. II. Muscle amino acids and energy-rich phosphates. Clin Nutr 1983; *2*:3–11.
15. Nordemar R, Lovgren O, Furst P, et al.: Muscle ATP content in rheumatoid arthritis—a biopsy study. Scand J Clin Lab Invest 1974; *34*:185.
16. Lipmann F. Metabolic generation and utilization of phosphate bond energy. Adv Enzymol 1941; *18*:99–162.
17. Atkinson DE, Walton GM. Adenosine triphosphate conservation in metabolic regulation. J Biol Chem 1967; *242*:3239–3241.
18. Muller P, Bergstrom J, Furst P, et al. Muscle biopsy studies in patients with moderate liver cirrhosis with special reference to energy-rich phosphagens and electrolytes. Scand J Gastroenterol 1984; *19*:267–272.
19. Moller P, Bergstrom J, Furst P, et al. Energy-rich phospha-

gens, electrolytes and free amino acids in leg skeletal muscle of patients with chronic obstructive lung disease. Acta Med Scand 1982; *211*:187–193.

20. Bergstrom J, Bostrom H, Furst P. Preliminary studies of energy-rich phosphagens in muscle from severely ill patients. Crit Care Med 1976; *4*:197.

Protein Metabolism

21. Kinney JM, Elwyn DH. Protein metabolism and injury. Ann Rev Nutr 1983; *3*:433–466.
22. Duke JH, Jorgensen SB, Broell JR, et al. Contribution of protein to caloric expenditure following injury. Surgery 1970; *68*:168–174.
23. Takala J, Klossner J. Branched chain enriched parenteral nutrition in surgical patients. Clin Nutr 1986; *5*:167–170.
24. Elwyn DH. Protein metabolism and requirements in the critically ill patient. Crit Care Clin, in press.
25. Keys A, Brozek J, Henschel A, Mickelsen O, Taylor HL. The Biology of Human Starvation. Vol. 1. Minneapolis, University of Minnesota Press, 1950: Chapter 20.
26. Insel J, Elwyn DH. Body composition. *In* Askanazi J, Starker P, Weissman C (eds). Fluid and Electrolyte Management in Critical Care. Boston, Butterworth, 1986.
27. Kinney JM, Duke JH Jr, Long CL, et al. Tissue fuel and weight loss after injury. J Clin Pathol 1970; *23*(Suppl 4):65–72.
28. Reifenstein EC Jr, Albright F, Wells SI. The accumulation, interpretation and presentation of data pertaining to metabolic balances, notably those of calcium, phosphorus, and nitrogen. J Clin Endocrinol 1945; *5*:367–395.
29. Elwyn DH. Nutritional requirements of adult surgical patients. Crit Care Med 1980; *8*:9–20.
30. Starker PM, LaSala PA, Askanazi J, et al. The influence of preoperative TPN on morbidity and mortality. Surg Gynecol Obstet 1986; *162*:569–574.
31. Goodman N, Ruderman NB. Starvation in the rat. I. Effects of age and obesity on organ weight, RNA, DNA and protein. Am J Physiol 1980; *239*:E269–E270.
32. Grant JP. Clinical impact of protein malnutrition on organ mass and function. *In* Blackburn GL, Grant JP, Young VR (eds). Amino Acids: Metabolism and Medical Application. Littleton, MA, Wright PSG, 1983: 347–358.
33. Rochester DF. Malnutrition and the respiratory muscles. Clin Chest Med 1986; *7*:91–99.
34. Weissman C, Askanazi J, Rosenbaum S, et al. Amino acids and respiration. Ann Intern Med 1983; *98*:41–44.
35. Bryan-Brown CW, Savitz MH, Elwyn DH, et al. Cerebral edema unresponsive to conventional therapy in neurosurgical patients with unsuspected nutritional failure. Crit Care Med 1973; *1*:125–129.
36. Russell DM, Prendergast PJ, Darby PL, et al. A comparison between muscle function and body composition in anorexia nervosa: the effect of refeeding. Am J Clin Nutr 1983; *38*:229–237.
37. Elwyn DH. Repletion of the malnourished patient. *In* Blackburn GL, Grant JP, Young VR (eds). Amino Acids: Metabolism and Medical Application. Littleton, MA, Wright PSG, 1983: 359–375.
38. Shaw SN, Elwyn DH, Askanazi J, et al. Effects of increasing nitrogen intake on nitrogen balance and energy expenditure in nutritionally depleted adults receiving parenteral nutrition. Am J Clin Nutr 1983; *37*:930–940.
39. Rowlands BJ, Giddings AEB, Johnston AOB, et al. Nitrogen-sparing effect of different feeding regimes in patients after operation. Br J Anaesth 1977; *49*:781–787.
40. Larsson J, Martensson J, Vinnars E. Nitrogen requirements in hypercatabolic patients. Clin Nutr (Special Suppl) 1984; *4*:0.4.
41. Long CL, Zikria BA, Kinney JM, et al. Comparison of fibrin hydrolysates and crystalline amino acid solutions in parenteral nutrition. Am J Clin Nutr 1974; *27*:163–174.
42. Andersen GH, Patel DG, Jeejeebhoy KN. Design and evaluation by nitrogen balance and blood aminograms of an amino acid mixture for total parenteral nutrition of adults with gastrointestinal disease. J Clin Invest 1974; *53*:904–912.

43. Vinnars E, Furst P, Hermansson IL, et al. Protein catabolism in the postoperative state and its treatment with amino acid solution. Acta Chir Scand 1970; *136*:95–109.
44. Fischer JE, Rosen HM, Eberd AM, et al. The effect of normalization of plasma amino acids on hepatic encephalopathy in man. Surgery 1976; *80*:77–91.
45. Cerra FB, Cheung NK, Fischer JE, et al. Disease-specific amino acid infusion (F080) in hepatic encephalopathy: a prospective, randomized, double blind, controlled trial. JPEN 1985; *9*:288–295.
46. Eriksson LS, Persson A, Wahren J. Branched chain amino acids in the treatment of chronic hepatic encephalopathy. Gut 1982; *23*:801–806.
47. Weser E. Nutritional aspects of malabsorption: short gut adaptation. Clin Gastroenterol 1983; *12*:443.
48. Grote AE, Elwyn DH, Takala J, et al. Nutritional and metabolic effects of enteral and parenteral feeding in severely injured patients. Clin Nutr 1987; *6*:161–167.
49. Carpentier YA, Askanazi J, Elwyn DH, et al. Effects of hypercaloric glucose infusion on lipid metabolism in injury and sepsis. J Trauma 1979; *19*:649–654.
50. Nordenstrom J, Carpentier YA, Askanazi J, et al. Free fatty acid mobilization and oxidation during total parenteral nutrition in trauma and infection. Ann Surg 1983; *198*:725–735.
51. Askanazi J, Carpentier YA, Elwyn DH, et al. Influence of total parenteral nutrition on fuel utilization in injury and infection. Ann Surg 1980; *191*:40–46.
52. Wilmore DW, Aulick LH, Mason AD Jr, et al. The influence of the burn wound on the local and systemic responses to injury. Ann Surg 1977; *186*:444–458.
53. Elwyn DH. Nutritional requirements of stressed patients. *In* The Society of Critical Care Medicine: Textbook of Critical Care. Philadelphia, WB Saunders, 1988.

Carbohydrate and Fat Metabolism

54. Cuthbertson DP. Observations on the disturbance of metabolism produced by injury to the limbs. Q J Med 1932; *1*:233–241.
55. Fellows IW, MacDonald IA, Bennett T, et al. The effect of undernutrition on thermoregulation in the elderly. Clin Scien 1985; *69*:525–532.
56. Carpentier YA, Jeevanandam M, Robin AP, et al. Measurements of glycerol turnover by infusion of nonisotopic glycerol. Am J Physiol 1984; *247*:E405–E411.
57. Nordenstrom J, Carpentier YA, Askanazi J, et al. Free fatty acid mobilization and oxidation during total parenteral nutrition in trauma and sepsis. Ann Surg 1983; *198*:725–735.
58. Askanazi J, Carpentier YA, Elwyn DH, et al. Influence of total parenteral nutrition on fuel utilization in injury and sepsis. Ann Surg 1980; *191*:40–46.
59. Wolfe RR, Shaw JHF, Durkot MJ: Effect of sepsis on VLDL kinetics: responses in basal state and during glucose infusion. Am J Physiol 1985; *248*:E732–E740.
60. Carpentier YA, Nordenstrom J, Askanazi J, et al. Relationship between rates of clearance and oxidation of 14C-Intralipid in surgical patients. Surg Forum 1979; *30*:72–74.
61. Robin AP, Askanazi J, Cooperman A, et al. Influence of hypercaloric glucose infusion on fuel economy in surgical patients: a review. Crit Care Med 1981; *9*:680–686.
62. Nordenstrom J, Jeevanandam M, Elwyn DH, et al. Increasing glucose intake during total parenteral nutrition increases norepinephrine excretion in trauma and sepsis. Clin Physiol 1981; *1*:525–534.
63. Hulman G, Fraser I, Pearson HJ, et al. Agglutination of Intralipid by sera of acutely ill patients. Lancet 1982; *2*:1426–1427.
64. Mayfield C, Nordenstrom J. Creaming and plasma clearance

rate of intravenous fat emulsion in critically ill patients. Clin Nutr 1984; *3*:93–97.

65. Jarstrand C, Berghem L, Lahnborg G. Human granulocyte and reticuloendothelial system function during Intralipid infusion. JPEN 1978; *2*:663–670.

66. Nordenstrom J, Jarstrand C, Wiernik A. Decreased chemotactic and random migration of leucocytes during Intralipid infusion. Am J Clin Nutr 1979; *32*:2416–2422.

67. Fraser I, Neoptolemos J, Darby H, et al. The effects of Intralipid and heparin on human monocyte and lymphocyte function. JPEN 1984; *8*:381–384.

68. Wiernik A, Jarstrand C, Julander I. Effect of Intralipid on mononuclear and polymorphonuclear phagocytes. Am J ClinNutr 1983; *37*:256–261.

69. Lattanzio A, Montemurro P, Pannarale O, et al. Increased production of procoagulant activity (tissue factor) by human peripheral blood monocytes after Intralipid infusion. Clin Nutr 1984; *3*:177–182.

70. Cooper RA, Arner EC, Wiley JS, et al. Modification of red cell membrane structure by cholesterol-rich lipid dispersions. J Clin Invest 1975; *55*:115–126.

71. Strunk RC, Kunke KS, Kolski GB, et al. Intralipid alters macrophage membrane fatty acid composition and inhibits complement (C2 synthesis). Lipids 1983; *18*:493–500.

72. Richelle M, Bury J, Kasry A, et al. In vitro exchanges of lipids and apoproteins between HDL and exogenous fat. (Abstract.) Clin Nutr 1987; *5*(Suppl):55.

73. Bury J, Rosseneu MY, Bihain BE, et al. Influence of an intravenous fat emulsion on the concentration and distribution of plasma apolipoproteins in man. (Abstract.) Clin Nutr 1987; *5*(Suppl):115.

74. Deckelbaum RJ, Eisenberg S, Granot E, et al. Core lipid exchange and lipoprotein in lipase in modelling human HDL. Arteriosclerosis 1982; *2*:437a.

75. Granot E, Deckelbaum RJ, Eisenberg S, et al. Core modification of human low-density lipoprotein by artificial triacylglycerol emulsion. Biochim Biophys Acta 1985; *833*:308–315.

76. Deckelbaum RJ, Richelle M, Kasry A, et al. Cholesterol ester enrichment of medium vs. long chain triglyceride emulsions via LDL and HDL in vitro. Arteriosclerosis 1985; *5*:536a.

39

THE BURNED PATIENT

PALMER Q. BESSEY / DOUGLAS W. WILMORE

The comprehensive management of a burned patient can be one of the most complicated and challenging problems encountered in clinical medicine. Superficially injured tissue must be treated to promote healing; deeper injuries require skin replacement. Injured skin loses its normal barrier and protection functions, and methods of management must be utilized to compensate for the altered skin function. In addition, unburned tissue must be preserved and optimal function maintained. Central to these tasks is the support of cellular metabolism. That is best accomplished by providing optimal cellular nutrition.

A burn is a physicochemical injury, usually involving coagulation necrosis of at least part of the skin or other epithelial tissue. Most commonly the injury is caused by heat, but it may also follow exposure to cold, chemicals, ionizing radiation, or electric current. If the burn involves the full-thickness of the skin—that is, necrosis through the dermis, an injury referred to as a third-degree of full thickness burn—the injured tissue must be removed and the deep tissues covered with a skin graft. This is performed by cutting or shaving a thin sheet of skin from an unburned area (split-thickness skin graft) and placing this on the wound to achieve coverage. If the burn involves only part of the thickness of the skin (partial-thickness burn), the wound will often heal spontaneously as new epidermis grows over the injured surface. Normal skin provides both a barrier to the loss of water from the deep tissues of the body and a barrier to the entrance of bacteria and other potentially noxious environmental agents into the body. Both of these important skin functions are lost after burn injury. Much of the care of burned patients involves maintaining proper fluid and electrolyte balance and controlling microbial growth and invasion via the burn wound.

Like most injuries, a burn elicits characteristic and predictable physiological and biochemical responses that collectively are referred to as the metabolic response to injury. An understanding of this injury response forms the basis of effective support of cellular metabolism and organ system function. In this chapter we will review our current understanding of the metabolic responses to burn injury. We will also outline principles of metabolic and nutritional support of burned patients. Because the responses to burn injury are qualitatively similar to the responses to other injuries, the discussions in this chapter could also apply to other injured and critically ill patients.

In the United States, approximately 150,000 persons die annually from injuries.[1] Trauma is the leading cause of death for persons between the ages of 1 and 44 years,[2] and it is the third leading cause of death for all ages. However, trauma is the major cause of years of life lost under age 65, and hence affects individuals with years of potential productivity ahead of them.[3] Burns are a severe form of traumatic injury and claim some 7000 lives annually.[2] Approximately two million persons seek medical attention for burns,[4] and some 100,000 require hospitilization.[2] The medical care of burn victims is complex, prolonged, costly, and imperfect. All but the most superficial burns result in scarring, which may be debilitating as well as deforming; the emotional repercussions of these injuries can be devastating. Fires exact high costs from society not only for the replacement and repair of damaged property, but also for the care of the burned victims of fires and for their lost productivity.

Fire prevention and safety have long been of concern to society. As a result of major public fire disasters, fire codes and certain safety measures have become law and are integrated into our daily lives.[5] Other measures have been proposed to further reduce burns and fire damage. These include installation of residential smoke detectors and fire alarms; use of flame-retardant materials for building construction, upholstery, and clothing; lowering the temperature of hot water; and manufacturing self-extinguishing cigarettes. The technology for these measures already exists, but the relative costs and benefits are still being debated. Furthermore, not all burn injuries are obviously preventable. Thus, care of the victims of burn injury, as well as victims of mechanical trauma, will continue to require major health care resources in the foreseeable future.

THE METABOLIC RESPONSE TO INJURY

Sir David Cuthbertson, a Scottish biochemist, was one of the first investigators to study the metabolic responses of injured patients in a systematic and quantitative way. Over 50 years ago he described the main features of the injury response that are still recognized today.[6] He emphasized that the injury response evolved with time. Two distinct phases could be identified[7] (Table 39–1). The first of these, the "ebb" phase, began immediately after injury and was characterized by a decreased oxygen consumption, lowered body temperature, and lethargy. If the victim survived, the ebb evolved into a "flow" phase, characterized by an increase in oxygen consumption, body temperature, and nitrogen excretion. The response to burn injury reflects this general phenomenon. The "ebb" is associated with burn shock. Perfusion is limiting. Clinical efforts are directed toward maintaining effective cardiovascular performance and tissue perfusion. The "flow" is a period of heightened cardiovascular and metabolic activity. Provision of substrate to support this hypermetabolism is a primary goal.

TABLE 39–1. Metabolic Response to Injury

Ebb Phase	Flow Phase
↓ Oxygen consumption	↑ Oxygen consumption
↓ Cardiac output	↑ Cardiac output
↓ Core temperature	↑ Core temperature
↑ Blood glucose	↑ Blood glucose—mild—flux increased
Normal glucose production	↑ Glucose production
↑ Lactate	Normal lactate
↑ Free fatty acids	↑ Free fatty acids—mild—flux increased
↑ Catecholamines, glucagon, cortisol	↑ Catecholamines, glucagon, cortisol
↓ Insulin	↑ Insulin
Insulin resistance	↑ Insulin resistance

Ebb Phase

BURN SHOCK

Shock can be defined as a clinical syndrome of acute onset usually characterized by systemic hypotension, signs of autonomic nervous system activity (sweating, peripheral cyanosis, tachycardia), and signs of inadequate cardiac output and tissue perfusion (oliguria, lethargy or restlessness, acidosis). Shock is seen commonly after burns and other types of injury and may be a cause of early death. The major conceptual advance in our understanding of the nature of shock following trauma was made by Alfred Blalock over 50 years ago.[8] He studied shock following a variety of injuries in experimental animals and demonstrated that loss of circulating blood volume was the recurrent cardinal feature. In addition to loss of blood (i.e., hemorrhage), loss of plasma volume into the injured tissues was also observed. The result of unchecked blood volume loss is reduction of cardiac output and diminished flow to the microcirculation. Oxygen delivery is impaired and tissue hypoxia results. Most cells of the body can tolerate anaerobic conditions for only a finite period of time before they cease to function and die. The main objective of resuscitation from shock following trauma is restoration of circulating volume to achieve adequate oxygen delivery to all tissues before irreversible deterioration of cellular function occurs. This is usually accomplished by vigorous blood and fluid replacement.

In burned animals Blalock observed the accumulation of plasma-like fluid in the soft tissues underneath the injured skin and an increase in plasma hemoglobin concentration.[9] He calculated that there had been a translocation of fluid from the vascular space to the soft tissues amounting to over one half of the circulating plasma volume. Although shock following other types of injuries is commonly due to hemorrhage, loss of plasma volume into the interstitial space to form "burn edema" is the major cause of burn shock.

Early studies of burn edema[10,11] demonstrated that the fluid had a high protein content (approximately one-half to two-thirds the protein concentration of plasma), and that the rate of edema formation was proportional to the extent of the body surface area that was burned. Thus, a mathematical formula for estimating the amount of fluid required for resuscitation based on the extent of burn injury was proposed.[12] Subsequently, other formulas were developed. All of these called for the administration of colloid- and sodium-containing fluids in amounts quantitatively related to the extent of the total body surface area injured. Because some studies suggested that alterations in capillary permeability to colloidal particles occurred in both burned and nonburned tissues for the first 24 hours post burn, one fluid regimen for the treatment of burn shock did not provide colloid during the first post-burn day, but called for the administration of crystalloid solutions only.[13]

EARLY METABOLIC RESPONSES

The dramatic fluid shifts early after burn injury dominate the clinical findings. Decreased circulating plasma volume initiates homeostatic mechanisms that reduce volume losses and preserve perfusion to major organs such as the brain and heart. Both pressure and volume receptors in the walls of the atria of the heart and of several major arterial trunks are stimulated and send afferent signals to the central nervous system. The resultant reflex sympathetic discharge leads to vasoconstriction in peripheral tissues (primarily skeletal muscle), thereby directing perfusion to more vital capillary beds. The juxtaglomerular apparatus of the kidney also senses the diminished circulating volume and falling pressure, and it contributes to generalized vasoconstriction via the renin-angiotensin system and to sodium and water conservation by the stimulation of aldosterone elaboration.

In additon to volume changes there may be other signals that elicit systemic responses early after burn injury. Hume and Egdahl studied adrenal elaboration of 17-OH steroids in response to injury in anesthetized dogs.[14] They divided all the tissues of the proximal hind leg except for the major vessels, nerve trunks, and bone. When a small burn was inflicted, they observed a prompt and dramatic rise in adrenal

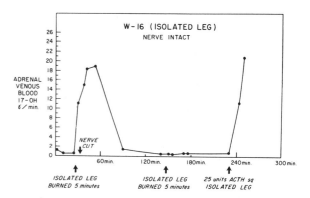

FIGURE 39–1. *Glucocorticoids are elaborated by the adrenal glands following an injury to an isolated leg that is attached to the body by only one artery, one vein, and one nerve. After the nerve is divided, the leg is reinjured, but there is no adrenocortical response. This demonstrates the importance of afferent sensory nerve stimulation in mediating glucocorticoid output. (From Hume DM, Egdahl RH. Ann Surg 1959; 150:697–712. Reproduced with permission.)*

steroid output (Fig. 39–1). They then divided the nerve trunks, and the adrenal steroid output returned to basal rates. They inflicted another burn, but there was no increase in steroid output. Adrenal responsiveness was confirmed with ACTH administration. This study documented the importance of neural afferent signals from the region of injury in initiating the adrenocortical response to injury. In other studies, Hume demonstrated that the afferent arm of this response involved peripheral nerves, spinal cord, medullary tissue, and midbrain. One of the more familiar neural signals following injury is pain, yet the perception of pain does not appear to be essential for the injury response. Kehlet and colleagues[15] studied many of the metabolic and hormone responses to elective operation. Under general anesthesia, when overt pain perception was absent, surgical patients demonstrated adrenal responses similar to those observed in injured patients. However, with epidural blockade (i.e., temporary spinal nerve blockage similar to afferent nerve section) these changes were much diminished or absent.

Thus, neural afferent signals that affect the central nervous system early after burn injury arise both from the site of injury and from central pressure and volume receptors stimulated by reduced circulating volume. In addition acidosis, which commonly occurs during periods of low perfusion, may stimulate central chemoreceptors and generate still other homeostatic adjustments. Furthermore, a variety of active humoral factors may be produced locally in the region of the burn injury. These include histamine, kinins,[16] prostaglandins,[17] and interleukin-1.[18] The role of these locally released compounds in mediating systemic responses is not defined. Immediately after experimental burn injury a decrease in cardiac output was observed before any major translocation of fluid could occur.[19] It was postulated that this represented a systemic effect of massive histamine release. However, in the classic studies of Hume and Egdahl[14] on the adrenocortical responsiveness of animals to injury, there was no response to a burn applied to an isolated, denervated leg even though vascular and lymphatic connections were intact, which suggested that local humoral factors did not produce major systemic effects in response to small injury.

The immediate effects of burn injury seem largely determined by the efferent activity of the sympathoadrenal axis. Markedly elevated concentrations of epinephrine and norepinephrine have been measured after injury,[20,21] and increased rates of discharge have been detected in sympathetic ganglia in experimental injury models. Glucose concentrations are elevated, in part owing to the stimulatory effects of catecholamines on glycogenolysis. Insulin concentrations are decreased relative to the glucose levels, owing to sympathetic inhibition of insulin production (alpha effect).[22] In addition, epinephrine can induce insulin resistance acutely in peripheral tissues.[23] Finally, free fatty acid levels are increased acutely following burn injury and these may also contribute to the peripheral insulin resistance observed.[24]

The adrenocortical response following injury in experimental animals is prompt.[14] In intact patients both urinary cortisol output and plasma concentrations have been observed to rise soon after injury.[25] This phenomenon is due to increased elaboration of ACTH from the anterior pituitary. The importance of this early cortisol response is not clear. It has been proposed that cortisol potentiates the effectiveness of catecholamines. Adrenalectomized animals have a high mortality from experimental injury and shock unless maintained on replacement glucocorticoids.[26]

Flow Phase

With successful resuscitation the "ebb" gradually gives way to the "flow" phase, usually some 36 to 48 hours after burn. The flow phase extends for days, weeks, or even months until the wounds are healed. It is during this period that metabolic and nutritional support figure prominently in overall management. The flow phase is characterized chiefly by hypermetabolism, by increased protein breakdown and loss of nitrogen from the body, and by alterations in carbohydrate metabolism. In addition there are changes in fluid and electrolyte balance that affect overall management.

HYPERMETABOLISM

Biochemical and physiological processes are inherently inefficient. A portion of the energy involved in those processes is lost as heat. Since humans maintain fairly constant body temperatures, heat generated by the body is equal to the heat lost in biochemical and physiological processes and is an indicator of overall metabolic activity. The metabolic rate is a measure of the heat lost from the body over time. In humans and other animals all energy utilized ultimately comes from the oxidation of organic fuels. Therefore the rate of heat production is related to oxygen consumption and carbon dioxide production. Metabolic rate may be determined directly by actually measuring the amount of heat lost from a subject over time (direct calorimetry), or it may be calculated based on measurements of oxygen consumption and carbon dioxide production (indirect calorimetry). Metabolic rates determined by these two techniques under basal conditions are comparable.[27] Indirect methods require less cumbersome and elaborate equipment than do direct methods and have been more widely utilized in the evaluation of critically ill patients. The relationship between metabolic rate (MR) oxygen consumption ($\dot{V}O_2$), and carbon dioxide production ($\dot{V}CO_2$)* (under both fasting and fed conditions is:[28]

$$MR\ (kcal/m^2/hr) = \frac{[3.9 \times \dot{V}O_2(1/min) + 1.1 \times \dot{V}CO_2(1/min)] \times 60(min/hr)}{Body\ surface\ area\ (m^2)}$$

The metabolic rate derived from gas exchange data should be determined under "basal" conditions—in the early morning after a 10- to 12-hour fast in a semi-darkened, quiet, thermoneutral environment, when the subject is rested, reclining, comfortable, calm, and familiar with the apparatus. This value is reproducible and predictable within ± 12 per cent[29] based on age, sex, and body size. If the metabolic rate of a burned patient is determined under basal conditions, it will be greater than that predicted based on the patient's age, sex, and preburn body surface area. Thus, the burned patient is said to be hypermetabolic. The degree of hypermetabolism is proportional to the severity of injury[30]—that is, to the amount of tissue injured. In burn victims this may be quantitated by the extent of body surface area that is burned. Metabolic rate under basal conditions increases with increasing burn size (Fig. 39-2).

Hypermetabolism is also associated with other injuries and critical illness, but massive burn injury elicits the most intense responses. Post-burn hypermetabolism reaches an upper limit of about twice predicted basal energy requirements. Most non-burn injuries elicit lesser responses, and elective operations are associated with only minor changes in the metabolic rate[30,31] (Fig. 39-3).

Hypermetabolic burned patients demonstrate

---

*There is a third term which is often included based on nitrogen excretion. It is small [− 3.3 × urea nitrogen (g/ml)], adjusting MR by only 2–3 per cent.

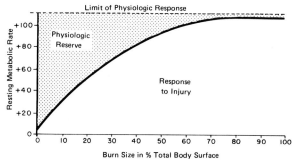

FIGURE 39–2. The intensity of the hypermetabolic response to injury is a function of the severity of the injury. Metabolic rate increases as a function of burn size up to a maximum of twice the predicted value. Patients with extensive injuries approach maximal responses and have limited physiological reserve with which to respond to additional stressors such as infection, hemorrhage, or even exposure to a cold environment. (From Wilmore DN. The Metabolic Management of the Critically Ill. New York; Plenum Medical, 1977: 118. Reproduced with permission.)

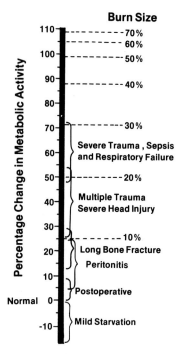

FIGURE 39–3. Burns and other critical illnesses increase whole-body metabolic activity under basal conditions in proportion to the severity of injury or disease. (Adapted from Wilmore DW. The Metabolic Management of the Critically Ill. New York, Plenum Medical, 1977: 33–36. Includes data from Clifton GL, Robertson CS, Grossman CS, et al. J Neurosurg 1984; 60:687–696.)

clinical signs of increased cardiac output, including a widened pulse pressure, mild tachycardia, and hyperdynamic peripheral pulses. Both cardiac output and whole-body oxygen consumption are proportional to burn size,[32] increasing to a maximum level. Regional oxygen consumption and blood flow are not so consistently related. Wilmore and associates[32] found that blood flow in an injured extremity was at least two times greater than flow to an uninjured extremity. Flow was proportional to the extent of the local burn on the extremity, and it appeared directed to the surface wound. Additional muscle blood flow measurements demonstrated that perfusion of skeletal muscle was comparable to that in normal individuals, not increased.[33] The oxygen consumption of the limb increased with *total* whole-body burn size and represented a fairly constant 6 per cent of the total body oxygen consumption. Extremity oxygen consumption was not related to the size of local limb injury. Hence, oxygen consumption in both injured and uninjured extremities in the same patient was similar. Thus, the differences in extremity blood flow could not be related to differences in regional oxygen requirements.

The oxygen consumption of other regional tissue beds also increases during the hypermetabolic response to burn injury.[34] The oxygen consumption of the kidney and splanchnic bed increases in concert with total body oxygen consumption. Splanchnic flow increases in proportion to total body flow (cardiac output.[35] In fact the increases in splanchnic and wound blood flow account in large part for the total increase in cardiac output. Renal blood flow correlates best with solute load, rather than with oxygen consumption.[35] From these and other data, it has been possible to partition both cardiac output and whole-body oxygen consumption among a variety of regional vascular beds[36] (Fig. 39–4).

In summary, hypermetabolism is a characteristic component of the response to burns and other injuries and critical illnesses. The degree of hypermetabolism is proportional to the severity of injury. The severity of a burn injury can generally be quantitated by the extent of body surface area that is burned. Hypermetabolism appears to be the result of a generalized increase in oxygen consumption by all major regional tissue beds. Cardiac output is also increased in proportion to injury severity, but regional blood flow is not consistently related to regional oxygen requirements.

ALTERATION IN BODY TEMPERATURE

Body temperature reflects the net balance between heat production and heat loss. Under normal circumstances it is regulated closely and maintained within a narrow range. Patients with burns or other injuries typically have an elevated body temperature even in the absence of clinical infection.[37] Heat production, measured as metabolic rate, is also increased in the burned patient. Heat is lost from nor-

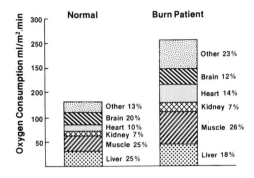

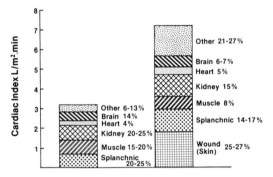

FIGURE 39–4. *The increase in oxygen consumption is a generalized response and can be seen in most regional vascular beds. However, most of the increase in blood flow is directed toward the wound, liver, and kidney. (From Bessey PQ. Parenteral nutrition and trauma. In Rombeau JL, Caldwell MD (eds). Clinical Nutrition. Vol 1. Philadelphia, WB Saunders, 1986. Adapted from Wilmore DW, Aulick LH. Surg Clin North Am 1978; 58:1173–1187.)*

mal individuals either as wet heat loss (evaporation) or as dry heat loss (radiation, direct contact with other objects, or convection). In the burned patient the normal barrier function of the skin is altered because of the surface injury. The major portion of the heat lost from the body of a burn victim is by the evaporative route. This varies directly with both the size of the injury and the ambient temperature. The elevated heat production was once considered to be a thermal regulatory response to increased evaporative water and heat loss from the surface wound. This was supported by original observations of Carl Moyer[38] and evidence gathered in animal studies.[39] Liljedahl and associates[40] realized the deleterious effects of a cool ambient temperature on burned patients and reported their clinical studies in 1968. A group of 11 patients with burns exceeding 20 per cent of their body surface area were treated in an environment of warm, dry air (32° C and a relative humidity of approximately 20 per cent). These patients were compared with another group of patients with burns of similar size who were exposed to normal ward temperatures of 22° C and relative humidity of 45 per cent. The patients treated in the warm, dry air showed substantial reduction in basal metabolic rate, increased rate of evaporation of water from the burn wound, rapid drying of the

burned surfaces, and smaller weight loss associated with the reduced metabolic rate.

A variety of subsequent studies, however, demonstrated that evaporative cooling of the burn wound does not appear to be the major metabolic stimulus of burned patients in a thermally neutral environment. Zawacki and associates were unable to demonstrate any consistent change in metabolic rates of burned patients in a thermally neutral environment after blocking evaporative water loss by wrapping the wound with a water-impermeable membrane.[41] In another study, oxygen consumption was determined in burned patients in a variety of ambient temperatures ranging from 19 to 33° C, and it was demonstrated that the decrease in metabolic rate that occurred as ambient temperature was elevated was related to burn size.[42] However, metabolic rate remained elevated when ambient temperature was increased up to and above thermal neutrality, suggesting that thermal regulatory factors in this warm environment were not the dominant stimulus of burn hypermetabolism, but the increased heat production was the consequence of an elevated metabolic state. This concept has been supported by subsequent investigations of burned patients studied for prolonged periods in warm environments (Table 39–2).

The interaction of evaporative water loss, ambient temperature, and hypermetabolism in the burned patient has yet another facet that must be considered. Burned patients are febrile, and it appears that thermoregulation in these patients occurs around an elevated central reference temperature.[43] They maintain above-normal surface and central body temperatures over a wide range of thermal environments (from 19 to 33° C). Because of the rise in "setpoint" temperature, these febrile burned patients prefer above-normal ambient temperatures (30 to 33° C) to achieve thermal comfort. In this warm environment, unburned skin remains relatively vasoconstricted as an additional means to satisfy the new hypothalamic reference temperature and maintain the febrile state. However, under these conditions of comfort, burned patients continue to maintain metabolic rates 1.5 to 2 times basal. Thus, while there may be thermal regulatory influences on burn hypermetabolism, the increased rate of heat

TABLE 39–2. Effect of Ambient Temperature on Metabolic Rate and on Core and Skin Temperatures

Ambient Temperature	Core Temperature °C	Skin Temperature °C	Metabolic Rate (kcal/m²/hr)
Normals			
21° (N=3)	36.7	30.0	41.2
25° (N=4)	36.8	31.4	35.6
33° (N=4)	36.8	34.2	36.3
Burn Patients (45% BSA)			
21° (N=9)	38.1	32.1	83.7
25° (N=20)	38.5	33.1	63.5
33° (N=20)	38.0	36.2	62.0

production is primarily determined by metabolic factors; that is, *burn hypermetabolism is temperature-sensitive, but not temperature-dependent.* However, this concept remains controversial; data collected by Caldwell and associates[44] in studying burned children of varying sizes (and, hence, various surface-to-mass ratios) suggest that dressings applied to the burn wound may reduce metabolic rate, presumably by reducing surface cooling. If these effects can be extrapolated to adult burned patients, then treating the burn wounds of these individuals with occlusive dressings while the patient is in a warm environment should markedly reduce the daily caloric requirements for weight maintenance. This result has not been observed over the past 7 years in a group of adult patients treated by excisional therapy and occlusive dressings in a warm environment; oxygen consumption and caloric requirements remain elevated throughout the post-traumatic course.

In normal individuals, approximately two thirds of the resting metabolic heat production occurs in the head and trunk. When oxygen consumption of visceral organs was determined in injured patients,[34] both splanchnic and renal oxygen consumption were elevated 75 to 100 per cent above resting normal levels. Peripheral oxygen consumption in injured and uninjured extremities of patients was unaffected by the local presence of a wound, but remained a relatively constant proportion of total body oxygen consumption (approximately 5 to 6 per cent of both hypermetabolic burned patients and normal controls). Thus, burn hypermetabolism appears to be a generalized or systemic response involving the entire body. Consequently, the general increase in body heat production appears to be distributed in a relatively normal fashion, approximately two thirds of the heat being produced in the visceral tissues and another one third in the extremities.

The specific mechanisms that may mediate the hypermetabolic response to injury will be discussed in detail later. However, calorigenic hormones generated by the sympathetic nervous system and adrenal medulla appear to have a major influence in post-traumatic hypermetabolism. Other hormones, particularly the counterregulatory agents, also seem essential to elicit all components of the injury response. The exact role of hormones, neurotransmitters, and other mediators in directing hypermetabolic responses remains unknown. A variety of biochemical reactions occur that cycle substrate and hence are energy-inefficient. Such reactions include the Cori cycle, the alanine-glutamine cycle, the increased synthesis and breakdown of protein, and the accelerated lipogenesis and lipolysis of body triglycerides. These and other biochemcial reactions contribute to increased heat production because of the accelerated utilization of energy.

ACCELERATED PROTEIN CATABOLISM AND NITROGEN LOSS

One of the most striking features of the metabolic response to injury is the marked muscle wasting that is observed in critically ill patients. This is associated with an increased urinary excretion of nitrogen and an acceleration of net protein breakdown. Cuthbertson first described this phenomenon in patients with long bone fractures.[37] Similar observations were made in this country by Howard and associates.[45] Detailed studies of nitrogen loss in burned patients were reported by Soroff and colleagues in 1961.[46]

Based on the associated urinary losses of phosphorus and sulfur and on the clinical observation of muscle wasting, Cuthbertson concluded that skeletal muscle was the major source of the nitrogen excreted.[6] Later studies utilizing a rat fracture model indicated that the increased nitrogen lost could not be accounted for just by the wasting of muscle that either was injured itself or was in the vicinity of the fracture.[47] Thus, nitrogen loss appeared to be a generalized, whole-body response to injury. These concepts have been supported by more recent data on the excretion of markers of skeletal muscle catabolism such as creatine, creatinine,[48] and Nτ-methyl (3-methyl) histidine.[49] As skeletal muscle protein undergoes degradation, these markers are released and excreted unchanged by the kidneys. Increased excretion of these markers has been observed in patients following burns,[50] trauma,[48,51] and infections,[52] thus reflecting increased proteolysis.

However, there are other potential sources of nitrogen loss from patients with burns and other injuries. These include eschar separation or excision, loss of blood or exudate from the wound, and the loss of muscle mass from disuse. Cuthbertson estimated that the amounts of nitrogen lost due to direct tissue injury, to wound exudate, and to generalized protein catabolism were roughly equivalent during the first 10 days following a burn.[53] Moore and co-workers measured the exudate nitrogen loss in burned patients throughout the post-burn course.[54] Exudate nitrogen accounted for as much as 25 to 30 per cent of the total nitrogen loss during the early post-burn period.

In his early studies Cuthbertson[6] observed that the time course of the nitrogen loss following injury was distinctive—excretion peaked several days after injury and gradually returned toward normal over several weeks. This pattern was similar to that of the increased metabolic rate—both nitrogen loss and hypermetabolism peaked shortly after injury and gradually returned toward normal. Soroff and colleagues[46] and later Wilmore[55] found a similar relationship in burned patients in additional studies. Metabolic rate and nitrogen excretion peaked in the early post-burn period. The return to basal values correlated with wound closure. This pattern is characteristic of the response to any injury.[56] However, the greatest losses are seen in severely burned patients (Fig. 39–5).

Protein turnover is an indicator of overall protein metabolic activity. It is determined utilizing tracer methodology and has been measured in a variety of

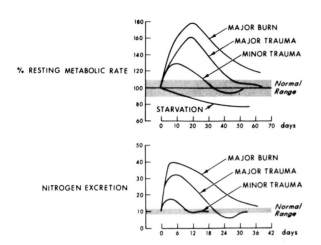

FIGURE 39–5. Hypermetabolism and nitrogen excretion are closely related following injury. They both reflect injury severity and return toward normal as the wounds heal. (Adapted from Kinney JM. Energy deficits in acute illness and injury. In Morgan AP (ed). Proceedings of a Conference on Energy Metabolism and Body Fuel Utilization. Cambridge, MA, Harvard University Press, 1966, p 774.)

critically ill patients. The interpretation of the data is based on the concept of a free amino acid pool *to which* nitrogen is added by both nitrogen intake and protein breakdown and *from which* nitrogen is removed by both nitrogen excretion and protein synthesis.[57] If the total amino acid nitrogen of the pool is constant, then turnover is the total amount of nitrogen that enters or leaves the pool. Protein turnover during the flow phase of the injury response is increased.[58] If turnover data are combined with measurements of nitrogen intake and excretion, rates of whole-body protein synthesis and catabolism may be estimated. These estimates indicate that protein catabolism is increased following injury,[59] but in the unfed patient synthesis rates remain normal. Synthesis will increase to approach or match catabolism when feeding is adequate. Levenson and co-workers[60] performed body compositional studies in rats following burn injury. They found that the incorporation of labeled amino acids into a variety of protein tissues after injury was equal to or greater than that in controls. In addition, when the animals were given labeled amino acid prior to injury, the loss of the label from protein after burn was more rapid than in controls. These data indicate that injury increases whole-body protein turnover in part by increasing the rate of protein breakdown and not suppressing the rate of protein synthesis.

AMINO ACID METABOLISM

Plasma concentrations of amino acids have been determined in a variety of critically ill and injured patients in an attempt to characterize a specific amino acid pattern associated with critical illness.

The findings have been variable. While some studies have found a generalized hypoaminoacidemia,[61] others have reported elevated concentrations of certain specific amino acids.[62–65] For example, elevated concentrations of phenylalanine, an essential amino acid that is not metabolized by muscle, have been reported following injury and critical illnesses. The concentration ratio of phenylalanine and tyrosine has been proposed as an indicator of the severity of muscle protein catabolism.[66] The branched-chain amino acids (BCAA)—leucine, isoleucine, and valine—are of particular interest because they are oxidized primarily in muscle,[67] unlike other amino acids that are metabolized mainly by the liver. Both elevated[62,68,69] and decreased[61,64] plasma BCAA concentrations have been reported following injury. The variation in the findings of these several investigations may be due to differences in analytical methodology, patient selection, or intercurrent treatment.[70]

Although amino acid concentrations in plasma are readily determined, they may not reflect quantitative alterations in the total amino acid pool. It has been estimated that as much as 80 per cent of the total body free amino acid pool is in skeletal muscle.[71] Concentrations of free amino acids in intracellular water may be as much as 30 times greater than plasma values.[72] Thus, the total skeletal muscle intracellular free amino acid pool of a 70-kg man would contain approximately 87 g of amino acids, whereas the total plasma pool would contain only 1.2 g. Based on muscle biopsy data from normal human subjects, the essential amino acids combined constitute 8.4 per cent of the total intracellular pool, whereas the single nonessential amino acid, glutamine, constitutes 61 per cent. Glutamine, glutamate, and alanine together constitute 79 per cent of the total free amino acid pool.

Although glutamine constitutes only about 6 per cent of muscle protein, it is a major constituent of the intracellular free amino acid pool. Following starvation, inactivity,[69] elective operation,[73] trauma,[74] and sepsis,[70] intracellular glutamine concentration falls (Fig. 39–6). Thus, a decrease in intracellular glutamine concentration seems to be a typical feature of the response to critical illness,[70] and it also appears to be a graded response[75] reflecting injury severity.

Associated with a decrease in intracellular glutamine, increased intracellular and plasma concentrations of phenylalanine, tyrosine, alanine, and the BCAA have been observed following injury.[70,73] This pattern of intracellular amino acid concentrations was little affected by intravenous nutrition.[76] During convalescence, the essential amino acid concentrations returned toward normal, but the decrease in intracellular glutamine persisted.[70]

The in vitro studies of Garber and co-workers[77] demonstrated that glutamine and alanine constitute as much as 70 per cent of the amino acids released

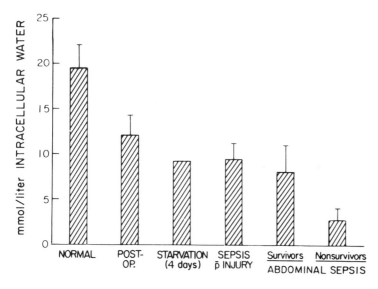

FIGURE 39–6. Skeletal muscle intracellular glutamine concentrations fall during critical illness. This response appears to be related to the degree of stress. (From Wilmore DW, Black PR, Muhlbacher F. Injured man: trauma and sepsis. In Winters RW (ed). Nutritional Support of the Seriously Ill Patient. New York, Academic Press, 1983: 33–52. Reproduced with permission.)

from skeletal muscle. Furthermore, this reflected the net rate of formation of alanine and glutamine from other amino acids.[78] The relative amounts of glutamine and alanine released depended on amino acid availability.

Aulick and Wilmore[79] measured femoral arterial and venous plasma concentrations of amino acids and blood flow in patients with major body surface area burns. From these determinations they calculated amino acid release from peripheral tissues. The net total release of amino acid nitrogen, based on the ten amino acids measured, was five times greater in the burned patients than in control subjects. Alanine was the only single amino acid that was significantly increased by itself between the two groups. Alanine release was related to burn size and oxygen consumption, not to the extent of leg burn (i.e., local injury). In companion studies[34] increased amino acid uptake across the splanchnic bed matched the accelerated peripheral release. Moreover, the uptake of alanine was increased three to four times over control values. These findings support the interpretation of the whole-body data and indicate that following injury skeletal muscle protein breaks down at an accelerated rate, releasing increased amounts of amino acids for transport to central tissues. Furthermore, this appears to be a generalized response of total-body skeletal muscle to critical illness.

ALTERATIONS OF CARBOHYDRATE METABOLISM

Hyperglycemia and impaired glucose tolerance following injury have long been recognized[80] and gave rise to the term "diabetes of injury." Although insulin concentrations may be disproportionately low acutely following burn injury, they are normal or elevated following resuscitation.[81] In addition, the insulin response to a glucose challenge is not impaired.[82] Under basal conditions glucose disappearance is increased following burn injury.[83] This increased glucose "flow" is proportional to injury severity and returns toward control values during convalescence.

Several investigators have documented increased rates of hepatic (endogenous) glucose production following injury.[34,84,85] Both lactate and alanine can serve as precursors for endogenous glucose production.[86] The hepatic uptake of these substances is increased following burn injury.[34] Lactate release from the periphery is proportional to local injury severity and is closely related to glucose uptake.[32] Both lactate release and glucose uptake in the periphery correlate well with blood flow but not with oxygen consumption, suggesting that the heightened blood flow delivers glucose to healing tissue for glycolytic metabolism to lactate, a process that does not require oxygen.

Under fasting conditions patients recovering from moderate injury have elevations of both plasma glucose and serum insulin concentrations (Table 39–3). However, the elevations are disproportionate, suggesting an alteration in normal glucose and insulin

TABLE 39–3. Basal Glucose and Insulin Concentrations (Mean ± SEM)

Subjects	Plasma Glucose mg/dl	Serum Insulin μU/ml
Normals (N = 49)	98 ± 1	12 ± 1
Trauma patients (N = 19)	104 ± 2	17 ± 2
P	<0.02	<0.01

interactions. Black and associates[87] quantitated these alterations in seriously injured patients utilizing glucose and insulin clamp techniques. Insulin was administered at a constant infusion, so as to achieve a variety of steady-state insulin concentrations. During the infusion, euglycemia was maintained by a glucose infusion. At all doses studied and at comparable insulin concentrations, total body glucose disposal was lower in patients than in normal controls (Fig. 39–7). When fixed hyperglycemia was achieved, an exaggerated insulin response was observed in the patients, but glucose disposal was significantly depressed. These studies provided quantitative evidence of post-traumatic insulin resistance. Brooks and co-workers[88] determined glucose uptake by uninjured forearm muscle under conditions of hyperinsulinemia and euglycemia. Uptake was lower in patients than in controls, demonstrating that peripheral tissue, principally skeletal muscle and fat, is a major site of insulin resistance following injury.

INTEGRATED RESPONSE TO INJURY

The metabolic alterations discussed above occur simultaneously. The wound appears to play a dominant role. The wound utilizes glucose for energy and also requires other substrates for wound healing. Blood flow to the wound is increased to meet these heightened demands, especially to deliver glucose. Glucose is metabolized to lactate and released. This process does not require oxygen. The oxygen

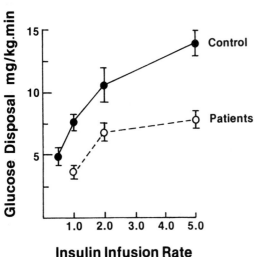

FIGURE 39–7. *Insulin-stimulated whole-body glucose disposal is lower in injured subjects than in controls. This insulin resistance cannot be reversed even at very high concentrations, indicating a post-receptor mechanism. (From Bessey PQ. Parenteral nutrition and trauma. In Rombeau JL, Caldwell MO (eds). Clinical Nutrition. Vol. 1. Philadelphia, WB Saunders, 1986. Adapted from Black PR, Brooks DC, Bessey PQ, et al. Ann Surg 1982; 196:420–435.)*

consumption of an injured extremity is not greater than that of an uninjured one.

The lactate is taken up by the liver and recycled to glucose. These processes require energy, which is presumably provided in part by fat oxidation,[89] and they contribute to the hypermetabolism observed. The liver also takes up alanine, which may be converted to new glucose, another energy-requiring process.

Uninjured skeletal muscle is a major source of alanine and other amino acids used for gluconeogenesis. Muscle protein breaks down at an accelerated rate. The amino acids are converted largely to alanine and glutamine and released into the circulation for transport to the liver. The carbon chain is converted to new glucose and the amino nitrogen to urea, which is excreted by the kidney. Glutamine may serve as a fuel for the energy metabolism of the gut,[90] in which it is converted to alanine. Also, glutamine may be transported to the kidney to serve as a buffer of increased acid excretion[91] associated with accelerated protein catabolism. Muscle does not take up glucose readily despite elevated insulin concentrations. Instead energy needs are met largely by fat oxidation.

The wound appears to have a principal, controlling role in this scheme (Fig. 39–8). The wound acts as a large arteriovenous shunt, robbing the host of blood supply. It also induces profound metabolic alterations. The host breaks down its own lean tissues, releasing amino acids which serve as precursors for acute-phase protein synthesis and wound repair and also as substrates for gluconeogenesis to support the wound's energy demands. The bigger the wound, the more intense is the metabolic response. As the wound heals, the heightened metabolic activity abates. Thus, burn wound closure is the single most important and definitive anticatabolic therapy.

REGULATION

The metabolic response to injury is graded and dose-dependent—it is proportional to the amount of tissue injured. How the wound or injury turns on the response and regulates it is largely unsettled. The classic studies of Hume and Egdahl[14] discussed above demonstrated the importance of neural afferent pathways in the initiation of systemic responses to injury. Thus, signals such as pain may initiate systemic responses early after injury—that is, during the ebb phase. However, the importance of neural afferent signals during the flow phase of the injury reponse is less clearly established. Wilmore and colleagues[92] applied lidocaine to burn wounds and made them anesthetic, but the patients remained hypermetabolic. A patient with quadriplegia who was burned did not demonstrate hypermetabolism until he developed an infection. Another patient with a major burn and brain death was not hypermetabolic. Dempsey,[93] Fried,[94] and co-workers

6 Carbon — 3 Carbon Flow — Catabolism of Injury

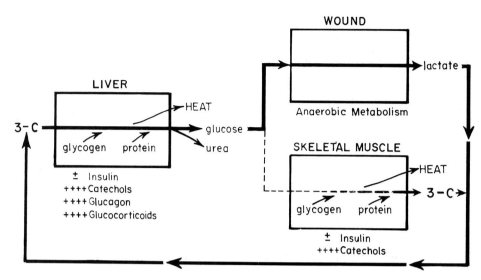

FIGURE 39–8. *The metabolic processes in the liver, wound, and skeletal muscle are closely interrelated following injury. (From Wilmore DW. The Metabolic Management of the Critically Ill. New York, Plenum Medical, 1977. Reproduced with permission.)*

studied patients with head injuries during barbiturate coma and found that metabolic rate and nitrogen excretion decreased toward predicted basal values during coma. It would appear that the central nervous system continues to have a regulatory role during the flow phase, but the mechanisms by which it communicates with the wound are not defined.

Several metabolically active humoral substances might also serve as afferent signals for the injury response. Prostaglandins, histamine, kinins, eicosanoids, and leukotrienes may be released from the burn wound and may have systemic as well as local effects. Endogenous pyrogen[95] and other leukocytic substances, now referred to as interleukin-1, are released by activated macrophages and may elicit fever and stimulate the synthesis of acute-phase proteins.[96]

Endotoxin has long been known to elicit many of the alterations observed in shock states.[97] Fish and Spitzer[98] have recently developed a model of chronic endotoxemia in rats. Compared with pair fed controls, the animals were hypermetabolic for several days.

The metabolic effects of local bacterial colonization of the burn wound were investigated by Aulick and co-workers[99] utilizing an animal model. Following a standard full-thickness burn, some wounds were seeded with gram-positive or gram-negative bacteria. A portion of these were treated with topical antimicrobial agents. Some animals developed invasive burn wound sepsis and bacteremia. The metabolic effects of infection appeared to parallel the severity of the local wound invasion and systemic infection. It is conceivable that endotoxin produced by the bacteria colonizing the burn wound is ab-

sorbed through the wound and contribute to the hypermetabolic response. Alternatively, endotoxin might be absorbed through gastrointestinal mucosa[100] rendered atrophic following injury and starvation.

The sympathoadrenal axis is one of the major effector limbs of the metabolic response to injury and serves as a link between the central nervous system and the endocrine organs. Many of the signs of shock represent autonomic overactivity. The catecholamines, particularly norepinephrine and epinephrine, are increased in proportion to the severity of injury.[21] In the flow phase the plasma concentrations of catecholamines may be persistently elevated.[55] Additionally, catechol turnover is markedly increased following burn injury.[101] Oxygen consumption[101] and metabolic rate[30] have been directly related to the urinary excretion of catecholamines. When alpha and beta blockade was achieved in burned patients, metabolic rate decreased significantly, although it did not return to control values.[30] This effect was not observed with alpha blockade alone. Porte and associates[22] have defined the influence of the sympathetic nervous system on the endocrine pancreas. The insulin response to glucose is reduced substantially with alpha stimulation, but it is enhanced with beta stimulation. Epinephrine infusion in low doses, having primarily beta effects, induced insulin resistance in uninjured forearm tissues.[23] However, amino acid release from skeletal muscle in vitro was reduced by epinephrine.[102]

Cortisol[25] and glucagon[103] are elevated following burn injury. The degree of elevation appears to be related to the extent of burn. Cortisol is known to be associated with glucose intolerance.[104] Patients with Cushing's syndrome have a reduced muscle mass and loss of protein from the skin. Owen and Cahill[105] administered hydrocortisone to starving obese patients and observed a decrease in urea excretion and an increase in ammonia excretion resulting in no net change in nitrogen loss. Glucagon promotes gluconeogenesis.[106] This effect may be overcome by increased concentrations of insulin.[107] Wolfe and colleagues[108] administered glucagon to fasting normal volunteers and observed a slight increase in nitrogen excretion primarily as urea. Net loss of nitrogen from peripheral tissue, however, did not increase.

Other hormones also appear to have a role in mediating the metabolic response to injury. Growth hormone is elevated following injury and in other "stress" states.[109] When administered exogenously, growth hormone may have an anabolic effect in burned patients.[110] Thyroid hormones may also be altered by injury,[111] but their role is unclear.[112]

Although alterations in the hormonal environment following injury have been well characterized, it has not been possible to ascribe all of the features of the injury response to the known actions of the individual hormones. Various "toxic factors" have been proposed to account for the catabolic response following injury. Baracos and co-workers[113] demonstrated that interleukin-1 induces in vitro skeletal muscle proteolysis via prostaglandin E_2 formation. Clowes and associates[114] have identified a polypeptide from the serum of septic patients that can also induce in vitro skeletal muscle proteolysis. It has been postulated that this may be a fragment of interleukin-1.[115] Tumor necrosis factor and cachectin[116] are other substances elaborated in inflammatory cells that are of current interest. At this time, the importance of these or other lymphokines in the catabolic response to injury is unclear.

Watters and colleagues[117] administered etiocholanolone, a steroidal agent known to stimulate interleukin-1 production, to normal volunteers. Although all of the subjects developed fever, leukocytosis, hypoferremia, and increased concentrations of acute phase proteins, they were not hypermetabolic and they remained in nitrogen equilibrium when fed a normally weight-maintaining diet. In contrast, Bessey and co-workers[118] measured the metabolic responses in normal subjects receiving a constant infusion of hydrocortisone, glucagon, and epinephrine for 3 days. The results were compared with paired measurements in the same subjects during a control saline infusion. The triple hormone infusion increased the concentrations of cortisol, glucagon, and epinephrine to levels observed in patients with mild-to-moderate injury. With that alteration in the hormonal environment, hypermetabolism, negative nitrogen and potassium balances, increased endogenous glucose production, insulin resistance, sodium retention, and leukocytosis were

observed. These changes occurred in the absence of a wound or other inflammatory focus. Unlike the subjects receiving etiocholanolone, those receiving the triple hormone infusion had little elevation in temperature and no decrease in serum iron or increase in C-reactive protein. However, when both etiocholanolone and the triple hormone infusion were administered, a combined response was observed[119] reflecting both additive and interactive effects.

The role of the hormonal environment in mediating accelerated post-traumatic skeletal muscle proteolysis was also investigated.[120] Following 3 days of the triple hormone infusion, intracellular skeletal muscle amino acid nitrogen was decreased, owing primarily to a fall in the glutamine concentration. Whole-blood amino acid concentration and forearm amino acid efflux were little affected. Thus, alteration of the hormonal environment by the triple hormone infusion was not a sufficient stimulus to induce all of the changes in skeletal muscle proteolysis observed following injury and critical illness. However, alteration of the endocrine environment following injury has modulated the protein catabolic response. For example, Hulton and associates[121] monitored hindleg amino acid efflux following abdominal operation in an animal model. The accelerated efflux of skeletal muscle amino acids observed postoperatively was greatly attenuated by administration of agents that achieved complete alpha and beta adrenergic blockade or by use of thoracic epidural anesthesia. Brandt and colleagues[122] have measured hormonal and protein catabolic responses following abdominal hysterectomy in patients receiving either general or high epidural anesthesia. Concentrations of cortisol and catecholamines were lower and nitrogen loss was attenuated in patients with epidural anesthesia compared with those with general anesthesia alone. Tsuji and associates[123] have reported similar findings. Thus, it appears that the post-traumatic hormonal environment is necessary but not entirely responsible for accelerated protein catabolism following injury.

The metabolic response to injury that is observed clinically appears to be the result of a variety of interacting and possibly synergistic influences. The central nervous system would appear to play a major coordinating role. Although the basis of the response may be the simultaneous elaboration of several hormones, other factors probably play a role also. Interleukin-1 and/or other lymphokines may affect temperature set point via prostaglandin synthesis in the CNS and also stimulate the other components of the "acute phase response." Acidosis or hypoxia if prolonged may lead to catabolic responses.[124] The contribution of the autolysis of injured tissue and hematoma and of disuse to the overall clinical response also remains to be defined.

METABOLIC SUPPORT OF THE BURNED PATIENT

Early Care

PRIORITIES OF MANAGEMENT

The immediate management of a patient with burn injury is the same as it would be for any other acutely injured or critically ill patient.[125] First priority is given to the detection and treatment of conditions that might be immediately life-threatening. Thus, the airway must be secured, effective ventilation achieved, and access to the circulation established—the "A-B-C's." The common objective of these early resuscitative measures is to assure adequate cellular oxygenation. Of all the constituents delivered to the microcirculation, oxygen is the most acutely limiting. A compromised airway, ineffective ventilation and oxygenation, or inadequate tissue perfusion will result in cellular hypoxia. If that persists, cellular dysfunction and cell death may ensue.

The airway may be compromised early because of the effects of inhalation injury. Upper airway obstruction may occur suddenly owing to edema, if there are burns of the oropharynx. Inhalation of toxic fumes may result in necrosis and sloughing of the bronchial mucosa with airway obstruction, or in extensive atelectasis and a resultant ventilation-perfusion abnormality. Patients with facial burns, singed nasal vibrissae, carbonaceous sputum, intra-oral or pharyngeal burns, or a history of being burned in a closed space are commonly presumed to have inhalation injury and are intubated early. High-flow oxygen is instituted to reduce the concentration of carboxyhemoglobin. Positive-pressure ventilation may be required to achieve adequate gas exchange.

FLUID RESUSCITATION OF BURN SHOCK

Large bore IV's are placed for the rapid administration of fluid and treatment of burn shock. Sodium-containing fluids and colloid are administered in amounts based on burn size. Cope and Moore[12] described a fluid management program in 1947 that was based on burn size and that became a prototype for all subsequent regimens. In addition they emphasized that the formulas provided only estimates of fluid requirements which should be adjusted upward or downward based on the patient's response.

Several formulas for the treatment of burn shock have been proposed since Cope and Moore's report[13,126–130] (Table 39–4). They are all effective. They differ in the amounts and the timing of the administration of crystalloid and colloid solutions. Several studies[131–133] have indicated that capillary permeability to colloidal sized particles is increased not only in the region of the burn but throughout the microcirculation. Thus, it has been argued that

colloid offers no advantage over crystalloid solutions in resuscitation during the first 24 hours post burn. However, Demling and associates[134] have reported that edema in *nonburned* tissue following burn of a 25 to 30 per cent of body surface area (BSA) in an animal model is due mainly to hypoproteinemia and not altered permeability. After 8 hours post burn it was possible to restore colloid osmotic pressure, thus reducing the volume needed for resuscitation.[135] Although some centers advocate the use of colloid in the first 24 hours of fluid resuscitation,[136] the issue remains controversial. A randomized clinical trial[137] demonstrated that resuscitation with electrolyte solution and colloid resulted in no long-lasting hemodynamic benefit compared with resuscitation with electrolyte solution alone. Furthermore, lung water gradually increased over a 7-day period in the patients resuscitated with the colloid regimen.

One commonly utilized formula is that recommended at an NIH Consensus Development Conference on the management of acute burn injuries.[130] It is simple, effective, and relatively inexpensive. Fluid requirements for the first 24 hours are estimated at 2 to 4 ml of lactated Ringer's solution per kilogram of body weight for each 1 per cent of BSA burned. One half of this volume is administered in the first 8 hours. The second half is administered over the next 16 hours. From 24 to 32 hours after the burn 0.3 to 0.5 ml of plasma or other colloid per kilogram is given for each 1 per cent BSA burn, and enough 5 per cent dextrose solution is given to maintain urine output without lowering serum sodium concentration excessively.

EXAMPLE. A 25-year-old truck driver lit a match to check the level of gasoline in his tank. He sustained 40 per cent BSA burns. His pre-burn weight was 80 kg and his height 74 inches (BSA = 2.06 m²). Estimate his fluid requirements for the first 48 hours post burn.

1. First 24 hours 2–4 ml/kg/%BSA × 80 kg × 40% burn = 6,400–12,800 ml lactated Ringer's
   Administer lactated Ringer's at 400–800 ml/hr for the first 8 hr post burn. Then administer fluid at 200–400 ml/hr for the next 16 hr (8–24 hr post burn).

2. Second 24 hours 0.3–0.5 ml/kg/%BSA × 80 × 40% burn = 960–1600 ml plasma.
   Administer over first 8 hr. Administer 5% dextrose in sufficient quantities to maintain urine flow of 30–50 ml/hr without lowering serum sodium concentration to <135 mEq/L.

The volumes of fluid calculated by this or any other formula are only estimates of the volumes required to maintain effective tissue perfusion. The response to therapy must be monitored closely. The

TABLE 39–4. Burn Fluid Resuscitation Regimens for the First 48 Hours Post Burn

Formula and Author	First 24 Hours		Second 24 Hours	
	Fluid	Amount	Fluid	Amount
Surface area formula	Plasma*	75 ml/% BSA burn	Plasma	37.5 mg/% BSA burn
Cope and Moore (1947)[12]	NS*	75 ml/% BSA burn	NS	37.5 ml/% BSA burn
Evans formula	Colloid*	1 ml/kg/% BSA burn	Colloid	0.5 ml/kg/% BSA burn
(50% BSA burn upper limit)	NS*	1 ml/kg/% BSA burn	NS	0.5 ml/kg/% BSA burn
Evans et al. (1952)[126]	D₅W	2000 ml	D₅W	2000 ml
Brooke Formula	Colloid*	0.5 ml/kg/% BSA burn	Colloid	0.25 ml/kg/% BSA burn
(50% BSA burn upper limit)	NS*	1 ml/kg/% BSA burn	NS	0.5 ml/kg/% BSA burn
Reiss et al. (1953)[127]	D₅W*	2000 ml	D₅W	1500–5000 ml
Hypertonic sodium solution (HSS)	HSS†	Maintain urine output—30 ml/hr	HSS	Maintain urine output 30 ml/hr
Monafo (1973)[129]	D₅W†	Maintain serum Na<165	D₅W	Maintain serum Na<165
			Oral fluid	Up to 3500 ml
Parkland formula	RL*	4 ml/kg/% BSA burn	Colloid	10–30 ml/kg
Baxter (1974)[14]			D₅W	2000 ml
Consensus formula	RL*	2.4 ml/kg/% BSA burn	Colloid	0.3 = 0.5 ml/kg/% BSA burn
Schwartz et al. (1979)[130]			D₅W	Maintain urine output and serum Na

BSA, body surface area; NS, 0.9% sodium chloride (Na = 154 mEq/L); Colloid, plasma, plasmanate, 5% albumin, hydroxyethyl starch, dextran; D₅W, 5% dextrose in water; HSS, sodium chloride and lactate (Na = 250 mEq/L); RL, lactated Ringer's solution (Na = 103 mEq/L).

*One half in first 8 hours.
†Two thirds in first 12 hours.

urine output is the most sensitive parameter. A urine flow of 30 to 50 ml/hr in adults or 0.7 to 1.0 ml/kg/hr in children usually indicates adequate perfusion. In that case the blood pressure is usually normal and there is a mild tachycardia. The central venous pressure is almost always low during the first 24 hours and is not a particularly useful parameter for judging the adequacy of early resuscitation. With adequate resuscitation there is usually only a moderate degree of metabolic acidosis and hemoconcentration.

If there has been significant inhalation injury, the lower limits of urine flow are usually selected as clinical goals in the hope that the rate of formation of lung edema will be minimized, should it occur. In the case of electrical injury, the fluid requirement will usually be significantly greater than that estimated from the surface burns alone, because of deep tissue injury. If myoglobinuria is present, fluid administration should be increased to achieve a urine output of 100 ml/hr to prevent tubular obstruction. If the urine does not clear readily, mannitol should be administered concurrently.

Clearly, the appropriate therapy for shock following burn injury is intravascular volume replacement. However, because of the loss of osmotic forces, volume replacement leads to an increase in edema formation. Pruitt and colleagues[138] measured plasma volume in patients with major burns (average 64 per cent of BSA) during resuscitation from burn shock, and calculated the rate of volume loss from the plasma compartment. Regression analysis of fluid loss on fluid administration showed that plasma volume was maintained or increased only if the rate of fluid administration was equal to or greater than 4.4 ml/kg/hr. Not surprisingly, volume resuscitation may nearly double a patient's extracellular fluid volume. Edema may be massive.

ELECTROLYTE BALANCE

Fluid resuscitation expands the extracellualr fluid compartment. If the resuscitation fluid is a balanced, "physiologic" salt solution, such as lactated Ringer's, electrolyte abnormalities are not commonly observed. Such solutions are slightly hypotonic with respect to sodium (130 mEq/L) and also contain potassium (4 mEq/L). The use of isotonic saline (0.9 per cent NaCl—154 mEq/L) for resuscitation may result in hyperchloremia and compound the metabolic acidosis associated with shock and inadequate tissue perfusion.[139]

Because of the apparent dominant importance of the sodium ion in resuscitation, Monafo and coworkers[129] used hypertonic sodium solutions (250 mEq/L) for burn shock therapy. They were able to reduce the total fluid volume required and consequent edema. The results with this approach were similar to those utilizing other formulas, but dangerous hypernatremia (serum Na > 165 mEq/L) was occasionally observed. Hypernatremia may also occur if large amounts of sodium bicarbonate have been administered to treat metabolic acidosis.

NUTRITIONAL SUPPORT

Nutritional support is not a major component of the early management of a patient with acute burn injury. Hyperglycemia is usually observed and glucose tolerance is markedly reduced, in part because of suppression of the pancreatic beta cell.[22] In addition, free fatty acid concentrations are elevated early after burn injury and may then compete with glucose for entry into the cell.[24] Energy substrate is not limited. The risk of reduced perfusion of the microcirculation is a critical reduction in oxygen delivery, leading to cellular hypoxia and ultimately to cell death. The best metabolic support is aggressive treatment of burn shock and support of cardiovascular performance.

Following a major burn intestinal motility is commonly impaired for several days, and nasogastric suction is routinely instituted. Intravenous nutrition is not usually provided during this early period when organ system function is so unstable. However, following resuscitation the administration of intravenous nutrients may be started. In his classic "life raft" studies Gamble[140] demonstrated that the daily urinary nitrogen loss could be reduced by simply providing up to 100 g of glucose. Glucose-containing solutions are begun during the second 24 hours post burn. McDougal and associates[141] further demonstrated that isotonic amino acids would reduce net nitrogen loss to the same degree as an isocaloric amount of glucose and that the two effects were additive. Thus, early after burn injury, when fluid requirements are often still high, peripheral vein feedings may be helpful in reducing net nitrogen loss until the gastrointestinal tract is functional again.

Support of the Hypermetabolic Patient

With successful resuscitation and restoration of circulating blood volume, the patient moves into the next phase of the injury response, the "flow" phase. This phase begins about 48 hours after injury and extends until wound closure occurs. Partial-thickness burns may heal spontaneously within 7 to 14 days. Full-thickness burns usually require skin grafting. Management of the patient during the flow phase is directed both toward care of the wound and toward care of the patient with a wound. Once the wound is closed, the intense metabolic activity of the flow phase subsides and the patient moves into a phase of gradual weight gain and restoration of lean tissue. Thus, expeditious closure of the wound is a primary goal in overall patient management.

Metabolic support of the hypermetabolic burned patient includes fluid and electrolyte management to maintain the volume and composition of the extracellular fluid, administration of red cells to maintain the oxygen carrying capacity of the blood, and adequate ventilation and gas exchange. Under these conditions tissue blood flow and oxygen delivery are not limited as they are during the ebb of burn shock. Metabolic alterations appear directed to providing sufficient energy and protein substrate for the healing wound. However, without provision of exogenous substrate the patient's energy stores and lean tissues may become depleted. The patient appears to "run out of gas" as sepsis and multiple system organ failure supervene, often leading to death. Thus, appropriate nutritional support in an effort to minimize the draft on body protein and energy stores is a major component of support of the patient with a healing burn wound.

FLUID REQUIREMENTS

Burn injury destroys the lipoprotein components of the skin. Associated with this biochemical disruption there is loss of the water vapor pressure barrier. The surface vapor pressure of normal skin is approximately 2 to 3 mm Hg. This increases to 25 to 35 mm Hg following a full-thickness burn injury.[142] This is similar to the vapor pressure of an open pan of water under identical environmental conditions of temperature and humidity. Thus, there is a marked increase in evaporative water loss following a burn. This component of insensible fluid loss is directly related to the extent of injury.[143] Ambient temperature affects surface temperature and also influences evaporative water loss. Evaporative loss increases as the hypermetabolic response peaks 7 to 10 days following injury and subsides as the wounds are re-epithelialized. The pulmonary component of insensible loss is usually less than 10 per cent of the total unless the patient is particularly febrile and hyperventilating. A satisfactory formula for estimating the volume of insensible water loss of patients with open wounds is:[143,144]

Insensible loss (ml/hr)

$$= (25 + \%\text{BSA burn}) \times \text{BSA (m}^2)$$

If the wounds are covered with dressings and creams that are not permeable to water, the water loss will be reduced. However, insensible water loss may be markedly increased in the patient cared for on an air-fluidized bed because of increased convection.

Following resuscitation the thermally injured patient requires fluid therapy to replace urinary and insensible losses. With the increased rate of tissue breakdown there is a marked osmotic load which may promote a high-volume urinary output even in the face of clinical dehydration. Because of the large sodium load administered during resuscitation, hypotonic or sodium-free fluids may be utilized to replace these losses.

EXAMPLE—CONTINUED. Calculate the water requirements of the patient described above.

3. Determine evaporative loss:
   Insensible loss (ml/hr)
   $$= (25 + 40) \times 2.06 \text{ m}^2$$
   $$= 134 \text{ ml/hr}$$
   $$= 3,216 \text{ ml/day}$$

4. Replace evaporative loss and urinary loss (1500 ml/day):
   Fluid requirements (ml/day)
   $$= 3216 + 1500$$
   $$= 4716 \text{ ml/day}$$
   $$= 197 \text{ ml/hr}$$

The serum sodium concentration is the most valuable guide for judging the adequacy of hydration in the burned patient. A value between 132 and 138 mEq/L usually indicates an adequate state of hydration. If serum Na rises, free water should be administered; if serum Na falls, free water should be restricted. The urine volume is an unreliable guide for assessing the adequacy of fluid therapy after the first 48 hours post burn because of the osmotic load delivered to the kidneys. Volume status may best be judged by clinical parameters (blood pressure, heart rate, and central pressures) in addition to careful maintenance of fluid intake and output records and daily body weight determinations (under the same conditions with dressings and splints removed).

In addition to water replacement, other extrarenal losses of fluid, such as nasogastric suction or diarrhea, should be replaced appropriately. Plasma may be administered to maintain colloid osmotic pressure. Finally, red blood cells may be required to maintain a hematocrit of 30 to 35 per cent or more, so as to assure adequate oxygen carrying capacity.

ELECTROLYTE REQUIREMENTS

Although sodium is conserved following injury, potassium losses are markedly increased,[145] in part as a result of renal mechanisms in which potassium is exchanged for sodium in the distal tubule. Because the extracellular potassium concentration is usually maintained within a narrow range, it may not be abnormal despite a marked deficit of total body potassium. The extracellular concentration is maintained by exchange of intracellular potassium for hydrogen ion. Thus, depletion of total body potassium is commonly associated with a metabolic alkalosis. Not uncommonly this is compounded by the loss of acid and chloride ion from the gastrointestinal tract. Burned patients may excrete as much as 150 to 300 mEq of potassium daily in the urine. This loss may be exacerbated if mafenide acetate (Sulfamylon), a carbonic anhydrase inhibitor, is used for topical antimicrobial therapy. Thus, 30 to 40 mEq of potassium chloride is usually added to each liter of intravenous fluid administered after the first 24 hours post burn.

Other electrolyte abnormalities may also occur following burn injury. Urinary excretion of magnesium is commonly increased in conjunction with osmotic diuresis.[146] In critically ill patients, magnesium excretion appears to be related to total nitrogen excretion as well as to intake.[147] Hypomagnesemia may interfere with the correction of metabolic alkalosis with potassium chloride replacement.[148] It may be necessary to provide calcium, phosphorus, zinc, and other trace metals, especially during nutritional support. Therapy should be guided by regular determinations of electrolyte concentration.

NUTRITIONAL SUPPORT

Goals. Hypermetabolism and increased protein catabolism result in an accelerated loss of lean body tissues. The consequences of acute lean tissue loss depend on its extent. If subjects of normal body composition lose less than 10 per cent of their body weight, little disability is observed.[149] An acute loss of 40 per cent of body weight is usually fatal.[150] Loss of between 10 and 40 per cent of weight is associated with increased debility and risk of morbidity and mortality.[151] Therefore a primary goal of nutritional support following burn injury is to limit weight loss during convalescence to less than 10 per cent of pre-burn weight.[152] For obese patients the goal would be to limit net weight loss to less than 10 per cent of ideal body weight.

In Benedict's classic study of starvation,[153] his subject lost 10 per cent of his body weight in 11 days. During the same time his metabolic rate *decreased* about 10 per cent also. Burned patients are hypermetabolic, and if totally starved could lose 10 per cent of their pre-burn lean weight in approximately 5 to 6 days. Patients invariably have a brief period of starvation immediately following a burn, but some nutritional support may be instituted safely within 24 ot 48 hours post burn.[141] Although hypocaloric feedings may slow the rate of net catabolism, the operational goal of nutritional support in burned patients is nutritional maintenance or balance.

Estimating Nutritional Requirements. To achieve nutritional maintenance, energy and nitrogen substrate (calories and protein) should be provided in amounts equivalent to the caloric requirements (energy expenditure or heat loss) and to the nitrogen losses of the patient. Post-burn hypermetabolism is a graded response—its intensity is a function of the severity of injury. Thus, total energy requirements may be estimated based on age, sex, body size, and severity of burn injury.

TABLE 39–5. Standard Metabolic Rates Under Basal Conditions

Age (Years)	Metabolic Rates (kcal/m²/hr)	
	Women	Men
1	53.0	53.0
5	48.4	49.3
10	42.5	44.0
15	37.9	41.8
20	35.3	38.6
25	35.2	37.5
30	35.1	36.8
35	35.0	36.5
40	34.9	36.3
45	34.5	36.2
50	33.9	35.8
55	33.3	35.4
60	32.7	34.9
65	32.2	34.4
70	31.7	33.8
75	31.3	33.2
80	30.9	33.0

Adapted from Fleisch A. *Helv Med Acta* 1951; *18*:23–44.

TABLE 39–6. Estimates of Daily Calorie Requirements for Burned Patients

Harris & Benedict[156]
  Men
    BMR (kcal/day) $= 66 + [13.7 \times weight (kg)] + [5 \times height (cm)] - [6.8 \times age (yrs)]$
  Women
    BMR (kcal/day) $= 665 + [9.6 \times weight (kg)] + [1.7 \times height (cm)] - [4.7 \times age (yrs)]$
    Requirements (kcal/day) $= BMR (kcal/day) \times [0.6637 \times (\% BSA burn)^{0.2717}] \times 1.25$
Curreri[158]
    Requirements (kcal/day) $= [25 \times weight (kg)] \times [40 \times \% BSA burn]$
McLaurin, Mason, et al.—USAISR[157]
    BMR (kcal/m²/hr)* $= 54.33782 - 1.19961 \times (age) (yrs) + 0.02548 \times (age)^2 - 0.00018 (age)^3$
    Requirements (kcal/day) $= BMR (kcal/m^2/hr) \times [2.33764 - 1.33764\ EXP\ (-0.0286 \times \% BSA\ burn)] \times BSA\ (m^2) \times 24$ (hr/day) $\times 1.25$.

*This value should be reduced 7 to 10% for women.

Several acceptable standards of basal metabolic rate are available. The standards of Fleisch[154] are based on an analysis of 24 published sets of "normal" values (Table 39–5). For a patient with a burn, the metabolic rate under basal conditions will be greater than predicted in proportion to injury severity. Figure 39–3 depicts the percentage increase in metabolic activity associated with burns of varying size. A "stress factor" may be determined and used to multiply the basal rate. After multiplying this value by body surface area (based on pre-burn height and ideal weight) and by 24 hours, an additional 20 to 25 per cent should be added to account for minimal hospital activity and the specific dynamic action (SDA) of feeding.[155] The resulting value is the estimated total daily caloric requirement.

This method of estimating energy requirements was proposed by Wilmore[155] and has been reliably used for nutritional assessment in a wide variety of critically ill patients. Another commonly employed technique is based on the equations of Harris and Benedict.[156] These provide estimates of basal metabolic activity and can be adjusted upward based on burn size[157] (Table 39–6). The formula proposed by Curreri and associates[158] is simpler than the others and is widely used for nutritional assessment in burned patients. McLaurin and co-workers[157] derived an exponential equation based on careful measurements of metabolic rates under basal conditions of a large number of burned men studied in an environmental chamber. This equation may be useful for clinicians who have access to a programmable calculator or computer.

The availability of portable metabolic carts with equipment that can measure oxygen consumption and carbon dioxide production of both spontaneously breathing and mechanically ventilated patients has led to the use of indirect calorimetry in the nutritional assessment of critically ill patients.[159,160] The measurements are usually made at a discrete time and must be adjusted to reflect 24-hour energy expenditure. The equation on page 675 may be used to calculate daily energy requirements. No "stress factor" would be required. If the patient were eating or receiving nutritional support during the measurement, an additional 5 to 10 per cent should be added to account for minimal hospital activity.[161] If there were no nutritional support, a factor of 1.2 to 1.25 should be used to account for the metabolic effects of nutrient processing and minimal activity. Estimates made using one of the empiric formulas or those based on gas exchange measurements are good guidelines for determining early nutritional goals. However, the efficacy of nutritional support should be monitored and the nutrient intake modified as appropriate (see below) throughout the post-burn course.

EXAMPLE—CONTINUED. Estimate the nutritional requirements of the patient described above (height 74 inches, weight 80 kg, BSA 2.06 m²).

5. The standard metabolic rate for a 25-year-old man is 37.5 kcal/m²/hr.

6. A 40 per cent body surface area burn would be expected to increase metabolic rate approximately 85 to 90 per cent. Thus, the "stress factor" for this patient would be 1.9, and his metabolic rate under basal conditions would be estimated to be 71.3 kcal/m²/hr.

7. His total basal caloric requirements would be 71.3 kcal/m²/hr $\times$ 2.06 m² $\times$ 24 hr/day = 3525 kcal/day.

8. This basal requirement should be increased 20 to 25 per cent:
Total caloric requirements $= 3525$ kcal/day $\times 1.25$
$= 4406$ kcal/day.

Protein (Amino Acid) Requirements. Duke and co-workers[162] demonstrated that 15 to 20 per cent of the daily energy expenditure is derived from protein. Thus, 15 to 20 per cent of the total caloric requirement should be provided as protein. The amount of protein would represent a nonprotein calorie to nitrogen ratio of 142:1 to 100:1.

EXAMPLE—CONTINUED

9. Of the total kcal required, 15 to 20 per cent should be provided as protein:
Protein calories $= 4400$ kcal/day $\times 0.17$
$= 740$ kcal/day

10. The caloric equivalent of protein is 4 kcal/g:
Protein requirement $= 749/4$
$= 187$ g

Non-protein Calories. Both carbohydrate and fat may be utilized as nonprotein energy sources. Glucose alone both in simple starvation[140] and following burn injury[141] has a pronounced protein-sparing effect. Long and associates[163] administered glucose and fat in a variety of combinations to burn patients receiving a fixed amount of protein. Glucose was much more effective than fat in reducing nitrogen excretion when provided in amounts less than the caloric requirement. Additional energy provided as fat or carbohydrate in excess of requirements did not further reduce nitrogen excretion. The nitrogen-sparing effect of carbohydrate was most pronounced with loads that provided less than about 60 per cent of the total caloric intake. Wolfe and colleagues[164] measured glucose oxidation in postoperative patients given different doses of dextrose intravenously. Following operation the infused glucose was oxidized when given in doses up to 7 mEq/kg/min. With larger doses lactate production increased, indicating increased rates of futile cycling. In companion studies[85,165] in burn patients, limitations in both glucose clearance and glucose oxidation were observed at glucose infusion rates as low as 4 mg/kg min. Black and co-workers[87] produced sustained constant hyperglycemia in controls and in nonseptic trauma patients. Whole-body glucose disposal increased steadily during the period of fixed hyperglycemia in the control studies (Fig. 39–9). This was associated with a steady increase in peripheral insulin concentration. When given a similar hyperglycemic challange, injured patients demonstrated an insulin response that was greater than that of controls. However, they were limited in their ability to dispose glucose. They quickly attained a maximum rate of glucose disposal which was independent of peripheral insulin concentration. This value, 6 to 7 mg/g/min, was similar to the level of maximum glucose oxidation determined by Wolfe.[85,164,165] In addition, this upper limit of disposal represented about 60 per cent of the patients' estimated caloric requirements, a value similar to the findings of Long and associates.[163]

When glucose was given to critically ill patients in amounts greater than estimated maintenance requirements, Askanazi and colleagues[166] found that metabolic demands and catecholamine excretion increased. Overfeeding appeared to be an additional stress for these patients. In addition, overfeeding resulted in increased ventilatory requirements.[167] Sheldon and associates[168] found that high glucose loads in patients receiving total parenteral nutrition were associated with bile stasis and liver dysfunction.

In summary, glucose has a marked beneficial effect on nitrogen economy following injury. However, there appears to be a limit to the effective utilization of carbohydrate as an energy source. When glucose composes more than 60 to 70 per cent of the total caloric requirement of a critically ill patient, it may

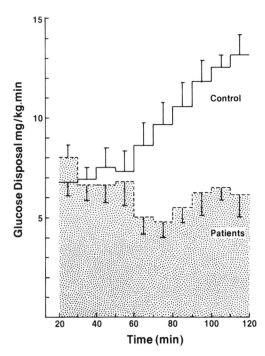

FIGURE 39–9. *Fixed hyperglycemia leads to increasing glucose disposal in normal subjects. Under the same conditions, injured patients appear to reach a maximum disposal rate despite high concentrations of insulin. (From Bessey PQ. Parenteral nutrition and trauma. In Rombeau JL, Caldwell MD (eds). Clinical Nutrition. Vol. 1. Philadelphia, WB Saunders, 1986. Adapted from Black PR, Brooks DC, Bessey PQ. Ann Surg 1982; 196:420–435.)*

exceed this limit and may lead to hyperglycemia and organ system dysfunction.

EXAMPLE—CONTINUED

11. 50 to 70 per cent of total calories should be provided as carbohydrate:
    Carbohydrate calories = 0.6×4406 kcal/day
    = 2644 kcal/day
12. The caloric equivalent of oral or enteral carbohydrate is 4 kcal/g. Intravenous dextrose is a monohydrate of glucose; its caloric equivalent is 3.4 kcal/g. Thus:
    Oral or enteral carbohydrate = 2644/4
    = 661 g/day;
    Intravenous glucose = 2644/3.4
    = 778 g/day.

The remaining total caloric requirement may be provided as carbohydrate or fat. Additional carbohydrate may be provided, but this will often be associated with hyperglycemia requiring exogenous insulin for control. Black and co-workers[87] were able to increase glucose disposal in euglycemic injured patients to a maximum of 9 to 10 mg/kg/min by infusing large doses of insulin. However, this may still be insufficient to meet the increased energy requirements of the burned patient.

Fat constitutes 40 to 50 per cent of calories in the normal North American diet and is a major caloric source in many of the commonly used enteral nutritional products. Lipid emulsions for intravenous administration are available for clinical use. Nordenstrom and co-workers[169] supported injured patients with parenteral nutrition in which glucose and fat composed roughly equal proportions of the total caloric load. The lipid emulsion was utilized as an energy source, but oxidation did not correlate with plasma clearance. Goodenough and Wolfe[170] provided 30 per cent of total calories to burned patients as fat and studied free fatty acid (FFA) and energy metabolism. Oxidation of lipid accounted for about 25 per cent of the energy expenditure, but most of the lipid oxidized appeared to come from endogenous stores. It was suggested that exogenous intravenous lipid is not directly utilized as an energy source, but rather serves to maintain endogenous fat stores. In the past the use of lipid emulsions has been associated with a variety of complications. However, with current products the incidence of these complications should be exceedingly rare,[171] especially if the infusion is administered slowly over 8 to 24 hours.

Feeding the Burned Patient

The goal of nutritional maintenance is achievable in virtually all patients utilizing readily available techniques and products. Once maintenance nutritional requirements have been estimated, a plan of nutritional support should be formulated for each patient. The quantity, composition, and type of nutritional support will vary from patient to patient depending on several individual factors, such as burn size, gastrointestinal function, glucose tolerance, fluid allowances, concurrent illness, and motivation. If the patient can and will eat, nutritional requirements may be met by a high-protein, high-calorie diet alone or in combination with enriched milkshakes or commercial supplements. Often the patient is unable to consume sufficient calories and protein to meet the heightened metabolic demands of the healing burn injury, particularly if the burn is large. In that case exogenous nutritional support must be provided as either enteral or parenteral feedings.

Enteral Feedings

If the gastrointestinal tract is functional, enteral feedings should provide as much of the total nutritional requirements as possible. The enteral route has several theoretical and practical advantages over the intravenous route.[100,172,173] It avoids a central venous line and its risks, and it is less costly. The absorption of nutrients by the portal system and delivery to the liver may support splanchnic metabolism better than intravenous feedings. In addition it may protect the mucosal barrier and lead

to a reduction of the intensity of the injury response.[100] Gastrointestinal motility is often reduced early after burn injury, but usually returns within 2 to 4 days. Occasionally the ileus will persist for several days, or will develop later in the post-burn course. This is often associated with organ system failure or sepsis.

Enteral feedings are commonly delivered through a soft, flexible, small-caliber (8 French) Silastic feeding tube. These tubes are weighted with tungsten. They are relatively easy to pass nasally into the stomach and are well tolerated. Occasionally the tube may curl up in the esophagus, or if the patient is obtunded, it may pass into the trachea. Thus, confirmation of proper tube position is required either by the return of gastric contents in a fully alert patient or by a chest or abdominal x-ray. The enteral formula is infused continuously at a slow rate. The gastric contents should be aspirated periodically to assure that gastric stasis has not developed and that the formula is not pooling in the stomach. The infusion rate should be increased slowly over 36 to 72 hours until full nutritional requirements are provided. If the infusion rate is increased rapidly, it may lead to nausea and vomiting or diarrhea. The tube may be placed in the duodenum to reduce the likelihood of vomiting and aspiration. In some cases gastric decompression can be maintained while duodenal feedings are administered.

A wide and ever-growing selection of enteral feeding preparations is available. These products differ in nutrient and electrolyte composition, caloric density, osmolality, and palatability. In addition, modular components are available. These may be utilized to compound a unique mixture of nutrients or to alter the composition of a standard formulation to meet specific patient requirements. The costs of these enteral products vary widely and may be further influenced by contractual agreements between the hospital or burn center and the manufacturers. The clinician should become familiar with the products available at his or her institution and their respective costs, so that he or she may provide appropriate enteral nutritional support in a cost-effective manner.

The burned patient has increased requirements for calories, nitrogen, and other nutrients as well as for fluids. In the metabolic management of a patient with a burn, these may be considered jointly or separately. Formulas with a caloric density of 1.5 to 2 kcal/ml will deliver the same nutrients in a smaller enteral fluid volume than more dilute formulas. However, in most cases the burned patient would require extra water provided intravenously, enterally, or by spontaneous oral intake. Supplementary vitamins and minerals are usually provided. These may be taken orally or administered via the feeding tube.

EXAMPLE—CONTINUED. On the morning of post-burn day 3, the patient's abdomen is soft and the bowel sounds are active. He reports passage of flatus. Formulate a plan for the nutritional management of the patient described above.

13. There is evidence of effective gastrointestinal function. Nutritional support may be started using the gastrointestinal tract. It is tempting to remove the nasogastric tube, begin liquids, and advance the diet as tolerated as one would for a patient following an elective operation. For some patients this would be appropriate. However, many patients, especially those with large burns or burns of the hands or face, will be unable to meet their nutritional requirements spontaneously for quite some time. If spontaneous oral intake is tried, the clinician should monitor nutrient intake closely and at the outset specify the conditions under which he would begin exogenous nutritional support so as to prevent excessive lean tissue erosion.

14. Alternatively, one could assume that the patient will be unable to meet his full nutritional requirements by spontaneous intake within an acceptable time period. One could then begin oral intake and enteral feedings simultaneously. For patients with extensive injuries or other conditions that could interfere with gastrointestinal tract motility, it is sometimes useful to begin enteral feedings utilizing the nasogastric tube that is already in place. It is more effective in aspirating the gastric contents than a small-bore feeding tube, and it will allow the clinician to watch for the development of gastric stasis more closely.

15. The enteral formula should be started slowly (20 to 30 ml/hr). If gastric residuals remain low, the infusion rate may be gradually increased over the next 48 to 72 hours until full nutritional requirements are met. The infusion is usually begun with an isotonic formula (1 kcal/ml). After this has been tolerated for 24 to 36 hours, a formula of higher caloric density or a special formulation may be used and increased to meet full nutritional requirements. However, if the volumes can be tolerated, the isotonic mixtures will provide a greater proportion of water than the more concentrated formulas. Isotonic preparations are available that provide between 14 and 17 per cent of the calories as protein. Approximately 4 liters of an isotonic formula would be required to meet this patient's needs. Alternatively his needs could be met with approximately 2 liters of a 2 kcal/ml formula, but extra water might also be required.

INTRAVENOUS FEEDINGS

If the gastrointestinal tract is unavailable for nutritional support because of a persistent ileus, a concurrent injury, intra-abdominal sepsis, or poor tolerance of enteral feedings, nutritional support should be provided intravenously. Because of the heightened nutritional requirements of the hypermetabolic burned patient, the goal of nutritional maintenance requires the use of hypertonic glucose and amino acid solutions. These solutions must be delivered into a vein with a high blood flow, usually a central vein, to minimize the risk of phlebitis, sclerosis, and thrombosis. To reduce the risk of contamination and bacteremia, the central line is placed under sterile conditions and utilized exclusively for intravenous nutrition. Critically ill burned patients typically require the administration of blood and blood products, intravenous fluids, and medications in addition to any intravenous feedings. Thus, venous access may be limited, especially if there have been extensive burns of the torso and upper extremities. Multi-lumen catheters are frequently utilized in burned and other critically ill patients. One of the side ports may be dedicated to the hypertonic nutrient solution, leaving the larger, distal port available for the administration of blood and blood products and the measurement of central venous pressure. Blood may be drawn for analysis from the distal lumen after interrupting the intravenous feeding solutions for several minutes. A high index of suspician concerning catheter-associated infection must be maintained in these critically ill patients with open wounds. If there is a "fever spike" the catheter should be changed. The catheter tip and a sample of blood should be sent for culture. In some centers all central lines are changed over a guide wire or to a new site every 3 to 5 days—even in the absence of clinical signs of infection.

Several different concentrations of intravenous dextrose, amino acid solutions, and fat emulsions are available to the pharmacist, so that the clinician has considerable flexibility in designing the parenteral nutrient mixture. The regimen should deliver the required amounts of calories and nitrogen in a fluid volume that is appropriate for the patient's cardiopulmonary and renal status. Unlike enteral formulas, the parenteral mixture requires the addition of appropriate amounts of electrolytes, minerals, and vitamins.

Solutions of glucose and amino acids have been the basis for intravenous feedings in the United States for 20 years. In this setting intravenous fat emulsion is useful to prevent fatty acid deficiency. When glucose and amino acids provide all of the calories and nitrogen required, one bottle of 10 per cent fat emulsion administered twice weekly suffices to prevent this metabolic complication. However, based on many of the considerations cited above, fat is being used increasingly as a regular caloric source. In addition, the cost of these emulsions has decreased markedly in the last several years. Fat emulsion may be administered continuously and "piggybacked" into the glucose and amino acid line at the catheter hub. Alternatively glucose, amino acid solution, and fat emulsion may be admixed in one container to supply the patient's nutrient needs for 24 hours.[174] In compounding these admixtures there is sufficient flexibility to allow for a wide variety of combinations of glucose, fat, and amino acid calories.

EXAMPLE—CONTINUED. The patient develops high gastric residual volumes and enteral feedings must be discontinued. Nasogastric suction is resumed. Outline a plan for nutritional support utilizing intravenous techniques.

16. The patient's nutritional requirements are 4400 total kcal/day provided in part by 180 to 190 g of protein. To provide maintenance nutritional support parenterally, central vein feedings must be utilized.

17. "Standard" TPN solutions typically contain 250 g of glucose and 42.5 g of amino acids per liter. Approximately 4.2 L of this solution (196 ml/hr) would ultimately be required to deliver the estimated protein needs. Usually the solution is started at a low rate (approximately 50 ml/hr) and increased over the course of 48 to 72 hours. A limiting factor is usually hyperglycemia. In this case approximately 3600 kcal from glucose (1050 g) would be delivered when the full protein requirements were also met. That would represent a glucose infusion rate of approximately 9.2 mg/kg/min, which would most likely result in marked hyperglycemia. Large doses of insulin would be required, but the blood glucose concentration could still remain elevated. 500 ml of 10 per cent lipid emulsion would be provided twice weekly. This approach would be adequate provided that hyperglycemia could be controlled and provided that there were no complications that might be related to the high glucose load, such as increased ventilatory requirements and pronounced hepatic dysfunction.

18. Alternatively, an approach utilizing both fat and glucose as nonprotein calorie sources could be employed. A 10 per cent amino acid solution and a 70 per cent glucose solution could be mixed in a ratio of 650 ml to 350 ml. Three liters of this mixture administered over 24 hours (120 ml/hr) would provide 182 g amino acids and 2330 kcal from glucose—53 per cent of total requirements. Another 1000 kcal could be provided by 500 ml of 20 per cent fat emulsion administered continuously over 24 hours at 21 ml/hr. This regimen would require a total volume of approximately 3500 ml, 700 ml less (16 per cent) than the glucose regimen. However, the resultant glucose load (6 mg/kg/min) would be 34 per cent less and should result in minimal or only moderate hyperglycemia. The glucose and amino acid solution would also be started at a low rate and gradually increased over 48 to 72 hours.

19. If the capability to compound a nutrient admixture were available, 70 per cent dextrose, 10 per cent amino acids, and 20 per cent fat emulsion could be combined into an admixture providing 60 per cent of the calories from dextrose, 17 per cent from amino acids, and 23 per cent from fat. Approximately 3200 ml of this mixture would provide 4000 kcal. The glucose load would be approximately 6.1 mg/kg/min. The daily amount of calories provided by the mixture could be increased over 3 to 4 days until full nutrient requirements were met.

20. Appropriate electrolytes and vitamins should be added daily. Although total body sodium is high, some sodium may be required to maintain tonicity. Potassium losses are generally large, and 100 to 200 mEq of potassium may be required. This may be included as phosphate salts, which will provide necessary phosphorus. In addition, the use of acetate salts may be advisable if there is a tendency toward hyperchloremic acidosis. Magnesium and calcium are also re-

quired in generous amounts. A multiple vitamin preparation and trace element solution are included to provide at least normal daily requirements. Increased amounts of vitamin C, vitamin A, and zinc may be beneficial.

21. As the patient improves and GI motility returns, attempts should again be made to institute enteral feedings. In practice several nutritional support modalities may be utilized during a patient's convalescence (Fig. 39–10). The important issue is that calorie and protein substrate and other nutrients are provided in sufficient quantities to meet nutritional requirements.

Although the hypermetabolic response to burn injury accounts for much of the erosion of lean tissue, the inactivity associated with critical illness may also play a part. Thus, early physical therapy, even while the patient is bedridden, may provide some metabolic benefit[175,176] in addition to its functional one. As the burned patient recovers and the size of the open wound is reduced, he or she generally becomes more active. It is often apparent too that despite aggressive nutritional support, there has been appreciable loss of muscle mass. For these reasons the level of nutritional support is not necessarily reduced during the patient's convalescence as the size of the open wound is reduced. The extra calorie and nitrogen substrate support repletion of lean tissue and increased physical activity. Patients are encouraged to be active and to eat.

Nutritional Support Following 40% BSA Burn in a 25 Year Old Man

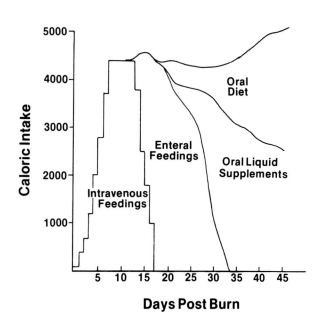

FIGURE 39–10. A variety of nutritional support modalities may be used during a patient's post-burn course. The major objective is to provide adequate energy and nitrogen substrate to meet the patient's heightened nutritional requirements.

Metabolic Monitoring

An important component in the management of any critically ill patients is a system for monitoring the adequacy and efficacy of therapy. The adequacy of fluid and electrolyte therapy is judged by careful intake and output records, by central venous pressure measurements and other clinical signs of cardiovascular performance, and by determination of the serum electrolyte concentrations. Monitoring is also important to judge the adequacy and efficacy of nutritional support.

Once the nutritional support regimen has been instituted, careful nutrient intake records should be maintained. These include the number of calories provided and the proportion of those calories contributed by carbohydrate, fat, and amino acids or protein. If a patient's nutritional needs are not being met, the nutritional support plan should be altered. In some particularly complicated cases or when convalescence is not progressing satisfactorily, further nutritional assessment may be helpful. Metabolic rate may be determined by indirect calorimetry using a metabolic cart (see page 688) or an alternative method. A simple one is the measurement of oxygen consumption utilizing a spirometer in a closed circuit. Alternatively, if a pulmonary artery catheter is in place, oxygen consumption may be calculated by multiplying the cardiac output (L/min) by the difference in systemic and pulmonary arterial (mixed venous) oxygen content (ml/dl).* However, this calculation will necessarily be imprecise because of the combined measurement errors. Although it is usually impossible to achieve completely basal conditions in the modern intensive care unit, several variables may be controlled. Nutrient intake may be stopped for several hours prior to measurement. The determination can be made in the early morning, and the patient kept quiet, comfortable, and warm. To calculate metabolic rate (MR) from O_2 consumption alone, a conversion factor of 4.86 kcal/L O_2 consumed may be used[177] (this assumes RQ = 0.85):

$$MR \text{ (kcal/hr)} = 4.86 \times V_{O_2} \text{ (L/min)} \times 60 \text{ (min/hr)}$$

The resulting rate should be within 3 per cent of the value that would be obtained if carbon dioxide production were also known. This value (kcal/hr) can be multiplied by 24 hr/day and 1.25 to determine total daily caloric requirements. If nutrient intake is in progress during the measurement, a factor of 1.05 to 1.10 should be used for activity alone.[161]

The clinical parameters commonly used to judge nutritional status—changes in body weight, serum albumin, and anthropometric parameters—are complicated by changes in the fluid compartments of the body.[178] The body weight of a burned patient may increase by 20 per cent or more with resuscitation in the first 24 hours. That represents an expansion of the extracellular fluid space and a positive sodium balance. As the patient recovers, body weight should decrease. Concentrations of serum albumin reflect neither total body protein content nor nitrogen balance[179] because of the marked extracellular fluid expansion. The serum albumin returns to normal after the wounds are covered and the patient is well. Anthropometric measurements will be influenced by the expanded extracellular fluid compartment as well.

Nitrogen balance techniques have long been used to judge the adequacy of nutrition. Although there are certainly limitations to these techniques and to their interpretation,[180,181] they are safe, simple, and inexpensive and can be performed in most centers. In addition, nitrogen equilibrium or positive balance has long been associated with recovery.

Determination of total nitrogen is not readily available in many clinical settings, but assays for urea nitrogen in blood and urine are commonly performed by the clinical laboratory. The most difficult part of the determination is to collect 24 hours' worth of urine. Once that is done, the chemical determinations are routine. Urinary loss of sodium, potassium, magnesium, phosphorus, and creatinine may be measured for balance approximations and calculations of creatinine clearance. Urea nitrogen composes 80 to 90 per cent of the total urinary nitrogen excretion under normal conditions. However, this proportion may be altered by a variety of factors. For example, in prolonged simple starvation urea nitrogen may constitute less than 50 per cent of the total.[182] A similar finding is seen after protein depletion.[181] In a group of injured patients on maintenance nutritional support that included both glucose and fat, urea nitrogen* was 80 per cent of total urinary nitrogen. Under normal conditions gastrointestinal and skin losses are thought to account for approximately 2 g of nitrogen per day. Gastrointestinal losses may be increased in the presence of diarrhea, nasogastric suction, or fistula drainage. Nitrogen loss from the burn wound varies over the course of treatment, but it may account for several grams per day.[54] Thus, during maintenance nutritional support, nitrogen loss may be estimated by:

$$N \text{ loss (g/day)} = [24 \text{ hr UUN (g/day)}/0.8] + 4 \text{ g}$$

and nitrogen balance calculated:

$$N \text{ balance (g/day)}$$
$$= [\text{protein intake (g/day)}/6.25] - N \text{ loss (g/day)}.$$

---

*O_2 content (ml/dl) = [Hemoglobin (g/dl) × O_2 saturation × 1.34 (ml/g)] + [0.003 × P_{O_2}]

*Determined by a widely used method that includes reaction with the enzyme urease and that measures both urea and ammonia nitrogen. Urea nitrogen alone accounted for 70 per cent of total urinary nitrogen.

Future Directions

The above approach to the nutritional support of burned patients can achieve the goal of nutritional maintenance in most cases. The effect of burn injury on metabolic and nutritional demands may be estimated reliably, and the required nutrients administered utilizing readily available products. Net weight loss can usually be limited to less than 10 per cent of pre-burn weight. This approach may also be adapted to other injured and critically ill patients.[173] In all cases energy and nitrogen substrate is provided to meet the increased requirements of the hypermetabolic patient.

Current investigations may modify this approach in the future. Improved understanding of regulatory mechanisms may lead to therapies that could alter the intensity or nature of the injury response and so modify the consequent metabolic demands. Studies of regional metabolism may identify altered requirements for specific nutrients in certain tissues. In some cases, specific modification of the composition of nutrient intake might have clinical benefit in certain disease states; treatment involving such modifications is known as disease-specific therapy.

The most notable example of disease-specific therapy for hypermetabolic patients has been the development of amino acid solutions enriched with the branched-chain amino acids (BCAA). Leucine, isoleucine, and valine and/or their alpha-keto analogues are thought to be important regulators of skeletal muscle protein metabolism. The BCAA undergo oxidative degradation primarily in skeletal muscle, unlike other amino acids which are largely metabolized in the liver.[67] Based on in-vitro data several investigators have suggested that the BCAA, especially leucine, are in-vivo regulators of protein turnover in skeletal muscle.[183] It has been proposed that if the BCAA were present in increased quantities they could attenuate net protein breakdown.[184] It has also been hypothesized that following injury or with sepsis there is an "energy fuel deficit" in skeletal muscle, presumably because of inhibition of glucose entry into cells or because of a limitation of fat as substrate.[185] In that view, net skeletal muscle protein breakdown occurs to provide amino acids as an oxidizable fuel source. In muscle the BCAA would be the preferred energy substrate. They could be transaminated with alpha-ketoglutarate and pyruvate ultimately to form alanine and glutamine for transport to the liver and kidney. The carbon skeletons of the BCAA could be oxidized in muscle to generate ATP. In accordance with this hypothesis, administration of exogenous BCAA in critically ill patients in excess of normal requirements could serve as an additional fuel source specifically for skeletal muscle, enhance protein synthesis, and thus spare the net catabolism of skeletal muscle protein.

A variety of studies have supported these hypotheses. Freund and associates[186] demonstrated that BCAA alone were as effective in achieving postoperative nitrogen equilibrium as a balanced amino acid solution. Desai and colleagues[187] demonstrated equivalent protein kinetics in postoperative patients randomly assigned to receive one of three amino acids differing only in the proportion of BCAA. Cerra and co-workers[188] reported an earlier appearance of positive nitrogen balance following operation or injury in patients receiving BCAA-enriched nutritional support than in patients receiving balanced amino acid formulations. This was thought to reflect an enhancement of protein synthesis rather than a suppression of protein degradation.[189] In addition, various immunological parameters, such as total lymphocyte count and reversal of skin test anergy, were improved. Cerra also found that these effects appeared to be related to the BCAA dose.[190] However, Bonau and colleagues[191] showed that the nitrogen-sparing effect depended more on the ratios of the individual BCAA than on the total amount.

In studies measuring intracellular muscle amino acid concentration following injury and sepsis, the BCAA concentrations were greater than normal.[70] They were increased still further with infection. Johnson and co-workers[192] compared the effects of BCAA-enriched solutions versus balanced mixtures utilizing a standardized catabolic animal model. Skeletal muscle uptake of BCAA was related to BCAA dose, but this effect was small and transitory. There were no differences in nitrogen balance or in skeletal muscle intracellular free amino acid concentrations. A study by Bower and associates[193] compared the effects of two BCAA-enriched solutions versus a balanced amino acid mixture in the nutritional support of septic surgical patients. In both study solutions the BCAA composed 45 per cent of the total, as compared with the control solutions in which only 25 per cent of the amino acids were BCAA. One of the study solutions had predominantly valine and the other predominantly leucine. Patients received the solutions for a 10-day study period. Nitrogen balance was marginally but statistically better in the groups receiving BCAA as compared with the control group on days 5, 7, and 10. Cumulative nitrogen balance appeared to be improved with the BCAA solutions, but the difference did not reach statistical significance. There was no difference in 3-methylhistidine excretion, indicating that there was no effect on skeletal muscle catabolic processes. All patients received insulin as required to maintain glucose in an acceptable range. However, the insulin requirements for patients receiving the high-leucine solution were significantly lower than for the high-valine group.

The development of amino acid solutions enriched with BCAA grew out of hypotheses concerning the mechanism of post-traumatic catabolic responses. The solutions have been utilized safely for up to 10 days and are at least as effective as balanced amino acid preparations in the nutritional support of patients with critical illness. However, the biochemical benefits reported to date have generally been small and transitory. No study has yet demonstrated a consistent effect on the patient's clinical course. Depending on local contractual arrangements, the cost of the specialized solutions may be five to six times that of conventional preparations.

Efforts to develop new and improved strategies to support patients following burns, trauma, sepsis, and other critical illness continue. Alexander and colleagues[194] reported the effects of altering lipid type in the enteral nutritional support of animals following a standard burn injury. Some animals received fish oil, which is rich in the eicosapentaenoic acids, while others received safflower oil, which is rich in linoleic acid. The animals receiving the fish oil had reduced hypermetabolic responses, better preservation of lean tissue, and improved immunological function.

The possible contributory role of the gastrointestinal tract to these hypercatabolic responses continues to be investigated. In an animal model, atrophy of the small bowel mucosa was observed early following burn injury, but this could be prevented by gavage feedings.[100] Preservation of mucosal mass was associated with reductions in post-traumatic responses. Furthermore, enteral stimulation enhanced gastrointestinal immune function in another study.[195] The absorption of endotoxin or the direct translocation of bacteria across the small bowel has been suggested as a contributing cause of organ system dysfunction in critical illness.[196,197] Thus, efforts to maintain small bowel integrity may have metabolic benefits.

As discussed above, glutamine is a principal intracellular amino acid that is commonly depleted with critical illness. Recent evidence suggests that intracellular glutamine may be an important determinant of muscle proteolysis. Following a standard operative procedure, the fall in skeletal muscle glutamine concentration predicted the degree of skeletal muscle proteolysis.[198] When intracellular glutamine concentration fell, amino acid efflux from skeletal muscle increased. When intracellular glutamine concentration was maintained, net efflux was reduced. These findings were consistent with observations in a cultured skeletal muscle cell line in which the addition of glutamine to the media resulted in inhibition of protein degradation.[199] Thus, efforts to preserve intracellular glutamine concentration might be of benefit. No commercially available amino acid solution for parenteral administration contains glutamine. In addition, most enteral products contain no appreciable amount of glutamine. This is due to the tendency of glutamine to decompose in solution. However, in short-term studies utilizing an animal model, postoperative intracellular glutamine concentrations were preserved when large quantities of amino acids were provided intravenously.[200] Finally, glutamine may be important for the maintenance of small bowel integrity. Souba and Wilmore demonstrated active update of glutamine by the gut following operation.[90] Thus, following injury, diminished muscle glutamine and the absence of glutamine in nutritional support might lead to loss of gut integrity, which could further amplify catabolic processes.

Attempts to modify the hormonal environment may have a beneficial effect in terms of post-traumatic catabolic responses, as discussed above. In addition, various anabolic compounds may be administered to stimulate lean tissue accretion and wound healing. Manson and Wilmore[201] achieved positive nitrogen balance in human volunteers receiving hypocaloric intravenous feedings by administering exogenous recombinant growth hormone. Improved epithelial growth was observed in a patient who sustained a major burn following pituitary ablation[202] when replacement growth hormone was administered. Brown and associates[203,204] applied epidermal growth factor topically to burns in animals and demonstrated accelerated healing. The use of these or other substances may have a marked effect on the healing wound and the efficient utilization of nutrients.

EPILOGUE

The burned patient presents one of the most demanding and complicated challenges in all of clinical medicine. We have reviewed many of the metabolic alterations that occur following burn injury, and we have outlined some approaches to the metabolic support of the burned patient. The dramatic responses observed begin at the time of burn injury and subside as the wounds heal. The open burn wound is a dominant controlling force. The most metabolically beneficial strategy of all is to close the wound.

References

1. Trunkey DD. On the nature of things that go bang in the night. Surgery 1982; 92:123–132.
2. Injury: magnitude and pharmacokinetics of the problem. *In* Committee on Trauma Research, Injury in America: A Continuing Public Health Problem. Washington, National Academy Press, 1985: 18–24.
3. Trunkey DD. Trauma. Sci Am 1983; 249:28–35.
4. Prevention of injury. *In* Committee on Trauma Research, Injury in America: A Continuing Public Health Problem. Washington, National Academy Press, 1985: 37–47.
5. Layton TR, Elhavge ER. US fire catastrophies of the 20th century. J Burn Care Rehab 1982: 3:21–28.
6. Cuthbertson DP. Observations on disturbance of metabolism produced by injury to the limbs. Q J Med 1932; 25:233–246.
7. Cuthbertson DP. Post-shock metabolic response. Lancet 1942; 1:433–437.
8. Blalock A. Experimental shock: the cause of the low blood pressure produced by muscle injury. Arch Surg 1930; 20:959–996.
9. Blalock A. Experimental shock. VII. The importance of

local loss of fluid in the production of low blood pressure after burns. Arch Surg 1931; *22*:610–616.

10. Cope O, Moore FD. A study of capillary permeability in experimental burns and burn shock using radioactive dyes in blood and lymph. J Clin Invest 1944; *23*:241–257.

11. Cope O, Graham JB, Moore FD, Ball MR. The nature of the shift of plasma protein to the extravascular space following thermal trauma. Ann Surg 1948; *283*:1041–1055.

12. Cope O, Moore FD. The redistribution of body water and fluid therapy of the burned patient. Ann Surg 1947; *126*:1010–1045.

13. Baxter CR. Fluid volume and electrolyte changes of the early postburn period. Clin Plast Surg 1974; *1*:693–709.

14. Hume DM, Egdahl RH. The importance of the brain in the endocrine response to injury. Ann Surg 1959; *150*:697–712.

15. Kehlet H, Brandt MR, Rem J. Role of neurogenic stimuli in mediating the endocrine-metabolic response to surgery. JPEN 1980; *4*:152–156.

16. Hayashi H, Yoshinago M, Koono M, et al. Endogenous permeability factors and their inhibitors affecting vascular permeability in cutaneous Arthus reactions and thermal injury. Br J Exp Pathol 1964; *45*:419–35.

17. Arthurson G. Prostaglandins in human burn wound secretion. Burns 1977; *3*:112–118.

18. Kupper TS, Deitch EA, Baker CC, et al.: The human burn wound as a primary service of interleukin-1 activity. Surgery 1986; *100*:409–414.

19. Moncrief JA. Effect of various fluid regimens and pharmacologic agents on the circulatory hemodynamics of the immediate postburn period. Ann Surg 1966; *164*:723–752.

20. Jaattela A, Alho A, Avikainen V, et al.: Plasma catecholamines in severely injured patients: a prospective study of 45 patients with multiple injuries. Br J Surg 1975; *62*:177–181.

21. Davies CL, Newman RJ, Molyneux SG, et al. The relationship between plasma catecholamines and severity of injury in man. J Trauma 1984; *24*:99–105.

22. Porte D Jr, Robertson RP. Control of insulin secretion by catecholamines, stress, and the sympathetic nervous system. Fed Proc 1973; *32*:1792–1796.

23. Bessey PQ, Brooks DC, Black PR, et al. Epinephrine acutely mediates skeletal muscle insulin resistance. Surgery 1983; *94*:172–177.

24. Randle PJ, Garland PB, Hales CN, et al. The glucose and fatty acid cycle. Its role in insulin sensitivity and the metabolic disturbance of diabetes mellitus. Lancet 1963; *1*:785–789.

25. Vaughan GM, Becker RA, Allen JP, et al. Cortisol and corticotrophin in burned patients. J Trauma 1982; *22*:263–273.

26. Ingle DJ. Permissive actions of hormones. J Clin Endocrinol Metab 1954; *14*:1272–1274.

27. Atwater WO, Benedict FG. Experiments on the metabolism of matter and energy in the human body. USDA Office of Experimental Stations Bulletin, Publication 1903: No. 136.

28. Ben-Porat M, Sideman S, Bursein S. Energy metabolism rate equation for fasting and postabsorptive subjects. Am J Physiol 1983; *244*:R764–769.

29. Dubois EF. Basal Metabolism in Health and Disease. Philadelphia, Lea & Febiger, 1936: 163–165.

30. Wilmore DW, Long JM, Mason AD Jr, et al. Catecholamines: mediators of the hypermetabolic response to thermal injury. Ann Surg 1974; *180*:653–669.

31. Wilmore DW. The Metabolic Management of the Critically Ill. New York: Plenum Medical, 1977: 33–35.

32. Wilmore DW, Aulick LH, Mason AD, et al. Influence of the burn wound on local and systemic responses to injury. Ann Surg 1977; *186*:444–458.

33. Aulick LH, Wilmore DW, Mason AD Jr, et al.: Muscle blood flow following thermal injury. Ann Surg 1978; *188*:778–782.

34. Wilmore DW, Goodwin CW, Aulick LH, et al. Effect of injury and infection on visceral metabolism and circulation. Ann Surg 1980; *192*:491–504.

35. Aulick LH, Goodwin CW, Becker RA, et al.: Visceral blood flow following thermal injury. Ann Surg 1981; *193*:112–116.

36. Wilmore DW, Aulick LH. Metabolic changes in burned patients. Surg Clin North Am 1978; *58*:1173–1187.

37. Cuthbertson DP. The disturbance of metabolism produced by bony and non-bony injury, with notes on certain abnormal conditions of bone. Biochem J 1930; *24*:1244.

38. Monafo WW. The Treatment of Burns, Principles and Practice. St. Louis, Warren H Green, Inc., 1971: 111.

39. Caldwell FT Jr, Osterholm JL, Sower ND, et al. Metabolic response to thermal trauma of normal and thyroprivic rats at three environmental temperatures. Ann Surg 1959; *150*:976–1988.

40. Barr PO, Birke G, Liljedahl SO, et al.: Oxygen consumption and water loss during treatment of burns with warm dry air. Lancet 1968; *1*:164–168.

41. Zawacki BE, Spitzer KW, Mason KD Jr, et al. Does increased evaporative water loss cause hypermetabolism in burn patients? Ann Surg 1970; *171*:236–240.

42. Wilmore DW, Mason AD Jr, Johnson DW, et al. Effect of ambient temperature on heat production and heat loss in burn patients. J Appl Physiol 1975; *38*:593.

43. Wilmore DW, Orcutt TW, Mason AD Jr, et al. Alterations in hypothalamic function following thermal injury. J Trauma 1975; *15*:697.

44. Caldwell FT Jr, Bowser BH, Crabtree JH. The effect of occlusive dressings on the energy metabolism of severely burned children. Ann Surg 1981; *193*:579–591.

45. Howard JE, Parson W, Stein K, et al. Studies on fracture convalescence. I: Nitrogen metabolism after fracture and skeletal operations in healthy males. Bull Johns Hopkins Hosp 1944; *75*:156–168.

46. Soroff HS, Pearson E, Artz CP. An estimation of the nitrogen requirements for equilibrium in burned patients. Surg Gynecol Obstet 1961; *112*:150–172.

47. Cuthbertson DP, McGirr JL, Robertson JSM. The effect of fracture of bone on the metabolism of the rat. Q J Exp Physiol 1939; *29*:13–25.

48. Threlfall CJ, Stoner HB, Galasko CSB. Patterns in the excretion of muscle markers after trauma and orthopedics surgery. J Trauma 1981; *21*:140–147.

49. Young VR, Munro HN. Nτ-Methylhistidine (3-methylhistidine) and muscle protein turnover; an overview. Fed Proc 1978; *37*:2291–2300.

50. Bilmazes C, Kien CL, Rohrbaugh DK, et al.: Quantitative contributors by skeletal muscle to elevated rates of whole-body protein breakdown in burned children as measured by 3-methylhistidine output. Metabolism 1978; *27*:671–676.

51. Williamson DH, Farrell R, Kerr A, et al.: Muscle protein catabolism after injury in man as measured by urinary excretion of 3-methylhistidine. Clin Sci Mol Med 1977; *52*:527–533.

52. Long CL, Schiller WR, Blakemore WS, et al. Muscle protein catabolism in the septic patient as measured by 3-methylhistidine excretion. Am J Clin Nutr 1977; *30*:1349–1352.

53. Cuthbertson DP. The physiology of convalescence after injury. Br Med Bull 1945; *3*:96–102.

54. Moore FD, Langohr JL, Ingebretsen M, et al. The role of exudate losses in the protein and electrolyte imbalance of burned patients. Ann Surg 1950; *132*:1–19.

55. Wilmore DW. Nutrition and metabolism following thermal injury. Clin Plast Surg 1974; *1*:603–619.

56. Kinney JM. Energy deficits in acute illness and injury. *In* Morgan AP (ed). Proceedings of a Conference on Energy Metabolism and Body Fuel Utilization. Cambridge, Harvard University Press, 1966: 174.

57. Picou D, Taylor-Roberts T. The measurement of total protein synthesis and catabolism and nitrogen turnover in infants on different amounts of dietary protein. Clin Sci 1969; 36:283–296.

58. Birkhahn RH, Long CL, Fitkin D, et al. Effects of major skeletal trauma on whole body protein turnover in man measured by L-[1,14C]-leucine. Surgery 1980; 88:294–308.

59. Kien CL, Young VR, Rohrbaugh DK, et al. Increased rates of whole body protein synthesis and breakdown in children recovering from burns. Ann Surg 1978; 187:383–391.

60. Levenson, SM, Pulaski EJ, del Guerico LRM. Metabolic changes associated with injury. In Zimmerman LM, Levine R (eds). Physiological Principles of Surgery. 2nd ed. Philadelphia, WB Saunders, 1964: 5–7.

61. Everson TC, Fritschel MJ. The effect of surgery on the plasma levels of the individual essential amino acids. Surgery 1952; 31:226–232.

62. Levenson SM, Howard JM, Rosen H. Studies of the plasma amino acids and amino conjugates in patients with severe battle wounds. Surg Gynecol Obstet 1955; 101:35–47.

63. LaBrasse EH, Beech JA, McLaughlin JS, et al. Plasma amino acids in normal humans and patients with shock. Surg Gynecol Obstet 1967; 125:516–520.

64. Cerra FB, Siegel JH, Border JR, et al. Correlations between metabolic and cardiopulmonary measurements in patients after trauma, general surgery, and sepsis. J Trauma 1979; 19:621–629.

65. McMenam RH, Birkhahn R, Oswald G, et al. Multiple systems failure: I. The basal state. J Trauma 1981; 21:99–114.

66. Wannemacher RW Jr. Key role of various individual amino acids in host response to infection. Am J Clin Nutr 1977; 30:1269–1280.

67. Adibi SA. Metabolism of branched chain amino acids in altered nutrition. Metabolism 1976; 25:1287–1302.

68. Wedge JH, DeCampos R, Kerr A, et al. Branched chain amino acids, nitrogen excretion and injury in man. Clin Sci Mol Med 1976; 50:393–399.

69. Askanazi J, Elwyn DH, Kinney JM, et al. Muscle and plasma amino acids after injury: the role of inactivity. Ann Surg 1978; 188:797–803.

70. Askanazi J, Carpentier YA, Michelson CB, et al. Muscle and plasma amino acids following injury: influence of intercurrent infection. Ann Surg 1980; 792:78–85.

71. Munro HN. Free amino acid pools and their role in regulation. In Munro HN (ed). Mammalian Protein Metabolism. New York, Academic Press, 1970: 299.

72. Bergstrom J, Fuerst P, Noree L-O, et al. Intracellular free amino acid concentration in human muscle tissue. J Appl Physiol 1974; 36:693–697.

73. Vinnars E, Bergstrom J, Fuerst P. Influence of the postoperative state on the intracellular free amino acids in human muscle tissue. Ann Surg 1975; 182:665–671.

74. Fuerst P, Bergstrom J, Chao L, et al. Influence of amino acid supply on nitrogen and amino acid metabolism in severe trauma. Acta Chir Scand (Suppl.) 1979; 494:136–138.

75. Wilmore DW, Black PR, Muhlbacher F. Injured man: trauma and sepsis. In Winters RW (ed). Nutritional Support of the Seriously Ill Patient. New York, Academic Press, 1983: 33–52.

76. Askanazi J, Fuerst P, Micheken CB, et al. Muscle and plasma amino acids after injury: hypocaloric glucose vs. amino acid infusion. Ann Surg 1980; 191:465–472.

77. Garber AJ, Karl IE, Kipnis DM. Alanine and glutamine synthesis and release from skeletal muscle. I: Glycolysis and amino acid release. J Biol Chem 1976; 251:826–835.

78. Garber AJ, Karl IE, Kipnis DM. Alanine and glutamine synthesis and release from skeletal muscle. II: The precursor role of amino acids in alanine and glutamine synthesis. J Biol Chem 1976; 251:836–843.

79. Aulick LH, Wilmore DW. Increased peripheral amino acid release following burn injury. Surgery 1979; 85:560–565.

80. Howard JM. Studies of the absorption and metabolism of glucose following injury. Ann Surg 1955; 141:311–326.

81. Allison SP, Hinton P, Chamberlain MJ. Intravenous glucose-tolerance, insulin, and free-fatty acid levels in burned patients. Lancet 1968; 2:1113–1116.

82. Wilmore DW, Mason AD Jr, Pruitt BA Jr. Insulin response to glucose in hypermetabolic burn patients. Ann Surg 1978; 183:314–320.

83. Wilmore DW, Mason AD Jr, Pruitt BA Jr. Alterations in glucose kinetics following thermal injury. Surg Forum 1975; 26:81–83.

84. Long CL, Spencer JL, Kinney JM, et al. Carbohydrate metabolism in man: effect of elective operations and major injury. J Appl Physiol 1971; 31:110–116.

85. Wolfe RR, Durkot MJ, Allsop JR, et al. Glucose metabolism in severely burned patients. Metabolism 1979; 28:1031–1039.

86. Ruderman MB. Muscle amino acid metabolism and gluconeogenesis. Ann Rev Med 1975; 26:245–258.

87. Black PR, Brooks DC, Bessey PQ, et al. Mechanisms of insulin resistance following injury. Ann Surg 1982; 196:420–435.

88. Brooks DC, Bessey PQ, Black PR, et al. Post-traumatic insulin resistance in uninjured skeletal muscle. J Surg Res 1984; 37:100–107.

89. Askanazi J, Carpentier YA, Elwyn DH, et al. Influence of total parenteral nutrition on fuel utilization in injury and sepsis. Ann Surg 1980; 191:40–46.

90. Souba WW, Wilmore DW. Postoperative alteration of arteriovenous exchange of amino acids across the gastrointestinal tract. Surgery 1983; 94:342–350.

91. Pitts RF. Renal regulation of acid base balance. In Physiology of the Kidney and Body Fluids. 3rd ed. Chicago, Year Book Medical Publishers, 1974: 217–241.

92. Wilmore DW, Taylor JW, Handler EW, et al. Central nervous system function following thermal injury. In Wilkinson AW, Cuthbertson DP (eds). Metabolism and the Response to Injury. Chicago, Year Book Medical Publishers, 1976: 274–286.

93. Dempsey DT, Guenter P, Crosby LO, et al. Barbiturate therapy and energy expenditure in head trauma. Presented at 42nd annual meeting of the America Association for the Surgery of Trauma, Colorado Springs, 1982.

94. Fried R, Dempsey D, Guenter P. Barbiturates improve nitrogen balance in patients with severe head trauma. (Abstract.) JPEN 1984; 8:86.

95. Bennett IL Jr, Beeson PB. Studies on the pathogenesis of fever: effect of injection of extracts and suspensions of uninfected rabbit tissues upon the body temperature of normal rabbits. J Exp Med 1953; 98:477–492.

96. Dinarello LA. Interleukin-1. Rev Infect Dis 1984; 6:51–95.

97. Young LS, Stevens P, Kaijser B. Gram-negative pathogens in septicemic infections. Scand J Infect Dis (Suppl.) 1982; 31:78–94.

98. Fish RE, Spitzer JA. Continuous infusion of endotoxin from an osmotic pump in the conscious, unrestrained rat: a unique model of chronic endotoxemia. Circ Shock 1984; 12:135–147.

99. Aulick LH, McManus AT, Mason AD Jr, et al. Effects of infection on oxygen consumption and core temperature in experimental thermal injury. Ann Surg 1986; 204:48–52.

100. Mochizuki H, Trocki O, Dominioni L. Mechanism of prevention of post-burn hypermetabolism and catabolism by early enteral feeding. Ann Surg 1984; 200:297–310.

101. Harrison TS, Seaton JF, Feller I. Relationship of increased oxygen consumption to catecholamine excretion in thermal burns. Ann Surg 1967; 165:169–172.

102. Garber AJ, Karl JE, Kipnis DM. Alanine and glutamine synthesis and release from skeletal muscle. IV. β-Adrenergic inhibition of amino acid release. J Biol Chem 1976; 251:851–857.

103. Wilmore DW, Lindsey CA, Moylan JA, et al. Hyperglucagonaemia after burns. Lancet 1974; 1:73–75.

104. Baxter JD, Forsham PH. Tissue effects of glucocorticoids. Am J Med 1972; 53:573–589.

105. Owen OE, Cahill GF. Metabolic effects of exogenous glucocorticoids in fasted man. J Clin Invest 1973; 52:2596–2605.

106. Felig P, Wahren J, Hendler R. Influence of physiologic hyperglucagonemia on basal and insulin-inhibited splanchnic glucose output in normal man. J Clin Invest 1976; 58:761–765.

107. Ferrannini E, DeFronze RA, Sherwin RS. Transient hepatic response to glucagon in man: role of insulin and hyperglycemia. Am J Physiol 1982; 242:E73–E81.

108. Wolfe RM, Culebras JM, Aoki TT, et al. The effects of glucagon on protein metabolism in normal man. Surgery 1979; 86:248–257.

109. Roth J, Glick SM, Cuatrecasas P, et al. Acromegaly and other disorders of growth hormone secretion. Ann Intern Med 1967; 66:760.

110. Wilmore DW, Moylan JA Jr, Bristow BF, et al. Anabolic effects of growth hormone and high calorie feedings following thermal injury. Surg Gynecol Obstet 1974; 138:875–884.

111. Becker RA, Wilmore DW, Goodwin CW, et al. Free T$_4$, free T$_3$, and reverse T$_3$ in critically ill, thermally injured patients. J Trauma 1980; 20:713–721.

112. Becker RA, Vaughan GM, Goodwin CW, et al. Plasma norepinephrine, epinephrine, and thyroid hormone interactions in severely burned patients. Arch Surg 1980; 115:439–443.

113. Baracos V, Rodeman HP, Dinarello CA, et al. Stimulation of muscle protein degradation and prostaglandin E$_2$ release by leukocytic pyrogen (interluekin-1): a mechanism for the increased degradation of muscle proteins during fever. N Engl J Med 1983; 308:553–558.

114. Clowes GHA, George BC, Villee CA, et al. Muscle proteolysis induced by a circulating peptide in patients with sepsis or trauma. N Engl J Med 1983; 308:545–552.

115. Dinarello CA, Clowes GHA Jr, Gordon HA, et al. Cleavage of human interleukin-1: isolation of a peptide fragment from plasma of febrile humans and activated monocytes. J Immunol 1984; 133:1332–1338.

116. Old LJ. Tumor necrosis factor (TNF). Science 1985; 230:630–632.

117. Watters JM, Bessey PQ, Dinarello CA, et al. The induction of interleukin-1 in humans and its metabolic effects. Surgery 1985; 98:298–305.

118. Bessey PQ, Watters JM, Aoki TT, et al. Combined hormonal infusion simulated the metabolic response to injury. Ann Surg 1984; 200:264–281.

119. Watters JM, Bessey PQ, Dinarello CA, et al. Both inflammatory and endocrine mediators stimulate host reponses to sepsis. Arch Surg 1986; 121:179–190.

120. Bessey PQ, Jiang Z-M, Johnson DJ, et al. Post-traumatic skeletal muscle proteolysis: the role of the hormonal environment, in press.

121. Hulton, N, Johnson DJ, Smith RJ, et al. Hormonal blockade modifies post-traumatic protein catabolism. J Surg Res 1985; 39:310–315.

122. Brandt MR, Fernandes A, Mordhorst R, et al. Epidural analgesia improves postoperative nitrogen balance. Br Med J 1978; 1:1106–1108.

123. Tsuji H, Shirasaka C, Asoh T, et al. Effects of epidural administration of local anaesthetics or morphine on postoperative nitrogen loss and catabolic hormones. Br J Surg 1987; 74:421–425.

124. Schrock H, Goldstein L. Interorgan relationships for glutamine metabolism in normal and acidotic rats. Am J Physiol 1981; 240:E519–E525.

125. Initial assessment and management. In Committee on Trauma, Advanced Trauma Life Support Course for Physicians— Student Manual. Chicago; American College of Surgeons, 1984: 5–14.

126. Evans EI, Purnell OJ, Robinett PQ, et al. Fluid and electrolyte requirements in severe burns. Ann Surg 1952; 135:804–817.

127. Reiss E, Stirman JA, Artz CP, et al. Fluid and electrolyte balance in burns. JAMA 1953; 152:1309–1313.

128. Moore FD. The body-weight burn budget: basic fluid therapy for the early burn. Surg Clin North Am 1970; 50:1249–1265.

129. Monafo W, Chuntrasakul C, Ayvazian VA. Hypertonic sodium solution in treatment of burn shock. Am J Surg 1973; 126:778–783.

130. Schwartz, SI, Baxter C, Burke JF, et al. Fluid resuscitation. In Shires GT, Black EA (eds). Consensus development conference: supportive therapy in burn care. J Trauma (Suppl) 1979; 11:864–877.

131. Arthurson C. Pathophysiologic aspects of burn syndrome with special reference to liver injury and alterations of capillary permeability. Acta Chir Scand (Suppl) 1961; 274:55–103.

132. Birke G, Liljedahl S-O, Plantin L-O, et al. Studies on burns: the distribution and losses through the wound of ^{131}I-albumin measured by whole-body counting. Acta Chir Scand 1968; 134:27–36.

133. Harms BA, Bodai BI, Kramer GC. Microvascular fluid and protein flux in pulmonary and systemic circulation after thermal injury. Microvasc Res 1982; 23:77–88.

134. Demling RH, Kramer G, Harms B. Role of thermal injury–induced hypoproteinemia in fluid flux and protein permeabilty in burned and nonburned tissue. Surgery 1984; 93:130–143.

135. Demling RH, Kramer GC, Gunther R, et al. Effect of nonprotein colloid on postburn edema formation in soft tissues and lung. Surgery 1984; 73:593–602.

136. Demling RH. Improved survival after massive burns. J Trauma 1983; 23:179–184.

137. Goodwin DW, Dohethy J, Lem V, et al. Randomized trial of efficacy of crystalloid and colloid resuscitation on hemodynamic response and lung water following thermal injury. Ann Surg 1983; 197:520–531.

138. Pruitt BA Jr, Mason AD Jr. Moncrief JA. Hemodynamic changes in the early postburn patient: the influence of fluid administration and of a vasodilator (hydralazine). J Trauma 1971; 11:36–46.

139. Shires GT, Hulman J. Dilution acidosis. Ann Intern Med 1948; 28:557–559.

140. Gamble JL. Physiological information gained from studies on life raft ration. Harvey Lect (1946–1947) 1950; 42:634–640.

141. McDougal WS, Wilmore DW, Pruitt BA Jr. Effect of intravenous isoosmotic nutrient infusions on nitrogen balance in critically ill injured patients. Surg Gynecol Obstet 1977; 145:408–414.

142. Wilson JS, Moncrief JA. Vapor pressure on normal and burned skin. Ann Surg 1965; 162:130–134.

143. Harrison HN, Moncrief JA, Duckett JW, et al. The relationship between energy metabolism and water loss from vaporization in severely burned patients. Surgery 1964; 56:203–211.

144. Zawachi BE, Divincent PC, Moncrief JA. The effect of topical Sulfamylon on the insensible water loss of burn patients. Ann Surg 1969; 169:249–252.

145. Pearson E, Soroff HS, Arney GK, et al. An estimation of the potassium requirements for equilibrium in burned patients. Surg Gynecol Obstet 1961; 112:263–273.

146. Juan D. Clinical review: The clinical importance of hypomagnesemia. Surgery 1982; 91:510–517.

147. Custer MD, Bessey PQ. Injury accelerates magnesium depletion. (Abstract.) South Med J 1986; 79:78.

148. Whang R, Flink EB, Dyckner T, et al. Magnesium depletion as a cause of refractory potassium repletion. Arch Intern Med 1985; 145:1686–1689.

149. Daws TA, Consolazio CF, Hilty SL, et al. Evaluation of cardiopulmonary function and work performance in man

during caloric restriction. J Appl Physiol 1972; 33:211–217.

150. Levenson, SM, Selfur E. Starvation: metabolic and physiological responses. *In* Fischer JE (ed). Surgical Nutrition. Boston, Little, Brown, 1983: 423–478.

151. Studley HO. Percentage of weight loss: a basic indicator of surgical risk in patients with chronic peptic ulcer. JAMA 1936; 106:458–460.

152. Wilmore DW, Kinney JM. Panel report on nutritional support of patients with trauma or infection. Am J Clin Nutr 1981; 34:1213–1222.

153. Benedict FJ. A Study of Prolonged Fasting. Publication No. 203. Washington, DC, The Carnegie Institution of Washington, 1915: 69–82.

154. Fleisch A. Le métabolisme basal standard et sa détermination au moyen du "Metabocalculator." Helv Med Acta 1951; 18:23–44.

155. Wilmore DW. The Metabolic Management of the Critically Ill. New York, Plenum Medical, 1977: 29–42.

156. Harris JA, Benedict FG. Biometric studies of basal metabolism in man. Publication No. 279. Washington DC, The Carnegie Institution of Washington, 1919.

157. McLaurin NK, Mason AD Jr, Goodwin CW, et al. Estimating energy requirements of burned patients: a comparative study. *In* US Army Institute of Surgical Research Annual Progress Report FY 1983. Fort Sam Houston, San Antonio, 1983: 278–290.

158. Curreri PW, Richmond, Marvin J, et al. Dietary requirements of patients with major burns. J Am Diet Assoc. 1974; 65:415–417.

159. Bartlett RH, Dechert RE, Mault JE, et al. Measurement of metabolism in multiple organ failure. Surgery 1982; 92:771–779.

160. Feurer IN, Mullen JL. Bedside measurement of resting energy expenditure and respiratory quotient via indirect calorimetry. Nutr Clin Prac 1986; 1:43–49.

161. Swinamer DL, Phang PT, Jones RL, et al. Twenty-four hour energy expenditure in critically ill patients. Crit Care Med 1987; 15:637–643.

162. Duke JH, Jorgensen SB, Broell JR, et al. Contribution of protein to caloric expenditure following injury. Surgery 1970; 68:168–174.

163. Long, JM, Wilmore DW, Mason AD Jr, et al. Effect of carbohydrate and fat intake on nitrogen excretion during total intravenous feeding. Ann Surg 1977; 185:417.

164. Wolfe RR, O'Donnell TF Jr, Stone MD, et al. Investigation of factors determining optimal glucose infusion rate in total parenteral nutrition. Metabolism 1980; 29:892–900.

165. Burke JF, Wolfe RR, Mullany CJ, et al. Glucose requirements following burn injury. Ann Surg 1979; 190:274–285.

166. Askanazi J, Carpentier YA, Elwyn DH, et al. Influence of total parenteral nutrition on fuel utilization injury and sepsis. Ann Surg 1980; 191:40–46.

167. Askanazi J, Elwyn DH, Silverberg PA, et al. Respiratory distress secondary to a high carbohydrate load: a case report. Surgery 1980; 87:596–598.

168. Sheldon GF, Peterson SR, Sanders R. Hepatic dysfunction during hyperalimentation. Arch Surg 1978; 113:504–508.

169. Nordenstrom J, Carpentier YA, Askanazi J, et al. Metabolic utilization of intravenous fat emulsion during total parenteral nutrition. Ann Surg 1982; 196:221–231.

170. Goodenough RD, Wolfe RR. Effect of total parenteral nutrition on free fatty acid metabolism in burned patients. JPEN 1984; 8:357–366.

171. Jeejeebhoy KN, Marliss EB. Energy supply in total parenteral nutrition. *In* Fischer JE (ed). Surgical Nutrition. Boston, Little, Brown, 1983: 645–662.

172. Matarese LE. Enteral alimentation. *In* Fischer JE (ed). Surgical Nutrition. Boston, Little, Brown, 1983: 719–755.

173. MacBurrey MM, Wilmore DW. Rational decision-making in nutritional care. Surg Clin North Am 1981; 31:571–582.

174. Brown R, Quercia RA, Sigman R. Total nutrient admixture: a review. JPEN 1986; 10:650–658.

175. Cuthbertson DP. Certain effects of massage on the metabolism of convalescing fracture cases. Q J Med 1932; 25:401–408.

176. Wheldon GD, Deitrick JE, Shorr E. Modifications of the effects of immobilization upon metabolic and physiologic functions of normal men by the use of an oscillating bed. Am J Med 1949; 6:684–711.

177. Peters JP, Van Slyke DD. Quantitative Clinical Chemistry: Interpretations. 2nd ed. Baltimore, Williams & Wilkins, 1946: 9.

178. Elwyn DH, Bryan-Brown CW, Shoemaker WC. Nutritional aspects of body water dislocations in postoperative and depleted patients. Ann Surg 1975; 182:76–85.

179. Starker PM, Gump FK, Askanazi J, et al. Serum albumin levels as an index of nutritional support. Surgery 1982; 91:194–199.

180. Margen S. Evaluation of efficacy. *In* Fischer JE (ed). Surgical Nutrition. Boston, Little, Brown, 1983:391–406.

181. Allison JB, Bird JWC. Elimination of nitrogen from the body. *In* Munro HN (ed). Mammalian Protein Metabolism (Vol 1). New York, Academic Press, 1964: 483–512.

182. Cahill GF Jr. Starvation in man. N Engl J Med 1970; 282:658–675.

183. Buse MG, Reid SS. Leucine: a possible regulator of protein turnover in muscle. J Clin Invest 1975; 56:1250–1261.

184. Freund H, Yoshimura N, Lunetta L, et al. The role of branched-chain amino acids in decreasing muscle catabolism in vivo. Surgery 1978; 83:611–618.

185. Ryan NT, Blackburn, GL, Clower GHA. Differential tissue sensitivity to elevated endogenous insulin levels during experimental peritonitis in rats. Metabolism 1974; 23:1081–1089.

186. Freund H, Hoover HC Jr, Atamian S, et al. Infusion of branched chain amino acids in postoperative patients: anticatabolic properties. Ann Surg 1979; 190:18–23.

187. Desai SP, Bistrian BR, Moldawer LL, et al. Whole-body nitrogen and tyrosine metabolism in surgical patients receiving branched-chain amino acid solutions. Arch Surg 1985; 120:1345–1350.

188. Cerra FB, Mazuski JE, Chute E, et al. Branched chains support postoperative protein synthesis. Surgery 1982; 92:192–199.

189. Cerra FB, Mazuski J, Chute E, et al. Branched chain metabolic support: a prospective randomized, double-blind trial in surgical stress. Ann Surg 1984; 199:286–291.

190. Cerra FB, Mazuski J, Teasley K, et al. Nitrogen retention in critically ill patients is proportional to branched chain amino acid load. Crit Care Med 1983; 11:775–778.

191. Bonau R, Ang S, Jeevanandam M, et al. High–branched chain amino acid solutions: relationship of composition to efficacy. (Abstract.) JPEN 1984; 8:622–627.

192. Johnson DJ, Kapadia CR, Jiang Z, et al. Branched-chain amino acid supplementation fails to reduce post-traumatic protein catabolism. Surg Forum 1984; 35:102–105.

193. Bower RH, Muggia-Sullam M, Vallgren S, et al. Branched chain amino acid-enriched solutions in the septic patient: a randomized, prospective trial. Ann Surg 1986; 203:13–20.

194. Alexander JW, Saito H, Ogle CK, et al. The importance of lipid type in the diet after burn injury. Ann Surg 1986; 204:1–8.

195. Alverdy J, Chi HS, Sheldon GF. The effect of parenteral nutrition in gastrointestinal immunity: the importance of enteral stimulation. Ann Surg 1985; 202:681–684.

196. Keller GA, West MA, Cerra FB, et al. Multiple systems organ failure: modulation of hepatocyte protein synthesis by endotoxin activated Kupffer cells. Ann Surg 1985; 201:87–95.

197. Deitch EA, Winterton J, Berg R. Thermal injury promotes bacterial translocation from the gastrointestinal tract in mice with impaired T-cell–mediated immunity. Arch Surg 1986; 121:97–101.

198. Johnson DJ, Jiang ZM, Colpys M, et al. Branched chain amino acid uptake and muscle free amino acid concentrations predict postoperative muscle nitrogen balance. Ann Surg 1986; 204:513–523.

199. Smith RJ. The role of skeletal muscle in interorgan amino acid exchange. Fed Proc 1986; 45:2172–2176.

200. Kapadia CR, Colpoys MF, Jiang ZM, et al. Maintenance of skeletal muscle intracellular glutamine during standard surgical trauma. JPEN 1985; 9:583–589.

201. Manson JM, Wilmore DW. Positive nitrogen balance with human growth hormone and hpocaloric intravenous feeding. Surgery 1986; 100:188–197.

202. Bessey PQ, Dimick AR. Thermal injury following pituitary ablation: the importance of growth hormone. In preparation.

203. Brown GL, Curtsinger LJ, Brightwell JR, et al. Human epidermal growth factor accelerates epithelialization of partial-thickness burns. Presented at the Annual meeting of the Association for Academic Surgery, Cincinnati, November 1985.

204. Brown Gl, Curtsinger, LH, Brightwell Jr, et al. Enhancement of epidermal regeneration by biosynthetic epidermal growth factor. J Exp Med 1986; 163:1319–1324.

40

THE SKELETAL SYSTEM

JOAN E. HARRISON / KENNETH G. McNEILL

Nutrition is of considerable importance in the growth and preservation of the skeleton. The skeletal system of the human body has two essential but quite different functions: to provide support for the body and to provide a reservoir for the storage of bone minerals. The support function includes the protection of vital organs (e.g., the brain and the spinal cord) and the mechanism for movement. However, the bone minerals, mainly calcium and phosphate, are required for many metabolic functions essential for life. For example, normal soft tissue concentrations of calcium are essential for muscle contractility, cell membrane permeability, hormone secretion, and hormone activity. If necessary, bone mineral will be removed from bone in order to maintain these vital metabolic functions, at the expense of the skeletal support functions. Thus a consideration of the role of nutrition in the development and preservation of the skeleton must include the effects on calcium and phosphorus metabolism.

Dietary calcium and phosphate are essential. Vitamin D is important for the regulation of calcium metabolism. Vitamin A, vitamin C, and a number of trace elements are also required for normal bone metabolism. Alterations in dietary protein can affect calcium metabolism, and several trace element pollutants can cause bone problems. To establish the optimal diet, it is necessary to understand the factors that regulate bone metabolism, the alterations that occur in abnormal situations, and the requirement for these various nutrients in health and in disease.

THE STRUCTURE OF BONE

Gross Features

Bone is well designed to provide maximum strength with minimum weight. For body support, the central skeleton consists of the spinal column, which transmits the main weight of the body to the long bones of the leg and thence to the ground via

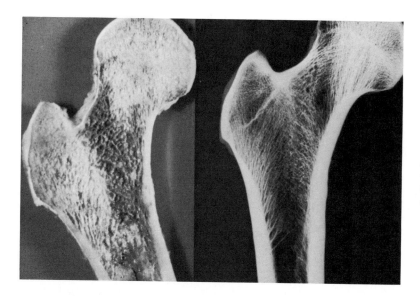

FIGURE 40–1. A section through the proximal end of the femur, seen by naked eye and by x-ray. The outer shell of cortical bone and the mesh of trabecular bone are visible; note particularly how trabecular bone is laid down along the lines of greatest horizontal and vertical stress. (From the collection of Dr. V. Fornasier.)

the bones of the foot. The long bones (Fig. 40–1) consist of an outer shell of dense bone, or cortical bone, and a central cavity containing a mesh of thin rods, trabecular bone, which connect to the outer cortical bone and to each other. In engineering terms, the cortical bone acts like the main I-beams of a structure, while the trabecular bone acts as the cross-bracing between the beams. In outer diameter, the long bone is smaller in the middle than at the ends, but the cortex is thicker in the middle. The trabecular bone is most obvious at the ends of the bones.

The structural analogy can be carried further. When a solid beam or plate is pushed from one side, as shown in Figure 40–2A, there are compressive forces in the outer layers on that side and extensive forces in the opposite outer layers, whereas the middle is largely neutral. For economy of material, it is possible to weaken the middle while maintaining the strength of the outer layers. This results in the ability to replace a solid beam by an I-beam (Fig. 40–2B), with the mass of material being on the outside. To meet stresses from all sides, the best structure is a hollow cylinder with some cross-bracing to give extra strength (Fig. 40–2C). This is just the shape of the

long bones, which have the cross-bracing supplied by the trabeculae. The bones are then able to cope with the sideways stresses put upon them by the tendons during muscular action.

To withstand the straight downward forces on the leg bones, for instance, the cortical bone has to be of a very mechanically strong material and, in particular, has to have a high compressive breaking stress, so that the bone will not crumble under the weight of the body. As shown in Table 40–1, its breaking strength is in fact much better than that of concrete, though not as good as that of steel.[1] Taking as an example the femur, for which the outer cylinder of bone has cross-sectional area of about 3 cm², the femur can support a straight downward force of 5×10^4 newtons, equal to that produced by a weight of 5 tons. Such forces are not met with under static conditions, but the breaking stress can be exceeded in traumatic accidents. For instance, if a stiff-legged parachute descent were made, limbs would be broken by the force associated with rapid deceleration; to reduce this force, the parachutist rolls as he lands, thus lengthening the contact time with the ground and reducing the instantaneous deceleration.

Buckling may be a greater cause of breakage than

FIGURE 40–2. A, If a metal sheet is pushed from one side, the further side will be extended while the front surface is in compression. There is a neutral plane with no stresses on it in the middle. B, The middle may then be thinned down for economy of mass, leaving an I-beam. C, If forces are from all directions, the preferred shape is a hollow cylinder (with possibly some internal cross-bracing).

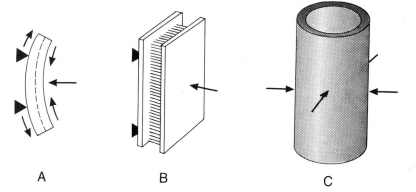

A

B

C

TABLE 40–1. *Breaking Strength of Bone and of Construction Materials*

	Compression Breaking Stress Newtons/mm²	Tensile Breaking Stress Newtons/mm²	Y* × 10² Newtons/ mm²
Hard steel	552	827	2000
Concrete	21	2	165
Cortical Bone	170	120	179
Trabecular Bone	2	—	0.8

*Young's modulus (measure of elasticity).

compression failure as a result of a straight downward force. A straw will bend in the middle if it is pushed down upon, rather than collapse like an accordion. To counteract such buckling in the bone, the mid-shaft is thickened so that it can withstand the applied stresses.

Mechanically one of the most vulnerable parts of the skeleton is the head of the femur. Here the main weight of the body is received by the femur but instead of this force being carried directly downward, the leg bones are about 5 cm outside the hip joint. This produces a large torque or shearing stress on the neck and head of the femur. To mitigate possible serious consequences of this stress, the trabecular bone in this region is so formed (Fig. 40–1) that it leads the stress down to the main shaft of the bone, in an analogous way to that in which flying buttresses on cathedrals lead downward the outward force due to the roof pushing against the walls, converting the outward force to a vertical thrust onto the ground and to internal stress in the stone.

The bones of the central skeleton, the vertebrae, ribs, and pelvis, in distinction to the long bones, are highly trabecular in nature. This provides greater flexibility or resilience, so that the bones can more readily withstand the repeatedly applied forces due to locomotion. However, the trabecular bone is more metabolically active than the cortical bone, and under adverse conditions the trabeculae may be lost preferentially. With no great amount of cortical bone to provide support, loss of trabeculae results in great loss of strength. With osteoporotic bone loss, for instance, a vertebra may collapse under the weight of the body above it (Fig. 40–3). Clearly, the lower vertebrae are mechanically more at risk than the upper ones.

Gross Structure

Bone consists of organic matrix, inorganic minerals, and cells. The matrix is 95 per cent collagen, and the remaining components of matrix contain protein polysaccharides (or glycosaminoglycans) and sialoproteins. The collagen fibers provide the mold in which the inorganic minerals are deposited as hydroxyapatite ($Ca_{10}[PO_4]_6[OH]_2$). The non-collagen proteins are believed to be important for the control of mineral deposition. The bone mineral provides 65 per cent of the total bone weight. Reinforced concrete has a similar arrangement of a poured filler on a preformed matrix, and in both cases the het-

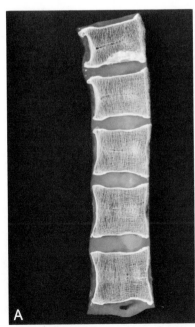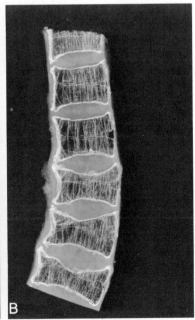

FIGURE 40–3. *In osteoporosis, vertebrae may collapse. A, X-ray of segment of the spine showing normal content of trabecular bone. B, X-ray of segment of the spine showing extensive loss of trabecular bone and collapsed vertebrae. Note the "codfish" appearance. (From the collection of Dr. V. Fornasier.)*

TABLE 40–2. *Mineral Constituents of Bone*

	As Per Cent of Bone Mass	Grams
Calcium	25.7	1146
Phosphate (PO₄)	34.5	1539
Carbonate (CO₃)	5.8	258
Sodium	0.65	29.0
Magnesium	0.32	14.4
Chloride	0.12	5.3
Fluoride	0.03	1.6
Potassium	0.02	0.8

Data from Pellegrino and Biltz.[2] Totals calculated based on a total bone mass of 4460 g.

erogeneous nature of the structural element helps the structural strength. Trace amounts of other ions (CO₃, Na, Mg, Cl) may exchange for apatite ions, affecting crystal size and shape (Table 40–2). Although it is known that the percentages of these various trace elements alter with age, the importance of their effects on crystallization is unclear.

Cellular Structure

Bone is a very active organ metabolically. The major cells producing this activity are the osteoclasts, which destroy ("chew away at") bone, the osteoblasts, which lay down new organic matrix, and the osteo-cytes, which maintain the integrity of mature bone (Fig. 40–4).

The osteoclasts are fully differentiated, multi-cleated, large cells that are instrumental in resorbing bone tissue. They are synthesized from cells of the hemopoietic tissue. The osteoclasts resorb bone by making and releasing enzymes that cause the actual resorption, with mineral and matrix always removed together.

After a resorption cavity has been formed, and while osteoclasts are still active in parts of it, osteo-blasts are formed on the new bone surface from primitive precursor cells and begin to lay down new matrix, or osteoid, which is subsequently mineral-ized.

After bone formation is complete, the osteoblast becomes imprisoned in the bone of its own making, and under these circumstances becomes an osteo-cyte. The osteocyte maintains the healthiness of mature bone and appears to be involved in the exchange of minerals between bone and soft tissue fluids.

Bone Growth and Remodeling

In embryo, the bone is initially laid down as cartilage, which is then mineralized. The calcified car-

METABOLISM

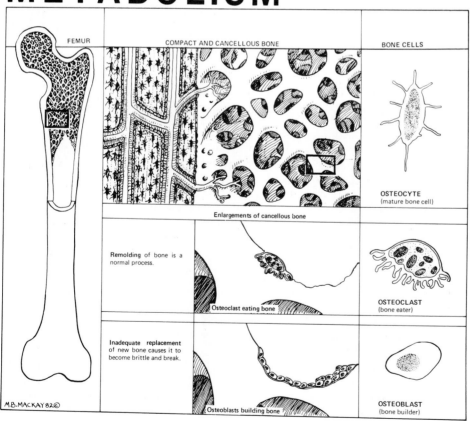

FIGURE 40–4. Diagrams of bone structure at different magnifications to illustrate terms of bone remodeling referred to in the text. (Courtesy of M.B. MacKay, Dept. of Art as Applied to Medicine, University of Toronto.)

tilage is vascularized and reorganized into bone; since the collagen of the new matrix is laid down in an irregular fashion (membranous bone), it has later to be reorganized into lamellar bone, as this type provides maximum strength.

During childhood bone undergoes extensive remodeling, with increase in length and outer diameter, thickening of the cortex, and enlargement of the marrow cavity. Growth in length occurs at the growth plates—the areas of cartilage at the ends of the long bones. On the distal sides of the growth plates, new cartilage is synthesized, while in the basal layers of the growth plate the old cartilage is vascularized and reorganized into new trabecular bone in the same way that bone is formed from cartilage in utero. The outer diameter of bone increases by the deposition of new bone on the subperiosteal (outer) surfaces, and the marrow cavity enlarges by resorption at endosteal (inner) surfaces. Trabecular bone is extensively remodeled in response to the enlarging bone and increasing body size. With the increasing thickness of cortical bone, reorganization from woven to lamellar bone takes place.

Haversian systems are formed in the dense cortical bone, providing a more adequate blood supply to the osteocytes enclosed within the bone. The haversian system consists of a cylinder of bone, positioned in the prevailing direction of the force, in which the collagen fibers are laid down in concentric layers around a central canal. The osteocytes in the haversian system are interconnected by canaliculae to each other and to the central canal.

With maturity, the cartilaginous growth plates fuse and longitudinal growth ceases. Throughout adult life, however, the other aspects of bone change continue but at a much slower rate. Thus subperiosteal new bone formation, endosteal resorption, and cortical and trabecular bone remodeling continue. The remodeling is focal. Each remodeling site is termed a bone modeling unit (BMU). At each BMU site bone is removed by osteoclasts, leaving a cavity; the osteoblasts are formed and synthesize new bone to replace that which was resorbed. In the cortex new haversian systems are formed and, on trabecular and endosteal bone surfaces, new layers of bone. In normal young adults, the volume of bone replaced in each BMU is relatively constant; the whole process takes 4 months. A volume of bone, about 100 μm in thickness, is resorbed over 1 month and then new bone matrix is deposited at a rate of about 1 μm/day. There is a delay of 10 days while the matrix matures prior to mineral deposition. This modeling process allows both bone repair and structural modification to meet changes in long-term forces. This focal remodeling can be compared to the process of replacing one brick of a structure at a time, allowing the building to remain functional during the repair process. With extensive physical activity, as in athletes, bone is strengthened by in-

creases in cortical and trabecular bone, while inactivity results in loss of bone mass.[3,4]

Bioelectrical Effects

Collagen fibers tend to be laid down in parallel lines, positioned to provide maximum strength. The mechanism for positioning the collagen fibers is believed to be governed by electrical forces engendered in the bone by pressure. Bone is piezoelectric; that is, when subjected to pressure the bone crystals will produce an electrical field (and correspondingly an external electric field will result in a distortion of the crystal). It is also known that free-floating collagen fibers will line up under the influence of an external electric field. It is hypothesized that remodeling of bone is programmed by additional stresses on the bone producing electric fields that cause collagen fibers to be laid down in such a way that the stress can be best resisted by the strengthened bone.[5]

Conversely, lack of stress, due to bed rest or to "weightlessness" in space flight, would result in a decrease in matrix formation and consequent loss of bone if resorption proceeds unhindered.

In practice extensive resorption is observed during the initial months of inactivity.[6] Possibly with inactivity there is reduced blood supply within the canaliculae as a result of lack of massaging of the blood flow within small vessels (compare the situation in veins). The lack of blood will cause devitalization of the bone tissue and its subsequent removal by osteoclasts. After some 6 months of inactivity, the rate of bone remodeling returns to the normal low rate: presumably a new steady state has been established at a reduced bone mass proportionate to the reduced forces applied to the bone.

CALCIUM AND PHOSPHATE METABOLISM AND HOMEOSTASIS

From the composition of bone, it is clear that calcium (Ca) and phosphorus (P) play important roles in the maintenance of the skeletal system. Both elements are common in the diet; it is certainly possible to have a diet that is Ca deficient, but it is difficult, with the modern Western diet, to have one which is P deficient. Indeed, it has been argued that dietary P is excessive and/or that the Ca/P ratio is too low.

Calcium Homeostasis

Almost all the calcium in the body is in bone (>99 per cent). The standard 70-kg man is stated to have 1000 g of Ca in him.[7] However, the small amounts of soft tissue Ca in intracellular (ICF) and extracellular (ECF) fluids are essential for many vital biological functions, and as a result the concentrations of Ca in soft tissue fluids have to be very carefully controlled. In blood the normal level is 2.5 mmol/L; changes outside the range of 2.2 to 2.6 will result in severe clinical conditions. The ionized calcium (Ca^{2+}) in plasma and ECF is 1.25 mmol/L with the remaining intravascular Ca largely bound to protein. Ca^{2+} in ICF is much lower, at about 1 μmol/L, and it is the changes in ICF Ca^{2+} concentrations that control such vital functions as muscle contractility, hormone secretions, and hormone responses. The tight regulation of ECF Ca^{2+} is maintained by parathyroid hormone (PTH), calcitonin, and the active vitamin D metabolite $1,25(OH)_2D$. These hormones, which will be discussed later, maintain Ca homeostasis by affecting Ca absorption, renal excretion, and bone mineral uptake (Fig. 40–5).

Thus bone plays an important role in maintaining Ca^{2+} soft tissue homeostasis. With insufficient calcium intake, homeostasis is maintained by resorption of bone mineral into the blood stream. Over short terms, for example overnight, loosely bound calcium is released and replaced the next day, but longer-term deficiency can lead to uncompensated loss of bone mineral. From the numbers given above, there are large stores of Ca in the bone, but a drain of 0.5 g per day would lead to a 30 per cent loss of bone mineral within 2 years.

Intestinal Calcium Absorption and Renal Excretion

Unlike the case of caloric nutrients and major electrolytes (Na, K, and Cl), intestinal absorption of calcium is incomplete. The caloric nutrients are completely absorbed and excess intake is stored as fat. With electrolytes, excess intake is excreted by the kidney. With Ca, however, intestinal absorption is regulated to meet body requirements and hormonal control of renal Ca excretion provides only fine tuning. Since calcium is relatively insoluble, excessive

intake and complete absorption would result in hypercalciuria and urinary stone formation or in abnormal soft tissue calcification. Bone appears to have only limited capacity to store excess mineral.

In normal adults, then, the absorbed calcium must equal the inevitable losses, which are about 0.3 g/day: endogenous losses into the intestine are about 0.15 g/day and a comparable amount is excreted via the kidney. Dietary calcium normally varies from 0.7 to 1.5 g/day, and the fractional absorption would then vary from about 20 to 45 per cent in order to replace the 0.3 g daily losses. The fractional absorption is increased with low dietary calcium intake, with increased need (as in growth, pregnancy, or lactation), and with excessive renal losses. Fractional rate of absorption is regulated by the synthesis of the active vitamin D metabolite. Materials in the gut itself may also affect absorption; bile salts increase calcium solubility, alginates may reduce absorption, and phytic acid may also play a part. Presumably the adaptive mechanism for Ca absorption will compensate for these nutrient effects.

The adaptation to calcium requirements operates only in response to long-term changes in body requirement. It is not concerned with preventing hourly fluctuations in soft tissue Ca^{2+} homeostasis. Following ingestion, the absorbed calcium is rapidly taken up into an exchangeable bone pool and then slowly released to soft tissue fluids as required to offset calcium losses during periods of fasting. Urinary Ca (about 0.15 g/day) represents a very small fraction (about 3 per cent) of the plasma calcium filtered by the renal glomeruli, while 97 per cent of the filtered load is resorbed by the renal tubules. Clearly, the kidney strives to conserve calcium and under normal conditions can play only a minor role in controlling hourly soft tissue homeostasis.

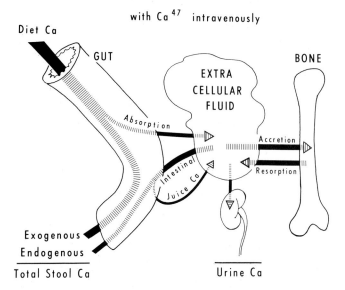

FIGURE 40–5. *Calcium goes from the gut to extracellular fluid, to bone, to kidney and, endogenously, back into the intestine.*

Phosphorus Metabolism

Phosphate is the major cation of apatite. A much higher percentage (30 per cent) of the total P of the body is outside the bone, however, than is the case with Ca. The extraosseous P exists largely as organic phosphate. The control of phosphorus metabolism differs from that of calcium metabolism, with less control at the gut and greater control at the kidney. Furthermore, soft tissue homeostasis is less rigid— the normal plasma level in adults ranges from 0.8 to 1.4 mmol/L. The average daily dietary intake is stated to be 2 g,[7] but it may be much larger if, for instance, drinks containing phosphate are taken. Of this phosphorus, about 70 per cent is absorbed through the gut and, in equilibrium, an equal absolute amount is excreted daily by the kidney. Renal P excretion represents 30 per cent of the total filtered load with 70 per cent resorbed by renal tubular cells. The kidneys play the major role in maintaining homeostasis. Once again, phosphate released with calcium from bone will influence plasma levels.

REGULATION OF BONE AND BONE MINERAL METABOLISM

Parathyroid hormone, calcitonin, and the active metabolites of vitamin D are involved primarily with the regulation of soft tissue calcium homeostasis. Their effects on bone are, therefore, primarily related to the transfer of mineral between bone and soft tissues. Growth hormone (through effects on release of somatomedin) and insulin have direct stimulating effects on bone growth, while glucocorticoids have complex effects involving bone growth and bone resorption. Thyroid hormone and sex hormones are known to affect bone metabolism in vivo, but their effects appear to be indirect. Also, there are a number of other systemic and local factors that either stimulate or inhibit bone growth.

Vitamin D

The active form of vitamin D is, in fact, a hormone,[8] but the term vitamin D continues to be used. The natural form of vitamin D, cholecalciferol or vitamin D_3, is produced in the skin by the influence of sunlight. Foods of animal origin may also contain cholecalciferol. Ergocalciferol or vitamin D_2, a synthetic analogue, is commonly added to food. It has a minor structural modification in the side chain from cholecalciferol, but the two forms are equally effective in man. In normal doses, vitamin D is not itself biologically active and undergoes further metabolism within the body. Vitamin D undergoes hydroxylation in the liver to 25(OH)D or calcidiol, and further hydroxylation in the kidney to either the active metabolite 1,25(OH)$_2$D (calcitriol) or 24,25(OH)$_2$D. Synthesis of calcidiol or 25(OH)D is not controlled, so that blood levels reflect levels of vitamin D intake. Calcidiol, carried in blood, is bound to a specific binding protein and, at normal blood levels, has no biological effect. The active metabolite, 1,25(OH)$_2$D, is a hormone: the synthesis of 1,25(OH)$_2$D in the kidney is tightly regulated to meet body requirements and it acts at target organs outside the kidney, on intestinal mucosa and on bone. Synthesis is stimulated by low plasma Ca^{2+} and by low plasma PO_4^{3-}. Plasma Ca and P are increased by enhancing the rates of Ca and P intestinal absorption and by increasing bone mineral resorption. 1,25(OH)$_2$D also heals the bone mineralization defect of vitamin D deficiency, but this effect may be secondary to improved plasma Ca and P homeostasis. PTH, which is secreted in response to hypocalcemia, stimulates synthesis of 1,25(OH)$_2$D, while the effect of hypophosphatemia is independent of PTH. Conversely, a rise in plasma Ca^{2+} and PO_4^{3-} inhibits synthesis of 1,25(OH)$_2$D and stimulates synthesis of 24,25(OH)$_2$D. The function of this latter metabolite is unclear.

Parathyroid Hormone

Parathyroid hormone (PTH) is produced in the parathyroid gland; its synthesis and secretion are stimulated by low plasma Ca^{2+} levels. Release of PTH into the blood stream results in an increased resorption of bone (with release of Ca and P to the blood) and in a slightly increased percentage of tubular resorption of Ca, but a decrease in tubular resorption of phosphate. PTH also stimulates increased production of 1,25(OH)$_2$D, which will increase intestinal absorption of Ca and P and further stimulates bone resorption. The effect of PTH on bone resorption is dependent on adequate levels of vitamin D activity. The overall result is an increase in plasma Ca together with a fall in P. The PTH supply is turned off when the Ca level returns to normal. Under normal steady state conditions, PTH will mobilize bone mineral resorption during periods of fasting, perhaps from areas adjacent to osteocytes, (in which case the process is called osteocytic osteolysis), and then the mineral will be replaced from mineral ingested with meals. Thus PTH is involved in the hourly control of soft tissue Ca^{2+} homeostasis, while adaptation of intestinal Ca absorption to meet long-term body requirements is controlled by synthesis of 1,25(OH)$_2$D, which is itself controlled by the mean daily levels of PTH activity that are required to maintain Ca^{2+} homeostasis. A net drain on bone mineral reserves, however, will result in stimulation of osteoclastic bone resorption (osteoclasts always remove both mineral and matrix) and replacement with new bone. Presumably, significant losses in bone mineral and altered bone structure stimulate the remodeling process, perhaps by disturbances in piezoelectrical effects.

It should be noted that the effect of PTH on renal tubular resorption of phosphorus, and thus of increasing renal P excretion, is essential in raising plasma Ca^{2+}. In resorption of bone mineral (and in increasing intestinal Ca and P absorption via $1,25(OH)_2D$ activity), plasma levels of both Ca and P would be increased. There is a tight reciprocal relationship between plasma levels of Ca and P: a rise in one ion is always associated with a fall in the other. Since plasma levels of Ca and P are normally maintained at supersaturation, a rise in either ion would exceed solubility, causing deposition of calcium phosphate or apatite. Thus, the effect of PTH on bone and gut would not raise plasma Ca unless the excess phosphate were removed.

Calcitonin

Calcitonin (CT) is a hormone produced in the C cells of the human thyroid. In lower vertebrates CT is produced in a distinct organ, the ultimo-branchial bodies. This hormone inhibits the resorption of bone, perhaps by reducing the effectiveness of osteoclasts. Plasma calcium levels appear to control production of CT; thus, whereas reduction of plasma Ca concentrations stimulates production of PTH, increase of plasma Ca stimulates production of CT and switching off of PTH.

Growth Hormone and Somatomedin

Growth hormone (GH) is secreted by the anterior pituitary. The classical effects of GH on bone growth are produced by the somatomedins. This group of peptides is synthesized in liver, kidney, and other tissues, and secretion is stimulated by GH. Somatomedin causes cell replication of many tissue cells including bone and cartilage cells, and also stimulates bone matrix synthesis.[9] Deficiency of GH causes dwarfism, while excess causes an increase both in the rate at which, and the extent to which, bone will grow. Excess GH causes giantism in children and acromegaly in adults. With acromegaly, the long bones widen and flat bones increase in size, affecting primarily the bones of the hands, feet, and jaw. As normal growth results in loss of bone from the endosteal surface and the need for remodeling of trabeculae which were anchored on this surface, there is a possibility that in adults excess growth hormone may result in a net thinning of the cortical bone and a loss of trabeculae. Both situations could lead to a loss of bone strength. If there is sufficient calcium in the diet, it appears that there is adequate replacement of bone and that strength is unimpaired.[10,11]

Insulin

Insulin is a hormone secreted by the islet cells of the pancreas and is responsible for controlling blood sugar. In vitro it stimulates bone collagen synthesis.[9] It also stimulates secretion of somatomedin by the liver and synthesis of the active vitamin D metabolite $1,25(OH)_2D$. Although osteoporosis is associated with diabetes, it is uncertain whether insulin deficiency is the direct cause of the bone loss (see page 718).

Corticosteroids

Cortisol and other corticosteroid hormones are secreted by the adrenal glands in response to stress and their primary function is to increase blood sugar. Corticosteroids also have anti-inflammatory properties and are used widely as treatments for diseases associated with immunological reactions; for example, with allergies such as asthma or in autoimmune disorders such as rheumatoid arthritis, systemic lupus, and ulcerative colitis. Excessive cortisol activity, either endogenously, as in Cushing's disease, or as a result of corticosteroid medication, is associated with bone loss. Corticosteroids inhibit intestinal Ca absorption, resulting in increased PTH activity and increased bone remodeling.[12] Corticosteroids also enhance the effects of PTH on bone.[13] In addition, corticosteroids stimulate somatomedin secretion by the liver and enhance the effects of somatomedin on bone; effects that would stimulate bone growth initially. However, corticosteroids also inhibit bone cell replication in vitro and, with prolonged exposure, inhibit bone growth.[9] Thus, in vivo prolonged excess corticosteroid results in increased bone resorption together with inhibition of new bone formation,[14] effects that would result in profound bone loss.

Thyroid Hormone

The general effect of thyroid hormone is to control the rate of metabolic activity in the body, and this is seen again in its effect on bone. Thyroid hormone has no direct effect on bone, but, like insulin and corticosteroids, stimulates secretion of somatomedin by the liver.[9] Hyperthyroidism makes the active bone modeling surface area much greater, both for resorption and formation. By itself this would not lead, except temporarily, to any change in overall bone tissue, but in addition there is a decrease in gastrointestinal absorption of calcium.[15] The result of this is a decrease in bone mass and weakening of bone. The increased rate of bone remodeling might enhance the effects of PTH on bone so that lower levels of PTH are required. This would affect the level of the active vitamin D metabolite (calcitriol), and therefore the absorption at the gut. In hypothyroidism the opposite is true—reduced turnover and increased gastrointestinal absorption, resulting in net bone gain.

Sex Hormones

Estrogens and androgens have no direct effect on bone,[9] but deficiencies of these hormones are associated with bone loss. The fact that the incidence of osteoporosis in women often occurs postmenopausally suggested many years ago that there was a relationship between sex hormones and bone. With the loss of sex hormones at menopause, more rapid bone loss occurs and estrogen supplements at menopause prevent this rapid bone loss.[16] However, estrogen therapy does not, over the long term, result in regaining of lost bone, but it can slow down postmenopausal bone loss. The known facts[17] are largely consistent with the idea that estrogen acts as a protector of bone against resorption (by making bone more resistant to PTH stimulation) and thus guards the female calcium reserves from the heavy calls made upon them in pregnancy and lactation. Estrogen is also associated with increased $1,25(OH)_2D$ activity and, secondarily, with increased intestinal Ca absorption. Possibly the increased $1,25(OH)_2D$ synthesis is secondary to higher PTH levels which would occur if bone were resistant to PTH activity. Estrogen also stimulates calcitonin secretion, inhibiting bone resorption.[18] Conversely, with losses of sex hormones following menopause, PTH levels fall as bone becomes more sensitive to PTH activity; secondarily, $1,25(OH)_2D$ synthesis is inhibited and intestinal absorption of calcium reduced. The reduction in calcitonin secretion would facilitate bone loss.

Nonhormonal Factors

Local and Systemic Growth Factors. Systemic growth factors have been isolated from fibroblasts (FGF), epidermis (EGF), and platelets (PDGF) and primarily stimulate osteoblast cell replication. Local bone-derived and cartilage-derived growth factors have been found to act like sometomedin to stimulate both cell replication and bone matrix synthesis.[9] There are also potent bone resorption factors. Osteoclast activating factor has been isolated from lymphoid cells and prostaglandins from bone and bone tumor cells.[9] These resorption factors may be responsible for the hypercalcemia associated with cancer.

Acidity. In addition to the role of bone as a reservoir for bone mineral, apatite can also be used as a buffer to maintain pH homeostasis. Thus systemic acidosis is associated with bone mineral resorption and negative calcium balance. Hyperparathyroidism is associated with systemic acidosis and may be, at least in part, the mechanism by which PTH stimulates bone mineral resorption.

Physical Activity. As stated above in the section on Bioelectrical Effects, the bone structure is maintained in response to the long-term forces put on it. With complete disuse there is profound bone loss, and, conversely, with a high degree of physical activity, as with Olympic athletes, a greater than average bone mass is produced.[3,4]

Summary

The complex nature of bone, its formation, its dynamic equilibrium, and the means of maintaining that equilibrium provide many opportunities for physiological errors to occur with resultant injury to the body as a whole. Specific diseases will be treated in the next section, but here we will review the kinds of things that can go wrong.

There can be deficiencies or excesses of calcium and phosphate and of other essential elements in the diet, and/or in the amount that passes through the gut wall. Insufficiency of vitamin D can prevent proper utilization of these elements, and insufficiency or excess of endogenous hormones such as PTH, calcitonin, or sex hormones can lead to a failure to maintain homeostasis. Kidney failure will have a profound effect on bone stability, as this organ controls not only Ca and P excretion but also the production of $1,25(OH)_2D$.

Any bone problem could lead to failure of any of the bone functions listed at the beginning. However, the bone has its set priorities, and appears to insist that the bone put its function as a chemical reserve as the first priority; to use its stores to maintain homeostasis at whatever cost to mechanical and support functions. Thus the bone problems that develop appear first in the mechanical functions of the bone, particularly in its support mode. That bones break too easily is a common symptom of bone disorder.

Many bone disorders result from organ dysfunction. In this book, we are primarily concerned with nutritional problems and their treatment, and many bone problems are not caused by nutritional defects. As a result, the discussions that follow concerning bone diseases and their treatment are selective, with emphasis being placed on nutritional aspects of disease and its management.

BONE PATHOLOGY AND PATHOGENESIS

There are four types of abnormal bone metabolism: (1) increased rate of bone remodeling or hyperactive bone, typically osteitis fibrosa, (2) defective mineralization or osteomalacia, (3) too much bone or osteosclerosis, and (4) too little bone or osteoporosis. Several of these metabolic abnormalities may simultaneously occur in the same individual. For example, too little bone may be associated with either the hyperactive or the normally hypoactive bone, while the mineralization defect of osteomalacia may be associated with either too little or too much bone. Nutrition can be the cause or a contributing factor in the development of these various types of abnormal bone metabolism.

Hyperactive Bone

In healthy young adults, bone remodeling is slow, about 3 per cent per year, with cortical bone remodeling at 2 per cent per year and trabecular bone more active at 10 per cent per year. An increase in the normal rate of bone remodeling is not necessarily deleterious. Provided that new bone completely replaces bone resorbed, the bone mass and bone strength will be preserved. However, if at each modeling site an imbalance exists between the amount resorbed and the amount of new bone formed, the rate of change in bone mass will depend on the rate of bone turnover. For example, during childhood bone growth is normally hyperactive with an increase in bone mass. Conversely, bone is hyperactive with profound bone loss during the initial months of complete paralysis. Hyperactive bone occurs in response to changes in the body's requirements for the bone support functions and also occurs in response to demands on bone mineral reserves.

PRIMARY HYPERPARATHYROIDISM

Parathyroid hormone is primarily responsible for raising soft tissue ionized calcium. In excess, PTH not only increases bone mineral resorption (osteocytic osteolysis) but also stimulates bone remodeling, that is, both osteoclastic bone resorption and osteoblastic new bone formation. Osteoclasts always remove both mineral and matrix, leaving a cavity which is subsequently filled with new bone; no significant bone mineral is ever removed leaving detectable unmineralized matrix. With new bone formation, however, there is a delay prior to matrix mineralization so that formation surfaces show a layer of osteoid, normally less than 10 μm in thickness, but with hyperparathyroidism, the unmineralized osteoid may be thicker than normal, suggesting either a delay in mineralization or an increased rate of osteoid deposition.[19] With primary hyperparathyroidism, in addition to the extensive remodeling, the bone may show a marked increase in primitive bone cells, termed "fibrous tissue," within the marrow cavity. This advanced stage of hyperparathyroid bone disease is called osteitis fibrosa cystica.

Although primary hyperparathyroidism causes hypercalcemia and hypercalciuria, it is not necessarily associated with a negative Ca balance and net loss in bone mass (see Fig. 40–10). PTH stimulates synthesis of the active vitamin D metabolite, $1,25(OH)_2D$, and, secondarily, hyperabsorption of Ca, which may offset the excessive urine losses. In a few cases, even increased bone mass or osteosclerosis has been reported.[20,21] Osteitis fibrosa may cause bone pain and tenderness, but more often the problems related to hypercalcemia and hypercalciuria cause the major complications, which are described in Chapter 19.

Treatment for primary hyperparathyroidism is surgical removal of the tumor or, in the case of hyperplasia, removal of three of the four hyperplastic glands. Following surgery, calcium supplements are usually prescribed to prevent postoperative hypocalcemia.

SECONDARY HYPERPARATHYROIDISM

Any situation tending to lower plasma and ECF Ca^{2+} will result in an increase in PTH secretion and an increase in rate of bone remodeling. PTH secretion is increased whenever the calcium intake is insufficient to meet calcium losses, causing a demand on bone mineral reserves to maintain soft tissue Ca homeostasis. Thus, inadequate dietary Ca or defective calcium absorption may result in insufficient absorbed Ca to meet normal or excessive calcium losses in urine and endogenous fecal excretion. In these situations, soft tissue Ca homeostasis will be preserved but hyperactive bone remodeling will result in net loss in bone mass. As with primary hyperparathyroidism, however, there are situations in which secondary hyperparathyroidism may be associated with a net gain in bone mass. This will be discussed further under Secondary Osteoporosis, below.

Osteomalacia and Rickets

Osteomalacia is characterized by defective or delayed mineralization of new bone. Histologically, the surfaces of bone are covered by abnormally thick, uncalcified osteoid. There is no failure in the production of bone tissue, but more than 50 per cent of the trabecular bone volume may remain unmineralized. In children, this mineralization defect is called rickets. In addition to the excessive osteoid, there is defective calcification in the basal layers of the cartilagenous growth plates, hypertrophy of the cartilage layer, and inhibition in longitudinal bone growth.

In children, the lack of calcification results in delayed growth and in weakening of the bones, which bend under the stress of the body's weight, resulting in bow legs or knock knees (Fig. 40–6). These deformities may last throughout life. The bone ends become enlarged, and this may be seen at the knees, wrists, and ankles. There may also be a muscle weakening, which, with the bone abnormalities, causes a waddling gait.

With onset of osteomalacia in adult life, the skeletal deformities do not occur; the symptoms are generally pain felt in the bones and weakness of the muscles. Together they make the sufferer very loath to move, and as a result he may be thought to be malingering. In children, radiology can readily demonstrate the rachitic features of widened and irregular demarcations of the epiphyseal growth plates. In adults, osteomalacia is not readily detected by radiology, but development of pseudofractures (also

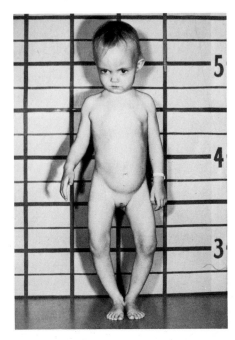

FIGURE 40–6. Vitamin D deficiency can result in rickets. In this case, the child has bow legs as a result of rickets. (From the collection of Drs. D. Fraser and S.W. Kooh.)

called Looser's zones or Milkman's fractures) is diagnostic. Pseudofractures are local decalcifications, a few millimeters wide, appearing on the side of or across a bone. Most commonly they occur in the upper part of the femur or the ribs.

VITAMIN D DEFICIENCY

Osteomalacia (including rickets) is caused by vitamin D deficiency, and can normally be cured by proper diet. The osteomalacic bone picture is usually associated with abnormal Ca and PO_4 homeostasis. With a mild degree of vitamin D restriction, serum Ca is normal, but serum P is reduced owing to secondary hyperparathyroidism while, with more severe deficiency, PTH is ineffective and hypocalcemia occurs. Mild osteomalacia, however, has been observed in bone biopsies in association with normal plasma Ca and P levels, but with low or undetectable levels of 25(OH)D.[22]

Since vitamin D can either be absorbed from the diet or made in the skin by the action of sunlight, both factors must be absent for there to be a deficiency. In cases in which sunlight is not available (for instance, to the bedridden) or inadequate, dietary vitamin D must be provided to compensate for the deficiency.

Because the need for vitamin D is well established, it is perhaps surprising that rickets is still a far from rare disease. Many reasons can be cited, however, ranging from residence in the north side of a highrise building, with consequent inability to put the child out in the sun in the winter, to food fads, to the failure of immigrants to recognize all the problems of a new land. Even in countries with plentiful sunshine, osteomalacia can be a problem as the inhabitants may carefully cover themselves to avoid exposure to the sun or stay indoors to avoid the heat.

In North America, osteomalacia and rickets is largely prevented by fortification with vitamin D_2 of dairy products and margarine. The recommended daily intake for children is 10 μg/day. Vitamin D deficiency can also occur, however, in spite of adequate dietary intake, if bowel disease causes malabsorption of fat and fat-soluble vitamins.

ABNORMAL VITAMIN D METABOLISM

Osteomalacia (or rickets) can also occur, in spite of adequate stores of vitamin D, as a result of defective metabolism of vitamin D. Physiological levels of vitamin D are not themselves biologically active; the vitamin undergoes hydroxylation at the liver and further hydroxylation in the kidney to produce the biological active metabolite, 1,25(OH)$_2$D.

Hereditary vitamin D–dependent rickets is a hereditary disorder developing in early childhood. Affected children show the classical features of vitamin D deficiency rickets, but the normal therapeutic doses of vitamin D (25 to 100 μg/day) are ineffective. The disease can be completely cured, however, by administration of the active metabolite, 1,25(OH)$_2$D, at a level of 1 μg/day. The disease is due to defective synthesis of this active metabolite. Vitamin D itself is also effective if given in massive doses of 1 to 2 mg/day. At these doses, vitamin D itself or the resulting high levels of 25(OH)D are also effective at the target tissues of gut and bone.

Acquired osteomalacia, due to abnormal vitamin D metabolism, is also associated with prolonged use of anticonvulsant drugs. These drugs appear to accelerate synthesis of 25(OH)D by the liver, quickly depleting vitamin D stores. The active metabolites themselves are not stored well in the body, so depletion of the precursor (vitamin D) results in depletion of the metabolites.[23] A moderate increase in vitamin D intake from 10 to 25 μg/day will cure the osteomalacia.

Severe liver disease might be expected to cause inadequate synthesis of 25(OH)D. Osteomalacia is associated with this disorder, but no evidence for defective 25(OH)D synthesis has been found.[24] The osteomalacia appears to be due to vitamin D deficiency secondary to malabsorption of fat and fatsoluble vitamins.

Similarly, osteomalacia or rickets is associated with end-stage renal failure where defective synthesis of 1,25(OH)$_2$D might be expected. Administration of 1,25(OH)$_2$D appears to correct the epiphyseal cartilage lesions of rickets but does not correct the bone mineralization defect, suggesting that multiple factors are involved in this situation.[25]

OSTEOMALACIA NOT RELATED TO LACK OF VITAMIN D ACTIVITY

Osteomalacia (or rickets) also can occur for reasons other than deficiency of vitamin D or its active metabolites.

Vitamin D–refractory rickets (or familial hypophosphatemia) is a sex-linked dominant hereditary disorder appearing in early childhood. It is characterized by persistent hypophosphatemia and severe bone deformities of rickets. Hypophosphatemic osteomalacia also occurs spontaneously in adults.

Phosphate supplements (4 g/day) appear to heal the epiphyseal cartilage lesions and improve longitudinal growth.[26] The excessive unmineralized osteoid of bone tissue, however, persists. The high doses of phosphate stimulate secondary hyperparathyroidism in response to the tendency toward hypocalcemia associated with high phosphate intake. The addition of small doses of $1,25(OH)_2D$ together with the phosphate supplements appears to be beneficial in preventing the secondary hyperparathyroidism. Adults with familial hypophosphatemia have osteosclerosis in spite of the persistent osteomalacia[27] (see Fig. 40–10).

FLUOROSIS

Osteomalacia is a characteristic feature of fluoride toxicity and in this situation the lesion is called fluorosis.[28] In addition to the extensive osteomalacia, there is excessive bone growth or osteosclerosis. Focal bone overgrowth or osteophyte formation at the place of insertion of tendons causes pain and stiffness of joints.

Fluoride (F) is readily absorbed and rapidly cleared from the plasma. More than 50 per cent of daily intake is incorporated into bone replacing the (OH) in apatite to form fluoroapatite. The remainder is excreted by the kidney. The fluoroapatite is more resistant to resorption than hydroxyapatite, a factor in the prevention of tooth decay. Fluoride also stimulates osteoblast and osteoclast activity. These effects of fluoride act directly on bone cells in vitro by mechanisms unknown. The reason for inhibition of bone mineralization causing osteomalacia is also obscure. Presumably the mineralization is only delayed, since prolonged fluoride stimulation also produces an increase in mineralized bone (Fig. 40–7).

In small quantities, fluoride is considered to be advantageous for the healthy growth of teeth in children, but in excess it can cause severe bone problems. These problems progress with increasing severity of the disease from vague pains to extreme sclerosis of the spine, with vertebrae fused together, ligaments ossified, spurs of new bone created, and bone reaching across between the radius and ulna.

The fluorosis may be the result of industrial processes, in which case the disease may show up in the workers and in the neighborhood, or it may be the result of natural excess fluoride in the water supply.

The degree of fluorosis is related to the concentration of fluorine in the bone ash. Normal values are around 1 to 4 mg F/g ash; mild histological and radiological changes are seen at levels above this range, while crippling fluorosis is associated with concentrations of more than 10 mg F/g ash. In terms of total bone fluorine, these figures translate to levels of 2.5 to 25 g F.

In industrial cases, correct management is the prevention of undue fluoride concentrations in the air and in dust by proper enclosure and ventilation, though it is appreciated that ventilation merely produces a dilute version for the neighborhood. In addition, medical tests should pick out any persons showing initial signs of fluorosis, and these should be taken off the job. In endemic situations, it may not be possible to ensure a fluoride-free water supply. In this case, reduction of the turnover time in the body would be beneficial. Meta-silicate of magnesium has been used to increase the fecal excretion of fluoride by 10 to 55 per cent.

Other Toxins. Osteomalacia has also been associated with other industrial pollutants or toxic substances.

Cadmium. A disease called itai-itai ("ouch, ouch") has been observed in Japanese exposed to cadmium environmentally.[29] The symptoms were bone pain and fractures, and histologically there was a bone picture of osteomalacia. Cadmium is largely retained in liver and kidney; significant levels in bone have not been reported. Since most patients also showed renal lesions with proteinuria and glycosuria, it is unclear whether cadmium affects bone metabolism directly or whether the bone disease is secondary to renal failure (see Renal Osteodystrophy, below).

Aluminum. Osteomalacia has also been reported in association with aluminum retention in bone. The association has been reported in renal osteodystrophy and in bone disease related to total parenteral nutrition.[30] These two disorders will be discussed in more detail later.

Vitamin D Toxicity. Excessive retention of vitamin D causes hypercalcemia, hypercalciuria, hyperphosphatemia, and renal damage due to calcific deposits in the kidneys. Curiously, with vitamin D toxicity, the bone histology shows osteomalacia together with osteosclerosis.[31] The mechanism by which this osteomalacic bone picture occurs is unclear.

Too Much Bone or Osteosclerosis

OSTEOPETROSIS

Osteopetrosis or marble bone disease is a hereditary disorder in which osteoclastic activity is defective. As a result, the extensive bone remodeling associated with bone growth is impaired. In its severe form, failure to enlarge the marrow cavity results in deficiency of the blood-forming elements of bone

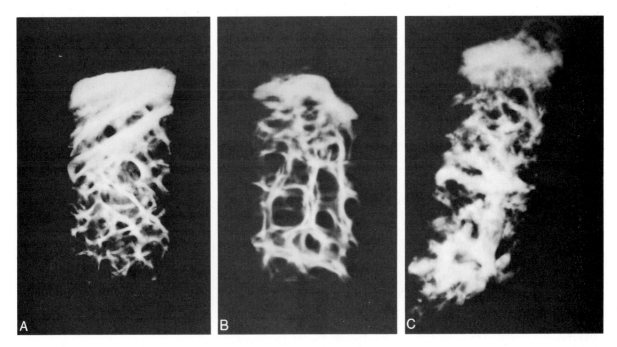

FIGURE 40–7. *X-rays of bone biopsy cores from iliac crest. A, Normal bone. B, Osteoporotic bone. C, Bone from an osteoporotic patient treated with NaF for 4 years. (From the collection of Dr. V. Fornasier.)*

marrow. In addition, failure to enlarge bone causes pressure effects on vital organs such as the brain and results in death in early childhood. With the more benign form, patients survive to maturity, but the lack of normal bone remodeling results in poor-quality bone, with recurrent fractures in spite of the excessive bone mass.

ACQUIRED OSTEOSCLEROSIS

Osteosclerosis is associated with other types of metabolic bone disease. As noted above, osteosclerosis is a common feature of prolonged fluoride toxicity (fluorosis) and of familial hypophosphatemia, conditions that are associated with the mineralization defect of osteomalacia. Osteosclerosis also occurs with renal osteodystrophy, the bone disease secondary to end-stage renal failure. Renal osteodystrophy has a mixed etiology and may show features of both osteomalacia and hyperparathyroidism. Typically, the sclerotic features affect predominantly trabecular bone of the spine, pelvis, and ribs, while features of excessive bone resorption affect the bones of the hand and the skull. Renal osteodystrophy is discussed further later in this chapter. Osteosclerosis and osteomalacia have also been reported with vitamin D toxicity.[31]

Too Little Bone Mass or Osteoporosis

Osteopenia may occur in association with osteomalacia or osteitis fibrosa (hyperparathyroidism), situations in which the calcium intake is insufficient to meet calcium losses and bone mineral reserves are depleted. The condition is called osteoporosis when there is no evidence of osteomalacia or osteitis and when the existing bone is essentially normal. Although the underlying disease is the reduction in bone mass, the diagnosis is usually made when the bone is so weakened that fractures occur with minimal trauma. Classic situations include breaking of the neck of the femur on stepping out of bed or spontaneous crushing of a vertebra resulting in loss of height and thoracic deformity (Fig. 40–8).

IDIOPATHIC OSTEOPOROSIS

Although there are many known causes of osteoporosis, in most cases no underlying cause can be identified. This idiopathic osteoporosis can affect persons of both sexes and of all ages, including children, but it occurs most frequently in older women (postmenopausal osteoporosis) and in the very elderly of both sexes (senile osteoporosis). Osteoporotic fractures are the most common problem of older women affecting an estimated 1 to 4 white women over the age of 60.

Those persons whose bones have weakened sufficiently that osteoporotic fractures (i.e., minimal trauma fractures) occur have on average 30 per cent less bone than normal young adults (Fig. 40–9). This indicates little "over-design" in the skeleton, that is, a very small safety factor in the engineering plans. In view of the fact that "what bone there is is good bone," and the high breaking stress of cortical bone, it implies that mechanical strength has been lost because of the loss of cross-bracing. Indeed, radio-

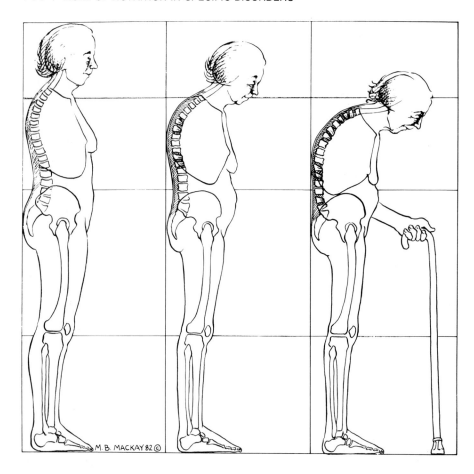

FIGURE 40–8. Progressive development of the "dowager's hump" with increasing osteoporotic fractures of the vertebrae. (Courtesy of M.B. MacKay, Dept. of Art as Applied to Medicine, University of Toronto.)

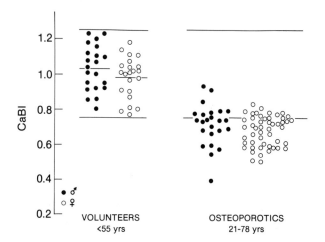

FIGURE 40–9. Osteoporotic patients have, on average, 30 per cent less bone mass than normal young adults. CaBI stands for calcium bone index; by definition, the average CaBI for normal young adults is 1.0. Note that, for both normals and osteoporotic patients, there is little difference in CaBI between the sexes although the only normalization made is that for body height and arm span. (Reprinted with permission from Harrison JE. In Cohn SH (ed). Non-Invasive Measurements of Bone Mass and Their Clinical Application. Copyright CRC Press, Inc., Boca Raton, FL.)

logically, the trabeculae are seen to be diminished and the bones that are predominantly trabecular are more likely to fracture—for instance, the distal ends of the radius, the proximal end of the femur, the ribs, and the vertebrae.

When the vertebrae are unable to take the stress, they collapse, often audibly. They may take up a typical "codfish" shape (see Fig. 40–3) indicative of the fact that the cortical sides of the vertebrae are still capable of holding weight, but that the absence of trabeculae weakens the central part. Complete collapse of vertebrae leads to a diminution in height of the individual and the characteristic upper thoracic deformity, "the dowager's hump," which is due to wedge-shaped fracturing (Fig. 40–8).

The diagnosis of osteoporosis prior to the onset of fractures is difficult. In agreement with the existing bone being essentially normal, all biochemical tests of bone and bone mineral metabolism are usually normal. Measurements of dietary intake and fecal and urinary losses of calcium may demonstrate a negative calcium balance, consistent with active bone loss; but with the normal low rate of bone remodeling, the daily losses (20 to 40 mg/day) would not exceed the accuracies of the measurements. A valid test of the only diagnostic abnormality, the reduced bone mass, is required. Conventional radiology provides qualitative information on bone mineral mass, but is unreliable unless the reduction is more than 30 to 50 per cent.

A noninvasive procedure for quantitation of bone mass is required.[32] Quantitation of cortical bone thickness has been made from hand x-rays. The density of forearm bone (radius and ulna) has been measured by x-ray or gamma photon absorptiometry. These methods, though probably accurate and reproducible enough, suffer from the major disadvantage that the bone measured is not that most at risk. Nor is it even of the type most at risk, for the long bones are largely cortical in nature, while the head of the femur and the vertebrae are trabecular. This mismatch is of particular importance because the rates of remodeling are very different in the two different types of bone; with more rapid changes in trabecular bone, measurements of cortical bone may not reflect trabecular bone status except after comparatively long times. Thus while both the radius and the vertebrae may be normal in unaffected persons, the radius may still show normal bone mineral content after the vertebrae have become significantly demineralized.

Dual photon absorptiometry (DP) and the more sophisticated technique of computed tomography (CT) should obviate these problems, as these procedures can be applied to quantitation of the vertebrae.

Direct measurement of total bone mineral can be made by in vivo neutron activation analysis (IVNAA). On exposure to neutrons, some of the ^{48}Ca isotope becomes converted to radioactive ^{49}Ca, which on decay emits a characteristic gamma ray of 3.2 MeV, which may be detected by sensitive equipment external to the body. Under standard conditions of irradiation and detection, the count obtained from these gamma rays is directly proportional to the stable calcium in the body and thus to the bone mineral content of the body. There is an advantage in measuring only the central part of the skeleton, since the peripheral skeleton contains much cortical bone, and being slower in changing its measurement dilutes the changes in the trabecular bone which is first affected. The central skeleton bone mineral measurement is useful for the diagnosis of osteopenia:[33] 75 per cent of patients with osteoporotic fractures have bone values below the normal range (Fig. 40–9). A few patients with hyperthyroidism, with primary hyperparathyroidism, and with osteomalacia have bone values within this osteoporotic range, while patients with familial hypophosphatemia have high values indicative of osteosclerosis (Fig. 40–10). Patients with severe renal osteodystrophy, however, have normal values owing to the combined effects of osteopenia and osteosclerosis (Fig. 40–10). Both methods, partial and total-body IVNAA, have been used in long-term studies of osteoporosis.[34,35] They have the great advantage that they really measure mineral content of a large part of the skeleton and thus are less affected by local changes in small portions of the skeleton.

These considerations of change of size of the individual bone suggest that one must be very careful in the use of such terms as bone density, bone mass per unit length, or bone volume. In osteoporosis, the cortex is thinned but, on the small scale, the density of the remaining cortical bone is normal. The density of the long bone as a whole is reduced, however, as the inner layers of cortex are replaced by marrow cavity. Conversely, the volume of cortical bone is reduced but the overall volume of the bone itself is largely unaffected. The effect of crushing would be to increase the apparent density of the vertebrae and of the mass per unit length, which could be misleading. Similarly, total body mass or cortical thickness or photon absorption can be misleading without normalization for body size. Clearly, a small normal person may have less bone mineral mass than a large person with osteoporosis—in fact, a 10 per cent difference in height is expected to be associated with a 30 per cent difference in bone mass, which, if lost by an individual, could result in osteoporotic fractures.[33]

Universal loss in bone mass with aging in both men and women and in all races has been demonstrated by all quantitative techniques. The age at onset and rate of loss measured vary depending on the quantitative procedure, but this universal loss in men is very slow, about 3 per cent per decade, and cannot, by itself, cause the 30 per cent reduction associated with osteoporotic fractures within the normal life span. With loss of female sex hormones following the menopause, women show an increased rate of bone loss of about 10 per cent per decade (Fig. 40–11). In women older than 60 years the rate of loss decreases. It is uncertain whether the osteoporotic fractures in the early postmenopausal years are caused by a higher than normal rate of postmenopausal bone loss or by the normal postmenopausal rate of loss superimposed on a suboptimal bone mass at the onset of the menopause. Thus postmenopausal osteoporotic fractures may be due to suboptimal skeletal development in childhood or to abnormal bone loss during young adult life. However, the CT measurements of trabecular bone of the vertebrae suggest that, at least in some cases, there is a large drop in trabecular bone following the menopause.[36]

Consistent with the definition of osteoporosis, 75 per cent of patients with osteoporotic fractures show the normal low rate of bone remodeling,[37] implying either very little or no active bone loss at the time of biopsy. Possibly these patients have developed the 30 per cent reduction in bone loss very slowly over a prolonged period of 20 to 30 years. Alternatively, the active disease process causing bone loss may have occurred at an earlier time and then subsided by the time the patient presents with osteoporotic fractures; a new steady state has been established, but with a reduced bone mass which is at risk of recurrent fractures. This situation occurs, for example, with disuse osteoporosis–during the initial 6 months following acute paralysis, bone histology shows hyperactive

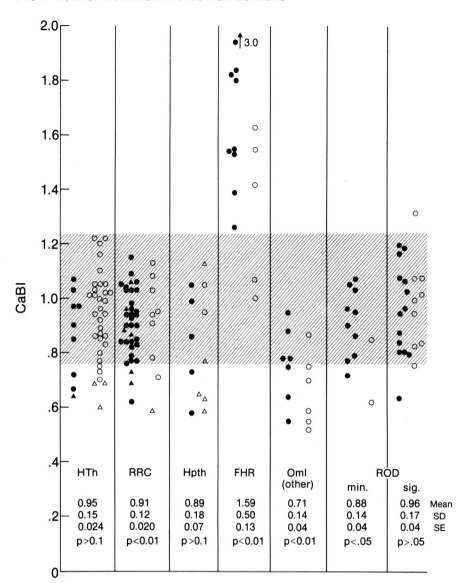

FIGURE 40–10. Calcium bone indices for a variety of diseases. HTh, hyperthyroid; RRC, idiopathic recurrent renal calculi; Hpth, hyperparathyroid; FHR, adults with familial hypophosphatemic rickets; Oml, other types of osteomalacia; ROD, renal osteodystrophy, minimal and significant. Solid figures represent men; open figures, women; triangles represent persons over 50 years of age. (Reprinted with permission from Harrison JE. In Cohn SH (ed). Non-Invasive Measurements of Bone Mass and Their Clinical Application. Copyright CRC Press, Inc., Boca Raton, FL.)

bone metabolism, and subsequently the bone picture returns to the normal low rate of bone remodeling but with osteoporotic bone mass. Similarly, during the more rapid bone loss following onset of menopause, the bone picture shows an increased rate of remodeling, while subjects more than 10 years postmenopausal have normal hypoactive bone associated with a slower rate of remodeling.

About 25 per cent of osteoporotic patients, however, do have hyperactive bone metabolism consistent with more active osteoporotic bone loss.[37] The response to treatment for these two distinct groups of patients would differ. With active disease causing rapid bone loss, treatments to suppress the rate of bone remodeling, that is, to inhibit PTH secretion, would be beneficial; but with only minimal bone loss or inactive disease, such treatments would have little effect.

In addition to aging and loss of female hormones at menopause, regional differences in the incidence of osteoporosis suggest that racial, occupational, nu-

tritional, or environmental factors also may be involved[38] (Fig. 40–12). Osteoporosis is more common in whites than in blacks and Asians, suggesting genetic factors. Since the integrity of bone is maintained by the long-term forces put on it, reduced physical activity may be an important factor in the age-related bone loss. Possible nutritional factors and environmental pollutants will be discussed in detail in following sections.

Juvenile Osteoporosis. Osteoporosis sometimes spontaneously appears in adolescents, and usually equally spontaneously disappears with maturity. The symptoms of this juvenile osteoporosis include nontraumatic fractures and bone pain. The patients have thin bones and may have vertebral collapse. Presumably (on the basis of the age), the disease is related to hormonal imbalance. Although symptomatic recovery occurs without treatment (and no treatment is known to hasten recovery), the subjects will retain the fracture deformity (e.g., loss of height). Curiously, bone mineral measurements of

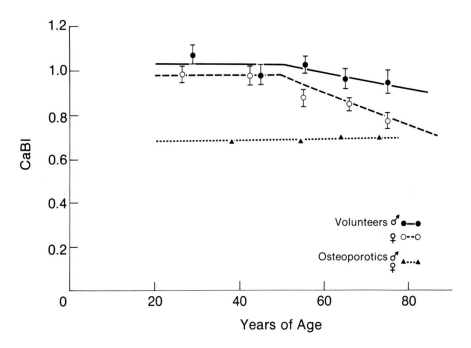

FIGURE 40–11. Cross-sectional data show, in volunteers, decreased CaBI values with age; in osteoporotic patients the CaBI values are independent of age. (Reprinted with permission from Harrison JE. Recent advances in osteoporosis: in vivo neutron activation analysis. Clin Invest Med 5[2/3]:161–162. Copyright 1982, Pergamon Journals, Ltd.)

the central skeleton reveal continued low bone mass (compared with normal persons with the same actual height).[39]

SECONDARY OSTEOPOROSIS

There are many known causes of osteoporosis—malnutrition, gastrointestinal diseases, renal disease, hormonal imbalances, drugs, and inactivity, anything that disturbs the normal homeostatic regulation of bone and bone minerals. Nutritional deficiencies of calcium, protein, vitamin C, and some trace elements (Cu, Mn, and Si) are known to cause osteoporosis. These will be discussed in more detail below. Similarly, organic bowel or liver disease causing malabsorption of essential nutrients will affect bone. A number of therapeutic drugs are known to affect bone metabolism directly or to inhibit calcium

absorption, for example, cortisone products, antacids, heparin, anticonvulsant drugs, and lithium treatment. Chronic alcoholism is associated with osteoporosis and may be related to malnutrition, to associated chronic liver disease, or, possibly, to inactivity. Osteoporosis may be associated with hormone excess, for example, hyperthyroidism (thyrotoxicosis), cortisol excess (Cushing's disease), or growth hormone excess (acromegaly), or with hormone deficiencies, such as sex hormone deficiencies (hypogonadism) or diabetes. Such endocrine disorders may be expected to affect bone metabolism, but bone loss does not necessarily occur.

Thyrotoxicosis. Thyrotoxicosis is a known cause of bone loss, but not all patients with excess thyroid function show such loss (Fig. 40–10). Indeed, in a series of 41 patients,[40] we found that the average

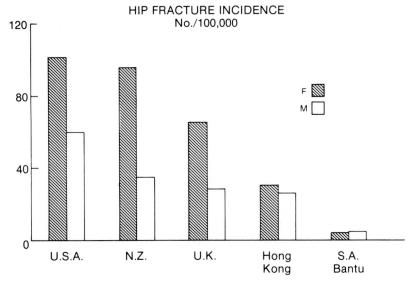

FIGURE 40–12. The incidence of hip fractures in the United States, New Zealand, the United Kingdom, and Hong Kong and among the Bantu population of South Africa. (Data from Gallagher et al.[38])

value of bone mineral (normalized for body size) was not different from that of normal individuals; however, 9 patients, 6 of whom were less than 55 years old, had significantly low values.

Excess thyroid hormone increases the rate of bone remodeling. As stated before, in the case of hyperparathyroidism, hyperactive bone will not cause a change in bone mass provided that new bone formation completely replaces bone resorbed at each remodeling site. If, however, there is a new loss in bone at completion of each site of remodeling, the hyperactive bone will accelerate the rate of bone loss. Thus hyperthyroidism will cause osteoporosis and atraumatic fractures in situations in which dietary Ca intake is inadequate, sex hormones are deficient (as in postmenopausal women), or physical activity is reduced.

With successful treatment for thyrotoxicosis, the bone loss can be reversed. We[40] have measured bone mass in 13 patients over 2 to 3 years following successful treatment with radioiodine. On average, the bone mass increased by 13 per cent, the greatest increases (up to 45 per cent) being obtained in patients with low bone masses prior to treatment. Thus, in fact, bone loss can be reversed by proper treatment of this secondary osteoporosis.

Diabetes. Diabetes is due to lack of insulin secretion. While osteoporosis has been associated with diabetes, the evidence of bone loss related to long-standing diabetes is not well established. In our study of 15 adults with juvenile-onset diabetes of more than 20 years duration and, in the majority of patients, with diabetic complications, the bone mass was reduced by only 5 per cent; only one patient had a bone mass below the normal range.[39]

Steroid-Induced Osteoporosis. Osteoporosis is a common problem resulting from prolonged high levels of steroid; these may be due to excess endogenous secretion of cortisol as in Cushing's disease, or to therapeutic use of steroid derivatives. Excess cortisol appears to disturb the normal tight coupling of bone resorption and formation by enhancing the effect of PTH on bone mineral mobilization and, at the same time, by inhibiting osteoblastic bone formation. For treatment with steroids, the doses should be kept as low as possible and measures to prevent or reduce bone loss should be considered. For example, dietary calcium supplements and, in postmenopausal women, estrogen supplements should be prescribed. Recent evidence suggests that pharmacological doses of vitamin D or its metabolites might be beneficial,[12] as vitamin D enhances Ca absorption and has been shown to counteract the inhibitory effect of cortisone on bone formation.[14]

Hypogonadism. Osteoporosis is associated with estrogen deficiency in women and with testosterone deficiency in men. Hormone replacement is beneficial in preventing bone loss, although complete reversal of osteoporotic bone loss has not been demonstrated. The mechanism of action is not understood, but sex hormones appear to have an indirect effect on bone metabolism since, in vitro, no direct effects have been demonstrated.

Disuse. Prolonged immobilization is known to cause profound bone loss and osteoporosis, probably owing to lack of the stimulation of weight-bearing and muscular action. After short-term disuse, as with astronauts or with wearing body casts during fracture repair, the bone loss can be reversed, but long-term disuse probably results in permanent loss.

TREATMENT OF OSTEOPOROSIS

A careful investigation for possible underlying causes of osteoporosis (discussed before) is essential. As in the case of thyrotoxicosis, successful treatment of the underlying disease can result in restoration of bone mass. For the majority of patients in whom no underlying cause can be identified, or in situations in which the underlying causes cannot be corrected, attention should be given to possible risk factors. Aging and genetic factors cannot be avoided, but advice on nutrition, exercise, and accident prevention is beneficial.

Calcium supplements (1 g/day of elemental Ca) are usually prescribed on the assumption that dietary intake or intestinal absorption is inadequate. Increased calcium intake will suppress PTH secretion and decrease the rate of bone remodeling. As noted above, this treatment may be beneficial for patients with hyperactive bone by inhibiting further bone loss but will have little effect on the majority of patients whose disease process appears to be inactive and who have hypoactive bone.

Estrogen is often prescribed for postmenopausal patients, since estrogen prevents the more rapid bone loss after menopause. To prevent the bone loss, however, the estrogen must be continued indefinitely, since bone loss will occur whenever the estrogen is discontinued. Long-term estrogen administration has been associated with endometrial cancer, but low-dose conjugated estrogen (0.625 mg/day) and cyclic therapy with progesterone appears to prevent this complication. Estrogen is most effective in patients in the initial postmenopausal period and is less useful in older patients in whom the rapid postmenopausal bone loss has subsided and a new steady state has been established.

At best, calcium and estrogen treatments will prevent further bone loss, but the bone mass will not be restored to normal (Fig. 40–13) and these osteoporotic patients will continue to suffer recurrent fractures. Many treatments have been tried in an effort to inhibit bone resorption or to stimulate new bone formation. However, with the tight coupling between bone resorption and new bone formation, any change in one parameter is followed by a compensatory change in the other, resulting in no net change in bone mass. Thus no long-term beneficial effects have been reported with prolonged admin-

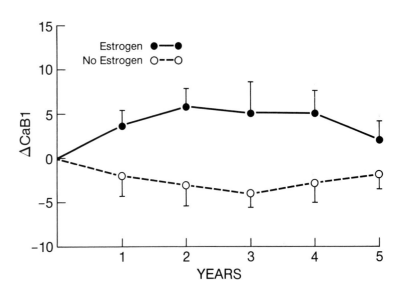

FIGURE 40–13. Patients with postmenopausal osteoporosis treated conventionally with calcium supplements (– – – –) show no increase in CaBI over 5 years. The use of estrogen together with calcium (———) is associated with a modest (6 per cent) increase in CaBI over 2 years, but the increase is not sustained.

istration of agents that inhibit bone resorption (calcitonin, phosphate, or diphosphonates) or with anabolic agents that stimulate bone formation. Effective treatment requires new bone formation to exceed bone resorption. In an effort to disturb in this direction the tight coupling between bone resorption and formation, cyclic treatments are currently under investigation. These sequentially stimulate sites of bone remodeling, inhibit the resorptive phase, and allow the normal amount of new bone to be formed. While such a therapeutic concept is interesting and, over the short term, some encouraging results have been reported,[41] it is possible that in the long term bone formation will continue to be coupled to the amount of bone resorbed.

However, net increase in bone mass or osteosclerosis is produced in a number of the clinical situations reported above, suggesting that bone loss with aging is not inevitable. Hyperparathyroidism, for example, is occasionally associated with osteosclerosis, and for this reason treatment for osteoporosis with long-term PTH administration is being investigated.[42] To date, however, fluoride treatment appears to be the most promising. Osteosclerosis is characteristic or prolonged fluoride toxicity (fluorosis), and fluoride treatment for osteoporosis has caused, in some but not all patients, significant increases in bone mass.[34,43,44] There are, however, some problems with fluoride treatment that need to be resolved before it can be recommended for routine use. The increases in bone mass are associated with the osteomalacic bone picture of fluorosis (Fig. 40–14), and it is not certain whether this abnormal new bone produces the required increase in bone strength. A decreased incidence of new fractures has been reported,[44] but further confirmation is required. Furthermore, in some cases, the fluorosis and the increases in bone mass are associated with skeletal symptoms of bone and joint pain and tenderness, suggesting fluoride overdose. Other adverse symptoms of nausea and abdominal distress also have occurred.

Results of fluoride treatment clearly demonstrate that osteoporotic bone loss can be reversed, but further investigation of the optimal fluoride treatment is required. With further experience, fluoride treatment may prove undesirable but, with evidence that osteoporotic bone loss can be reversed, it is very possible that an alternative treatment that is safe and effective can be found.

In addition to specific medication, patients will benefit by supportive and rehabilitative measures. Activity undoubtedly plays a role in the development of osteoporosis. With the onset of fractures, however, the related pain and fear of new fractures result in further reduction in activity. Exercise, as appropriate, is essential. Group exercise programs appear to be particularly beneficial in providing both rehabilitation and peer group morale.

Mixed Bone Pathology

RENAL OSTEODYSTROPHY

Abnormal bone metabolism is a common complication of end-stage renal failure. Owing to the multiple factors involved in this disease, all four manifestations of abnormal bone metabolism may occur in varying degrees. With progressive loss of renal function, the excretion of excess phosphate absorbed from the diet is impaired. The subsequent rise in serum phosphate and an associated tendency for serum Ca to fall results in secondary hyperparathyroidism. PTH maintains serum Ca and PO_4 homeostasis predominantly by increasing renal phosphate excretion (reducing renal tubular resorption of PO_4). PTH also increases renal tubular resorpton of Ca and stimulates bone remodeling, causing osteitis fibrosa.

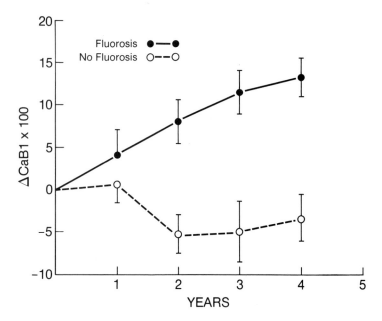

FIGURE 40–14. *Treatment with NaF for post-menopausal osteoporosis produced, over 4 years, an increase in CaBI of 14 per cent in patients in whom the osteomalacic picture of fluorosis is obtained. Without fluorosis, no improvement in bone mass was observed.*

With loss of renal function, synthesis of $1,25(OH)_2D$ is impaired, resulting in reduced Ca absorption and subsequent osteomalacia. Administration of $1,25(OH)_2D$ does not, however, cure the osteomalacia;[25] this is evidence that deficiency of this active D metabolite is not the only cause of this osteomalacia.

The retention of phosphate is usually reduced by administration of phosphate binders (or antacids); aluminum-containing antacids are usually prescribed. Owing to impaired renal clearance, abnormal aluminum retention may occur; this is reported to be an additional cause of the osteomalacia.[30] Retention of pollutants such as cadmium and fluoride may also contribute to the osteomalacia; osteomalacia due to trace element toxicity is not likely to respond to $1,25(OH)_2D$ treatment.

Both osteosclerosis and osteopenic fractures also may occur. There are many possible factors contributing to the osteopenia. In addition to the osteitis and osteomalacia, these subjects have chronic anemia, the inactivity of chronic ill health, and possible protein depletion due to dietary protein restriction. The osteosclerosis is not understood, but, as noted above, it is associated with hyperparathyroidism and with fluorosis.

TOTAL PARENTERAL NUTRITION AND BONE DISEASE

Total parenteral nutrition (TPN) is a life-saving procedure for patients with organic bowel disease that precludes adequate caloric intake. More than 2000 patients are maintained on TPN; most are able to lead a normal active life. Some patients with prolonged TPN, however, have developed abnormal bone metabolism; the reason for this is not understood.[45]

The features of the skeletal disorder include bone pain and fractures, hypercalcemia, hypercalciuria, and marked negative calcium balance together with low levels of serum PTH and $1,25(OH)_2D$. Despite adequate intake of vitamin D and normal levels of plasma $25(OH)D$, the bone histology shows osteomalacia; and, curiously, on withdrawal of vitamin D from TPN solutions the osteomalacia heals. However, no significant improvement in bone mineral mass has been observed in association with the healing of the osteomalacia, and indeed further bone loss and further fractures have occurred.[46]

Aluminum toxicity also has been suggested as a cause of the osteomalacia. Aluminum is a contaminant of the protein hydrolysate used in some TPN solutions. However, the osteomalacic picture has also developed when synthetic amino acids were used as the only source of protein. Other pollutants, for example, iron, strontium, and cadmium, have been sought but not found in significant levels in TPN solutions.

Although vitamin D toxicity can produce a similar picture of osteomalacia[31] together with hypercalcemia and hypercalciuria, normal serum levels of $25(OH)D$ do not suggest vitamin D toxicity. In this TPN situation, either the bone is abnormally sensitive to normal vitamin D intake or normal levels of vitamin D enhance some other underlying cause of the bone disorder.

PAGET'S DISEASE

Paget's disease is a benign tumor of bone. It is therefore not a metabolic bone disease, but is commonly included in the differential diagnosis of osteopenia and fractures. As with malignancy, its incidence increases rapidly with age, with cases being uncommon below age 40. Slightly more men than women get the disease.

The symptoms may simply be continuing slight pain. One patient of ours presented because his disease was so painful that, at 80 years old, he could no longer play tennis. The disease is characterized by very rapid turnover of bone in a localized region, and this location, being highly vascularized, can become so warm that the hand is involuntarily removed when touching it. The rapid turnover of bone may be accompanied by remodeling of the shape of the affected bone, giving rise to lateral bowing of a tibia or enlargement of the skull. The new bone laid down will be of the "woven" type, and there may be weakening of the bone at the affected site resulting in fractures. Pseudofractures, similar to those noted in osteomalacia, may also be present, though in the case of Paget's disease they will be in clearly abnormal bone. The rapid turnover is also accompanied by increased levels of alkaline phosphatase in the blood and increased urinary hydroxyproline.

Treatment is directed to reducing the rate of remodeling by administration of calcitonin, diphosphonate, or mithramycin. These agents inhibit bone resorption, and thus break into the cycle of resorption and apposition characteristic of the disease. Serum alkaline phosphatase and urinary hydroxyproline decrease as would be expected from the reduction of the rate of turnover. With diphosphonates an osteomalacic bone picture may be produced,[47] whereas with calcitonin, in the doses used, no deleterious effects have been observed.[48]

NUTRITIONAL CONSIDERATIONS

Dietary Calcium and Phosphate

It is well established that insufficient dietary calcium to meet body requirements will cause reduced bone mass; this calcium-deficient osteoporosis is associated with hyperactive bone due to secondary hyperparathyroidism. To prevent calcium deficiency, dietary calcium must be sufficient to replace inevitable losses in urine and losses by endogenous gastrointestinal excretions; additional calcium is required to support bone growth in childhood, fetal growth during pregnancy, and increased losses during lactation. In adults, the recommended Ca intake of more than 700 mg/day should be more than sufficient to meet the inevitable losses of about 300 mg/day.

Nutritional surveys[49] indicate, however, that the normal dietary intake of calcium in North American adults, and particularly in women, is below the recommended level; the mean value falls from 630 to 530 mg/day for women between 19 and 64 years of age. Furthermore, the ability to adapt to a reduced dietary intake of calcium appears to be progressively less efficient with aging. Thus, inadequate dietary calcium may be a causative factor in age-related bone loss. Current knowledge indicates that even the recommended Ca levels for adults of 700 mg/day are too low. Heaney et al.[50] have carried out calcium balance studies on perimenopausal women ingesting diets that reflected their normal daily nutrient intakes. In premenopausal women they found, on average, losses of body calcium with diet calcium intakes less than 1000 mg/day and, in postmenopausal women, calcium intakes less than 1500 mg/day. Premenopausal women with a low dietary intake of Ca, 500 mg/day, lost on average about 30 mg/day of skeletal Ca, equivalent to a total bone mineral loss of 1 per cent per year. In the early postmenopausal period, however, the same level of dietary Ca was associated with twice as much bone mineral loss. Estrogen supplements at the menopause prevent the accelerated bone loss but calcium supplements, at least over the short term (2 years), appear to have a similar beneficial effect.

It should be noted that adequate dietary Ca is a life-long requirement. Development of optimal bone mass during childhood and preservation of the skeletal mass during early adult life is just as important as preventing or reducing bone loss with aging. Osteoporotic fractures occur whenever the bone mass and bone strength are insufficient to withstand normal forces placed on them. With suboptimal bone mass at maturity, less than average age-related bone loss is required to produce a bone mass at risk of osteoporotic fractures. The population study of Matkovic et al.[51] has provided further evidence for the beneficial effects of life-long high intake of dietary calcium. In their study, a reduced rate of age-related bone loss and a reduced incidence of hip fractures were observed in a Yugoslavian community on a high Ca intake compared with a neighboring community on a low Ca intake. However, other factors should also be considered, since in this study, even for the population on a diet low in Ca, the incidence of hip fractures was well below that reported for the total population of the United States.[38]

As a preventative measure against age-related bone loss, increased intake of dietary Ca in both the pre- and postmenopausal periods would appear advisable; certainly levels of the currently established guidelines (700 mg/day) should be encouraged, and an argument can be made that these guidelines are too low, particularly for postmenopausal subjects. It should be noted, however, that the high levels recommended by Heaney et al.[50] (i.e., 1000 mg/day for premenopausal women and 1500 mg/day for postmenopausal women) are not entirely logical. For normal young adults in a steady state situation (i.e., without added requirements during pregnancy and lactation), the current recommended guidelines of daily Ca intake of 700 mg/day should be more than sufficient to offset inevitable losses of 300 mg/day. With losses of sex hormones after the menopause, women do undergo a period of more rapid bone loss, but this adverse effect of sex hormone deficiency appears to be primarily a net increase in bone mineral resorption, and only secondarily a reduction in intestinal absorption. The situation with estrogen withdrawal appears analogous to that of acute disuse, although to a less severe degree. In the initial phase of acute paralysis, there is profound bone loss, hypercalciuria, and secondarily reduced intestinal Ca absorption. There is no evidence that Ca supplements prevent the bone loss, and in patients with hypercalciuria, such supplementation would be harmful.

The excess phosphate together with the relatively low dietary calcium was considered a further contributing factor to age-related bone loss. Animal studies have provided evidence to support this possibility,[52,53] but in the clinical situation excess phosphate does not appear to have a deleterious effect.[50]

Despite the lack of convincing evidence for the requirement of calcium supplementation in normal pre- and postmenopausal women, it appears to be a reasonable recommendation. There is no evidence that Ca supplements are harmful (except in disorders associated with hypercalciuria). With aging, there would be an increased incidence of diseases associated with inhibition of Ca absorption, and in these situations additional dietary Ca would be helpful. Patients with gastrointestinal disorders of achlorhydria, gastrectomy, partial small bowel resection, mucosal atrophy, or lactose intolerance would benefit from additional dietary Ca. Similarly, with drug therapy, such as corticosteroids, antacids, anticonvulsant drugs, and some antibiotics, dietary Ca should be increased. It must be emphasized, however, that hypercalcemia and hypercalciuria are contraindications to excess dietary calcium because, in these situations, it increases the risk of kidney and soft tissue calcification. Hypercalciuria occurs as a result of rapid bone loss that is not secondary to deficient Ca intake; for example, bone loss associated with primary hyperparathyroidism, hyperthyroidism, some types of cancer, vitamin D toxicity with paralysis, or immobilization. Additional dietary calcium for patients with these disorders would be harmful.

Protein and Other Caloric Nutrients

Adequate dietary protein is essential for the development and preservation of the organic matrix of bone. The common North American diet, however, is high in protein, so that, with normal bowel function, protein malnutrition is an unlikely cause of osteoporosis. On the other hand, excessively high protein intake appears to have a deleterious effect on bone mass. Volunteers fed protein diets of 100 g/day for many months showed increased urinary Ca excretion without compensatory increases in intestinal Ca absorption.[54] Heaney et al.[50] also reported in perimenopausal women an increase in urinary Ca

losses equivalent to a loss in bone mass of 1 per cent per year on a diet containing protein 50 per cent above the average intake of 70 g/day. This deleterious effect of excess protein is not understood but may be related to the increased acid load or to increased sulfate from metabolism of the sulfated aminoacids. Moderation in dietary protein would appear to be advisable, although limited protein intake (e.g., in a strict vegetarian diet) is not encouraged.

For preservation of bone mass, total caloric restriction, as in weight reduction programs, is not necessarily beneficial. Age-related osteoporosis is more common in thin women than in overweight subjects.[55] Body weight and particularly muscle mass may be beneficial in maintaining bone strength because they put additional force on the skeleton. There is also the suggestion that fat stores are useful in the postmenopausal subjects, as fat stores synthesize estrogen derivatives from androgens secreted by the adrenal glands.[56] Certainly severe weight reduction seen, for example, with anorexia nervosa is detrimental presumably due to a related loss of ovarian function.

Vitamins

Adequate intakes of vitamins A, D, and C are essential for normal bone metabolism, but there is no convincing evidence that increased intake of these vitamins is of any additional value.

VITAMIN D

Complete vitamin D deficiency causes the classic bone picture of osteomalacia with hypocalcemia and hyperphosphatemia associated with "functional hypoparathyroidism." Mild vitamin D deficiency may cause a bone picture and serum biochemistry indistinguishable from secondary hyperparathyroidism. Limited intake of vitamin D over a prolonged period together with inadequate dietary Ca or reduced intestinal absorption of Ca may contribute to the development of osteoporosis.[57]

Children are stated to require 2.5 to 5 μg/day of vitamin D, although the recommended level of intake is 10 μg/day. A similar intake is recommended in adults during periods of additional bone mineral requirements (e.g., pregnancy and lactation). During normal periods of a steady state, adults are believed to require about 5 μg/day, although there are no data to support this value. Much of the daily vitamin D requirement can be met by synthesis in the skin, but in northern countries (and conversely southern countries in the southern hemisphere) fortification of food with vitamin D is helpful. There is, however, increasing evidence that, with aging, some degree of vitamin D deficiency is not uncommon. Some 5 per cent of patients investigated for osteoporosis are found to have osteomalacia on bone biopsy, and a larger number have hyperkinetic bone history consistent with secondary hyperparathyroidism.[22] This vitamin D deficiency in the geriatric population may be related to reduced exposure to sunlight and avoidance of vitamin D–fortified foods. In addition, some degree of vitamin D malabsorption may be more common with aging.

Vitamin D status can be determined by measurement of plasma levels of 25(OH)D: the normal range is 35 to 100 nmol/L, and levels below this range are indicative of inadequate vitamin D status. As a preventative measure, however, a generalized increase in the use of vitamin D supplementation might be recommended, since there is a large safety factor with toxic levels of vitamin D being about 100 times the basal requirements. Certainly, vitamin D deficiency should be avoided and, for all age groups, 10 μg/day of vitamin D/day from all sources should be adequate to maintain appropriate plasma levels of 25(OH)D.

Megadoses of vitamin D are toxic, producing hypercalcemia, hypercalciuria, and soft tissue calcification. The daily doses for symptomatic toxicity vary on an individual basis and are usually between 600 and 2500 μg. The toxicity is due to the direct effect of $25(OH)_2D$ which increases in plasma proportional to the excess dietary vitamin D intake. Excess vitamin D is stored in fat so that toxic plasma levels of 25(OH)D, and related hypercalcemia, will persist for many weeks after vitamin D withdrawal. High doses of 25(OH)D and $1,25(OH)_2D$ will also produce the typical features of vitamin D toxicity but, with these metabolites, toxicity subsides more quickly (within 1 week of 25(OH)D, and within a few days of $1,25(OH)_2D$ withdrawal). Vitamin D toxicity occurs occasionally in individuals ingesting megavitamins but, more commonly, occurs with pharmacological doses of vitamin D or D metabolites for treatment of hypoparathyroidism, renal osteodystrophy and various types of resistant rickets, since effective vitamin D doses for treatment of these disorders are in the subtoxic range.

Supraphysiological doses of vitamin D, 25(OH)D and $1,25(OH)_2D$ for treatment of osteoporosis have been investigated but with no consistent beneficial effects, and possibly with adverse effects. These treatments were used primarily to enhance intestinal Ca absorption and, for this effect, subtoxic doses are required. The classic features of vitamin D toxicity are well documented, but subclinical toxicity is more difficult to detect; it may cause mild hypercalciuria without hypercalcemia and also may result in renal or arterial calcification. In any event, no improvement in osteoporotic bone mass has been reported with any of the vitamin D treatments, and in some studies further bone loss has been reported.[58] A recent study using $1,25(OH)_2D$ treatment[59] reported reduced incidence of further osteoporotic fractures, but, without further experience, the use of pharmacological doses of vitamin D or D metabolites for prevention or treatment of osteoporosis is not recommended.

VITAMIN A—RETINOL

Vitamin A is essential for normal bone remodeling. In growing animals vitamin A deficiency results in extensive bone overgrowth and failure of the normal marrow cavity enlargement. Conversely, excess vitamin A causes profound resorption of cartilage and bone. Retinol appears to enhance release of proteolytic enzymes involved in the solubilization of cartilage and bone matrix.[60] Adequate levels of vitamin A are essential, but hypervitaminosis A is detrimental.

VITAMIN C—ASCORBIC ACID

It has been recognized for a long time that vitamin C, a natural constituent of citrus fruits, is essential for normal bone formation. Vitamin C deficiency is the cause of scurvy, a condition of osteoporotic bone with loss of teeth and failure to repair fractures. In British ships, scurvy used to be a common problem among sailors and was eliminated by the provision of lime juice—a practice that led to the term "limey" for British sailors. The vitamin is essential for collagen synthesis. Clearly, an adequate intake of vitamin C is essential. Again, however, there is no evidence that excess doses of vitamin C have any additional benefit.

Trace Elements

ESSENTIAL TRACE ELEMENTS

Copper, manganese, zinc, and silicon are essential for normal bone metabolism.[61,62] Copper deficiency causes an osteoporotic bone picture with thin cortices and fractures. The existing bone is of normal composition, but osteoblast activity is reduced. The deficiency results in reduced activity of copper-containing enzymes essential for collagen synthesis.

Manganese deficiency also decreases the activity of some enzymes involved in cartilage production, causing retarded bone growth with shortening and bowing of the legs.

Zinc is known to be essential in such functions as wound healing, but zinc deficiency also affects bone growth, presumably by inhibition of collagen and matrix synthesis.

Silicon also is essential for normal collagen formation.

In the average North American diets, these essential trace elements are normally present in sufficient quantities, but supplements may be required with diseases causing a malabsorption syndrome. They are also essential requirements of total parenteral nutrition.

FLUORIDE

Fluoride is not considered an essential trace element, but the value of fluoride in the prevention of age-related bone loss requires further consideration. Toxic doses of fluoride (> 20 mg/day) over prolonged periods of time are known to cause the osteosclerotic picture of fluorosis, and comparable fluoride doses have been shown to reverse bone loss of osteoporotic patients (see Treatment of Osteoporosis, earlier in this chapter). It is possible that life-long intake of fluoride, well below toxic levels, may have a beneficial effect in prevention of age-related osteoporosis.

Fluoride at 1 ppm (about 2 mg/day) is commonly added to the water supply since, at this concentration, the incidence of dental caries is reduced without development of dental mottling or the osteosclerotic manifestations of fluorosis. The value of life-long intake at this low level of fluoride on preservation of bone mass is unknown, but in individuals with fluoride levels above 3 ppm the incidence of osteoporotic fractures is reported to be significantly reduced as compared with that in individuals whose fluoride levels are below 1.0 ppm.[63] Similar conclusions have been reached in other studies.[64] It is of interest that fluoride is reported to be beneficial in the prevention of soft tissue calcification[63] as well as in the preservation of bone mass and bone strength. In rat studies, fluoride inhibits renal and aortic calcification.[65,66] In one population study,[67] but not in others,[64,68] fluoride levels in drinking water were negatively correlated with the incidence of death due to cardiovascular disease. Clearly, there is now sufficient evidence to suggest that life-long intake of fluoride is beneficial, but much more research is required to establish optimal levels since excessive amounts are undoubtedly toxic.

DRUGS

Osteoporosis has been associated with alcohol abuse,[69] excessive caffeine intake,[50] and smoking.[54,55,70,71] It is uncertain whether these drugs have direct effects on bone or merely reflect reduced intake of dietary Ca, other forms of malnutrition or reduced physical activity. Without further knowledge, however, moderation in the use of these drugs should be encouraged.

Summary

Nutrition plays an important role in the prevention or treatment of skeletal disease. In addition to total calories and sufficient protein, adequate intake of the bone minerals (Ca and PO_4), vitamins A, D and C, and essential trace elements (Cu, Mn, Zn, and Si) are required for normal bone metabolism. In diseases affecting intestinal absorption (or malabsorption), increased intake of these nutrients might be required. For the preventon of age-related osteoporosis, the current recommended guidelines for dietary calcium may be too low, while the excessive intake of phosphate in the standard North American diet does not appear to be deleterious. Although increased dietary calcium is recommended for the prevention of bone loss, it must be noted that, with clinical problems associated with hypercalcemia or hypercalciuria, such treatment can be harmful. The current recommendations for vitamin D intake in children and pregnant women probably should be extended to include the total population or at least the female population, but there is no evidence to support the use of pharmacological doses of any of the vitamins. In addition to the essential trace elements, fluoride appears to be beneficial, although the current level of fluoride supplementation in drinking water (1 ppm) may not be optimal. Excessive intakes of protein, caffeine, alcohol, or nicotine should be discouraged.

It should be noted, however, that our understanding of bone metabolism and the role of nutrition in health and disease is far from complete. With further research, some of the dogma of today may well be discarded.

References

1. Cameron JR, Skofronick JG. Medical Physics. New York, John Wiley, 1978.
2. Pellegrino ED, Biltz RM. The composition of human bone in uremia. Medicine 1965; 44:397–418.
3. Nilsson BE, Westlin NE. Bone density in athletes. Clin Orthop 1971; 77:179–182.
4. Nilsson BE, Anderson SM, Havdrup T, et al. Ballet-dancing and weight-lifting—effects on BMC. Am J Roentgenol 1978; 131:539–553.
5. Bassett CAL. Biophysical principles affecting bone structure. In Bourne GH (ed). The Biochemistry and Physiology of Bone. 2nd ed. New York, Academic Press, 1971: 1–76.
6. Harris WH, Heaney RP. Skeletal renewal and metabolic bone disease. N Engl J Med 1969; 280:193–202, 253–259, 303–311.
7. Report on the Task Group on Reference Man. International Commission on Radiological Protection. No. 23. Oxford, Pergamon Press, 1975.
8. DeLuca HF, Schnoes HK. Vitamin D: recent advances. Ann Rev Biochem 1983; 52:411–439.
9. Canalis E. The hormonal and local regulation of bone formation. Endocrinol Rev 1983; 4:62–77.
10. Riggs BL, Randall RV, Wahner HW, et al. The nature of the metabolic bone disorder in acromegaly. J Clin Endocrinol Metab 1972; 34:911–918.
11. Doyle FH. Radiologic assessment of endocrine effects on bone. Radiol Clin North Am 1967; 5:289–302.
12. Hahn TJ. Corticosteroid-induced osteopenia. Arch Intern Med 1978; 138:882–885.
13. Ng B, Hekkelman JW, Heersche JNM. The effect of cortisol on the adenosine 3',5'-monophosphate response to parathyroid hormone of bone in vitro. Endocrinology 1979; 104:1130.
14. Tam CS, Wilson DR, Hitchman AJW, et al. Protective effect of vitamin D_2 on bone apposition from the inhibitory action of hydrocortisone in rats. Calcif Tiss Int 1981; 33:167–172.
15. Swaminathan R, Care AD. The effect of thyroxine administration on intestinal calcium absorption and calcium binding protein activity in the chick. Calcif Tiss Res 1975; 17:257–261.
16. Lindsay R, Hart DM, Aitken JM, et al. Long term prevention

of postmenopausal osteoporosis by estrogen. Lancet 1976; *1*:1038–1041.

17. Heaney RP, Recker RR, Saville PD. Menopausal changes in calcium balance performance. J Lab Clin Med 1978; *92*:953.

18. Stevenson JC. Regulation of calcitonin and parathyroid hormone secretion by estrogens. Maturitas 1982; *4*:1–7.

19. Tam CS, Wilson DR, Harrison JE. The effect of parathyroid extract (PTE) on bone apposition and the interaction between parathyroid hormone and vitamin D. J Min Electro Metab 1980; *3*:74–80.

20. Aitken RE, Kerr JL, Lloyd HM. Primary hyperparathyroidism with osteosclerosis and calcification in articular cartilage. Am J Med 1964; *37*:813–820.

21. Templeton AW, Jaconette JR, Ormond RS. Localized osteosclerosis in hyperparathyroidism. Radiology 1962; *78*:955–957.

22. Parfitt AM, Gallagher JC, Heaney RP. Vitamin D and bone health in the elderly. Am J Clin Nutr 1982; *36*:1014–1031.

23. Hahn TJ, Birge SJ, Sharp CR, et al. Phenobarbital-induced alterations in vitamin D metabolism. J Clin Invest 1972; *51*:741–747.

24. Recker RR, Maddrey W, Herlong F, et al. Primary biliary cirrhosis and alcoholic cirrhosis as examples of chronic liver disease associated with bone disease. *In* Frame B, Potts JT Jr (eds). Clinical Disorders of Bone and Mineral Metabolism. Amsterdam, Excerpta Medica, 1983: 227–231.

25. Coburn JW, Sherrard DJ, Ott SA, et al. Use of active vitamin D sterols in end-stage renal failure. *In* Frame B, Potts JT Jr (eds). Clinical Disorders of Bone and Mineral Metabolism. Amsterdam, Excerpta Medica, 1983: 263–272.

26. Glorieux FH. Diagnosis and management of hypophosphatemic disorders. *In* Frame B, Potts JT Jr (eds). Clinical Disorders of Bone and Mineral Metabolism. Amsterdam, Excerpta Medica 1983: 438–446.

27. Harrison JE, Cumming WA, Fornasier V, et al. Increased bone mineral content in young adults with familial hypophosphatemic vitamin D refractory rickets. Metabolism 1976; *25*:33–40.

28. Schlatter CH. Metabolism and toxicology of fluorides. *In* Courvoisier B, Conath A, Baud CA (eds). Fluoride and Bone. Bern, Hans Huber, 1978: 1–21.

29. Murata I, Hirono T, Saeki Y, et al. Cadmium enteropathy, renal osteomalacia ('itai itai' disease in Japan). Bull de la Societe Internationale de Chirurgie 1970; *29*:34–42.

30. Coburn J, Kanis J, Popovtzer M, et al. Pathophysiology and treatment of uremic bone disease. Calcif Tissue Int 1983; *35*:712–714.

31. Ham AW, Lewis MD. Hypervitaminosis D rickets: the action of vitamin D. Br J Exp Path 1934; *15*:228–234.

32. Cohn SH (ed). Non-Invasive Measurements of Bone Mass and Their Clinical Application. Boca Raton, FL, CRC Press, 1981: 5–50.

33. Harrison JE, McNeill KG, Hitchman AJ, et al. Bone mineral measurements of the central skeleton by in vivo neutron activity analysis for routine investigation of osteopenia. Invest Radiol 1979; *14*:27–34.

34. Harrison JE, McNeill KG, Sturtridge WC, et al. Three year changes in bone mineral mass of postmenopausal osteoporotics based on neutron activity analysis of the central third of the skeleton. J Clin Endocrinol Metab 1981; *52*:751–758.

35. Chesnut CH, Nelp WD, Baylink DJ, et al. Effect of methandrostenolone on postmenopausal bone wasting as assessed by changes in total body mineral mass. Metabolism 1977; *26*:267–277.

36. Genant HK, Cann CE, Ettinger G, et al. Quantitative computed tomography of vertebral spongiosa: a sensitive method for detecting early bone loss after oophorectomy. Ann Intern Med 1982; *97*:699–705.

37. Meunier PJ, Brianson D, Vignon E. Effects of combined therapy with sodium fluoride–vitamin D–calcium on vertebral fracture risk and bone histology in osteoporosis. *In* Deluca HF, Frost HM, et al. (eds). Osteoporosis—Recent Advances in Pathogenesis and Treatment. Baltimore, University Park Press, 1981: 449–456.

38. Gallagher JC, Melton LF, Riggs BL, et al. Epidemiology of fractures of the proximal femur in Rochester, Minnesota. Clin Orthop Rel Res 1980; *150*:163–171.

39. Harrison JE. Personal observations.

40. Bayley TA, Harrison JE, McNeill KG, et al. Effect of thyrotoxicosis and its treatment on bone mineral and muscle mass. J Clin Endocrinol Metab 1980; *50*:916–922.

41. Rasmussen H, Bordier P, Marie P, et al. Effect of combined therapy with phosphate and calcitonin on bone volume in osteoporosis. Metab Bone Dis Rel Res 1980; *2*:107–111.

42. Reeve J, Meunier PJ, Parsons JA, et al. Anabolic effect of human parathyroid hormone fragment on trabecular bone in involutional osteoporosis: a multicentre trial. Br Med J 1980; *280*:1340–1344.

43. Briancon D, Meunier RJ. Treatment of osteoporosis with fluoride, calcium and vitamin D. Orthop Clin North Am 1981; *12*:629–648.

44. Riggs BL. Effect of the fluoride/calcium regimen on vertebral fracture occurrence in postmenopausal osteoporosis. N Engl J Med 1982; *306*:446–450.

45. Shike M, Sturtridge WC, Tam CS, et al. A possible role of vitamin D in the genesis of parenteral-nutrition-induced metabolic bone disease. Ann Intern Med 1981; *95*:560–568.

46. Harrison JE, Jeejeebhoy KN, and the Bone and Mineral Metabolism Unit. The Effect of TPN on Bone Mass. Presented at the Metabolic Bone Disease in Total Parenteral Nutrition Symposium, Deerfield, IL, June, 1982.

47. Bijvoet OLM. Bisphosphonate treatment for Paget's disease of bone. *In* Frame B, Potts JT Jr (eds). Clinical Disorders of Bone and Mineral Metabolism. Amsterdam, Excerpta Medica 1983: 389–394.

48. de Deuxchaisnes CN. Do calcitonins help Paget's disease? *In* Frame B, Potts JT Jr (eds). Clinical Disorders of Bone and Mineral Metabolism. Excerpta Medica 1983: 384–388.

49. U.S. Department of Agriculture, Consumer Nutrition Center. Food and Nutrient Intakes of Individuals in 1 Day in the United States, Spring 1977. Nationwide Food Consumption Survey 1977–78, preliminary report No. 2. Hyattsville, MD, USDA, 1980.

50. Heaney RP, Gallagher JC, Johnston, et al. Calcium nutrition and bone health in the elderly. Am J Clin Nutr 1982; *36*:986–1013.

51. Matkovic V, Kostial K, Simonovic I, et al. Bone status and fracture rates in two regions of Yugoslavia. Am J Clin Nutr 1979; *32*:540–549.

52. Draper HH, Bell RR. Nutrition and Osteoporosis. *In* Draper HH (ed). Advances in Nutritional Research. Vol 2. New York, Plenum, 1979: 79–106.

53. Spencer H, Kramer L, Osis D, et al. The effect of phosphorus on the absorption of calcium on the calcium balance in man. J Nutr 1978; *108*:447–457.

54. Linkswiler HM, Joyce CL, Arand CR. Calcium retention of young adult males as affected by level of protein and calcium intake. Trans NY Acad Sci 1974; *36*:333–400.

55. Daniell HW. Osteoporosis of the slender smoker—vertebral compression fractures and loss of metacarpal cortex in relation to postmenopausal cigarette smoking and lack of obesity. Arch Intern Med 1976; *136*:298.

56. Heaney RP. Osteoporosis. *In* Bronner F, Coburn JW (eds). Disorders of Mineral Metabolism, Vol. 3. New York, Academic Press, 1981: 67–119.

57. Nordin BEC, Horseman A, Marshall DH, et al. The treatment of postmenopausal osteoporosis. *In* Barzel US (ed). Osteoporosis II. New York, Grune & Stratton, 1978: 183–204.

58. Christiansen C, Christensen MS, Rodbro P, et al. Effect of 1,25-dihydroxy-vitamin D_3 in itself or combined with hormone treatment in preventing postmenopausal osteoporosis. Am J Clin Invest 1981; *11*:305–309.

59. Gallagher JC, Riggs BL, Recker R, et al. The effect of calcitriol on patients with postmenopausal osteoporosis with special reference to fracture frequency. Osteoporosis Program and Abstracts, NIH Consensus Development Conference, 1984: 52.

60. Reynolds JJ. Skeletal tissue in culture. *In* Bourne GH (ed). The Biochemistry and Physiology of Bone. 2nd ed. New York, Academic Press, 1972; *1*:69–126.

61. Bronner F, Coburn JW. Disorders of Mineral Metabolism. Vol. 1, Trace Minerals. New York, Academic Press, 1981.
62. Underwood EJ. Trace Elements in Human and Animal Nutrition. 4th ed. New York, Academic Press, 1977.
63. Bernstein DS, Sadowsky N, Hegsted DM, et al. Prevalence of osteoporosis in high- and low-fluoride areas in North Dakota. JAMA 1966; 198:499–504.
64. Nixon JM, Carpenter RG. Mortality in areas containing natural fluoride in their water supplies, taking account of socioenvironmental factors and water hardness. Lancet 1974; 2:1068–1071.
65. Harrison JE, Hitchman AJW, Hasany SA, et al. The effect of fluoride on nephrocalcinosis in rats. Clin Biochem 1985; 18:109–113.
66. Luoma H, Nuuja T. Caries reduction in rats by phosphate, magnesium and fluoride additions to diet with modifications of dental calculus and calcium of the kidneys and aorta. Caries Res 1977; 11:10–108.
67. Masironi R. Cardiovascular mortality in relation to radioactivity and hardness of local water supplies in the USA. Bull WHO 1970; 43:687–697.
68. Schroeder HA, Kraemer LA. Cardiovascular mortality, municipal water, and corrosion. Arch Environ Health 1974; 28:303–311.
69. De Vernejoul MC, Bielakoff J, Herve M, et al. Evidence for defective osteoblastic function. Clin Orthop Rel Res 1983; 179:107–115.
70. Heaney RP, Gallagher JC, Johnston CC, et al. Calcium nutrition and bone health in the elderly. Am J Clin Nutr 1982; 36:986–1013.
71. Lindsay R. The influence of cigarette smoking on bone mass and bone loss. In DeLuca HF, Frost HM, Jee WSS, et al. (eds). Osteoporosis—Recent Advances in Pathogenesis and Treatment. Baltimore, University Park Press, 1981: 481 (Abstract).

41

NUTRIENTS AND BRAIN FUNCTION

LYDIA A. CONLAY

For many years physicians have understood that food consumption affects the body, yet many are less familiar with the mechanisms by which dietary constituents influence brain function. Brain function can be affected by nutrient precursors of neurotransmitters. The amino acids tryptophan and tyrosine, and the compound choline are the biochemical precursors of serotonin, the catecholamines, and acetylcholine.[1-3] These neurotransmitter precursors cross the blood-brain barrier and increase the synthesis of their respective neurotransmitter products, thereby affecting a wide variety of physiological processes.[1-5] This review discusses the biochemistry of the precursor-neurotransmitter relationships, the physiological effects of neurotransmitter precursors, their therapeutic applications in the treatment of specific disorders, and the mechanisms by which other nutrient compounds may alter precursor uptake and thus affect neurotransmitter synthesis.

GENERAL CONCEPTS OF PRECURSOR CONTROL

Biochemical Criteria

Neurotransmitters are divided by chemical structure into three general categories: (1) amines (catecholamines, serotonin, acetylcholine, and histamine); (2) peptides (opiates, substance P, thyrotropin releasing factor, etc.); and (3) nonessential amino acids and their metabolites (glycine, GABA or gamma-aminobutyric acid, and glutamate).[1-3] In order for neurotransmitter synthesis to be increased by neurotransmitter precursors, several conditions must be satisfied.[1-3] First, the neurotransmitter's nutrient precursor must cross the blood-brain barrier and gain entry into the neuron. Second, the neuron must be able to generate more product when exposed to more of its precursor substrate. Third, the neurotransmitter product must not feed back to inhibit its own synthesis.

The effects of dietary presursors on neurotransmitter synthesis have been characterized almost exclusively in neurons of the amine group. The precursors for amine neurotransmitters cross the blood-brain barrier and other cell membranes by facilitated diffusion, through specific macromolecule carrier transport systems.[4] In addition, the enzymes that catalyze amine neurotransmitter synthesis are not saturated with substrate at normal tissue concentrations. Since the enzymatic binding sites are not occupied, the addition of more precursor substrates generates more of the neurotransmitter product.[1-3,5] Finally, feedback inhibition has not been described in vivo for serotonin or acetylcholine, and appears unimportant in rapidly firing catecholamine-containing cells.[1-3,5]

Peptide-containing neurons do not fit the biochemical criteria for precursor control. The rate-limiting step in peptide synthesis involves the coupling of transfer RNA to its specific amino acid.[6] The enzymes catalyzing this reaction have high substrate affinities in the brain: they are fully saturated even at low amino acid concentrations.[6] Therefore, the addition of more amino acid does not increase the concentration of amino acid bound to its respective transfer RNA, nor does it generate more of its peptide product.[1-3]

Data relating precursor concentration to the synthesis of nonessential amino acids and their metabolites are scarce. Some neurons in this category seem to increase neurotransmitter release when exposed to more precursor (for example, administration of the amino acid threonine increases spinal cord glycine concentration[7]), though the physiological sequelae of precursor administration in this class of neurons are unknown. These neurotransmitters are also components of metabolic pathways: their concentrations in neurons are 1000 to 2000 times higher than that of most other neurotransmitters. Present technology cannot separate metabolic pools from neurotransmitter pools; hence, precursor effects in this group of compounds are difficult to quantitate.[1,3]

Precursors of Amine Neurotransmitters

Serotonin is formed from the amino acid tryptophan.[1-3] Like serotonin, tryptophan has been reported to increase the tolerance to a painful stimulus, elevate mood, and decrease sleep latency.[8-14] Tryptophan is a large neutral amino acid, and it shares the blood-brain-barrier carrier system with other amino acids of similar chemical structure: tyrosine, valine, leucine, isoleucine, and methionine.[15] Since these amino acids compete for the same brain uptake system, tryptophan uptake is determined not only by the plasma tryptophan concentration, but also by the plasma concentration of the other large neutral amino acids that compete with it for the brain uptake system. This is expressed as the plasma ratio of tryptophan to the other large neutral amino acids (tryptophan/LNAA, or trp/phe + tyr + val + ileu + leu + met, or the "tryptophan ratio").[4,15]

The tryptophan/LNAA ratio may be increased by increasing the ratio's numerator (by the administration or consumption of tryptophan), or by decreasing the ratio's denominator (the other large neutral amino acids).[4,15,16] For example, carbohydrate consumption evokes insulin secretion, and insulin promotes degradation of the branched-chain amino acids (valine, leucine, and isoleucine) in muscle, thus decreasing the blood concentrations of large neutral amino acids.[16] Insulin, therefore, increases the plasma tryptophan/LNAA ratio by decreasing the ratio's denominator, thus increasing brain tryptophan levels even though no tryptophan has been consumed.[16]

The rate-limiting enzyme in serotonin synthesis is tryptophan hydroxylase. This enzyme is unsaturated with, and limited by the availability of, tryptophan at physiological concentrations.[1-3,5] Therefore, the administration or consumption of tryptophan, or other treatments that increase the tryptophan/LNAA ratio, may increase serotonin synthesis in brain.[16]

Catecholamines (norepinephrine, epinephrine, and dopamine) are formed from the amino acid tyrosine. Like the catecholamines, tyrosine has been reported to influence a wide variety of physiological functions such as cardiovascular function, prolactin secretion, and mood.[17-25] Tyrosine is derived either directly from the diet, or from hepatic metabolism of the amino acid phenylalanine.[1] It occupies the same large neutral amino acid carrier system within the blood-brain barrier as tryptophan.[1,4] Just as the tryptophan/LNAA ratio determines brain tryptophan uptake, so does the tyrosine to large neutral amino acid ratio (tyrosine/LNAA), instead of the plasma tyrosine concentration alone.[4,15]

The rate-limiting enzyme in catecholamine synthesis is tyrosine hydroxylase. Like tryptophan hydroxylase, this enzyme is unsaturated with its amino acid substrate, tyrosine, at normal concentrations.[5,26] However, unlike the tryptophan-serotonin relationship, the administration of tyrosine does not always increase catecholamine synthesis. In resting catecholamine-containing cells, tyrosine hydroxylase is affected by end product inhibition and is unsaturated with its cofactor, tetrahydrobiopterin, so tyrosine administration under these conditions does not increase catecholamine synthesis.[1,3] When a catecholamine-containing neuron fires frequently, the tyrosine hydroxylase enzyme is phosphorylated, inducing kinetic changes that increase its saturation with cofactor and remove it from end product inhibition.[26] Therefore, tyrosine administration to frequently firing catecholamine-containing neurons generates more of the catecholamine product.[1,2,5] Since catecholamine-containing neurons in the central nervous system modulate a wide variety of physiological function, depending on the conditions, some neurons will be quiescent, while others will be firing frequently. Tyrosine's effects are specific for the frequently firing catecholamine group(s).[1–3]

Acetylcholine is formed from the compound choline. Cholinergic neurons transmit signals for motor neurons, preganglionic sympathetic neurons, and certain neurons in the central nervous system (CNS), particularly those involved in memory and awareness.[1–3,27] Choline can be synthesized in liver and brain; however, the major portion of circulating choline is derived from dietary lecithin, a choline-containing phospholipid found in high concentration in cell membranes from fish, liver, and eggs.[27] Capillary endothelia composing the blood-brain barrier contain a facilitated diffusion carrier system for choline similar to that for the large neutral amino acids, and allow equilibration of choline between plasma and brain.[28] Choline acetyltransferase is the enzyme that limits the rate of acetylcholine synthesis, but the factors regulating this enzyme's activity in brain are not well studied.[3,27] Nonetheless, the consumption of choline or its naturally occurring parent compound lecithin can increase the release of acetylcholine from neurons within the central nervous system.[29,30] Choline probably does not increase acetycholine in plasma, since circulating acetylcholine is rapidly hydrolyzed by circulating cholinesterase.[30]

In humans, choline administration causes a body odor reminiscent of rotten fish: bacteria in the gut degrade choline to trimethylamine. This problem has been circumvented by administering choline as its parent compound lecithin, which is also the naturally occurring source of choline found in body membranes.[3] Pure (80 per cent phosphatidylcholine) sources of lecithin are available for clinical trial, but lecithins sold at health food stores often contain less than 20 per cent phospatidylcholine, even though they are called "phosphatidylcholine."

INFLUENCES OF NEUROTRANSMITTER PRECURSORS

Pain

Pain is the most urgent of human symptoms. It represents a diagnostic and therapeutic challenge for physicians, and an enormous financial burden for health care systems around the world.[31] Recent research suggests that tryptophan, a dietary amino acid, produces pain relief in some chronic pain patients by increasing the synthesis of the neurotransmitter serotonin.[8–11] Tryptophan may therefore represent a new and relatively innocuous approach to the management of the unfortunate patients of chronic pain.

In animals, an increase in brain serotonin causes analgesia.[32] Likewise depletion of this neurotransmitter, either pharmacologically (with serotoninergic neurotoxins) or with surgical denervation, decreases the pain threshold.[32,33] In rats, diets deficient in tryptophan result in an increased pain sensitivity; the injection of tryptophan returns the animals to normal.[34]

Tryptophan increased pain tolerance in normal humans in two studies.[8,11] In 30 volunteers subjected to electrical stimulation of dental pulp, tryptophan (2 g/day) significantly increased pain tolerance levels, although it exerted little effect on the pain perception threshold when compared with placebo in a double-blind fashion.[8] In eight healthy men subjected to a thermal stimulus on the forearm, tryptophan (50 mg/kg) also reduced the sensitivity to pain in a placebo-controlled, double-blind study.[11] Like morphine, tryptophan had an effect that was specific for moderately intense stimuli, as opposed to nonpainful or maximally painful intensities.[11]

Serotonin potentiates the effects of morphine; likewise, depletion of this neurotransmitter has been reported to decrease the effectiveness of opiate analgesics.[9] Hosobuchi et al. found that tryptophan (3 g/day) reversed the tolerance of opioid analgesia produced by stimulation of the central gray matter.[35] In another study, tryptophan loading (4 g/day) for several weeks reversed the opiate tolerance in five patients tolerant to opiate analgesics (as defined by their inability to obtain relief after 30 mg of intravenous morphine).[36] Four of the five patients obtained relief from pain at half their daily morphine doses.[36] King reported that 3 g/day of tryptophan restored sensory deficits and relieved the pain that reappeared following chordotomy and rhizotomy, surgical procedures used to treat chronic pain patients.[10]

In 30 patients with chronic maxillofacial pain (temporomandibular joint pain-dysfunction syndrome; trigeminal, atypical facial, or migranous neuralgia; and phantom tooth pain), Dewart et al. reported the effects of tryptophan on pain relief and mood using a placebo-controlled, double-blind design.[37] After 1 month of therapy, tryptophan (3 g/day) alleviated the chronic maxillofacial pain when compared with placebo. No significant differences were noted in the psychological tests administered for depression, though subjective estimates of both depression and anxiety declined after intake of the amino acid.[37]

Depression

Depression is usually treated with drugs that increase brain catecholamine release: the tricyclics block catecholamine reuptake, whereas monoamine oxidase inhibitors block their degradation. Since drugs that increase catecholamines benefit patients with depression, Gelenberg et al. studied the effects of tyrosine in patients with depression.[38–40] In several studies they noted improvement in certain indices of depression such as the Hamilton depression rating scale in patients taking tyrosine when compared with depressed patients taking placebo.[38–40]

Although some forms of depression are associated with abnormalities of norepinephrine release, other forms of depression may involve serotonin. Indeed, the original monoamine theory of depression postulated a defect in central serotonergic neurotransmission.[41] This theory is supported by studies demonstrating reduced concentrations of 5-hydroxyindoleacetic acid, a serotonin metabolite, in the cerebrospinal fluid of depressed patients[42] and low brain serotonin concentrations in depressed patients who commit suicide.[43] Furthermore, many of the drugs used to treat depression (such as monoamine oxidase inhibitors) have similar effects on serotonergic and noradrenergic neurotransmission. Tryptophan administration to manic-depressive patients has variable effects, although those with low tryptophan/LNAA ratios in blood seemed to respond.[12] It is, however, also possible that large doses of tryptophan could exacerbate depression by competing with tyrosine for entry into brain, thereby resulting in lower levels of brain tyrosine and norepinephrine.[1,2]

Memory

Cholinergic neurons influence memory in both animals and man.[1,3] Choline-deficient diets exacerbate the age-related diminution of memory in mice, and choline-rich diets improve memory in older mice.[42] In humans, memory is impaired by scopolamine, a cholinergic receptor blocker, but is restored by physostigmine (which inhibits acetylcholinesterase, and thus increases the acetylcholine content in the synapse).[45]

Choline administration may also alter memory in humans; it decreases the number of trials needed to memorize lists,[46] and may diminish deficits in short-term memory that are associated with Alzheimer's disease or with aging.[47] Many open label studies using choline and its parent compound lecithin in memory disorders have been published, and three studies have shown clinical improvement with double-blind, placebo-controlled protocols.[47,48] In the first, 5 of 5 patients exhibited significant improvement in testing by mental status questionnaire after 2 weeks of consuming choline bitartrate.[47] However, these same authors were unable to confirm this finding in a subsequent larger study.[49] In the second study, 7 of 11 patients showed a 50 to 200 per cent improvement in "long-term storage" after 2 to 8 weeks of lecithin.[50] In the third study, lecithin was found to have little effect in 51 patents with Alzheimer's disease.[51] However, when grouped according to therapy compliance, the "poor compliers" performed significantly better on self-care psychological

tests when taking lecithin than when taking placebo. Thus, the "poor compliers" may represent a subgroup of Alzheimer's patients more likely to respond to lecithin (i.e., with either more advanced disease, or perhaps a specific type of yet-undifferentiated Alzheimer's disease).[51] The effectiveness of acetylcholine precursors in significantly improving memory function awaits more well-controlled clinical trials. Lecithin does raise plasma choline on a long-term basis, but does not appear to have a dramatic therapeutic effect.

Parkinson's Disease

Parkinson's disease is caused by the destruction of dopaminergic neurons in the brain's *corpus striatum*, thus resulting in a deficiency in the release of the neurotransmitter dopamine. It is treated with a catecholamine precursor, L-dopa (tyrosine is converted to dopa, and dopa is converted to dopamine). However, L-dopa bypasses the rate-limiting tyrosine hydroxylase step, and may be enzymatically converted to dopamine in many sites throughout the body (the amino acid decarboxylase enzyme is contained in a variety of tissues). This lack of specificity may be related to some of the side effects associated with chronic L-dopa therapy.[1,3]

Unlike L-dopa, tyrosine is converted to dopamine only in cells that contain tyrosine hydroxylase—namely, catecholaminergic neurons like those in the striatum and the adrenal glands.[1–3] As discussed previously, tyrosine affects frequently firing neurons, thus possibly providing greater specificity and potentially fewer side effects in the treatment of Parkinson's disease. Growdon and Melamed reported increases in cerebrospinal fluid concentrations of tyrosine and the dopaminergic metabolite homovanillic acid after tyrosine administration to parkinsonian patients.[52] These results indicate that the amino acid enters the human brain and increases the release of dopamine, the neurotransmitter deficient in Parkinson's disease. In 33 patients with various stages of Parkinson's disease tyrosine treatment benefitted 10 of the mildly affected patients, but was ineffective in patients in whom the disease was more advanced.[53] Tyrosine's lack of effectiveness in the advanced stages of Parkinson's disease may be explained by animal experiments. Tyrosine increased dopamine release (as measured by the dopaminergic metabolites homovanillic acid and dihydroxyphenylacetic acid) in rats with partial nigrostriatal lesions, whereas it had no effect in totally lesioned or unlesioned striata.[54] In the latter cases, catecholaminergic neurons either were destroyed, or were not firing rapidly, and therefore did not increase dopamine synthesis when exposed to additional tyrosine. In the partially lesioned rats, the remaining neurons probably increased firing in order to compensate for the lesion, thus leading to tyrosine-dependent dopamine synthesis. In patients with Parkinson's disease, variations in the clinical response to L-dopa may thus be related to differences in the number of surviving nigrostriatal neurons.[54]

Blood Pressure Control

The effects of *catecholamines* on blood pressure (BP) are determined by the location of the neurons from which they are released. In the spinal cord, catecholamines may excite sympathetic preganglionic neurons and thus increase sympathetic outflow.[55–57] Conversely, neurons from the A_1 catecholamine group (in the brain) excite inhibitory neurons in the vasomotor area of the brain stem, thus causing BP to decrease.[58,59] It is therefore possible in a given situation to predict the group of neurons most likely to fire frequently. For example, during hypotension, neurons that mediate increases in sympathetic activity release catecholamines onto blood vessels, the heart, and sympathetic preganglionic neurons in the spinal cord.[60] In hypotension, the neurons that decrease BP remain quiescent. Conversely, during hypertension, catecholamine-containing neurons from vasodepressor areas in the brain stem fire frequently, presumably in an attempt to decrease BP towards normal.[56] In hypertension, neurons that mediate increases in sympathetic activity are quiescent. Since the firing frequency of each of the respective catecholamine-containing groups is determined by BP (i.e., hypotension or hypertension), and since tyrosine increases catecholamine synthesis only in neurons that are frequently firing, BP determines tyrosine's vasoactive effect.

During hemorrhage, sympathoadrenal neurons fire frequently in order to increase BP, shunt blood to the vital organs, and vasoconstrict the site of injury.[60] During hemorrhagic shock intravenous administration of 100 mg/kg of tyrosine increased BP in rats and dogs by an average of 60 per cent.[17,22] Tyrosine's effects were mediated through an increase in catecholamine synthesis: tyrosine was ineffective in animals pretreated with carbidopa, which inhibits peripheral catecholamine synthesis, or with phentolamine, an alpha receptor blocker.[61] Under certain circumstances, tyrosine can be decarboxylated to form tyramine, an indirect-acting sympathomimetic amine. However, tyrosine's pressor effects during hypotension do not result from tyramine formation.[62]

In animals with hypertension, tyrosine administration decreases BP.[18–20] In rats, the BP decrease parallels an increase in brain stem norepinephrine release, suggesting that tyrosine decreases BP by increasing catecholamine synthesis and release in brain stem vasodepressor noradrenergic neurons.[19] The simultaneous administration of another large neutral amino acid (valine) that competes with tyrosine for entry into the brain blocks tyrosine's antihyper-

tensive effect.[19] Diets augmented with tyrosine have been shown to decrease BP in hypertensive rats, and also to delay the onset of hypertension in the spontaneously hypertensive rat model.[21] Though it is likely that tyrosine acts by increasing catecholamine synthesis and release in brain stem vasodepression neurons, the possibility that tyrosine acts via its conversion to tyramine has not been excluded. Tyramine indirectly releases catecholamines, and intraventricular injection of tyramine has been reported to decrease BP in hypertensive animals.[63]

Unfortunately, tyrosine is the least soluble amino acid (followed closely by tryptophan). In order to dissolve the large amounts required for intravascular administration, it must be administered as a derivative such as the methylester form (used in most studies) or as a dipeptide. Such derivatives are not presently approved for human use.

Thus, tyrosine is specific for frequently firing neurons. It increases BP during hypotension by increasing catecholamine synthesis in peripheral sympathoadrenal cells, and decreases BP during hypertension by increasing brain stem catecholamine synthesis and release.

Choline administration increases urinary catecholamine excretion in animals.[64] Biochemical evidence implicates an increase in acetylcholine release from sympathetic preganglionic neurons, which in turn increase the firing of sympathetic postganglionic fibers releasing catecholamines. Acetylcholine, released from preganglionic sympathetic neurons, induces tyrosine hydroxylase in the postganglionic catecholaminergic neurons located in sympathetic ganglia.[65] Choline, like acetylcholine, also activates this enzyme in sympathetic ganglia. Its effects are blocked by atropine, or by preganglionic surgical denervation, suggesting that choline acts by increasing sympathetic preganglionic acetylcholine release.[66] Thus, choline's availability may influence sympathetic function.

Choline is itself a weak muscarinic agonist. However, the plasma concentration (approximately 1 mmol) necessary to occupy peripheral muscarinic receptors is 20 to 100 times normal. No changes in cardiovascular parameters have been reported to date in patients receiving large doses of choline or lecithin used to treat disorders such as Alzheimer's disease or tardive dyskinesia.[3]

The effects of *tryptophan* on BP were examined by Sved et al.[67] In hypertensive animals, L-tryptophan decreased BP by an average of 30 mm Hg. Valine blocked the effects (presumably by competing for brain uptake), as did an inhibitor of serotonin synthesis, parachlorophenylalanine, which inhibits tryptophan hydroxylase. Tryptophan's effects, however, may not reflect an increase in serotonin synthesis, as might have been predicted by the tryptophan-serotonin relationship. D-Tryptophan also increased brain serotonin release (as indicated by the serotonin metabolite 5-hydroxyindoleacetic acid) similarly to

L-tryptophan, but did not alter BP in hypertensive rats.[68] The fact that tryptophan's effects on BP are not stereospecific suggests that the amino acid may be converted to another compound that indirectly releases serotonin. Tryptophan may be converted to such compounds, called kyalurenins.[68]

Ventricular Arrhythmias

Sudden death syndrome claims as many as 450,000 lives per year.[69] Since autopsies frequently do no demonstrate acute myocardial lesions in these patients, the syndrome may represent an electrical accident (such as ventricular fibrillation, or VF) instead of chronic, irreversible myocardial damage.

Signals from the central nervous system affect cardiac irritability. For example, one's chances of sudden death are doubled during the first 6 months following the death of a spouse, and patients with coronary artery disease exhibit an increased number of extrasystoles (accompanied by ST segment depression) while speaking before a group.[70] Though these changes may represent ischemia resulting from an increase in myocardial oxygen demand secondary to an increase in BP and heart rate, evidence suggests that sympathetic activity directly affects myocardial vulnerability as well.

Stellate ganglion stimulation induces VF in 60 per cent of dogs subjected to electrical stimulation of the right ventricle[71] (this experimental model is used to study cardiac vulnerability[72]). In the absence of stellate ganglion stimulation, fibrillation does not occur. Likewise, pharmacological manipulations that mimic sympathetic activation decrease the threshold for, or increase the susceptibility to, ventricular arrhythmias. Norepinephrine infusion (in animals whose BP was held constant by exsanguination) decreases the threshold for VF by almost 50 per cent.[73] On the other hand, reflex reductions in sympathetic activity from constriction of the thoracic aorta, or from the BP elevation following phenylephrine infusion, increases the VF threshold by 49 per cent.[74] Thus, in the dog model increases in sympathetic neural activity increase the susceptibility to ventricular arrhythmias, while decreases in sympathetic tone exert a protective effect.

As discussed earlier, drugs that stimulate release of catecholamines or mimic their postsynaptic effects in the brain stem decrease sympathetic outflow. Just as clonidine reduces sympathetic outflow by a central action,[75,76] Rotenberg et al. found that it also decreases the susceptibility to VF.[77] Scott et al. tested the effects of tyrosine on VF in dogs and observed that tyrosine increased the VF threshold in a dose-related manner.[78] Its protective effect was blocked by the concomitant administration of the large neutral amino acid, valine.[78] (Though the change was not statistically significant, valine seemed to decrease the threshold when administered alone in the six

dogs studied.) Tyrosine's effects in humans remain to be tested.

Serotonin agonists decrease the susceptibility to VF.[79] Likewise, the administration of the serotonin precursor 5-hydroxytryptophan in combination with a monoamine oxidase (MAO) inhibitor (which inhibits the breakdown of both serotonin and catecholamines) decreases sympathetic activity. (Tryptophan is converted to 5-hydroxytryptophan, which in turn forms 5-hydroxytryptamine, or serotonin.)[80] L-Tryptophan, in the presence of carbidopa (which prevents serotonin formation in the peripheral nervous system) and an MAO inhibitor, increased the threshold for VF by approximately 50 per cent.[81] However, in the absence of the drug pretreatments, L-tryptophan caused no significant change in the threshold. Though treatments modifying brain serotonin affected cardiac vulnerability, it is necessary to pretreat animals with both carbidopa and an MAO inhibitor in order to observe the antiarrhythmic effect. Because several drugs, each with substantial side effects of their own, must be used in combination with tryptophan, its practical application in the treatment of human arrhythmias seems unlikely.

Sleep

Tryptophan decreases both sleep latency (the time to sleep) and waking time when administered orally in 1-g doses.[13,14] Hartman has summarized over 40 human studies concerning tryptophan's effects.[13,14] They are potentiated by carbohydrate, which decreases the concentrations of the competing large neutral amino acids. When 20 mg of tryptophan is added to Similac infant formula, newborns enter both quiet and active sleep sooner than controls.[82]

POSSIBLE EFFECTS OF NON-PRECURSOR NUTRIENTS ON NEUROTRANSMISSION

Non-Precursor Large Neutral Amino Acids

As previously discussed, tyrosine and tryptophan share a transport protein within the blood-brain barrier with the other large neutral amino acids—leucine, isoleucine, valine (the branched-chain amino acids), and methionine.[1-4] Though these components do not form neurotransmitters themselves, they block brain uptake of tyrosine and tryptophan, and may thereby indirectly affect neurotransmitter synthesis. For example, valine blocks the ability of both tyrosine and tryptophan to decrease BP in hypertensive animals, as well as tyrosine's beneficial effect on ventricular arrhythmias.[19,67,78]

Commercially available hyperalimentation solutions contain very small quantities of tyrosine and tryptophan as compared with the other large neutral

TABLE 41–1. *Large Neutral Amino Acid Ratios in Human Plasma and Commercially Available Amino Acid Mixtures*

	Tyrosine/LNAA's	Tryptophan/ LNAA's
Plasma (fasting)	0.081 ± 0.006	0.11 ± 0.03
Freamine III	0	0.04
Travisol R	0.017	0.06
Aminosyn	0.016	0.05

These commercially available mixtures are 8.5 per cent parenteral solutions. They contain only about a quarter of the normal ratio of tyrosine and half of the normal ratio of tryptophan to the other large neutral amino acids.

amino acids, and branched-chain enriched solutions contain even less (Table 41–1). When administered to humans, commercial amino acid solutions alter the tryptophan/LNAA and tyrosine/LNAA ratios,[83] and the simultaneous administration of competing LNAA's such as valine may block the effects of circulating tyrosine and tryptophan. The possible effects of these solutions on neurotransmission in humans have not yet been examined.

Choline is also absent in parenteral nutrition solutions. Indeed, as of 1984, the only choline-deficient state known in man is parenteral nutrition, in which plasma choline concentrations are significantly lower than controls after 14 days of therapy.[84] The effects of choline deficiency on neurotransmission have not yet been addressed.

Alpha-methyldopa also shares the large neutral amino acid carrier. Administration of this antihypertensive drug with a protein-rich meal (which elevates the competing large neutral amino acids) decreases its brain uptake, as well as its antihypertensive action.[85]

ASPARTAME

A new artificial sweetener, aspartame (Nutrasweet, Equal) is a dipeptide composed of phenylalanine and aspartic acid. The phenylalanine in this sweetener is transported into the brain by the large neutral amino acid carrier shared with tyrosine and tryptophan, and can be hydroxylated to form tyrosine.[4] Consumption of 32 mg/kg—the dose estimated to replace the average daily sugar consumption of a person in the United States—has been shown to double the ratio of phenylalanine to the other large neutral amino acids in the plasma of human subjects.[86]

In rats equivalent doses of aspartame increased both the plasma tyrosine/LNAA ratio and brain tyrosine concentration, suggesting that the sweeteners might have physiological effects similar to those of tyrosine.[87]

Tyrosine decreases BP in hypertensive rats; and aspartame likewise had a similar antihypertensive effect (200 mg/kg aspartame lowered BP by an average of 20 mm Hg systolic).[88] These findings suggest that not only aspartame but also other peptides that are degraded to amino acid precursors of neurotransmitters may exert physiological effects by selectively altering neurotransmitter synthesis.

CONCLUSIONS

Naturally occurring dietary constituents, the precursors for neurotransmitters, exert physiological effects and may be useful to treat disorders involving specific neutrotransmitter abnormalities. Neurotransmitters influenced by precursor availability share certain common features. In each instance, the administration of precursor (tyrosine, tryptophan, or choline) increases its plasma concentration, facilitates entry into the brain, and increases its availability for conversion to the parent neurotransmitter. The resulting increase in neurotransmitter synthesis may affect a variety of conditions such as circulation, mood, pain perception, memory, and neurological function.[1–3]

Neurotransmitter precursors have several advantages over currently available synthetic drugs. First, they are naturally occurring substances. They circulate normally in the blood, and the body's metabolic pathways have withstood the tests of evolution.

TABLE 41–2. *Summary of Neurotransmitters, Their Precursors, Pharmacological Effects, and Disorders for Which They Have Been Proposed as Therapeutic Agents*

Neurotransmitter	Precursor	Proposed As Therapy for:	References
Serotonin	Tryptophan	Chronic pain	8–11
		Decreases opiate tolerance	35, 36
		Depression	12
		Sleep disorders	13, 14
Norepinephrine	Tyrosine	Hypertension	18*, 19*, 20*, 21*
		Hypotension	22*, 61*, 62*
		Sudden death syndrome	78*
		Depression	24, 25, 38–40
		Hyperprolactinemia	23
Acetylcholine	Choline	Alzheimer's disease	47–51

*Animal studies.

Second, they are water-soluble compounds; toxic concentrations are therefore less likely to accumulate in body tissues. Finally, precursor administration increases product formation only in neurons that normally convert the precursor to its neurotransmitter product; this specificity might be expected to decrease potential side effects as compared with those of synthetic drugs.

The ability of neurotransmitter precursors to alter physiological functions is important from several perspectives. First, precursors constitute a novel and apparently innocuous approach to the therapy of disorders involving neurotransmission. (Table 41–2 summarizes the present experimental uses of precursors in specific disorders.) Second, administered parenteral amino acid solutions may themselves alter brain function by blocking the uptake of tyrosine and tryptophan, and therefore by decreasing the synthesis of the catecholamines and serotonin. Finally, the availability of neurotransmitter precursors, as estimated by plasma levels, may aid in the prediction of a patient's response to a specific situation.

ACKNOWLEDGMENT

The author wishes to acknowledge Dr. Richard Wurtman, who discovered the link between foods and thought.

References

1. Wurtman RJ, Hefti F, Melamed G. Precursor control of neurotransmitter synthesis. Pharmacol Rev 1981; *32*:315–335.
2. Wurtman RJ. Nutrients that modify brain function. Sci Am 1982; *246*:50–59.
3. Conlay LA, Zeisel SH. Neurotransmitter precursors and brain function. Neurosurgery 1982; *10*:524–529.
4. Pardridge WM, Oldendorf WH. Transport of metabolic substrates through the blood-brain barrier. J Neurochem 1977; *28*:5–12.
5. Carlsson A, Lindqvist M. Dependence of 5HT and catecholamine synthesis on concentrations of precursor amino acids in rat brain. Naunyn Schmiedebergs Arch Pharmacol 1978; *303*:157–164.
6. Barra HS, Unates LE, Sayavedra MS, et al. Capacities of binding amino acids by tRNAs from rat brain and their changes during development. J Neurochem 1972; *19*:2287–2297.
7. Maher TJ, Wurtman RJ. L-Threonine administration increases glycine concentrations in the rat central nervous system. Life Sci 1980; *26*:1283–1286.
8. Seltzer S, Stoch R, Marcus R, et al. Alteration of human pain thresholds by nutritional manipulation and L-tryptophan supplementation. Pain 1982; *13*:385–393.
9. Seltzer S, Marcus R, Stoch R. Perspectives in the control of chronic pain by nutritional manipulation. Pain 1981; *11*:141–148.
10. King RB. Pain and tryptophan. J Neurosurg 1980; *53*:44–52.
11. Lieberman HR, Corkin S, Spring BJ, et al. Mood, performance, and pain sensitivity: changes induced by food constituents. J Psychiat Res 1983: *17*:135–146.
12. Moller SE, Kirk L, Fremming KH. Plasma amino acids as an index for subgroups in manic depressive psychosis: correlation to the effect of tryptophan. Psychopharmacology 1976; *49*:205–213.
13. Hartman E. Tryptophan and sleep: who responds to L-tryptophan. Proceeds of Third World Congress of Biological Psychiatry, 1983.
14. Hartman E. Effects of L-tryptophan on sleepiness and sleep. J Psychiat Res 1983; *17*:107–114.
15. Fernstrom JD, Faller DV. Neutral amino acids and the brain: changes in response to food ingestion. J Neurochem 1978; *30*:1513–1538.
16. Fernstrom JD, Wurtman RJ. Brain serotonin content: increase following ingestion of carbohydrate diet. Science 1971; *174*:1023–1025.
17. Conlay LA, Maher TJ, Wurtman RJ, et al. Tyrosine's vasoactive effect in the dog shock model depends on the animal's starting BP. J Neurol Trans 1983; *58*:69–74.
18. Bresnahan MR, Hatzinikolaw P, Brunner HR. Effect of tyrosine infusion in normotensive and hypertensive rats. Am J Physiol 1980; *239*:H206–H209.
19. Sved AF, Fernstrom JD, Wurtman RJ. Tyrosine administration reduces blood pressure and enhances brain norepinephrine release in spontaneously hypertensive rats. Proc Natl Acad Sci USA 1979; *76*:3511–3514.
20. Yamori YM, Fujiwara M, Horie R, et al. The hypotensive effect of centrally administered tyrosine. Eur J Pharmacol 1980; *68*:201–204.
21. Osumi Y, Tanka C, Takaori S. Levels of tyrosine and tryptophan in the plasma and brain of spontaneously hypertensive rats. Jpn J Pharmacol 1974; *24*:715–720.
22. Conlay LA, Maher TJ, Wurtman RJ. Tyrosine increases blood pressure in hypotensive rats. Science 1981; *212*:559–560.
23. Sved AF, Fernstrom JD, Wurtman RJ. Tyrosine administration decreases serum prolactin in chronically reserpenized rats. Life Sci 1979; *25*:1293–1300.
24. Gelenberg AJ, Wojcik JD, Growdon JH, et al. Tyrosine in the treatment of depression. Am J Psychiatry 1980; *137*:622–623.
25. Goldberg IK. L-Tyrosine in the treatment of depression. Lancet 1980; *2*:364.
26. Lovenberg W, Bruckswick EA, Hanbauer I. ATP, cyclic AMP, and magnesium increase the affinity of rat striatal tyrosine hydroxylase for its cofactor. Proc Natl Acad Sci USA 1978; *72*:2955–2958.
27. Zeisel SH. Dietary choline: biochemistry, physiology, and pharmacology. Ann Rev Nutr 1981; *1*:95–121.
28. Cornford EM, Braun LD, Oldendorf WH. Carrier-mediated blood-brain transport of choline and certain choline analogs. J Neurochem 1978; *30*:299–308.
29. Hirsch MJ, Growdon JH, Wurtman RJ. Relations between dietary choline or lecithin intake, serum choline levels, and various metabolic indices. Metabolism 1978; *27*:953–960.
30. Cohen EL, Wurtman RJ. Brain acetylcholine: increase after systemic choline administration. Life Sci 1975; *16*:1095–1102.
31. Bonicer JJ. Pain Research and Therapy: Past and Current Status and Future Needs. Pain Discomfort and Humanitarian Care. New York, Elsevier/North-Holland, 1980.
32. Skil H, Liebiskind JC. Monoaminergic mechanisms of stimulation-induced analgesia. Brain Res 1975; *94*:279–296.
33. Harvey JA, Lints C. Lesions in the medial forebrain bundle: relationship between pain sensitivity and telencephalic content of serotonin. J Comp Physiol Psychol 1971; *74*:28–36.
34. Lytle LD, Mersing RB, Fisher L, et al. Effects of long-term corn consumption on brain serotonin and the response to electric shock. Science 1975; *190*:692–694.
35. Hosobuchi Y. Tryptophan reversal of tolerance to analgesia induced by central grey stimulation. Lancet 1978; *2*:47.
36. Hosobuchi Y, Lamb S, Bascom D. Tryptophan loading may reverse tolerance to opiate analgesics in humans. A preliminary report. Pain 1980; *9*:161–169.
37. Dewart D, Seltzer S, Pollack R, et al. The effects of tryptophan on chronic pain. J Psychiat Res 1983; *17*:181–186.

38. Gelenberg AJ, Wojcik JD, Gibson CJ, et al. Tyrosone for depression. J Psychiat Res 1983; 17:175–180.

39. Gelenberg AJ, Wurtman RJ. L-Tyrosine in depression. Lancet 1981; 2:863–864.

40. Gelenberg AJ, Wojcik JD, Sved AF, et al. Tyrosine for the treatment of depression. Am J Psychiat 1980; 137:622–623.

41. Coppen A. The biochemistry of affective disorders. Br J Psychiatry 1967; 113:1237–1264.

42. Van Praag HM, Korf J. Serotonin metabolism in depression: clinical application of the probenecid test. Int Pharmacopsychiatry 1974; 9:35–51.

43. Shaw DW, Camps FE, Eccleston EG. 5-Hydroxytryptamine in the hindbrain of depressive suicides. Br J Psychiatry 1967; 113:1407–1411.

44. Bartus RT, Dean RL, Boas AJ, et al. Age-related changes in passive avoidance retention: modulation with dietary choline. Science 1980; 209:301–303.

45. Drachman DA. Memory and cognitive function in man: does the cholinergic system have a specific role? Neurology (NY) 1977; 27:783–790.

46. Sitaram N, Weingartner H, Gillin JC. Human serial learning: enhancement with arecoline and choline and impairment with scopolamine. Science 1978; 201:274–276.

47. Boyd WD, Graham-White J, Blackwood G, et al. Clinical effects of choline in Alzheimer senile dementia. Lancet 1977; 2:711.

48. Fovall P, Dysken MW, Lazarus LW, et al. Choline bitartrate treatment of Alzheimer-type dementias. Commun Psychopharmacol 1980; 4:141–145.

49. Zeisel SH, Reinstein D, Corkin S, et al. Cholinergic neurons and memory. Nature 1981; 293:187–188.

50. Hu R, Vroulis G, Smith RC. Effects of lecithin on memory and behavior in Alzheimer's type dementia. In Abstracts of the Gerontology Society of America, 33rd Scientific Meeting, 1980: 128.

51. Levy R, Little A, Chuaqui P, Reith M. Early results from a double-blind, placebo-controlled trial of high-dose phosphatidyl choline in Altzheimer's disease. (Letter.) Lancet 1983; 1:987–988.

52. Growdon JH, Melamed E. Effects of oral L-tyrosine administration on homovanillic acid levels in patients with Parkinson's disease. Neurology 1980; 30:396–398.

53. Growdon JH, Melamed E, Logue M, et al. Effects of oral L-tyrosine administration on CSF tyrosine and homovanillic acid levels in patients with Parkinson's disease. Life Sci 1982; 30:827–832.

54. Melamed E, Hefti F, Wurtman RJ. Tyrosine administration increases striatal dopamine release in rats with partial nigrostriatal lesions. Proc Natl Acad Sci USA 1980; 464:4305–4309.

55. Chalmers JP, Petty MA, Reid JL. Participation of adrenergic and noradrenergic neurons in central connections of arterial baroreceptor reflexes in the rat. Circ Res 1979; 45:516–522.

56. Haeusler G. Cardiovascular regulation by central adrenergic mechanisms and its alteration by hypotensive drugs. Circ Res 1975; 36:223–232.

57. Taylor DG, Brody MG. Spinal adrenergic mechanisms regulating sympathetic outflow. Circ Res 1976; 38(6 Suppl 2):10–20.

58. Struyker HAJ, Smeets GMW, Brouwer GM, et al. Hypothalamic alphaadrenergic receptors in cardiovascular regulation. Neuropharmacology 1974; 13:837–846.

59. Laubie M, Delbarre B, Bogaievsky D, et al. Pharmacological evidence for a central sympathomimetic mechanism controlling blood pressure and heart rate. Circ Res 1976; 38(6 Suppl 2):35–41.

60. Chen Su. Role of the sympathetic nervous system in hemorrhage. Physiol Res 1967; 47:214–239.

61. Conlay LA, Maher TJ, Wurtman RJ. Tyrosine increases catecholamine synthesis during hypotension. Brain Res 1985; 333:81–84.

62. Conlay LA, Maher TJ, Wurtman RJ. Tyrosine is not converted to tyramine during hypotension. Life Sci 1984; 35:1210–1212.

63. Shalita B, Dikstein S. Central tyramine prevents hypertension uninephrectomized DOCA-saline treated rats. Experimentia 1977; 33:1430–1431.

64. Scally MC, Ulus IH, Wurtman RJ. Choline administration to the rat increases urinary catecholamines. J Neural Trans 1978; 43:103–112.

65. Ulus IH, Hirsch MJ, Wurtman RJ. Transynaptic induction of adrenal tyrosine hydroxylase activity by choline: evidence that choline administration increases cholinergic transmission. Proc Nat Acad Sci USA 1977; 74:798–800.

66. Ulus IH, Arslan Y, Tanrisever Y, et al. Postsynaptic effects of choline administration. In Barbeau A, Growdon JH, Wurtman RJ (eds). Nutrition and the Brain. Vol 5. New York, Raven Press, 1979.

67. Sved AF, Van Itallie CM, Fernstrom JD. Studies on the antihypertensive effect of L-tryptophan. J Pharm Exp Ther 1982; 221:329–333.

68. Wolf WA, Kuhn DM. Effects of L-tryptophan on blood pressure in normotensive and hypertensive rats. J Pharm Exper Ther 1984; 230:324–329.

69. Lown B, Wolf M. Approaches to sudden death from coronary heart disease. Circulation 1971; 44:130–142.

70. Taggart P, Parkinson P, Carruthers M. Cardiac responses to thermal, physical, and emotional stress. Br Med J 1972; 3:71–76.

71. Verrier RL, Thompson PL, Lown B. Ventricular vulnerability during sympathetic stimulation: role of heart rate and blood pressure. Cardiovasc Res 1974; 8:602–610.

72. Matta RS, Verrier RL, Lown B. The repetitive extrasystole as an index of vulnerability to ventricular fibrillation. Am J Physiol 1976; 230:1461–1466.

73. Verrier RL, Rabinowitz SH, Lown B. Vagal and adrenergic interactions and ventricular electrical stability. Clin Res 1975; 23:212A.

74. Verrier R, Calvert A, Lown B. Effect of acute blood pressure elevation on the ventricular fibrillation threshold. Am J Physiol 1974; 226:893–897.

75. Haeusler G. Central alpha adrenoceptors involved in cardiovascular regulation. J Cardiovasc Pharmacol 1982; 4:572–576.

76. Haeusler G. Further similarities between the action of clonidine central activation of the depressor baroreceptor reflex. Naunyn Schmiedebergs Arch Pharmacol 1974; 285:1–14.

77. Rotenberg FA, Verrier RL, Lown B, et al. Effects of clonidine on vulnerability to fibrillation in the normal and ischemic canine ventricle. Eur J Pharmacol 1978; 47:71–79.

78. Scott NA, DeSilva RA, Lown B, et al. Tyrosine administration decreases vulnerability to ventricular fibrillation in the normal canine heart. Science 1980; 211:727–729.

79. Blatt CM, Rabinowitz SH, Lown B. Central serotonergic agents raise the repetitive extrasystole threshold of the vulnerable period of the canine ventricular myocardium. Circ Res 1979; 44:723–730.

80. Baum T, Shropshire AT. Inhibition of efferent sympathetic nerve activity by 5-hydroxytryptophan and centrally administered 5-hydroxytryptamine. Neuropharmacology 1975; 14:227–233.

81. Rabinowitz SH, Lown B. Central neurochemical factors related to serotonin metabolism and cardiac ventricular vulnerability for repetitive electrical activity. Am J Cardiol 1978; 41:516–522.

82. Yogman MW, Zeisel SH, Roberts C. Assessing effects of serotonin precursors on newborn behavior. J Psychiat Res 1983; 17:123–134.

83. Landel A, Meguid MM, Chang CR, et al. Effects of TPN of varying amino acid composition on brain neurotransmitter precursors. (Abstract.) Am J Clin Nutr 1982; 35:19.

84. Sheard NS, Tayak JA, Bistran BR, et al. Plasma choline concentrations in humans fed parenterally. Am J Clin Nutr 1986; 43:219–224.

85. Zavisca F, Wurtman RJ. Effects of neutral amino acids on

the anti-hypertensive action of methyldopa in spontaneously hypertensive rats. J Pharm Pharmacol 1978; *30*:60–62.

86. Wurtman RJ. Neurochemical changes following high-dose aspartame with dietary carbohydrate. N Engl J Med 1983; *309*:597.

87. Yokogoshi H, Roberts CH, Caballero B, et al. Effects of aspartame and glucose administration on brain and plasma levels of large neutral amino acids and brain 5-hydroxyindoles. Am J Clin Nutr 1984; *40*:1–7.

88. Maher TJ, Wurtman RJ. High doses of aspartame reduce blood pressure in spontaneously hypertensive rats. New Engl J Med 1984; *309*:1125.

IV

NUTRITIONAL SUPPORT

42

THE FUNCTIONAL BASIS OF ASSESSMENT

K.N. JEEJEEBHOY

It is common experience that health and vigor do not correlate with body mass nor with visible muscularity. Thus, long-distance runners are characteristically gaunt in appearance but have extremely efficient cardiovascular, respiratory, and musculoskeletal systems. They often have better function than heavier or "more developed" persons. In order to study function, in contradistinction to body mass (composition), as a measure of nutritional status, there has been developed an objective measure of muscle function. The hypothesis has been tested that functional changes precede those of body composition during starvation and correspondingly are corrected earlier during refeeding. These results have been compared with those of more traditional methods of assessment such as levels of liver-produced plasma proteins and degrees of immunocompetence to skin testing.

A review of some functional consequences of malnutrition, including the evidence for the statements just made, seems best approached by considering the effects of malnutrition on three separate and vital organ functions, namely (1) hepatic secretory protein function, (2) immunocompetence, and (3) skeletal muscle function.

HEPATIC SECRETORY PROTEINS

A variety of proteins, including pre-albumin, albumin, transferrin, ceruloplasmin, and retinol-binding protein, are synthesized by the liver and secreted into the plasma.[1] Nutrient supply is critical for the maintenance of the polysomal aggregation required for optimum synthesis of these proteins, which are exported from the liver, and it has been clearly established that total hepatic protein and RNA levels decline during fasting.[2,3] Hence in conditions of deficient nutrient input, it might be expected that the plasma concentration of albumin and other plasma proteins secreted by the liver, namely transferrin and retinol-binding protein, would decline. Albumin is the most abundant of these proteins, and human serum contains 35 to 45 g/L. In the hepatocyte, it is not native albumin that is formed but a series of precursors, the first of which is known as prepro-albumin, which differs from native albumin by 24 additional amino acid residues. It takes 25 to 30 minutes for a molecule of albumin to be synthesized by the polysomes and secreted into the plasma. Albumin is not stored in the hepatocyte, but continuously secreted into the plasma at an estimated rate of 17 g per day, and turned over with a half-life of approximately 20 days.

The rate of decline in the serum levels of any of these proteins, due to reduced synthesis, is proportional to the rate of turnover (i.e., inversely proportional to half-life). Hence a protein with a short half-life (e.g., prealbumin—12 hr) is more sensitive to nutrient deprivation than albumin, which has a long half-life.[4,5] Although a low serum albumin level may indicate depletion of visceral protein, changes in its synthesis will not alter its circulating levels rapidly because of the protein's long half-life. Several clinical studies have demonstrated that serum albumin does not respond to short-term changes in protein and energy intake, compared with pre-albumin and retinol-binding protein, the levels of which change more rapidly in response to both dietary restriction and refeeding. Unfortunately a fall in the levels of circulating proteins is not specifically due to nutrient deficiency. The plasma levels of these proteins critically depend on liver function. Altered liver function due to septicemia and underlying liver disease may account for low serum albumin levels even when nutrients are available in sufficient quantities. In addition, excessive protein losses (e.g., protein-losing enteropathy) may cause a fall in circulating levels simply because of the bulk loss of protein in excess of synthesis.[6] Thus one of the intrinsic difficulties in using the plasma concentration of these hepatic secretory proteins in the assessment of nutritional status is the problem of separating the effects of actual nutrient deprivation from those of a disease process. In conclusion, nutrient deficiency per se cannot be adequately assessed by measuring plasma protein levels, and low protein levels do not necessarily mean a lack of nutrients.

IMMUNODEFICIENCY

Malnutrition is the commonest cause of secondary immunodeficiency. This alteration in immune function affects almost all facets of host resistance, and as a result, infection is one of the most frequent complications of undernutrition. Cell-mediated immune response is affected early and severely by undernutrition. In malnutrition it has been demonstrated that the proportion and absolute numbers of T cells are decreased,[7] the function of T helper cells is impaired, and T cell differentiation may be retarded because of reduction in thymic inductive hormones.[8]

In addition to impaired cell-mediated immunity, the complement system, opsonic function of plasma, and polymorphonuclear cell function may also be altered in severe malnutrition. Recently the phagocytic role of a high-molecular-weight glycoprotein, fibronectin, has been emphasized. Fibronectin is found in blood and tissue fluid as well as in association with basement membranes, connective tissue, and the extracellular matrix of many cells.[9–12] The site of synthesis of the opsonically active plasma fibronectin is yet to be found. In tissue culture, fibronectin is actively produced by vascular endothelial cells, fibroblasts and hepatocytes, and some macrophages.[9,10,12] Plasma fibronectin is known to aid the phagocytic function of macrophages such as the Kupffer cell. Multiple organ failure in the septic patient may be related to Kupffer cell dysfunction mediated by plasma opsonic fibronectin deficiency.[13] This deficiency has also been noted in patients with major burn injury[14] and during starvation in rats.[13] Deficiency of plasma opsonic fibronectin in septic injured patients can be reversed by intravenous infusion of fibronectin-rich fresh plasma cryoprecipitate.[15] The levels of opsonic fibronectin are sensitive to disturbed nutrition, and thus host defense mechanisms may be impaired in malnutrition by fibronectin deficiency.

Severe undernutrition also alters serum immunoglobulins. Serum immunoglobulin G (IgG) concentration is usually elevated, although rarely it may be low,[16] particularly in low-birth-weight marasmic infants. Secretory immunoglobulin A (IgA) and mucosal antibody responses to viral antigens are usually reduced. This may be due to a reduction in IgA-producing plasma cells, reduced synthesis of secretory component, or decreased T cell function.[17]

Selected nutrient deficiencies can also alter immune function. Zinc deficiency is associated with lymphoid atrophy and decreased delayed cutaneous hypersensitivity.[18] Iron and magnesium deficiencies can impair in vitro immune function testing and are associated with an increased incidence of certain infections.[19] As well, deficiencies of pyridoxine, folic acid, vitamin A, and vitamin E may result in impaired cell-mediated immunity and reduced antibody responses.[20]

The most common form of in vivo testing of immunocompetence in hospitalized patients is delayed cutaneous hypersensitivity (DCH) to known recall antigens. The common antigens tested by intradermal injection include mumps, *Candida*, streptokinase-streptodornase, purified protein derivative (PPD), dinitrochlorobenzene (DNCB), and, in pediatrics, diphtheria toxoid. At least three antigens are injected intradermally on the forearm and read at 24 and 48 hours. Greater than 10 mm of induration is considered positive, and a patient is considered anergic if he does not react to any of the three antigens. Meakins et al.[21] showed that increased post-operative infection and decreased survival were seen in patients with absent delayed cutaneous hypersensitivity. They considered the cause of such anergy to be malnutrition. However, it is well known that a number of factors other than undernutrition can suppress DCH.[22] These factors, noted below, must be taken into account before abnormal responses to skin testing are attributed to malnutrition alone.

1. *Infections.* Sepsis due to viral,[23,24] bacterial,[25] and granulomatous infections[26] can suppress normal DCH. Therefore, it is not surprising that it has been found that simply draining the site of infection may reverse anergy.[27]

2. *Metabolic disorders.* Uremia,[28,29] cirrhosis,[30,31] hepatitis,[32,33] inflammatory bowel diseases,[34-36] and sarcoidosis[37-39] are known to suppress normal DCH. It appears that trauma alone in the absence of malnutrition can produce anergy.[40] The same is true of burns[41] and hemorrhage.[42,43]

3. *Malignant disease.* Anergy or depressed DCH has been noted in patients with solid tumors.[22] Also, chemotherapy[44] and radiotherapy[45-47] are known to impair DCH.

4. *Drugs.* Many commonly used drugs affect DCH, including steroids,[48,49] immunosuppressants,[50] cimetidine,[51-53] coumadin,[54] and perhaps aspirin.[55]

5. *Surgery and anesthesia.* General anesthesia alone, even in the absence of surgery, can depress immune function and change DCH.[56]

Clearly abnormalities in DCH in the hospitalized patient are nonspecific, and do not necessarily reflect a state of nutrient deficiency. Hence the view that increased morbidity or mortality associated with reduced DCH is due only to malnutrition per se is incorrect, and the evidence that absence of DCH is a major cause of increased morbidity or mortality is equivocal. It may be that stress, with elevation of steroid levels, present in many diseases and in malnutrition, is a common pathway resulting in depressed skin test response.

SKELETAL MUSCLE FUNCTION

Wasting of muscle is an obvious effect of severe malnutrition, and this has led to the use of anthropometric measurements, including limb muscle circumference, to assess malnutrition. Based on the assumption that a positive nitrogen balance indicates muscle anabolism, a positive nitrogen balance has been used as an index of the beneficial effects of nutritional support. In animal experiments (with growing rats) and in young children, nitrogen retention and growth are obvious effects of optimum nutritional intake. This observation has been applied to malnourished adult humans (nongrowing) who have been considered potentially able to "regrow" the lost tissue.

It is true that patients receiving long-term home total parenteral nutrition (TPN) have been shown to gain body weight and nitrogen; this is in contrast to the results in those receiving short- and intermediate-term nutritional intervention, in whom despite an adequate intake of nitrogen and calories, little or no increase in total body nitrogen has been seen in a variety of patients receiving TPN in hospital over several weeks.[57] If, however, the nitrogen intake is markedly increased, then some gain in nitrogen is observed.[58] Despite the lack of any gain or the very modest gain in nitrogen, nutritional support does indeed appear to improve outcome in the form of reduced complications and mortality after a period of support so short that body composition can hardly be altered. For example, it has been shown that support with amino acids and support with calories both resulted in equivalent sparing of body nitrogen, but the latter was associated with more rapid wound healing and fewer complications.[59] It has also been shown that patients with reduced plasma protein levels and absent delayed cutaneous hypersensitivity had increased postoperative morbidity, which was improved by a 7-day course of preoperative nutritional support.[60] However, the same investigators noted that improvement was not associated with a change or improvement in the very indices used to predict the presence of malnutrition (Prognostic Nutritional Index). Other investigators have demonstrated that a 10-day period of preoperative nutritional support altered morbidity and mortality following surgery in patients with gastrointestinal carcinoma.[61]

Thus the good outcome does not correlate with the very modest changes in body composition. The data suggest that the reversal of the adverse effects of malnutrition is not based on improvement of the traditional parameters of nutrition, such as gain in body nitrogen or a demonstrated increase in muscle mass or in plasma proteins. Concordant with this discrepancy is the observation that global clinical assessment is at least equivalent to, and in some respects better than, individual objective traditional measurements of nutritional status in predicting outcome.[62]

On the basis of the foregoing evidence, there are grounds for suspecting that functional abnormalities in adult (nongrowing) humans may not be the result of simple loss of lean tissue and also that patients may recover from these disorders before any such lean tissue is regained.

To investigate this area we have done a series of three studies using objective measurements of muscle function in relation to nutritional deprivation and refeeding in humans and in an animal model.

Muscle Function Tests

We have examined a function that could be measured objectively, namely the muscle contraction-relaxation characteristics (in contrast to pure force) and endurance. Muscle function was chosen because it is of vital importance; changes in the ability to contract and relax quickly and reduced endurance may alter respiratory function and lead to respiratory failure in critically ill patients.

It has been shown consistently that the ratio of potassium to sodium content in the body is altered in malnutrition.[63,64] Such changes could affect the intracellular electrolyte content (and thus the responsiveness of muscle), so that muscle function might be altered before these changes could be detected by whole-body measurements. Thus during a period of deficient nutrient intake, changes in muscle function might well precede detectable changes in structure or composition. Through an objective study of muscle function in response to deficient nutrient intake, we could, in theory, define the commencement of functional impairment.

HUMAN STUDIES

There are problems in testing for muscle strength and fatigue. The straightforward approach would be to have the patient exercise, measuring performance on a treadmill or bicycle. Obviously this is not possible with seriously ill patients, and, furthermore, the result depends on previous training and motivation. Of more importance is the fact that during the initial phases of contraction, the nerve impulses are rapid. As high-frequency fatigue sets in, the impulse rate slows. Thus voluntary contraction has an inbuilt reserve mechanism that does not allow the demonstration of early abnormality. To avoid these obstacles it was necessary to use a more controlled and objective method of stimulating the muscle that did not depend on voluntary effort by the patient. The method chosen involved electrical stimulation of the ulnar nerve at the wrist and measurement of the contraction-relaxation characteristics of the adductor pollicis muscle in the right hand.

The techniques for objective muscle testing were originally described by Merton[65] and more recently have been modified by Edwards.[66,67] It has also been shown that the measurement of muscle function as described by Merton and Edwards will give the same results when muscles as diverse as the adductor pollicis, quadriceps, sternomastoid, and diaphragm are tested.[68] The similarity of the results from diverse muscles allows us to consider the function of the adductor pollicis as representative of muscle function in general. In preliminary studies it was confirmed that the diaphragmatic changes in malnutrition do mirror those in the adductor pollicis. Thus the studies described below may be thought of as representative of a more vital muscle mass such as the diaphragm. The function of the adductor pollicis muscle in the right hand was measured by stimulating the ulnar nerve at the wrist with an electrical unidirectional square wave impulse of 75 to 100 microsecond duration. The stimulus was of a supramaximal voltage (range: 80 to 120 volts) and at frequencies increasing from 10 to 100 Hertz. Simultaneous EMG records documented constant supramaximal nerve stimulation (Fig. 42–1).

This technique involved minor discomfort but not pain. When the motor nerve to a muscle is stimulated at a voltage at least 20 per cent greater than that needed to achieve a maximum mechanical or electrical response ("supramaximal nerve stimulation"), all muscle fibers are made to contract. The force generated depends on the frequency of stimulation and whether the muscle is fresh or fatigued. Absolute forces vary among individuals depending on body size and muscular training. However, the force obtained at different stimulation frequencies expressed as a percentage of the maximal force produced by electrical stimulation (force-frequency curve) is reproducible and comparable among individuals. Electrical stimulation of the ulnar nerve at 10, 20, 30, 50, and 100 Hz with 15- to 30-second

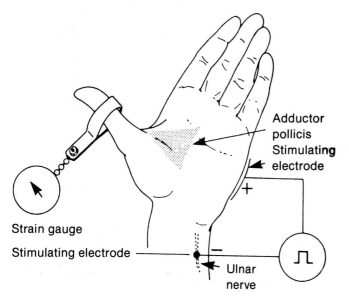

FIGURE 42–1. *Relative positions of the stimulating electrode, strain gauge, and adductor pollicis muscle during skeletal muscle function testing. (From Edwards RHT. Clin Sci Mol Med 1977; 52:283–290. Reproduced with permission.)*

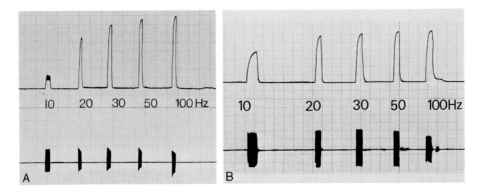

FIGURE 42–2. *Force of contraction at different stimulation frequencies. The force of contraction with electrical stimulation at 10, 20, 30, 50, and 100 Hz. The malnourished patient (B) shows an increased force at 10 Hz expressed as a percentage of the force at 100 Hz compared with the normal subject (A). The lower tracing in each graph shows the surface electromyograph (EMG) demonstrating constant nerve stimulation. (From Lopes J, Russell DM, Whitwell J, et al. Am J Clin Nutr 1982; 36:602–610. © 1982, Am J Clin Nutr, American Society for Clinical Nutrition. Reproduced with permission.)*

intervals between the stimuli was performed (Fig. 42–2). This procedure was repeated to test for reproducibility. The effects of post-tetanic potentiation were standardized by a fixed order of testing. In normal healthy subjects at low-frequency stimulation, the muscle responds as single twitches that generate a small percentage of the maximum force. As the stimulus frequency increases, the twitches start to fuse and the force increases. Above 20 Hz the muscle is tetanized, and above 50 Hz the force is equal to the maximum voluntary force. The shape of this frequency curve is the same for different muscles and the same in all normal individuals. In the malnourished patient, tetany occurs at a lower stimulation frequency with potentiation of the muscle force. There is also a loss of force at high-frequency stimulation, so that the force at 10 Hz expressed as a percentage of the force at 100 Hz (F_{10}/F_{max}) is increased.

Muscle relaxation rate was determined after a brief tetanic stimulation (1 to 2 seconds) at 30 Hz (Fig. 42–3). Maximal relaxation rate (MRR) is calculated from the gradient of the initial phase of relaxation.[69] MRR is expressed as the percentage of force lost per 10 milliseconds. Although relaxation rate from voluntary isometric quadriceps contractions does increase with the force of contraction, electrically stimulated contractions producing increasing forces do not significantly change the MRR. Malnutrition results in significant slowing of the MRR of the adductor pollicis.

Endurance was tested with continuous electrical stimulation at 20 Hz for 30 seconds' duration, and the percentage of force lost in 30 seconds was noted (Fig. 42–4). Malnutrition resulted in significant muscle fatigue during this prolonged stimulation.

ANIMAL STUDIES

Barbiturate-anesthetized 8-week-old male Wistar rats had the gastrocnemius muscle freed with an intact blood supply and its nerve supply isolated. The body and hind limbs of the animal were immersed in modified Liley's solution kept at 37° C. The same measurements were made as in the human, but at frequencies from 0.5 to 200 Hz, and the effects of stimulating the sciatic nerve on the contraction characteristics of the gastrocnemius muscle

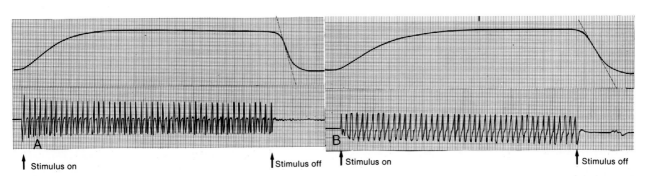

FIGURE 42–3. *Maximal relaxation rate (MRR). The force of contraction (and EMG recording) after a brief tetanic stimulation at 30 Hz. The MRR is calculated from the gradient of the initial phase of relaxation, and is slower in the malnourished patient (B) compared with the normal subject (A). (From Lopes J, Russell DM, Whitwell J, et al. Am J Clin Nutr 1982; 36:602–610. © 1982, Am J Clin Nutr, American Society for Clinical Nutrition. Reproduced with permission.)*

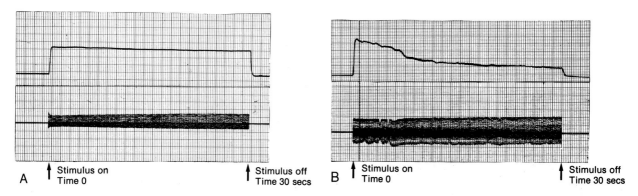

FIGURE 42–4. *Muscle endurance. The force of contraction (and EMG recording) at 20 Hz stimulation for 30 seconds. There is significant muscle fatigue in the malnourished patient (B) compared with the normal subject (A). (From Lopes J, Russell DM, Whitwell J, et al. Am J Clin Nutr 1982; 36:602–610. © 1982, Am J Clin Nutr, American Society for Clinical Nutrition. Reproduced with permission.)*

were noted. Simultaneously biopsies were taken from the contralateral gastrocnemius.

Effect of Malnutrition and Nutritional Support

Specific abnormalities in muscle function were observed in 10 patients with a variety of gastrointestinal disorders.[70] All patients had clinical and biochemical features of severe nutritional depletion. Three discrete abnormalities of muscle function were noted: (1) altered force-frequency pattern with an increased force at 10 Hz stimulation expressed as a percentage of the maximal force (increased F_{10}/F_{max}), (2) slower maximal relaxation rate, and (3) increased muscle fatiguability. To test the hypothesis that the functional abnormalities are purely due to nutritional deprivation and precede detectable alterations in body composition, six morbidly obese subjects were studied initially and after 2 weeks of a 400 kcal/day diet, again after an additional 2 weeks of fasting, and finally after 2 weeks of refeeding.[71] Significant changes in muscle contraction-relaxation characteristics were noted after the 2 weeks of hypocaloric dieting, and even more profound changes of decreased MRR and increased muscle fatiguability were noted after the 2 weeks of fasting. Oral refeeding resulted in restoration of all muscle function parameters to normal within 2 weeks (Figs. 42–5 to 42–7).

To reinforce the findings with obese subjects, six patients with primary anorexia nervosa were studied at a time of severe nutritional depletion, and then sequentially during strictly supervised oral refeeding.[72] This study confirmed that pure protein-calorie malnutrition was associated with profound changes in muscle function, that after 4 weeks of oral refeeding muscle endurance and maximal relaxation rate were normal, and that by 8 weeks of refeeding all parameters were normal (Figs. 42–8 to 42–10).

In order to confirm that the observations in hu-

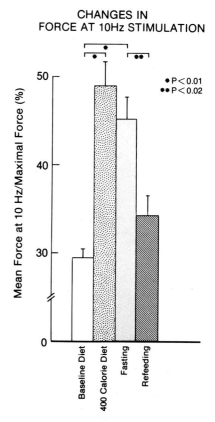

CHANGES IN
FORCE AT 10Hz STIMULATION

* P < 0.01
** P < 0.02

FIGURE 42–5. *The bar graphs represent the mean ± SEM force at 10 Hz stimulation expressed as a percentage of the maximal force. The brackets above the graphs indicate the significant changes during the study. (From Russell DM, Leiter LA, Whitwell J, et al. Am J Clin Nutr 1983; 37:133–138. © 1983, Am J Clin Nutr, American Society for Clinical Nutrition. Reproduced with permission.)*

CHANGES IN
MAXIMAL RELAXATION RATE (MRR)

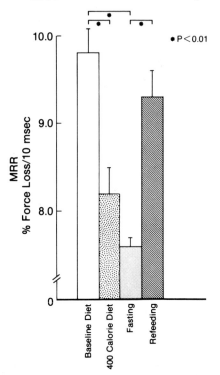

FIGURE 42–6. *Mean ± SEM maximal relaxation rate. The brackets above the bar graphs indicate the significant changes during the study. (From Russell DM, Leiter LA, Whitwell J, et al. Am J Clin Nutr 1983; 37:133–138. © 1983, Am J Clin Nutr, American Society for Clinical Nutrition. Reproduced with permission.)*

mans were clearly related to nutritional deprivation, we studied the same functional parameters, together with metabolic analysis of muscle biopsies, in rats acutely deprived of nutrients or chronically underfed (as compared with pair-fed animals). This animal model produced similar changes in skeletal function as assessed by stimulating the sciatic nerve and measuring the function of the gastrocnemius muscle. It also allowed us to analyze muscle composition in order to understand better the mechanisms responsible for changes in muscle function in malnutrition.

Correlation of Objective Measurements of Body Composition and Muscle Function

The starved obese humans did not lose significant amounts of TBK or TBN, nor was there a significant change in creatinine-height index at a time when abnormalities of muscle function were obvious.[71] Conversely, during refeeding these subjects rapidly lost muscle fatiguability and had normal contraction-relaxation characteristics at a time when there was no significant increase in lean body components or in body weight.

In the anorexic patients, gross muscle fatigue and abnormal function were present at baseline.[72] However, it was noted that these patients had normal plasma proteins at that time (Table 42–1). Initially they had marked loss of lean body mass and of total body nitrogen and potassium. When they were refed, muscle fatigue disappeared within 4 weeks and all functional abnormalities were resolved by 8 weeks of refeeding when the creatinine-height index was still very low at 67 per cent and TBN had risen by only 13 per cent (Table 42–2). Interestingly, while the TBK and body fat had risen proportionately more during this period, they were still well below the level expected for their height. Despite an incomplete return to normal body composition, clinically these patients had restored their ability to exercise and function.

Muscle Biopsy Analysis in Malnutrition

In obese patients, fasting resulted in Type II fiber atrophy.[73] In animals, 2 to 5 days of fasting resulted in an increase in slow-twitch oxidative fibers (Type I), but prolonged hypocaloric dieting resulted in the appearance of fibers depleted in both myosin and Na-K ATPase, a fiber type not normally seen. De-

CHANGES IN
MUSCLE FATIGUABILITY

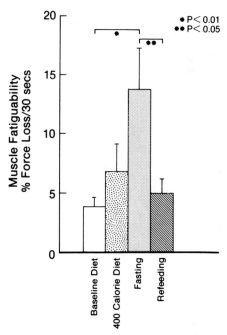

FIGURE 42–7. *Mean ± SEM muscle fatiguability. The brackets indicate the significant changes during the study. (From Russell DM, Leiter LA, Whitwell J, et al. Am J Clin Nutr 1983; 37:133–138. © 1983, Am J Clin Nutr, American Society for Clinical Nutrition. Reproduced with permission.)*

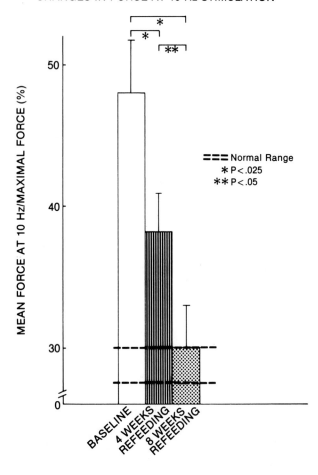

CHANGES IN FORCE AT 10 Hz STIMULATION

=== Normal Range
* P<.025
** P<.05

FIGURE 42–8. Mean ± SEM force at 10 Hz stimulation expressed as a percentage of the maximum. The brackets indicate the significant changes during refeeding. (From Russell DM, Prendergast PJ, Darby PL, et al. Am J Clin Nutr 1983; 38:229–237. © Am J Clin Nutr, American Society for Clinical Nutrition. Reproduced with permission.)

FIGURE 42–9. Mean ± SEM maximal relaxation rate. The brackets indicate the significant changes during refeeding. (From Russell DM, Prendergast PJ, Darby PL, et al. Am J Clin Nutr 1983; 38:229–237. ©Am J Clin Nutr, American Society for Clinical Nutrition. Reproduced with permission.)

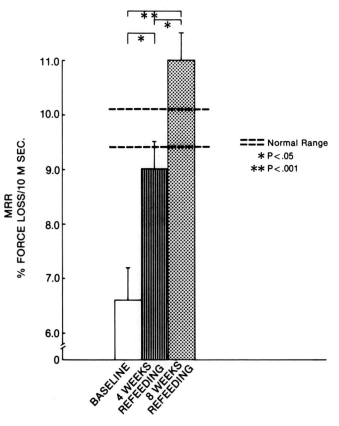

CHANGES IN MAXIMAL RELAXATION RATE

=== Normal Range
* P<.05
** P<.001

CHANGES IN MUSCLE FATIGUABILITY

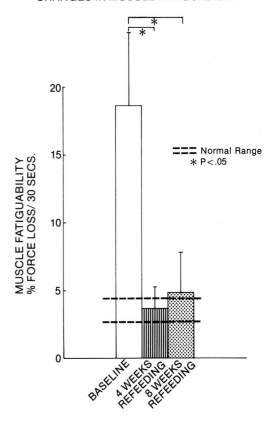

FIGURE 42–10. *Mean ± SEM muscle fatiguability. The brackets indicate the significant changes during refeeding. The dotted lines represent the previously reported normal range. (From Russell DM, Prendergast PJ, Darby PL, et al. Am J Clin Nutr 1983; 38:229–237. © Am J Clin Nutr, American Society for Clinical Nutrition. Reproduced with permission.)*

spite these very different fiber type patterns, the muscle function abnormalities and fatiguability were similar with nutritional deprivation.

The most striking findings during hypocaloric dieting and fasting in both humans and rats were an increase in the total water content and an increase in both the intracellular concentration and total ionic content of muscle sodium and calcium. In contrast, total potassium, magnesium, chloride, and phosphate remained normal. Other notable changes were a fall in the ATP/ADP ratio and a rise in the lactate/pyruvate ratio in hypocalorically fed rats and in humans.

Phosphofructokinase fell with short-term fasting, while succinate dehydrogenase and acyl CoA dehydrogenase remained normal or rose, suggesting a change to more oxidative fibers with early starvation.[74] However, prolonged hypocaloric feeding was followed by a reduction in phosphofructokinase, succinate dehydrogenase, and acyl CoA dehydrogenase.

These studies demonstrated a lack of relationship between changes in lean body mass and body function. It is clear that the loss or restoration of lean body mass is not essential for the occurrence of the corresponding changes in muscle contraction-relaxation characteristics and endurance properties. Our findings are consistent with the somewhat similar data concerning morbidity and mortality mentioned earlier.[60,61] Thus one may well question whether the demonstration of malnutrition should depend on

changes in lean body mass, and conversely whether the restoration of lean body mass and improved nitrogen balance constitute the gold standards for good nutritional support. Our results indicate that the failure to restore body nitrogen, observed in earlier studies, does not negate the possibility that such support may have restored function.

What then are the possible causes of the improved function noted? An obvious explanation for slow relaxation is loss of fast-twitch fibers (Type II). However, there are several reasons for doubting this hypothesis. First, it has been shown that the contraction characteristics are the same for many different muscles of completely different fiber composition.[68] Second, these functional effects of short-term fasting (associated with maintenance of oxidative enzyme activity) are the same as after prolonged hypocaloric feeding (when all enzymes are reduced). Third, histochemical examination showed that the fiber type, after prolonged hypocaloric feeding, is unlike Type I.

In contrast, the most consistent finding was one of an increase in intracellular sodium and calcium in all situations associated with increased fatigue, slower relaxation, and a rise in the percentage of maximum force attained at lower frequencies—another way of expressing slower relaxation. It may be recalled that in striated muscle, the regulation of the cellular calcium content is critical for its kinetic properties.[75] In ventricular myocardial muscle fibers, membrane currents are dependent on the sodium and calcium influx and efflux during depolarization

TABLE 42–1. Changes in Standard Parameters of Nutritional Assessment in Anorexic Patients during Refeeding

	Total Body Weight	Lean Body Weight*	% Body Fat*	Serum Albumin	Serum Transferrin	Creatinine-Height Index	Lymphocyte Count	DCH
	kg	kg	%	g/dl	µg/dl	%	mm³	No. Anergic Patients
A. Baseline	39.0±3.9	33.5±3.2	14.0±0.5	4.0±0.1	170±44	49.7±7.4	1845±252	5/6
B. 2 weeks refeeding	41.1±3.6	34.9±3.1	15.0±0.7	4.2±0.4	228±45	57.7±6.1	1747±220	—
C. 4 weeks refeeding	43.4±3.7	36.6±3.1	15.7±0.8	4.4±0.3	215±38	64.9±3.4	2013±315	3/6
D. 6 weeks refeeding	44.8±3.8	37.7±2.9	16.8±0.8	4.5±0.3	243±41	63.4±4.1	1727±262	—
E. 8 weeks refeeding	46.5±4.4	38.6±3.4	17.1±1.0	4.4±0.3	245±50	67.0±7.7	1810±222	1/6
P value AC	<0.001	<0.001	<0.05	ns†	<0.01	ns	ns	ns
AE	<0.001	<0.001	<0.01	ns	<0.005	ns	ns	<0.025
CE	<0.01	<0.01	ns	ns	ns	ns	ns	ns

*Calculated from anthropometric measurements.
†ns, not significant.
From Russell DM, Prendergast PJ, Darby PL, et al. Am J Clin Nutr 1983; 38:229–237. © 1983, Am J Clin Nutr, American Society for Clinical Nutrition. Reproduced with permission.

TABLE 42–2. *Conventional Measures of Body Composition in Patients with Anorexia Nervosa*

	Total Body Nitrogen*	Total Body Potassium†	Creatine-Height Index	Body Fat‡
	kg	*mmol*	*%*	*%*
Baseline	1.21 ± 0.11	1590 ± 179	49.7 ± 7.4	14 ± 0.5
4 wks refed	1.33 ± 0.10	1897 ± 205	64.9 ± 3.4	15.7 ± 0.8
8 wks refed	1.37 ± 0.10	2103 + 179	67.0 ± 7.7	17.1 ± 1.0

*Predicted normal on the basis of height and armspan = 1.70 ± 0.08 kg.[76]
†Normal in our institution = 2462 ± 359 mmol.
‡Average for a woman considered to be 24%. Values calculated from anthropometric measurements.

and repolarization. Clearly the accumulation of intracellular muscle calcium will reduce the muscle relaxation rate and alter the contraction characteristics. This accumulation can also interfere with mitochondrial function and may explain the increased intracellular lactate/pyruvate ratio. Calcium accumulation may occur because it cannot be pumped out. The process of calcium efflux is energy dependent, and thus calcium accumulation may be a sensitive index of reduced cell energy reserves—and indeed the creatine phosphate/ATP ratio is reduced. It is of interest that branched-chain amino acids provide energy for muscles, and so protein may have a special role in this regard rather than simply as a means of accumulating nitrogen.

Obviously while many interesting avenues need confirmation and exploration, there is sufficient evidence to suggest that in the adult human, the adverse functional effects of malnutrition cannot be equated to, nor quantitated by, a simple loss of lean body mass. Furthermore, restoration of body function cannot be equated to "regrowth" of lean body mass assessed by a gain in body nitrogen or the attainment of a positive nitrogen balance. Clearly the changes in cellular energy resulting in changes in cellular electrolytes at a time of functional impairment need further study.

Thus it becomes increasingly apparent that simply attempting to give nutritional support for the purpose of increasing lean body mass or body nitrogen is neither necessary nor desirable on a short-term basis. In such patients the ulimate object should be better function and clinical outcome.

References

1. Gitlin D, Gitlin JD. Fetal and neonatal development of plasma proteins. *In* Putman FW (ed). The Plasma Proteins. Structure, Function and Genetic Control. Vol 2. 2nd ed. New York, Academic Press, 1975: 263–319.
2. Shafritz DA. Molecular hybridization probes for research in liver disease: studies with albumin cDNA. Gastroenterology 1979; 77:1335–1348.
3. Rothschild MA, Oratz M, Schreiber SS. Albumin synthesis. *In* Javitt NB (ed). Liver and Biliary Tract Physiology I. Int. Rev. Physiol. Vol. 21, Baltimore: University Park Press, 1980: 249–274.
4. Shetty PS, Jung RT, Watrasiewicz KE, et al. Rapid-turnover transport proteins: an index of subclinical protein-energy malnutrition. Lancet 1979; 2:230–232.
5. Young GA, Collins JP, Hill GL. Plasma proteins in patients receiving intravenous amino acids or intravenous hyperalimentation after major surgery. Am J Clin Nutr 1979; 32:1192–1199.
6. Jeejeebhoy KN. Cause of hypoalbuminaemia in patients with gastrointestinal and cardiac disease. Lancet 1962; 1:343–348.
7. Chandra RK. Rosette-forming T lymphocytes and cell-mediated immunity in malnutrition. Br Med J 1974; 3:608–609.
8. Chandra RK. Serum thymic hormone activity in protein-energy malnutrition. Clin Exp Immunol 1979; 38:228–230.
9. Yamada KM, Olden K. Fibronectin: adhesive glycoproteins of cell surface and blood. Nature (London) 1978; 275:179–184.
10. Saba TM, Jaffe E. Plasma fibronectin (opsonic glycoprotein): its synthesis by vascular endothelial cells and role in cardiopulmonary integrity after trauma as related to reticuloendothelial function. Am J Med 1980; 68:577–594.
11. Mosher DF, Proctor RA, Grossman JE. Fibronectin: role in inflammation. Advances in Inflammation Research 1981; 2:187–207.
12. Ruoslahti E, Engvall E, Hayman E. Fibronectin: current concepts of its structure and function. Collagen Res 1981; 1:95–128.
13. Saba TM, Dillon BC, Lanser ME. Fibronectin and phagocytic host defence: relationship to nutritional support. JPEN 1983; 7:62–68.
14. Lanser ME, Saba TM, Scovill WA. Opsonic glycoprotein (plasma fibronectin) levels after burn injury: relationship to extent of burn and development of sepsis. Ann Surg 1980; 192:776–782.
15. Scovill WA, Saba TM, Blumenstock FA, et al. Opsonic alpha₂ surface binding glycoprotein therapy during sepsis. Ann Surg 1979; 188:521–592.
16. Chandra RK. Immunocompetence as a functional index of nutritional status. Br Med Bull 1981; 37:89–94.
17. Chandra RK. Nutritional deficiency and susceptibility to infection. Bull WHO 1979; 57:167–177.
18. Dreizen S. Nutrition and the immune response—a review. Int J Vitam Nutr Res 1978; 49:220–228.
19. Chandra RK, Dayton DH. Trace element regulation of immunity and infection. Nutr Res 1982; 2:721–733.
20. Biesel WR, Edelman R, Nauss K, et al. Single-nutrient effects on immunological functions. JAMA 1981; 245:53–58.
21. Meakins JL, Pietsch JB, Bubenick O, et al. Delayed hypersensitivity: indicator of acquired failure of host defences in sepsis and trauma. Ann Surg 1977; 186:241–250.
22. Twomey P, Ziegler D, Rombeau J. Utility of skin testing in nutritional assessment: a critical review. JPEN 1982; 6:50–58.
23. Reed WP, Olds JW, Kisch AL. Decreased skin-test reactivity associated with influenza. J Infect Dis 1972; 125:398–402.

24. Mangi RJ, Niederman JC, Kelleher JE, et al. Depression of cell-mediated immunity during acute infectious mononucleosis. N Engl J Med 1974; 291:1149–1153.

25. Mitchell AG, Nelson WE, LeBlanc TJ. Studies in immunity. V. Effect of acute diseases on the reaction of the skin to tuberculin. Am J Dis Child 1935; 49:695–702.

26. Bullock WE. Studies of immune mechanisms in leprosy. N Engl J Med 1968; 278:298–304.

27. Meakins JL, Christou NV, Shizgal HM, et al. Therapeutic approaches to anergy in surgical patients. Ann Surg 1979; 190:286–296.

28. Wilson WEC, Kirkpatrick CH, Talmage DW. Suppression of immunologic responsiveness in uremia. Ann Intern Med 1965; 62:1–14.

29. Bansal VK, Popli S, Pickering J, et al. Protein-calorie malnutrition and cutaneous anergy in hemodialysis maintained patients. Am J Clin Nutr 1980; 33:1608–1611.

30. Straus B, Berenyi M, Ming-Huang J, et al. Delayed hypersensitivity in alcoholic cirrhosis. Dig Dis 1971; 16:509–516.

31. Fox RA, Scheuer PF, Sherlock S, et al. Impaired delayed hypersensitivity in primary biliary cirrhosis. (Abstract.) Gut 1968; 9:729.

32. Toh BH, Roberts-Thomson IC, Matthews JD, et al. Depression of cell-mediated immunity in old age and the immunopathic diseases, lupus erythematosus, chronic hepatitis and rheumatoid arthritis. Clin Exp Immunol 1973; 14:193–202.

33. Snyder N, Bessoff J, Dwyer JM, et al. Depressed delayed cutaneous hypersensitivity in alcoholic hepatitis. Dig Dis 1978; 23:353–358.

34. Meyers S, Sachar DB, Taub RN, et al. Anergy to dinitrochlorobenzene and depression of T-lymphocytes in Crohn's disease and ulcerative colitis. Gut 1976; 17:911–915.

35. Sachar DB, Taub RM, Ramachandar K, et al. T and B lymphocytes and cutaneous anergy in inflammatory bowel disease. Ann NY Acad Sci 1976; 278:565–572.

36. Thayer WR, Fixa B, Komarkova O, et al. Skin test reactivity in inflammatory bowel disease in the United States and Czechoslovakia. Dig Dis 1978; 23:337–340.

37. Jones JV. Development of sensitivity to dinitrochlorobenzene in patients with sarcoidosis. Clin Exp Immunol 1967; 2:477–487.

38. Chusid EL, Shah R, Siltzbach LE. Tuberculin tests during the course of sarcoidosis in 350 patients. Am Rev Respir Dis 1971; 104:13–21.

39. Goldstein RA, Janicki BW, Mirro J, et al. Cell-mediated immune responses in sarcoidosis. Am Rev Respir Dis 1978; 117:55–62.

40. Meakins JL, McLean AP, Kelly R, et al. Delayed hypersensitivity and neutrophil chemotaxis: effect of trauma. J Trauma 1978; 18:240–247.

41. Hiebert JM, McGough M, Rodeheaver G, et al. The influence of catabolism on immunocompetence in burned patients. Surgery 1979; 86:242–247.

42. Pietsch JB, Meakins JL, MacLean LD. The delayed hypersensitivity response: application in clinical surgery. Surgery 1979; 82:349–355.

43. Ota DM, Copeland EM, Corriere JN, et al. The effects of nutrition and treatment of cancer on host immunocompetence. Surg Gynecol Obstet 1979; 148:104–111.

44. Boeva M, Donchev T, Markova R, et al. Delayed hypersensitivity reactions in patients with breast cancer. Neoplasma 1978; 25:733–736.

45. Campbell AC, Hersey P, MacLennan ICM, et al. Immunosuppressive consequences of radiotherapy and chemotherapy in patients with acute lymphoblastic leukemia. Br Med J 1973; 2:385–388.

46. Cosimi AB, Brunstetter FH, Kemmerer WT, et al. Cellular immune competence of breast cancer patients receiving radiotherapy. Arch Surg 1973; 107:531–535.

47. Wara WM, Phillips TL, Wara DW, et al. Immunosuppression following radiation therapy for carcinoma of the nasopharynx. Am J Roentgenol 1975; 123:482–485.

48. Bovornkitti S, Kangsadal P, Sathirapat P, et al. Reversion and reconversion rate of tuberculin skin reactions in correlation with the use of prednisone. Dis Chest 1960; 38:51–55.

49. MacGregor RR, Sheagren JN, Lipsett MB, et al. Alternate-day prednisone therapy. N Engl J Med 1969; 280:1427–1431.

50. Mailbach H, Epstein WL. Immunologic responses of healthy volunteers receiving azathioprine (Imuran). Int Arch Allergy 1965; 27:102–109.

51. Avella J, Binder HJ, Madsen JE, et al. Effect of histamine H2-receptor antagonists on delayed hypersensitivity. Lancet 1978; 1:624–626.

52. Goodwin JS. Cimetidine and delayed hypersensitivity. (Letter.) Lancet 1978; 1:934.

53. Bicks RO, Rosenberg EW. Reversal of anergy in Crohn's disease by cimetidine. Lancet 1980; 1:552–553.

54. Edwards RL, Rickles FR. Delayed hypersensitivity in man: effects of systemic anticoagulation. Science 1978; 200:541–543.

55. Yazici H, Saville PD, Chaperon ED. Aspirin suppression of delayed hypersensitivity. Clin Res 1974; 22:645a.

56. Bruce DL, Wingard DW. Anesthesia and the immune response. Anesthesiology 1971; 34:271–282.

57. Jeejeebhoy KN, Baker JP, Wolman SL, et al. Critical evaluation of the role of clinical assessment and body composition studies in patients with malnutrition and after total parenteral nutrition. Am J Clin Nutr 1982; 35:1117–1127.

58. Greenberg GR, Jeejeebhoy KN. Intravenous protein-sparing therapy in patients with gastrointestinal disease. JPEN 1979; 3:427–432.

59. Young GA, Hill GL. A controlled study of protein-sparing therapy after excision of the rectum. Ann Surg 1980; 192:183–191.

60. Mullen JL, Buzby GP, Matthews DC, et al. Reduction of operative morbidity and mortality by combined preoperative and postoperative nutritional support. Ann Surg 1980; 192:604–613.

61. Muller JM, Dienst C, Brenner U, et al. Preoperative parenteral feeding in patients with gastrointestinal carcinoma. Lancet 1982; 1:68–71.

62. Baker JP, Detsky AS, Wesson DE, et al. Nutritional assessment: a comparison of clinical judgment and objective measurements. N Engl J Med 1982; 306:969–972.

63. Shizgal HM. The effect of malnutrition on body composition. Surg Gynecol Obstet 1981; 152:22–26.

64. Forse RA, Shizgal HM. Assessment of malnutrition. Surgery 1980; 88:17–24.

65. Merton PA. Voluntary strength and fatigue. J Physiol 1954; 123:553–564.

66. Edwards RHT. Physiological analysis of skeletal muscle weakness and fatigue. Clin Sci Mol Med 1978; 54:463–470.

67. Edwards RHT, Young A, Hosking GP. Human skeletal muscle function: description of tests and normal values. Clin Sci Mol Med 1977; 52:283–290.

68. Moxham J, Morris AJR, Spiro SG, et al. Contractile properties and fatigue of the diaphragm in man. Thorax 1981; 36:164–168.

69. Wiles CM, Young A, Jones DA, et al. Relaxation rate of constituent muscle-fibre types in human quadriceps. Clin Sci Mol Med 1979; 56:47–52.

70. Lopes J, Russell DM, Whitwell J, et al. Skeletal muscle function in malnutrition. Am J Clin Nutr 1982; 36:602–610.

71. Russell DM, Leiter LA, Whitwell J, et al. Skeletal muscle function during hypocaloric diets and fasting: a comparison with standard nutritional assessment parameters. Am J Clin Nutr 1983; 37:133–138.

72. Russell DM, Prendergast PJ, Darby PL, et al. A comparison between muscle function and body composition in anorexia nervosa: the effect of refeeding. Am J Clin Nutr 1983; 38:229–237.

73. Russell DM, Walker PM, Leiter LA, et al. Metabolic and structural changes in muscle during hypocaloric dieting. Am J Clin Nutr 1984; 39:503–513.

74. Russell DM, Atwood HL, Whittaker JS, et al. The effect of

fasting and hypocaloric diets on the functional and metabolic characteristics of rat gastrocnemius muscle. Clin Sci 1984; *67*:185–194.

75. Reuter H, Scholz H. A study of the ion selectivity and the kinetic properties of the calcium dependent slow inward current in mammalian cardiac muscle. J Physiol 1977; *264*:17–47.

76. Harrison JE, McNeill KG, Strauss AS. A nitrogen index—total body protein normalized for body size—for diagnosis of protein status in health and disease. Nutr Res 1984; *4*:209–224.

NUTRITIONAL OPTIONS

C. RICHARD FLEMING / JENNIFER NELSON

The past 20 years have witnessed the evolution of clinical nutrition into a bona fide specialty. The acceptance that protein-calorie malnutrition contributes to increases in morbidity and mortality made viable the organized efforts at nutritional support. Attempts at correcting protein-calorie malnutrition in patients who were compromised by infection, trauma, or end-organ failure received the first real impetus when in 1968 the effectiveness of central parenteral nutrition (CPN) was established.[1] The use of CPN has become more refined after studies on nutrient administration and utilization, nutrient-nutrient interactions, and trace nutrients. Furthermore, the use of specific solutions for specific patients (e.g., branched amino acids for trauma victims) appears to be well supported by research findings. The availability of safe isotonic fat emulsions has made it possible to administer many more calories in smaller volumes through either central or peripheral veins.

The sophistication of enteral nutrition has been accompanied by improved feeding tubes, a plethora of commercial formulas, and increasing information on the utilization of nutrients when delivered by tube perfusion in both health and disease.

The increasing data base and commercialization of nutritional support have, in general, had a positive impact on the delivery of nutritional support. However, the ready access to commercial preparations and companies created to assist in delivering nutritional supplies to patients in the hospital and at home have made it easy to practice "reflex" nutritional support without much thought as to patients' needs or of simpler remedies.

Our objectives in this chapter are to discuss (1) the general assessment prior to selecting the nutritional option, (2) the relative merits of enteral versus parenteral nutrition, (3) enteral nutrition, and (4) parenteral nutrition.

GENERAL ASSESSMENT

A thorough history and physical examination by an experienced clinician is usually adequate to detect the presence or absence of protein-calorie malnutrition,[2] and, if needed, to make the selection of the safest and most cost-effective means of supplying the nutrition. The history should elicit the presence or absence of weight loss and the time frame in which the weight loss occurred. The causes of weight loss may be evident by eliciting symptoms of anorexia, oral ulcers, altered taste or smell, early satiety, dysphagia, postprandial abdominal pain, and diarrhea. An inquiry about dietary habits may yield information that otherwise would not be volunteered, such as the intake of unorthodox diets, multiple drugs with the potential for drug-nutrient interactions, and unfounded nutritional supplementation. The popularity of nutritional supplements has been perpetuated by health food stores and preventive nutrition magazines that imply that better health is likely after consumption of such supplements. We often warn our patients against excessive doses of fat-soluble vitamins, especially vitamins A and D. However, we have usually not worried about the potential for significant toxicity from water-soluble vitamins. A recent report describes seven adults who developed ataxia and severe nervous system dysfunction after high doses of vitamin B_6 (pyridoxine).[3] These patients consumed 2 to 6 g of pyridoxine per day for 4 to 40 months, compared with the minimal daily requirement for adults of 2 to 4 mg/day. All of these patients improved after withdrawal of the pyridoxine. This report should alert us to inquire specifically about dietary supplements, and in particular vitamins, since most patients will not think to mention vitamins when asked about medications.

Intolerances to specific foods may be present, and some will have a physiological basis. For example, most patients who are not of Northern European origin are deficient in intestinal lactase.[4] Persons deficient in lactase may have malabsorption of as much as 50 per cent of ingested lactose, which then enters the colon and acts osmotically to retain water. Variable amounts of cramping, diarrhea, borborygmi, and flatus result. Some lactase-deficient patients will be labeled as having irritable bowel syndrome before the correct diagnosis is made. More recently, Anderson et al. described impressive increases in breath hydrogen, indicative of malabsorbed carbohydrate, in 17 of 18 healthy subjects after ingesting 100 g of wheat starch in the form of macaroni or bread made from all-purpose white flour.[5]

It is extremely important to inquire about alcohol consumption, because alcoholics may take 30 to 60 per cent of their total calories as ethanol. Twenty ounces (600 ml) of 86-proof liquor represents about 1400 kcal, approximately one half of the normal daily caloric requirement. Malnutrition may result in chronic alcoholics because ethanol replaces dietary nutrients, particularly carbohydrate and vitamins, and because malabsorption or maldigestion (or both) result from alcohol-induced hepatic, pancreatic, and small bowel dysfunction.[6]

Knowledge about the functional capacity of the gastrointestinal tract is essential. A review of past surgical records will provide information about previous resections or bypasses, the remaining segments and length of bowel, the status of the residual gut, and the presence or absence of the ileocecal valve. Careful measurements of urinary, stool, and fistula volumes may provide clues as to the source of deficiency states. For example, there is usually an excellent correlation between stool volume and zinc losses.[7] A patient with 1 L of stool per day may lose 10 mg or more of zinc in the stool. Therefore, zinc deficiency may be common in patients with inflammatory bowel disease or short bowel syndrome.[8,9]

The physical examination should include accurate measurements of weight and height on the same scale and in the same circumstance (e.g., early morning in hospital gown and bare feet) that will be used throughout a hospitalization. The presence of a fever and tachycardia often provides the first clue to a catabolic state that will demand greater nutritional needs. Careful inspection may provide signs of muscle wasting, edema, depleted fat stores, decubitus ulcers, and the presence of altered anatomy such as enterocutaneous fistulas that should influence the type of nutritional support that is selected. Clues as to the presence of specific deficiencies may include neuropathies (B-complex vitamins), combined systems disease (vitamin B_{12}), perifollicular hemorrhage (vitamin C), carpal-pedal spasm (calcium), soft tissue hemorrhage (vitamin K), glossitis and spoon nails (iron), acrodermatitis (zinc), and eczematoid dermatitis (essential fatty acids).

Sensitive means of measuring body composition such as neutron activation are not readily available and are therefore not practical for the day-to-day assessment of nutritional status. The objective criteria for evaluating nutritional status include measurements of visceral proteins (albumin, transferrin, pre-albumin, retinol binding protein), anthropometrics (weight-for-height, triceps skinfold, midarm circumference), skeletal protein (ratio of 24-hour urinary creatinine to height) and muscle degradation (urinary 3-methylhistidine). However, these measurements lack specificity and sensitivity for a given patient on the initial evaluation. They are most useful when longitudinally monitoring the effectiveness of nutritional intervention.

ENTERAL VERSUS PARENTERAL NUTRITION

The status of the intestinal tract is the most important consideration that guides one in selecting enteral or parenteral nutrition. The intestinal tract should always be used as long as it is patent and healthy. An adequate length of small bowel absorptive surface must be present. Some patients with an extremely shortened small bowel can manage with enteral nutrition if the colon is in continuity. Impaired gastrointestinal motility from either a transient condition (e.g., postoperative paralytic ileus) or a diffuse motility disorder (e.g., chronic idiopathic intestinal pseudo-obstruction) usually makes it difficult to achieve maintenance nutrition via the enteral route. Diffuse inflammatory diseases of the intestines such as radiation enteritis and Crohn's disease often impair enteral nutrition even though the lumen is patent and the motility apparently adequate. These patients often have so much postprandial pain that they voluntarily limit their intake.

Enteral nutrition is necessary in order to maintain morphological and functional integrity of the gut. Animals that are nourished parenterally without enteral feedings show a decrease in mucosal mass and enzyme activity and fail to exhibit adaptive changes after small bowel resections.[10,11] Thus, there are advantages in attempting to maintain some enteral nutrition in patients receiving parenteral nutrition as their dominant source of nutrition.

Many patients who present with nutritional management problems will declare themselves as either those who will not eat[12] or those who cannot eat.[13]

Patients Who Will Not Eat

Some of the most difficult patients to manage are those who will not eat even though their intestinal tracts are healthy. Anorexia in association with depression, drugs, or malignancy is very prevalent. The use of antidepressants, withdrawal of medications suspected of causing anorexia, or resection of a malignancy may markedly improve appetite and food intake. However, the anticholinergic effects of some antidepressants may cause dryness of the mouth and make eating unpleasant.

In other cases, the issues become much more complex and involve the social aspects of eating. For instance, the lonely geriatric patient may eat well when encouraged in the hospital but lose the incentive to eat after returning home. Many older patients will have poor eyesight, poorly fitting dentures, or impaired smell and taste that make eating laborious. These patients will restrict their intake unless someone makes a conscious effort to help them.

Some cancer patients have altered taste sensations that result in decreased food intake. They often have elevation of the taste threshold for sweets, so that a higher concentration of sugar will be necessary in order for cancer patients to enjoy their foods. Other patients with cancer lose their desire for red meats and many complain that meat has a bad or rotten taste. At the same time, they often tolerate poultry and fish protein quite well.

In general, patients who will not eat can be helped by treating their underlying disease or condition and encouraging foods of their choice and, if necessary, liquid nutritional supplements. If this approach is unsuccessful, enteral nutrition via a nasogastric or intestinal tube or the use of peripheral parenteral nutrition (PPN) will often provide adequate nutrition.

Patients Who Cannot Eat

There are some patients in whom attempts at enteral nutrition will fail. Examples include patients with bowel obstructions, proximal enterocutaneous fistulas, and hyperemesis gravidarum. Patients who are comatose or who have lost the ability to initiate swallowing (e.g., brain stem strokes or myasthenia gravis) can be fed by tube feedings with careful attention directed to the risk of aspiration.

Although we commonly think of parenteral and enteral nutrition as being mutually exclusive, PPN and enteral nutrition are often used together as an attractive alternative to central parenteral nutrition (CPN). This less invasive technique was as effective as central parenteral nutrition in reversing protein-calorie malnutrition and minimizing complications in young malnourished children beginning treatment for advanced neuroblastoma or Wilms' tumor.[14]

A small group of patients will become dependent on either tube enteral or parenteral nutrition and will be transferred to their home following proper instruction for self-administration. Home enteral nutrition is 10 to 20 times less expensive than home parenteral nutrition (HPN) and is associated with far fewer complications.[15] Furthermore, many patients with incurable cancer or neurological disability who would not be considered for home parenteral nutrition in most centers can usually be managed on home enteral nutrition. Therefore, at least in theory, patients should never be given a choice between home enteral nutrition and HPN. HPN should be restricted to those gut failure patients in whom all attempts at enteral nutrition have failed and for whom additional intestinal surgery or drugs seem unlikely to restore the gut function for enteral nutrition.

ENTERAL NUTRITION

It is assumed that patients will be fed with solid food if there is no contraindication. Stable but malnourished hospitalized patients with intact gastrointestinal tracts absorb calories, nitrogen, electrolytes (Na, K, Cl) and minerals (P, Ca, Mg) as efficiently from solid food as from predigested monomeric or polymeric diets.[16] Liquid formulas can often supplement the regular diets of hospitalized patients, especially if their caloric intakes are marginal. By replacing meal beverages such as tea, coffee, or water with a 240-ml glass of a formula containing 1 kcal/ml, one will increase the daily caloric intake by 720 kcal.

Enteral nutrition as it is used in patients who will not or cannot eat is essentially synonymous with the use of commercially prepared liquid formulas that are usually given through tubes.

Evolution of Tube Feeding

The earliest accounts of tube feedings were of Egyptians who used cloysters or rectal alimentation.[17] In 1793 John Hunter described the techniques of tube feeding similar to what we know today.[18] He described the passing of a tube through the mouth into the stomach prior to each meal that was made of "fresh eel skin . . . and whale bone." A "bladder" served as an administration flask from which a formula consisting of "jellies, eggs, water, sugar, milk, and wine" was delivered. The use of tube feedings did not become widespread, however, and there were limited publications on the subject for the next 100 years. In 1879 Newington, an Assistant Medical Officer, suggested that passing a tube through the nose was preferred over oral intubation for forced feeding.[19] He described a feeding instrument consisting of three tubes, two for inserting through each nostril, while the third could be affixed to a funnel. Major advances in the past century in the development of nutritional formulas have paralleled the improved equipment for administering the feedings. The space program prompted the search for nutritional support that would alleviate problems with food storage, preparation, and fecal waste disposal. The efforts resulted in the development of a powdered elemental diet[20] that offered: (1) compactness—one cubic foot of powder provided all nutritional needs for a 154-pound astronaut for 1 month; (2) easy preparation—addition of water eliminated "crumbs," which in a weightless state were potentially a major problem; (3) nutrient flexibility—the nature of the powder allowed alterations of each nutrient; and (4) low bulk—mitigated the problem of disposal of solid fecal waste.

Sophisticated feeding tubes and delivery systems have simplified tube enteric feedings. One can now choose from a large number of tubes with different diameters and lengths and the presence or absence of weighted ends and insertion stylets. These have allowed either gastric or intestinal feeding with fewer complications and greater patient comfort.

Another major advancement in the delivery of enteral feedings has been the development of feeding pumps. Pumps allow controlled rates of administration, and some offer "fail-safe" mechanisms in the form of alarms and automatic shutoffs. Pump-assisted feeding has decreased the time required of hospital personnel to closely monitor and administer the tube feedings. In the home, pumps assure more safety and allow the convenience of nighttime feedings while providing the patient a more normal lifestyle during the day.

Nutritional Formulations

A wide variety of commercially prepared formulas are currently available that have different sources and concentrations of protein, carbohydrate, and fat. Consequently, they differ in caloric density, calorie-to-nitrogen ratio, electrolyte and mineral content, and osmolality. Commercial products offer many distinct advantages over hospital- or home-blended mixtures, including a known nutrient composition, controlled osmolality and consistency, ease in preparation and storage, bacteriological safety, and cost.

Tables 43–1 to 43–6 display the nutrient contents of some of the commonly used commercial formulas. Data were derived from manufacturers' analysis and are presented on the basis of nutrients per 1000 ml. The volumes needed to assure 100 per cent of the recommended dietary allowance (RDA) for vitamins should be noted and supplements provided as needed.

These liquid diets are often categorized as monomeric, polymeric, special formulas, and supplemental nutrient sources.

Monomeric or elemental diets are composed of low-molecular-weight nutrients and require minimal digestive and absorptive capability (Table 43–1). Protein sources include short-chain peptides and amino acids. Carbohydrates are oligosaccharides, sucrose, and glucose, while fat sources usually consist of medium-chain triglycerides and small amounts of essential fatty acids. The fat content ranges from 1 to 12 per cent of total calories. Monomeric diets have minimal residue because of the efficient absorption of the nutrients provided in an elemental form. Because of the small molecular weight of the nutrients, the products are hyperosmolar, and osmotic diarrhea is one of the more common side effects. In addition, the low fat content leaves the formulas without much taste, and they frequently have to be administered through a tube because of poor compliance by patients. The taste can be improved by adding flavor packets, but the flavoring may also increase osmolality.

The major advantage of the elemental diets, namely, the elemental composition which requires minimal digestion, has been refuted by studies showing that absorption from small peptides may occur at equivalent rates or more efficiently than absorption of the equivalent free amino acids.[21,22]

Polymeric formulas are composed of intact proteins, complex carbohydrates, and variable amounts of fat, residue, and lactose. The osmolality of polymeric formulas is usually lower than elemental diets and the fat content is greater, allowing for better-tasting solutions. Tables 43–2 to 43–4 provide information on some of the more commonly used polymeric formulas.

These formulas are usually classified as lactose-free diets, milk-based diets, and blenderized whole

TABLE 43–1. Monomeric ("Elemental") Formulations

Characteristics: Minimal residue, lactose-free, assimilated readily with little or no digestion
Protein—predigested (hydrolyzed protein, di- and tripeptides and/or crystalline amino acids)
Fat—small amount of essential fatty acids with or without medium chain triglycerides
Hyperosmolar
Poor palatability—designed primarily for tube feeding

Formula	Caloric density (Kcal/ml)	Protein g (% Kcal)	Fat g (% Kcal)	Carbohydrate g (% Kcal)	N:Non-protein Kcal	mOsm/kg	Sodium mg/mEq	Potassium mg/mEq	Volume (ml) to Meet Vitamin Requirements except K	Protein Sources	Fat Sources	Carbohydrate Sources
Vivonex (Norwich-Eaton)	1.0	20 (8%)	1.4 (1%)	230 (91%)	1:281	550	468/20.4	1172/30.0	1800	L-Amino acids	Safflower oil (100%)	Glucose oligo-saccharides
Vivonex HN (Norwich-Eaton)	1.0	46 (18%)	0.9 (1%)	210 (81%)	1:125	810	529/23.0	1173/30.0	3000	L-Amino acids	Safflower oil (100%)	Glucose oligo-saccharides
Vivonex TEN (Norwich-Eaton)	1.0	38 (15%)	3.0 (2.5%)	206 (82%)	1:149	630	460/20.0	782/20.0	2000	L-Amino acids (33% BCAA)	Safflower oil (100%)	Maltodextrins, modified cornstarch
Vital HN (Ross)	1.0	42 (17%)	11 (9%)	185 (74%)	1;125	460	467/20.3	1333/34.1	1892	Whey, soy, and meat protein hydrolysates, free amino acids	Safflower oil (60%) MCT oil (40%)	Hydrolyzed cornstarch, sucrose
Criticare HN (Mead-Johnson)	1.06	37.5 (14%)	3.3 (3%)	222 (83%)	1:148	650	634/27.6	1323/33.8	1892	Casein hydroly-sates, peptides, amino acids	Safflower oil (100%)	Maltodextrins, cornstarch
Travasorb HN (Travenol)	1.0	45 (18%)	13 (12%)	175 (70%)	1:126	560	920/40.0	1170/30.0	2000	Lactalbumin peptides	Sunflower oil (60%) MCT oil (40%)	Glucose oligo-saccharides
Travasorb STD (Travenol)	1.0	30 (12%)	13 (12%)	190 (76%)	1:202	560	920/40.0	1170/30.0	2000	Lactabumin peptides	Sunflower oil (60%) MCT oil (40%)	Glucose oligo-saccharides

Contents per 1000 ml unless otherwise specified.

foods. Lactose-free diets, the most commonly used polymeric preparations, have variable caloric densities and osmolalities of 1 to 2 kcal/ml and 300 to 740 mOsmol, respectively. The fat content is usually between 30 to 40 per cent of total calories; however, there are a few such diets with only 1 per cent of total calories as fat (e.g., Precision HN and Precision Low Residue, Sandoz).

Blenderized diets are made from natural whole foods and contain all nutrients and fiber found in table food, including lactose in some instances. The high viscosity of the blenderized formulas frequently negates the use of small-bore nasogastric tubes. Instead, one has to rely on larger-bore tubes and frequently the use of a feeding pump to assure delivery of the desired volume.

Special formulas are products designed for patients with specific medical conditions. Table 43–5 details the contents of some of the more commonly used special formulas. In patients with hepatic encephalopathy associated with chronic liver disease, the use of formulas high in branched-chain amino acids (leucine, isoleucine, and valine) and low in aromatic amino acids (phenylalanine, tyrosine, tryptophan, and methionine) may increase the ratio of serum branched-chain amino acids (BCAA) to aromatic amino acids (AAA). Some studies that tested the benefit of orally administered BCAA preparations in patients with hepatic encephalopathy showed that the encephalopathy was not ameliorated even though the BCAA/AAA ratios were usually increased.[23,24] One study evaluated Hepatic-Aid (Kendall-McGaw) by comparing a 50 g casein diet with 20 g casein/30 g Hepatic-Aid per day in a crossover study.[23] Although the casein/Hepatic-Aid regimen in four malnourished cirrhotics with encephalopathy maintained nitrogen balance similar to casein alone and altered amino acid profiles towards normal, the encephalopathy did not improve. Erickson et al. treated seven patients with hepatic encephalopathy of 6 months duration or longer by supplementing their diets with 30 g BCAA or placebo during two 14-day crossover periods.[24] No improvement in the encephalopathy was appreciated when patients received the BCAA as determined by clinical appraisal, psychometric testing, and electroencephalograms. More recently, a randomized study comparing increasing amounts of dietary protein with an oral BCAA enriched amino acid solution showed that the patients given BCAA supplements achieved positive nitrogen balance as often as those given the equivalent amount of only dietary protein without inducing encephalopathy as frequently.[25]

Patients with chronic renal failure may benefit from the use of formulas containing nitrogen in the form of essential amino acids and histidine.[26] If renal failure patients are receiving maintenance hemodialysis, 1.2 g of protein per kilogram of body weight primarily of high biological value protein and 35 kcal/kg of body weight should be adequate.[27]

TABLE 43–2. Polymeric Formulas—Lactose-Free

Characteristics: Moderate to low residue
Protein—intact; semipurified isolates; high molecular weight; derived from casein salts or egg white solids
Carbohydrate—starches, maltodextrins; glucose oligosaccharides; corn syrup solids
Fat—contributes greater percentage of calories; corn oil; soy oil; as well as MCT
Osmolality—isomolar as well as hyperosmolar
Palatable

Formula	Caloric Density (Kcal/ml)	Protein g (% Kcal)	Fat g (% Kcal)	Carbohydrate g (% Kcal)	N:Nonprotein Kcal	mOsm/kg	Sodium mg/mEq	Potassium mg/mEq	Volume (ml) to Meet Vitamin Requirements except K	Protein Sources	Fat Sources	Carbohydrate Sources
Hypercaloric												
Sustacal HC (Mead-Johnson)	1.5	61 (16%)	58 (34%)	190 (50%)	1:134	650	840/37	1480/38	1200	Sodium and calcium caseinates	Soybean oil	Corn syrup solids, sucrose
Isocal HCN (Mead-Johnson)	2.0	75 (15.%)	91 (40%)	225 (45%)	1:145	690	800/35	1400/36	1500	Sodium and calcium caseinates	Soybean oil (70%), MCT (30%)	Corn syrup solids
Ensure Plus HN (Ross)	1.5	63 (17%)	50 (30%)	200 (53%)	1:125	650	1184/51	1818/47	947	Sodium and calcium caseinates	Corn oil	Hydrolyzed corn starch, sucrose
Ensure Plus (Ross)	1.5	55 (15%)	53 (32%)	200 (53%)	1:146	600	1141/50	2325/60	1600	Sodium and calcium caseinates	Corn oil	Corn syrup solids, sucrose
Magnacal (Chesebrough-Ponds)	2.0	70 (14%)	80 (36%)	250 (50%)	1:154	590	1000/44	1250/32	1000	Sodium and calcium caseinates	Soy oil	Maltodextrin, sucrose
TwoCal HN (Ross)	2.0	83 (17%)	90 (40%)	216 (43%)	1:126	740	1052/46	2316/59	950	Sodium and calcium caseinates, soy protein isolates	Corn oil, MCT	Hydrolyzed cornstarch, sucrose
Normal Caloric												
Osmolite (Ross)	1.06	37 (14%)	38 (31%)	145 (55%)	1:153	300	634/28	1013/26	1887	Sodium and calcium caseinates, soy protein isolate	MCT (50%), corn oil and soy oil (50%)	Hydrolyzed cornstarch
Isocal (Mead-Johnson)	1.06	34 (13%)	44 (37%)	132 (50%)	1:167	300	530/23	1320/34	1887	Sodium and calcium caseinates, soy protein isolate	Soy oil (80%), MCT oil (20%)	Maltodextrin
Precision Isotonic (Sandoz)	0.96	29 (12%)	30 (28%)	144 (60%)	1:183	300	770/34	960/25	1560	Egg albumin	Soy oil	Glucose oligosaccharides, sucrose
Ensure (Ross)	1.06	37 (14%)	38 (31%)	145 (55%)	1:153	450	845/37	1564/40	1887	Sodium and calcium caseinate, soy protein isolate	Corn oil	Hydrolyzed corn starch
Travasorb Liquid (Travenol)	1.06	35 (14%)	35 (32%)	136 (55%)	1:154	488	738/32	1266/33	1896	Sodium and calcium caseinate, soy protein isolate	Corn oil	Sucrose, corn syrup solids
Precision LR (Sandoz)	1.1	26 (10%)	1.6 (1%)	248 (89%)	1:239	530	700/30	888/22	1710	Egg albumin	Soy oil	Maltodextrin, sucrose
Normal Caloric and High Nitrogen												
Precision HN (Sandoz)	1.05	44 (17%)	1.3 (1%)	216 (82%)	1:125	525	980/43	910/23	2850	Egg albumin	Soy oil	Maltodextrin, sucrose
Ensure HN (Ross)	1.06	44 (17%)	37 (30%)	141 (53%)	1:125	470	930/40	1564/40	1321	Sodium and calcium caseinate, soy protein isolate	Corn oil	Corn syrup, sucrose
Osmolite HN (Ross)	1.06	44 (17%)	37 (30%)	141 (53%)	1:124	310	930/40	1564/40	1321	Sodium and calcium caseinate, soy protein isolate	Corn oil (50%) MCT oil (50%)	Hydrolyzed corn starch, sucrose
Isotein HN (Sandoz)	1.2	68.5 (23%)	34 (25%)	156 (52%)	1:86	300	620/27	1070/27	1770	Delactosed lactalbumin	Soybean oil (N/A), MCT (N/A)	Maltodextrin, monosaccharides
Sustacal Liquid (Mead-Johnson)	1.0	61 (24%)	23 (21%)	140 (55%)	1:79	625	938/41	2085/54	1080	Sodium and calcium caseinate, soy protein isolate	Soy oil	Sucrose, corn syrup

Contents per 1000 ml unless otherwise specified.

TABLE 43–3. Polymeric Formulas—Lactose-Containing

Characteristics: Moderate to low residue; milk base; designed as oral supplement
Protein—intact; semipurified isolates; high molecular weight
Carbohydrate—lactose, sucrose, corn syrup solids
Hyperosmolar
Palatable

Formula	Caloric Density (Kcal/ml)	Protein g (% Kcal)	Fat g (% Kcal)	Carbohydrate g (% Kcal)	N:Nonprotein Kcal	mOsm/kg	Sodium mg/mEq	Potassium mg/mEq	Volume (ml) to Meet Vitamin Requirements except K	Protein Source	Fat Sources	Carbohydrate Sources
Carnation Instant Breakfast (Travenol)	1.1	60 (21%)	36 (29%)	136 (50%)	1:92	677–715	966/42	2808/72	1373	Nonfat milk, soy protein, sodium caseinate	Milk fat	Sucrose, corn syrup solids, lactose (96 gm)
Meritene Liquid (Sandoz)	0.96	58 (24%)	32 (30%)	111 (46%)	1:79	505+	880/38	1600/45	1200	Concentrated skim milk	Corn oil	Corn syrup solids, sucrose, lactose (55 gm)
Meritene Powder (Sandoz)	1.06	69 (26%)	35 (29%)	119 (45%)	1:71	690	1100/48	2800/72	1040	Nonfat dry milk, whole milk	Milk fat	Lactose (104 gm), sucrose, corn syrup solids
Sustacal powder (Mead-Johnson)	1.33	77 (24%)	34 (22%)	180 (54%)	1:80	700–1010	1200/54	3400/87	800	Nonfat milk	Milk fat	Lactose (86 gm), sucrose, corn syrup solids
Sustagen (Mead-Johnson)	1.7	111 (24%)	16 (8%)	312 (68%)	1:77	1100	1270/55	3380/87	1030	Nonfat milk, whole milk, calcium caseinate	Milk fat	Lactose (96 gm), corn syrup solids, glucose

Contents per 1000 ml unless otherwise specified.

Supplemental nutrient sources are products that provide one or more nutrients and are not nutritionally complete. These products should be added to solid food or formulas in order to more closely meet nutritional requirements. Supplemental nutrient sources include carbohydrates, fats, and proteins (Table 43–6).

Access to the Intestinal Tract

Enteral nutrition may be accomplished by voluntary oral intake of food, diet plus supplemental formulas, a commercial formula alone by mouth, or tube feeding. Attention to personal preferences, tolerances, and quality of preparation all contribute to making meals well received. However, if the patient is unable to meet daily requirements in this manner, liquid formulas should be provided. Voluntary consumption of liquid formulas as a sole source of nutrition is indicated only for short-term nutritional support. If an enteral formula diet is to be continued, administration through a tube usually becomes necessary.

Tube feedings may be accomplished via several routes, which may be chosen depending on the anticipated duration of feeding, the condition of the gastrointestinal tract (e.g., esophageal obstruction, prior gastric or small bowel resections), and the potential for aspiration. Access to the gut can be accomplished at the bedside (nasogastric tube, percutaneous needle pharyngostomy, or percutaneous endoscopic gastrostomy) or in the operating room (gastrostomy or jejunostomy).

Transnasal. Nasal intubation for gastric or intestinal feeding is the simplest and most commonly

TABLE 43–4. Polymeric Formulas—Blended Foodstuffs

Characteristics: Contain nondigestible residue; ± lactose; require intact bowel function
Protein, fat, carbohydrate—based on blended mix of food
Not intended for oral use

Formula	Caloric Density (Kcal/ml)	Protein g (% Kcal)	Fat g (% Kcal)	Carbohydrate g (% Kcal)	N:Nonprotein Kcal	mOsm/kg	Sodium mg/mEq	Potassium mg/mEq	Volume (ml) to Meet Vitamin Requirements	Protein Sources	Fat Sources	Carbohydrate Sources
Complete Regular (Sandoz)	1.07	43 (16%)	43 (36%)	128 (48%)	1:131	405	1300/56	1400/36	1500	Beef puree, nonfat dry milk	Beef puree, corn oil	Maltodextrins, vegetables, lactose (24 gm), fruit
Complete Modified (Sandoz)	1.07	43 (16%)	37 (31%)	140 (53%)	1:131	300	670/29	1400/36	1500	Beef puree, calcium caseinate	Beef puree, corn oil	Maltodextrins, vegetables, fruit
Vitaneed (Chesebrough-Ponds)	1.0	35 (14%)	40 (36%)	125 (50%)	1:154	310	500/22	1250/32	2000	Beef, sodium, and calcium caseinates	Soy oil, beef puree	Maltodextrins, puree fruit and vegetables

Contents per 1000 ml unless otherwise specified.

TABLE 43–5. Special Formulas

Characteristics: Formulated to meet nutrient requirements for patients with specific medical conditions

Formula	Caloric Density (Kcal/ml)	Protein g (% Kcal)	Fat g (% Kcal)	Carbohydrate g (% Kcal)	N:Nonprotein Kcal	mOsm/kg	Sodium mg/mEq	Potassium mg/mEq	Volume (ml) to Meet Vitamin Requirements except K	Protein Sources	Fat Sources	Carbohydrate Sources
Hepatic Hepatic-Aid II (Kendall-McGaw)	1.1	44 15%	36 27.7%	169 57.3%	148:1	560	<345/<15	<234/<6	—	Amino acids—high branched chain amino acids (46%), low aromatic amino acids	Partially hydrogenated soy oil	Maltodextrins, sucrose
Travasorb Hepatic (Travenol)	1.1	29.1 10.6%	14 12%	209 77.4%	211:1	690	445/19	1140/29	2100	Amino acids—high branched chain amino acids (50%), low aromatic amino acids	MCT, sunflower oil	Glucose oligosaccharides, sucrose
Renal Amin Aid (Kendall-McGaw)	2.0	19 4.0%	47.1 21.2%	366 75%	830:1	1095	<345/<15	<234/<6	—	Essential amino acids and histidine	Partially hydrogenated soy oil	Maltodextrins, sucrose
Travasorb Renal (Travenol)	1.35	23 6.9%	18 12%	271 81.1%	363:1	590	0/0	0/0	2100	Essential amino acids plus nonessential amino acids	MCT, sunflower oil	Glucose oligosaccharides, sucrose
Stress Stresstein (Sandoz)	1.2	70 23%	28 20%	170 57%	97:1	910	650/28	1100/28	2000	Branched chain amino acids (44%) plus essential amino acids	MCT, soy oil	Maltodextrin
Traum-Aid HBC (Kendall-McGaw)	1.0	55 22%	13 12%	165 66%	102:1	675	533/23	1166/30	3000	High branched-chain amino acids (50%) plus essential and nonessential amino	MCT, soy oil	Maltodexrin
Trauma-cal/Fulfil (Mead-Johnson)	1.5	82 22%	68 41%	143 38%	89:1	550	1200/52	1400/36	2000	Branched chain amino (23%) plus essential and nonessential amino acids	MCT, soy oil	Corn syrup, sucrose
Pulmocare (Ross)	1.5	63 17%	92 55%	106 28%	125:1	490	1310/57	1902/49	960	Sodium and calcium caseinates	Corn oil	Sucrose, hydrolyzed cornstarch

Contents per 1000 ml unless otherwise specified.

used approach for tube feeding. Patients tolerate well the soft, small-diameter tubes. The placement of long, weighted tubes into the duodenum is possible, but some tubes have to be placed through the pylorus under fluoroscopic guidance. Table 43–7 provides details on some of the commonly used feeding tubes.

Gastrostomy. Conventional gastrostomies require a surgical procedure, often with the use of general anesthesia; for high-risk patients the morbidity and mortality are high. Major complication rates of surgical gastrostomies are 2.5 to 16 per cent and mortality rates 1 to 6 per cent.[28–32] In a review of 147 patients with Stamm gastrostomies, 23 complications were noted—9 major and 14 minor—for an incidence of 16 per cent.[33]

Percutaneous endoscopic placement of a gastrostomy has many advantages. It can be performed at the bedside with minimal or no sedation in patients who are severely compromised by their underlying disease.[34] In 150 consecutive patients receiving endoscopic gastrostomy, there was only a 10 per cent morbidity and there were no procedure-related deaths.[35] Complications included minor wound infections in seven patients, extrusion of the tube in three, partial separation of the gastrostomy from the abdominal wall in one patient, and gastrocolic fistula in one adult and one child.

Combining gastrostomy as access, with insertion of a jejunal feeding tube permits gastric decompression while the formula is delivered into the jejunum. It should minimize the risk of aspiration; in one assessment, there were no documented episodes of aspiration in 45 patients managed with this tube and only three (7 per cent) major complications.[36]

Jejunostomy. Enthusiasm has been generated for the needle catheter jejunostomy, which is placed at the time of laparotomy.[37] Indications for the placement of the needle catheter jejunostomy include preoperative malnutrition for which postoperative nutritional support is planned, emergency or elective major upper abdominal operations, and the anticipated need for postoperative chemotherapy or radiation therapy.[37,38] The intrajejunal feedings minimize the risk of vomiting and aspiration from the infusions and do not necessarily interfere with oral intake. It avoids parenteral nutrition in some patients with a functioning small bowel associated with obstruction or reduced motility in the stomach.

TABLE 43–6. Supplemental Nutrient Sources

Characteristics: Add specific nutrients
Not nutritionally complete

Formula	Caloric Density Kcal/ml	Protein g (% Kcal)	Fat g (% Kcal)	Carbohydrate g (% Kcal)	N:Nonprotein Kcal	mOsm/kg	Sodium mg/mEq	Potassium mg/mEq	Protein Sources	Fat Sources	Carbohydrate Sources
Carbohydrate											
Polycose (Ross)	2.0 (3.8 Kcal/g)	—	—	500 (100%)	—	850	700/30	60/1.5	—	—	Hydrolysis of corn starch
Moducal (Mead-Johnson)	2.0 (3.8 Kcal/g)	—	—	500 (100%)	—	725	360/16	20/0.6	—	—	Maltodextrin
Fat											
MCT Oil (Mead-Johnson)	7.7 (8.3 Kcal/g)	—	927 (100%)	—	—	—	—	—	—	Fractionated coconut oil	—
Microlipid (Chesebrough-Ponds)	4.5	—	500 (100%)	—	—	60	—	—	—	Safflower oil	—
Protein											
Casec (Mead-Johnson)	1.0 (3.7 Kcal/g)	238 (95%)	5 (5%)	0 (0%)	—	—	410/18	27/0.7	Calcium caseinate	—	—
RDP (Navaco)	1.0 (3.6 Kcal/g)	209 (84%)	11 (10%)	14 (6%)	—	—	640/28	2300/58	Whey protein	—	—
Pro Mod (Ross)	1.0 (4.2 Kcal/g)	179 (71%)	21.4 (19%)	24 (10%)	—	—	460/21	2300/59	Whey protein	—	—
Propac (Chesebrough-Ponds)	1.0 (4.0 Kcal/g)	192 (77%)	20 (18%)	13 (5%)	—	—	580/25	1300/33	Whey protein	—	—

Contents per 1000 ml unless otherwise specified.

TABLE 43–7. Feeding Tubes for Enteral Nutrition

Feeding Tube	Manufacturer	French Gauge	Composition	Features
Argyle Quest Duo-Tube	Argyle Division Sherwood Medical St. Louis, MO	5, 6, 8, 10, 12, 14, 16	Silicone Polyvinyl chloride	Silicone or mercury (1 g) weighted tip. Removable plastic outer sheath for placement. 42-inch length.
Cartmill Tube	Impra Inc. Tempe, AZ	8	Silicone	Silicone bolus tip. External spring sheath for placement. 48-inch length.
Dobbhoff	Biosearch Medical Products, Inc. Somerville, NJ	8	Polyurethane	Mercury or tungsten (7 g) weighted bolus tip. Insertion stylet included. 43-inch length. Hydrophylic coating.
Entriflex	Biosearch Medical Products, Inc. Somerville, NJ	6, 8, 10, 12	Polyurethane	Mercury or tungsten (3 g) weighted bolus tip. Insertion stylet included. 36- and 43-inch length. Hydrophylic coating.
Keofeed	IVAC San Diego, CA	6, 8, 12, 14.6, 18.0	Polyurethane	Tungsten (varies) weighted tip. Insertion stylet included. 36- and 43-inch length. Prelubricated.
Travasorb	Travenol Lab., Inc, Deerfield, IL	8	Polyurethane	Tungsten (3 or 5 g) weighted tip. Insertion stylet included. 45-inch length. Prelubricated.
Vivonex	Norwich-Eaton Pharmaceuticals Norwich, NY	8	Polyurethane	Tungsten weighted tip. Does not need stylet for insertion. 45-inch length.
Moss Tube	Norwich-Eaton Pharmaceuticals Norwich, NY	18	—	Nasoesophagogastric decompression tube with duodenal feeding tube.
K-Tube	Midwest Metabolic Support Group Chicago, IL	9.6	—	Surgically placed jejunal tube with Dacron cuff for anchoring to abdominal wall.
Vivonex Jejunostomy Kit	Norwich-Eaton Pharmaceuticals Norwich, NY	5	—	Surgically placed jejunal tube and kit includes all equipment needed for placement.

Administration of Enteral Formula Feedings

Prior to initiating feedings, several issues need to be addressed, including the rate of infusion, osmolality of formulas, and continuous versus intermittent feedings. We usually begin by perfusing only 25 ml/hour, regardless of whether it is given through a nasogastric or enterostomy tube. We then increase by 25 ml/hour increments as tolerated until our goals are achieved. If the intestinal tract is normal, one can usually increase to maintenance needs within 48 hours. In patients who have a shortened or diseased small bowel, we generally start with isotonic diets that provide 1 kcal/ml. Although we suspect that this regimen is still best for those with compromised small bowel function, evidence exists that starter regimens in patients with normal gut function may not be justified. Keohane et al. randomly assigned 118 patients with normal bowel function to one of three treatment regimens that varied with respect to osmolality and nitrogen content.[39] The formulas were given by continuous 24-hour infusions through a nasogastric tube. Some patients received the maintenance nitrogen needs from the first day, whereas others were given increasing amounts over the first 4 days until the same maintenance formula was reached. The patients who received their complete maintenance needs (hypertonic, polymeric diet that provided 12 g of nitrogen and 1900 kcal) on the first day did not have more gastrointestinal side effects than the patients who received isotonic formulas or who had the polymeric formula gradually increased to full strength over 4 days. Diarrhea was related only to concurrent antibiotic treatment and not to hypertonicity or rate of infusion. Better nitrogen intakes and balances resulted from the complete hypertonic polymeric diet being started on the first day.

The decision as to whether continuous or intermittent feedings should be used depends on the therapeutic goal. Continuous infusion of nutrients is the preferred technique if enteral formulas are to provide all or most of the patient's nutrition, whereas intermittent feedings suffice if the enteral formulas are to serve only as supplements. We generally use a pump-controlled perfusion of enteral nutrition over a 24-hour period and cycle the feedings to a 10- to 12-hour nocturnal infusion. As in patients on CPN, the metabolic complications are decreased and nutrient utilization increased when the nutrition is given at a steady rate. These advantages of the continuous infusion become even more pronounced in patients with inflammatory bowel disease, short bowel syndrome, or radiation enteritis who, in general, do not tolerate tube feedings as well as patients with normal gastrointestinal function.

Intermittent feedings are well tolerated by many patients. The total quantity of formula needed for a 24-hour period is divided into equal portions and the required fractions are administered among 4 to 6 feedings. Each feeding is usually administered by gravity over a 20- to 40-minute period. Examples of these schedules are as follows:

Slow	240 ml/40 minutes	(6 ml/min)
Moderate	240 ml/30 minutes	(8 ml/min)
Regular	240 ml/20 minutes	(12 ml/min)

Major advantages to the intermittent feeding schedule is that it is cheaper and requires minimal equipment; however, it must be more closely monitored than the pump-assisted technique. We discourage the use of bolus feedings or the rapid administration of 300 to 400 ml of formula through a syringe. Although this method is frequently used in hospitals and nursing homes, the risk of aspiration and gastrointestinal side effects is probably great enough to discourage its use.

Complications

The most frequent complications associated with tube feedings are minimized through proper formula selection, controlled administration, and careful monitoring.

Mechanical problems are often associated with the tube and its position. Gastric erosions are more likely to occur when one uses large-diameter tubes.[40] Such tubes may also reduce the competency of the lower esophageal sphincter, thereby increasing the risk of gastroesophageal reflux and aspiration.[41] Tubes that are smaller in diameter (e.g., 8 or 9 French) and more pliable are associated with less irritation and better tolerance. However, small-lumen tubes are more likely to become occluded, usually from residual of the feedings or particulate matter from pulverized medications (or both) administered through the tube. To prevent obstruction, the tubes should be irrigated with 20 to 50 ml of water or cranberry juice every 8 to 12 hours and whenever the feeding is interrupted.[42] Also, only liquid forms of medication should be administered through small tubes. Displacement of nasogastric tubes can be disastrous and can be avoided if care is taken during intubation. Placement of the radiopaque tube can be confirmed by a chest x-ray, auscultating over the left upper quadrant of the abdomen after instillation of air through a syringe, or by aspiration of gastric contents. Enterostomy feedings may be complicated by leakage of intestinal contents with skin erosions, wound infection, and tube dislodgment.[43]

Gastrointestinal side effects of tube feedings include delayed gastric emptying, nausea, vomiting, cramping abdominal pain, and diarrhea. Vomiting and pulmonary aspiration are potentiated when gastric emptying is delayed. The risk of vomiting and aspiration can be lessened by elevating the patient's head at a 30-degree angle,[44] positioning the tube beyond the pylorus,[45] and checking for gastric residual. The residual should not exceed the amount infused during the preceding hour. If the residual is excessive, the feeding should be held and the residual rechecked in 1 hour. If large-volume residuals persist, a reduction in formula concentration or rate (or both) may alleviate the problem.

Diarrhea in a patient on enteral formula feedings can result from lactase deficiency, concomitant antibiotic treatment,[46] infectious diarrhea from contaminated formulas,[47] and excessive osmotic loads. Diarrhea that persists during the administration of formula feedings may lessen with the reduction in the rate or concentration of solution; however, we usually use antidiarrheal agents in hopes of maintaining optimal delivery of nutrients. The continuous pump-controlled perfusion system is generally associated with fewer gastrointestinal symptoms.

The potential for metabolic complications is the same as in patients on CPN and consists of excesses and deficiencies of almost every nutrient. Of 100 patients who were tube fed, 30 to 40 per cent experienced at least one metabolic complication, with hyperkalemia (in 40 per cent of patients with complications), hyponatremia (31 per cent), hypophosphatemia (30 per cent), and hyperglycemia (29 per cent) being the most common.[48] In another report, 43 per cent of 83 patients required modification of the enteral formulas in order to meet their fluid and electrolyte requirements.[49]

Fluid and electrolyte imbalances may readily occur in patients who have altered sensorium and cannot communicate their thirst sensation. Of 100 tube-fed patients, 10 per cent experienced manifestations of dehydration and hypernatremia secondary to free water loss.[50] Conversely, some patients with head injuries develop hyponatremia from inappropriate secretion of ADH, and the excessive water retention may prove harmful. Patients with congestive heart failure, cirrhosis, and renal failure are other examples of patients who cannot handle large salt and water loads.

Home Enteral Nutrition

With changing health care patterns resulting in shortened hospital stays, there has been increased emphasis on home care. Home care statistics estimate that about 7500 patients receive home enteral nutrition. It is also estimated that home nutritional therapy represents one of the most rapidly growing segments of home care, with a projected growth rate of 25 to 30 per cent annually.[51]

The need for assuring quality nutritional support has received attention. In late 1984, the Health Care Financing Administration produced guidelines governing financial coverage for home enteral and parenteral nutrition.[52] This policy outlined criteria for patient eligibility, the services and products that would be covered, the documentation that must be maintained, and the process by which the program would be administered. In 1985, the American Society for Parenteral and Enteral Nutrition published "Standards for Nutritional Support—Home Patients." These standards reflect "minimal acceptable levels of care to be subscribed to by home health care providers."[53]

In spite of this, there is an absence of information pertaining to the effectiveness of home enteral nutrition. In one report, Nelson et al. followed 144 home enteral patients over the course of one year.[54] Average duration of therapy for this patient population was 4½ months; at the end of the year 75 remained active on tube feeding, 30 resumed an oral diet, 38 expired, and 1 patient required parenteral nutritional support. A survey of this patient population revealed that of 53 patients remaining active on enteral nutritional support, 44 (82 per cent) were able to follow and tolerate their prescribed enteral program consistently. These patients subsequently maintained or improved body weight.

It is also thought that tube feeding is a simple procedure with few complications. This same study revealed that it is common for home patients to experience problems in maintaining access or with tolerance (Table 43–8). Although most complications were resolved at home, many others required more extensive attention at the physician's office, treatment in an emergency room, or admission to a hospital.

The benefits of nutritional support for patients who are considered terminal is controversial. Since most of these patients have malignancies or progressively deteriorating neurologic diseases, it was of interest to survey their opinions regarding home enteral therapy. When asked to describe their quality of life prior to initiation of home enteral nutritional support, 41 patients (77 per cent) reported that their quality of life was less than good. Each was also asked to describe the impact of home enteral nutrition on his or her quality of life. Of the 53 patients who participated in our survey, half (27) reported that home enteral support improved daily living, and 21 patients (39 per cent) reported maintenance of quality of life. Many patients commented that home tube feedings allowed return of a more normal life-style despite the demands that the therapy placed on their daily routine. Six patients (12 per cent) reported that home tube feeding resulted in deterioration in quality of life. Several of these patients reported being overwhelmed with the demands of tube feedings, and that such demands offset the benefits of the therapy.

It can be seen that although tube feeding is thought to be a simple procedure with few complications, problems with access and tolerance do occur. Although tube feeding can favorably affect perceived quality of life it can also impose overwhelming demands on the individual. These factors must be considered in selection of candidates for home enteral nutrition. Regular follow-up of these patients is also necessary.

TABLE 43–8. *Frequency of Reported Problems in 53 Home Tube-Fed Patients—Percent Resolution in Home or with Outside Intervention*

	No. of Patients with Problem	Total No. of Incidents	Percent Resolved			
			Home	MD Office	Emergency Room	Hospitalization
Access problems						
Tube blockage	33	36	67	16	14	3
Tube dislocation	33	39	36	13	31	20
Tube replacement	31	37	22	24	41	13
Site irritation/infection	29	34	65	32	3	0
Equipment malfunction	18	18	100	0	0	0
	53*	164	52†	19	20	9
Tolerance problems						
Diarrhea	31	31	84	16	0	0
Nausea/vomiting	25	25	80	12	8	0
Fullness/distention	21	21	81	10	0	9
Gas	21	21	90	10	0	0
Constipation	17	17	88	12	0	0
Regurgitation	13	13	92	8	0	0
	53*	128	85†	12	1	2

*Fifty-three patients reported one or more problems with the feedings.
†Percent of total problems reported.

PARENTERAL NUTRITION

The terminology used to describe parenteral nutrition is confusing, and there is no uniformly accepted nomenclature in the parenteral nutrition literature. Hyperalimentation, total parenteral nutrition, peripheral hyperalimentation, and protein-sparing therapy are commonly used terms which do not convey the same meaning to all readers. For purposes of this chapter, we will use the term central parenteral nutrition (CPN) to mean the use of a large-diameter central vein through which to administer hypertonic formulas. Peripheral parenteral nutrition (PPN) means the use of small-diameter peripheral veins to infuse isotonic or hypotonic nutrients.

Figure 43–1 shows a flow chart that can help one decide what type of parenteral nutrition to use for a specific patient. The patient's current nutritional status is of prime importance in helping decide the type of parenteral therapy. For the patient who is well nourished, the therapeutic goal is to preserve lean body mass. As an example, PPN is usually used in healthy patients following elective surgery if resumption of oral intake is anticipated in less than 1 week. On the other hand, the patient with pre-existing protein-calorie malnutrition will usually need CPN in order to restore and maintain lean body mass. Although attempts at aggressive restorative parenteral nutrition can be made through the peripheral vein, the task is much easier with hypertonic nutrients given through a large central vein.

Peripheral Parenteral Nutrition (PPN)

The availability of safe fat emulsions has made PPN an attractive means to provide parenteral nu-

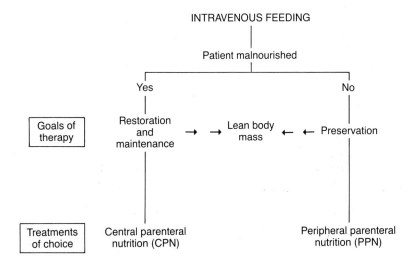

FIGURE 43–1. *Flow chart depicting intravenous treatment of choice based on pre-treatment nutritional status (presence or absence of protein-calorie malnutrition).*

trition. The isotonic fat emulsions are available in 10 per cent and 20 per cent solutions, making it possible to meet many patients' basic nutritional needs by use of PPN alone. Table 43–9 details how a 70-kg patient can have his basic caloric and protein nutritional needs met in 3.5 L of fluid when 50 per cent of total calories are given as fat. Unfortunately, PPN is usually more difficult to maintain because of frequent episodes of phlebitis of superficial arm veins and infiltrations of solutions into subcutaneous tissue. Also, malnourished patients who need nutritional support the most are those who are least likely to have adequate peripheral veins for PPN.

A basic solution of 5 per cent dextrose in water with potassium chloride and vitamins has been a mainstay for patients requiring only a few days of nutrition. Two liters of 5 per cent dextrose in water (100 g of dextrose), as compared with fasting, decreases urinary nitrogen losses by approximately 50 per cent.[55] The addition of another 100 g of dextrose (total of 200 g dextrose) each day resulted in little additional nitrogen preservation; therefore, it was recommended that 150 g of intravenous dextrose per day be given to the average elective surgical patient. Although there will be considerable loss of nitrogen during the 3- to 5-day postoperative period when patients are nil per os (NPO), they can rapidly replete stores when oral intake is resumed.

The term "protein-sparing therapy" should refer to the administration of any nutrient that will reduce nitrogen excretion and improve nitrogen balance, including 5 per cent dextrose in water. However, the concept of protein-sparing therapy is thought by most to mean the use of synthetic amino acids alone or amino acids plus hypotonic dextrose and additives (vitamins and minerals). The replacement of dextrose calories with isocaloric amounts of amino acids alone will improve nitrogen balance by 50 per cent.[56] Although it was initially thought that the addition of glucose to the amino acids, with greater insulin release, would blunt this apparent advantage of giving only amino acids, it is now apparent that the addition of hypotonic glucose to amino acids has the same effect as giving the amino acids alone. Thus, the protein-sparing effect of amino acids alone or amino acids with hypocaloric dextrose is due to the amino acids themselves rather than substrate-hormone interactions (e.g., insulin or glucagon re-

sponses). When amino acids are given through peripheral veins, the nitrogen balance is directly proportional to the amount of infused amino acids. Greenberg et al. showed that a positive nitrogen balance was possible with hypocaloric infusions in malnourished patients if the rate of amino acid infusion was about 2 g/kg ideal body weight per day.[57]

Central Parenteral Nutrition (CPN)

The use of CPN has provided a yardstick with which to compare other nutritional therapies. The use of the superior vena cava has permitted administration of ample calories, mainly as dextrose, without exceeding daily fluid tolerance levels.

Catheter Placement and Care. A catheter is inserted into a large-caliber central vein. This procedure is done at the patient's bedside, using sterile technique. The infraclavicular approach to the right subclavian vein is usually used in adults. The catheter tip is threaded into the superior vena cava to rest just above the right atrium. The needle guard is applied and the catheter is sutured to the skin. Antiseptic ointment is placed around the catheter exit site on the skin and a nonocclusive dressing is applied. A chest x-ray confirms the position of the catheter in the superior vena cava before the CPN solutions are begun.

Meticulous care of the catheter is necessary. Dressings are changed three times a week, using the same aseptic techniques that were followed when the catheter was inserted. A final filter is inserted between the intravenous tubing and catheter and is changed daily. Small-pore filters (0.22 μ size) serve as an effective bacterial and fungal filter. Larger-pore filters are designed to filter only particulate matter. An infusion pump is used to control the rate of infusion. Except under extraordinary circumstances, the catheter should not be used for other intravenous solutions such as blood, albumin, and drugs. Also, central venous pressure measurements should not be performed through the line.

Nutrients. The basic nutrients for CPN are carbohydrates, amino acids, fat emulsions, electrolytes and metals, trace elements, and vitamins.

CARBOHYDRATE. Dextrose is a safe and efficiently used caloric source. Solutions of alcohol, sorbitol, xylitol, and fructose have all been tried and are no longer used because of side effects.

PROTEIN. Synthetic crystalline amino acids are available in concentrations of 5 to 10 per cent, with and without electrolytes. The amino acid preparations usually consist of two thirds nonessential amino acids and one third essential amino acids. They are very efficiently used; the mean nitrogen retention when 1 g/kg/day of the 10 per cent amino acid mixture was given was equivalent to high biological value protein given orally.[58,59]

FAT. Intravenous fat solutions are available as

TABLE 43–9. Example of Peripheral Parenteral Nutrition (70-kg Patient)

Nutrient	kcal	Protein (g)	Volume (L)
Fat (20%)	1000		0.5
Amino acids (8.5%)	510	128	1.5
Dextrose* (10%)	510		1.5
	2020	128	3.5

This formulation would usually be given as 3 L of 500 ml of 8.5% amino acids and 500 ml of 10% dextrose, plus electrolytes, minerals, and vitamins and 0.5 L of a 20% fat emulsion.

*Anhydrous dextrose, caloric value of 3.4 kcal/g

emulsions of soybean or safflower oils, egg lecithin phospholipid, and glycerol. Ten and 20 per cent concentrations of isotonic fat emulsions can be administered with PPN or CPN. Fat emulsions are usually added "piggyback" into the main intravenous line leading from the bottle containing dextrose and amino acids. However, companies have recently provided the technology that allows one to mix dextrose, amino acids, and fat emulsions (3-in-1 system) in the same bag. A controlled study comparing the mixture of dextrose, amino acids, and fats with the conventional system of dextrose and amino acids in one bottle and the fat emulsion in another found a significantly higher rate of catheter occlusions with the former.[60] All patients on CPN should receive at least enough fat (e.g., 1 to 1.5 L of 10 per cent fat emulsion for the average adult) each week to prevent biochemical evidence of essential fatty acid deficiency.

ELECTROLYTES. Single-package electrolyte solutions added to parenteral nutrition solutions will meet most patients' needs. There are exceptions when alterations are needed, such as in patients with cardiac, hepatic, or renal diseases.

TRACE ELEMENTS. Additives of either single or multiple trace elements are available. Solutions with three or four trace elements added are usually satisfactory; however, patients with cholestasis should have copper omitted,[61] and patients with large stool or fistula losses may lose zinc in excess of what the standard formula will replace.[7]

VITAMINS. There are vitamin preparations with both water-soluble and fat-soluble vitamins. Vitamin K is not routinely added, but it can be supplemented either orally or parenterally. Vitamin requirements in patients receiving CPN have not been studied as carefully as most other nutrients.

Nonprotein Energy. The use of dextrose as the only nonprotein energy source in CPN solutions is associated with several problems. The infusion of dextrose in excess of that which is readily oxidized results in net synthesis of body fat and water accumulation.[62,63] Complications observed in patients receiving excessive glucose are fatty liver and mild elevations in serum amino transferases and alkaline phosphatase values[64,65] and, in patients on respirators, an increase in carbon dioxide production with only a minimal increase in oxygen consumption.[66,67] Also, biochemical evidence of essential fatty acid deficiency (triene:tetraene ratio > 0.4) develops in approximately 10 days after fat-free CPN is begun.[68]

The dual energy system (dextrose and fat) appears more efficient than glucose alone in repleting protein and avoiding water retention. Macfie et al. randomly assigned 32 patients on 50 kcal/kg/day to either hypertonic dextrose alone or to a combination of glucose and fat with 60 per cent of nonprotein energy given as fat.[69] Although both groups gained significant weight, patients on glucose alone gained only fat and water, whereas patients on glucose and fat gained body protein without significant gains of fat and water. This advantage of using the dual energy system in all patients must be weighed against the disadvantage of the added expense of the fat emulsions.

Patient Monitoring. Daily records should include weight, and fluid intakes and outputs. Urine samples are tested for glucose. Prior to starting CPN, values for serum electrolytes, creatinine, aminotransferase, alkaline phosphatase, bilirubin, total protein, albumin, glucose, magnesium, zinc, and copper should be measured. Serum electrolytes are measured twice in the first week, and the entire chemistry profile is repeated at the end of 1 week of CPN. As the patient's condition stabilizes, tests are repeated less frequently. Measurements of urinary and fecal nitrogen are needed to determine nitrogen balance; however, they are not necessary for the average uncomplicated patient receiving CPN. The measurement of visceral proteins with short half-lives (e.g., pre-albumin and retinol binding protein) confirms protein synthesis. Since the half-life of albumin is approximately 19 days, one should not expect a rapid rise in albumin levels. A CPN flow chart placed on the front of the patient's chart serves to maintain a continuous record of blood chemistry results, the intake-output record, and daily weights which will allow early recognition of evolving deficiencies or excesses.

Indications. All patients for whom a combination of enteral nutrition and PPN is inadequate for longer than 1 week are candidates for CPN. The therapeutic goal in using CPN should be formulated prior to its initiation. A time frame for treatment should be considered. For instance, some severely malnourished but stable patients with inflammatory bowel disease will receive 2 weeks or more of CPN prior to an elective operation, whereas others will have CPN for only a few days prior to more urgent surgery and CPN will be continued into the postoperative period until it is obvious that the patient can ingest and absorb enough nutrients.

Many chapters in this book deal with the use of CPN in specific diseases or conditions. Our remarks will highlight only selected conditions for which CPN is commonly used in order to demonstrate its effectiveness.

Inflammatory Bowel Disease. CPN is most often used in patients with inflammatory bowel disease (IBD) as an adjunct to surgery or conventional medical treatment; however, it occasionally is used as primary therapy for patients with gut failure from extensive Crohn's disease. Patients with Crohn's disease usually respond better to CPN and bowel rest than do patients with ulcerative colitis, and patients with Crohn's enteritis respond better than patients with Crohn's colitis.

A randomized controlled trial of CPN and bowel rest was reported in patients with acute colitis, most of whom had chronic ulcerative colitis (CUC).[70] Patients in the control group were fed an ad lib oral diet, and the treatment group received CPN and bowel rest. Controls and CPN-treated patients were taking comparable amounts of corticosteroids. Half of each group required surgery during the same hospitalization. Of those not requiring surgery, the time required of medical treatment to induce clinical remission was comparable in the two groups. Thus, there was no difference in the outcome in the control and CPN groups with regard to frequency of surgery or duration of medical treatment. Retrospective reviews and this one controlled study suggest that the addition of CPN and bowel rest will not prompt clinical remission more often than the use of corticosteroids and hospitalization alone. These reports should not, however, discourage the use of CPN to reverse malnutrition in patients with ulcerative colitis in whom enteral nutrition is impossible or inadequate.

A clinical trial that randomized CPN and other intravenous nutritional therapies suggested that CPN may improve surgical results following proctocolectomy.[71] The patients undergoing proctocolectomy, half of whom had inflammatory bowel disease, received one of three intravenous solutions: balanced amino acids (85 to 127 g daily) without another caloric source, conventional CPN, and controls who received only an intravenous saline solution. Nitrogen and potassium losses were prevented in patients treated with amino acids or CPN. The major difference was that patients receiving CPN had significantly fewer postoperative complications than either the controls or those given amino acid infusions. Eighty per cent of the CPN-treated patients were home with complete perineal wound healing by 4 weeks, compared with only 40 per cent of patients in the control group and 30 per cent in the amino acid group who had healed their wounds during the same period.

Patients with Crohn's disease have a greater nutritional liability than patients with CUC, because the small bowel is frequently involved in Crohn's disease. A randomized, controlled trial comparing CPN and bowel rest with other therapies (e.g., prednisone alone, enteral nutrition of liquid formulas, PPN plus oral food) in patients with Crohn's disease has not been reported. Allowing for differences in author's definitions of clinical remission, uncontrolled data suggests that 60 to 70 per cent of patients with Crohn's disease will undergo an initial, in-hospital remission, but only 40 to 50 per cent of those followed for 3 months after CPN is stopped remain in remission.[72]

Muller et al. treated 30 consecutive patients with complicated Crohn's disease with 12 weeks of CPN and bowel rest.[73] No medications were given. Although surgery was initially avoided in 25 of 30 patients, the cumulative relapse rate was 60 per cent after 2 years and 85 per cent after 4 years. This was compared with the results of resection, obtained

from a 10-year period before CPN was begun at the same hospital, showing the cumulative recurrence rates after CPN to be four times higher than after resection.

Lochs et al. randomly assigned 20 malnourished patients with Crohn's disease to one of two groups.[74] One group was placed on CPN and complete bowel rest, while the other group was allowed to eat while receiving CPN. There was no significant difference between the two regimens in that the disease activity was decreased and the nutritional status improved comparably in both groups. It should be noted, however, that the food given these patients was a low-residue diet and liquid formulas rather than an ad lib selected diet.

The use of CPN and bowel rest in patients with fistulas from Crohn's disease has been disappointing, and surgery should not be delayed unnecessarily in the hope that the fistulas will permanently close. Those fistulas that do close will usually recur following resumption of oral intake. Many such patients require CPN and bowel rest for restoration of adequate nutrition during the perioperative period.

Growth failure in the child or adolescent with Crohn's disease is very difficult to treat. The use of steroids and surgery is controversial in restoring growth. Good nutritional management ($\geq$ 75 to 100 kcal/kg/day and 2 g protein/kg/day) has usually reversed the growth arrest and many patients have demonstrated "catch-up" growth. Although aggressive enteral nutrition is preferred, one occasionally has to resort to CPN in the hospital or home.[75]

Gastrointestinal Fistulas. CPN and bowel rest decrease the volume as well as modify the content of upper gut secretions and may facilitate closure of fistulas by correcting protein depletion, thus facilitating healing. Fistulas that are unlikely to close with the use of CPN and bowel rest alone are those that have an obstruction distal to the fistula, are associated with intra-abdominal infections, or arise from Crohn's disease, radiation damage to the intestine, or malignancy.

Before the introduction of CPN, the morbidity rate in patients with high-output enterocutaneous fistulas arising from the proximal small bowel was approximately 50 per cent. Complications that were encountered included fluid and electrolyte losses (78 per cent), malnutrition (61 per cent), and generalized peritonitis (67 per cent).[76] With the addition of CPN, malnutrition and electrolyte imbalances have been minimized. Comparison of results before and after the availability of CPN in the treatment of fistulas is enlightening. Table 43–10 compares the results from two large series reported 9 years apart, one before the use of CPN and the other after CPN was routinely included in the management of patients with fistulas. Chapman et al. supplied suboptimal nutrition by hypotonic dextrose and protein hydrolysates through peripheral veins and blenderized formulas given through tubes placed distal to

TABLE 43–10. Nutritional Management of Gastrointestinal Fistulas

	Calories and Protein Peripheral Vein*	Bowel Rest and TPN†
Nonsurgical closure (%)	—	70
Surgical closure (%)	58	92
Mortality (%)	45	6
Time (days)	60	35

*Data from Chapman et al.[73]
†Data from MacFadyen et al.[74]

the origin of the fistulas.[77] MacFadyen et al. used CPN and bowel rest to meet patients' requirements.[78] Mortality rates in the pre-CPN and CPN patients were 45 and 6 per cent, respectively. Seventy per cent of the CPN-treated patients had their fistulas close without surgery, and 92 per cent of fistulas closed after CPN plus surgery. The average time between initiation of CPN and closure of the fistula in the study by MacFadyen et al. was 35 days, approximately half of the time spent in the hospital in the patients described by Chapman et al. The use of CPN and bowel rest is certainly not the only reason patients with intestinal fistulas now have less morbidity and mortality. In addition to better nutritional support, there have been advances in intensive care nursing, antibiotics, and surgical efforts that have contributed to the improvement. Nonetheless, the ability to maintain excellent nutrition while decreasing intestinal secretions and fistula drainage has to be, if not the most important, one of the most important contributions to the management of fistulas.

Short Bowel Syndrome. Patients who have had a large resection of the small intestine require CPN and bowel rest until stool losses become predictable and, it is hoped, manageable. Most patients with short bowel syndrome can absorb 40 to 60 per cent of their calories[79,80] and if they eat often enough, they can sustain themselves with oral calories. However, many patients with short bowel syndrome become chronically depleted of fluid and electrolytes if the colon has been resected along with most of the small intestine. These patients often require an indwelling permanent catheter, which is used more for fluid and electrolytes than for calories.

Complications. The major complications encountered in patients on CPN are infections, catheter-related mechanical problems, and metabolic abnormalities.

Infections. Patients who require CPN have many reasons for their host defense mechanisms to be impaired, including protein-calorie malnutrition, hypophosphatemia, corticosteroid treatment, chemotherapy, and radiation therapy. The use of broad-spectrum antibiotics increases the likelihood of fungal infections.

The incidence of catheter related-sepsis in most hospitals where CPN is quality controlled is between 3 and 7 per cent.[81,82] When strict aseptic technique was used in catheter insertion and maintenance, as judged by an independent observer, catheter-related sepsis dropped to 3 per cent, compared with 20 per cent when breaks in technique were observed.[82]

The recognition of infections in patients on CPN is sometimes difficult because most will have other reasons to be febrile. A low-grade temperature as might be seen in patients with Crohn's disease or pancreatitis is not as suggestive of a catheter-related infection as is the fever spike that occurs in a previously afebrile patient. When a patient receiving CPN who had been afebrile becomes febrile, one should (1) remove the CPN bottle and administration set but keep the catheter open with a dextrose solution, (2) culture the CPN solution and blood drawn from a peripheral line for bacteria and fungi, and (3) search for other sources of infection. If no other source of infection can be found and if fever persists, blood should be drawn from the catheter for culture, the catheter should be removed, and its tip should be cultured. If the fever subsides shortly after removal of the catheter, it was probably caused by bacterial or fungal contamination of the line.

Mechanical Catheter Problems. The infraclavicular route of most central venous line placements is only a few centimeters above the apex of the lung; therefore, a misguided catheter may result in pneumothorax. The catheter may lodge in the jugular vein and cause a chemical phlebitis when CPN is infused; the importance of obtaining a chest x-ray prior to initiating CPN is punctuated by this rare complication. Air embolism may occur if the junction between the catheter and CPN line becomes disconnected. All such connections should be tightly taped or have a Luer lock. Fatal air embolism has also occurred when the CPN bottle was changed, stressing the importance of having the patient hold his breath on inspiration while changing the bottles and tubing as well as during placement of the catheter.[83] Central venous thrombosis is a well recognized complication of plastic catheters. The belief that silicone rubber catheters are less thrombogenic was supported by the finding that thrombosis occurred in only 4 per cent of patients who received them.[84] The use of intravenous heparin as prophylaxis against thrombosis reduces the risk of thrombus formation on the central venous catheter,[85] but it is uncertain whether the advantage of reducing thrombus around the catheter is worth the risk of hemorrhagic complications that could occur if heparin was used in all patients receiving CPN. Other major dangers of central catheters include hemothorax, chylothorax, pericardial tamponade, arteriovenous fistula, and brachial plexus injury.

Metabolic Complications. The metabolic complications associated with CPN are legend. The nutritional needs of each patient are different, so metabolic complications are best avoided by assessing each patient's need before starting CPN and then monitoring the clinical status and blood chemistries on a regular basis. The major metabolic complications are listed in Table 43–11.

Normal persons metabolize glucose at rates varying between 0.4 and 1.2 g/kg/hour. Some patients on CPN, including victims of trauma and patients in the postoperative period, will have glucose intolerance. Excessive total dose or rate of glucose infusion may result in hyperglycemia, glycosuria, osmotic diuresis, and, occasionally, hyperosmolar nonketotic coma.[86] Rebound hypoglycemia, following sudden cessation or interruption of CPN, is a potential problem; however, symptomatic hypoglycemia is very uncommon. Patients on CPN while under anesthesia are at particular risk of prolonged hypoglycemia because the sympathomimetic response may not be appreciated.

Hypercalcemia can result from infusion of excessive quantities of calcium or from vitamin D toxicity.[87] Pancreatitis[88] and hypercalciuria with nephrolithiasis[89] have been observed to be associated with acute hypercalcemia produced by excessive calcium or vitamin D in CPN infusions.

Hypophosphatemia was a particularly dangerous complication which occurred more commonly before phosphate was routinely added to the commercially available CPN preparations. It usually occurs in severely malnourished patients who are given excessive amounts of CPN to which phosphorus has not been added in amounts that are adequate to meet the requirements for the metabolism of the infused glucose and amino acids. An intravascular to intracellular shift of phosphate results. Patients experience paresthesias, weakness, confusion, convulsions, and death.[90,91] Associated with the hypophosphatemia is a reduction in erythrocytic 2,3-diphosphoglycerate, which results in increased affinity of hemoglobin for oxygen and less oxygen released to peripheral tissues. There are also reductions in ATP content of red blood cells, white cells, and platelets, which are causally related to hemolytic anemia, impaired chemotactic, phagocytic, and bactericidal functions of granulocytes, and shortened platelet survival,[92,93] respectively.

Patients receiving CPN without added zinc show declines in plasma zinc at rates of 6 to 10 μg/dl/week.[94] Eventually, they may develop evidence of biochemical and clinical zinc deficiency. Clinically, alopecia and acrodermatitis may appear;[95] the rash has a predilection for the nasolabial and perineal areas. Clinical zinc deficiency usually occurs in the anabolic state when the patient is gaining weight and the requirements for zinc are increased.[96] A low serum level of alkaline phosphatase, a zinc metalloenzyme, may return to normal or above normal with zinc replacement.

Copper deficiency in patients on long-term CPN may present as neutropenia, leukopenia, and anemia.[97,98] The anemia may be normocytic-normochromic or hypochromic-microcytic. The daily requirement for copper in patients on CPN is 300 μg per day in patients without diarrhea and 400 to 500 μg per day with diarrhea or increased fluid losses through gastrointestinal stomas or fistulas.[99]

Chromium potentiates insulin at target organs, perhaps in the form of the "glucose tolerance factor." Two isolated case reports have documented unusual glucose intolerance in patients on home parenteral nutrition which responded to chromium supplementation.[100,101]

Selenium deficiency and fatal cardiomyopathy have occurred in patients on home parenteral nutrition (HPN).[102,103] Selenium levels and glutathione peroxidase activities were extremely low in blood prior to death and in solid tissues at autopsy. Glutathione peroxidase is a selenium-dependent enzyme necessary for lipid peroxidation. The fatal cardiomyopathies resembled Keshan's disease, a cardiomyopathy seen in children and pregnant women in China which is associated with selenium deficiency and has nearly been eliminated by selenium supplementation.

Vitamin A deficiency with impaired dark field adaptation has occurred in patients on CPN, but it requires many months because of the large amount of vitamin A stored in the liver. Clinically, it presents

TABLE 43–11. Major Metabolic Complications in Patients Receiving Total Parenteral Nutrition

	Presentations
Nutrient Excess	
Glucose	Hyperglycemia, polyuria, polydipsia
Amino acids	Hyperammonemia in patients with liver disease
	Azotemia in renal failure
Calcium	Hypercalcemia, pancreatitis, renal stones
Vitamin D	Hypercalcemia, osteopenia, long bone pain
Nutrient Deficiencies	
Copper	Neutropenia, anemia, scorbutic bone lesions, $\downarrow$ ceruloplasmin
Zinc	Nasolabial and perineal acrodermatitis, alopecia, $\downarrow$ T cell function, $\downarrow$ alkaline phosphatase
Chromium	Glucose intolerance
Selenium	Myalgias, cardiomyopathy, $\downarrow$ glutathione peroxidase
Molybdenum	Amino acid intolerance, tachycardia, tachypnea, central scotomas, irritability, $\downarrow$ uric acid
Essential fatty acids	Eczymoid dermatitis, $\uparrow$ 20:3/20:4
Vitamin A	Night blindness, $\downarrow$ dark field adaptation
Vitamin E	In vitro platelet hyperaggregation and H_2O_2-induced RBC hemolysis
Biotin	Dermatitis, alopecia, hypotonia
Thiamine	Wernicke's encephalopathy

as night blindness. Possible causes include interruption of an enterohepatic cycle for vitamin A, adherence to glass or tubing during storage of premixed parenteral solutions, and a deficiency of zinc, which in animals appears to block mobilization of vitamin A from the liver.[104]

Morphological evidence for osteomalacia in patients on HPN has been accompanied by intermittent hypercalcemia, hypercalciuria, and negative calcium balance.[105,106] Serum phosphorus and 25-hydroxy-vitamin D levels were normal and parathyroid hormones were appropriate for the serum calcium values. Surprisingly, symptoms subsided, morphology improved, and urinary calcium losses were decreased when vitamin D was removed from the solutions.[107] Vitamin D may be a major factor in the cause of metabolic bone disease in patients on long-term CPN; however, many patients with short bowel syndrome will have had chronic malabsorption of calcium and vitamin D and osteopenia before CPN was begun. More recently, it has been proposed that there is a causal relationship between the osteopenia and the increased concentrations of aluminum in bone and in the protein hydrolysates that were infused.[108]

In vitro platelet hyperaggregation and hydrogen-peroxide–induced red cell hemolysis have been linked to vitamin E deficiency during TPN.[109] Since the requirement for vitamin E is directly proportional to the amount of dietary fat, the needs of vitamin E will increase if intravenous fat is used on a regular basis.

Biotin responsive dermatitis and alopecia have been reported in an infant[110] and an adult[111] on CPN. The newer vitamin preparations contain biotin.

Home Parenteral Nutrition

Patients were first managed with home parenteral nutrition (HPN) approximately 15 years ago. Many individuals have benefitted from this advance in the care of patients with gut failure. The basic principle of HPN is to infuse the nutrients during an overnight period and encourage patients to pursue normal activities during the day. Because of the complexity of the overall condition of most patients receiving such treatment, most centers have organized their efforts with a multispecialty team consisting of physicians, nurses, pharmacists, dieticians, and social workers. The involvement of industry as intermediary suppliers to patients has greatly facilitated the transition from hospital to home and decreased significantly the time and detail required of hospital pharmacies. Although the increasing involvement of industry has facilitated the management of HPN patients, the major responsibility for the success of HPN still resides with patients and the HPN care team.

Two major ingredients for HPN are the venous access and the delivery system. The most popular form of venous access has been a Silastic catheter that is tunneled subcutaneously down the anterior chest wall from the venous entry site in the infra-clavicular area to exit at the mid to lower sternal area. The external segment of the catheter contains a Luer lock through which heparin is placed in the catheter in the morning when the infusion is stopped. Attempts to avoid the external catheter segment for patients has led to trials with an implantable central venous access disc. The cosmetic advantage of having the disc totally concealed has been offset thus far by mechanical problems and patients' dislike of inserting a needle into the disc every night.

Table 43–12 lists the most common causes for gut failure that prompt the use of HPN. The nutritional repletion of patients on HPN is gratifying. Ideal body weight is usually achieved; the mean weight gain in adult patients treated for 3 months or longer (mean 29 months) was 13 kg.[112] Measurements of visceral protein and serial 24-hour urinary creatinine-to-height ratios confirmed nitrogen repletion. Also, body composition studies have confirmed repletion of both fat and lean body mass. Seventy-five per cent of patients on HPN have clearly been rehabilitated and return to gainful employment, school, or homemaking activities.[112,113] Although nutritionally repleted, 25 per cent remain disabled by their primary disease or jejunostomy care. Once patients on HPN are dismissed from hospital, they usually can remain out of hospital. In a representative year, 83 per cent of patients either remained out of hospital or required only one hospitalization, and only 20 per cent of the admissions were for HPN complications or modifications, whereas 80 per cent of the admissions were for complications of the primary disease.[112]

Although the dangers of HPN are great, the complication rates have been acceptable. Thirty-three per cent of HPN patients experienced sepsis at some time during the course of their treatment. However, only one infection occurred for every 6.2 patients years of HPN.[112] Most of the infections have been due to *Staphylococcus aureus* or *Candida* sepsis. The most common mechanical problem is damage to the external segment of the catheter, which is easily repaired in the outpatient department by the use of a

TABLE 43–12. Intestinal Failure: Candidates for Home Parenteral Nutrition

Absolute decrease in absorptive surface
Short bowel syndrome
Relative decrease in absorptive surface
Crohn's disease
Radiation enteritis
Refractory sprue
Motor failure
Pseudo-obstruction
Miscellaneous
Chronic adhesive obstructions
Intestinal lymphangiectasia

catheter repair kit. Catheter occlusion is surprisingly rare and can usually be managed by instillation of streptokinase into the catheter. Patients on long-term HPN are more likely to develop unusual metabolic complications such as deficiencies in chromium, vitamins A and E, and selenium.

HPN has radically altered our attitude toward the treatment of gut failure patients. Some patients who heretofore died or faced the prospect of repeated and prolonged hospitalizations can maintain excellent nutrition and resume a good quality of life. Until small bowel transplants or small bowel pacemakers to slow transit and increase absorption prove successful in humans, HPN remains the treatment of choice in patients with severe short bowel syndrome.

References

1. Dudrick SJ, Wilmore DW, Vars HM, et al. Long-term total parenteral nutrition with growth, development, and positive nitrogen balance. Surgery 1968; 64:134–141.
2. Baker JP, Detsky AS, Wesson DE, et al. Nutritional assessment: a comparison of clinical judgement and objective measurements. N Engl J Med 1982; 306:969–972.
3. Schaumburg H, Kaplan J, Windebank A, et al. Sensory neuropathy from pyridoxine abuse: a new megavitamin syndrome. N Engl J Med 1983; 309:445–448.
4. Newcomer AD, McGill DB. Clinical importance of lactase deficiency. (Editorial.) N Engl J Med 1984; 310:42–43.
5. Anderson IH, Levine AS, Levitt MD. Incomplete absorption of the carbohydrate in all-purpose wheat flour. N Engl J Med 1981; 304:891–892.
6. Hurt RD, Higgins JA, Nelson RA, et al. Nutritional status of a group of alcoholics before and after admission to an alcoholism treatment unit. Am J Clin Nutr 1981; 34:386–392.
7. Wolman SL, Anderson GH, Marliss EB, et al. Zinc in total parenteral nutrition: requirements and metabolic effects. Gastroenterology 1979; 76:458–467.
8. Fleming CR, Huizenga KA, McCall JT, et al. Zinc nutrition in Crohn's disease. Dig Dis Sci 1981; 26:865–870.
9. McClain C, Soutor C, Zieve L. Zinc deficiency: a complication of Crohn's disease. Gastroenterology 1980; 78:272–279.
10. Levine GM, Deren JJ, Steiger E, et al. Role of oral intake in maintenance of gut mass and disaccharide activity. Gastroenterology 1974; 67:975–982.
11. Feldman EJ, Dowling RH, McNaughton J, et al. Effects of oral versus intravenous nutrition on intestinal adaptation after small bowel resection in the dog. Gastroenterology 1976; 70:712–719.
12. Gastineau CF, DeWys W, Martin MJ, et al. The patient who won't eat. Dialogues in Nutrition 1976; 1(1):1–8, by Health Learning Systems Inc, Bloomfield, NJ.
13. Darby WJ, Balint J, Bloch A, et al. The patient who can't eat. Dialogues in Nutrition 1976; 1(2):1–11, by Health Learning Systems Inc, Bloomfield, NJ.
14. Rickard KA, Foland BB, Detamore CM, et al. Effectiveness of central parenteral nutrition versus peripheral parenteral nutrition plus enteral nutrition in reversing protein-energy malnutrition in children with advanced neuroblastoma and Wilms' tumor: a prospective randomized study. Am J Clin Nutr 1983; 38:445–456.
15. Chrysomilides SA, Kaminski MV. Home enteral and parenteral nutritional support: a comparison. Am J Clin Nutr 1981; 34:2271–2275.
16. Heymsfield SB, Bleier MNS, Witmire L. Nutrient bioavailability from nasojejunally administered enteral formulas: comparison to solid food. Am J Clin Nutr 1984; 39:243–250.
17. Pareira MD, Conrad EJ, Hicks W, et al. Therapeutic nutrition with tube feeding. JAMA 1954; 156:810–816.
18. Hunter J. A case of paralysis of the muscles of deglutition, cured by an artificial mode of conveying food and medicines into the stomach. Transactions of the Society for Improvement of Medical Chirurgical Knowledge 1793; 1:182–188.
19. Newington T. Feeding by the nose. Lancet 1879; 1:83.
20. Winitz M, Graff J, Gallagher N, et al. Evaluation of chemical diets as nutrition for man-in-space. Nature 1965; 205:741–743.
21. Adibi SA. Intestinal absorption of amino acids and peptides. Viewpoints Dig Dis 1978; 10:1–4.
22. Matthews DM, Adibi SA. Peptide absorption. Gastroenterology 1976; 71:151–161.
23. McGhee A, Henderson JM, Millikan WJ, et al. Comparison of the effects of Hepatic-Aid and a casein modular diet on encephalopathy, plasma amino acids, and nitrogen balance in cirrhotic patients. Ann Surg 1983; 197:288–293.
24. Eriksson LS, Persson A, Wahren J. Branched-chain amino acids in the treatment of chronic hepatic encephalopathy. Gut 1982; 23:801–806.
25. Horst D, Grace N, Conn H, et al. Comparison of dietary protein with an oral branched chain–enriched amino acid supplement in chronic portal-systemic encephalopathy: a randomized controlled trial. Hepatology 1984; 4:279–287.
26. Abel RM. Parenteral nutrition in the treatment of renal failure. In Fischer JE (ed). Total Parenteral Nutrition. Boston, Little, Brown, 1976: 143–170.
27. Kluthe R, Luttgen FM, Capetianu T, et al. Protein requirements in maintenance hemodialysis. Am J Clin Nutr 1978; 31:1812–1820.
28. Gallagher MW, Tyson KRT, Ashcraft KW. Gastrostomy in pediatric patients: an analysis of complications and techniques. Surgery 1973; 74:536–539.
29. Haws EB, Sieber WK, Kiesewetter WB. Complications of tube gastrostomy in infants and children: 15-year review of 240 cases. Ann Surg 1966; 164:284–290.
30. Connar RG, Sealy WC. Gastrostomy and its complications. Ann Surg 1956; 143:245–250.
31. Campbell JR, Sasaki TM. Gastrostomy in infants and children: an analysis of complications and techniques. Am Surg 1974; 40:505–508.
32. Holder TM, Leape LL, Ashcraft KW. Gastrostomy: its use and dangers in pediatric patients. N Engl J Med 1972; 286:1345–1347.
33. Wasiljew BK, Ujiki GT, Beal JM. Feeding gastrostomy: complications and mortality. Am J Surg 1982; 143:194–195.
34. Larson DE, Fleming CR, Ott BJ, et al. Percutaneous endoscopic gastrostomy. Mayo Clin Proc 1983; 58:103–107.
35. Ponsky JL, Gauderer MWL, Stellato IA. Percutaneous endoscopic gastrostomy. Review of 150 cases. Arch Surg 1983; 118:913–914.
36. Rombeau JL, Twomey PL, McLean GK et al. Experience with a new gastrostomy-jejunal feeding tube. Surgery 1983; 93:574–578.
37. Page CP, Carlton PK, Andrassy RJ, et al. Safe, cost-effective postoperative nutrition: defined formula diet via needle-catheter jejunostomy. Am J Surg 1979; 138:939–945.
38. Moore EE, Dunn EL, Jones TN. Immediate jejunostomy feeding: its use after major abdominal trauma. Arch Surg 1981; 116:681–684.
39. Keohane P, Attrill H, Love M, et al. Starter regimes significantly impair enteral nutrition—a double blind controlled trial. (Abstract.) JPEN 1984; 8:95.
40. Seigle RL, Rabinowitz JG, Sarasohn C. Intestinal perforation secondary to nasojejunal feeding tubes. Am J Roentgenol 1976; 126:1229.
41. Hayhust E, Wyman M. Morbidity associated with prolonged

use of polyvinyl feeding tube. Am J Dis Child 1975; *129*:72–74.

42. Cataldi-Betcher EL, Seltzer MH, Slocum BA, et al. Complications occurring during enteral nutrition support: a prospective study. JPEN 1983; *7*:546–552.

43. Torosian MH, Rombeau JL. Feeding by tube enterostomy. Surg Gynecol Obstet 1980; *150*:918–927.

44. Steffee WP, Krey SH. Enteral hyperalimentation for patients with head and neck cancer. Otolaryngol Clin North Am 1980; *13*:437–448.

45. Chernoff R. Enteral feedings. Am J Hosp Pharm 1980; *37*:65–74.

46. Kaminski MV, Freed BA. Enteral hyperalimentation: prevention and treatment of complications. Nutritional Support Services 1981; *1*:29–35.

47. White WT, Acuff TE, Sykes TR, et al. Bacterial contamination of enteral nutrient solution: a preliminary report. JPEN 1979; *3*:459–461.

48. Vanlandingham S, Simpson S, Daniel P, et al. Metabolic abnormalities in patients supported with enteral tube feeding. JPEN 1981; *5*:322–324.

49. Freed BA, Hsia B, Smith JP, et al. Enteral nutrition: frequency of formula modification. JPEN 1981; *5*:40–45.

50. Kubo W, Grant M, Walike B, et al. Fluid and electrolyte problems in tube fed patients. Am J Nurs 1976; *76*:912–916.

51. Rucker BB, Holmstedt KA. Institutional research report. Home Infusion Therapy Industry, Hambrecht and Quist Incorporated, 1984.

52. Parver JD. Reimbursement for Parenteral and Enteral Nutrition. Silver Spring, MD, American Society for Parenteral and Enteral Nutrition, January, 1985.

53. Standards for Nutrition Support—Home Patients. Silver Spring, MD, American Society for Parenteral and Enteral Nutrition, January, 1985.

54. Nelson JK, Palumbo PJ, O'Brien PC. Home enteral nutrition: observations of a newly established program. Nutr Clin Pract 1986; *1*:193–199.

55. Steffee WP. Malnutrition in hospitalized patients. JAMA 1980; *244*:2630–2635.

56. Greenberg GR, Marliss ER, Anderson GH, et al. Protein-sparing therapy in the post-operative patient: effects of added hypocaloric glucose or lipid. N Engl J Med 1976; *294*:1411–1416.

57. Greenberg GR, Jeejeebhoy KN. Intravenous protein-sparing therapy in patients with gastrointestinal disease. JPEN 1979; *3*:427–432.

58. Anderson GH, Patel DG, Jeejeebhoy KN. Design and evaluation by nitrogen balance and blood aminograms of an amino acid mixture for total parenteral nutrition of adults with gastrointestinal disease. J Clin Invest 1974; *53*:904–912.

59. Patel D, Anderson GH, Jeejeebhoy KN. Amino acid adequacy of parenteral casein hydrolysate and oral cottage cheese in patients with gastrointestinal disease as measured by nitrogen balance and blood aminogram. Gastroenterology 1973; *65*:427–437.

60. Messing B, Beliah M, Girard-Pipau F, et al. Technical hazards of using nutritive mixtures in bags by cyclical intravenous nutrition: comparison with standard intravenous nutrition in 48 gastroenterological patients. Gut 1982; *23*:297–303.

61. Fleming CR, Dickson ER, Baggenstoss AH. Copper and primary biliary cirrhosis. Gastroenterology 1974; *67*:1182–1187.

62. Smith RC, Burkinshaw L, Hill GL. Optimal energy and nitrogen intake for gastroenterological patients requiring intravenous nitrogen. Gastroenterology 1982; *82*:445–452.

63. Wolfe RR, Allsop JR, Burke JF. Glucose metabolism in man: responses to intravenous glucose infusion. Metabolism 1979; *28*:210–220.

64. Lindor KD, Fleming CR, Abrams A, et al. Liver function values in adults receiving total parenteral nutrition. JAMA 1979; *241*:2398–2400.

65. Grant JP, Cox CE, Kleinman LM, et al. Serum hepatic enzyme and bilirubin elevations during parenteral nutrition. Surg Gynecol Obstet 1977; *145*:573–580.

66. Askanazi J, Rosenbaum SH, Hyman AI. Respiratory changes secondary to the high carbohydrate loads of TPN. JAMA 1980; *243*:1444–1447.

67. Askanazi J, Nordenstrom J, Rosenbaum SH. Nutrition for the patient with respiratory failure: glucose vs fat. Anesthesiology 1981; *54*:373–377.

68. Fleming CR, Smith LM, Hodges RE. Essential fatty acid deficiency in adults receiving total parenteral nutrition. Am J Clin Nutr 1976; *29*:976–983.

69. Macfie J, Smith RC, Hill GL. Glucose or fat as a nonprotein energy source? A controlled clinical trial in gastroenterological patients requiring intravenous nutrition. Gastroenterology 1981; *80*:103–107.

70. Dickinson RJ, Ashton MG, Axon ATR, et al. Controlled trial of intravenous hyperalimentation and total bowel rest as an adjunct to the routine therapy of acute colitis. Gastroenterology 1980; *79*:1199–1204.

71. Collins JP, Oxby CB, Hill GL. Intravenous aminoacids and intravenous hyperalimentation as protein-sparing therapy after major surgery. A controlled clinical trial. Lancet 1978; *1*:788–791.

72. Bengoa JM, Rosenberg IH. Parenteral nutrition in gastrointestinal disease. Adv Intern Med 1983; *28*:363–385.

73. Muller JM, Keller HW, Erasmi H, et al. Total parenteral nutrition as the sole therapy in Crohn's disease—a prospective study. Br J Surg 1983; *70*:40–43.

74. Lochs H, Meryn S, Marosi L, et al. Has total bowel rest had a beneficial effect in the treatment of Crohn's disease? Clin Nutr 1983; *2*:61–64.

75. Strobel CT, Byrne WJ, Ament ME. Home parenteral nutrition in children with Crohn's disease: an effective management alternative. Gastroenterology 1979; *77*:272–279.

76. Edmunds LH Jr, Williams GM, Welch CE. External fistulas arising from the gastrointestinal tract. Ann Surg 1960; *152*:445–469.

77. Chapman R, Foran R, Dunphy JE. Management of intestinal fistulas. Am J Surg 1964; *108*:157–164.

78. MacFadyen BV, Dudrick SJ, Ruberg RL. Management of gastrointestinal fistulas with parenteral hyperalimentation. Surgery 1973; *74*:100–104.

79. Woolf GM, Miller C, Kurian R, et al. Diet for patients with a short bowel: high fat or high carbohydrate. Gastroenterology 1983; *84*:823–828.

80. Ovesen L, Chu R, Howard L. The influence of dietary fat on jejunostomy output in patients with severe short bowel. Am J Clin Nutr 1983; *38*:270–277.

81. Goldmann DA, Maki DG. Infection control in total parenteral nutrition. JAMA 1973; *223*:1360–1364.

82. Ryan JA Jr, Abel RM, Abbott WM. Catheter complications in total parenteral nutrition: a prospective study of 200 consecutive patients. N Engl J Med 1974; *290*:757–761.

83. Green HL, Nemir P Jr. Air embolism as a complication during parenteral alimentation. Am J Surg 1971; *121*:614–616.

84. Ross AHM, Griffith CDM, Anderson JR, et al. Thromboembolic complications with silicone elastomer subclavian catheters. JPEN 1982; *6*:61–63.

85. Brismar B, Hardstedt C, Jacobson S, et al. Reduction of catheter-associated thrombosis in parenteral nutrition by intravenous heparin therapy. Arch Surg 1982; *117*:1196–1199.

86. Ashworth CJ Jr, Sacks Y, Williams LF Jr. Hyperosmolar hyperglycemic nonketotic coma: its importance in surgical problems. Ann Surg 1968; *167*:556–560.

87. Greene HL. Vitamins in total parenteral nutrition. Drug Intell Clin Pharm 1972; *6*:355–360.

88. Manson RR. Acute pancreatitis secondary to iatrogenic hy-

percalcemia: implications of hyperalimentation. Arch Surg 1974; *108*:213–215.

89. Adelman RD, Abern SB, Halsted CH. Nephrolithiasis in a patient on total parenteral nutrition. (Abstract.) J Clin Nutr 1975; *28*:420.

90. Sand DW, Pastore RA. Paresthesias and hypophosphatemia occurring with parenteral nutrition. (Abstract.) J Clin Nutr 1975; *28*:420.

91. Silvis SE, Paragas PD Jr. Paresthesias, weakness, seizures, and hypophosphatemia in patients receiving hyperalimentation. Gastroenterology 1972; *62*:513–520.

92. Yawata Y, Hebbel RP, Silvis S. Blood cell abnormalities complicating the hypophosphatemia of hyperalimentation: erythrocyte and platelet ATP deficiency associated with hemolytic anemia and bleeding in hyperalimented dogs. J Lab Clin Med 1974; *84*:643–653.

93. Craddock PR, Yawata Y, VanSanten L. Acquired phagocyte dysfunction: a complication of the hypophosphatemia of parenteral hyperalimentation. N Engl J Med 1974; *290*:1403–1407.

94. Fleming CR, Hodges RE, Hurley L. A prospective study of serum copper and zinc levels in patients receiving total parenteral nutrition. Am J Clin Nutr 1976; *29*:70–77.

95. McClain CJ, Souter C, Steele N, et al. Severe zinc deficiency presenting with acrodermatitis during hyperalimentation: diagnosis, pathogenesis, and treatment. J Clin Gastroenterol 1980; *2*:125–131.

96. Kay RG, Tasman-Jones C, Pybus J. A syndrome of acute zinc deficiency during total parenteral alimentation in man. Ann Surg 1976; *183*:331.

97. Dunlap WM, James GW III, Hume DM. Anemia and neutropenia caused by copper deficiency. Ann Intern Med 1974; *80*:470–476.

98. Vilter RW, Bozian RC, Hess EV. Manifestations of copper deficiency in a patient with systemic sclerosis on intravenous hyperalimentation. N Engl J Med 1974; *291*:188–191.

99. Shike M, Roulet M, Kurian R, et al. Copper metabolism and requirements in total parenteral nutrition. Gastroenterology 1981; *81*:290–297.

100. Jeejeebhoy KN, Chu RC, Marliss EB, et al. Chromium deficiency, glucose intolerance, and neuropathy reversed by chromium supplementation, in a patient receiving long-term total parenteral nutrition. Am J Clin Nutr 1977; *30*:531–538.

101. Freund H, Atamiam S, Fischer JE. Chromium deficiency during total parenteral nutrition. JAMA 1979; *241*:496–498.

102. Johnson RA, Baker SS, Fallon JT. An occidental case of cardiomyopathy and selenium deficiency. N Engl J Med 1981; *304*:1210–1212.

103. Fleming CR, Lie JT, McCall JT, et al. Selenium deficiency and fatal cardiomyopathy in a patient on home parenteral nutrition. Gastroenterology 1982; *83*:689–693.

104. Howard L, Chu R, Reman S, et al. Vitamin A deficiency from long-term parenteral nutrition. Ann Intern Med 1980; *93*:576.

105. Shike M, Harrison JE, Sturtridge WC, et al. Metabolic bone disease in patients receiving long-term total parenteral nutrition. Ann Intern Med 1980; *92*:343–350.

106. Klein GL, Ament ME, Bluestone R, et al. Bone disease associated with total parenteral nutrition. Lancet 1980; *2*:1041–1044.

107. Shike M, Sturtridge WC, Tam CS, et al. A possible role of vitamin D in the genesis of parenteral-nutrition-induced metabolic bone disease. Ann Intern Med 1981; *95*:560–568.

108. Ott SM, Maloney NA, Klein GL, et al. Aluminum is associated with low bone formation in patients receiving chronic parenteral nutrition. Ann Intern Med 1983; *98*:910–914.

109. Thurlow PM, Grant JP. Intravenous fat and vitamin E deficiency. (Abstract.) JPEN 1981; *5*:568.

110. Mock DM, DeLorimer AA, Liebman WM. Biotin deficiency: an unusual complication of parenteral nutrition. N Engl J Med 1981; *304*:820–823.

111. McClain CJ, Baker H, Onstad GR. Biotin deficiency in an adult during home parenteral nutrition. JAMA 1982; *247*:3116–3117.

112. Fleming CR, Beart RW Jr, McGill DB, et al. Fate of gut failure patients on home parenteral nutrition (HPN). (Abstract.) Gastroenterology 1983; *84*:1154.

113. Wolfe BM, Beer WH, Hayashi JT, et al. Experience with home parenteral nutrition. Am J Surg 1983; *146*:7–14.

Index

Page numbers *in italics* indicate a figure; page numbers followed by the letter t indicate a table.